# *Essentials of Critical Care Nursing*

## Nursing Management of Neurological Alterations



## Nursing Management of Renal Alterations



## Nursing Management of Gastrointestinal Alterations



## Nursing Management of Endocrine Alterations

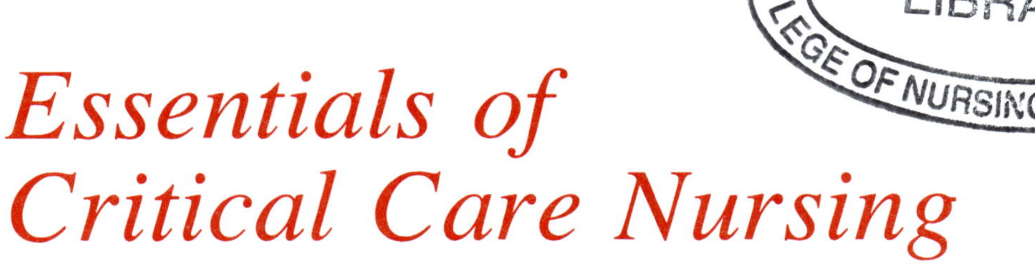

# Essentials of Critical Care Nursing

Linda Diann Urden, DNSc, RN, CNA
Director, Nursing Support Programs
Children's Hospital
San Diego, California

Joseph Kevin Davie, MSN, RN
Dean, School of Nursing
The Long Island College Hospital
Brooklyn Heights, New York
Diagnosis Review Committee
North American Nursing Diagnosis Association
St. Louis, Missouri

Lynne Ann Thelan, MN, RN
Critical Care Consultant
San Diego, California

*with 170 illustrations*

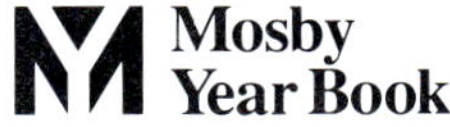

Mosby
Year Book

St. Louis Baltimore Boston Chicago London Philadelphia Sydney Toronto

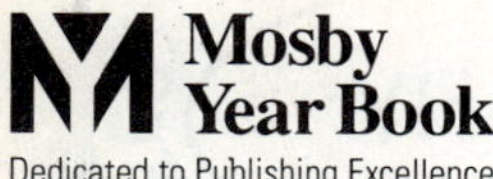

Dedicated to Publishing Excellence

Acquisitions Editors: Don Ladig, Terry Van Schaik
Developmental Editor: Jeanne Rowland
Project Manager: John A. Rogers
Production Editor: Catherine M. Vale
Production: Jeanne Genz
Designer: Jeanne Wolfgeher
Cover Illustration: Matthew Henke



Printed in the United States of America.

Mosby–Year Book, Inc.
11830 Westline Industrial Drive
St. Louis, MO 63146

**Library of Congress Cataloging in Publication Data**

Essentials of critical care nursing / [edited by] Linda Diann Urden,
Joseph Kevin Davie, Lynne Ann Thelan.
p. cm.
Includes bibliographical references and index.
ISBN ~~0-8016-5223-5~~
1. Intensive care nursing. I. Urden, Linda Diann. II. Davie, Joseph Kevin. III. Thelan, Lynne A.
[DNLM: 1. Critical Care—nurses' instruction. WY 154 E786]
RT120.I5E83 1992
610.73'61—dc20
DNLM/DLC
for Library of Congress

91-25801
CIP

92 93 94 95 96 GW/VH/VH 9 8 7 6 5 4 3 2 1

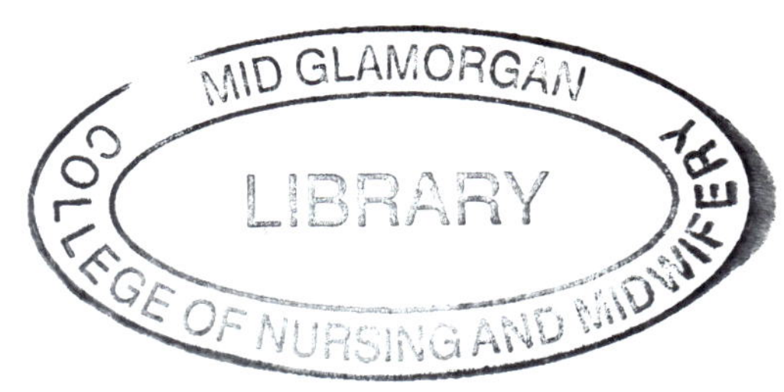


To our family and friends for their patience and support on "not another book!"

**LDU JKD LAT**

# Contributors

**Jennifer N. Bloomquist,** MN, RN
Cardiothoracic Clinical Nurse Specialist
VA Medical Center
San Diego
San Diego, California
*Chapter 7*

**Joy Boarini,** MSN, RN, CETN
Professional Education Manager
Hollister, Inc.
Libertyville, Illinois
*Chapters 18 and 19*

**Karen Brasfield,** MSN, RN, CNN
Instructor of Nursing
Point Loma Nazarene College
San Diego, California
*Chapters 16 and 17*

**Dorothy J. Brundage,** PhD, RN, FAAN
Associate Professor of Nursing
School of Nursing
Duke University
Durham, North Carolina
*Chapter 4*

**Ruth Bryant,** MSN, RN
Director, Enterostomal Therapy Nursing Education Program
Abbott-Northwestern Hospital
Minneapolis, Minnesota
*Chapters 18 and 19*

**JoAnn M. Clark,** MSN, RN
Professor of Nursing
Grossmont College
San Diego, California
*Chapters 20 and 21*

**Kathleen S. Crocker,** MSN, RN, CNA, CNSN
National Director of Nursing
Critical Care America
Westborough, Massachusetts
*Unit 10*

**Joseph Kevin Davie,** MSN, RN
Dean, School of Nursing
The Long Island College Hospital
Brooklyn Heights, New York
Diagnosis Review Committee
North American Nursing Diagnosis Association
*Chapters 1, 4-6, 13-15, 18, 19, and 22 and Unit 10*

**Katherine M. Fortinash,** MSN, RN, CS
Professor and Certified Clinical Specialist
Adult Psychatric–Mental Health Nursing
Grossmont College
San Diego, California
*Chapter 4 and Unit 10*

**Jane Frein,** MN, RN
Director of Nursing Services
Arroyo Grande Community Hospital
Arroyo Grande, California
*Chapter 3*

**Sheana Whelan Funkhouser,** MN, RN
Doctoral Student
School of Nursing
University of California-Los Angeles
Los Angeles, California
*Chapter 7*

**Judith R. Heggie,** MN, RN
Associate Chief of Nursing Services Education
San Diego VA Medical Center
San Diego, California
*Unit 10*

**Jacqueline Kartman,** MS, RNC, CCRN
Critical Care Clinical Nurse Specialist
Lutheran Hospital-La Crosse
La Crosse, WI
*Chapter 5 and Unit X*

**Christine Kennedy-Caldwell,** PhD, RN, CNSN
Assistant Clinical Professor
Department of Family Health Care Nursing
School of Nursing
University of California-San Francisco
San Francisco, California
*Chapters 18 and 19*

**Gere Harris Lane,** MSN, MEd, RN, GNP
Director, Medical-Surgical Services
The Cheshire Medical Center
Keene, New Hampshire
*Chapters 10, 11, and 12*

**Mary Lough,** MS, RN, CCRN
Critical Care Educator
Sequoia Hospital
Redwood City, California
Assistant Clinical Professor
School of Nursing
University of California-San Francisco
San Francisco, California
*Chapter 7*

**Martha J. Love,** MN, RN, CCRN
Cardiovascular Clinical Nurse Specialist
San Diego VA Medical Center
San Diego, California
*Chapter 7*

**Mary Courtney Moore,** MSN, RN, RD, CNSN
Doctoral Candidate
Vanderbilt University
Nashville, Tennessee
*Chapter 6*

**Mimi O'Donnell,** MS, RN, CCRN
Cardiovascular Clinical Nurse Specialist
Massachusetts General Hospital
Boston, Massachusetts
*Chapter 8*

**Thomas W. Oertel,** MSN, RN
Assistant Professor
Grossmont College
San Diego, California
*Chapters 23 and 25*

**Angela Palomo,** MN, RN
Clinical Nurse Specialist-Cardiac Surgery
University Hospital
Denver, Colorado
*Chapter 9*

**Jeanne Raimond,** MSN, RN, CCRN
Faculty, Department of Nursing
Grossmont College
San Diego, California
*Unit 10*

**Judith Hartman Ruekberg,** MSN, RN
Coordinator-Pulmonary Rehabilitation
San Diego Rehabilitation Institute
San Diego, California
*Chapter 12*

**Kathleen M. Stacy,** MS, RN, CCRN
Critical Care Clinical Specialist
Tri-City Medical Center
Oceanside, California
*Chapter 24*

**Lynne A. Thelan,** MN, RN
Critical Care Consultant and Lecturer
San Diego, California
*Chapters 10, 11, and 12, and Unit 10*

**Linda D. Urden,** DNSc, RN, CNA
Director, Nursing Support Programs
Children's Hospital
San Diego, California
*Chapters 2, 3, 7-9, 13-17, and 20-25*

**David Unkle,** MSN, RN, CCRN, CEN
Transplant Coordinator
Delaware Valley Transplant Program
Philadelphia, Pennsylvania
*Chapter 22*

**Helen R. Vos,** MS, RN, CNRN
Director, Clinical Projects
University of California-San Diego Medical Center
San Diego, California
*Chapters 13, 14, 15, and 22*

**Evelyn Wasli,** DNSc, RN
Emergency Psychiatric Response Division
Commission of Mental Health Services
Washington, D.C.
*Chapter 4*

# Preface

A dominant theme of this book is nursing diagnosis and management. The book is organized around alterations in dimensions of human functioning that span biopsychosocial realms. We have gone beyond the traditional physiologic focus of critical care texts and incorporated chapters on the following:

- Nursing process
- Ethical and legal issues
- Patient and family education
- Sleep alterations
- Nutritional alterations
- Psychosocial alterations

The power of a research-based practice has been incorporated into nursing interventions. To foster critical thinking and decision making, a boxed "menu" of nursing diagnoses complete with specific etiologic, related, and risk factors accompanies each medical disorder discussion and directs the learner to the section in the book where appropriate nursing management is detailed.

Organizationally, the book is composed of 10 major units. The chapter content of Unit I, *Foundations of Critical Care Nursing,* forms the basis of practice regardless of the physiologic alterations of the critically ill patient. The book may be studied in any sequence; however, it is recommended that Chapter 1, *The Nursing Process,* be studied first because it clarifies the major assumptions on which the entirety of the book is based.

Unit II, *Common Problems in Critical Care,* examines perennial critical care practice problems and is divided into three chapters: *Psychosocial Alterations, Sleep Alterations,* and *Nutritional Alterations.*

Unit III, *Cardiovascular Alterations;* Unit IV, *Cardiopulmonary Alterations;* and Unit V, *Neurological Alterations,* are each structured by the following chapters:

- Assessment and Diagnostic Procedures
- Disorders
- Therapeutic Management

Unit VI, *Renal Alterations;* Unit VII, *Gastrointestinal Alterations;* and Unit VIII, *Endocrine Alterations,* are each structured by the following chapters:

- Assessment and Diagnostic Procedures
- Disorders and Therapeutic Management

Unit IX, *Multisystem Alterations,* addresses disorders that affect multiple body systems and necessitate discussion as a separate category. Unit IX includes four chapters:

- Trauma
- Disseminated Intravascular Coagulation
- Septic Shock
- Anaphylaxis

Unit X, *Nursing Management Plans,* contains the core of critical care nursing practice presented in nursing process format: signs and symptoms, nursing diagnosis, outcome criteria, and interventions. The Nursing Management Plans are cross-referenced throughout the text with "Nursing Diagnosis and Management" boxes.

Finally, two appendixes have been included that contain extremely useful information for all students and practitioners of critical care. Appendix A, *North American Nursing Diagnosis Association's (NANDA) Taxonomy I Revised,* contains all diagnostic labels approved at the Ninth Conference on the Classification of Nursing Diagnoses in 1990. These categories are organized into the nine human response patterns of the profession's official taxonomic structure. Appendix B, *Advanced Cardiac Life Support (ACLS) Guidelines,* presents the American Heart Association's decision trees for use in treating life-threatening dysrhythmias and administering emergency drugs and defibrillation during cardiopulmonary resusitation.

*Essentials of Critical Care Nursing* represents a commitment on *our* part to bring you the best of essential elements of critical care nursing practice. A commitment on *your* part to develop a comprehensive research-based critical care speciality practice is not a simple one, nor one casually made. This is precisely, however, our challenge to you now.

*Linda Diann Urden*
*Joseph Kevin Davie*
*Lynne Ann Thelan*

# Acknowledgements

The talent, hard work, and inspiration of many people have produced *Essentials of Critical Care Nursing*. We appreciate the assistance of our Executive Editor, Don Ladig, and Developmental Editor, Jeanne Rowland, who have helped us transform our book into a reality. Their creativity, expertise, availability, and generosity of time and resources have been invaluable to us during this endeavor. We are also grateful to Catherine Vale, Production Editor, for her scrupulous attention to detail. We are again proud of the association we share with the extraordinary people at Mosby–Year Book, Inc.

## Use of the "Nursing Diagnosis and Management" boxes:

Each body system unit (Units III through VIII) opens with a chapter that covers clinical assessment, laboratory tests, and other diagnostic procedures related to disorders of the body system being discussed. A disorders chapter then discusses etiology and pathophysiology, reviews assessment and diagnosis, briefly covers therapeutic management, and finally discusses nursing care for each disorder presented. Completing each unit is a therapeutic management chapter, which describes therapeutic interventions specific to the body system along with nursing care related to the interventions.

"Nursing Diagnoses and Management" boxes accompany each presentation of nursing care and list nursing diagnoses related to the particular disorder or therapeutic measure being discussed. Following each diagnosis listed in the box is a page reference to Unit X, where the reader will find the nursing management plan related to that nursing diagnosis. Unit X, "Nursing Management Plans," provides a plan correlated with each of the nursing diagnoses used in this text.

# Contents

# Detailed Contents

## UNIT X

# Nursing Management

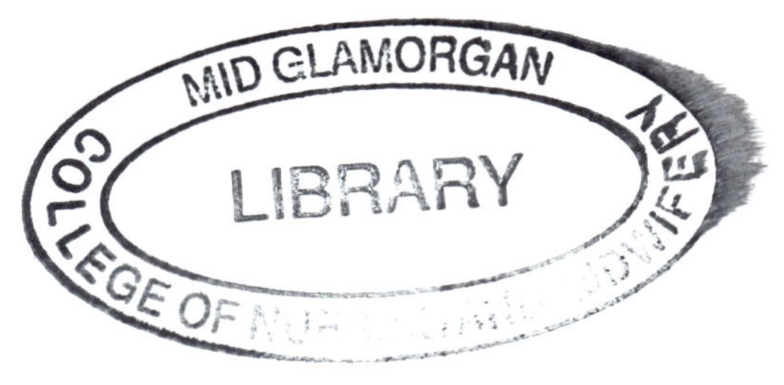


UNIT I

# FOUNDATIONS OF CRITICAL CARE NURSING PRACTICE

CHAPTER 1

# The Nursing Process

## CHAPTER OBJECTIVES

- *Define nursing diagnosis.*
- *Differentiate the methods of stating actual and high-risk nursing diagnoses.*
- *Formulate nursing diagnosis statements from the North American Nursing Diagnosis Association (NANDA) list of approved diagnoses, their etiologic/related factors, and defining characteristics.*
- *Designate nursing actions capable of resolving actual and high-risk nursing diagnoses in critically ill adults.*
- *Identify the two tasks associated with the evaluation phase of the nursing process.*
- *Propose a relationship between the phases of the nursing process and such professional practice issues as reimbursement for nursing services, allocation of nursing manpower and professional autonomy.*

## KEY TERMS



## THE NURSING PROCESS

The **nursing process** is a method for making clinical decisions. It is a way of thinking and acting in relation to the clinical phenomena of concern to nurses. Classically, the nursing process comprises five phases or dimensions: data collection, nursing diagnosis, planning, implementation, and evaluation. The nursing process is a systematic decision making model that is cyclical, not linear (Fig. 1-1). By virtue of its evaluation phase, the nursing process incorporates a feedback loop that maintains quality control of its decision-making outputs.

The nursing process is indeed a method for solving clinical problems, but it is not merely a problem-solving method. Similar to a problem-solving method, it offers an organized, systematic approach to clinical problems. Unlike a problem-solving method, the nursing process is continuous, not episodic. The nursing process doesn't become activated only in the face of an identified problem, and then deactivated when the problem is resolved. The five phases constitute a continuous cycle throughout the nurse's moment-to-moment data interpretation and management of patient care. Kritek[18] describes the phases of the nursing process as being not only continuous but "interactive"; in other words, all phases operate and influence each other and the patient simultaneously. Fig. 1-2 illustrates this interactive nature of the nursing process, wherein each phase is represented by a line that intersects with the others and converging at a point in time to which the nurse attends.[18]

Why a nursing process? Why a systematic method for approaching, analyzing, and managing clinical problems? Because it yields sound decisions. And it grooms the novice critical care practitioner for expert practice by necessitating organized thinking and maximizing the nurse's analytic skills.

### Data Collection: Organizational Frameworks

By virtue of nursing's unique orientation and commitment to holism, nurses collect an enormous amount of data about a patient's biopsychosocial health status. By virtue of a vast array of technophysiological monitoring devices, critical care nurses process an additional layer of data in the form of physiological parameter measurements. Consequently, in the process of assembling this data base, the critical care

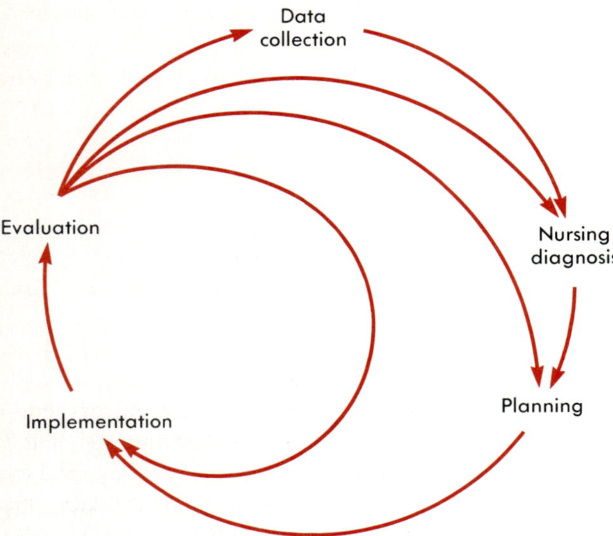


***Fig. 1-1*** The cyclic nature of the nursing process.

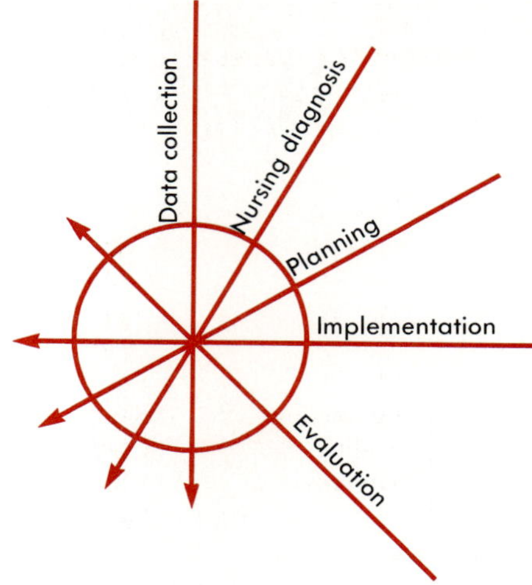


***Fig. 1-2*** The interactive nature of the nursing process.

nurse needs some place to file the information as it is collected. Ideally, this storage system would contain compartments, which could keep the data separated and organized. Such a system is called an **organizational framework**. Organizational frameworks also serve as guides for assessment, and their compartments consist of headings corresponding to the attributes the nurse accepts as constituting the nature of humans, health, illness, and nursing. In this way, the framework helps guide the identification of diagnoses that are within the domain of nursing.

Organizational frameworks are neither new nor unique to nursing. Traditionally, nursing used medicine's organizational framework for the collection and organization of data, but as nursing's knowledge base and conceptual orientation became increasingly differentiated and complex, the biological mechanistic scheme of medicine was found to be insufficiently comprehensive for its use by nurses as a tool for holistic assessment. The organizational framework for generalist medical practice, and two frameworks for nursing practice are shown in Table 1-1.

Organizational frameworks are necessary to process the volume of information nurses accrue in the assessment of a patient. Frameworks facilitate diagnostic reasoning (discussed later in this chapter) by guiding data collection and organizing it into manageable parts. Organizing incoming information in this way increases its availability for retrieval and facilitates subsequent identification of relationships among the data.

The selection of any one framework over another, as long as it is designed to organize nursing data, is an individual choice.

## Nursing Diagnosis

The concept of **nursing diagnosis,** a process whereby nurses interpret assessment data and apply standardized labels to health problems they identify and anticipate treating, is rapidly evolving in clinical and educational settings. Not coincidentally, this evolution is taking place parallel to the overall process of professionalization of nursing. Critical attention is currently being focused on aspects of nursing practice and education that either foster or inhibit the establishment of the discipline of nursing as a profession.

A traditional reliance on the language and therapeutics of other sciences is inhibiting the establishment of nursing as a free-standing profession. Efforts to identify and name the conditions that nurses study and treat, on the other hand, foster nursing's professional identity by clarifying its distinct services to society and providing a vehicle for the building of its science.

### Historical development of nursing diagnosis

***Pre–North American Nursing Diagnosis Association (NANDA) era.*** Diagnosis by nurses of health problems amenable to their treatment is not new. There is evidence that this activity spans nursing's history. During the Crimean War, Florence Nightingale identified and treated such health problems as alterations in comfort and nutrition, fear, anxiety, and potential for injury.[14] In fact, Nightingale, by her writings, teachings, and example, set the precedent for the scrupulous data collection and goal-directed planning of care that today characterizes the practice of nursing.

The term *nursing diagnosis* first appeared in the literature in the 1950s. Gordon points out that along with the genesis of this term, a fundamental change in the process whereby nurses moved from data collection to care planning began to occur: a pause in which the data collected are analyzed and grouped, the signs and symptoms of a suspected health problem identified, a possible cause uncovered, and the diagnostic conclusion stated. Only *then* was care planning begun.[14]

Historically, nursing interventions tended to be disjointed

***Table 1-1*** Comparison of selected organizational frameworks

| Medicine | Nursing | |
|---|---|---|
| BODY SYSTEMS | NANDA TAXONOMY II | FUNCTIONAL HEALTH PATTERNS |
| Cardiovascular | Exchanging | Health perception–health management |
| Respiratory | Communicating | Nutritional-metabolic |
| Neurological | Relating | Elimination |
| Endocrine | Valuing | Activity-exercise |
| Metabolic | Choosing | Sleep-rest |
| Hematopoietic | Moving | Cognitive-perceptual |
| Integumentary | Perceiving | Self-perception–self-concept |
| Gastrointestinal | Feeling | Role-relationship |
| Genitourinary | Knowing | Sexuality-reproductive |
| Reproductive | | Coping–stress tolerance |
| Psychiatric | | Value-belief |

and episodic. The nurse often looked on each piece of assessment data as separate, discrete entities, neither seeking nor perceiving relationships among groups of symptoms. Intervention strategies were planned and carried out in relation to what were considered to be series of independent findings. For example, if soft tissue swelling, frequent infections, and delayed healing were observed in a patient, it is likely these would be interpreted and managed separately, that is, interventions slated to reduce swelling, some to avoid or control infection, and others to promote healing. Consider the gains if the nurse instead considers the possibility of a relationship among these symptoms, uncovers a cause, and organizes a treatment plan corresponding to the diagnosis, Altered Nutrition: Less Than Body Protein Requirements.

With nursing diagnosis as a component of our decision-making methods, we necessarily become more systematic in the collection and interpretation of data and accomplish a change in the substance of our clinical operations, from symptom management to problem solving.

***NANDA era.*** Prompted initially by a need to clarify the nurse's role and to distinguish it from that of other health professionals in their own practice setting, two faculty members at St. Louis University, Kristine Gebbie and Mary Ann Lavin, called together the First National Conference on the Classification of Nursing Diagnoses in 1973.[13] The group organized around the task of identifying, standardizing, and classifying health problems treated by nurses. This conference has heralded a now-international professional movement. The organization, now known as the *North American Nursing Diagnosis Association (NANDA),* consists of nurse theorists, nurse researchers, nurse educators, and advanced and grass roots clinicians.

The impetus for the work of NANDA and its scientific sessions derives from the necessity of establishing a vocabulary that specifically reflects the treatment domain of nursing practice. In addition to it being requisite to nursing's status as a profession, such a vocabulary serves to coordinate communication among nurses in relation to the health problems they are observing and treating, and is as much for purposes of social policy as it is, says Carpenito, for "clarifying nursing for nurses."[9]

Approved nursing diagnoses are listed in Appendix B of this book. Though not included in the appendix, accompanying each diagnosis are possible causative factors (etiologic/related factors) and the signs and symptoms of the health problem (defining characteristics). These are used by the nurse to help formulate the diagnostic statement and tailor it to the individual patient characteristics and circumstance.

An "approved" nursing diagnosis is one accepted by NANDA as having been refined to the point of clinical usefulness and approved for beginning clinical validation through formal research methods. Practitioners using approved nursing diagnoses, their etiologies, and defining characteristics are in fact participating in the preliminary testing of the diagnoses as they relate to the health problems described by the diagnostic labels. NANDA actively seeks input from practicing nurses regarding the development and refinement of nursing diagnoses. The Association publishes guidelines for submitting new diagnoses to its Diagnosis Review Committee, and direct input into the proceedings of the biennial conferences is possible through membership and participation in NANDA and any of its regional associations.

The immediate goals of NANDA include (1) further validation and refinement of existing diagnoses and their etiologies and defining characteristics, (2) the generation of new diagnoses, (3) the incorporation of a category of wellness diagnoses that describes patients' strengths and potential for growth, (4) the development of NANDA's Taxonomy II Revised, and (5) the incorporation of approved diagnoses into the tenth revision of the World Health Organization's *International Classification of Diseases.*

**Definitions of nursing diagnosis.** No single definition of nursing diagnosis is sufficiently comprehensive to convey its identity as a concept, a skill, and an international professional movement. Basic to any definition is the recognition that nursing diagnosis exists both as part of a process—the nursing process—and is a process unto itself—the diagnostic reasoning process.

Several of the most enduring definitions of nursing diagnosis are found in the box on p. 6 and includes the new working definition adopted by NANDA at the ninth conference in 1990. Key terms emerging from these definitions are *conclusion, judgment, inference, person's response,* and *actual* or *potential health problem.*

A nursing diagnosis is a conclusion the nurse reaches

### DEFINITIONS OF NURSING DIAGNOSIS

*Gebbie and Lavin:* The judgment or conclusion that occurs as a result of nursing assessment.[13]

*Mundinger:* A statement of a person's response to a situation or illness which is actually or potentially unhealthful and which nursing intervention can change in the direction of health.[22]

*Aspinall:* A process of clinical inference from observed changes in the patient's physical or psychological condition.[3]

*Gordon:* Actual or potential health problems which nurses, by virtue of their education and experience, are capable and licensed to treat.[14]

*Shoemaker:* A clinical judgment about an individual, family or community which is derived through a deliberate, systematic process of data collection and analysis. It provides the basis for prescriptions for definitive therapy for which the nurse is accountable. It is expressed concisely and it includes the etiology of the condition when known.[27]

*NANDA:* A clinical judgment about individual, family, or community responses to actual or potential health problems/life processes. Nursing diagnoses provide the basis for selection of nursing interventions for which the nurse is accountable.

after collecting and analyzing data relative to the patient's biopsychosocial health status. It is a professional judgment in that, in addition to the collection and analysis of data, interpretations are made by the nurse about the meaning and significance of these findings both individually and collectively. This conclusion, this judgment, forms the basis for nursing action: intervention.

The term **inference** is useful in defining nursing diagnosis because it emphasizes the tentative and assumptive nature of diagnoses. Webster's Collegiate Dictionary defines inference as the "process of arriving at a conclusion by reasoning from evidence" and warns that "if the evidence is slight the term comes close to *surmise*.[31] In recognizing that elements of both judgment and inference are part of nursing diagnosis, one can appreciate the need to limit or control the influence of bias on the part of the diagnostician and in the act of diagnosing so that the diagnostic conclusion reached is as logical and factually based as possible. Inference in the context of diagnostic reasoning is discussed in greater detail later in this chapter.

The person's response to health and illness situations constitutes the focus, or phenomenon, of concern to nurses, and it is the object of nurses' diagnostic activities. In 1980, the American Nurses' Association (ANA) issued *Nursing: A Social Policy Statement*, which defined the nature and scope of the profession as follows: "Nursing is the diagnosis and treatment of human responses to actual or potential health problems."[2] Actual or potential health problems to which nurses direct their diagnosis and treatment, then, are human responses—human responses to the health challenges encountered in birth, illness, wellness, growth and development, and death.

The most essential and distinguishing feature of any nursing diagnosis is that it describe a health condition *primarily resolved by nursing interventions or therapies*. There is, however, some difficulty in applying this criterion to the broad spectrum of health problems that nurses have historically, do currently, and will in the future identify and treat. The boundaries of nursing and those, particularly, that it shares with other health professions, are dynamic and not at once easily delineated.[2]

To assist in clarifying the boundaries of nursing and provide a framework for the development and classification of nursing diagnoses, the ANA outlines the following categories of health problems, the treatment of which lies within the profession's domain[9]:

1. Self-care limitations
2. Impaired functioning in areas such as rest, sleep, ventilation, circulation, activity, nutrition, elimination, skin, sexuality, and the like
3. Pain and discomfort
4. Emotional problems related to illness and treatment; life-threatening events; or daily life experiences, such as anxiety, loss, loneliness, and grief
5. Distortion of symbolic functions, reflected in interpersonal and intellectual processes, such as hallucinations
6. Deficiencies in decision making and ability to make personal choices
7. Self-image changes required by health status
8. Dysfunctional perceptual orientations to health
9. Strains related to processes that occur during life such as birth, growth and development, and death
10. Problematic affiliative relationships

Although the above categories are not in themselves nursing diagnoses, standardization of diagnostic labels developed from within this framework helps to ensure a discipline-specific perspective for the intervention activities of professional nurses.

**Nursing diagnosis in critical care.** Currently there is controversy regarding the application of nursing diagnosis in critical care.[11,17,26,29] The appropriateness of critical care nurses contending that they diagnose and treat phenomena such as decreased cardiac output, impaired pulmonary gas exchange, and altered tissue perfusion is disputed, although some of the strongest reservations appear to have come from nurses outside the critical care specialty.

In addition to the scientific and general assembly sessions of the biennial NANDA Conference, the American Association of Critical-Care Nurses (AACN) and Marquette University have cosponsored national conferences addressing nursing diagnosis in critical care and the professional issues from which it is inseparable.

For clarity, the position taken in this book is one of inclusion versus exclusion: all phenomena—physiological, psychological, and social—of concern to critical care nurses and the object of their treatment are represented by nursing diagnoses throughout this text. The factors contributing to their development (their etiologic factors) are modifiable by nursing intervention.

Kritek[18] asserts that the categorization of nursing diagnoses as *independent* or *collaborative* constitutes a political distinction, not a conceptual one. If this designation is desired, however, it can be easily superimposed by the practitioner.

**Formulating nursing diagnosis statements.** *PES format.* There are three distinct components to a nursing diagnosis statement. The format for documenting these components is called the PES format, where:

P = *Problem.* This is a concise statement of the patient's actual or potential human response to the health state and is also called a *diagnostic label* or *category label.* Problem statements come from the list of approved nursing diagnoses. An example is Impaired Skin Integrity.

E = *Etiology.* This is a specification of the source(s) from which the health problem is thought to arise, also called *related* or *contributing factors.* The **etiology** of a problem is its cause (to the extent that cause and effect can be known or shown). A nursing diagnosis may be, and often is, based on several etiological factors. These factors, whether they are psychological, biological, environmental, circumstantial, or interpersonal, interact to produce the health problem. Each diagnostic label has accompanying listings of possible causative factors. Examples of etiological factors for the diagnosis Impaired Skin Integrity are *shearing forces, physical immobilization,* and *nutritional deficit.*

S = *Signs and symptoms.* These are observed, reported, or measured biopsychosocial findings that serve as supporting evidence of the diagnosis, also called the **defining characteristics** or *manifestations.* Defining characteristics are listed for each diagnostic label. Examples of defining characteristics for the diagnostic label Impaired Skin Integrity are *disruption of skin surface* and *destruction of skin layers.*

When communicating nursing diagnoses, either verbally or in writing, nurses customarily link the PES components with words that indicate the direction of the relationship between the problem, its etiologic factors, and defining characteristics. The problem and etiology are linked with the indicator *related to* and the defining characteristics are linked by the indicator *as evidenced by.* To illustrate documenting diagnostic statements in this way, a diagnosis of Pain would be written:

> Pain *related to muscle spasm as evidenced by (patient statements) "8/10," "sharp knifelike pain," and (nurse observations) guarding behaviors, tightened brow, tachycardia.*

Additionally, it is common practice to abbreviate *related to* and *as evidenced by* as *R/T* and *AEB,* respectively. A diagnosis of Constipation would be written:

> Constipation *R/T immobility, fluid volume deficit, AEB no BM × 5 days, hypoactive bowel sounds, straining at stool.*

***Guidelines for use of the list of approved nursing diagnoses.*** It is important to recognize that classification of the phenomena to which a profession addresses itself is a sizable and ongoing task. The development and refinement of nursing's nomenclature of health problems is in its earliest stages and subject to much revision based on the research and clinical reports presented and reviewed at each of NANDA's conferences and by the Diagnosis Review Committee. Work on existing diagnoses is also incomplete. Several have etiologies and defining characteristics yet to be developed, making clinical use difficult and frustrating. Other diagnoses may be deleted from the approved list from conference to conference. Such changes are both necessary and usual in the process of taxonomy development. One has only to look at the system of names describing health problems treated by physicians not many years ago (for example, chilblains, consumption, dropsy) to appreciate nursing's progress to date.

**GUIDELINES FOR PROBLEMS (P)**

*Definitions of health problems.* Many diagnoses have accompanying definitions to better explain the health problem. These definitions are important for the student of nursing diagnosis to consider, because they clarify more about the problem than is apparent from the label alone. For example, the definitions accompanying the diagnoses Fear and Anxiety draw a particularly useful distinction between the two problems: Fear is an emotion that has an identifiable source or object that the patient validates, whereas Anxiety is an emotion whose source is nonspecific or unknown to the patient. Other good examples of such definitions accompany the diagnoses Social Isolation, Powerlessness, Altered Parenting, and Ineffective Family Coping.

Until definitions accompany all approved diagnoses, it will be important for nurses collaborating in care to establish consensus about the meaning and scope of the health problems stated.

*Making diagnostic labels specific.* Some nursing diagnoses need accompanying qualifiers or specifiers based on the characteristics of the health problem as it manifests itself in a particular patient. For example, the diagnosis Fear needs specification as to the object of the patient's particular fear, such as death, pain, disfigurement, or malignancy. Similarly, the diagnosis Knowledge Deficit needs specification about the content of the deficiency, such as use of incentive spirometer, counting the pulse rate, or respiratory muscle strengthening exercise. Below is a list of nursing diagnoses needing specification, each with an example of a particular patient circumstance so specified:

Fear: *Postoperative Pain*

Knowledge Deficit: *Self-Monitoring of Oral Anticoagulation Therapy*
Altered *Peripheral* Tissue Perfusion
Altered Nutrition: Less than Body *Potassium* Requirements
Altered Nutrition: More Than Body *Calorie* Requirements
Self-Care Deficit: *Bathing and Feeding*
(Note: this diagnosis needs even further specification as to the functional level classification.)
Noncompliance: *Prescribed Activity Restrictions*

#### GUIDELINES FOR ETIOLOGIC/RELATED FACTORS (E)

*Making etiologies specific.* In many instances, etiologic factors are broad categories or examples needing to be made specific based on characteristics of the problem and the patient being treated. For example, one of several possible etiologies for the diagnosis Fluid Volume Excess is *compromised regulatory mechanism*. Considering this the cause of the fluid excess in a particular patient, the nurse would need to specify which regulatory mechanism and in what way compromised (for example, inappropriate ADH secretion by the neurohypophysis) before the diagnosis could be formally stated (leaving aside the question as to whether this problem is treatable by nurses or would need referral).

Several etiologies needing to be made specific are listed below, along with examples of such specification in parentheses:

Situational crisis (recent diagnosis of terminal illness)
Psychological injuring agent (hurtful relationship, verbal abuse)
Developmental factors (developmental arrest, extremes of age)

*Nursing diagnoses as etiologies.* Nursing diagnostic labels may rightfully serve as etiologies for other diagnoses. Examples are Anxiety R/T knowledge deficit, and Activity Intolerance R/T decreased cardiac output.

*Etiologies as the focus of treatment.* The treatment plan formulated for a given diagnosis must include interventions aimed at resolution or management of the etiologic factors as well as the health problem. In fact, in some instances nursing treatment will be directed exclusively at the etiology of a problem, with the logical expectation that, if the causative factors are reduced in influence, the problem should begin to be resolved. This will be especially true in instances where a nursing diagnosis has as its etiology another nursing diagnosis. Consider treatment approaches to the diagnosis Ineffective Breathing Pattern R/T high abdominal incision pain. Predictably little effectiveness would be shown were the interventions to be focused solely on reviewing the rationale for slow, deep, symmetrical breathing; demonstrating the technique; and encouraging the patient in its performance without some plan for manipulation of the pain variable.

*Medical diagnoses as etiologies.* Because, as previously mentioned, the etiology of a nursing diagnosis becomes a focus of intervention in the treatment of the overall problem, citing a medical condition or diagnosis as the etiology is conceptually inadvisable if the problem statement is to retain its identity as a health problem primarily resolved by nursing therapies. And yet many problems of concern to critical care nurses and amenable to their treatment *are* consequent to medical conditions. Examples are the Ineffective Airway Clearance that results from chronic obstructive pulmonary disease (COPD), and Sensory-Perceptual Alterations resulting from coronary artery bypass graft surgery. In these instances, the nurse should isolate those aspects of the contributing pathological state that are modifiable by nursing intervention, and cite these factors as etiologic; for instance, Ineffective Airway Clearance R/T thick tracheobronchial secretions, respiratory muscle weakness, and knowledge deficit: effective cough and hydration techniques; and Sensory-Perceptual Alterations R/T sensory overload, sensory deprivation, and sleep pattern disturbance. These problem statements are more clearly worded and provide a much sharper focus for nursing intervention.

#### GUIDELINES FOR DEFINING CHARACTERISTICS [SIGNS AND SYMPTOMS] (S)

*Making defining characteristics specific.* As with problem statements and statements of etiology, defining characteristics cited for diagnoses are in nonspecific form and often need to be modified to reflect the particular situation presented by the patient being diagnosed. For example, the diagnosis Impaired Gas Exchange has as one of its possible defining characteristics *abnormal blood gases*. In the nurse's formulation of this diagnostic statement for clinical use, the specific blood gas value used to diagnose the problem should be cited in the statement (for example, $PO_2$: 54 mm Hg and/or $Pco_2$: 50 mm Hg) versus the nonspecific symptom category, abnormal blood gases.

Several defining characteristics are cited below in nonspecific form, with accompanying examples of proper specification:

Respiratory depth changes (hypoventilation)
Blood pressure changes (hypotension)
Autonomic responses (dilated pupils, tachycardia)
Altered electrolytes (hypokalemia)
Change in mental state (confusion, obtundation, apprehension)

*Major or critical defining characteristics.* Major or critical defining characteristics are designated signs and/or symptoms that *must be present for the health problem to be considered present.* Major defining characteristics, when applicable, must be present in the nurse's assessment profile to diagnose the corresponding health problem with any degree of certainty. For example, the diagnosis Unilateral Neglect has as its major defining characteristic *consistent inattention to stimuli on affected side*. It is essential, then, that this characteristic be present in the patient's situation (in addition, perhaps, to several other noncritical signs) for the diagnosis of this problem. The assignment of major or critical status to a defining characteristic is based on research or extensive clinical experience in which the signs and symptoms of a health problem are tested for their ability to most reliably predict the presence of the diagnosis and can therefore be used with confidence by the nurse diagnostician.

**GUIDELINES FOR DIAGNOSING HIGH-RISK STATES**

*Determining a risk-state for diagnosis.* Predicting a potential health problem in a given patient involves an estimation of probability. The potential for an event, or pattern of response, to occur can truly be said to exist in almost any situation. Consider the high-risk health problems facing the postoperative patient. This risk state includes High Risk for Noncompliance with the rehabilitative regime, High Risk for Body Image Disturbance, High Risk for Sleep Pattern Disturbance, High Risk for Ineffective Airway Clearance, High Risk for Constipation, and High Risk for Aspiration to name only a few. To state each of these diagnoses on a treatment plan without regard for probabilities and develop desired patient outcomes and interventions for each is pointless.

What needs to occur is an appraisal of the patient's health status and the identification of risk factors that place him or her at higher risk for the health problem than the general population. For example, all persons recovering from abdominal surgery have High Risk for Constipation because of the effects of general anesthesia and narcotic analgesics, manipulation of abdominal viscera, and postoperative immobility. All nurses have a tacit understanding of this risk, and monitoring and intervention are carried out to avert the problem as part of routine nursing care, hence no need to state the problem.* A patient is at higher risk than the general population of postoperative patients if there is, for example, a history of dependence on laxatives, fluid volume deficit, prolonged immobility, or noncompliance with nursing prescription for ambulation. The diagnosis indicating this potential and its risk factors would be stated so that additional and/or more intensified interventions, over those that are routine, can be planned.

*Stating high-risk diagnoses.*† Several of the approved diagnoses address potential dysfunctional states and cite defining characteristics as risk factors. Examples of such diagnoses are:

Altered Nutrition: High Risk for More Than Body Requirements
High Risk for Aspiration
High Risk for Disuse Syndrome
High Risk for Infection
High Risk for Impaired Skin Integrity
High Risk for Injury
High Risk for Poisoning
High Risk for Suffocation
High Risk for Trauma
High Risk for Violence

In addition to those diagnoses formally listed as high risk, any diagnosis from the approved list can be stated as a high-risk problem by simply adding the modifier *high risk for* to the label. For example, Self-Esteem Disturbance can be written High Risk for Self-Esteem Disturbance by virtue of there being risk factors present but not yet the actual health problem.

High-Risk nursing diagnoses have only two parts to the statement: the *health problem at risk* and the *risk factors.*[14] An example is High Risk for Ineffective Individual Coping, risk factors: malignant biopsy results, absence of interpersonal support system, and history of alcohol abuse.

***Diagnostic reasoning.*** **Diagnostic reasoning** is the process through which the nurse moves to arrive at a nursing diagnosis. Like any process, it is often orderly and systematic. However, unlike a process, not all of its factors and operations exist in our conscious awareness. The challenge of refining one's diagnostic reasoning is to bring into awareness the factors and operations that influence the process and are necessary in arriving at an accurate "answer," or diagnosis. Four key components of diagnostic reasoning are collecting and organizing the data base, cues, inferences, and validating inferences.

**COMPONENTS**

*Collecting and organizing the data base.* Collecting and organizing a data base was discussed earlier in this chapter, under Data Collection.

*Cues.* A **cue** is a piece of information, a raw fact. Nurses notice and seek cues regarding patients' health status and functioning. Sweaty palms, restlessness, and a heart rate of 102 beats/min are cues. In the process of diagnostic reasoning, cues are the units of information that are collected and recorded for later analysis.

*Inferences.* An *inference* is the assignment of meaning to cues. A nursing diagnosis is an example of an inference. When individual cues are clustered and interpreted collectively, they begin to assume an identity either the same as or different from what each represented individually. Sweaty palms, restlessness, and a heart rate of 102 beats/min, when interpreted as a cluster, can now mean anxiety, shock, fear, or pain.

Inferences are created, whereas cues exist. The process of creating inferences from cues, therefore, carries with it the risk of error in logic. If the cues sweaty palms, restlessness, and a heart rate of 102 beats/min were grouped and interpreted in a patient who also manifested gurgling respiratory sounds and a rapid, shallow breathing pattern—and these additional cues were overlooked or ignored by the person assigning meaning to the cluster—the inference would be erroneous, the more probable inference now being ineffective airway clearance. Nursing diagnoses are inferences, and the defining characteristics are the cues that lead to these inferences.

*Validating inferences.* Once a diagnostic inference is formulated, the nurse will develop and implement a treatment plan designed to resolve or reduce the problem represented

* No need to state the problem on an individualized nursing care plan; however, this potential problem should be on record in a standards of care manual or standardized care plan.

† NOTE: In 1992 *potential* nursing diagnoses will thenceforth be called *high-risk* nursing diagnoses. The term *high risk* will be applied throughout the remainder of this text.

by that inference. Erroneous inferences carry an obvious implication in terms of potential patient harm resulting from treatment of a nonexistent health problem or from treatment withheld for a missed diagnosis: nursing malpractice. Consequently, it is essential to seek validation of diagnostic inferences before implementing treatment.

Four approaches to the validation of inferences are recommended. The first is to consult with an authoritative source. This may be a clinical nurse specialist, nurse educator, a textbook, or published research, for example. Seek confirmation of the logical and scientific integrity of your diagnostic statement. Second, reexamine the cues: Could the ones in this diagnostic statement support any other diagnosis or only the one chosen? Could the cues from the data base felt *not* to be a part of the cluster supporting this diagnosis belong to some other cluster, or could several of them, together with cues supporting this diagnosis, suggest an altogether different diagnosis? Third, nurses should validate inferences with the patient. Nurses may share with the patient the cluster of cues identified and what is represented. Patients often have remarkable insight into what underlies their patterns of response and can be of great resource in validating the nurse's conclusions. Additionally, people benefit significantly from having their situations reflected back to them. Indeed, collaborating with the patient in this way may be all the intervention that is necessary. Fourth is to seek evidence of the reliability of the diagnostic inference from within the appropriate reference group. Do most professional peers conclude the same explanation for the available cues?

These approaches are workable strategies for seeking validation of diagnostic inferences before the institution of treatment; however, the only way to achieve or confirm validation of a diagnosis is to treat the problem and evaluate the outcome. If favorable and predicted outcomes result, strong evidence exists that the problem and its etiology and defining characteristics were accurately inferred.

**SOURCES OF DIAGNOSTIC ERROR.** Currently there is much scientific curiosity within the nursing profession regarding the diagnostic reasoning process, strategies effective in increasing diagnostic accuracy, and sources of diagnostic error. Many of the principles identified through research thus far have come from studying differences in the diagnostic strategies employed by experts and those used by novices.[5,6,8,30] The following discussion will focus only on the most common type of diagnostic error, *the inferential leap,* and several of its sources. For more in-depth examinations of the skills of clinical problem solving and decision making, the reader is referred to Gordon, Carnevali, Tanner, and Benner.

*Inferential leap.* As the term implies, the inferential leap involves a jump to a conclusion based on premature termination of the data gathering/data analysis phase of the nursing process. Numerous studies have shown that this jump to an erroneous conclusion is most frequently made because not all of the variables were known or examined at the time the inference was formulated.[5,8,30] Interestingly, the novice often closes the *search* for cues prematurely, whereas the expert will more often prematurely terminate the *analysis* of cues.

The novice may close the search for cues prematurely because of a lack of understanding of the scope of the problem to be diagnosed. Diagnoses such as Disturbance in Self-Concept and Ineffective Individual Coping are reported to be at the highest level of abstraction among nursing diagnoses and are therefore more difficult to fully grasp, let alone discriminate from other diagnostic possibilities.[20] The expert has an advantage in this regard by virtue of a greater breadth of experience, both with the label and the clinical presentation of patients demonstrating the problem.

Additionally, the novice will often halt the collection of data and conclude a diagnosis prematurely because of a discomfiture with uncertainty. The erring expert will, however, occasionally rely too heavily on knowledge from previous experience, which can foster a tendency to stereotype patients and their health alterations, thereby obscuring vital relationships among assessment data.[8]

**Professional advantages of nursing diagnosis.** Baer has assembled from the literature the following statements in advocacy of nursing diagnosis. They are presented here to highlight the advantages nursing diagnosis brings to the profession.

Nursing diagnosis

- Assists in organizing, defining, and developing nursing knowledge
- Aids in identifying and describing the domain and scope of nursing practice
- Focuses nursing care on the patient's response to problems
- Prescribes diagnosis-specific nursing interventions that should increase the effectiveness of nursing care
- Facilitates the evaluation of nursing practice
- Provides a framework for testing the validity of nursing interventions
- Provides a standardized vocabulary to enhance intraprofessional and interprofessional communication
- Prescribes the content of nursing curricula
- Provides a framework for developing a system to direct third-party reimbursements for nursing services
- Indicates specific rationales for patient care based on nursing assessment
- Leads to more comprehensive and individualized patient care[4]

In summary, nursing diagnoses are standardized labels that represent clinical judgments made by professional nurses and describe health problems resolved primarily by nursing therapies. Nursing diagnosis focuses nursing assessment and intervention on the human response to altered health states, thus constituting a unique, distinct, and imperative component to critical health care. Nursing diagnosis is mandated as part of competent registered nurse criteria by many state Nurse Practice Acts, as well as constituting the core of the ANA's formal definition of nursing.

## Planning

Two things are accomplished in the planning phase of the nursing process: (1) patient **outcome criteria** are established and (2) *nursing interventions* are selected.

**Outcome criteria.** Outcome statements consist of highly specific indicators that will be used by the nurse in the evaluation phase as criteria that either (1) the actual problem has been resolved or reduced, or (2) the high-risk problem has not occurred. An outcome statement is a projection of the expected influence that the nursing intervention will have on the patient in relation to the identified problem. Though often confused, statements of expected patient outcome are *not* patient goals or nursing goals, nor should they describe nursing interventions.

As shown in Fig. 1-3, outcome criteria for an *actual* problem are developed from the signs and symptoms of the nursing diagnosis. In other words, the assessment findings that were used to certify the existence of a diagnosis should also be used to establish its resolution or improvement. For example:

| *Nursing diagnosis* | *Outcome criteria* |
|---|---|
| Ineffective Breathing Pattern R/T respiratory muscle fatigue | $P_{CO_2} \leq 45$ |
| | RR ≤ 20 at rest |
| AEB-$P_{CO_2}$ = 52 | |
| -RR = 28 | |

Outcome criteria for *high-risk* problems differ only in that, being a two-part statement, signs and symptoms will be absent from the diagnostic statement. Fig. 1-4 illustrates how the outcome criteria are developed from what would be the signs and symptoms of the high-risk problem *were it to become actual*. For example:

| *Nursing diagnosis* | *Outcome criteria* |
|---|---|
| High Risk for Aspiration | Lungs clear to auscultation |
| RISK FACTORS: | Absence of blue tinge to tracheal aspirate |
| Endotracheal tube | |
| Continuous intraenteral feedings | Afebrile |
| Decreased level of consciousness | $SvO_2 \geq 94\%$ |

Outcome criteria should be measurable, desirable, and—given full consideration to the resources of the patient and those of the nurse—attainable.

Measurable outcome criteria consist of patient behaviors, statements, and/or physiological parameters that are recognizable on their occurrence. Many of the phenomena critical care nurses diagnose and treat are readily measurable, such as adequacy of ventilation, cardiac output, and tissue perfusion. Many, however, are not readily measurable and thus present a challenging task to care planning in general and outcome criteria development specifically. Phenomena such as anxiety, powerlessness, body image, and coping involve the patient's subjective perception and, as such, elude the nurse's quantification. Outcome statements such as "less anxiety," "perceives personal power," or "copes effectively" represent favorable goals for nursing interventions but offer little in the way of criteria against which successful patient attainment can be measured. Again, here it is helpful to consider the signs and symptoms of the problem being treated and to modify them to reflect a situation in which the problem is absent or reduced. Several examples are:

| *Signs and symptoms* | *Outcome criteria* |
|---|---|
| "Why is it I have no say in any of this?" | Patient makes five decisions regarding his or her care |
| Distracted, preoccupied | Maintains eye contact throughout interactions |
| Looks away during stoma care | Visually regards stoma |

Outcome statements are made further measurable by indicating the date and time of anticipated attainment. Projecting outcome attainment seems in some situations to be an arbitrary exercise, such as predicting the date or hour for the return of clear lung fields. The importance of this aspect of outcome criteria development lies however in the fact that a specific deadline for evaluation of outcome attainment has been designated. Evaluating attainment of the outcome at designated intervals ensures that certain problems do not persist beyond acceptable time periods (such as Altered Peripheral Tissue Perfusion, Urinary Retention, and Pain) and that modification of the treatment approach occurs regularly. The outcome criteria applied throughout this text purposefully do not include date and time projection for attainment as this should be a reflection of actual, not hypothetical, patient characteristics.

The desirability and attainability of patient outcome cri-

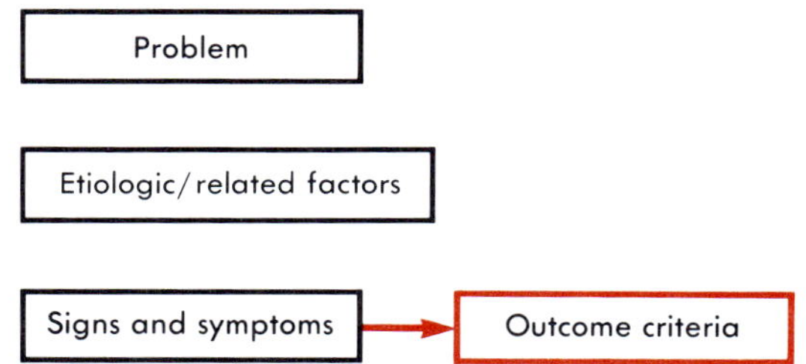


***Fig. 1-3*** Developing outcome criteria for an actual problem.

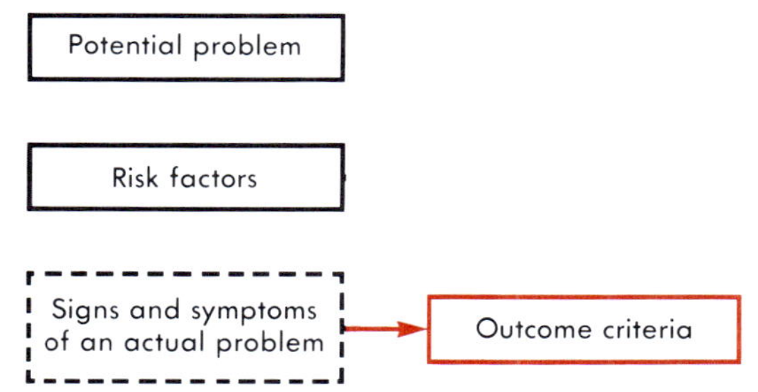


***Fig. 1-4*** Developing outcome criteria for a high-risk problem.

***Table 1-2*** Correct and incorrect outcome criteria statements

| Nursing diagnosis | Incorrect outcome | Correct outcome |
|---|---|---|
| Fluid volume deficit | Improved hydration<br>Patient will be offered 100 cc fluid q 2 hr | Systolic blood pressure ≥100 mm Hg<br>24 hr fluid intake ≥body surface area fluid requirements<br>Skin turgor ≤3 seconds |
| Decreased cardiac output | Hemodynamic stability | Cardiac index 2.5-4.0 |
| Potential for thrombophlebitis* | Patient will be taught active leg exercises<br>Patient will perform active leg exercises 10 × q 1 hr | No calf tenderness<br>No ankle swelling |
| Pain | Patient will have a reduction in pain | Pain ≤"4/10" 10 minutes after IV narcotic |
| Powerlessness | Patient will perceive greater control over situation | Patient will make five decisions regarding his or her care |

*Not an approved diagnosis.

teria is another important aspect of planning nursing management. Individual patient baseline, patterns, and nurse and patient resources are the dominant considerations given to a projection of desired outcome, versus normative values. An example of an undesirable outcome is "RR <16 at rest" for a patient with an unmodifiable chest wall restriction. "Absence of pain" in a patient with a sternotomy incision is also an undesirable target for early postoperative intervention. Examples of outcome criteria that are unattainable (and therefore undesirable) are "$P_{CO_2}$ <40" in a patient who chronically retains carbon dioxide and "no anxiety" preoperatively for open heart surgery (see Table 1-2 for examples of correct and incorrect outcome criteria statements for assorted nursing diagnoses).

Developing outcome criteria statements has particular relevance to critical care nursing, because they describe, in measurable terms, the effects or results of critical care nursing. And they communicate the influence nursing intervention has in preventing, resolving, or improving various health states and provide a basis for justifying the allocation and reimbursement of professional nursing resources.

**Nursing intervention**

***The power of nursing intervention.*** Interventions are the power of nursing and a distinct strength of this text. Also known as *nursing orders* or *nursing prescriptions,* interventions constitute the treatment approach to an identified problem. Interventions are selected to satisfy the outcome criteria and prevent or resolve the nursing diagnosis.

A common shortcoming of nursing interventions, as much in the literature as in individual practice, is the prescription of very vague, weak, nonsubstantive nursing actions. By definition, a nursing diagnosis is a health problem that nurses treat. *Treatment* implies producing a change in a situation, not merely maintaining equilibrium. And *prescribe* connotes recommending a course of action, not simply supporting an existing regimen. Intervention strategies that consist solely of monitoring, measuring, checking, obtaining physician orders, documenting, reporting, and notifying do not fulfill criteria for the treatment of a problem. Nursing intervention for nursing diagnoses should designate therapeutic activity that assists the patient in moving from one state of health to another. The growing body of research-based independent nursing therapies should be liberally applied to treatment plans for nursing diagnoses in critical care. Exciting advances in nurse management of such phenomena as ventilation-perfusion inequalities, excessive preload and afterload, increased intracranial pressure, and sensory-perceptual alterations associated with critical illness afford the critical care nurse the opportunity to incorporate potency into treatment plans.

***Focus for interventions.*** As discussed earlier in this chapter, interventions have the greatest impact when they are directed at the etiologic/related factors of the diagnosis (Fig. 1-5) or, in the case of a high-risk problem, the risk factors (Fig. 1-6). This stipulates that the etiologic factors of a problem be modifiable by nursing. To achieve the most favorable patient outcome, the multiple etiologic factors of a problem should be studied carefully and interventions selected to modify each.

***Specificity of interventions.*** Planned interventions should provide clarity, specificity, and direction to the spectrum of nurses implementing care for a patient. Statements such as "check vital signs" and "measure I and O" provide no real direction to nursing care and are therefore quite useless. Instead, "monitor for heart rate elevations 30 beats/min over baseline" and "look for 24 hr positive fluid balances" are preferable.

Include a brief rationale as part of intervention statement where this would enhance understanding of the treatment maneuver. For example, "change position dynamically q2hr, *to best match ventilation with perfusion.*" Rationales are *italicized* throughout the care planning sections of this book.

Medically delegated actions, such as administering med-

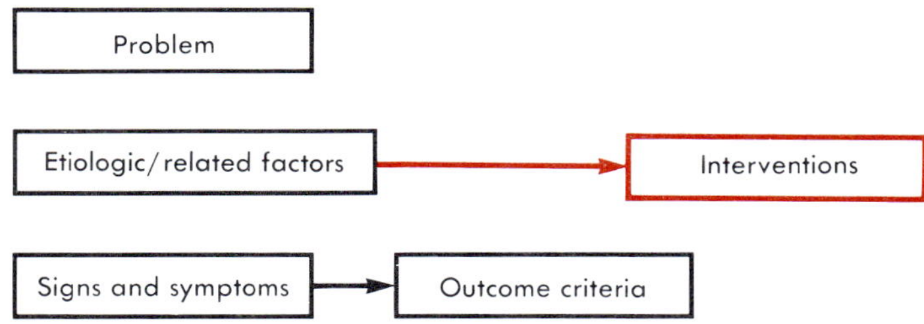


***Fig. 1-5*** Developing interventions for an actual problem.

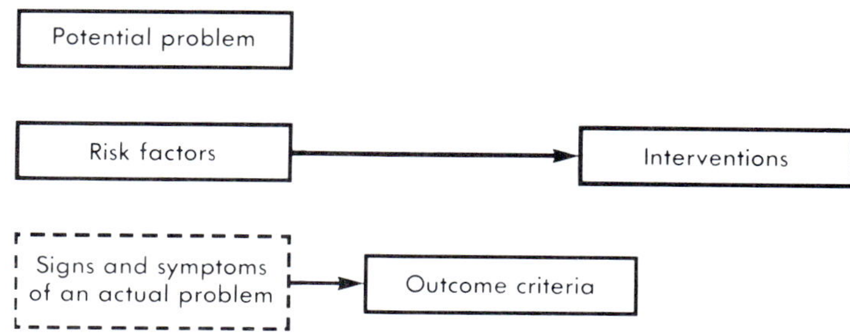


***Fig. 1-6*** Developing interventions for a high-risk problem.

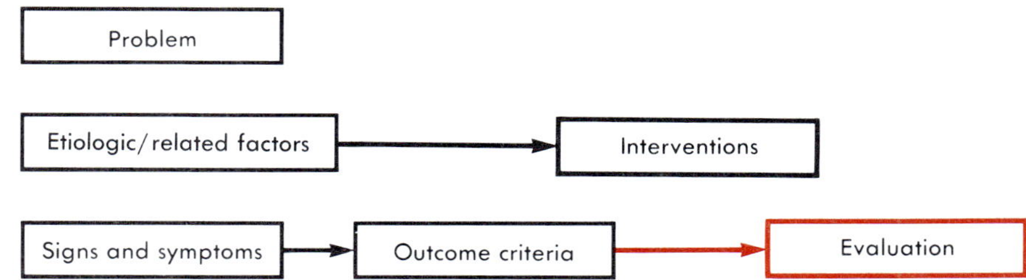


***Fig. 1-7*** Evaluating an actual problem.

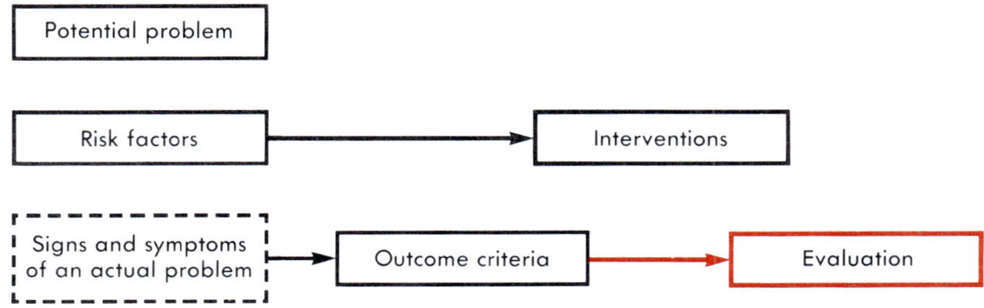


***Fig. 1-8*** Evaluating a high-risk problem.

ications and initiating ventilator setting changes, should be included in the interventions but with the emphasis placed clearly on the assessments and judgments the nurse makes in evaluating their effectiveness, patient tolerance, safety, dosage, titration, and discontinuance. In critical care there is no such thing, for example, as "administer nitroprusside as ordered." Adequate specificity of nursing orders has been achieved when one is reasonably certain that a nurse unfamiliar with the patient can review the treatment plan and implement the kind of care intended by the primary nurse or case manager.

### Implementation

Implementation is the action component of planning. It is the phase of the nursing process in which the nursing treatment plan is carried out. Data collection and evaluation are continuous throughout this phase.

### Evaluation

Evaluation of attainment of the expected patient outcomes occurs formally at intervals designated in the outcome criteria. Informal evaluation occurs continuously. Fig. 1-7 and Fig. 1-8 illustrate how evaluation is conducted in relation to the outcome criteria for actual and high-risk problems, respectively. There are two components to the evaluation phase of the nursing process. First, the nurse should compare the patient's current state with that described by the outcome criteria: Are his breath sounds clear and equal bilaterally? Is the tidal volume of his spontaneous respirations >500 cc, as they were projected to be by this point in time? An evaluation of nursing effectiveness is done by commenting on the extent to which a predicted outcome has been attained.

Second, the nurse should query: If not, why not? Is it too soon to evaluate? Should implementation of the plan be continued for 24 hours longer and then reevaluated? Should the interventions be intensified; perhaps increase the frequency of respiratory muscle strengthening exercises? Are the outcome criteria impractical for this patient? Is the validity of the nursing diagnosis questionable? Are more data needed? Specific recommendations are then proposed which include either continuing implementation as outlined or returning to the data collection, nursing diagnosis, planning, or implementation phase of the process.

The evaluation phase and the activities that take place within it is perhaps the most important dimension of the nursing process (see Fig. 1-1). Evaluation of patient progress against a standard of nursing care incorporates accountability into the process—accountability to the standard of care. Lack of progress in outcome attainment or lack of progress in problem solving is readily identified and kept in check, and alternate solutions can then be proposed.

#### REFERENCES


1. American Association of Critical-Care Nurses: Demonstration project, Newport Beach, Calif, 1988, The Association.
2. American Nurses' Association: Nursing: a social policy statement, Kansas City, Mo, 1980, The Association.
3. Aspinall NJ: Nursing diagnosis: the weak link, Nurs Outlook 24:433, 1976.
4. Baer CL: Nursing diagnosis, Top Clin Nurs 5:89, 1984.
5. Benner P: From novice to expert: excellence and power in clinical nursing practice, Menlo Park, Calif, 1984, Addison-Wesley.
6. Benner P and Tanner C: How expert nurses use intuition, Am J Nurs 87:23, 1987.
7. Carnevali DL: Nursing care planning: diagnosis and management, Philadelphia, 1983, JB Lippincott Co.
8. Carnevali DL, and others: Diagnostic reasoning in nursing, Philadelphia, 1984, JP Lippincott Co.
9. Carpenito LJ: Nursing diagnosis: application to clinical practice, Philadelphia, 1989, JB Lippincott Co.
10. Cosier RA and Alpin JC: Intuition and decision-making: some empirical evidence, Psychol Rep 51:275, 1982.
11. Davie JK: Independent and interdependent/collaborative nursing practice, Newsletter of the Southern California Nursing Diagnosis Association 5:3, 1988.
12. Dreyfus H and Dreyfus S: Mind over machine: the power of human intuition and expertise in the era of the computer, New York, 1985, Free Press.
13. Gebbie KM and Lavin MA: Classification of nursing diagnoses: proceedings of the first national conference, St Louis, 1975, Mosby—Year Book, Inc.
14. Gordon M: Nursing diagnosis: process and application, St Louis, 1991, Mosby—Year Book, Inc.
15. Guzzetta CE, and others: Clinical assessment tools for use with nursing diagnoses, St Louis, 1989, Mosby—Year Book, Inc.
16. Guzzetta CE, and others: Unitary person assessment tool: easing problems with nursing diagnoses, Focus Crit Care 15:12, 1988.
17. Kim M: The dilemma of physiological problems: without collaboration, what's left?, Am J Nurs 85:281, 1985.
18. Kritek PB: Generation and classification of nursing diagnoses: toward a theory of nursing, Image J Nurs Sch 10:33, 1978.
19. Kritek PB: Nursing diagnosis in perspective: response to a critique, Image J Nurs Sch 17:3, 1985.
20. Kritek PB: Advantages and limitations of using nursing diagnostic categories as a framework for nursing practice research. Audiotape transcription: Debate at the National Teaching Institute of American Association of Critical-Care Nurses, Anaheim, Calif, May 1986.
21. Kritek PB: Development of a taxonomic structure for nursing diagnoses: a review and an update. In Hurley ME, editor: Classification of nursing diagnoses: proceedings of the sixth conference, St Louis, 1986, Mosby—Year Book, Inc.
22. Mundinger MO: Nursing diagnoses for cancer patients, Cancer Nurs 1:122, 1978.
23. Munhall PL and Oiler CJ: Nursing research, Norwalk, Conn, 1986, Appleton-Century-Crofts.
24. Prescott PA, Dennis KE, and Jacox AK: Clinical decision-making of staff nurses, Image J Nurs Sch 19:56, 1987.
25. Rew L: Intuition in decision-making, Image J Nurs Sch 20:150, 1988.
26. Roberts SL: Physiologic nursing diagnoses are necessary and appropriate for critical care, Focus Crit Care 15:42, 1988.
27. Shoemaker J: Essential features of a nursing diagnosis. In Kim MJ, McFarland G, and McLane A, editors: Classification of nursing diagnoses: proceedings of the fifth national conference, St Louis, 1984, Mosby—Year Book, Inc.
28. Smith SK: An analysis of the phenomenon of deterioration in the critically ill, Image J Nurs Sch 20:12, 1988.
29. Tanner C: Overview. Symposium on nursing diagnosis in critical care, Heart Lung 14:423, 1985.
30. Tanner C, and others: Diagnostic reasoning strategies of nurses and nursing students, Nurs Res 36:358, 1987.
31. Webster's New Collegiate Dictionary, ed 9, Springfield, Mass, 1986, Merriam-Webster, Inc.
32. Wescott MR: Antecedents and consequences of intuitive thinking. Final report to US Department of Health, Education & Welfare, Poughkeepsie, New York, 1968, Vassar College.

CHAPTER 2

# Ethical and Legal Issues

## CHAPTER OBJECTIVES

- *Relate the ethical theories of consequentialism and formalism to decision making in critical care.*
- *Discuss ethical principles as they relate to the critical care patient.*
- *Describe what constitutes an ethical dilemma.*
- *List steps for making ethical decisions.*
- *Identify legal and professional obligations of critical care nurses.*
- *Describe the elements of several torts that might result from critical care nursing practice.*
- *Delineate types of liability.*

## KEY TERMS

morals, p. 15
ethics, p. 16
consequentialism, p. 16
autonomy, p. 16
beneficence, p. 17
nonmaleficence, p. 17
distributive justice, p. 18
quality of life, p. 19
ethical dilemma, p. 20
ethical decision making, p. 20
tort, p. 22
negligence, p. 23
malpractice, p. 23
personal liability, p. 25
vicarious liability, p. 25
res ipsa loquitur, p. 25
borrowed servant, p. 25

## CRITICAL CARE NURSING PRACTICE: ETHICAL OVERVIEW

There has been a revolution in health care in the last 50 years as the result of new technologies and treatments that were used during World War II. Issues that require ethical decisions about treatments, therapies, and life support are found in all health care settings and are most evident in technologically advanced critical care units. A multiplicity of factors surrounds ethical decisions and has an impact on both the health care recipient and the health care provider: autonomy, philosophical views of health and life, moral and ethical beliefs, societal trends, cultural background, legal directives, health care costs, and bureaucratic constraints.

The most common ethical issues that occur in critical care units are those of foregoing treatment and allocating the scarce critical care unit resource. Historically, the critical care professionals believed that life had to be maintained at all costs and that death signified the failure of medicine and technology. More recently, long-term prognosis in terms of quality of life has replaced the earlier emphasis on sanctity of life as a major factor in ethical decision making.

The critical care nurse is confronted with moral and ethical conflicts on a frequent, sometimes daily, basis and is the health care professional who is most involved with all persons affected by the decision.[37,62] It is essential that the critical care nurse has an understanding of professional nursing ethics and ethical theories and principles and that she or he is able to use a decision-making model to guide nursing actions.[61] The purpose of this chapter is to provide the reader with an overview of ethical theories and principles and professional nursing ethics. An ethical decision-making model will be described and illustrated. Finally, recommendations will be given about methods to discuss ethical issues in the critical care setting.

## MORALS AND ETHICS

### Morals Defined

The word **moral** is derived from the Latin *moralis*, which is defined as "good or right in conduct or character . . . making the distinction between right and wrong . . . principles of right and wrong based on custom."[27] Morals are the "shoulds," "should nots," "oughts," and "ought nots" of actions and behaviors and have been related closely to sexual mores and behaviors in Western society. Religious and cultural values and beliefs largely mold one's moral thoughts and actions. Morals form the basis for action and provide a framework for evaluation of behavior.

### Ethics Defined

The word **ethics** is derived from the Greek *ethos,* which is defined as "the system or code of morals of a particular person, religion, group, or profession . . . the study of standards of conduct and moral judgment."[27] The term ethics is sometimes used interchangeably with the word morals. However, ethics is more concerned with the "why" of the action rather than with whether the action is right or wrong, good or bad.[54] Ethics implies that an evaluation is being made that is theoretically based on or derived from a set of standards. *Normative ethics* is the division of ethics that focuses on "norms or standards of behavior and value and their ultimate application to daily life"[24] with an emphasis on evaluation for purposes of guiding moral action. *Bioethics* incorporates all aspects of life but most frequently refers to health care ethics and the application of ethical principles to individual cases.

## ETHICAL THEORIES

Philosophers have described ethical theories to be the combination of thinking processes, related principles, and rationales. The approach is normative, because it attempts to provide a basis for action. There are two traditional ethical theories that will be briefly discussed in this chapter: teleological and deontological.

### Teleological Theory (Consequentialism)

The focus of **consequentialism** is on the consequence of an action. There is an obligation for individuals to provide the greatest amount of happiness for the greatest number or the least amount of harm to the greatest number. The underlying assumption is that harm and benefit can be weighed and measured and that the outcome will demonstrate a good over evil for most people.[17] According to Fowler, utilitarian ethics is the most important teleological theory for use in health care today.[24] Two common aphorisms summarize the utilitarianism approach: "the greatest good for the greatest number" and "the end justifies the means."[54]

### Deontological Theory (Formalism)

The focus of the deontological approach to ethical problems is on the rules that determine the rightness or wrongness of the action.[24,64] Immanuel Kant, a German philosopher, has been credited with the formulation of this approach. Democratic principles or laws are stressed and universality is the basis for decisions.[64] Past moral or ethical judgments are considered, and value is assigned to significant relationships, commitments, and promises. Actions are independently assessed for their own value, and the consequences are not part of the decision.[33]

The aphorism inherent in formalism is "the end does not justify the means." Decisions based on formalism are normally congruent with one's strong sense of duty when acting out of principle regardless of consequences.[32,35] Strict adherence to rules, policies, and standards may stifle creativity and examination of alternatives in the fast paced health care environment of today.

## ETHICAL PRINCIPLES

There are certain ethical principles that were derived from classic ethical theories that are used in health care decision making.[33] Principles are general guidelines that govern conduct, provide a basis for reasoning, and direct actions.[17] The six ethical principles that will be discussed in this chapter are autonomy, beneficence, nonmaleficence, veracity, fidelity, and justice.

### Autonomy

The concept of **autonomy** appears in all ancient writings and early Greek philosophy. Immanuel Kant described an ethical person as one who is guided and motivated in response to one's own inward obedience, free from coercion, desire, or fear of future consequences.[31] Persons are not to be treated as a means to an end but rather as an end themselves.[26] In health care, autonomy can be viewed as the freedom to make decisions about one's own body without the coercion or interference of others. Autonomy is a freedom of choice or a self-determination that is a basic human right. It can be experienced in all human life events.

The obligation for health care professionals is to respect the values, thoughts, and actions of patients and not to let their own values or morals influence treatment decisions.[13,39] Fry described this as a respect for the "unconditional worth of the individual."[26] Often there is a conflict between the values of the patient and the health care professionals when dealing with life-sustaining matters in critical care. Miller suggested that any conflict can be "resolved by taking a firm line on autonomy: any autonomous decision of a patient must be respected."[39]

The critical care nurse is often "caught in the middle" in ethical situations and promoting autonomous decision making is one of those situations. As the nurse works closely with patients and families to promote autonomous decision making, another crucial element becomes clear. Patients and families must have all of the information about a certain situation to make a decision that is best for them. Not only should they be given all of the information and facts, but they must also have a clear understanding of what was presented. This is where the nurse is a most important member of the health care team—that is, providing more information, clarifying points, reinforcing information, and providing support during the process.

### Beneficence

The concept of doing good and preventing harm to patients is a *sine qua non* for the nursing profession. However, the ethical principle of **beneficence,** which requires that one promote the well-being of patients, points to the importance of this duty for the health care professional. According to Davis and Aroskar, the principle of beneficence presupposes that harms and benefits are balanced, leading to positive or beneficial outcomes.[17]

Murphy described the ethical mandate of the nurse as being different from that of the physician in some aspects of care. Because nurses diagnose and treat human responses to health problems, it is they who deal most closely with quality of life issues.[41] In these situations, the nurse is obligated to act different from the physician, whose duty is to preserve life at all means.

In approaching issues related to beneficence, there is frequently conflict with another principle, that of autonomy. *Paternalism* exists when the nurse or physician makes a decision for the patient without consulting or including the patient in the decision process. *Paternalism* is "making people do what is good for them" and "preventing people from doing what is bad for them."[31] Jameton[31] described two types of paternalists: strong paternalists who make decisions for obviously competent persons and weak paternalists who make decisions for persons who are mentally or physically unable to make their own decision.

Traditional health care has been based on a paternalistic approach to patients. Many patients are still more comfortable in deferring all decisions about care and treatment to their health care provider. Active involvement by various organizations and agencies regarding health care has demonstrated a trend toward the public's need and desire for more information about health care and alternative treatments and providers. Paternalism, or maternalism in the case of female providers, may always be a possibility in the health care setting, but enlightened consumers are changing this practice of health care professionals.

In the critical care setting, there are many instances and possibilities for paternalistic actions by the nurse. Postoperative care, which is designed to assist the patient with a quick recovery, is a good example of paternalistic action by the nurse. Encouraging the patient to turn, cough, and deep breathe and increasing activity in the form of dangling, sitting in a chair, and ambulating are all paternalistic when the patient is in pain, sleep deprived, and wanting to be left alone. However, there are times when the priorities of benefits and harms must be balanced. In this instance, the duty to do no harm, which is the next principle to be discussed, takes precedence over paternalistic actions. When there are conflicts in ethical principles, one must weigh all of the benefits and choose the best one.[17]

### Nonmaleficence

The ethical principle of **nonmaleficence,** which dictates that one prevent harm and remove harmful situations is a *prima facie* duty for the nurse.[17] Thoughtfulness and care are necessary, as is balancing risks and benefits, which was discussed earlier with beneficence. Beneficence and nonmaleficence are on two ends of a continuum and are often carried out differently, depending on the views of the practitioner. A practitioner using a utilitarian approach will consider long-term consequences and the good to society as a whole. The practitioner operating from a deontological basis will consider the principle and its effect on the single individual in the situation.

Such complex situations as quality of life versus sanctity of life are always difficult to analyze in the critical care setting as well as in non–critical care settings. Flynn described such decisions as withholding and withdrawing treatments as being based on not one ethical principle alone, but rather on a balance of all ethical principles so that the most appropriate moral decision can be made.[22] Nonmaleficence should serve as the guide for practice of health care professionals.[33]

### Veracity

Veracity or truth-telling is an important ethical principle that underlies the nurse-patient relationship. In 1860 Florence Nightingale described veracity with patients: "Far more now than formerly does the medical attendant tell the truth to the sick who are really desirous to hear it about their own state."[45] Nightingale's philosophy was not agreed on by other health care providers of the time (that is, physicians), but she was sensitive to the needs of patients who sought information about their own conditions.

Veracity is important in soliciting informed consent, so that the patient is aware of all potential risks and benefits from specific treatments or their alternatives. Once again, the critical care nurse can be in the middle of a situation where all of the facts and information about a particular treatment option are not disclosed. Sometimes information has been given accurately but has been delivered with bias or in a way that is misleading. In this case and other instances with veracity, the ethical principle of autonomy has been violated.[4]

Are there ever any situations in which nurses should lie to patients? This subject was discussed in depth by Schmelzer and Anema[53] who posed that nurses make many value judgments in their daily practice, some of which are made after careful consideration and some of which are made quickly with minimal thought. Veracity is also related closely to the principle of beneficence in which the nurse must consider whether the lie will benefit the patient and if so, how. They stressed the importance of designating lies as negative benefits when comparing them with the positive benefits of the truth.

When faced with a veracity dilemma, one should analyze the personal abilities, values, and beliefs of the patient. All possible options and truthful alternatives should be examined. The long-term effects of a lie may be the loss of credibility of the nurse with the patient, the need for additional "cover-up" lies, and stress to the nurse who told the lie. Schmelzer and Anema concluded that "nurses should be committed to telling the truth and, when faced with situations where they are tempted to lie, should instead seek alternative actions based on honesty."[53] This principle should guide all areas of practice for the nurse, that is, colleague relationships, employee relationships, as well as the nurse-patient relationship.

### Fidelity

Another ethical principle that is closely related to autonomy and veracity is fidelity. Fidelity, or faithfulness and promise-keeping to patients, is also a *sine qua non* for nursing. It forms a bond between individuals and is the basis of all relationships, both professional and personal. Regardless of the amount of autonomy that patients have in the critical care areas, they are still quite dependent on the nurse for a multitude of types of physical care and emotional support. A trusting relationship that establishes and maintains an open atmosphere is one that is very positive for all involved.

As do all the other principles, fidelity extends to the family of the critical care patient. When a promise is made to the family that they will be called if an emergency arises or that they will be informed of other special events, the nurse should make every effort to follow through on the promise. Not only will fidelity be upheld for the nurse-family relationship, but there will also be a positive reflection on the nursing profession as a whole and on the institution in which the nurse is employed.

*Confidentiality* is one element of fidelity that is based on traditional health care professional ethics. According to Veatch and Fry,[59] the nursing and medical professions have established ethical codes that allow no patient-centered reasons for breaking the principle of confidentiality. Confidentiality is described as a right whereby patient information can only be shared with those involved in the care of the patient. An exception to this guideline might be when the welfare of others is at risk by keeping patient information confidential. Again in this situation, the nurse must balance ethical principles and weigh risks with benefits. Special circumstances, such as mandatory reporting laws, will guide the nurse in certain situations.

*Privacy* has also been described as inherent in the principle of fidelity. It may be closely aligned with confidentiality of patient information and a patient's right to privacy of his or her person, such as maintaining privacy for the patient by pulling the curtains around the bed or making sure that he or she is adequately covered.

### Justice/Allocation of Resources

The principle of justice is often used synonymously with the concept of allocation of scarce resources. Contrary to the belief of many people, health care is not a right guaranteed by the Constitution of the United States. Rather, *access* to health care should be provided to all people. With escalating health care costs, expanded technologies, an aging population with its own special health care needs, and (in some instances) a scarcity of health care personnel, the question of health care allocation becomes even more complex.[40,51]

The application of the justice principle in health care is concerned primarily with allocation of goods and services, which is termed **distributive justice.** According to Jameton, distributive justice appears at three levels of health care: national policies and budget, state or local distribution of resources, and distribution in the individual health care settings.[31] Traditionally, six criteria for making decisions about allocation of resources have been used.[31,34] Distribution has been based on:

- Equality for all persons
- Individual merit
- Societal contributions
- Availability in an open market
- Individual need
- Similar treatment for similar cases

**Equality for all persons.** Equality for all persons has been a traditional stance of health care and has been evidenced in ethical codes and in the practices of professionals. With equality, all persons are given equal treatments and resources, such as access to health care, technologies, specialists, personnel to perform necessary care and treatment, and support for physical and emotional needs during the process.

**Individual merit.** Distribution of services based on individual merit has not been a traditional practice of health care professionals and is an area that may be subtle to observe. Individual merit might be based on that which has already been achieved or that which is expected to occur in the future, such as in the case of an infant or child or a person who may have potential for success in some endeavor. Basically, the issue at hand is whether this type of person deserves a particular treatment. The decision is based on values that are subjective and not driven by a set of rules or principles.

**Societal contribution.** Decisions based on the societal contribution of the individual examine the worth of that individual in society and are subjective and value based. Using this as a framework for making decisions causes the elderly, the young, persons who have conditions that are socially undesirable such as alcoholism or mental diseases, and those who are handicapped to a degree that makes them very dependent to be considered to not have worth to society.

**Free market acquisition.** Justice determined by free market acquisition is guided by money and what individuals can acquire with their money. Persons both in the past and in the present who have unlimited money are able to receive the ultimate in services and are able to quickly search for and find services to meet their needs and desires. They are usually limited only by the technologies and services available. However, when time is not crucial, money will pay for technologies or services that can be developed if there is money to support such efforts.

**Individual need.** Jameton described individual need as most applicable to health care in deciding allocation of resources.[31] The dilemma arises when one considers one individual's need for heart transplantation or other technologies versus the possibility of using those resource dollars for early education on preventing heart disease for many people.

**Similar treatment for similar cases.** The concept of similar treatment for similar cases expands on the concept of equality and applies the same basic principle at the societal level. However, consideration of contribution to society is also inherent in this method of decision. For instance, criteria may be established that designate that all who have a certain condition and who are under a certain age will be given the treatment, surgery, or service. This allows equal access of all who meet those criteria but disallows others who do not meet the criteria. Decisions based on this standard cover groups of people, whereas decisions based on individual need hold only for that one person.

## ALLOCATION OF SCARCE RESOURCES IN CRITICAL CARE

According to Engelhardt and Rie[20]:

> It is impossible to discover a concrete view of a just system of health care allocation. . . . At best, moral arguments will be able to establish a range of acceptable models. As a result, moral justifiable concrete system for providing health care is secured through common agreement, rather than through rational arguments alone.

There have been reductions in federally funded health care programs and a leveling off of monies for health care research funds from previous years. Resources available for health needs are no longer unlimited, as they previously appeared to be. It has become evident that both resource allocation and allocation decisions will become inevitable and may appear in forms of public policies and guidelines.[21] Allocation will be discussed in two areas: allocation of technologies and treatments and allocation of health care energy.

### Allocation of Technologies and Treatments

Marsden[36] described health care professionals as dealing with the needs of their current patients and families, not as anticipating future patients' needs. Health care providers may be required to act based on rules and regulations that are in conflict with their code of ethics or ethical principles. Discussions of the moral and ethical dilemmas inherent in organ procurement and transplantation are liberally demonstrated in the literature.[7,9,10,19,36,42]

Other technologies found in critical care that were considered experimental only a few years ago are the intraaortic balloon pump (IABP),[6] the left ventricular assist device (LVAD), and the artificial heart.[47] Essential in the use of all technologies and critical care treatments are veracity, autonomy, and informed consent,[6] which have been discussed earlier in this chapter. In cases in which research protocols are used with patients in the critical care units, all ethical principles apply.[18]

**Quality of life** is an issue that should be considered when examining the use of technologies. It is an area that is very personal and value laden and one that will be different for all involved and dependent on the content. O'Mara[47] described quality of life having dual dimensions of both objectivity and subjectivity. Objectivity examines the person's functionability, whereas subjectivity analyzes his or her psychosocial state. He stated that an evaluation of quality of life issues can only take place after one has received the technology and "lived" that "new" life.

### Allocation of Health Care Energy

Of all hospital beds in the United States, 6% to 10% are designated as critical care, which reflects a higher proportion than in any other country.[32] Knaus stated that "access to an expensive and complex resource like intensive care can never be absolute."[32] Critical care nurses are faced with rationing of critical care beds and nursing staff on a daily basis. Strengths and weaknesses of the staff must be balanced with the needs of the patient. Orientation and other special circumstances—such as designation for charge nurse, trauma nurse, and code nurse—must be taken into consideration when scheduling staff and making out assignments. Any inexperienced staff, float staff, or registry staff must be given appropriate orientation and backup during the shift.

There is frequently a triage system for critical care units that is called on when there are more admissions than available beds. The critical care nurse is instrumental in assisting the medical director to determine patient selection for transfer, if appropriate. Some hospitals use a set of standards, criteria, or guidelines for determining patient admission and transfer to and from critical care areas.

## ETHICS AS A FOUNDATION FOR NURSING PRACTICE

Traditional theories of professions have included a code of ethics as the basis for the practice of professionals. The moral foundation of nursing has been discussed in the literature by various authors who describe the unique relationship of the professional nurse with the patient, which establishes a caring, trusting approach.[14,16,48,63] It is by adherence to a code of ethics that the professional fulfills an obligation for quality practice to society.

According to Curtin,[15] nursing ethics is concerned with duties that are assumed by nurses and with the consequences of decisions that affect patients, colleagues, society, and the nursing profession. A professional ethic is based on three elements: the professional code of ethics, the purpose of the profession, and the standards of practice of the profession. The need for the profession and its inherent promise to provide certain duties form a contract between nursing and society. The code of ethics developed by the professionals is the delineation of its values and relationships with and among members of the profession and society. The professional standards describe specifics of practice in a variety of settings and subspecialties. Each element is dynamic, and ongoing evaluations are necessary as societal expectations change, technologies increase, and the profession evolves.

### Nursing Code of Ethics

The American Nurses' Association (ANA) provides the major source of ethical guidance for the nursing profession. According to the preamble of the *Code for Nurses*, "When individuals become nurses, they make a moral commitment to uphold the values and special moral obligations expressed in their code."[2] The 11 statements of the Code are found in the box below. They are based on the underlying assumption that nursing is concerned with protection, promotion, and restoration of health; prevention of illness; and the alleviation of suffering of patients.[2]

The *Code for Nurses* was adopted by the ANA in 1950 and has undergone revisions over the years. It provides a framework for the nurse in ethical decision making and provides society with a set of expectations of the profession. The Code is "not open to negotiation in employment settings, nor is it permissible for individuals or groups of nurses to adapt or change the language of this code."[2] The ANA also suggests that the requirements of the Code may not be in concert with the law and that it is the nurse's obligation to uphold the Code because of the societal commitment inherent in nursing.

#### CODE OF ETHICS FOR NURSES

1. The nurse provides services with respect for human dignity and the uniqueness of the client, unrestricted by considerations of social or economic status, personal attributes, or the nature of health problems.
2. The nurse safeguards the client's right to privacy by judiciously protecting information of a confidential nature.
3. The nurse acts to safeguard the client and the public when health care and safety are affected by the incompetent, unethical, or illegal practice of any person.
4. The nurse assumes responsibility and accountability for individual nursing judgments and actions.
5. The nurse maintains competence in nursing.
6. The nurse exercises informed judgment and uses individual competence and qualifications as criteria in seeking consultation, accepting responsibilities, and delegating nursing activities to others.
7. The nurse participates in activities that contribute to the ongoing development of the profession's body of knowledge.
8. The nurse participates in the profession's efforts to implement and improve standards of nursing.
9. The nurse participates in the profession's efforts to establish and maintain conditions of employment conducive to high quality nursing care.
10. The nurse participates in the profession's effort to protect the public from misinformation and misrepresentation and to maintain the integrity of nursing.
11. The nurse collaborates with members of the health professions and other citizens in promoting community and national efforts to meet the health needs of the public.



## ETHICAL DECISION MAKING IN CRITICAL CARE

In general, ethical cases are not always clear-cut or black and white, but rather arise in settings and circumstances that involve innumerable side issues and distractions. The most common ethical dilemmas encountered in critical care are foregoing treatment and allocating the scarce resource of critical care. But how does one know that a true ethical dilemma exists?

### What Is An Ethical Dilemma?

Before the application of any decision model, a decision must be made about the existence of a true ethical dilemma. Thompson and Thompson[54] delineated the following criteria for defining moral and **ethical dilemmas** in clinical practice:

1. Awareness of different options
2. An issue with different options
3. Two or more options with true or "good" aspects and the choice of one over the other compromises the option not chosen

Krekeler asserted that ethical situations arise when "the moral decision of one person conflicts with the moral decision of another. Both decisions may be good for each individual in question and undoubtedly are made according to their traditional values."[33] What complicates this process is when there is a third person involved, as is the case in most treatment care decisions in the critical care areas.

### Steps in Ethical Decision Making

To facilitate the ethical decision process, a model or framework must be used so that all involved will consistently and clearly examine the multiple ethical issues that arise in critical care. Steps in **ethical decision making** are listed in the box on p. 21.

**Step one.** First, the major aspects of the medical and health problem must be identified. In other words, the scientific basis of the problem, potential sequelae, prognosis, and all data relevant to the health status must be examined.

**Step two.** The ethical problem must be clearly delineated from other types of problems. Systems problems, that is, those resulting from failures and inadequacies in the organization and operation of the health care facility and the

**STEPS IN ETHICAL DECISION MAKING**

1. Identify the health problem.
2. Define the ethical issue.
3. Gather additional information.
4. Delineate the decision maker.
5. Examine ethical and moral principles.
6. Explore alternative options.
7. Implement decisions.
8. Evaluate and modify actions.

health care system as a whole, are often misinterpreted as being ethical issues. Occasionally, a social problem that stems from conditions existing in the community, state, or country as a whole are also confused with ethical issues. Social problems can lead to a systemic problem, which can constrain responses to ethical problems.

**Step three.** Although categories of necessary additional information will vary, whatever is missing in the initial problem presentation should be obtained. If not already known, the health prognosis and potential sequelae should be clarified. Usual demographic data, such as age, ethnicity, religious preferences, and educational and economic status, may be considered in the decision process. The role of the family or extended family and other support systems needs to be examined. Any desires that the patient may have expressed either in writing or in conversation about treatment decisions are essential to obtain.

**Step four.** The patient is the primary decision maker and autonomously makes these decisions after receiving information about the alternatives and sequelae of treatments or lack of treatments. However, in many ethical dilemmas, the patient is not competent to make a decision, as occurs when he or she is comatose or otherwise physically or mentally unable to make a decision. It is in these situations that surrogates are designated or court appointed, because the urgency of the situation requires a quick decision. Although the decision process and ultimate decision are more important than who makes the decision, delineating the decision maker is an important step in the process.[54]

Others who are involved in the decision should also be identified at this time, such as family, nurse, physician, social worker, clergy, and any other members of disciplines having close contact with the patient. The role of the nurse should be examined. There may not be a need for a nurse decision; rather the nurse may provide additional information and support to the decision maker.

**Step five.** Personal values, beliefs, and moral convictions of all involved in the decision process should be known. Whether actually achieved through a group meeting or through personal introspection, values clarification facilitates the decision process. Professional ethical codes of the nurse and physician will serve as a foundation for future decisions. At this time, legal constraints or previous legal decisions for circumstances at hand will need to be assessed and acknowledged.

General ethical principles need to be examined in relation to the case at hand. For instance, are veracity, informed consent, and autonomy promoted? Beneficence and nonmaleficence will be analyzed as they relate to the patient's condition and desires. Close examination of these principles will reveal any compromise of ethical or moral principles for either the patient or the health care provider and assist in decision making.

**Step six.** After the identification of alternative options, the outcome of each action must be predicted. This analysis helps one to select the option with the best "fit" for the specific situation or problem. Both short-range and long-range consequences of each action must be examined, and new or creative actions should be encouraged. Consideration should also be given to the "no action" option, which is also a choice.[54]

**Step seven.** When a decision has been reached, it is usually after much thought and consideration, and there is rarely complete agreement among all interested persons.[54] Krekeler described following the action until the actual results of the decision can be seen.[33] Fowler stated that the decision may need to be modified to meet legal or policy requirements.[25]

**Step eight.** Evaluation of an ethical decision serves to both assess the decision at hand and use it as a basis for future ethical decisions. If outcomes are not as predicted, it may be possible to modify the plan or to use an alternative that was not originally chosen.

## STRATEGIES FOR PROMOTION OF ETHICAL DECISION MAKING

The complexity of health care and frequent ethical dilemmas encountered in clinical practice demand the establishment of mechanisms to address ethical issues found in hospitals and health care facilities. Four types of mechanisms will be discussed briefly in this chapter: institutional ethics committees, inservice and education, nursing ethics committees, and ethics rounds and conferences.

### Institutional Ethics Committees (IECs)

Although not required by law, many health care facilities have developed IECs as a way to review ethical cases that are problematic for the practitioner. The three major functions of IECs are education, consultation, and recommendation to policy-making bodies.

IECs are very often committees comprising executive medical staff. Membership may include staff physicians, administrators, legal counsel, nurses, social workers, clergy, and community public volunteers. To fulfill its requirement for consultation, the committee must include members that not only have expertise, but also are representative of various groups. Regardless of the type of committee model, consultation and support becomes available to the practitioners.

### Inservice and Education

Basic education about ethical principles and decision making is an important first step in facilitating ethical decision making among nursing staff in the critical care area. It is important for nurses to examine their own values, beliefs, and moral convictions. The ANA *Code for Nurses* should be known and used by nurses in their daily clinical practice. Treatment choices for patients and ethical issues involving patients, nurses, and medical colleagues should be explored and discussed in the classroom setting where there are no time constraints or extraneous distractions to interrupt the decision process.

### Nursing Ethics Committees

Nursing ethics committees provide a forum in which nurses can discuss ethical issues that are pertinent to nurses at the individual, unit, or department level.[3,23] Unlike the IEC, which involves treatment choices of patients, the nursing committee may or may not involve a patient situation. Depending on the specific goals of the committee, it can also serve as a resource to nursing staff, make recommendations to a policy-making body about a variety of professional issues, or actually formulate policies. It may also serve to educate the department on ethical and professional issues. Membership usually comprises representatives from all major clinical areas or divisions, educators, clinical nurse specialists, administrators, and other specialty staff. Some departments such as critical care may have their own unit or division committee.

### Ethics Rounds and Conferences

Ethics rounds at the unit level on patients in the unit can be done by nurses on a weekly or otherwise established basis. Rounds educate the staff to problems and serve to be "preventive" when facilitated appropriately.[25] During the discussions, potential problems may be identified early, and actions taken to decrease or prevent a future problem. An individual patient ethics conference can be scheduled to include only the nursing staff or to include a multidisciplinary group to discuss unit issues. A patient ethics conference may either function as a liaison with the IEC or as an end in itself.

## CRITICAL CARE NURSING PRACTICE: LEGAL OBLIGATIONS OVERVIEW

The scope of critical care nursing practice has been defined by the American Association of Critical-Care Nurses (AACN), as follows[1]:

> Critical care nursing practice is a dynamic process, the scope of which is defined in terms of the critically ill patient, the critical care nurse and the environment in which critical care nursing is delivered; all three components are essential elements for the practice of critical care nursing. The critically ill patient is characterized by the presence of real or potential life-threatening health problems and by the requirement for continuous observation and intervention to prevent complications and restore health. The concept of the critically ill patient includes the patient's family and/or significant others. The critical care nurse is a registered professional nurse committed to ensuring that all critically ill patients receive optimal care.

In *Nursing, A Social Policy Statement,* the American Nurses' Association (ANA) defines nursing as the diagnosis and treatment of human responses to actual or potential health problems. "Critical care nursing is that speciality within nursing which deals specifically with human responses to life-threatening problems."[1]

These definitions raise several pertinent legal and professional concerns[12]:

1. The critical care nurse has legal obligations to the patient, the critical care setting, and the environment.
2. Both definitions speak to the fact that the nurse deals with life-threatening health problems. In this context, nursing mistakes are more likely than those made in situations that are not life-threatening to cause significant injuries, if not death, to a patient. Risk of suit is high.
3. The nurse is obligated to provide continuous observation and intervention.
4. The patient includes more than the individual for whom care is being provided; the family or significant other must also be cared for.
5. The nurse is licensed by the state and has legal obligations to the public to perform her or his duties safely.
6. The nurse's goal is to provide optimal care. This type of care is a professional obligation and is distinguishable from a reasonable level of care, which is the legal standard of care.
7. Critical care nursing is a specialty. Therefore the nurse's legal obligations are those of a specialist, one with special knowledge and skill. These obligations involve a higher standard of care.

These areas of concern are the focus of this chapter. Following a discussion of the types of liabilities and the law and legal processes that have an impact on critical care nursing, the nurse's duty of reasonable care, obligations of state licensure, and special patient care issues will be discussed.

## LIABILITY AND RESPONSIBILITY

When a nurse takes a position in a critical care unit, a special relationship is created between patient and nurse and employer and nurse. Every state has a law that requires that a special course of study be taken, successfully completed, and an examination passed for one to practice nursing. A registered nursing position requires state registration and licensure as a registered nurse. The act of licensure creates a legal relationship between the nurse and the state.

### Civil and Tort Liability

The area of civil law is divided into many categories, two of which are torts and contracts. A **tort** is a type of civil wrong, meaning that the dispute resulted from an occurrence

### CLASSIFICATION OF TORTS

| Intentional torts | Unintentional torts | Quasi-intentional torts |
|---|---|---|
| Assault | Negligence | Defamation |
| Battery | Malpractice | Slander |
| False imprisonment | Abandonment | Libel |
| Trespassing | | Invasion of privacy |
| Infliction of emotional distress | | |

between private entities or individuals (referred to as parties to the dispute), and the wrong is the type that society does not consider criminal or a wrong against society as a whole. The *law of contracts* contains a set of rules governing the creation and enforcement of agreements between two or more parties (again, entities or individuals).

There are three types of torts. The box above catalogues the classifications of tort law and gives selected examples within each category. *Intentional torts* involve an intent and an act. The intent is not a malicious one; rather, it is the intent to achieve a particular outcome and consequence. Assault, battery, false imprisonment, trespassing, and infliction of emotional distress are all examples of intentional torts. In each of these torts, there is a specific act that is required. In *assault*, the act is any behavior that places the plaintiff (the one being wronged who later sues) in fear or apprehension of an offensive contact. The person being sued for wronging another in civil law is referred to as the defendant. *Battery* is the unlawful or offensive touching of another's physical being. *False imprisonment*, another intentional tort, involves isolating another against his or her will. There are two types of *trespassing*—one type involves a person's land; the other involves his or her personal property. These acts are defined as unauthorized entry onto land of another or unauthorized handling of another's personal property. In addition, the law protects a person's interest in peace of mind through the tort, *infliction of mental or emotional distress*. The act here, however, must be one of extreme misconduct or outrageous behavior.

*Unintentional torts* involve mistakes in nursing practice that lead to harm, including negligence, malpractice, and abandonment. **Negligence** is the failure to meet an ordinary standard of care, resulting in injury to the patient (here again, the allegedly injured person is referred to as the plaintiff). **Malpractice,** a type of negligence, is professional misconduct, illegal or immoral conduct, or a lack of reasonable skill, which leads to harm. A more complete outline of the elements of these two torts will follow. *Abandonment* is a type of negligence in which a duty to give care existed, was totally ignored, and resulted in harm to a patient. It is the absence of care and the failure to respond to a patient that can give rise to an allegation of abandonment.

*Quasi-intentional torts* protect interests one has in his or her reputation and privacy; defamation (including slander and libel) and invasion of privacy are both quasi-intentional torts. *Defamation* is actually made up of two torts, *slander* (oral defamation) and *libel* (written defamation). Defamation is not just saying or writing words that injure one's reputation or good name. The words must be communicated to another, and if the words are true this may provide a defense against a defamation lawsuit. *Invasion of privacy* is another type of tort that involves a violation of a person's right of privacy. Nurses can invade another's privacy by revealing confidential information without authorization or by failing to follow the patient's health care decisions. Ways in which nurses can avoid torts are listed in the box below.

### Administrative and Licensure Law

A second type of law and legal process in which nurses have been involved is *administrative law*. This area of law governs the nurse's relationship to the government, either state or federal. Administrative law involves the rules of the government's activities in regulating health care delivery

### WAYS TO AVOID TORTS

1. Assure patients, as far as possible, that the nursing care is part of an acceptable treatment plan.
2. Ask patients for their consent before giving care (in addition, many hospital policies require that the nurse validate that the patient's physician has also received consent for medical treatment—this will be discussed more in a later section).
3. Determine if and when the patient needs self-protection or needs to be restrained to protect others from harm and take steps to protect the patient or others by following established protocols, hospital policies, and state regulations governing the use of restraints.
4. Handle the patient's personal effects in a safe, secure manner and follow hospital policies about patient valuables.
5. Avoid extreme, outrageous behavior by delivering care according to generally accepted standards of care.
6. Identify when a duty exists, know what the duty consists of, and provide nursing care that meets that expected duty.
7. Document the care that was delivered and participate in other activities that decrease the chance of patient harm and a subsequent lawsuit.
8. State opinions of another's reputation only when objectively substantiated or privileged.
9. Respect another's privacy and autonomy and maintain a confidential relationship with the patient.

and practice. Generally, there are several sections of the government that are involved in regulatory activities.

A state has the power to regulate nursing because the state is responsible for the health, safety, and welfare of its citizens. Therefore establishing minimum standards of nursing practice, education, and competence is an acceptable state activity. The state legislatures create the laws governing nursing practice, and a unit of the state government within the executive branch of government is responsible for the enforcement of nursing laws. This unit is often called the state board of nursing. However, states do vary. This is another important reason that nurses must seek advice from counsel licensed to practice law within their own states.

For administrative law, the rules of investigation and procedure differ from civil law and criminal law. Each type of law has its own rules of procedure and evidence. Examples of disputes between the state and nurses will be provided below.

## NEGLIGENCE AND MALPRACTICE

As defined earlier, negligence is an unintentional tort involving a failure (through either an act or a failure to act) to meet a standard of care, causing patient harm. Malpractice is negligence by a member of a profession in which the defendant is held accountable for a standard of care involving special knowledge and skill. These torts have several elements, all of which the plaintiff has the burden of proving.

### Definition of Elements

Most legal scholars itemize four elements of negligence and malpractice, including:

1. Duty and standards of care
2. Breach of duty
3. Causation
4. Injury or damages

A *duty,* or legal obligation, must be one recognized by law, requiring the actor to conform to a certain standard of conduct, for the protection of others against unreasonable risks.[60] The critical care nurse's legal duty is to act in a reasonable and prudent manner, as any other critical care nurse would act under similar circumstances. The standard is that of a critical care nurse, one with special knowledge and skill in critical care. The standard is one that is owed at the time the incident occurred, not at the time of litigation. In most jurisdictions, the standard is a regional or even national standard, as opposed to a local, community standard.

*Breach of duty* involves a failure on the actor's part to conform to the standard required. *Causation,* the third element, involves proving that the actor's breach was reasonably close or causally connected to the resulting injury. This is also referred to as *legal cause,* or *proximate cause.*

The fourth element, *injury*, must involve an actual loss or damage to another or his or her interests. There are different types of damages that a plaintiff may claim, such as compensatory or punitive. Patient injury can range in value, depending on what happened to the patient. The plaintiff must produce evidence of the damages and their value. If the nurse breaches a standard of care, which leads to injury, the plaintiff must show what amount of money will compensate for his or her injuries. The goal of the compensation is to provide the amount of money that will place the plaintiff back in the position he or she was in before the injury occurred.

Because critical care nurses deal with life-threatening patient care situations, patient injury could be severe, such as death. If this does occur, the nurse may be held accountable for the patient's death and also for the resulting loss to family members. All states have survival or wrongful death acts. Under these statutes, a lawsuit can be brought if the death was the result of a negligent act.

The box above enumerates specific examples of critical care nurse actions that involved actual lawsuits. In these cases, the nurse's action was the center of the lawsuit, but in few instances was the nurse actually sued. Whether the nurse is actually sued depends on the situation and who else is responsible for the nurse's actions.

Overall, nursing negligence cases have involved failures in relation to six general categories, which are found in the box on p. 25.

**SAMPLE OF CRITICAL CARE NURSING ACTIONS INVOLVED IN NEGLIGENCE SUITS**

- Failure to advise physician and/or supervisor of changes in patient's health status
- Failure to monitor patients
- Failure to adhere to protocols for monitoring oxygen levels
- Failure to adequately assess postoperative status
- Failure to respond to alarms
- Using malfunctioning equipment
- Refusing to provide supplemental oxygen when the ventilator could not be promptly reattached
- Allowing inappropriate use of the IV infusion equipment to extensively infuse fluids extravascularly
- Failure to monitor, recognize infiltration, and discontinue IV therapy
- Failure to recognize signs of intracranial bleeding
- Failure to investigate patient's complaint of pain and discover hematoma under blood pressure cuff

### Types of Liability and Legal Doctrines

In tort and civil law, there are several rules of liability under which the nurse's actions may be examined, and responsibility defined. Types of liability include:

1. Personal
2. Vicarious: *respondeat superior*
3. Corporate

**COMMON AREAS OF NURSING NEGLIGENCE**

- Administration of treatments
- Medications
- Communication
- Supervision of patients
- Incorrect or inappropriate postoperative treatment, which can result in infections
- Foreign objects left in patient during surgery

4. Other special doctrines, such as *res ipsa loquitur,* temporary or borrowed servant, and captain of the ship

**Personal liability** means that each individual is responsible for his or her own actions. This includes the critical care nurse, the supervisor, the physician, the hospital, and the patient. Each has responsibilities that are uniquely his or her own. The opposite of personal liability is personal immunity. For some health care situations, Congress or state legislatures have determined that nurses do not have personal liability and are therefore immune from liability.

Generally, however, mandated reported statutes include personal immunity provisions. For example, state child abuse statutes provide that a nurse who makes a good faith report will not be liable for making that report. Or, physicians and hospitals that are mandated to report communicable diseases to state or federal authorities are immune from liability for good faith reporting in a confidential manner. Also, nurses who render voluntary emergency care to a stranger are immune from liability for negligence under state good samaritan laws. Finally, federally employed nurses are immune from liability for negligence under the Federal Tort Claims Act.[56]

These personal immunities are not a guarantee of not being sued; rather, they are defenses for the nurse should the nurse be sued. The nurse-defendant must show how the immunity applies to her or his situation, and if so shown, the case against the nurse is dismissed.

**Vicarious liability** is sometimes referred to as employer liability. Under the doctrine of *respondeat superior,* an employer is responsible and liable for an employee's acts that are performed within the scope of the employee's employment. In critical care, the nurse is usually an employee of a hospital, but nurses may be independent contractors to the hospital through critical care nursing businesses. If the latter is the case, the nurse is not an employee of the hospital, so the hospital is not vicariously liable for the nurse's actions. Critical care nurses who are hospital employees are given work assignments and provided equipment and supplies to perform those assignments by the employer's agent, a supervisor. In fact, the hospital is responsible for the patient census and staffing in the critical care unit. Because of these responsibilities, the hospital-employer is responsible for the employee's performance within parameters that the employer determines. It would be unfair to hold the individual nurse solely responsible for patient care, which the nurse only partially controls.

*Corporate liability* is the liability that attaches to the corporate entity itself (in this case, the hospital) for its own decisions, such as patient census and staffing, budget, and hiring practices. These are corporate decisions for which the hospital is independently responsible.

There are other special doctrines, such as **res ipsa loquitur,** temporary or borrowed servant, and captain of the ship, which may apply to the critical care nurse and the critical care unit. The doctrine of *res ipsa loquitur* literally means "the thing speaks for itself." It is a doctrine that allows the plaintiff to introduce evidence of harm and imply negligence from the fact that the harm occurred. In this case, the type of injury incurred by the plaintiff is one that does not occur without someone's being negligent.

For example, negligence can be implied when muscle damage results from body positioning when applying restraints. Or negligence can be implied from a foreign object left in a patient's abdomen following surgery. The plaintiff must show that someone among the defendants was in exclusive control of the action that caused the injury. The burden of proof is shifted to the defendants to show how none of them was negligent.

The doctrines of *temporary or* **borrowed servant** and *captain of the ship* apply when the plaintiff argues that the physician is responsible for the nurse's actions, even though the nurse is an employee of the hospital and not the physician. If it can be shown that the nurse acted under the direction and control of the physician, it is possible that the physician may be accountable for the nurse's actions. These doctrines, however, are not applied very often.

## NURSE PRACTICE ACTS

Every state has legislation that defines the legal scope of nursing practice and defines unprofessional conduct, conduct that may lead to investigation and disciplinary action by the state.

Generally, state law contains two definitions of nursing: one for the registered (or professional) nurse and one for the licensed practical (or vocational or technical) nurse. These definitions determine titles that may be used by nurses, the scope of nursing practice, and requirements for entering the nursing profession. In some states advanced registered nursing practice, prescriptive authority for some nurses, and third party reimbursement are also statutorily defined.

How critical care nursing practice fits within these legal definitions can be revealed by comparing the professional definitions and the job description of a nurse with the state law in the jurisdiction. In this way, nurses can avoid or defend themselves against allegations of practicing medicine without a license. The scope of medical practice is also statutorily defined, and in most states a physician is given broad discretion to delegate tasks to others. For critical care nurses, proper medical delegation may occur through written protocols or standing orders that exist for the critical care area.

These orders must be written, dated, and signed by the physician. They should be updated regularly, and the old orders should be kept with other older unit documents in archives. The nurse must be adequately prepared to perform each aspect of the protocol and is personally liable for performing each order in a reasonable and prudent manner under the circumstances. Protocols and standing orders should be established with formal recognition of the roles of hospital administration and nursing and medical staffs.

The state also defines unprofessional conduct and establishes mechanisms for enforcement of these rules. *Misconduct* generally includes fraud in obtaining a license or registration; negligence; incompetence; criminal acts; practicing while impaired (chemically, physically, or mentally); having been found guilty of misconduct in another jurisdiction; and violating the nursing practice act, including any specific regulations, such as improper delegation of nursing responsibilities. A particular government unit is assigned to the investigation and the follow-up of complaints of nurses' misconduct. Complaints, reported both voluntarily and mandatorily, are initiated by patients, hospitals, other state agencies, or the criminal justice system. State investigators have broad powers and may conduct interviews and review and copy hospital charts and personnel files.

*Chemical impairment* is a frequent cause of nurses' licenses being revoked. In some states, an impaired nurse may avoid disciplinary action by voluntarily surrendering her or his license in exchange for entering a rehabilitation program. This should be done with the advice of counsel (the nurse's own counsel). Generally, this option is available in the states that have it as long as no patient has been harmed because of the nurse's impaired practice.

## SPECIAL PATIENT CARE ISSUES

There are many patient care issues that arise in critical care nursing. Critical care nurses manage some of the most complex, acute care in some of the most vulnerable situations for both nurses and patients alike. Questions often arise about consent, withholding or withdrawing of treatment, and organ procurement.

### Consent and Informed Consent

Generally, patient consent is always an essential component of health care, including critical care. However, some exceptions do exist. For example, in life-threatening, emergency situations, patients give implied consent to treatment that will remove the threat to their lives. Consent as a legal doctrine recognizes the right of a patient to control his or her own body, privacy, and autonomy. As early as 1914, a court ruled that every adult of sound mind has a right to determine what shall be done with his or her own body (including consent and the right to refuse treatment), and a surgeon who performs an operation without consent commits an assault, for which he or she is liable in damages.

Although consent can be either verbal or written, most hospital policies require that it be confirmed in writing that a patient agreed to treatment after being informed, that the patient agreed voluntarily, and that the patient was legally competent to agree to the treatment. These are the basic elements of consent and informed consent doctrines: voluntary, informed, and competent (having legal capacity). Consent is a process, not just the signing of a form.

Policies should set forth who should obtain the consent, how and when the consent should be obtained, and the documentation requirements. Obtaining the patient's consent is the responsibility of the patient's treating physician, who should explain the proposed procedure or treatment. However, if the treatment is going to be done by a specialist, that person, the one most knowledgeable about the risks and benefits of the procedure, should obtain the consent.

It is not advisable to delegate the physician's responsibility for obtaining the patient's consent to the hospital or its nursing staff.[38] Generally, though, critical care nurses may be given the task by their witnessing the signature of the patient and documenting that the consent form was completed. As in any witnessing role, one can be called on later to state her or his knowledge of the situation.

If the nurse has any doubts or questions about the patient's consent, those doubts should be discussed with the patient's physician and with the nursing supervisor. Hospitals are liable (under corporate liability doctrine) for injuries that result from their failure to rectify incompetent, unsafe practice of any member of its staff, employee or nonemployee. Once the nurse has told her or his supervisor, the hospital is alerted to a problem that it is obligated to investigate.

### Refusing Treatment

The right to consent and informed consent includes the right to refuse treatment. In most circumstances a competent adult's decision to refuse even life-sustaining treatment must be honored. There are a few situations in which the right to refuse treatment is not honored. These include, but are not limited to situations in which:

1. The treatment relates to a contagious illness that threatens the health of the public (for example, immunizations are required, even over religious objections, if the community danger is extreme)
2. The innocent third parties will suffer (for example, a mother's wish to refuse a blood transfusion was overruled to save the mother for her 9-month-old infant; these cases are often decided on a case-by-case basis, and legal counsel should always be sought)
3. The refusal violates ethical standards (for example, a Massachusetts court held that a hospital was not required to compromise its ethical principles by following a patient's decision but must cooperate in the transfer of the patient to a hospital that was willing to cooperate[8]; how-

ever, a New Jersey court ruled the opposite. A patient indicated that she did not want to be fed if she became incapacitated; the hospital opposed this. The court upheld the patient's right and refused to order her transfer)[30]

4. Treatment must be instituted to prevent suicide and to preserve life (courts have clearly indicated, however, that terminally ill and/or comatose patients with no hope of recovery do not intend suicide when they refuse treatment)

When patients refuse treatment, complex ethical, legal, and practical problems arise. Hospitals should have specific policies to guide nurses in these areas. Ethics committees, case conferences, and careful medical and legal evaluation can provide direction on how to proceed.

**Tools for indicating wishes.** Patients themselves can provide clear direction by preparing in advance written documents that specify their wishes. Tools for indicating wishes include the living will and durable power of attorney. To be effective in a jurisdiction, both of these tools must be statutorily or judicially recognized. The *living will* specifies that if certain circumstances occur, such as terminal illness, the patient will decline specific treatments, such as cardiopulmonary resuscitation. The living will does not cover all treatment. For example, in some states nutritional support may not be declined through a living will. The *durable power of attorney* is a tool through which a patient designates a spokesperson, someone who will speak for the patient if he or she becomes unable to speak on his or her own. Both the living will and the durable power of attorney have statutory requirements, such as number of witnesses and the time for which the document is effective.

Critical care nurses whose patients have these or other tools should follow the policies that the hospital has about them. For example, special sections are set aside for these tools in the patient's medical record. Risk management staff or specialists, the administration, and legal counsel should review them and answer any questions nurses have about implementing them. Most statutes, for example, have immunity provisions, which protect nurses from liability for following the patient's wishes in good faith.

**Working with substituted decision makers.** A person identified by a patient as holding his or her durable power of attorney is authorized to speak for that patient. In some situations, a patient may have a legal guardian. This person is appointed by the court following a formal determination by the court that the patient is legally incompetent. A few states have family consent laws that allow relatives of adults who do not have decision making capabilities to make legally binding decisions on behalf of those patients without a formal judicial proceeding.[46] New York has yet another option—specific legislation has been enacted entitled *Orders Not to Resuscitate*.[44] Under this law, if two physicians decide a patient does not have the capability to consent, a surrogate decision maker can be selected from a priority list established by the law. This can be done without a formal judicial determination of the patient's legal competency.

In fact, the only way an adult loses legal competency is through a formal judicial proceeding. And even after a formal proceeding determines that a patient should be involuntarily committed, the patient still has important rights in treatment decisions, such as the right to refuse antipsychotic medications.

The first step in working with substitute decision makers is to be assured that they have the authority to speak for the patient. This authority should be documented in the patient's chart. Clearly identifying who speaks for the patient is important for the patient's care and for respect of the patient's privacy. If the patient's surrogate has authority to speak on the patient's behalf, then nurses avoid allegations of invasion of privacy and breach of confidentiality, because the surrogate is an authorized person, entitled to knowledge of private facts and information about the patient.

### Withholding and Withdrawing Treatment

As indicated earlier, an adult has the right to refuse treatment, even treatment that sustains life. This right means that the critical care nurse may participate in withholding or withdrawing treatments. Initially, the distinction between withholding and withdrawing treatments was considered important, but that is no longer the case. These health care decisions become most complex when patients lose capacity to personally make their own decisions.[49]

**Orders not to resuscitate and other orders.** Hospital policies that discuss orders to withhold or withdraw treatment should exist in all critical care units. For example, orders not to resuscitate, commonly referred to by nurses as DNR (do not resuscitate) orders, should be governed by written policies, including, but not limited to, the following:

1. DNR orders should be entered in the patient's record with full documentation by the responsible physician about the patient's prognosis, the patient's agreement (if he or she is capable), or the family's concurrence (for incapacitated patients).
2. DNR orders should have the concurrence of another physician, designated in the policy.
3. Policies should specify that orders are reviewed periodically (some policies require daily review).
4. Patients with capacity must give their informed consent.
5. For patients without capacity, that incapacity must be thoroughly documented, along with the diagnosis and prognosis, and family agreement.
6. Judicial intervention before writing a DNR order is usually indicated when the patient's family does not agree, or there is uncertainty or disagreement about the patient's prognosis or mental status.
7. Policies should specify who is to be contacted and notified within the hospital administration.

Other orders to withhold or withdraw treatment may involve mechanical ventilation, dialysis, nutritional support, hydration, and medications, such as antibiotics. The legal and ethical implications of these orders for each patient must be carefully considered. Hospitals should have written policies on all orders to withhold or withdraw treatment. Policies must cover how decisions will be made; who will decide; and what the roles of patient, family, health care providers, and the institution will be. Policies must be developed that take into consideration state laws and judicial opinions, such as those governing neglect or abuse of patients.[50]

### Organ Procurement

Critical care nurses are often involved in organ procurement for donation and transplantation. State and federal laws regulate this area. For example, before an organ can be procured, a patient must first be declared dead. State laws and regulations define death. Traditionally, death was defined as cessation of circulation and respiration; today, laws define death to include irreversible cessation of all functions of the entire brain, including the brain stem. Laws state that a determination of death must be made in accordance with accepted medical standards and is deemed to have occurred when the determination of death is completed. In the critical care unit, a physician determines that death has occurred for all legal purposes, including organ procurement.[5,11,52]

The federal law on organ transplants establishes a national network of procurement centers, encourages and funds coordination of organ donation, and prohibits the sale of organs. It is unlawful for any person to knowingly acquire, receive, or otherwise transfer any human organ for valuable consideration for use in human transplantation if the transfer affects interstate commerce. Any person violating this law shall be fined not more than $50,000 or imprisoned not more than 5 years, or both.[57]

The state law governing organ procurement is referred to as the Uniform Anatomical Gift Act.[55] Each state has adopted a variation of this uniform statute. Generally, the law provides that any individual of sound mind and over 18 years of age may donate any part or all of his or her body. In most states, the individual's decision in this regard cannot be overruled after death by a family member. However, in some states family members can do this.[28,43] State law also specifies who else may donate, who may receive the anatomical gift, and how the gift is made; state law also includes restrictions. For example, the physician who determines time of death may not participate in the removal or transplantation of organs.

To increase the availability of organs, state and federal laws and regulations have been passed that require hospitals to ask patients or their family members about organ donation. From the federal level, under Medicare regulations, hospitals participating in Medicare or Medicaid must establish written protocols for the identification of potential donors. From the state level, through amendments to the anatomical gift act, hospital administrators must establish a policy to ask patients or their family members to make an organ donation. These policies should specify clearly the nurse's involvement in organ procurement, how it is to be carried out, and what documentation requirements exist.

## SUMMARY

The emergence of critical care as a specialty and the introduction of sophisticated technological innovations into critical care units have had a great impact on health care professional practices. Ethical dilemmas and legal risks are encountered daily in the practice of critical care. The criticality of the situation and speed that is required to make decisions often prevent practitioners from gaining insight into the desires, values, and feelings of patients. The practitioner is often left with no clear ethical or legal guidelines, particularly in the fast-paced modern critical care unit.

Critical care nurses have been urged by their professional association to ensure the delivery of safe nursing care to patients. To that end, their standards of care include being cognizant of "causes of action" for which the nurse may be liable. By using an ethical decision-making process, the rights of the patient will be protected, and logical analysis of the case will lead to a decision that is made in the best interests of the patient.

#### REFERENCES


1. American Association of Critical-Care Nurses: Position statement: definition of critical care nursing, Newport Beach, Calif, 1984, The Association.
2. American Nurses' Association: Code for nurses with interpretive statements, Kansas City, Mo, 1985, The Association.
3. Aroskar M: Institutional ethics committees and nursing administration, Nurs Econ 2:130, 1984.
4. Aroskar M: Fidelity and veracity: questions of promise keeping, truth telling, and loyalty. In Fowler M and Levine-Ariff J, editors: Ethics at the bedside, Philadelphia, 1987, JB Lippincott Co.
5. Bailey L: Organ transplantation: a paradigm of medical progress, Hastings Center Report 20:24, 1990.
6. Birkholz G: IABP: legal and ethical issues, Dimens Crit Care Nurs 4:285, 1985.
7. Bouressa G and O'Mara R: Ethical dilemmas in organ procurement and donation, Crit Care Nurs 10:37, 1987.
8. Brophy v New England Sinai Hospital, 497 N.E. 2d 626 (Mass 1986).
9. Caplan A: Ethical and policy issues in the procurement of cadaver organs for transplantation, New Engl J Med 311:981, 1984.
10. Caplan A: Equity in the selection of recipients for cardiac transplants, Circulation 75:10, 1987.
11. Capron A: The burden of decision, Hastings Center Report 20:36, 1990.
12. Carr M: Legal aspects of standards of practice, Dimens Crit Care Nurs 8:111, 1989.
13. Childress J: The place of autonomy in bioethics, Hastings Center Report 20:12, 1990.
14. Cooper M: Convenantal relationships: grounding for the nursing ethic, ANS 10:48, 1988.
15. Curtin L: Ethics in nursing practice, Nurs Manage 19:7, 1988.
16. Dallery A: Professional loyalties, Holistic Nurs Prac 1:64, 1986.
17. Davis A and Aroskar M: Ethical dilemmas and nursing practice, Norwalk, Conn, 1983, Appleton-Century-Crofts.
18. Davison R and Davison L: Medical experimentation: ethics in high technology, Crit Care Nurse 10:27, 1987.
19. Engelhardt T: Shattuck lecture—Allocating scarce medical resources and the availability of organ transplantation, New Engl J Med 311:66, 1984.

20. Engelhardt T and Rie M: Intensive care units, scarce resources, and conflicting principles of justice, JAMA 255:1159, 1986.
21. Evans R: Health care technology and the inevitability of resource allocation and rationing decisions. Part 1. JAMA 249:2047, 1983.
22. Flynn P: Questions of risk, duty, and paternalism: problems in beneficence. In Fowler M and Levine-Ariff J, editors: Ethics at the bedside, Philadelphia, 1987, JB Lippincott Co.
23. Fost N and Cranford R: Hospital ethics committees, JAMA 253:2687, 1985.
24. Fowler M: Introduction to ethics and ethical theory: a road map to the discipline. In Fowler M and Levine-Ariff J, editors: Ethics at the bedside, Philadelphia, 1987, JB Lippincott Co.
25. Fowler M: Piecing together the ethical puzzle: operationalizing nursing ethics in critical care. In Fowler M and Levine-Ariff J, editors: Ethics at the bedside, Philadelphia, 1987, JB Lippincott Co.
26. Fry S: Autonomy, advocacy, and accountability. In Fowler M and Levine-Ariff J, editors: Ethics at the bedside, Philadelphia, 1987, JB Lippincott Co.
27. Guralnik D, editor: Webster's new world dictionary of the American language, New York, 1981, Simon and Schuster.
28. Hardwig J: What about the family? Hastings Center Report 20:5, 1990.
29. The Hastings Center: Guidelines on the termination of life-sustaining treatment and the care of the dying, Briarcliff Manor, NY, 1987, The Center.
30. In re Requena, 517 A. 2d 869 (NJ App Div 1986).
31. Jameton A: Nursing practice, the ethical issues, Englewood Cliffs, NJ, 1984, Prentice Hall.
32. Knaus W: Rationing, justice, and the American physician, JAMA 255:1176, 1986.
33. Krekeler K: Critical care nursing and moral development, Crit Care Nurs 10:1, 1987.
34. Levine-Ariff J: Justice and the allocation of scarce nursing resources in critical care nursing. In Fowler M and Levine-Ariff J, editors: Ethics at the bedside, Philadelphia, 1987, JB Lippincott Co.
35. Luckenbill-Brett J and Stuhler-Schlag M: Mandatory reporting: legal and ethical issues, J Nurs Admin 17:32, 1987.
36. Marsden C: Ethical issues in a heart transplant program, Heart Lung 14:495, 1985.
37. McCann J: Ethics in critical care nursing, Crit Care Clin North Am 2:1, 1990.
38. McDonald, Meyer, Essig: Health care law, section 18.03 [2] [2] (1987).
39. Miller B: Autonomy and the refusal of lifesaving treatment, Hastings Center Report 11:22, 1981.
40. Munoz E and others: Diagnosis-related groups, costs, and outcome for patients in the intensive care units, Heart Lung 18:627, 1989.
41. Murphy C: The changing role of nurses in making ethical decisions, Law Medicine and Health Care 12:173, 1984.
42. Murray T: Gifts of the body and the needs of strangers, Hastings Center Report 17:30, 1987.
43. New York public health law, section 4301 (3) (McKinney's 1987).
44. New York public health law 2960-2978 (McKinney's 1988).
45. Nightingale F: Notes on nursing, Toronto, 1969, Dover Publications, Inc.
46. Northrop C: Nursing practice and the legal presumption of competency, Nurs Outlook 36:112, 1988.
47. O'Mara R: Dilemmas in cardiac surgery: artificial heart and left ventricular assist device, Crit Care Nurs 10:48, 1987.
48. Packard J and Ferrara M: In search of the moral foundation of nursing, ANS 10:60, 1988.
49. Pohlman K: Cruzan by Cruzan v Harmon, Focus Crit Care 16: 487, 1989.
50. Pohlman K: DNR? CPR? Focus Crit Care 16:224, 1989.
51. Reigle J: Resource allocation decisions in critical care nursing, Nurs Clin North Am 24:1009, 1989.
52. Rodgers S: Legal framework for organ donation and transplantation, Nurs Clin North Am 24:837, 1989.
53. Schmelzer M and Anema M: Should nurses ever lie to patients? Image J Nur Sch 20:110, 1988.
54. Thompson J and Thompson H: Bioethical decision-making for nurses, Norwalk, Conn, 1985, Appleton-Century-Crofts.
55. 8A Uniform Law Acts [ULA] (1983).
56. 28 United States Code Sections 2671-2680 (1986).
57. 42 United States Code Section 274e (1986).
58. US Congress, Office of Technology Assessment: Life-sustaining technologies and the elderly, OTA-BA-306, Washington, DC, July 1987, US Government Printing Office.
59. Veatch R and Fry S: Case studies in nursing ethics, Philadelphia, 1987, JB Lippincott Co.
60. William Prosser, Law of torts 143 (4th ed, West 1971).
61. Wlody G: Ethical issues in critical care: a nursing model, Dimens Crit Care 9:224, 1990.
62. Wlody G and Smith S: Ethical dilemmas in critical care, Focus Crit Care 12:41, 1985.
63. Yarling R and McElmurry B: The moral foundation of nursing, ANS 8:63, 1986.
64. Young S: The nurse manager: clarifying ethical issues in professional role responsibility, Pediatr Nurs 13:430, 1987.

# CHAPTER 3

# Patient and Family Education

## CHAPTER OBJECTIVES

- *Adapt and apply teaching-learning theory to the critical care setting.*
- *Describe the stages of adaptation to illness and the implications of each for the patient teaching plan.*
- *Perform a learning needs assessment.*
- *Construct a teaching plan for a patient in the critical care unit.*
- *Discuss four methods of instruction and the appropriateness of each to the critical care setting.*

## KEY TERMS

noncompliance, p. 31
teaching-learning process, p. 32
stages of adaptation to illness, p. 32
motivation and readiness to learn, p. 33
methods of teaching, p. 35
procedural information, p. 38
sensory information, p. 38

Persons entering the health care system bring with them unique medical, social, and educational histories that affect their interactions with health care providers. When a patient is admitted to the hospital with an acute or critical problem, it is often the result of a failure to manage and maintain his or her own health. In addition, the illness often creates new requirements in the areas of health management and self-care that must be practiced by the patient during recovery and sometimes for a lifetime. This chapter presents theory related to health promotion and criteria through which a patient's health maintenance skills can be assessed. Compliance and noncompliance with the health care plan are discussed. Finally, the role of patient education in the critical care unit is covered.

## HEALTH PROMOTION IN THE CRITICAL CARE SETTING

Nurses in the critical care areas usually focus on the life-threatening physiological problems of their patients. Constraints of time and the necessity to prioritize care have limited health promotion activities of the critical care nurse. However, in the current climate of health care, with hospitalized patients more acutely ill and generally in the hospital for a shorter time, the role of health promotion in the hospitals and in the critical care areas must be examined.

Hospitalization may be the patient's first encounter with health care professionals and health promotion information. The nurses with whom the patient interacts have the potential to influence perceptions about future health care practices.[19] If health teaching, role modeling, effective communication, and skilled nursing care are combined in the experience of the critically ill patient, the patient may begin to identify his or her continuing role in health maintenance as recovery continues and discharge nears. Families, too, can benefit from health promotion activities during the hospitalization, and valuable information concerning the family environment to which the patient will return can be gained during health promotion assessment and teaching.[28] Creative nursing strategies that combine the holistic, long-term goals of health promotion with the critical short-term goals and behaviors in the critical care setting can add an important and satisfying aspect to the care of the acutely ill.

### Factors Influencing Health Practices

Assessment of factors influencing an individual's health practices provides information regarding the patient's overall health status and the effectiveness of the methods used to maintain health. This information provides insight into the patient's perceived health status, the importance he or she places on health, and the level of his or her commitment to health maintenance. Careful assessment in this area also identifies actual or potential health problems or risks that are unrelated to the reason for admission but may adversely

### NURSING HISTORY OF HEALTH PERCEPTION AND MANAGEMENT

How has the patient's general health been?
Has the patient had any other illnesses in the past year, including colds and minor illnesses?
What are the most important things the patient does to keep healthy? Do these things make a difference? Include folk remedies if appropriate.
Does the patient use cigarettes, alcohol, or drugs? Are appropriate self-screening examinations performed (e.g., regular breast self-examinations for women)?
In the past, has the patient found it easy to follow the advice of health professionals?
Are there financial, social, cultural, or geographical barriers to access to proper health care?
What caused this illness? What actions were taken when the symptoms were noticed? What were the results of those actions?
What things are most important to the patient while in the hospital? How can the staff be most helpful?

affect recovery or future self-care. For this reason, the nursing assessment in the critical care unit should include information related to these primarily nonacute health patterns. The patient's health perceptions provide some guidance in the planning of care in the critical care unit and in later stages of recovery. The care plan and teaching plan in the critical care unit should take into consideration individual differences in these beliefs. Refer to the nursing management of Altered Health Maintenance on p. 439.

The box above gives general information about health perception and management that should be obtained during the nursing history gathered for the assessment.[24] This assessment should be carried out as soon after admission as the patient's condition allows.

## NONCOMPLIANCE

Compliance is defined as "the extent to which a person's behavior coincides with medical or health advice."[23] This concept and that of noncompliance are generally discussed in reference to the chronically ill patient whose care and treatment regimen continues past hospitalization and requires commitment and energy by the patient and family. The use of the nursing diagnosis of **Noncompliance**, however, refers to the individual who wants to comply, but the presence of certain factors prevents him or her from doing so.[11] Using this definition, noncompliance issues concerning the hospitalized patient and the short-term problems of compliance with the medical and nursing treatments in the critical care unit can be considered. Thus the nurse can concentrate on identifying, reducing, or eliminating the factors that affect the patient's ability to comply with treatment. Nursing management of Noncompliance is found on p. 440.

### Factors Influencing Compliance

**Alteration in cognition.** Patients may be noncompliant because they do not know the reason for or the importance of the recommended behaviors. This group of patients includes those who, for whatever reason, do not want information that would lead to compliance. In addition, patients may have false or inaccurate information on which they are basing their behaviors. Some hold to folk beliefs that interfere with their motivation to follow the prescribed medical treatments. Any disturbance in thought processes such as memory loss, inability to concentrate, and inability to solve problems or to follow directions can affect compliance. This very often occurs in the critical care areas because of side effects of pain medications, sleep deprivation, sensory overload, anxiety, or neurological deficits. Nurses must also consider the patient's ability to read, write, and understand the language and any real or potential visual or hearing deficits.

**Alteration in perception.** Beliefs, feelings, and values may affect compliance. Psychological and emotional responses to illness are often seen in the critical care areas and can adversely affect the patient's ability to comply. For example, the defense mechanism of denial, although serving a useful purpose in protecting the patient from unmanageable levels of anxiety, allows him or her to discount the illness, its severity, or the need for cooperation with health care personnel or for making lifestyle changes. Depression, anger, or fear can also establish barriers to compliant behavior, as can a conflict in values. In this case, the patient agrees with the desirability of a behavior, but the necessary time, money, or energy resources are not available, or the goals are low priority. Finally, some patients agree with the need to comply but feel unable to make the required changes. This is often seen as a return to habitual behaviors despite the attempt to change.

**Inadequacies in the social system.** Factors related to the patient's environment, including significant others, job, community, religious beliefs, and material resources, may affect the ability to comply with treatment. The support of significant others may be the important determinant in the patient's compliance, especially in long-term compliance.[23] Inadequate financial resources may be a barrier to compliance (for example, an individual on a fixed income who has been prescribed a very expensive medication). Adequate financial resources, however, do not ensure compliance. Geographical and transportation difficulties may also affect the ability to comply in some cases.

**Deficits in the health care system.** Health care system deficits that may affect compliance include a treatment regimen that is perceived by the patient as too complex or unmanageable, the failure of the system to provide specific and complete instructions, and a patient–health provider relationship that is not supportive and mutually respectful. It is therefore necessary to examine the system and the caregivers as possible factors in patient compliance.

## PATIENT EDUCATION

The education of the patient and family is now universally accepted as an important nursing function in all settings of practice. Nowhere is this more important than in the critical care unit, which is often foreign and very threatening to the patient, who depends on the nurses to provide the information necessary to survive in this environment. In addition, nursing has a legal and ethical responsibility to meet standards of care related to patient education. These standards include identifying the patient's and family's learning needs, assessing their readiness to learn, teaching the appropriate content, documenting the teaching plan as part of the nursing care plan, and evaluating and documenting the results of the patient teaching.[42] The basis for all educational activities for patients and families is the belief that they have the right to information regarding diagnosis, treatment, and prognosis in terms that are understandable to them.[32,41] Part of this belief is that rational individuals can, on some level, understand all but the most technical aspects of their care.[44,50] It also involves the knowledge that each patient is unique, learns in a unique way, and has motivation and skill in applying new knowledge that differs from that of other patients. These individual differences are the reasons for varied responses to the same teaching strategies.[41]

Traditional views of teaching and learning involve the idea of providing information (teaching) that causes a lasting change in behavior (learning).[10] Effectiveness of the educational interaction is measured by the specific objectives that are met. If the nurse in the critical care setting limits measurement of teaching effectiveness to long-term behavior changes, many critical educational activities necessary for the well-being of the patient will be judged failures. It may be more appropriate to expand the view of successful educational outcomes to not only long-term behavior change but also to less concrete but equally valuable outcomes such as decreased anxiety or greater participation in self-care. This approach recognizes that there are real and valuable aspects of learning that cannot be easily measured by objective criteria. It does not negate the fact that in many situations written measurable objectives are necessary and useful, but it does mean that they should not be the sole measures of educational success.[7] A good example of this is the interaction that occurs when a patient is taught about the cardiac monitor on admission to the critical care unit. In teaching the reason for and function of this equipment, the nurse not only increases the patient's knowledge about cardiac monitoring but may also decrease his or her anxiety about the critical care setting, thereby promoting rest and healing. Refer to the nursing management plans on Knowledge Deficit on p. 441.

Along with a belief in the patient's right to know, the patient's right not to know must also be recognized in some cases. It must be respected in those cases in which patients prefer not to learn about their illnesses. Simple basic information about monitors and unit policy, for example, usually suffices in these cases. Indeed, more information than can be processed and integrated can greatly increase anxiety and may result in slower recovery.[10,44] Individuals have the right to accept, adopt, or reject the information provided in educational encounters, however frustrating this may be to the nurse.[10]

### THE TEACHING-LEARNING PROCESS

1. Assessment of the need to learn
2. Assessment of readiness to learn
3. Setting of objectives
4. Teaching-learning activities
5. Evaluation and reteaching if necessary

### Teaching-Learning Process

The **teaching-learning process** used in the health care setting can be defined as a set of activities organized and structured to maximize the results for the patient and to minimize the amount of time and effort on the part of the health care practitioner.[6] It can be divided into the five steps summarized in the box above. These steps can be closely related to the nursing process. Table 3-1 shows the application of the nursing process to the teaching-learning process in the care of the critically ill patient.

**Assessment.** The assessment step in patient teaching involves gathering a data base to assist the nurse in meeting the patient's and family's learning needs.[6] It is a vital part of any successful teaching plan. Among the components of this assessment in the critical care unit are identification of the various stressors present, assessment of biopsychosocial issues and adaptation to illness, and an examination of motivation and readiness to learn. In reality, these issues are often related to one another and cannot be assessed as separate entities. For ease of illustration, however, they are discussed separately.

***Physical assessment.*** A physical assessment will yield information about physiological reactions to stress. The following factors should be considered: Is the patient in pain or some other type of distress? What is his or her level of consciousness and orientation? Has he or she been sedated? Is the patient hypoxic or hypercapnic? Are the heart rate, blood pressure, cardiac output, and perfusion adequate? Can the patient see and hear? These questions add to the data base for formulation of an effective teaching plan.

***Psychological assessment.*** The psychological assessment is also important in determining the patient's ability to respond to the teaching-learning experience. A very important factor is the patient's stage in adaptation to illness during the time teaching is undertaken. The general characteristics of the **stages of adaptation to illness** are outlined in Table 3-2 with corresponding applications for the teaching-learning process. Salient points are reviewed here. It

***Table 3-1*** Application of the nursing process to the teaching-learning process

| Nursing process | Teaching-learning process |
|---|---|
| Assessment | Physiological<br>Psychological<br>Environmental<br>Sociocultural<br>Assessment of physiological and psychological stress response<br>Physiological<br>Heart rate<br>Blood pressure<br>Peristalsis<br>Mental acuity<br>Blood glucose<br>Dilated pupils<br>Psychological<br>Anxiety<br>Depression<br>Panic<br>Withdrawal<br>Denial<br>Hostility<br>Regression<br>Frustration<br>Assessment of readiness to learn |
| Nursing diagnosis and plan | Identification of specific knowledge deficit<br>Identification of causes and associated factors<br>Identification of expected outcomes and behavioral objectives<br>Development of teaching plan |
| Nursing intervention | Teaching-learning activities and experience |
| Evaluation | Evaluation and documentation of effectiveness of teaching-learning process<br>Measurement of knowledge gain<br>Measurement of behavior changes |

should be noted that each individual moves at his or her own pace through the stages, and it is not uncommon to skip or move back and forth through the stages.

**DISBELIEF AND DENIAL.** The first response to acute illness is generally disbelief and denial. The shock and threat of the condition or illness are so great that the patient denies the condition's existence and severity in an attempt to ease the emotional impact or to conserve energy by avoiding the work of worrying. Although this response has some psychological benefit for the patient, it acts as a barrier to learning. Patients who do not believe they are ill or do not believe their condition will affect their lives will have little motivation to learn. During this stage it is acceptable for the nurse to allow denial if it does not put the patient in danger. Teaching should be focused on the present, and comments referring to the future should be avoided.

**DEVELOPING AWARENESS.** After a few days, the denial mechanism usually breaks down, and the patient moves into the stage of developing awareness. This can occur while the patient is still in the critical care unit. At this time, a patient may respond with anger or guilt. If these emotions are turned inward, he or she may experience depression. If emotions are expressed outwardly, behavior may be hostile toward persons and things in the environment, including the nurse. Teaching during this time should continue to be oriented to the present but may relate more to the disease process, which is now recognized by the patient. He or she is still too anxious to learn and assimilate lists of facts but may be interested in the meaning of symptoms and treatments as they relate to his or her experience at the moment.

**REORGANIZATION.** The third stage of adaptation to illness is reorganization. At this time the patient has begun to work through the anger and guilt and to reorganize his or her self-concept and relationships with others consistent with the acceptance of the sick role. During this time the nurse should teach whatever the patient wants to learn, thus helping the patient to achieve the reorganization necessary to move on to adaptation. Some patients, especially those in the critical care unit for several weeks, may experience this stage during the stay in the unit.

**RESOLUTION AND IDENTITY CHANGE.** The final stages of adaptation are resolution and identity change. They occur late in recovery, even as late as the sixth week in the case of a patient with a myocardial infarction.[37] During these times the patient is more receptive to teaching based on objectives and to learning about long-term needs. Group instruction that includes the spouse and significant others can be an effective method at this time. These stages will rarely be reached during the critical care stay but may be identified by nurses working in step-down or telemetry units.

The nurse should consider that the family go through the stages of adaptation to their loved one's illness as well. Family members may or may not progress at the same rates as the patient, so teaching strategies may need modification to ensure meeting the individual needs of both the patient and the significant others.

***Assessment of motivation and readiness to learn.*** Evaluation of **motivation and readiness to learn** are important parts of the teaching-learning assessment. They are more difficult to measure and assess than the other variables discussed. One well-known and important theory describing human behavior motivation is Maslow's hierarchy of needs, which provides background for the discussion of motivation to learn.

Maslow described a number of needs that were postulated as motivating all behavior. According to this theory, human beings have a number of needs that are interrelated and hierarchical. In other words, the lower-level needs must be met before higher-level needs can emerge and be satisfied. The following needs were identified as basic to human mo-

***Table 3-2*** Teaching-learning process in adaptation to illness

| Stage of adaptation | Characteristic patient response | Implications for teaching-learning process |
|---|---|---|
| Disbelief | Denial | Orient teaching to present.<br>Teach during other nursing activities.<br>Reassure patient about safety.<br>Explain all procedures and activities clearly and concisely. |
| Developing awareness | Anger | Continue to orient teaching to present.<br>Avoid long lists of facts.<br>Continue to foster development of trust and rapport through good physical care. |
| Reorganization | Acceptance of sick role | Orient teaching to meet patient needs.<br>Teach whatever patient wants to learn.<br>Provide necessary self-care information. Reinforce with written material. |
| Resolution | Identification with others with same problem; recognition of loss | Use group instruction.<br>Use patient support groups and visits by recovered patients with same problem. |
| Identify change | Definition of self as one who has undergone change and is now different | Answer patient's questions as they arise.<br>Recognize that as basic needs are met more mature needs will arise. |

tivation: physiological needs, safety and security, love and belongingness, self-esteem, and self-actualization.[34] The physiological needs are the most basic and powerful, and if they are not at least minimally met, higher-level needs will not become apparent.

The need to know and understand are among the highest-level needs.[34] During a time of critical illness, a patient's energy is often consumed by the lower-level physiological and safety needs, and it would be impossible for the patient to attend to learning interactions. Attempting to teach a patient who fears for his or her life and safety is of little use unless the patient is being taught that he or she is safe and in no immediate danger of dying. Once the lower-level needs are met and the patient feels out of danger, he or she will have more resources to devote to learning and meeting higher-level needs.

Factors that motivate behavior change related to preventive health practices also influence a patient's motivation to learn about health and health practices in the hospital setting. The assessment of readiness and motivation to learn, then, should include information about individual perceptions and perceived benefits and barriers.

***Assessment of external barriers.*** Patient barriers to learning related to physiological, emotional, and motivational factors have been identified. To structure a successful teaching-learning experience in a critical care area, the nurse must also carefully assess the environmental and iatrogenic barriers that affect the interaction. Bright lights, unpleasant odors, unfamilar noises, and untidy surroundings can distract patients and add to cognitive impairment. Control of these factors can facilitate the learning process. Factors that cannot be controlled should be explained to the patient to alleviate anxiety and facilitate a trusting relationship between patient and nurse.

Finally, the nurse should examine possible barriers to learning that he or she brings to the interaction. Nurses have been found to set up barriers both consciously and unconsciously to the patient's learning and understanding.[37] The use of medical terms that are not understood by the patient and the use of language inappropriate to the patient's educational level are examples of ways in which nurses may adversely affect the teaching-learning process.[16] There may also be a failure to set aside time just for teaching, resulting in hurried and fragmented sessions. Nonverbal cues on the part of the nurse, such as glancing at the clock or breaking eye contact, may interrupt patient interactions. The manner in which the teaching sessions are planned and executed can have as important an effect on patient learning as the material presented.

## The Teaching-Learning Experience

Once the process of the initial educational assessment is completed, the nurse will have an adequate data base from which to determine a teaching plan and decide on appropriate teaching methods. Patient teaching and nursing care are, in many ways, inseparable. Patients are educated in many informal interactions with the nurse, and knowledge gained greatly fosters patient understanding and well-being. Educational opportunities can be present during various nursing care activities such as bathing and administration of medication. Each encounter with the patient and family should be viewed as a teaching opportunity. There are times, however, during the acute care experience when more formal or structured educational experiences are in order. For this reason, a discussion of objectives, methods, evaluation of the teaching-learning experience, and some suggested content for education in the critical care setting follow.

**Objectives.** Objectives state the desired behaviors expected from the learning process.[41] They are based on the patient's learning needs and serve as a guide for the teaching-learning process. Objectives are written in behavioral terms that are measurable and are stated in terms of what the patient is to learn, rather than what the nurse is to teach. Terms such as to know, understand, be familiar with, realize, and appreciate are open to many interpretations and are difficult to measure. Rather, active verbs such as to *identify, state, list, describe,* or *demonstrate* should be used, because they are readily understood by all and easily lend themselves to evaluation.

Both long-term and short-term objectives are appropriate; in many cases it takes days, weeks, or even months of repetition and practice for a new skill to be mastered. A nurse in the critical care setting should not hesitate to identify goals that are long-term. Often it is appropriate to begin the teaching early and continue to evaluate it later in the hospitalization. Standardized plans can be useful resource materials in developing a teaching plan but must not take the place of individualized, specific objectives designed for each patient.

**Teaching methods.** The three basic **methods of teaching** are lecture, discussion, and demonstration.[10] The choice of method depends on the material to be taught.

***Lecture.*** Lecture is the presentation of information in a highly structured format to a group. In this method the teacher provides a great deal of material but may not provide ample opportunities for teacher-learner interaction. Although this method can be used for patient teaching in outpatient settings, it is not a good choice for hospitalized patients and is inappropriate for acutely ill individuals.

***Discussion.*** Discussion is less structured than lecturing and allows an exchange and feedback between the teacher and learner. The teacher can adapt the material to meet the needs of the individual or group. The discussion approach is probably most useful when learning should result in behavior change or in development of an attitude.[10] Discussion groups can be effective with hospitalized patients when a group with similar problems and at similar stages of adaptation can be gathered. Individual discussion with patients and families is appropriate and valuable during the acute phase of illness because it allows them to express their feelings and interpretations. This approach is the ideal way to teach about sensitive issues such as resuming sexual activity after myocardial infarction.[10]

***Demonstration.*** Demonstration involves acting out a procedure while giving appropriate explanations to provide the learner with a clear idea of how to perform a task. The patient can then practice the skill and be given feedback about his or her performance. This method is often used in the acute care setting such as when coughing and deep breathing or taking one's own pulse is taught.

***Other methods of instruction.*** In addition to the three basic methods just presented, several other approaches to delivering or augmenting information in a patient teaching program are available. They include commercially prepared or custom-designed printed materials, bedside videotape programs, and computer-assisted patient education programs. Computer programs, relatively new to health education, have been used in community-based education programs, in hospital waiting rooms or designated teaching rooms, and, in some cases, at the bedside with microcomputers on transportable carts.[4] These programs allow the learner to set the program pace and are generally presented in an attractive, colorful format.[14]

Written materials can be very useful tools in patient and family education. They allow repetition and reinforcement of content and provide basic information in printed form for reference at a later time. To be useful, however, the content must be accurate and current, and the patient and family must be able to read and understand it.[29]

In recent years the use of educational videotapes at the bedside or in group settings has gained increasing popularity. The use of videotapes, however, should not be considered a substitute for individualized patient teaching, and it is most effective when it is promoted by staff as reinforcing other educational activities.[15,36] Staff should preview the tapes before showing them to patients to ensure the accuracy and appropriateness of the content and to assess the best way to introduce and reinforce the material.

Teaching the critically ill patient may require modification of traditional teaching methods and strategies. In critical care units, patient goals are generally short-term and objectives are concrete. Teaching should be kept brief and concise and should be in terms the patient can understand. The many stressors of illness and critical care and the effects of sedation and other drugs may cause the patient to require frequent repetitions and reinforcement of information. This is to be expected with the critically ill person and is not considered failure of the teaching experience. Each educational interaction between patient and nurse is of value, despite the fact it often will not result in long-term behavior change. Nurses should remember that family members are also stressed and may forget pertinent information that has been provided about visiting hours, unit policies, and how to contact a staff member for information about the patient. It is helpful to provide them with written information to supplement and reinforce verbal instructions.[9,20]

**Evaluation.** Traditionally, the teaching-learning process has been evaluated by measurable behavior changes, in other words, how well the predetermined objectives were met. This evaluation is appropriate for some teaching in critical care, but often the traditional criteria do not apply. If the teaching meets a momentary need, the effect may not be measurable or quantifiable but is no less valuable and successful. The effectiveness of teaching can also be measured by observation of subtle changes in patients such as signs of relaxation when the information provided decreases anxiety.

### Teaching in the Critical Care Setting

**Timing.** Determination of the content presented in the critical care unit will depend on the patient's clinical and emotional status and will vary with each patient. The nurse prioritizes learning needs based on the assessment as soon as possible. The teaching should be guided by the patient and family—that is, teach what they want to know when they want to know it. If the patient's questions and concerns are left unanswered during this time of high anxiety, the unmet needs will serve as a block to further communication and prevent the patient from focusing his or her energy appropriately.

**Content.** Although the specific content taught will vary, depending on the condition for which the patient was admitted, there are certain areas that should be covered with any patient who is conscious. Environmental factors in a critical care unit can be frightening to patients and should be explained as soon as possible. Cardiac monitors, oxygen equipment, indwelling lines and catheters, frequent laboratory tests, and checking vital signs may cause the patient undue anxiety unless their purpose or function is understood. The reason for procedures, as well as their associated sensations or discomfort, should be briefly explained. This information may not be retained and may require several repetitions, but it will assist in decreasing anxiety and providing a sense of control for the moment.

Most of the time it is appropriate to give information about the illness or diagnosis in the critical phase of care. The nurse must often interpret and explain information provided by physicians. Despite the denial often present, some patients want to know about their illness, prognosis, complications, and reason for admission to the critical care unit.

It is important for the nurse to remember that the entire experience of the critical care unit, although routine for the staff, is frightening for the patient who may be confronting mortality for the first time. Questions should be answered as honestly, compassionately, and sensitively as possible and should be followed by supportive care as necessary.

**Preoperative teaching and preparation for procedures.** Two specific instances in which patient teaching in the critical care area is especially important are in preparing the patient for surgery with preoperative teaching and preparing patients for other stressful medical procedures, which are performed often in critical care units.

Critical care nurses are in a position to positively influence many aspects of recovery and patient outcome through implementation of a carefully planned preoperative teaching program when the patient's condition and situation allows. Patient benefits from preoperative teaching include quicker return of functional capacity, prevention of postoperative complications, increased self-esteem, decreased anxiety, decreased hospitalization costs, and a decrease in immediate and residual pain.[21] Whenever possible, families should be included in the teaching session to decrease their anxiety and to foster a feeling of support for the family unit.[21]

Although specific content for preoperative teaching sessions depends on the patient's physical and psychological condition, the specific operative procedure, and the time

#### Teaching Plan for the Patient Taking Warfarin (Coumadin)

Education of the patient taking an anticoagulant medication is important to reassure the patient, secure compliance, and minimize risks.

During the critical care unit stay, limit teaching to simple statements such as "This is Coumadin. It is a blood thinner."

During the hospitalization the following points should be covered:

- Basic physiology of coagulation
- Action of warfarin
- Importance of taking the medication exactly as prescribed and at the same time each day
- Importance of regular laboratory work
- Use of dosage calendar to verify dosage and schedule
- Use of Medic-Alert or some other system of identification
- Recognition of following signs and symptoms of bleeding to be reported:
  - Prolonged bleeding from cuts
  - Nosebleeds
  - Bleeding gums
  - Hemoptysis or hematemesis
  - Spontaneous bruising
  - Red or black stools
  - Red or dark brown urine
  - Prolonged headache, severe abdominal pain, or backache
- Use of electric razor only
- Application of 5 to 10 minutes of pressure to cuts
- Notification of all health care providers, including dentists, of anticoagulation medication
- Avoidance of aspirin and aspirin-containing products
- Impact of diet on warfarin therapy:
  - Maintenance of steady diet is important.
  - Vitamin K affects anticoagulation.
  - Foods high in vitamin K (fish, green leafy vegetables) must be avoided.
  - Fasting or prolonged diarrhea should be reported.
  - Alcoholic beverages may alter clotting time; drink only with physician's approval.
- Possibility of drug interactions (suggest having all prescriptions filled at the same pharmacy)

Provide wallet identification card and printed material to reinforce learning.

## Teaching Plan for the Patient Undergoing Coronary Artery Bypass Surgery

### PREOPERATIVE PHASE

During the preoperative educational interactions, the nurse should assess the patient's and family's levels of anxiety and their effect on the ability or desire to learn. The preoperative education should be individualized to prepare the patient appropriately for the surgery, to educate him or her about postoperative care, and to minimize anxiety. Before the teaching-learning experience, the nurse:

- Assesses the patient's level of anxiety and desire to learn about the upcoming surgery.
- Individualizes the preoperative teaching plan, based on assessment findings.

The following content may be included in the preoperative teaching session:

- Review of the coronary artery bypass graft (CABG) procedure
- Time leaving room for surgery, length of surgery
- Location of family waiting area
- Surgical preparation and shave
- Nothing by mouth after midnight
- What to expect when awakening from anesthesia
- Sights and sounds of the recovery room and/or critical care unit
- Tubes and drains: chest tubes, hemodynamic monitoring lines, Foley catheter, intravenous lines, pacemaker wires (if appropriate), endotracheal tube
- Inability to speak with endotracheal tube in place
- Discomfort to expect from incisions, availability of pain medication
- Coughing and deep breathing practice
- Use of incentive spirometer
- When family can visit, how long, how often
- Usual length of critical care unit stay

In addition to this content, the nurse:

- Reassures patient that many staff members and much activity around bedside is normal and does not indicate complications.
- Elicits and answers any specific questions patient and family have at that time.
- Determines specific needs and desires for day of surgery (e.g., patient needs hearing aid or glasses as soon as possible).
- Meets with the family alone to offer support and address concerns they may not wish to voice to the patient.

### CRITICAL CARE UNIT PHASE

During the critical care unit phase, education is designed to meet immediate needs and reduce anxiety. The following are examples of content appropriate for this time:

- Basic explanation of bedside equipment
- Review of tubes and drains
- Turning, coughing, deep breathing
- Use of incentive spirometer
- Use of oxygen equipment
- Orientation to time, place, situation
- Explanation of procedures
- Basic purpose of medications
- Explanation of normal progression in early postoperative period
- Basic range-of-motion exercises (e.g., ankle circles, point and flex)

During this phase, the nurse also:

- Reassures patient and family of normal progression.
- Repeats and reinforces information as necessary.
- Answers questions as they arise.
- Begins early to prepare patient for transfer to prevent transfer anxiety.
- Determines family learning needs and addresses them together with patient or in separate teaching sessions as appropriate.

### STEP-DOWN UNIT PHASE

After transfer from the critical care unit, the patient's and family's educational needs increase. Short daily educational sessions should be planned to cover the following content:

- Basic pathophysiology of coronary artery disease
- Review of surgical procedure
- Risk factors for coronary artery disease
- Upper-extremity range of motion exercises
- Dietary recommendations (salt- and fat/cholesterol-modified diet)
- Taking of own pulse
- Recognition and treatment of angina (use of nitroglycerin)

During this phase, the nurse also:

- Uses audiovisual materials in teaching sessions or as reinforcement of content.
- Provides printed take-home materials outlining important content.
- Answers questions as they arise.

### DISCHARGE TEACHING

Before discharge, the following content should be covered with the patient and family:

- Activity guidelines
- Lifting restrictions
- Incisional care
- Possibility of patient being extremely fatigued or depressed after discharge
- Guidelines for return to work, driving, sexual activity
- Medication safety and administration

Before discharge, the nurse also:

- Reassures patient that ups and downs are normal.
- If necessary, reassures patient and family that likelihood of cardiac emergencies at home is small.
- Provides printed material for further study by patient and family.
- Answers questions as they arise.
- Provides phone number for patient or family to call when further questions arise.

available for teaching, these general topics should be considered when planning the teaching session: preoperative medications and treatments such as enemas, skin preparation, urinary catheters, and intravenous catheters; the experience of anesthesia; postoperative treatments, including coughing, deep breathing, use of incentive spirometer, pain medications, tubes, drains, and dressings; and information about arrangements for care of the family during surgery and their sources of information about the patient's progress and condition. Whenever possible, the session should be private and unhurried to allow ample time for questions and emotional support of the patient and family.

Patients in critical care units experience many stressful medical procedures during the course of their care, including radiological procedures, placement of vascular access or monitoring devices, intubation, suctioning, spinal taps, and many others. Educational and psychological preparation for these procedures can decrease anxiety and increase patient cooperation with care. Two types of information can be offered to patients in preparation for procedures. **Procedural information** refers to what will be done, when and where it will happen, and who will provide the service. **Sensory information** refers to what the patient should expect to feel during and after the procedure.[49] When time permits, allowing the patient to ask questions, see equipment that will be used, and practice movements or body positions that will be required can be very helpful in reducing anxiety. In addition, teaching the patient basic relaxation techniques such as deep breathing or guided imagery can be effective in helping patients relax during a stressful or uncomfortable procedure.[22,49] When these procedures must occur on an emergent basis without time for patient preparation, the nurse should explain what happened and why as soon as the patient has stabilized and is able to understand the information.

**Transfer from the critical care unit.** Transfer from the critical care unit can be an anxiety-producing time for the patients. During the stay in the unit, constant interaction with the nurse, monitoring devices, and controlled environment has offered security to the patient. Transfer from that environment can destroy the sense of security and create acute anxiety.[44] To avoid this anxiety, nurses should prepare patients for imminent or eventual transfer, that is, teach toward transfer.[2] To do this, the nurse should point out early in the stay that the patient will be there only temporarily until his or her condition is improved and stable, and these improvements should be made known to the patient on an ongoing basis. As the time for transfer approaches, careful explanations can reassure patients and families that close observation and monitoring are no longer necessary. When possible, tubes, machines, and equipment used in the critical care unit, which the patient may see as important to his or her survival, should be removed gradually rather than discontinued all at once. This will alleviate feelings of dependence on equipment.

At the time of transfer, patients can be told how care will change and what changes in activity, self-care, and visiting hours to expect. The critical care unit nurse should accompany the patient to the new floor and introduce the new staff members to the patient. The patient can be told that a complete report on his or her condition will be given and that nursing care needs at this stage of recovery will be met in the new setting. Family members should be contacted and informed of the transfer. The care plan and teaching plan developed in the critical care area should accompany the patient to the floor and the new nurses informed about current short-term and long-term goals and the patient's progress. Although careful preparation and planning for transfer are always desirable, a patient may be transferred unexpectedly to make room for a more critically ill admission. When this situation occurs, the patient to be moved from the unit must be notified and prepared for the possibility of a quick transfer. Tangible evidence of improvement such as improvement in vital signs, fewer medications, or fewer tubes can be helpful in pointing out advances in condition before unplanned transfers.

## SAMPLE TEACHING PLANS

Examples of teaching plans appropriate for the acutely ill patient begin in the boxes on pp. 36-37, including suggested content and time frames for teaching.

## SUMMARY

This chapter has outlined and discussed theory and assessment of health perception and health management issues important in the care of the critically ill patient, as well as the role of health promotion in the acute care setting. Factors influencing patient compliance have been identified, and strategies for optimizing patient compliance have been suggested. Finally, the role of patient education in the critical care area has been reviewed. A detailed educational assessment has been outlined, suggestions for content and teaching methods appropriate to the critical care area have been offered, and sample teaching plans provided.

### REFERENCES

1. American Nurses' Association: A social policy statement, Kansas City, Mo, 1980, The Association.
2. Appel-Hardin S: Maintaining continuity of care: transferring patients from the CCU, Crit Care Nurs 9:92, 1990.
3. Becker MH and others: Some influences on program participation in a genetic screening program, Community Health 1:3, 1975.
4. Bell JA: The role of microcomputers in patient education, Comput Nurs 4(6):255, 1986.
5. Bertakis KD: An application of the health belief model to patient education and compliance: acute otitis media, Fam Med 18(6):347, 1986.
6. Billie DA: The teaching-learning process. In Billie DA: Practical approaches of patient teaching, Boston, 1981, Little, Brown & Co., Inc.
7. Billie DA: Process oriented patient education, Dimens Crit Care Nurs 2:2, 1983.
8. Boyd MD: A guide to writing effective patient education materials, Nurs Management 18(7):56, 1987.
9. Burke LE: Learning and retention in the acute care setting, Crit Care Q 4:3, 1981.

10. Burke LE and Scalzi CC: Education of the patient and family. In Underhill S and others: Cardiac nursing, Philadelphia, 1982, JB Lippincott Co.
11. Carpenito L: Nursing diagnosis: application to clinical practice, Philadelphia, 1988, JB Lippincott Co.
12. Devine EC and Cook TD: Clinical and cost-saving effects of psychoeducational interventions with surgical patients: a meta-analysis, Res Nurs Health 9:89, 1986.
13. Doak L and Doak C: Patient comprehension profiles: recent findings and strategies, Patient Coun Health Educ 3:101, 1980.
14. Dobberstein K: Computer-assisted patient education, Am J Nurs 87(5):697, 1987.
15. Durand RP and Counts CS: Developing audio-visual programs for patient education, Am Neph Nurs Assoc 13(3):158, 1986.
16. Eaton S, Davis G, and Brenner P: Discussion stoppers in teaching, Nurs Outlook 25(9):578, 1977.
17. Edelman C and Milio N: Health defined: promotion and specific protection. In Edelman C and Mandle CL: Health promotion throughout the lifespan, ed 2, St Louis, 1990, Mosby–Year Book, Inc.
18. Elsberry NL and Sorensen ME: Using analogies in patient teaching, Am J Nurs 86(10):1171, 1986.
19. Flynn JB and Griffin PA: Health promotion in acute care settings, Nurs Clin North Am 19(2):239, 1984.
20. Foster DS: Written reinforcement for teaching, MCN 11(5):347, 1986.
21. Fox V: Patient teaching—understanding the needs of the adult learner, AORN 44(2):234, 1986.
22. Frenn M, Fehring R, and Kartes S: Reducing the stress of cardiac catheterization by teaching relaxation, Dimens Crit Care Nurs 5(2):108, 1986.
23. Gerber KE: Compliance in the chronically ill: an introduction to the problem. In Gerber KE and Nehemkis A: Compliance—the dilemma of the chronically ill, New York, 1986, Springer-Verlag New York, Inc.
24. Gordon M: Nursing diagnosis: process and application, New York, 1982, McGraw-Hill Book Co.
25. Gruber-Wood R and Mandel C: Health promotion and the individual. In Edelman C and Mandle CL: Health promotion throughout the lifespan, ed 2, St Louis, 1990, Mosby–Year Book, Inc.
26. Guzzetta CE: Can critically ill patients be taught? In Billie DA: Practical approaches to patient teaching, Boston, 1981, Little, Brown & Co, Inc.
27. Informational needs of families of intensive care unit patients, Quality Rev Bull 12:1, 1986.
28. Keeling AW: Health promotion in coronary care and step down units: focus on the family—linking research to practice, Heart Lung 17(1):28, 1988.
29. Lange J: Developing printed materials for patient education, Dimens Crit Care Nurs 8:250, 1989.
30. Lindeman CA: Influencing recovery through preoperative teaching, Heart Lung 2(4):515, 1973.
31. Lindeman CA and Van Aernam B: Nursing intervention with the presurgical patient—the effects of structured and unstructured preoperative teaching, Nurs Res 20(4):319, 1971.
32. Lipetz M and others: What is wrong with patient education programs? Nurs Outlook 38:184, 1990.
33. Murdaugh C: Barriers to patient education in the coronary care unit, Cardiovasc Nurs 18(6):31, 1982.
34. Narrow B: Patient teaching in nursing practice, Salt Lake City, 1978, John Wiley & Sons, Inc.
35. Nehemkis AM and Gerber KE: Compliance and the quality of life. In Gerber KE and Nehemkis AM: Compliance—the dilemma of the chronically ill, New York, 1986, Springer-Verlag New York, Inc.
36. Neilsen E and Sheppard MA: Television as a patient education tool: a review of its effectiveness, Patient Educ Coun 11:3, 1988.
37. Nite G and Willis F: The coronary patient: hospital care and rehabilitation, New York, 1964, Macmillan, Inc.
38. Novak J: The social mandate and historical basis for nursing's role in health promotion, J Prof Nurs 4(2):80, 1988.
39. Pender NJ: Health promotion in nursing practice, Norwalk, Conn, 1982, Appleton-Century-Crofts.
40. Provine R: The challenge of patient education in critical care, Crit Care Nurs 6(2):22, 1986.
41. Rosenthal K: Multimethod teaching modules, Dimens Crit Care Nurs 8:310, 1989.
42. Smith E: Patient teaching—it's the law, Nursing 87, 17(7):67, 1987.
43. Solomon S and Schwegman-Melton K: Structured teaching and patient understanding of informed consent, Crit Care Nurs 7(3):74, 1987.
44. Storlie F: Patient teaching in critical care, New York, 1975, Appleton-Century-Crofts.
45. Streiff LD: Can clients understand our instructions? Image: J Nurs Schol 18(2):48, 1986.
46. Surgeon General: Healthy people: the Surgeon General's report on health promotion and disease prevention, Washington, DC, 1980, Department of Public Health and Human Service.
47. Theirer J and others: Standards for nursing care of the critically ill, Englewood Cliffs, NJ, 1981, Reston Publishing Co.
48. Thompson J and others: Clinical nursing, ed 2, St Louis, 1989, Mosby–Year Book, Inc.
49. Williams CL and Kendall PC: Psychological aspects of education for stressful medical procedures, Health Educ Q 12(3):135, 1985.
50. Wingate S: Post-MI patient's perceptions of their learning needs, Dimens Crit Care Nurs 9:112, 1990.

UNIT

# II

# COMMON PROBLEMS IN CRITICAL CARE

CHAPTER 4

# Psychosocial Alterations

## CHAPTER OBJECTIVES

- *Describe the theoretical basis of self-concept and its related nursing diagnoses: body image disturbance, self-esteem disturbance, altered role performance, powerlessness, and hopelessness.*
- *Identify situations that increase the risk of disturbances of self-concept.*
- *Given a situation in which a patient experiences a self-concept alteration, match relevant interventions with expected outcomes.*
- *Discuss the following coping strategies as they relate to the critically ill patient: relaxation techniques, biofeedback, and psychotherapy.*
- *List and discuss factors that enhance coping.*
- *Discuss the importance of social support for the critically ill patient.*
- *Describe the needs and coping mechanisms of families of critically ill patients.*
- *Conduct a nursing interview that assesses the sexual concerns of patients with cardiovascular or chronic lung disease.*
- *Formulate nursing diagnoses for a patient whose sexual activity is compromised because of cardiovascular or chronic lung disease.*
- *Assist patients in correlating expended sexual energy with comparable MET equivalents.*
- *Facilitate opportunities for patients and partners to experience physical contact as a precursor to healthy sexual expression.*

## KEY TERMS

body image, p. 43
self-esteem, p. 44
powerlessness, p. 46
hopelessness, p. 47
cognitive appraisal, p. 48
relaxation techniques, p. 49
biofeedback, p. 49

## SELF-CONCEPT ALTERATIONS

The human self-concept comprises attitudes about oneself; perceptions of personal abilities, body image, and identity; and a general sense of worth. Included in this section are discussions of the nursing diagnoses of disturbances in self-concept, that is, body image disturbance, self-esteem disturbance, altered role performance, powerlessness, and hopelessness. The nursing diagnosis personal identity disturbance, included as a subcomponent of the human self-concept by the North American Nursing Diagnosis Association (NANDA), is omitted because it is not yet sufficiently developed for useful application to clinical practice. The four subcomponents of the human self-concept appear in Fig. 4-1.

### Body Image Disturbance

**Body image** is the mental picture an individual has of his or her body and its physical functioning at any given time. It is based on past and present perceptions and includes one's attitudes and feelings about one's body. The body image develops over time from internal-sensation postural changes, contact with people and objects in the environment, emotional experiences, and fantasies.[107] Although the body image is a stable part of the self-concept, it changes over time; it is influenced by cognitive growth and physical changes in the body. Fisher[32] suggested that body experiences can be dampened or minimized, or they can be magnified to the point where they are the center of attention. He also described the *body boundary,* the demarcation between the self and the environment and the pattern of body awareness. The latter refers to the variation in attention given to different parts of the body; more attention is given to the parts that have symbolic significance or that are currently being threatened.

A change in the body's appearance, structure, and/or function necessitates a change in the body image. Such changes may be caused by disease, trauma, or surgery. The cause of body image disturbance may be biophysical, cognitive-perceptual, psychosocial, cultural, or spiritual. Body image disturbances arise when the person fails to perceive

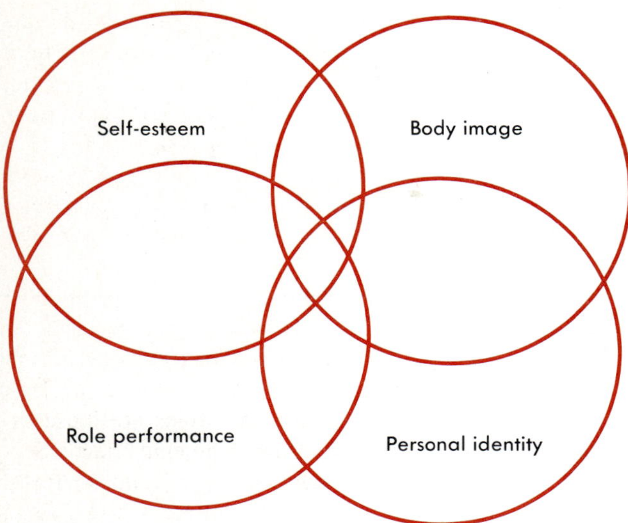


***Fig. 4-1*** Four subcomponents of the human self-concept (NANDA).

or adapt to the changed body. Such disturbances are manifested by verbal or nonverbal response to the actual or perceived change in appearance, structure, or function. A patient admitted to a surgical intensive care unit after a traumatic amputation may awake to find his or her leg missing with no prior knowledge of the loss. Reliving the accident and receiving explanations about the need for the amputation are priorities for such a patient. The critical care nurse must begin the process of helping the patient live with this alteration. Interventions by the nurse and others on the health team focus on helping the person manage the physical changes and the changes in the psychosocial areas affected. Helping the person recognize, accept, and live with the resultant change requires recognition that self-esteem and role performance may also be affected. See p. 443 for the nursing management of Body Image Disturbance.

Body image has received considerable attention in the nursing literature.* This body of knowledge forms the basis for interventions with patients experiencing the losses associated with altered body image. Body image may also be altered by the need to incorporate a prosthetic device or a donated body part.[88]

The meaning of the alteration (appearance, structure, or function) varies with the individual. What is lost? What value is placed on it? What did the body part or function enable the person to enjoy or accomplish? What disability results? The values of the culture are important; wholeness, independence, and attractiveness are important in society today. The person's ability to cope, the responses from others significant to him or her, and the help available to him or her and the family are important factors in the outcome of body image disturbances.

*References 6, 13-15, 19, 73, 87, 90.

### Self-Esteem Disturbance

**Self-esteem** develops as a part of self-concept through the reflected appraisals of significant others. The way in which such information is interpreted is probably more important than the content. Self-esteem is only partly related to material, economic, or social conditions. The need for self-esteem is a part of the hierarchy of human needs postulated by Maslow.[67] Having high self-esteem helps one deal with the environment and face more easily the maturational and situational crises of life. A low self-regard impairs one's ability to adapt. Overall, the goal is to maintain a high positive regard for oneself in the midst of ever-changing views of oneself. This goal, when met, contributes to the quality of life of the individual. Persons with a well-developed self-esteem are at less risk for disturbances of self-esteem than those with poorly developed self-esteem.

Disturbances in self-esteem arise when a person experiences a decrease in self-worth, self-respect, and self-approval or self-confidence. Causative factors of the decrease include repeated negative interactions with significant others, as well as cognitive-perceptual difficulties. Low self-esteem may be manifested by (1) inability to accept positive reinforcement, (2) lack of follow-through, (3) nonparticipation in therapy, (4) not taking responsibility for self-care (self-neglect), (5) self-destructive behavior, and (6) lack of eye contact.

Self-esteem is an important concept for nurses and other health professionals. It has been studied frequently in a variety of contexts.* Nurses have a significant impact on patients who are experiencing illness. Refer to the nursing management of Self-Esteem Disturbance on p. 442. When the illness is critical, a patient's self-esteem level may be imperiled. Perhaps the patient caused the accident that injured him or her and others, including family members. Perhaps he or she was under the influence of alcohol or drugs. Perhaps he or she will be subject to arrest if he or she survives. Perhaps he or she will lose his or her job or be unable to return to his or her previous occupation. The nurse who expresses negative reactions to a patient, either openly or covertly, will reinforce a patient's low self-esteem. An aloof, insensitive, or superficial relationship with a patient who has acquired immunodeficiency syndrome (AIDS), for example, can cause the patient to feel rejected, humiliated, and stigmatized.[127]

Antonucci and Jackson[3] pointed out that, although a link between self-esteem and mental illness has been confirmed, the link with physical health is not clear. Self-esteem level may be an outcome, a predisposing factor, or an insulating factor in situations involving physical health. In their study of self-esteem and physical health, self-esteem was lower

*References 3, 23, 24, 27, 44, 76, 77, 91, 105, 113.

as the severity of the health problem increased, as the perception of ill health increased, and as the degree of disability increased. The study stresses the need for awareness that patients with health problems probably have a lower self-esteem that may negatively affect behavior during illness.

The antecedents of self-esteem were the focus of Coopersmith's book.[23] He identified four major factors that contribute to the development of self-esteem:

1. The amount of acceptance and concern from significant persons in one's life.
2. The successes in one's past and one's status and position in the world.
3. The values and aspirations to which one commits oneself.
4. The manner in which one responds to devaluing experiences.

Basic self-esteem as described by Crouch and Straub[25] is that which is established early in life and, once firmly established, is relatively unchanging. They also described a functional level of self-esteem that varies from day to day according to ongoing evaluations of interactions. Such self-esteem may be more or less than the basic self-esteem. The functional level can be changed in response to interventions of the person himself or herself, the family, co-workers, or health professionals. Functional self-esteem may be increased through individually oriented, short-term approaches that attempt to improve the person's view of his or her worth.

In old age, a person faces loss of autonomy that may lower self-esteem. Changes in the expectations of others for one's behavior and capacity may occur. Losses related to health alterations and sensory impairment related to aging, dependency, retirement, and deaths of friends and family may affect self-esteem. If nurses are impatient with performance deficits, the patient may feel inadequate and guilty. If patients are treated as children, they may believe themselves burdens and react with resentment. Failure to include them in decision making may cause them to feel useless and rejected. On the other hand, people with a strong sense of self-worth are likely to be adjusted, happy, and competent.

Defensive self-esteem attempts to defend against the person's perception of a gap between his or her real self and his or her ideal self. High self-esteem is associated with a low need for social approval, comfort with intimacy and self-disclosure, and the ability to acknowledge personal failures. Rubin[105] discussed the loss of self-esteem that accompanies the loss of control of functioning in relation to time and place. This loss is associated with a decrease in self-esteem. A sense of shame accompanies this private judgment of failure.

A person's level of self-esteem is an important factor in the response to a critical illness, and behavior during illness may be negatively affected by lowered self-esteem. The patient with severe burns may interpret the avoidance behavior of nurses and family who are appalled by the appearance of the patient and the odor in his or her room as a devaluation of himself or herself. He or she may refuse to cooperate with the treatment regimen and may judge himself or herself a failure and be unable to see a future in which he or she will return to a productive life. Anticipatory interventions that assist the staff and family in their care of the patient would help to avoid such a situation.

### Altered Role Performance

Interactions with others that create and modify roles are an important part of the self-concept. The roles one chooses reflect one's beliefs and feelings. Persons have primary, secondary, and tertiary roles. Primary roles are those associated with gender, age, and developmental stage. Secondary roles are those of daughter, sister, and so forth. Tertiary roles are those assumed by choice such as scout leader or churchgoer. Illness, when it occurs, disrupts secondary and tertiary roles.

Role performance alterations are those problems that arise when a person experiences difficulties in making life transitions. Causative factors include lack of significant role models, inability to learn new roles because of life transitions, and cognitive-perceptual difficulties. Altered role performance may be manifested by (1) change in self-perception of role, (2) denial of role, (3) change in others' perception of role, (4) conflict in roles, (5) changes in physical capacity to resume role, (6) lack of knowledge of role, and (7) change in usual patterns of responsibility.

Role transitions occur in patients with critical illness. Role change in the transition from wellness or chronic illness to acute illness is a concern for the critical care nurse because role transitions mean changes in role relationships, expectations, or abilities and can be major concerns for the critically ill patient.

The rapid and potentially drastic changes that accompany critical illness may seriously interfere with role performance. The male patient after a myocardial infarction wonders about his role as husband, breadwinner, and careerist. The psychosocial needs of the patient in such a situation depend on age, gender, occupation, family roles, previous experience with illness, suddenness of onset, extent of illness, and prognosis. Nurses are frequently involved with situations that include alterations in role performance in individuals and families.

The patient may be unable to meet the demands of such changes and thus experience role insufficiency.[78] The use of role supplementation is an approach nurses can use in such a situation. As described by Meleis,[78] this intervention involves both preventive and therapeutic efforts. Using communication and interaction with patient and family, information or experience is conveyed that increases the awareness of the new roles and interrelationships necessary because of the role transition. For example, role insufficiency may be displayed in behaviors that reflect fear of moving from the critical care unit to the intermediate care unit. A variety of nursing activities can anticipate and facilitate this transition. See the nursing management of Altered Role Performance on p. 444.

### Powerlessness

The concept of **powerlessness** may be defined as the perceived inability to influence or control an outcome. Powerlessness as a nursing diagnosis is defined as the perception of the individual that one's own action will not significantly affect an outcome. Powerlessness is a perceived lack of control over a current situation or immediate happening. Unrelieved powerlessness may result in hopelessness, which is discussed in the next section.

The causes of powerlessness include factors in the health care environment, interpersonal interactions, illness-related regimen, and a lifestyle of helplessness. A severe level of powerlessness may be manifested by verbal expressions of having no control or influence over the situation, verbal expressions of having no control or influence over the outcome, verbal expressions of having no control over self-care, depression over physical deterioration that occurs despite the patient's compliance with regimens, and apathy. Moderate levels of powerlessness may be reflected by nonparticipation in care or decision making when opportunities are provided; expressions of dissatisfaction and frustration over inability to perform previous tasks and/or activities; not monitoring progress; expression of doubt about role performance; reluctance to express true feelings, fearing alienation from caregivers; passivity; inability to seek information about care; dependence on others that may result in irritability, resentment, anger, and guilt; and no defense of self-care practices when challenged. Low powerlessness may be reflected in passivity. Both actual and perceived control over present or impending events are important.

Most people expect to have the power to participate in making decisions that affect them. Feelings of powerlessness are avoided if possible. When patients feel their choices are limited, they may act against their own best interests.[49] Given enough frustration, any exercise of control—even one with negative outcomes (such as signing out of the hospital against medical advice [AMA])—can become attractive.

Individuals vary in the amount of control they prefer.[102] A patient may feel power, but he or she may or may not desire it. Important variables in this regard are the illness; values, traits, attitudes, and past experiences; the hospital setting; and social displacement. Personality, age, religion, occupation, income, residence, and race may all be pertinent factors. Apparently there is an increase in variability in the amount of control preferred as people age. Rodin[102] pointed out that giving a person more control than desired may result in negative outcomes: stress, worry, self-blame. The critical care unit routines may oppose or preclude any control by the patient. The person to whom control is important should be helped to continue to control as many areas of life as possible. On the other hand, a patient must be given the opportunity to choose not to control.

One explanation of this variable interest in control is the concept of *locus of control*. This idea of expectancy of control developed by Rotter[104] has been particularly helpful in explaining the variability of responses of people to similar situations. The locus of control is a personality characteristic, a relatively stable tendency to perceive events and outcomes as within or outside one's control regardless of the situation.

The Internal-External Locus of Control Scale developed by Rotter is useful in assessing this personality trait. A person with an internal locus of control tends to believe that events are under one's personal control. A person with an external locus of control, however, tends to believe that events are related to chance, fate, or powerful others. Situations exist in which the person with an internal locus of control has made serial lifestyle changes based on medical advice and then has experienced a major illness, typically a myocardial infarction. This experience forces him or her to believe that his or her own actions will not (because they have not) significantly affect the outcome. Repeated or significant experiences with illness may reinforce belief in an external locus of control for people who originally possessed an internal locus of control. Nursing interventions that support the power or influence the individual does wield help prevent an all-encompassing sense of powerlessness.

Another aspect of powerlessness is *learned helplessness*. Seligman[109] suggested that repeated experiences with uncontrollable events result in diminished motivation, lessened ability to perceive success, and increased emotionality. Interventions suggested to prevent or reverse learned helplessness include opportunities to exert control.

In the critical care unit, threats to a patient's control include the unusual signs and symptoms of his or her illness and inadequate knowledge about the situation.[101] The disease process and the personal, psychological, and social situation interact to affect the patient's perception of control or lack of control. If control is defined as the ability to determine the use of time, space, and resources, admission to a critical care unit strips away control to varying extents. Patients no longer can decide about physical care, socializing, or privacy. They are under the close scrutiny of the nurses and physicians and have decreased physical strength.

On admission persons lose their independent status. They become patients. Use of clothes and other personal belongings is usually restricted in a critical care unit. Patients cannot decide who enters the room, who provides personal care, or who intrudes with painful treatments. The hospital rules usually are not open to modification. Patients may feel anxious because they are separated from a familiar environment, have restrictions on visitors, and must depend on others for their care. They may fear death or permanent loss of function and may feel guilty if they have contributed to the cause of the illness or injury. They may resent the invasion of their privacy. By virtue of their experiences of critical illness and care, people may lose sight of areas of influence they retain over themselves because so much control is taken from them.

The extent of powerlessness is determined by the situation. Critically ill patients generally have experienced a rapid onset of illness without time to acquire the illness role. A sense of powerlessness in such situations is not unexpected. Poor interactions with the health care providers may make the situation worse. Patients may react aggressively, may try bargaining, or may refuse to comply with diagnostic and treatment regimens.

Powerlessness in acutely ill persons is related to (1) the uncertainty of the outcome, (2) the strange, threatening, overwhelming experience in the critical care unit, including diagnostic and treatment events, and (3) the lack of knowledge about the situation. The nurse has a primary role in preventing and alleviating the perception of personal powerlessness in the patient and family. (Refer to the nursing management of Powerlessness on p. 445.)

### Hopelessness

**Hopelessness** is a subjective state in which an individual sees limited or no alternatives or personal choices available and is unable to mobilize energy on his or her own behalf. To help clarify this nursing diagnosis, a definition of hope is included—a feeling that what is wanted will happen, that desire is accompanied by anticipation or expectation.[123] Most people agree that an element of hope must be maintained no matter how hopeless things appear. Hope is a force that helps one survive. It is an attitude toward the future, and it occupies a key position between the present and future. The absence of hope is a serious situation.

Causative factors related to hopelessness include (1) prolonged activity restriction, creating isolation, (2) a failing or deteriorating physiological condition, (3) long-term stress, (4) abandonment, and (5) a lost belief in transcendent values or God.

Hopelessness is defined in terms of negative expectations concerning oneself and one's future life.[7] Motivation is lost; a decision is made not to want anything, to give up, and not to try to get something. The future seems dark, vague, and uncertain.

Hope often arises in the presence of crisis. The idea of giving up is vigorously resisted. The help of others in the situation supports the patient's belief. Hope wards off despair, mental anguish, disorganization, helplessness, and hopelessness.

Hopelessness can take control and immobilize the patient. The sense of impossibility can block attempts to change the situation. A system of negative expectancies about oneself and the future may result in a sense of overwhelming defeat. The hopeful person can imagine a future and that the storm will pass. The hopeless one gives up.

Jones[52] pointed out that one tends to find what one expects in interactions with others. Processing information is selective. Expectancies cause an individual to act in ways that elicit behaviors that can be interpreted as confirming those expectancies, even when such expectancies are mistaken. This response is the behavioral confirmation of an expectancy, the self-fulfilling prophecy. This idea is important in instances of hopelessness. Staff members may feel helpless when patients do not respond to their care; they may label patients as hopeless. Patients recognize this attitude and react to confirm this expectancy by giving up. Engel[31] identified the "giving up—given up" syndrome and included hopelessness as one component. Other components included a depreciated self-image; lack of gratification from roles and role relationships; interference with continuity of the past, present, and future; and reawakened painful memories. The acutely ill individual is highly susceptible to such a situation. Persons may give up hope, believing that they have been given up by others—a self-fulfilling prophecy.

Illness influences hopelessness by threatening internal resources (one's ability to cope) and external resources (one's perceptions of who can help). A patient's autonomy, self-esteem, independence, strength, and integrity may be at risk.

The critically ill patient is a multiproblem patient. Nurses and physicians are tempted to focus on the crisis and overlook the patient in his or her totality. The critical care unit is noisy and frightening; it increases the patient's sense of vulnerability and the fear of death. The patient's degree of hopelessness is related to the perception and duration of his or her powerlessness. Thus feelings of hopelessness are not uncommon in critical care units. Therefore it is important to foster a realistic sense of hope. Science has progressed and can accomplish many things. Even if long-term survival is not likely, patients can be helped to plan to live the remaining life to the fullest. The critical care nurse must try to feel hopeful and identify some aspect of the situation in which hope is warranted, no matter how grave the situation, and must try to channel feelings toward some positive outcome, even the hope of a peaceful death (see the nursing management of Hopelessness on p. 446).

## COPING ALTERATIONS

### The Critical Care Experience

Wong,[128] a psychiatrist, wrote of his personal experience as a patient in a critical care unit. He described "losing connection" with the world and having no sense of time or sleep. He was immobile, experienced pain, and was attached to a ventilator, urinary catheter, gastric tube, intravenous (IV) lines, and chest tubes. A growing awareness of the tubes and lines entering his body helped him to get in touch with his sense of self. He realized his loss of control over himself and his world. He used humor and denial and became alert to indications of improvement of his body functions as each mechanical support was removed. Then, in a state of hypomania (excessive emotion, elation, and motor activity) he discussed his work and made plans to return to the job in 2 weeks. He was surprised at the pain he experienced during his first meal. He fought to be rational but experienced hallucinations.

## COMMON COPING STRATEGIES

1. Seek information; get guidance.
2. Share concern; find consolation.
3. Laugh it off; change emotional tone.
4. Forget it happened (suppression).
5. Keep busy; distract yourself.
6. Confront the issue; act accordingly.
7. Redefine the problem; take a more optimistic view.
8. Resign yourself; make the best of what cannot be changed.
9. Do something, anything, perhaps exceeding good judgment.
10. Review alternatives; examine consequences.
11. Get away from it all; find an escape.
12. Conform, comply; do what is expected or advised.
13. Blame or shame someone or something such as a spouse, the job.
14. Ventilate; feel emotional release.
15. Deny as much as possible.

People cope with the critical care experience in many ways, and a complete listing of strategies would be impossible. Weisman[124] identified 15 common coping strategies, which are found in the box above. The nurse supports her or his patients as they question their experiences, that is, what they feel, hear, see; as they wonder what their caregivers and significant others think of them; as they express their needs and wants against what they can realistically expect of themselves or others; and as they learn new skills and adapt old ones. The nurse is essential to patients' overall understanding and acceptance of the critical care experience. Refer to the nursing management of Ineffective Individual Coping on p. 447 and Anxiety on p. 448.

### Coping Theories

The reactions of patients to the critical care unit are varied as are the theories that explain feelings, thoughts, and behaviors of persons in such situations. Eisendrath[30] used Erikson's developmental theory to explain the psychosocial repression of individuals in the critical care unit, and Roberts[100] applied Piaget's theory of cognitive development to the egocentric behavior of the critically ill adult.

Other writers have focused on the emotional responses experienced by patients. Shine[110] described cardiac patients' reactions in terms of anxiety, that is, its manifestations, its undesirable physiological effects, and its frequent sources. Thomas[119] described the loneliness of the individual, and Quinless[99] wrote of the helplessness, powerlessness, hopelessness, and anxiety experienced in the critical care unit. Behavior has also been described as a manifestation of a psychiatric disorder, that is, the psychopathology of trauma patients,[111] and the "overload depression" of patients in the critical care unit.[12]

Coping as a concept offering interpretation of feeling, thought, and experience resulting in behavior after a stress-producing situation is presented in this section to offer further understanding of the patient and his behavior. Coping has been defined as "efforts to master conditions of harm, threat, or challenge when a routine or automatic response is not readily available."[83] Two models describing the process involved in coping—cognitive appraisal and conflict theory of decision making—are presented to assist the nurse in choosing interventions that are realistic and effective.

**Cognitive appraisal theory.** Lazarus and colleagues [34-36,59,61-63] have developed a dynamic multivariate multiprocess of stress and coping. Cognitive appraisal and coping are mediating processes between the person-environment encounters and the immediate and long-term outcomes.

**Cognitive appraisal** is the process that the individual uses to evaluate his or her encounters with the environment. If the environment is considered endangering, impairing, diminishing, or overwhelming to his or her resources and well-being, stress is interpreted. *Primary appraisal* refers to the evaluation of what is at stake—is there benefit or harm to his or her values, self-esteem, goals, or commitments? The *secondary appraisal* identifies actions to take, or the coping options. Together, these appraisals determine whether the interaction or encounter with the environment is threatening, with a chance of harm or loss, or challenging, with a chance of benefit or mastery.

Coping refers to "the person's cognitive and behavioral efforts to manage (reduce, minimize, master, or tolerate) the internal and external demands of the person-environment transaction that is appraised as taxing or exceeding the person's resources."[35] This definition focuses on the coping process: what the person thinks and does, what comes first, second, and so on. Its concerns are with the situational context of the demand—what the demand is itself, the resources available, the constraints, and the time involvement. Coping is not considered good or bad, effective or ineffective, successful or unsuccessful, reality oriented or defensive. The coping efforts are significant in and of themselves.

Coping generally encompasses two functions: (1) regulation of emotions (emotion-focused coping) and (2) alteration in the person-environment encounter (problem-focused coping).

**Conflict theory model of decision making.** The conflict theory model of decision making proposed by Janis and Mann[46,48] examines the decision and coping patterns associated with responses to threats such as life-threatening illnesses. Five patterns were identified: uncomplicated inertia, defensive avoidance, unconflicted change, hypervigilance, and vigilance.

***Uncomplicated inertia.*** Uncomplicated inertia, or immobilization and inactivity, is related to misjudgment that stems from ignorance about the threat at hand, for example, illness, treatment, or procedure. This pattern can easily be changed by providing correct information about the threat and associated actions.

***Defensive avoidance.*** A person who demonstrates defensive avoidance is either placing responsibility for decision making on another, procrastinating in making a decision or action, rationalizing a choice that is the least harmful, or ignoring threatening symptoms. Correction can occur as the person experiences hope about a positive outcome from the information and receives reassurances from the staff. For example, the patient questions that his or her doctor knows what to do in his or her case; the nurse encourages the patient to decide for himself or herself and assures the patient that he or she has the ability to do so.

***Unconflicted change.*** Unconflicted change is displayed when a person consents to do anything and everything the health care providers say and does not show any sign that he or she is worried, does not understand, or does not know what to do. When information is provided, the patient is selectively inattentive and afterwards is angry, feels he or she has been misled, and is not cooperative.

Providing too much knowledge about what will occur and developing overconfidence lead to the "work of worrying." During this time, the patient experiences anticipatory fear, rehearses what will occur, reassures himself or herself, and develops expectations for self and others. If this work of worrying cannot be done because of a pattern of suppressing the anticipatory fear, because the event was totally unexpected or accidental, because warnings were not given, or because reassurances were over-encouraging, then the individual cannot work through his or her emotional state.

***Hypervigilance.*** Individuals may experience a near panic state when faced with danger, and they subsequently manifest hypervigilance coping patterns. During these periods full or complete information is not sought, and decisions to act are made impulsively. The person is emotionally excited and cognitively restricted, has a short memory span, oversimplifies or ignores complicating factors, and often repeats words and phrases over and over.

Janis[46] asserted that hyperviligance coping patterns were frequently used by critical care patients. Patients who have experienced "near misses" (for example, had a cardiac arrest), observed activities in the unit with other critical patients, or have a worsening condition have an increased probability of having a hypervigilance pattern. Lack of time to find a way to escape the danger and perceived impending loss or death predispose the patient to its use.

The environment itself also adds to the probability of hypervigilance because of environmental factors such as invasive and monitoring lines and equipment that restrict movement. Physical symptoms may include pain, nausea, dizziness, hypothermia or hyperthermia, and altered mental status caused by analgesics. Sensory deprivation or overload are other conditions that may lead to hypervigilance. Examples in critical care are the continuous noise of machines and alarms, bright lights, repetitive questions, multiple caregivers and staff, and frequent procedures and treatments. The timing of the stress event (for example, frequent around-the-clock disturbances) also leads to hypervigilance.

Use of an alternative coping pattern is encouraged by giving the patient meaningful explanations of what has happened and what will be occurring in the future. The patient needs encouragement and reassurance that he or she has the ability to cope and that support is available to him or her. In addition, actions can be taken to reduce hospital and critical care restrictions and to approximate normal daily activity.

***Vigilance.*** The vigilance pattern is characterized by examining the situation for appropriate goals, carefully gathering information, assimilating information, examining possible consequences of actions, and planning action strategies. By using this pattern, the person has three basic beliefs: (1) the decision he or she is making involves risk, (2) the solution can be potentially satisfying, and (3) sufficient time will be available before a choice is made. For example, when faced with a decision about consenting to a coronary angiogram, the patient knows that there is risk involved, that he or she can gain the satisfaction of knowing whether he or she has coronary disease, and (in the case of a nonemergent elective procedure) that he or she will have time to consider the decision.

### Coping Interventions

Moos and Schaefer[85] described five major tasks that form the basis for treatment of patients in stressful situations: (1) establishing personal meaning for the crisis, (2) confronting the demands and reality of the crisis, (3) maintaining relationships with family and helpers, (4) managing emotions aroused by the crisis, and (5) sustaining a positive self-image. These goals can be achieved by the patients through the use of processes such as self-regulation, cognitive appraisal, coping with the emotional arousal, and decision making.

**Relaxation techniques. Relaxation techniques** produce a decrease in pulse, breathing rate, blood pressure, anxiety, and pain. Benson[9] offered four components necessary for the relaxation response to occur: quiet environment, passive attitude, mental capability, and a comfortable position. Benson's technique involves maintaining a comfortable position with eyes closed in a quiet place, relaxing all of the muscles, beginning with the toes and moving to the head, becoming aware of breathing and focusing on it, and maintaining this state of relaxation for 10 to 20 minutes.

**Biofeedback. Biofeedback** is closely associated with relaxation techniques and is used to monitor the responses of the body as the individual attempts to exert control over these responses. Miller[80] offered examples of the use of feedback response and relaxation techniques in critical care. After administration of pain medication, the patient is instructed in the use of relaxation techniques. The change from focusing on the pain to focusing on the breathing pattern and chest movement is a diversion that helps to reduce pain. Information is given to the patient about changes in the heart rate that occur as the result of his or her efforts. By using these techniques, the patient can learn to relax, monitor the state of tension, and divert his or her thoughts as a way to reduce pain and manage stress.

Wilson-Barnett[125] reviewed 43 studies on intervention to reduce stress responses over a 20-year period. Information, particularly sensory information, was found significantly to reduce anxiety and promote recovery. Positive reappraisal regarding selected concerns was more effective in reducing stress than general information about the stressors. Moss[86] reported that providing patient and family preoperative instruction is an effective method for decreasing fear and anxiety.

**Psychotherapy.** Brief psychotherapy, which focuses primarily on processing the painful event with a qualified psychotherapist, is another approach to the treatment of stress. Bellak, Leopold, and Siegel[8] described an exploration with patients of the meaning of surgery, anesthesia, possibility of death, and secondary gains of the surgery. Owen and Harrision[93] also used brief psychotherapy to examine stress and fears of patients who had experienced cardiac arrest. Psychodynamic considerations after heart surgery might include reducing hostility, widening sources of pleasure, stressing the value of relaxation, or developing less competitive and perfectionist attitudes.[41]

Crisis intervention, conceptualized by Aguilera and Messick,[1] is a form of brief psychotherapy. During this process an assessment is made of the person's perception of the precipitating event, what support systems are available, and what coping mechanisms might be helpful. Based on this assessment, an action plan is developed. Interventions are related to the skill of the therapist and involvement and capabilities of the patient. Interventions may include assisting the patient with an intellectual understanding of the crisis, exploring feelings, helping him or her to identify coping mechanisms, and assisting him or her to reestablish social support.

Slaby and Glicksman[112] specified 40 principal factors related to adaptation to life-threatening illnesses such as cancer, heart disease, and near-fatal trauma. Those factors specifically related to enhancing coping are listed in the following box.

### FACTORS ENHANCING COPING

#### PATIENT

- Patient and family's knowledge of the illness and treatment
- Awareness of the relationship of past experiences and conflicts to anger being experienced with current stress
- Use of age-appropriate adaptive mechanisms
- Obtaining care from person of one's own choosing
- Acknowledging psychological pain and seeking relief
- Receiving support from someone else who has the illness
- Identifying stages of adaptation, i.e., denial, anger, acceptance
- Tolerating dependence on others for care and assistance
- Finding strength and meaning in the experience

#### HEALTH CARE PROFESSIONALS

- Giving truthful information to the patient as changes in illness and treatment occur
- Demonstrating a positive, rational view of the illness, treatment, and prognosis
- Providing ways for the patient to express self-control and autonomous decision making
- Emphasizing the strengths and capabilities of the patient
- Recognizing that denial is an adaptive phase during illness
- Collaborating with the patient and family on care and treatments
- Allowing time—particularly time to mourn loss of body function or capabilities

**Families and social support.** The family is part of the patient's primary social support system and, as such, demands the attention and concern of the critical care nurse. Pearlmutter and colleagues[95] described the needs of families of critical care patients at various stages. Families should be immediately reassured that the reactions they are experiencing do not imply incompetence but are felt by others in similar situations. They should be given explanations of policies and procedures and should be told that there will always be qualified staff to care for their loved ones. Further contacts are necessary to demonstrate respect and acceptance for the family's reactions such as hostility, sadness, and withdrawal; to listen to complaints and problems without invoking fear of reprisal; and to assist in the grief process. Finally, the family needs assistance during the transition from the critical care unit to a step-down or general medical-surgical unit. During this time separation, loss of support, development of new relationships, and adjustment to a new environment and staff serve as new stressors to families.

Nine coping mechanisms of critically ill patients were identified by King and Gregor[54,55]: (1) turning to others for support, (2) remaining close to loved one, (3) review of events, (4) information seeking, (5) intellectualization, (6) rehearsal of potential future situations, (7) minimizing the situations, (8) repetition, and (9) hope. Questions to assess coping are listed in the box on p. 51. Nursing interventions to assist the family may consist of developing a helping relationship, listening, providing information, fostering hope, providing realistic expectations and goals, and assisting in an evaluation of previously used coping strategies.

Gaglione[39] identified behaviors of families of patients in the coronary care unit. Shock and disbelief were early responses, followed by anxiety, the need to be useful, the need to know that the patient is receiving the good care, and the need for emotional support. Informational, physical, and spiritual needs were only minimally mentioned.

### COPING ASSESSMENT QUESTIONS

#### CURRENT SITUATION

1. What is the nature of the threat, i.e., is it threatening to life, goals, values, or self-esteem, or to the ability to manage or cope?
2. What is the meaning of the event in terms of the past, present, and future?
3. What abilities, skills, and resources are available to meet the threat?
4. Is there an available support system?

#### COPING BEHAVIORS

1. What is the nature and range of emotion-focused behaviors?
2. What is the nature and range of cognitive-focused behaviors?
3. What are the effects of the current situation on self-esteem?
4. What are the effects of the coping behaviors on relationships with others?
5. Are there conflicts between values, beliefs, and needs?
6. How may the coping behavior affect the desired outcome?

## SEXUALITY ALTERATIONS

### Sexual Expression

Sexual expression at its best is more than just attainment of coitus and orgasm. It also encompasses love, warmth, sharing, and touching between people and an emotional union of hearts and minds, all of which transcend purely physical pleasure. It is the culmination and coming together within the individual of biological, psychological, and cultural influences that result in sex-role behavior or sexual expression of self.[22]

Sensuality, although a necessary component of sexual fulfillment, does not in itself reflect sexual activity. It refers to the pleasure one derives through the senses such as touch, smell, sight, and sound, which enhance the total sexual experience.

### Assessment of Sexual Activity Intolerance

Most sources agree that critical care nurses should seize the earliest opportunity to teach patients and their partners about myocardial infarction and how to recognize and manage the different types of chest pain and control the symptoms of fatigue, dyspnea, and rapid heart rate during times such as sexual activity. Since chest pain is the most frightening symptom, the nurse needs to begin by teaching patients the specific language that describes the characteristics of the various types of chest pain. In this way he or she can help patients differentiate chest wall pain from anginal pain and anginal pain from the pain of myocardial infarction. The nurse can then assist patients and partners in connecting each type of pain with its probable cause, symptoms, duration, and mode of prevention and treatment. She or he can instruct patients how to monitor changes in breathing and heart rates and to determine if they are within normal parameters in relation to the amount of energy expended. The nurse can alert patients to be aware of thoughts that may invoke anxious feelings that can contribute to the physical symptoms and then demonstrate strategies to reduce anxiety. "Thoughts that attempt to fight chest pain are more likely to increase anxiety than are those that go beyond the immediate pain experience and focus on the idea that the pain will quickly pass."[98]

The nurse needs to inform patients and partners that some or all of these symptoms may occur during sex, partly because the work load of the damaged cardiac muscle increases to provide the oxygen needed to satisfy the body's demands for energy. Also, anxiety could arouse the nervous system into provoking or sustaining the physical symptoms.[96,98]

*Angina pectoris* is the chest pain associated with myocardial ischemia. Patients with ischemia have an imbalance of regional myocardial perfusion in relation to the demand for myocardial oxygenation. This transient imbalance is precipitated by conditions that increase the heart rate such as exercise, anger, anxiety, or postural changes. The location of the pain may be substernal or extrathoracic (neck, jaw, shoulder, arm) and may include variable degrees of discomfort. Patients who experience anginal pain during sexual activity may benefit from the prophylactic use of nitroglycerin, the use of long-acting nitrate preparations, or the use of beta-blocking agents such as propranolol. Some types of anginal pain may be experienced as indigestion or a toothache. Since anginal pain is precipitated by activities and exercise, it is relieved within minutes by rest or the use of nitroglycerin.

*Myocardial infarction (MI)* involves cellular damage and death of a portion of the cardiac muscle as a result of prolonged ischemia of more than 30 to 45 minutes. Permanent cessation of contractile function occurs in the necrotic or infarcted area. The degree of ventricular dysfunction depends on the size, location, collateral circulation, compensatory mechanisms, and function of the uninvolved myocardium. The patient suffering from myocardial infarction typically experiences severe, prolonged chest pain, frequently associated with sweating, nausea, vomiting, and a feeling of impending doom. If symptoms of chest pain, chest tightness, or severe shortness of breath persist, sexual activities must cease, and the physician must be notified immediately. Hospitalized patients should be instructed that this type of pain can always be treated with narcotic-analgesics.[96]

*Chest wall pain* is caused by a "tightening" of the chest wall muscles, which generally results from poor posture and is exacerbated by anxiety. "Hunching" of the back during sexual intercourse can strain the chest wall muscles and produce dyspnea. Patients should be taught to decrease anxiety by focusing on the idea that the pain will pass versus attempting to fight the pain. Dyspnea can be controlled by straightening the back and performing slow, deep-breathing exercises. Patients can learn to associate anxiety-producing thoughts such as fear of recurrent myocardial infarction and/or death with the occurrence of chest wall pain and recognize that such thoughts exacerbate otherwise normal symptoms of activity intolerance. Once patients successfully master relaxing the chest wall muscles, the cessation of pain will afford them confidence and control during sexual activity and will help them better distinguish between the three types of chest pain.[98]

### Psychological Factors Affecting Sexual Function

Many authorities agree with the substantial evidence that recovery from myocardial infarction can be viewed from a psychological as well as biological perspective.

> The meaning one ascribes to one's heart in human terms encompasses a multitude of emotions and feelings such as love, courage, sympathy, affection and survival itself. The heart and its attributes are romanticized throughout literature, music and the art world, to the extent that the very thought of it failing is to reduce it to the mere organ that it is and to bring one face to face with mortality.[98]

Several authorities document the following psychological fears experienced by postmyocardial infarct patients and their partners[50]:

1. Sudden death will occur from exertion.
2. Sexual activity will impose physical difficulties in sexual function.
3. Heart attack is a "warning" that the aging process reflects a deterioration of sexual capacity.
4. Excitement and orgasm will cause another heart attack.

A study[84] was designed to demonstrate the influence of a brief marriage enrichment relationship skills training program (ME-RSTP) on marital satisfaction and quality of life in couples in the recovery phase of cardiovascular disease. It was established that adequate adaptation to life-threatening and lifestyle-threatening illness required that couples draw on previous relationship skills and coping styles honed from many years of marriage and past experience with stressful situations. It was concluded that only couples whose relationship skills and coping styles were inadequate to meet the demands of adapting to physical illness would truly benefit from such a program. Sexual counseling, no matter how well-intentioned, is not for everyone.

Couples who find in each other "a confidant—one with whom a person can have a close intimate relationship— . . . will be better able to sustain intimacy and satisfy the emotional needs of the relationship, in illness, as they did in health."[18] Interactive strategies for couples are delineated in the box above.

**Assessment of sexual concerns.** Myocardial infarct patients who are at high risk for sexual dysfunction because of psychological concerns may be identified early in the critical care unit. Refer to the nursing management of Sexual Dysfunction on p. 450 and Altered Sexuality Patterns on p. 453.

One study by Sulman and Verhaeghe[117] revealed there are two distinct groups of patients in need of sexual counseling.

*Group I* patients demonstrate grieving behaviors such as poor appetites, saddened affects, and passive resistance to treatment and exercise regimen. These patients can develop growing anxiety or depression as a result of exaggerated concern about the effect of the illness on their sexual integrity and self-esteem and may require psychiatric consultation.

*Group II* patients demonstrate angry, "bullying" behaviors such as being uncooperative and noncompliant to treatment in a belligerent manner. These patients may deny the extent of their illness by continuing to smoke and work while in the hospital and threatening to resume sexual relations at a dangerous pace on discharge. They generally exhibit difficulty in absorbing important information about their illess and frequently verbalize their eagerness for discharge with impatience and frustration.

This same study stipulates that, occasionally, male myocardial infarction patients will verbalize sexually explicit comments interspersed with humor, jokes and "adolescent" type behaviors directed at the staff or visitors. This is considered a "normal" means by which some patients cope with the fear of sexual dysfunction and threat of death. The denial

#### INTERACTIVE STRATEGIES

1. Provide privacy for patient and partner. This illustrates respect and consideration.
2. Demonstrate how they can comfort, touch, and hold each other. Explain the equipment so that they are not intimidated by it.
3. Begin slowly, with less personal topics, to build trust and rapport. Discuss topics such as diet, medications, and breathing treatments.
4. Bring in topics such as activities and discuss restrictions that this illness may impose on them (e.g., housework, gardening, playing golf).
5. Ask patient if he or she has any concerns about how these restrictions may affect sexual relations as well. If it is expressed that sex has not played a big part in the lives of the patient and partner for years but that they are still close in many ways, there is no need to pursue the subject. Simply move on to other areas. If a sexually active lifestyle is revealed, proceed to step 6.
6. Determine if the patient feels that the disease has affected, or may affect, his or her sexual activity and to what extent.
7. Ask whether he or she would like to continue sexual relations but is concerned or anxious about the shortness of breath that accompanies the sex act.[20]

is considered adaptive as long as they *comply* with the treatment and exercise program. In dealing with this personality type, the nurse is advised to ignore the content of the conversation and "go along with the intent" in a light exchange of banter, as long as it allows the patient to cope in a healthy manner.

### Exercise Physiology and Patient Education

Experts suggest that during the acute phase of hospitalization (first 3 to 4 days) the critical care nurse should inform the patient and partner that walking, running, sex, and other activities will be possible and can be regained gradually through participation in a progressive cardiac rehabilitation program. Eighty percent of postcoronary patients can resume sexual relations 2 to 4 weeks after discharge (4 to 8 weeks after MI), as long as there is no history of complications (50% are uncomplicated) and if exercise can be tolerated to the extent of raising the heart rate to approximately 110 to 120 beats per minute (bpm) without precipitating angina or severe shortness of breath. Exercise tolerance can be ascertained by formal testing such as the use of a calibrated bicycle ergometer or a submaximal treadmill test.[40,84]

Although sexual intercourse is one of the most physically demanding exercises, conjugal sexual activity in middle-aged males (and females) with uncomplicated cardiac pathology invokes only modest physiological exertion with maximal cardiac stress lasting only 10 to 15 seconds. Sexual activity, including coitus and orgasm, can be compared in terms of oxygen consumption and work load of the heart to activities equal in energy expenditure. Activity progression is based on METs, a term used to describe the energy expenditure for many activities. A MET is a metabolic equivalent that can be assigned to activities regardless of a person's weight. One MET represents the energy expenditure of a person at rest and equals approximately 3.5 ml of oxygen per kilogram of body weight per minute.[2]

Most patients will need to perform three to four MET-level activities when they return home, and hospitals gear exercise programs toward that goal. Some of the activities that are considered comparable in oxygen consumption and energy expenditure to sexual activity, including coitus and orgasm, are as follows[2]:

1. Climbing two flights of stairs (20 steps in 10 seconds) without difficulty (this task is considered by experts to be the most standard test).
2. Taking a brisk walk (3 to 4 METS equal 4.8 km or 2½ mph).
3. Performing ordinary tasks in many occupations and recreations such as pushing a light power mower or pulling a light golf bag cart (Table 4-1).

Authorities[71,92,106] cite four danger signals that may indicate that sexual intercourse is causing physiological problems because of increased work load of the heart beyond the patient's endurance and should be ceased and a physician notified immediately: (1) dyspnea or increased heart rate that lasts longer than 5 minutes after intercourse, (2) extreme fatigue the day after intercourse, (3) insomnia after intercourse, and (4) chest pain during intercourse that is unrelieved by vasodilators, cessation, rest, and/or use of relaxation and breathing techniques.

Sexual activities such as hugging, kissing, and embracing should begin in the critical care unit to prepare for the more strenuous activity of sexual intercourse and to provide a more natural transition to sex for the patient and partner. Continuation of intimacy in illness also maintains healthy sensual relations between couples, which promotes overall wellness. Some patients may find it reassuring to attempt masturbation (3 to 4 METs) before intercourse for these same reasons.[58]

Patients also need information about the medications that act to decrease cardiac work load, because they may be prescribed by the physician for use before intercourse to prevent chest pain.[4,71]

It is also important for nurses to inform patients about medications that can alter or interfere with sexual function and performance. Sometimes simply adjusting the dose of some drugs can ameliorate the problem.

A commonly shared perception has been that during the sex act the partner with the heart disease should assume the dependent or "patient-on-bottom" position. However, experts have reported no significant difference in either heart rate or blood pressure when healthy men were studied while they engaged in sexual intercourse in either position.[84]

Patients with coronary artery disease who can perform a comparable level of activity without symptoms can safely resume sexual activity as long as they *avoid* sex in the following situations:

- After a heavy meal—food and/or drink disrupts cirulatory efficiency and diverts blood flow from the heart and great vessels to the gut.[29]
- For at least 3 hours after alcohol ingestion—alcohol, even in small amounts, decreases cardiac index and stroke index in patients with heart disease[70]; avoid heavy drinking.[29]
- Positions requiring isometric exertion—they are more apt to increase the heart rate or precipitate dysrhythmias.[71,114]
- Anal intercourse—this could cause vagal stimulation and bradycardia.
- Extreme room temperatures—extreme hot or cold can add stress on the heart.
- When fatigued or during an emotional outburst—rest is beneficial before intercourse; and work load on the heart is increased during extreme tiredness, and there is increased stress on the heart during a highly emotional state.[70]

### Patient with Severe Heart Disease

Physical activity in general does not tend to induce ventricular tachycardia in patients whose conditions are well-controlled; but for the patients with severe heart disease, possible heart failure is a problem, and symptoms of angina,

***Table 4-1*** Approximate metabolic cost of activities

| | Occupational | Recreational |
|---|---|---|
| 1½-2 METs* | Desk work | Standing |
| 4-7 ml $O_2$/min/kg | Auto driving† | Walking (strolling 1.6 km or 1 mile/hr) |
| 2-2½ kcal/min (70-kg person) | Typing | Flying,† motorcycling† |
| | Electric calculating machine operation | Playing cards† |
| | | Sewing, knitting |
| 2-3 METs | Auto repair | Level walking (3.2 km or 2 miles/hr) |
| 7-11 ml $O_2$/min/kg | Radio, television repair | Level bicycling (8.0 km or 5 miles/hr) |
| 2½-4 kcal/min (70-kg person) | Janitorial work | Riding lawn mower |
| | Typing, manual | Billiards, bowling |
| | Bartending | Skier,† shuffleboard |
| | | Woodworking (light) |
| | | Powerboat driving† |
| | | Golf (power cart) |
| | | Canoeing (4 km or 2½ miles/hr) |
| | | Horseback riding (walk) |
| 3-4 METs | Brick laying, plastering | Walking (4.8 km or 3 miles/hr) |
| 11-14 ml $O_2$/min/kg | Wheelbarrow (45.4 kg or 100-lb load) | Cycling (9.7 km or 6 miles/hr) |
| 4-5 kcal/min (70-kg person) | Machine assembly | Horseshoe pitching |
| | Trailer-truck in traffic | Volleyball (6-person, noncompetitive) |
| | Welding (moderate load) | Golf (pulling bag cart) |
| | Cleaning windows | Sailing (handling small boat) |
| | | Fly-fishing (standing with waders) |
| | | Horseback riding (sitting to trot) |
| | | Pushing light power mower |
| 4-5 METs | Painting, masonry | Walking (5.6 km or 3½ miles/hr) |
| 14-18 ml $O_2$/min/kg | Paperhanging | Cycling (12.9 km or 8 miles/hr) |
| 5-6 kcal/min (70-kg person) | Light carpentry | Table tennis |
| | | Golf (carrying clubs) |
| | | Dancing (foxtrot) |
| | | Badminton (singles) |
| | | Tennis (doubles) |

Modified from Fox SM, Naughton JP, and Gorman PA: Mod Concs Cardiovas Dis 41:6, 1972.
NOTE: Includes resting metabolic needs.
*MET is the energy expenditure at rest, equivalent to approximately 3.5 ml $O_2$/kg body weight/minute.
†A major excessive metabolic increase may occur because of excitement, anxiety, or impatience during some of these activities, and a physician must assess his or her patient's psychological reactivity.

fatigue, and dyspnea must be considered warning signals. For these patients it is difficult to allay the fear of an impending episode of ventricular tachycardia and possible death.[6]

Experts suggest more investigation into the effect of sexual intercourse in provoking episodes of ventricular tachycardia. Since reliable data do not exist for this category of patient, guarantee of safe sexual experience cannot be made.[70]

Loss of physical capacity is frequently perceived as a severe threat to self-esteem and concepts of masculinity or femininity (body image). Without appropriate counseling, the patient may well transfer these negative feelings to other areas of life such as work, recreation, and the parenting role. The nurse should be aware of the possibility of the patient's developing overwhelming anxiety or depression and should seek psychiatric consultation if necessary.[106]

### Patient with Chronic Lung Disease

Another commonly seen group of patients who may have sexual dysfunction as a result of activity intolerance and shortness of breath are patients with chronic lung disease, for example, chronic obstructive pulmonary disease (COPD), cancer of the lung, or bronchiectasis. Because of the advanced age of some of these patients, the nurse should review the medical history carefully for other possible causes of sexual dysfunction unrelated to the respiratory problem such as excessive alcohol intake, renal disease, hypertension, diabetes mellitus, or use of medications. The history may uncover long-standing sexual problems that existed before the chronic respiratory illness. Such variables would alter the focus of the approach to sexual counseling.[20]

Anxiety caused by the shortness of breath is the most common complaint of patients with respiratory disease. The fear is so great that all physical activity, including sex, is avoided, often resulting in a decreased desire for sex and subsequent feelings of worthlessness and isolation. The desire for intimacy and close contact is also diminished because of the coughing, sputum production, and foul mouth odor that accompany respiratory disease.[57]

Nurses can reduce their own anxiety by increasing their knowledge about respiratory disease and sexuality and by recognizing the importance of sexual expression regardless of age, illness, disability, and course of treatment.

## REFERENCES


1. Aguilera DG and Messick JM: Crisis intervention: theory and methodology, ed 6, St Louis, 1989, Mosby–Year Book, Inc.
2. American College of Sports Medicine: Guidelines for graded exercise testing and exercise prescription, ed 2, Philadelphia, 1980, Lea & Febiger.
3. Antonucci TC and Jackson JS: Physical health and self-esteem, Fam Commun Health 6(4):1, 1983.
4. Baggs J: Nursing diagnosis: potential sexual dysfunction after myocardial infarction, Dimens Crit Care Nurs 5(3):178, 1986.
5. Barrier D and others: Practice: a family assessment tool for family medicine. In Christie-Seely J, editor: Working with the family in primary care: a systems approach to health and illness, New York, 1984, Praeger.
6. Baxley KO and others: Alopecia: effect on cancer patient's body image, Cancer Nurs 7(6):499, 1984.
7. Beck AT and others: The measurement of pessimism: the hopelessness scale, J Couns Clin Psychol 42(6):861, 1974.
8. Bellak L, Leopold R, and Siegel H: Handbook of intensive, brief and emergency psychotherapy, Larchmont, NY, 1984, CPJ, Inc.
9. Benson H: The relaxation response. In Monat A and Lazarus RS, editors: Stress and coping: an anthology, ed 2, New York, 1985, Columbia University Press.
10. Bonham PA and Cheney AM: Concept of self: a framework for nursing assessment. In Chinn P, editor: Advances in nursing theory development, Rockville, Md, 1983, Aspen Systems Corp.
11. Boycoff SL: Strategies for sexual counselling of patients following a myocardial infarction, Dimens Crit Care Nurs 8(6):368, 1989.
12. Bronheim HE and others: Depression in the intensive care unit, Crit Care Med 13:985, 1985.
13. Brown MS: Distortions in body image in illness and disease, New York, 1977, John Wiley & Sons, Inc.
14. Brown MS: Normal development of body image, New York, 1977, John Wiley & Sons, Inc.
15. Brundage DJ and Broadwell DC: Altered body image. In Phipps WJ and others, editors: Medical-surgical nursing: concepts and clinical practice, ed 4, St Louis, 1990, Mosby–Year Book, Inc.
16. Campbell ML: Sexual dysfunction in the COPD patient, Dimens Crit Care Nurs 6(2):70, 1987.
17. Carpenito L: Nursing diagnoses: application to clinical practice, Philadelphia, 1989, JB Lippincott Co.
18. Cassels C, Eckstein A, and Fortinash K: Retirement: aspects, response, and nursing implications, J Gerontol Nurs 7(6):335, 1981.
19. Champion VL, Austin JK, and Tzeng O: Assessment of relationships between self-concept and body image using multivariate techniques, Issues Mental Health Nurs 4(4):299, 1982.
20. Cohelo A and others: Treadmill testing in patients with recurrent sustained ventricular tachycardia, Circulation 64:IV, 1981.
21. Combs AW and Snygg D: Individual behavior: a perceptual approach to behavior, New York, 1959, Harper & Row, Publisher.
22. Cooper D: Sexual counseling of the patient with chronic lung disease, Focus Crit Care 13(3):18, 1986.
23. Coopersmith S: The antecedents of self-esteem, San Francisco, 1967, WH Freeman & Co.
24. Cormack D: Geriatric nursing: a conceptual approach, Oxford, 1985, Blackwell Scientific Publications, Ltd.
25. Crouch MA and Straub B: Enhancement of self-esteem in adults, Fam Commun Health 6(4):65, 1983.
26. Dennis KE: Patients' control and the information imperative: clarification and confirmation, Nurs Res 39(3):162, 1990.
27. Driever MJ: Problems of low self-esteem. In Roy C, Sr, editor: Introduction to nursing: an adaptation model, Englewood Cliffs, NJ, 1976, Prentice-Hall, Inc.
28. Driever MJ: Theory of self-concept. In Roy C, Sr, editor: Introduction to nursing: an adaptation model, Englewood Cliffs, NJ, 1976, Prentice-Hall, Inc.
29. Ebersole P and Hess P: Toward healthy aging, human needs, and nursing response, ed 3, St Louis, 1989, Mosby–Year Book, Inc.
30. Eisendrath SJ: Psychological concepts in the care of intensive care unit patients, Int J Psychosomat 31:8, 1984.
31. Engel GL: A life setting conducive to illness: the giving up–given up syndrome, Ann Intern Med 69:293, 1968.
32. Fisher S: Body experience in fantasy and behavior, New York, 1970, Appleton-Century-Crofts.
33. Foa EB and Kozak MJ: Emotional processing of fear: exposure to corrective information, Psychol Bull 99:20, 1986.
34. Folkman S and Lazarus RS: Stress process and depressive symptomatology, J Abnorm Psychol 95:107, 1986.
35. Folkman S and others: Appraisal, coping, health status, and psychological symptoms, J Pers Soc Psychol 50:571, 1986.
36. Folkman S and others: Dynamics of a stressful encounter: cognitive appraisal coping and encounter outcomes, J Pers Soc Psychol 50:992, 1986.
37. French JRP, Jr and Raven BH: Bases of social power. In Cartwright D, editor: Studies in social power, Ann Arbor, Mich, 1959, University of Michigan Press.
38. Frenn M, Fehring R, and Kartes S: Reducing the stress of cardiac catheterization by teaching relaxation, Dimens Crit Care Nurs 5:108, 1986.
39. Gaglione KM: Assessing and intervening with families of CCU patients, Nurs Clin North Am 19:427, 1984.
40. Gould L and others: Cardiac effects of a cocktail, JAMA 218:1799, 1971.
41. Heller S and Kornfeld D: Psychiatric aspects of cardiac surgery, Adv Psychosom Med 15:124, 1986.
42. Hellerstein HK and Friedman EH: Sexual activity and the postcoronary patient, Arch Intern Med 125:987, 1970.
43. Higgins CA: The AICD: a teaching plan for patients and families, Critic Care Nurse 10(6):69, 1990.
44. Hirst SP and Metcalf BJ: Promoting self-esteem, J Gerontol Nurs 10(2):72, 1984.
45. Janis IL: Adaptive personality changes. In Monat A and Lazarus RS, editors: Stress and coping: an anthology, ed 2, New York, 1985, Columbia University Press.
46. Janis IL: Coping patterns among patients with life-threatening diseases. In Speilberger CD and Sarason I, editors: Stress and anxiety: a source book of theory and research, New York, 1986, Hemisphere Publishers.
47. Janis IL: Stress inoculation in health care: theory and research. In Monat A and Lazarus RS, editors: Stress and coping: an anthology, ed 2, New York, 1985, Columbia University Press.
48. Janis IL and Mann L: Decision-making: a psychological analysis of conflict, choice and commitment, New York, 1977, Free Press.
49. Janis IL and Rodin J: Attribution, control, and decision-making: social psychology and health care. In Stone GC and Adler NC, editors: Health psychology—a handbook, San Francisco, 1979, Jossey-Bass, Inc, Publishers.
50. Johnson BS: Psychiatric mental health nursing, adaptation and growth, Philadelphia, 1986, JB Lippincott Co.
51. Johnson SJ: Ten ways to help the family of a critically ill patient, Nursing 86 16:50, 1986.

52. Jones EE: Interpreting interpersonal behavior: the effects of expectancies, Science 234:41, 1986.
53. Kim MJ, McFarland GK, and McLane AM: Pocket guide to nursing diagnoses, ed 4, St Louis, 1990, Mosby–Year Book, Inc.
54. King KB: Psychological aspects of critical care, Heart Lung 14:579, 1985.
55. King SL and Gregor FM: Stress and coping in families of the critically ill, Crit Care Nurs 5:48, 1985.
56. Kolodny RC and others: Textbook of human sexuality for nurses, Boston, 1979, Little, Brown & Co.
57. Krajicek MJ: Developmental disability and human sexuality, Nurs Clin North Am 17:173, 1982.
58. Kravetz H: Sexual counseling for the patient with chronic lung disease, Sexual Medicine Today 17(3):377, 1981.
59. Lazarus RS: Psychological stress and the coping process, New York, 1966, McGraw-Hill Book Co.
60. Lazarus RS: The costs and benefits of denial. In Monat A and Lazarus RS, editors: Stress and coping: an anthology, ed 2, New York, 1985, Columbia University Press.
61. Lazarus RS and Folkman S: Coping and adaptation. In Gentry WD, editor: The handbook of behavioral medicine, New York, 1984, Guilford.
62. Lazarus RS and Folkman S: Stress, appraisal and coping, New York, 1984, Springer-Verlag New York, Inc.
63. Lazarus RS and others: Stress and adaptational outcomes: the problem of confounded measures, Am Psychol 40:770, 1985.
64. Lee JM: Emotional reactions to trauma, Nurs Clin North Am 5(4):577, 1970.
65. Leventhal H and Nerenz DR: A model for stress research with some implications for the control of stress disorder. In Meichenbaum D and Jaremko ME, editors: Stress reduction and prevention, New York, 1983, Plenum Publishing Corp.
66. Martinez C: Nursing assessment based on Roy adaptation model. II. Self-concept. In Roy C, Sr, editor: An introduction to nursing: an adaptation model, Englewood Cliffs, NJ, 1976, Prentice-Hall, Inc.
67. Maslow AH: Motivation and personality, New York, 1954, Harper & Row, Publisher.
68. Masters W and Johnson V: Human sexual response, Boston, 1966, Little, Brown & Co.
69. Masters W and Johnson V: Human sexual inadequacy, Boston, 1970, Little, Brown & Co.
70. Mayou R, Foster A, and Williamson B: Psychosocial adjustment in patients 1 year after myocardial infarction, J Psychosom Res 22:447, 1978.
71. McCauley K and others: Learning to live with controlled ventricular tachycardia: utilizing the Johnson Model, Heart Lung 13(6):633, 1984.
72. McCloskey JC: How to make the most of body image theory in nursing practice, Nurs 76 6(5):68, 1976.
73. McFarland GK and McCann J: Self-perception–self concept. In Thompson JM and others, editors: Mosby's manual of clinical nursing, ed 2, St Louis, 1989, Mosby–Year Book, Inc.
74. Meichenbaum D: Stress inoculation training, New York, 1985, Pergamon Press.
75. Meichenbaum D and Novaco R: Stress inoculation: a preventive approach. In Speilberger CD and Sarason I, editors: Stress and anxiety: a source book of theory and research, New York, 1986, Hemisphere Publishers.
76. Meisenhelder JB: Self-esteem: a closer look at clinical interventions, Int J Nurs Stud 22(2):127, 1985.
77. Meisenhelder JB: Self-esteem in women: the influence of employment and perception of husband's appraisals, Image: J Nurs Schol 18(1):8, 1986.
78. Meleis AI: Role insufficiency and role supplementation: a conceptual framework, Nurs Res 24(4):264, 1975.
79. Meleis AI: The evolving nursing scholarliness. In Chinn PL, editor: Advances in nursing theory development, Rockville, Md, 1983, Aspen Systems Corp.
80. Miller BK: Teaching biofeedback techniques in critical care, Dimens Crit Care Nurs 4:314, 1985.
81. Miller JF: Coping with chronic illness: overcoming powerlessness, Philadelphia, 1983, FA Davis Co.
82. Miller JF: Development and validation of a diagnostic label: powerlessness. In Kim MJ, McFarland GK, and McLane AM, editors: Classification of nursing diagnoses: proceedings of the fifth national conference, St Louis, 1984, Mosby–Year Book, Inc.
83. Monat A and Lazarus RS: Stress and coping: some current issues and controversies. In Monat A and Lazarus RS, editors: Stress and coping: an anthology, ed 2, New York, 1985, Columbia University Press.
84. Moore K, Folk-Lightly M, and Nolen MJ: The joy of sex after a heart attack, Nurs 77 7(6):52, 1977.
85. Moos RH and Schaefer JA: Life transitions and crises. In Moos RH and Schaefer JA, editors: Coping with life crises: an integrated approach, New York, 1986, Plenum Publishing Corp.
86. Moss RC: Overcoming fear: a review of research on patient, family instruction, AORN J 43:1107, 1986.
87. Murray RLE: Symposium on the concept of body image, Nurs Clin North Am 7(4):593, 1972.
88. Muslin HL: On acquiring a kidney, Am J Psychiatry 127:1185, 1971.
89. Nemec ED, Mansfield L, and Kenneley J: Heart rate and blood pressure responses during sexual activity in normal males, Am Heart J 92:274, 1976.
90. Norris CM: The professional nurse and body image. In Carlson C and Blackwell B, editors: Behavioral concepts and nursing intervention, ed 2, Philadelphia, 1978, JB Lippincott Co.
91. Norris J and Kunes-Connell M: Self-esteem disturbance, Nurs Clin North Am 20(4):745, 1985.
92. O'Shea MD: An evaluation of a marriage enrichment and relationship skills training program (ME-RSTP) for couples coping with heart disease, doctoral dissertation, Atlanta, 1984, Georgia State University.
93. Owen PM and Harrison JW: Brief psychotherapy after survival from cardiac arrest, Heart Lung 14:18, 1985.
94. Panzarine S: Coping: conceptual and methodological issues, Adv Nurs Sci 7:49, 1985.
95. Pearlmutter DR and others: Models of family centered care in one acute care institution, Nurs Clin North Am 19:173, 1984.
96. Phipps WJ and others: Medical-surgical nursing: concepts and clinical practice, ed 4, St Louis, 1990, Mosby–Year Book, Inc.
97. Price SA and Wilson LM: Pathophysiology, ed 3, New York, 1986, McGraw-Hill Book Co.
98. Puksta NS: All about sex . . . after a coronary, Am J Nurs 77:602, 1977.
99. Quinless F: Assessing the client with acute cardiovascular dysfunction, Top Clin Nurs 8:45, 1986.
100. Roberst SL: Piaget's theory reapplied to the critically ill, Adv Nurs Sci 2:61, 1980.
101. Roberts SL: Behavioral concepts and the critically ill patient, ed 2, Norwalk, Conn, 1986, Appleton-Century-Crofts.
102. Rodin J: Aging and health: effects of the sense of control, Science 233:1271, 1986.
103. Rogers CR: Client-centered therapy: its current practice, implications, and theory, Boston, 1951, Houghton-Mifflin Co.
104. Rotter JB: Generalized expectancies for internal versus external control of reinforcement, Psychol Monogr 80(1):1, 1966.
105. Rubin R: Body image and self-esteem, Nurs Outlook 16:20, 1968.
106. Runions J: A program for psychological and social enhancement during rehabilitation after myocardial infarction, Heart Lung 14(2):117, 1985.
107. Salkin J: Body ego technique, Springfield, Ill, 1973, Charles C Thomas, Publisher.

108. Scalzi C, Burke L, and Greenland S: Evaluation of an inpatient educational program for coronary patients, Heart Lung 9:46, 1980.
109. Seligman ME: Helplessness: on depression, development and death, San Francisco, 1975, WH Freeman & Co.
110. Shine KI: Anxiety in patients with heart disease, Psychosomatics 25:27, 1984.
111. Silverman JJ and others: Surgical staff recognition of psychopathology in trauma patients, J Trauma 25:544, 1985.
112. Slaby AE and Glicksman AS: Adapting to life-threatening illness, New York, 1985, Praeger Publishers.
113. Stanwyck DJ: Self-esteem through the life span, Fam Commun Health 6(4):11, 1983.
114. Stein RA: The effect of exercise training on heart rate during coitus in the post-myocardial infarction patient, Circulation 55:738, 1977.
115. Sullivan HS: Conceptions of modern psychiatry, Washington, DC, 1946, William A White Psychiatric Foundation.
116. Sullivan HS: The interpersonal theory of psychiatry, New York, 1953, WW Norton & Co, Inc.
117. Sulman JY and Verhaeghe N: Myocardial infarction patients in the acute care hospital: a conceptual framework for social work intervention, Soc Work Health Care 11:1, 1986.
118. Thoits PA: Social support as coping assistance, J Consult Clin Psychol 54:416, 1986.
119. Thomas SA: Reducing loneliness in critical care, Dimens Crit Care Nurs 5:68, 1986.
120. Ueno M: The so-called coition death, Jpn J Legal Med 17:333, 1952.
121. Volden C and others: The relationship of age, gender and exercise practices to measures of health, lifestyle and self-esteem, Appl Nurs Res 3(1):20, 1990.
122. Watts RJ: Dimensions of sexual health, Am J Nurs 79:1572, 1979.
123. Webster's new world dictionary of the American language, Cleveland, 1966, The World Publishing Co.
124. Weisman AD: The coping capacity: on the nature of being mortal, New York, 1984, Human Sciences Press.
125. Wilson-Barnett J: Interventions to alleviate patients' stress: a review, J Psychosom Res 28:63, 1984.
126. Wishnie MA, Hackett TP, and Cassem N: Psychological hazards of convalescence following myocardial infarction, JAMA 215:1291, 1971.
127. Wolff PH and Colletti MA: AIDS: getting past the diagnosis and on to discharge planning, Crit Care Nurs 6(4):76, 1986.
128. Wong N: Psychological aspects of physical illness, Bull Menninger Clin 48:273, 1984.
129. World Health Organization: Education and treatment in human sexuality: the training of health professionals, Tech Rep 572, Geneva, 1975, The Organization.
130. Zalar MK: Role preparation for nurses in home sexual functioning, Nurs Clin North Am 17(3):152, 1982.

CHAPTER 5

# Sleep Alterations

## CHAPTER OBJECTIVES

- *State the stages of sleep.*
- *Explain three physiological effects that occur during rapid eye movement (REM) sleep.*
- *Describe desynchronized sleep and its primary effects.*
- *Describe the changes in sleep resulting from the aging process.*
- *State the two major methods that accurately measure sleep.*
- *Define dysfunctional sleep.*
- *Define circadian desynchronization.*
- *Name three commonly prescribed critical care medications that decrease REM sleep.*
- *Describe common symptoms of sleep deprivation.*
- *Identify four interventions for sleep pattern disturbance related to fragmented sleep.*
- *Name two interventions for sleep pattern disturbance related to circadian desynchronization.*



William Shakespeare early recognized the therapeutic value of sleep: "O sleep, o gentle sleep, nature's soft nurse!" Patients admitted to critical care units, because their critical illnesses require frequent treatments and 24-hour intensive monitoring, will probably suffer an alteration in sleep pattern. Henderson[20] described the inability to rest and sleep as "one of the causes, as well as one of the accompaniments of disease." Bahr[2] stated, "The phenomenon of sleep has the potential for relieving an individual of stress and responsibility when a break is needed to recharge the person's spirit, mind and body; or, it can remain maddeningly aloof when it is needed most." A lack of sleep can have disastrous results for the critically ill patient. The critical care nurse can promote recovery and healing through facilitating sleep for patients. To do this, the nurse must understand the physiology of normal sleep and recognize events that can potentially disrupt sleep in the critical care environment. The purpose of this chapter is to familiarize the reader with the phenomenon of sleep and the types of sleep pattern disturbances that may occur in critical care and to describe the assessment of **sleep pattern disturbance** in critically ill patients.

## PHYSIOLOGY OF SLEEP

Sleep has been defined as "a state of unconsciousness from which a person can be aroused by appropriate sensory or other stimuli."[15] Adults normally spend approximately one third of their lives asleep. Research involving the simultaneous monitoring of the **electroencephalogram** (EEG), **electrooculogram** (EOG), and **electromyogram** (EMG) has shown that there are two distinct stages of sleep: *REM (rapid eye movement) and NREM (non–rapid eye movement).*[14]

### NREM Sleep

**NREM sleep** is divided into four stages (NREM 1 through 4), which are associated with progressive relaxation. NREM stage 1 is a transitional stage, with the EEG being similar to that seen in the awake state. See Figs. 5-1 and 5-2 for a comparison of EEG patterns of subjects that were either awake or asleep. Stage 1 is the lightest level of sleep, lasting

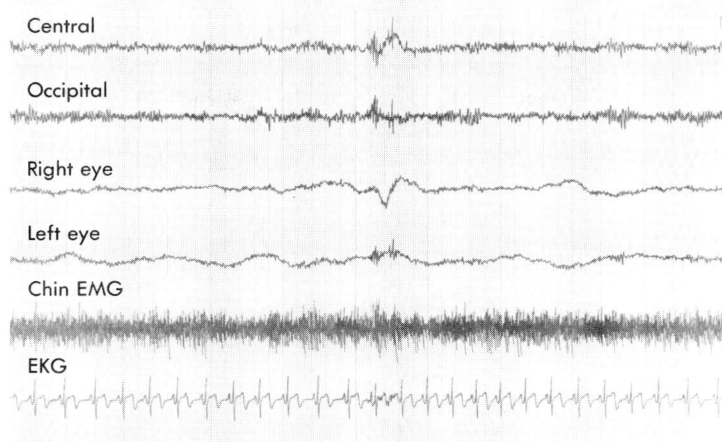


***Fig. 5-1*** Awake.

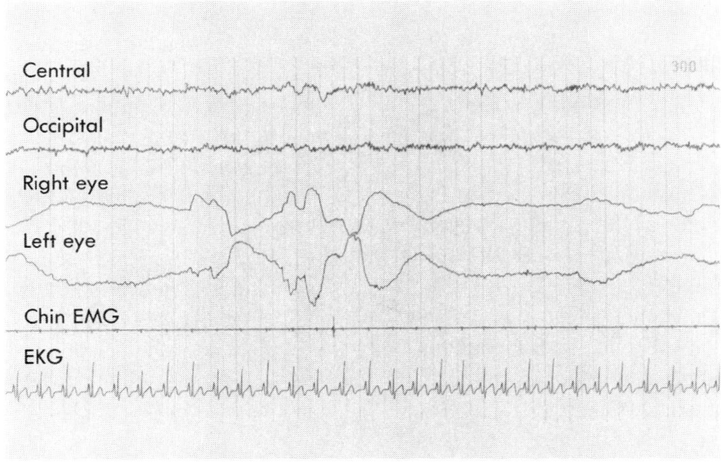


***Fig. 5-2*** REM sleep.

only 1 to 2 minutes. This stage is characterized by aimless thoughts, a feeling of drifting, and frequently, myoclonic jerks of the face, hands, and feet. The individual is easily awakened during this stage.[15]

NREM stage 2 differs from stage 1 in that the background wave frequency on the EEG is slower with *sleep spindles* (characteristic waveforms) superimposed and high voltage spikes known as K-complexes. This stage lasts from 5 to 15 minutes, during which time the individual becomes more relaxed but is still easily awakened. Stages 1 and 2 in the average young adult constitute 50% to 60% of the total sleep time.[2]

Stages 3 and 4 are characterized by large, slow-frequency delta waves on the EEG and are primarily differentiated by the relative percentage of these waves.[5] Random stimuli do not arouse the individual from these deepest levels of sleep. The length of time spent in stages 3 and 4 varies from 15 to 30 minutes and constitutes approximately 20% of the total sleep time. During NREM sleep, the EOG gradually slows and eye movements cease. The EMG also declines, indicating profound muscle relaxation; however, it does not reach the low levels that it does in REM sleep.[46] The parasympathetic nervous system predominates during NREM sleep. The cardiac and respiratory rates, the metabolic rate, and the blood pressure decrease to basal levels. Thus the supply/demand ratio of coronary blood flow is likely to improve.[19]

In addition, during slow wave sleep, growth hormone (GH) is secreted by the anterior pituitary and functions to promote protein synthesis while sparing catabolic breakdown. Elevated GH and other anabolic hormones, such as prolactin and testosterone, imply that anabolism is taking place during NREM stage 4, particularly in tissues with a high protein content. Thus activities associated with NREM stage 4 include protein synthesis and tissue repair, such as the repair of epithelial and specialized cells of the brain. NREM dreams are often realistic and thoughtlike, rarely in color, and often similar to a recent activity. These dreams are generally more difficult to remember than REM dreams.[48] NREM sleep, then, is a time of energy conservation.

### REM Sleep

**REM,** or *paradoxical,* **sleep** constitutes 20% to 25% of the total sleep time in the young adult.[46] This type of sleep is paradoxical in that some areas of the brain are quite active during REM sleep, while other areas are suppressed. During REM sleep, there are bursts of eye movements seen on the EOG that are often associated with periods of dreaming. The EMG becomes essentially flat, indicating immobility and functional paralysis of the skeletal muscles. The cerebral cortical activity increases during REM so that the EEG resembles one taken during the waking state[14] (see Fig. 5-2). During REM sleep, the individual is more difficult to awaken than in any other stage of sleep.[46] In this regard, REM sleep can be thought of as a "dissociative state."

The sympathetic nervous system predominates during REM sleep. Oxygen consumption increases, and cardiac output, blood pressure, heart rate, and respiratory rate may become erratic.[45] An increase in premature ventricular contractions (PVCs) and tachydysrhythmias associated with respiratory pauses may occur during REM sleep.[48] Serum cholesterol and antidiuretic hormone levels increase, and perfusion to the gray matter in the brain doubles.[5] The dreams of REM sleep tend to be colorful, vivid, and implausible, often containing an element of paralysis.[44] REM sleep filters information stored from the day's activities, sifting the important from the trivial, helping to psychologically integrate activities such as problem solving.[46] REM sleep seems to facilitate emotional adaptation to the physical and psychological environment and is needed in large quantities after periods of stress or learning.[47] The adequacy of sleep is judged by the relative periods of time spent in each of the stages of sleep.[5]

REM sleep, like the other stages of sleep, is essential to physiological and psychological well-being. REM sleep is of great importance to nurses because as the patient is entering this stage of sleep, the nurse may notice a change in vital signs and become concerned that the patient's condition is worsening. If the nurse increases the monitoring of the patient, adjusts drips, and measures vital signs in response to this perceived change in condition, she or he may awaken the patient. Thus the patient may not get the REM sleep he or she needs. Further research must address the ways in which the nurse can assess sleep and all of its stages without unnecessarily disrupting the patient from the much needed REM sleep. An accurate knowledge of sleep will assist nurses in monitoring patients safely.

### Cyclic Aspects

At the onset of sleep, the individual normally progresses through repetitive cycles beginning with NREM stages 1 through 4 and then back again to stage 2. From stage 2, the individual enters REM. Stage 2 is then reentered, and the cycle repeats (Fig. 5-3). These cycles occur at approximately 90-minute intervals, so that four to five cycles are normally completed in the sleep period. Early in the sleep period, NREM predominates. During the end of the sleep period, REM periods tend to be of longer duration than those of NREM sleep.[5]

The rhythmic nature of sleep is not unique. The body experiences rhythms in temperature, blood pressure, heart rate, respiratory rate, and hormone secretion. This cyclic 24-hour rhythm has been termed the circadian rhythm. Sleep normally occupies the low phase of the circadian rhythm, while wakefulness and activity normally occupy the higher phase.[47]

The cyclic nature of sleep and wakefulness is thought to be regulated by neurotransmitters. Excitation of an area in the pons called the locus ceruleus stimulates neurons to secrete norepinephrine, a major neurotransmitter of the sympathetic nervous system. Norepinephrine along with dopamine and epinephrine are believed to play a role in the waking process. Excitation of the raphe nuclei in the pons and the medulla leads to natural sleep. These cells secrete serotonin, a neurotransmitter that is therefore thought to be associated with the inducement of sleep.[15]

In addition to their role in the sleep-wake cycle, the catecholamine neurotransmitters are postulated to play a role in the cycles of REM and NREM sleep. Norepinephrine and dopamine secreted by the locus ceruleus and dorsal

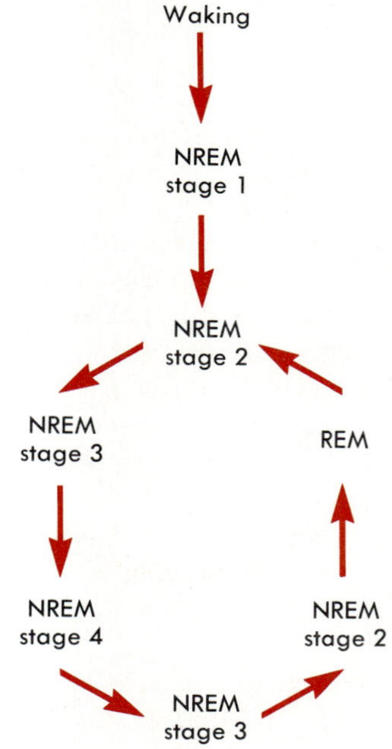


*Fig. 5-3* The cyclic nature of sleep.

raphe nuclei of the brainstem fire more slowly during REM sleep ("REM off" cells). In contrast, the major neurotransmitter of the parasympathetic nervous system, acetylcholine (ACh), is secreted more rapidly from the gigantocellular tegmental field (FTG) in the reticular formation during the initiation of REM ("REM on" cells). A negative feedback mechanism is theorized to be responsible for REM-NREM cycling in sleep. Thus both of the major neurotransmitters of the autonomic nervous system are hypothesized to play important roles in the cyclical regulation of sleep, including both the sleep-wake cycle and REM-NREM cycles.[31]

It is interesting to note that the neurotransmitters dopamine and serotonin are major determinants of mood and affect. The changes in mood and affect in persons with sleep deprivation and desynchronization may partially be explained by the functioning of these transmitters. It is also interesting to note in light of the major role of neurotransmitters in sleep that sleep disorders are frequently seen in psychiatric illness; that is, early morning awakenings are classically found with major depressive disorders that are thought to be biochemically induced.

The sleep-wake cycle follows the circadian rhythm in a 24-hour cycle synchronized with other biological rhythms.[5] Nighttime sleep is the normal pattern for most adults. To prepare the body for sleep, serotonin is cyclically released at around 8 PM. Conversely, adrenocorticotrophic hormone (ACTH), corticotropin-releasing hormone (CRH), and cortisol all normally peak in the early morning hours to prepare the individual for the day's stresses. If a person is deprived of sleep, especially the deeper stages, these hormones will still be released, but at times that may or may not coordinate approximately with the stresses he or she is about to face. Thus an abnormal sleep pattern will compromise the patient's ability to cope with the stress of critical illness, thereby possibly complicating his or her recovery.[45] When sleep occurs during the low phase of the circadian rhythm, circadian synchronization is present. Sleep that occurs during normal waking hours is out of phase or desynchronized (Fig. 5-4). Desynchronized sleep is rated as poor-quality sleep and causes a decreased arousal threshold; therefore frequent awakenings are more likely. Irritability, restlessness, depression, anxiety, and decreased accuracy in task performance are characteristic effects of desynchronized sleep.[48] Resynchronization with the circadian rhythm must occur whenever sleep has become desynchronized for the individual to establish a normal sleep-activity pattern. Although variable among individuals, the resynchronization process is thought to require a minimum of 3 days with a consistent sleep-wake schedule. During resynchronization, the individual often feels fatigued and unable to perform all of his or her activities of daily living.[48]

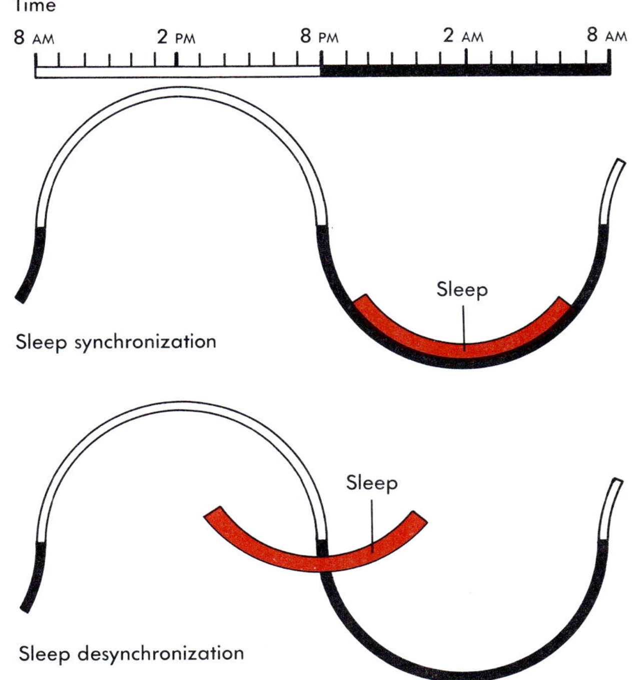


***Fig. 5-4*** Sleep synchronization and desynchronization with circadian rhythm.

## SLEEP CHANGES WITH AGE

Of the factors that influence the quality of sleep, age is one of the most prominent. The sleep of a normal infant is divided into two types. The first is characterized by no eye or body movements and regular respirations. The second type is associated with eye and body movements and a predominant suck reflex. The first type of sleep develops into NREM sleep and the latter into REM sleep. The infant, unlike the adult, goes from wakefulness directly into REM sleep. By approximately 3 months of age, the full-term infant develops the normal adult pattern of falling from wakefulness into NREM sleep.[8] Infants spend a relatively large proportion of their sleep time in REM sleep. For the full-term newborn this percentage is approximately 40% to 50% of total sleep time.[42]

As the biological systems change during the normal aging process, stress is placed on the human system, and the delicate mechanism of sleep is altered.[26] Hayter,[17] in a study of 212 healthy, noninstitutionalized older adults aged 65 to 93, found extreme variability in the sleep behaviors of different subjects within age-groups. Sleep behaviors between men and women had few differences, though women did report more difficulty getting to sleep and more frequent use of sleep aids than did men. The number of daytime naps and nighttime awakenings and variability in sleep behaviors increased with age. By age 75, the number of naps and length of naptime increased, resulting in a gradual increase in the total sleep time. Therefore both the time needed to fall asleep and the amount of time spent in bed increased with age.

The number of awakenings increases significantly, from one or two to as many as six per night; thus the elderly experience an increase in the total duration of NREM stage

1 sleep and an increase in the number of shifts into stage 1. The duration of stage 2 sleep changes very little; however, awakenings from stage 2 sleep become more frequent. NREM stage 3 tends to be normal. The duration of NREM stage 4, however, declines rapidly so that by age 50 it is reduced by 50%. Little or no stage 4 sleep may be found in 25% of the population in the sixth decade of life.[50] Stage 4 sleep is virtually absent in old age, and the proportion of REM begins to decline in relation to total sleep time.[35] The circadian rhythm in the elderly appears to shift to the earlier part of the night so that distribution of REM sleep throughout the night is unusually uniform.[2] These changes, along with more fragmentation and frequent long periods of wakefulness at night, cause the elderly to perceive an impairment in their quality of sleep.

Advanced age involves losses: of functional capabilities, friends, spouse, and material belongings.[8] Because these losses can lead to depression, a state that is relatively common in the older population, the relationship between depression and sleep disturbance is important for the nurse to consider when working with the elderly. These losses, by disrupting the psychological state of the elderly patient, may also compound existing sleep difficulties.

## SLEEP CHANGES WITH CHRONIC ILLNESS

Chronic illnesses, common in the elderly, tend to increase the frequency and severity of sleep disorders. Illnesses that commonly affect sleep are arthritis, angina pectoris, chronic obstructive pulmonary disease (COPD), congestive heart failure, diabetes mellitus, peptic ulcers, alcoholism, parkinsonism, thyroid disorders, altered sensory perceptions, and depression. Both situational stress and long-term anxiety are causes of disrupted and restless sleep.[46]

## ASSESSMENT OF SLEEP PATTERN DISTURBANCE

Assessment of the patient on admission to the critical care unit should include a description of the normal sleep pattern, including awakenings, naps, normal bedtime and waking time, and customary habits that enhance sleep (for example, number of pillows, extra blankets, bedtime rituals, and medications); any recent changes in the patient's normal pattern resulting from the acute illness; recent and past history of sleep disturbances; the severity, duration, and frequency of the problem; and history of chronic illnesses and physical conditions that may disturb sleep, such as COPD, bronchial asthma, bronchitis, arthritis, nocturnal angina, hyperthyroidism, hypertension, duodenal ulcer, or reflux esophagitis and nocturia. The patient's response to the critical care environment should be assessed, along with the noise level in the patient's immediate environment. The critical care nurse should elicit history of snoring because of its relationship to sleep apnea and sleep disturbances. One effective way to assess the quality of the patient's sleep is for the nurse to ask how his or her sleep in the hospital compares to sleep at home. Because of the extreme variations in sleep behaviors, individual differences must be recognized, and a flexible, individualized plan of care formulated to promote rest and sleep. Sleep, like pain, is a multidimensional process with considerable individual variations making the assessment of sleep a difficult process. For this reason, both qualitative and physiological indices are needed to measure sleep.[13] The scientific standard for the measurement of sleep is the polysomnogram (PSG). While the PSG is considered a medical diagnostic and research tool, the nurse can employ it to validate the results of observational and perceptual tools used to measure sleep. In normal healthy individuals, a high correlation exists between the person's subjective assessment of sleep recorded on a sleep log or questionnaire and PSG data.[1] However, in hospitalized persons this correlation does not always exist.[23]

Another problem in the measurement of sleep is that nurses' observations of patients' sleep have demonstrated both overestimation and underestimation of sleep when compared to PSG recordings. When a tool with specific sleep criteria was used, however, the amount of time a patient actually spent awake during the night (a measure of sleep efficiency) was valid when compared to PSG data.[13]

Sleep efficiency is an important sleep variable—it is defined as the proportion of actual sleep time in the total sleep period. Usual adult sleep efficiency is 95% of actual sleep time, whereas in multisystem trauma patients in the critical care area, it may be as low as 65%.[13]

For patients most at risk for a sleep pattern disturbance (for example, patients with invasive monitoring, those requiring hourly or more frequent assessments and interventions, patients whose illness will require an extended stay in critical care, or patients exhibiting initial signs of sleep deprivation), the nurse's keeping a sleep chart for 48 to 72 hours may assist in assessing actual quantity of sleep in addition to assessing necessary and unnecessary wakenings. The sleep chart should include the date and time, whether the patient was awake or asleep, and any procedures for which it was necessary to awaken the patient. A 24-hour flow sheet such as is common in critical care units could have an area for documentation of sleep. Just as nurses document other data relevant to the patient's recovery, sleep periods of more than 90 minutes in duration and total sleep time should be recorded and evaluated. Refer to the box below for the nursing management of sleep alterations.

**Nursing Diagnoses and Management**

***Sleep alterations***

Sleep pattern disturbance related to fragmented sleep and/or circadian desynchronization, p. 455

### Dysfunctional Sleep

In the acutely ill patient, the amount, quality, and consistency of sleep may all decrease. Total sleep deprivation rarely occurs outside the experimental setting; however, in the critical care unit sleep is often interrupted or fragmented, which alters the normal stages and cycles and produces dysfunctional sleep. With frequent interruptions in sleep, the patient spends a larger proportion of time in the transitional stages (that is, NREM stages 1 and 2) and less time in the deeper stages of sleep (NREM stages 3 and 4 and REM). Thus patients may suffer a decrease in total sleep time (TST) if they do not receive their usual amount of sleep, and they may also experience selective deprivation of the deeper stages of sleep.[45]

### Circadian Desynchronization

**Circadian desynchronization** or disruption is another form of sleep pattern disturbance that may affect critically ill patients. The loss of rhythmicity may result from external stressors, which then alters the timing relationships of neural, hormonal, and cellular systems. Animals and humans respond to stressors such as surgery, immobilization, and pain with increased levels and altered timing of adrenal and other hormones.[12] Farr[12] reported that circadian levels; the timing of temperature, blood pressure, and heart rate; and urinary excretion of catecholamines, sodium, and potassium were altered following surgery in hospitalized patients. Nurses should closely observe patients for signs and symptoms of such alterations and anticipate problems such as poor responses to physiological challenges, disruption of sleep, gastrointestinal disturbances, decreased vigilance and attention span, and malaise. Nursing interventions that maintain normal rhythmicity of the day-night cycle, such as opening window blinds, placing clocks and calendars within the patient's view, and allowing the patient to retire and rise at familiar times should be encouraged. Attention should be given to minimizing disruption during rest periods.[32]

## PHARMACOLOGY AND SLEEP

Patients hospitalized in critical care units often receive pharmacological therapy, which may affect their quality of sleep and compound sleep disturbances. The critical care nurse should be aware of the effects that commonly used

***Table 5-1*** Common drugs that affect sleep

| Drug | Effect on sleep | Comments |
|---|---|---|
| **BARBITURATES** | | |
| Amobarbital<br>Pentobarbital<br>Secobarbital | Increase NREM 2<br>Suppress REM | Not considered drugs of choice because of toxicity and long-lasting effects.<br>Often patients experience rebound insomnia, restless sleep, and frequent dreaming and nightmares when drugs are discontinued. |
| Phenobarbital | Facilitates NREM 4<br>Decreases REM in doses greater than 200 mg | REM rebound (increased REM in subsequent sleep) after withdrawal of phenobarbital. |
| **BENZODIAZEPINES** | | |
| Diazepam | Increases NREM 1<br>Decreases NREM 3 and 4<br>Decreases REM | NREM suppression is not dose related.<br>REM suppression is dose related.<br>May increase sleep apneic episodes. |
| Flurazepam | Increases total sleep time<br>Decreases NREM 2, 3, and 4<br>Decreases REM | Conflicting reports about effects on sleep.<br>Long half-life may produce daytime drowsiness. |
| Midazolam hydrochloride | No reports available as yet | |
| Triazolam | Decreases sleep latency (time it takes to get to sleep)<br>Decreases awakenings<br>Increases total sleep time | Drug has a short half-life.<br>Should not be used for a prolonged time because of decreased effectiveness. |
| **MISCELLANEOUS** | | |
| Chloral hydrate | Thought to be an effective sedative that does not disrupt sleep | Drug has a short half-life, and some reports of nightmares.<br>Increased daytime drowsiness. |
| Chlordiazepoxide<br>Methaqualone | Minimally disrupt sleep | |
| Morphine sulfate | Decreases NREM 3 and 4<br>Decreases REM | Results in increased spontaneous arousals and overall lighter sleep. |

drugs have on sleep. In fact, hypnotic drugs have been found to promote the lighter stages of sleep (that is, NREM stage 2) and may, paradoxically, be the cause of night terrors, hallucinations, and agitation in the elderly.[5] This is an area that has great potential for nursing research.

Barbiturates and sedative-hypnotic and analgesic medications may compound sleep disorders by further decreasing NREM stages 3 and 4 and REM sleep. Amobarbital, secobarbital, and pentobarbital reduce REM and increase NREM stage 2 sleep. Phenobarbital facilitates stage 4 NREM but decreases REM in doses greater than 200 mg. *REM rebound* (discussed later in this chapter) has been documented after the patient is withdrawn from phenobarbital therapy.[45]

Diazepam increases NREM stage 1 and reduces both NREM stages 3 and 4 and REM. REM suppression depends on the dose, with the larger doses leading to greater suppression. Flurazepam hydrochloride may be an effective hypnotic if administered in dosages equaling less than 60 mg/day. However, the long half-life of flurazepam may lead to morning drowsiness and may increase sleep apneic episodes in susceptible persons. Chloral hydrate has been shown to be an effective sedative that does not simultaneously disrupt sleep. Chlordiazepoxide and methaqualone also minimally disrupt sleep. Triazolam is effective for short-term use in increasing the total sleep time and decreasing the number of nocturnal awakenings, although it decreases REM sleep during the first 6 hours of sleep. These REM changes have been predominantly noted in young adults. An early morning "hangover" may occur with triazolam, and rebound insomnia may occur in the first 2 nights following discontinuation of the drug.[6] Morphine increases spontaneous arousals during sleep and shortens the sleep time by reducing both REM and NREM stages 3 and 4, resulting in overall lighter sleep.[50]

The prolonged half-life of medications, coupled with altered metabolism or decreased excretion of the drug resulting from renal or liver disease that may occur in the elderly, can cause the effects of sedatives to continue into the daytime, leading to confusion and sluggishness. Sedative and analgesic medications should not be withheld, but rather, drugs that minimally disrupt sleep should be used to complement comfort measures with dosages reduced gradually as the medication is no longer necessary. It is the responsibility of the critical care nurse to assess the need for sedative and analgesic medication, to administer them in the most effective manner to promote sleep, and to monitor their effectiveness (Table 5-1).

## SLEEP DEPRIVATION

Much of what is known about the function of sleep has been learned from observations made when people are deprived of sleep in the laboratory setting. Both physiological and psychological symptoms of sleep deprivation have been reported.[6] (See the box above.) These symptoms may be, but are not always, associated with the length of sleep deprivation. The symptoms vary among individuals with such factors as age, premorbid personality, motivation, and environmental factors.[14]

**Selective REM deprivation** leads to irritability, apathy, decreased alertness, and increased sensitivity to pain. Continued loss of REM sleep may lead to perceptual distortion and significant disturbance in mental-emotional function, often within 72 hours of REM deprivation. Manifestations of sleep deprivation range from disorientation and restlessness to frank auditory and visual hallucinations, with personality changes including withdrawal and paranoia.[14]

**Selective NREM deprivation** is less well studied, but it appears that fatigue is the primary result of NREM deprivation.[50] Because of the renewal, repair, and conservation functions of NREM sleep, deprivation impairs the immune system and depresses the body's defenses, rendering the individual vulnerable to disease.[46]

The critical care environment affects both the quantity and quality of sleep the critically ill patient receives. The patient admitted to a critical care unit is bombarded with combined sensory overload and deprivation and unfamiliar sights, sounds, people, and perceptions. Such environmental conditions have been shown to be of primary importance in sleep deprivation in the critical care unit. Dlin, Rosen, and Dickstein[9] showed the chief deterrents to sleep in the critical care unit in order of importance were activity and noise, pain and physical condition, nursing procedures, lights, vapor tents, and hypothermia. Woods and Falk[49] found that 10% to 17% of noises in the critical care unit were of a level capable of arousing patients from sleep (greater than 70 decibels).

Using EEGs, Hilton[21] documented quantity and quality of sleep of nine patients in a respiratory critical care unit. Total sleep time ranged from 6 minutes to 13.3 hours. Only 50% to 60% of the sleep occurred at night, and no patients had complete sleep cycles. NREM stage 1 sleep predominated, to the deprivation of all other stages. Significant deprivation of restorative sleep (NREM stages 3 and 4) was demonstrated by only 4.7% to 10.5% of sleep time being

### EFFECTS OF SELECTIVE SLEEP DEPRIVATION

**SYMPTOMS OF NREM SLEEP DEPRIVATION**

Fatigue
Anxiety
Increased illness

**SYMPTOMS OF REM SLEEP DEPRIVATION**

Restlessness
Disorientation
Combativeness
Delusions
Hallucinations

spent in these stages (normally 30% to 35%). Sleep-disturbing events validated by EEG were mainly staff and environmental noise, which occurred on the average of every 20 minutes. Quality and quantity of sleep were reported as poor in all subjects. Nightmares, hallucinations, restlessness, or other behavioral changes were observed in 60% of the patients in the sample.

Psychological stresses and fear associated with the critical care environment and critical illness make it difficult for patients to relax and fall asleep. Fear and stress precipitate sympathetic nervous system stimulation, which decreases the arousal threshold and results in frequent awakenings and sleep stage transitions.[45]

The relationship between sleep deprivation and delirium in the critical care unit has been shown to be significant.[10] In a study of 62 patients in critical care units and surgical critical care units who ranged in age from 16 to 70 years, Helton, Gordon, and Nunnery[18] correlated mental status alterations (disorientation, combativeness, hallucinations, paranoia, and delusions) and sleep deprivation. A 33% increase in mental status alterations was found in severely sleep-deprived patients, defined as those who received less than 50% of their normal sleep time.

Mortality is higher in critical care patients who exhibit symptoms of psychosis or delirium.[33] Perhaps persons experiencing hallucinations and paranoia (the most severe consequences of sleep deprivation) are in fact dreaming in the awake state. This hypothesis remains to be verified by research; however, caution needs to be taken in diagnosing a previously nonconfused elderly patient as having organic mental disorder (OMD) until the possibility of sleep deprivation has been ruled out.

"There is substantial evidence to support the fact that 4 days of sleep deprivation results in a decreased production of ATP, the critical energy substance. Sleep returns this balance to normal."[11] An understanding of the stages of sleep and the effects of sleep deprivation assists the nurse in evaluating the quantity and quality of sleep her or his patients receive.

## RECOVERY SLEEP

When an individual is sleep deprived, the changes in physiological and psychological performance can be reversed through **recovery sleep.** Rosa, Bonnet, and Warm[43] found that recall returned to baseline with 4 to 8 hours of recovery sleep after 40 to 64 hours of total sleep deprivation.

Deprivation of REM and NREM stage 4 results in rebounds in an attempt to compensate for "debts." The phenomenon of *REM rebound* occurs following selective REM deprivation. In an attempt to make up for lost REM and NREM stage 4 sleep, REM and NREM stage 4 periods quantitatively increase in the sleep periods following the deprivation. NREM stage 4 sleep is preferentially restored first, presumably because of its anabolic function. Because REM sleep is replenished last, it is more likely that REM debts will occur. REM rebound can exacerbate angina, dysrhythmias, duodenal ulcer pain, or sleep apneic episodes.[45] When a patient is exhibiting any of these symptoms and has had a period of sleep deprivation, REM rebound should be considered when determining the cause. Although the symptoms of angina, dysrhythmias, duodenal ulcer pain, and sleep apnea are treated as usual, further REM deprivation should be avoided.

### REFERENCES


1. Baekeland F and Hoy P: Reported vs. recorded sleep characteristics, Arch Gen Psychiatry 24:548, 1971.
2. Bahr R: Sleep-wake patterns in the aged, J Gerontol Nurs 9(10):534, 1983.
3. Berman TM and others: Sleep disorders: take them seriously, Patient Care 23(11):85, 1990.
4. Beyerman K: Etiologies of sleep pattern disturbance in hospitalized patients. In Classification of Nursing Diagnoses: Proceedings of the Seventh Conference, St Louis, 1987, Mosby–Year Book, Inc.
5. Biddle C and others: The nature of sleep, J Am Assoc Nurse Anesthetists 58(1):36, 1990.
6. Brewer MJ: To sleep or not to sleep: the consequences of sleep deprivation, Crit Care Nurse 5(6):35, 1985.
7. Culver BH: Pulmonary responses to sleep, Resp Care 34(6):510, 1989.
8. Davis-Sharts J: The elder and critical care: sleep and mobility issues, Nurs Clin North Am 24(3):755, 1989.
9. Dlin B, Rosen H, and Dickstein K: The problems of sleep and rest in the intensive care unit, Psychosomatics 12:155, 1971.
10. Dootson S: Critical care: sensory imbalance and sleep loss, Nurs Times 86(35):26, 1990.
11. Fabijan N and Gosselin M: How to recognize sleep deprivation in your ICU patient and what to do about it, Can Nurse 4:20, 1982.
12. Farr LA, Campbell-Grossman C, and Mack JM: Circadian disruption and surgical recovery, Nurs Res 37(3):170, 1988.
13. Fontaine DK: Measurement of nocturnal sleep patterns in trauma patients, Heart Lung 18(4):402, 1989.
14. Freemon F: Sleep research, Springfield, Ill, 1972, Charles C Thomas, Publisher.
15. Guyton AC: Medical physiology, ed 6, Philadelphia, 1981, WB Saunders Co.
16. Hartmann E: The sleeping pill, London, 1978, Yale University Press.
17. Hayter J: Sleep behaviors of older persons, Nurs Res 32(4):242, 1983.
18. Helton M, Gordon S, and Nunnery S: The correlation between sleep deprivation and ICU syndrome, Heart Lung 9(3):464, 1980.
19. Hemenway J: Sleep and the cardiac patient, Heart Lung 9(3):453, 1980.
20. Henderson V: Basic principles of nursing care, New York, 1969, Macmillan Publishing Co.
21. Hilton B: Quantity and quality of patient's sleep and sleep disturbing factors in a respiratory intensive care unit, Adv Nurs 1:453, 1976.
22. Johnson SE: Sleep pattern disturbance: defining characteristics observable in practice. In Classification of Nursing Diagnoses: Proceedings of the Eighth Conference, St Louis, 1989, Mosby–Year Book, Inc.
23. Kavey NB and Altshuler KZ: Sleep in herniorrhaphy patients, Am J Surg 138:682, 1979.
24. Kedas A and others: A critical review of aging and sleep research, West J Nurs Res 11(2):196, 1989.
25. Kinney M and others: Identifying critical defining characteristics of nursing diagnoses using magnitude estimation scaling, Res Nurs Health 12(6):373, 1989.
26. Lerner R: Sleep loss in the aged: implications for nursing practice, J Gerontol Nurs 8(6)323, 1982.
27. Levy RD and others: Negative pressure ventilation: effects on ventilation during sleep in normal subjects, Chest 95(1):95, 1989.
28. Littrell K and others: Promoting sleep for the patient with a myocardial infarction, Crit Care Nurse 9(3):44, 1989.

29. Locsin RC: Sleeplessness among the elderly, Rehab Nurs 13(6):340, 1988.
30. Martin LL: Obstructive sleep apnea: preventing complications, Dimens Crit Care Nurs 8(2):83, 1989.
31. Mendelson W: Human sleep, New York, 1987, Plenum Publishing Co.
32. Monjan AA: Sleep disorders of older people: report of a consensus conference, Hosp Community Psychiatry 41(7):743, 1990.
33. Noble M: Communication in the ICU: therapeutic or disturbing, Nurs Outlook 27:195, 1979.
34. Orr WC and others: Persistent hypoxemia and excessive daytime sleepiness in chronic obstructive pulmonary disease (COPD), Chest 97(3):583, 1990.
35. Pacini C and Fitzpatrick J: Sleep patterns of hospitalized and nonhospitalized aged individuals, J Gerontol Nurs 8(6):327, 1982.
36. Parish JM and others: Cardiovascular effects of sleep disorders, Chest 97(5):1220, 1990.
37. Pollack CP and others: Sleep problems in the community elderly as predictors of death and nursing home placement, J Community Health 15(2):123, 1990.
38. Reimer M: Sleep pattern disturbance: nursing interventions perceived by patients and their nurses as facilitating nocturnal sleep in hospital. In Classification of Nursing Diagnoses: Proceedings of the Seventh Conference, St Louis, 1987, Mosby–Year Book, Inc.
39. Reimer M: Sleep pattern disturbances related to neurological dysfunction, AXON 10(3):65, 1989.
40. Remmers JE: Sleeping and breathing, Chest 97(3):77S, 1990.
41. Roberts A: Senior systems . . . older patients and their medication . . . sleep and sleep difficulties in later life, Nurs Times 86(11):61, 1990.
42. Roffwarg HP, Muzio JN, and Dement WC: Ontogenetic development of the human sleep-dream cycle, Science 152:604, 1966.
43. Rosa R, Bonnet M, and Warm J: Recovery of performance during sleep following sleep deprivation, Psychophysiology 20:152, 1983.
44. Salamy JG: Sleep: some concepts and constructs. In Williams RL and Karacan I, editors: Pharmacology of sleep, New York, 1976, John Wiley & Sons.
45. Sanford S: Sleep and the cardiac patient, Cardiovasc Nurs 19(5):19, 1983.
46. Schirmer M: When sleep won't come, J Gerontol Nurs 9(1):16, 1983.
47. Sebilia A: Sleep deprivation and biological rhythms in the critical care unit, Crit Care Nurse 3:19, 1981.
48. Taub J: Acute shifts in the sleep-wakefulness: effects on performance and moods, Psychosom Med 36(2):164, 1974.
49. Woods N and Falk S: Noise stimuli in the acute care area, Nurs Res 23:144, 1974.
50. Wotring K: Using research in practice, Focus 9(5):34, 1982.

CHAPTER 6

# Nutritional Alterations

## CHAPTER OBJECTIVES

- *Describe the adverse effects of nutritional impairments on critically ill patients.*
- *Assess the nutritional status of critically ill patients.*
- *Participate with other health care team members in designing an effective nutrition support program for a patient in the critical care unit.*
- *Identify complications of nutrition support and nursing measures for prevention and treatment of these complications.*
- *Recognize nutritional alterations commonly associated with cardiovascular, pulmonary, neurological, fluid and renal, gastrointestinal, and endocrine systems.*
- *Develop a nutrition teaching plan for a critically ill patient.*

## KEY TERMS

triceps skinfold. p. 68
kwashiorkor, p. 69
marasmus, p. 69
total parenteral nutrition, p. 75
cardiac cachexia, p. 78

## NUTRITIONAL ASSESSMENT AND SUPPORT

### The Starvation Process

Extreme underfeeding or starvation of a healthy adult results in an initial decline in metabolic rate, which serves to protect the body from excessive tissue catabolism. Early in starvation, serum glucose levels drop by 10% to 15%. This drop causes a decrease in insulin release and an increase in glucagon, which in turn results in an increase in the following processes: glycogenolysis (glycogen breakdown), lipolysis (fat breakdown), and gluconeogenesis (catabolism of amino acids to produce glucose). There are limitations in the ability of body carbohydrate and fat stores to provide metabolic fuel for the body. Glycogen stores are essentially used up within a few hours of fasting. Although fat reserves are almost unlimited in many adults, not all body tissues can utilize fat. Initially, tissues such as the brain, peripheral nervous system, leukocytes, and erythrocytes depend solely on glucose. Although some of these tissues are eventually able to adapt so that they rely primarily on ketone bodies derived from fats, some (such as the erythrocytes) continue to utilize glucose, which can only be supplied by protein.

When stress (for example, major surgery, trauma, burns, or infection) accompanies starvation, sympathetic stimulation triggers the release of the catecholamines norepinephrine and epinephrine. These catecholamines increase the metabolic rate and thus the amount of catabolism required to provide sufficient fuel for the body. This can rapidly exacerbate the deterioration that accompanies starvation.

Prolonged starvation can be detrimental. Skeletal muscle catabolism weakens and debilitates the patient. Wasting of the diaphragm and intercostal muscles, for instance, impairs the ability to breathe deeply and may contribute to development of atelectasis and pneumonia. Even more serious is the loss of visceral proteins such as serum proteins, immunoglobulins, and leukocytes. These proteins have critical roles, including the transport of some nutrients to the cells, maintenance of immunocompetence, and maintenance of plasma oncotic pressure.

Surveys of hospitalized patients have revealed that 12%

to 48% of them show signs of malnutrition or starvation at admission.[15,37,38] Critically ill patients are especially vulnerable, with more than 40% of these patients being malnourished at the time of admission.[10] An even more ominous finding is that the nutritional status of more than two thirds of medical patients hospitalized for 2 weeks or longer deteriorates during hospitalization.[38] Patients who are hospitalized for longer than 2 weeks tend to be the sickest patients, and some of the nutritional deterioration may be ascribed to the severity of their illnesses. Other possible contributing factors include lack of communication among the nurses, physicians, and dietitians responsible for the care of these patients; frequent diagnostic testing, which causes patients to miss meals or to be too exhausted for meals; medications and other therapies that cause anorexia, nausea, or vomiting and thus interfere with food intake; or inadequate use of tube feedings or total parenteral nutrition to maintain the nutritional status of these patients.

When protein and calorie intake are inadequate for more than a few hours, existing body proteins will be broken down to meet the body's needs. Even when the individual has large fat reserves, catabolism of body proteins will occur. Unlike fat, proteins can provide the amino acids that are needed for tissue synthesis and repair and can also provide a significant source of glucose. The well-nourished individual tolerates a few days of starvation when not exposed to stress, but a patient with trauma, surgery, burns, or infection, along with inadequate nutritional intake will have accelerated catabolism. An already undernourished patient exposed to stress (for example, a cancer patient with anorexia and weight loss who undergoes surgery) will be especially vulnerable.

Malnutrition is an ominous finding among the very ill. Undernourished patients are three times as likely as well-nourished patients to have major surgical complications.[37] Wound dehiscence, decubitus ulcers, sepsis, and pulmonary infections are more common among the undernourished. Hospital stays of medical patients with evidence of malnutrition are approximately two thirds longer than those of well-nourished patients, and mortality is three times greater.[38]

## Nutritional Assessment

Nutritional assessment is a multistep process involving the collection and evaluation of pertinent information from the patient's diet and medical history, physical examination, and laboratory values. The assessment can be performed by a designated member of the health care team, such as the dietitian or the nurse, or it can be a team effort.

**History.** Information about dietary intake and significant variations in weight are vital parts of the history. A change of 10% or more in body weight during the past year or 5% to 6% during the last 3 months is usually considered significant. Dietary intake can be evaluated in several ways, including a diet record, a 24-hour recall, and a diet history. The diet record, a listing of the type and amount of all foods and beverages consumed for some period of time (usually 3 days), is useful for evaluating the patient's intake in the critical care setting if there is a question of the adequacy of intake. However, it tends to reveal little about the patient's habitual intake before the illness or injury. The 24-hour recall of all food and beverage intake is easily and quickly performed, but it, too, may not reflect the patient's usual intake and thus has limited usefulness. The diet history consists of a detailed interview about the patient's usual intake, along with social, familial, cultural, economic, educational, and health-related factors that may affect intake. Although the diet history is time consuming to perform and may be too stressful for the acutely ill patient, it provides a wealth of information about food habits over a prolonged period and provides a basis for planning specific patient teaching, if changes in eating habits are desirable.

**Physical assessment**

***Anthropometric measurements.*** Obtaining anthropometric or body measurements, of which height and weight are the most important, is the first step in physical evaluation. If at all possible, height and weight should be measured, rather than obtained through patient or family report. Skinfold measurements, another anthropometric parameter, provide an estimate of body fat, which is helpful in diagnosing obesity and malnutrition. The **triceps skinfold** is the most commonly used (Fig. 6-1). The triceps skinfold (TSF) is measured at the midpoint of the upper arm, which is located by taking half the distance between the olecranon and acromion. The TSF is obtained by grasping the skin and subcutaneous tissue at the back of the arm about 1 cm from the midpoint. Special calipers are then applied to the skinfold at the midpoint, and the skinfold reading is taken

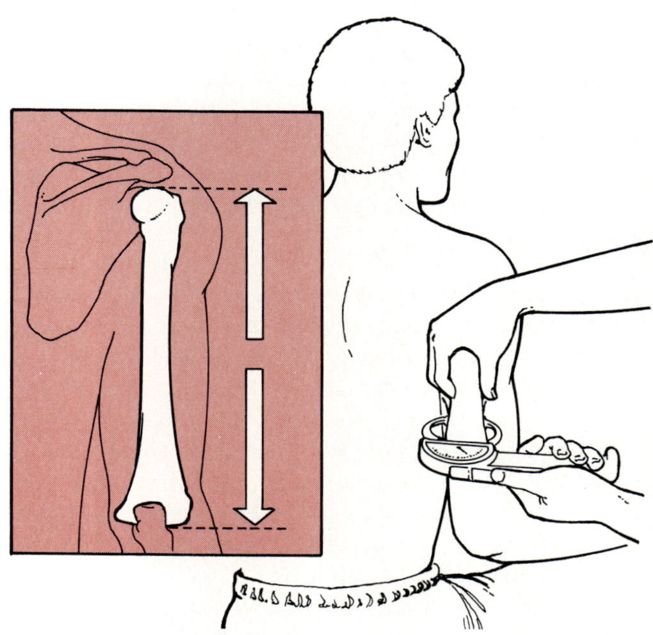

***Fig. 6-1*** Measuring the triceps skinfold.

***Table 6-1*** Physical findings in specific nutritional alterations

| Finding | Possible deficiency | Possible excess of |
|---|---|---|
| **HEAD AND NECK** | | |
| Hair loss | Protein, zinc, biotin | Vitamin A |
| Dull, dry, brittle hair; loss of hair pigment | Protein | |
| Conjunctival and corneal dryness | Vitamin A | |
| Blue sclerae | Iron | |
| Pale conjunctiva | Iron | |
| Gingivitis | Vitamin C | |
| Cheilosis or angular stomatitis (lesions at corners of mouth) | Vitamin $B_2$ | |
| Glossitis | Niacin, folate, vitamin $B_{12}$, other B vitamins | |
| Hypogeusia (poor sense of taste), dysgeusia (bad taste) | Zinc | |
| **SKIN AND NAILS** | | |
| Dry, scaly | Vitamin A, zinc, essential fatty acids | Vitamin A |
| Follicular hyperkeratosis (resembles gooseflesh) | Vitamin A | |
| Eczematous lesions | Zinc | |
| Petechiae, ecchymoses | Vitamin C or K | |
| Poor wound healing | Protein, zinc, vitamin C | |
| Koilonychia (spoon-shaped nails) | Iron | |
| **ABDOMEN** | | |
| Hepatomegaly | Protein | Vitamin A |
| **MUSCULOSKELETAL AND EXTREMITIES** | | |
| Muscle wasting | Calories | |
| Edema | Protein, vitamin $B_1$ | |
| Paresthesias | Vitamins $B_1$, $B_6$, $B_{12}$, biotin | |

to the nearest millimeter. Skinfold measurements are best performed by specially trained nurses and dietitians, because the measurements tend to vary greatly when performed by inexperienced personnel.

***Physical examination.*** A thorough physical examination is an essential part of nutritional assessment. Table 6-1 lists some of the more common findings that may indicate an altered nutritional state. It is especially important for the nurse to check for signs of muscle wasting, loss of subcutaneous fat, skin or hair changes, and impairment of wound healing.

**Laboratory data.** A wide range of diagnostic tests can provide information about nutritional status. Those most often used in the clinical setting are described in Table 6-2. As the table emphasizes, there are no perfect diagnostic tests for evaluation of nutrition, and care must be taken in interpreting the results of the tests.

**Evaluating nutritional assessment findings and determining nutritional needs.** It is rare for a patient to exhibit a lack of only one nutrient. Usually nutritional deficiencies are combined, with the patient lacking adequate amounts of protein and calories and possibly vitamins and minerals. A common form of combined nutritional deficit among hospitalized patients is protein-calorie malnutrition. Protein deficits, sometimes referred to as **kwashiorkor,** are evidenced by low levels of the serum proteins albumin, transferrin, and prealbumin; low total lymphocyte count; impaired immunity; loss of hair or hair pigment; edema; and an enlarged, fatty liver. Calorie deficits, termed **marasmus,** are recognizable by weight loss, a decrease in skinfold measurements, loss of subcutaneous fat, muscle wasting, and low levels of creatinine excretion. Since protein-calorie malnutrition weakens musculature, increases vulnerability to infection, and can prolong hospital stays, the health care team should diagnose this serious disorder as quickly as possible so that appropriate nutritional intervention can be implemented.

Nutritional assessment provides a basis for estimating nutritional needs. Table 6-3 demonstrates methods that are frequently used in estimating the calorie and protein needs of patients.

### Administering Nutrition Support

**Enteral nutrition support.** The enteral route is the preferred method of feeding whenever possible, because this route is generally safer, more physiological, and much less expensive than parenteral feeding. There are a variety of enteral feeding products, some of which are designed to meet the specialized needs of very sick patients. Some products can be consumed orally, but many of the specialized ones are so unpalatable that they are solely reserved for

***Table 6-2*** Nutritional assessment by laboratory tests

| Area of concern | Possible deficiency | Comments |
|---|---|---|
| **SERUM PROTEINS** | | |
| *Decrease of serum albumin, transferrin (iron transport protein), or thyroxine-binding prealbumin | Protein | These proteins are produced in the liver, depressed in hepatic failure, and are falsely low in fluid volume excess and elevated in volume deficit. Albumin has long half-life (14-20 days) and is slow to change in malnutrition and repletion; transferrin has a half-life of 7-8 days, but levels increase in iron deficiency, and prevalence of iron deficiency limits usefulness in diagnosing protein deficits; prealbumin half-life is 2-3 days, levels fall in trauma and infection |
| **HEMATOLOGICAL VALUES** | | |
| Anemia (decreased Hct, Hgb) | | Hct and Hgb are falsely low in fluid volume excess and falsely high in fluid volume deficit |
| Normocytic (normal MCV, MCHC) | Protein | |
| Microcytic (decreased MCV, MCH, MCHC) | Iron, copper | |
| Macrocytic (increased MCV) | Folate, vitamin $B_{12}$ | |
| Total lymphocyte count (TLC) = WBC × % lymphocytes | | |
| TLC <1200 $mm^3$ | Protein | Decreased in severe debilitating disease |
| **URINARY CREATININE** | | |
| Creatinine excretion <17 mg/kg/day (women), <23 mg/kg/day (men) | Protein (reflects lean body mass) | Difficult to collect accurate 24-hr urine; wide variation in creatinine excretion from day to day; levels decline with age as percentage of lean body mass declines |
| **NITROGEN BALANCE†** | | |
| Negative values | Protein, calories (during calorie deficit, protein is metabolized to provide calories) | Negative values occur when more nitrogen is excreted than is consumed (reflects inadequate intake or increased needs); positive values occur when more is consumed than lost (e.g., during nutrition repletion, growth, or pregnancy); normal healthy adults excrete exactly what they consume. Limitations: difficult to collect accurate 24-hr urine; retention of nitrogen does not necessarily mean that it is being used for tissue synthesis |

*Evaluation of at least one of these is a part of almost every nutritional assessment.
†Protein is 16% nitrogen. Thus nitrogen balance = [24-hr protein intake (g) × 0.16] − [24-hr urine nitrogen (g) + 4g]. The 4 g is an estimate of fecal, skin, and other minor losses.

tube feeding. Table 6-4 provides more information about the major categories of products.

***Oral supplementation.*** For patients who can eat and have normal digestion and absorption, but simply cannot consume enough regular foods to meet caloric and protein needs, oral supplementation may be necessary. Patients with mild to moderate anorexia, burns, or trauma sometimes fall into this category. To improve intake and tolerance of supplements, the critical care nurse should:

1. Collaborate with the dietitian to choose appropriate products and allow the patient to participate in the selection process if possible. Milk shakes made with ice cream and half-and-half; powdered milk added to cereal and fluid milk; and instant breakfast are often more palatable and economical than commercial supplements. However, intolerance of lactose (milk sugar) is common among adults, especially blacks, Orientals, American Indians, and Eskimos. Furthermore, many disease processes (for example, Crohn's

***Table 6-3*** Estimating nutritional requirements

**ESTIMATING CALORIC NEEDS**

1. Calculate basal energy expenditure (BEE). This is the energy needed for basic life processes such as respiration, cardiac function, and maintenance of body temperature.
   Women: BEE = 655 + (9.6 × W) + (1.7 × H) − (4.7 × A)
   Men: BEE = 66 + (13.7 × W) + (5 × H) − (6.8 × A)
   W = Current weight in kg; H = Height in cm; A = Age in yr
2. Multiply BEE by an appropriate activity factor.

| Level of activity | Multiply BEE by |
|---|---|
| Bed rest | 1.2 |
| Light (e.g., sedentary office work) | 1.3 |
| Moderate (e.g., nursing) | 1.4 |
| Strenuous (e.g., manual labor) | 1.5 or more |

3. Multiply by an appropriate stress factor to meet the needs of the ill or injured patient.

| Type of stress | Multiply the value obtained in step 2 by |
|---|---|
| Fever | 1 + 0.13/°C elevation above normal (or 0.07/°F) |
| Pneumonia | 1.2 |
| Major injury | 1.3 |
| Severe sepsis | 1.5-1.6 |
| Major burns | 1.8-2 |

**ESTIMATING PROTEIN NEEDS**

Protein needs vary with degree of malnutrition and stress.

| Condition | Multiply desirable body weight (kg) by |
|---|---|
| Healthy individual or well-nourished elective surgery patient | 0.8-1 g protein |
| Malnourished or catabolic state (e.g., sepsis, major injury, burns) | 1.2-2+ g protein |

**Example of calculation of needs**

A 38-year-old male patient with pelvic, rib, and long-bone fractures; pneumothorax; and a ruptured spleen following a motor vehicle accident. Height 180 cm (5′11″), current weight 81.8 kg (180 lb), desirable weight 72.7 kg (160 lb).

**Energy needs**

1. BEE = 66 + (13.7 × 81.8) + (5 × 180) − (6.8 × 38) = 1829 calories/day
2. Energy needs for bed rest = 1829 calories × 1.2 = 2195 calories/day
3. Energy needs for injury = 2195 calories × 1.3 = 2853 calories/day

**Protein needs** = 72.7 kg × 1.5 g = 109 g/day

---

disease, radiation enteritis, and severe gastroenteritis) are associated with lactose intolerance. Individuals with this problem experience abdominal cramping, bloating, and diarrhea after lactose ingestion and may require commercial lactose-free supplements.

2. Serve commercial supplements well chilled or on ice, because this improves flavor.

3. Advise patients to sip formulas slowly, consuming no more than 240 ml over 30 to 45 minutes. These products contain easily digested carbohydrates. If formulas are consumed too quickly, rapid hydrolysis of the carbohydrate in the duodenum can contribute to dumping syndrome, characterized by abdominal cramping, weakness, tachycardia, and diarrhea.

4. Record all supplement intake separately on the intake and output sheet so that it can be differentiated from intake of water and other liquids.

***Enteral tube feedings.*** Tube feedings are used for patients who have at least some digestive and absorptive capability but are unwilling or unable to consume enough by mouth. Patients with profound anorexia and those experiencing severe stress (for instance, major burns or trauma) that greatly increases their nutritional needs often benefit from tube feedings. Individuals who require elemental formulas or the specialized formulas for altered metabolic conditions (see Table 6-4) usually require tube feeding because the unpleasant flavors of the free amino acids, peptides, or protein hydrolysates used in these formulas are very difficult to mask.

**Table 6-4** Characteristics of enteral formulas

| Formula type | Examples of formulas | Oral or tube feeding | Nutritional problem | Clinical examples |
|---|---|---|---|---|
| Complete diet with intact protein and LCT*† (some contain blended foods) | Ensure and Osmolite (Ross), Sustacal and Isocal (Mead Johnson Nutritional), Meritene and Compleat (Sandoz), Entrition (Biosearch). For fluid restriction: Magnacal (Sherwood Medical), Isocal HCN (Mead Johnson Nutritional), TwoCal HN (Ross) | Some are suited to both (e.g., Ensure), some primarily to oral (Sustacal, Meritene), and some primarily to tube feeding (Compleat, Osmolite, Isocal) | Inability to ingest food<br>Inability to ingest enough food to meet needs | Oral or esophageal cancer<br>Coma<br>Anorexia resulting from chronic illness<br>Burns or trauma |
| Elemental diets‡ | Criticare HN (Mead Johnson Nutritional), Vital High Nitrogen (Ross), Reabilan (O'Brien), Vivonex and Vivonex T.E.N. (Norwich Eaton), Travasorb HN (Clintec Nutrition) | Tube feeding | Impaired digestion and/or absorption<br>Hypoalbuminemia | Pancreatitis<br>Inflammatory bowel disease<br>Radiation enteritis<br>Short bowel syndrome<br>Malnutrition |
| **SPECIALIZED DIETS FOR METABOLIC ALTERATIONS** | | | | |
| Diets high in essential amino acids, low in nonessential amino acids | Amin-Aid (Kendall McGaw), Travasorb Renal (Clintec Nutrition) | Both (especially tube) | Renal failure | Undialyzed end stage renal disease |
| Diets high in branched chain amino acids, low in aromatic amino acids | Hepatic-Aid II (Kendal McGaw), Travasorb Hepatic (Clintec Nutrition) | Both (especially tube) | Hepatic failure | Impending hepatic coma |
| Diets high in branched chain amino acids§ | Stresstein (Sandoz), TraumaCal (Mead Johnson Nutritional), Traum-Aid HBC (Kendall McGaw) | Both (especially tube) | Stress | Trauma and injury<br>Sepsis |

*LCT = Long-chain triglycerides or fat, used in formulas for patients with no digestive or absorptive abnormality.
†Some of these formulas contain lactose. If the patient has a lactose intolerance, the dietitian can recommend an appropriate lactose-free formula.
‡Contain "predigested" nutrients: protein in the form of amino acids and/or peptides or protein hydrolysates, fat as medium chain triglycerides (which require less emulsification by bile salts and enzymatic digestion than LCT) or minimal fat, and easily digested carbohydrates (no lactose).
§Branched-chain amino acids (leucine, isoleucine, and valine) contain a branch in their carbon chain structure. They are required for protein synthesis, but they are especially important because they serve as a valuable energy source following injury.

**LOCATION AND TYPE OF FEEDING TUBE.** Whether temporary tubes (nasogastric or nasoduodenal/nasojejunal) or more permanent ones (gastrostomy or jejunostomy) are used depends largely on the length of time that feedings are anticipated to be needed. Usually 3 months or longer constitutes long-term feedings. However, the patient who is extremely agitated or confused or for some other reason does not tolerate nasal intubation may require a permanent tube earlier. In addition, the advent of the percutaneous gastrostomy tube, which can be inserted with local anesthesia, has made gastrostomy increasingly popular, even in patients who do not require long-term feeding.

The site for intubation is also determined by patient need. Nasoduodenal, nasojejunal, or jejunostomy tubes are most often used when there is danger of pulmonary aspiration, because the pyloric sphincter provides a barrier which appears to lessen the risk of regurgitation and aspiration.[25] Jejunostomy tubes have the added advantage of being able to bypass an upper gastrointestinal (GI) obstruction.

**SUMMARY OF NURSING CARE.** The nurse's role in delivery of tube feedings usually includes insertion of the tube, if a temporary tube is used; maintenance of the tube; administration of the feedings; prevention of complications associated with this form of therapy; and participation in assessment of the patient's response to tube feedings. Assessment of response will be discussed later in this chapter.

Critical care nurses are usually familiar with tube insertion, and therefore this topic will not be discussed in depth here. However, transpyloric passage of tubes deserves special mention. Tubes with mercury, stainless steel, or tungsten weights on the proximal end are often used when transpyloric tube placement is desired, in the belief that the weight will encourage transpyloric passage of the tube or that the weight will help the tube maintain its position once it passes into the bowel. Two groups of investigators, however, have independently noted that unweighted tubes are just as likely as weighted ones to migrate through the pylorus.[19,29] Furthermore, weighted tubes appear to offer no advantage over unweighted ones in regard to remaining in place.[29,34] Because the weights increase manufacturing costs and sometimes cause discomfort while being inserted through the nares, unweighted tubes may be preferable. One technique that has been shown to promote transpyloric passage of tubes is the administration of metoclopramide hydrochloride before tube insertion. Administering the drug after the tube's proximal tip is already in the stomach is much less effective.[18,40]

Maintenance of the tube includes regular irrigation of the tube to maintain patency, skin care around the insertion site, and mouth care. The newer small-bore (usually 8 French) "nonreactive" tubes made of polyurethane, silicone rubber, and similar materials are much more comfortable for the patient than the older polyethylene or polyvinylchloride tubes (usually 12 to 16 French), and patient complaints of discomfort[11] and nasal and skin erosion have decreased with the use of the nonreactive tubes. Unfortunately, these small tubes tend to clog readily. Regular irrigation helps to prevent tube occlusion. Generally, 30 to 60 ml of irrigant every 3 to 4 hours or after each feeding is appropriate. The volume of irrigant may have to be reduced during fluid restriction. The irrigant is usually water, but other fluids such as cranberry juice or cola beverages are sometimes used in an effort to reduce the incidence of tube occlusion. However, cranberry juice is inferior to, and cola beverages appear no better than, water for irrigating tubes.[24] Furthermore, once a tube has occluded, cranberry juice and cola are of little use in clearing the occlusion. In vitro studies[21,27] have shown that pancreatic enzymes, and sometimes papain (an enzyme from fresh papaya, commonly used in meat tenderizers), can be effective in clearing occlusions, but no reports exist about the safety and efficacy of enzymes in clearing occlusions in the clinical setting. Polyurethane tubes clog less readily than silicone rubber, an important consideration for the nurse in selecting a feeding tube.[24]

The skin around the tube should be cleaned at least daily, and the tape around the tube replaced whenever loosened or soiled. Secure taping helps to prevent movement of the tube, which may irritate the nares or skin or result in accidental dislodgement of the tube. Dressings are used initially around gastrostomy insertion sites. The dressing should be changed daily and the skin cleansed with half-strength hydrogen peroxide. If leakage of gastric fluid occurs around a gastrostomy tube, the skin can be protected with karaya.

To prevent dryness of the mouth (a common complaint during tube feeding), the patient should be encouraged to breathe through the nose as much as possible, drink and eat as much as desired (if compatible with the patient's nutrition orders), suck sugarfree candies or chew sugarfree gum (if allowed), and perform regular mouth care. If the patient is unconscious or otherwise unable to perform mouth care, the nurse should do it or should enlist the family in performing it. Patients often report that they can "taste" the tube feedings, and frequent mouth care will clear the palate of unpleasant flavors from the formula, as well as cleaning the teeth, tongue, and oral mucous membranes.

Careful attention to administration of tube feedings can prevent many complications. Very clean techniques in the handling and administration of the formula can help prevent bacterial contamination and a resultant infection. Routinely monitoring the patient's gastric residuals (especially if feedings are delivered into the stomach) can prevent gastric distention, which could cause patient discomfort, vomiting, and pulmonary aspiration. The schedule for delivery of feedings is also important. Tube feedings may be administered intermittently or continuously. Intermittent feedings are best suited to those patients who are disoriented and attempt to remove the feeding tube when they are alone. Bolus feedings, which are intermittent feedings delivered rapidly into the stomach or small bowel, are likely to cause distention, vomiting, and dumping syndrome with diarrhea. Instead of using bolus feedings, nurses should gradually drip intermittent feedings, with each feeding lasting 20 to 30 minutes

*Table 6-5* Nursing management of enteral tube feeding complications

| Complication | Contributing factor(s) | Prevention/correction |
|---|---|---|
| Pulmonary aspiration | See the nursing management plan "High Risk for Aspiration," p. 476 | |
| Diarrhea | Medications with GI side effects (antibiotics, which can alter gut flora, are common culprits,[17] but others include digitalis, laxatives,[33] magnesium-containing antacids, and quinidine) | Evaluate the patient's medications to determine their potential for causing diarrhea, consulting the pharmacist if necessary; if the possibility of pseudomembranous colitis is ruled out, consult with the physician about adding pectin (a soluble fiber that may result in formation of firmer stools) to the formula or the use of antidiarrheal medications |
| | Hypertonic formula or medications (e.g., oral suspensions of antibiotics, potassium, or other electrolytes),[28] which cause fluid to be drawn into the gut to dilute the hypertonic load | Consult the physician about using continuous feedings (if feedings are currently intermittent) or diluting or slowing tube feedings temporarily; dilute enteral medications well |
| | Malnutrition (hypoalbuminemia impairs absorption by decreasing plasma oncotic pressure; malnutrition also results in loss of intestinal microvilli, reducing brush border enzymes needed for digestion, as well as the absorptive area[4]) | Consult with the physician about using an elemental formula, which may be more readily absorbed by the malnourished patient,[3] and utilizing continuous feedings[39,41] |
| | Cold formula[14] | Allow formula for intermittent feeding to come to room temperature before use (usually formula warms sufficiently during continuous infusions so that there is no need for prewarming.) |
| | Bacterial contamination[6] | Use scrupulously clean technique in administering tube feedings; keep opened containers of formula refrigerated and discard them within 24 hr; discard enteral feeding containers and administration sets every 24 hr[2]; hang formula no more than 4-8 hr unless it comes prepackaged in sterile administration sets; be especially careful with feedings given to patients being fed transpylorically or those receiving cimetidine or antacids, because these patients lack the normal antibacterial barrier of the stomach's hydrochloric acid[9] |
| | Fecal impaction with seepage of liquid stool around the impaction | Perform a digital rectal examination to rule out impaction; see guidelines for prevention of constipation (below) |
| Constipation | Low residue formula, creating little fecal bulk | Consult with the physician regarding the use of fiber-containing formula (e.g., Enrich [Ross], Compleat [Sandoz]), although this is not possible if the patient requires an elemental diet; consult with the physician about adding bran or bulk-type laxatives to the patient's regimen |
| | Inadequate fluid intake | Check patient's fluid intake to see that it totals 50 ml/kg/day, unless there is need for fluid restriction |
| Tube occlusion | Giving medications via tube (medications may physically plug the tube or may coagulate the formula, causing it to clog the tube)[7,22] | If medications must be given by tube, avoid use of crushed tablets; consult with the pharmacist to see whether medications can be dispensed as elixirs or suspensions; irrigate tube with water before and after administering any medication; never add any medication to the tube feeding formula unless the two are known to be compatible |
| | Sedimentation of formula | Irrigate tube every 4-8 hr during continuous feedings and after every intermittent feeding |

***Table 6-5*** Nursing management of enteral tube feeding complications—cont'd

| Complication | Contributing factor(s) | Prevention/correction |
|---|---|---|
| Gastric retention | Delayed gastric emptying resulting from neural impairment or serious illness (e.g., diabetic gastroparesis, trauma) | Measure gastric residual at least every 4-6 hr or before every feeding; consult with physician regarding use of transpyloric feedings, temporary reduction of formula volume, or metoclopramide hydrochloride to stimulate gastric emptying; encourage patient to lie in right lateral position frequently, unless contraindicated |

or longer, to promote optimal assimilation. Regardless of how slowly intermittent feedings are given, however, continuous feedings are usually better absorbed by patients who have compromised digestion or absorption. Even patients who might be expected to have normal GI function, such as those with burns or trauma, have been shown to absorb the feedings better, tolerate larger volumes of formula, and experience less diarrhea with continuous feedings than with intermittent ones.[13] Therefore, continuous feedings are usually preferable for very sick patients.

**PREVENTION AND CORRECTION OF COMPLICATIONS.** Some of the more common and serious complications of tube feeding are pulmonary aspiration, diarrhea, constipation, tube occlusion, and delayed gastric emptying. Delayed gastric emptying limits the amount of feeding that the patient can tolerate and thus interferes with adequate nutrition support. Nursing management of these problems is detailed in Table 6-5.

**Total parenteral nutrition. Total parenteral nutrition** (TPN) refers to the delivery of all nutrients by the intravenous route. TPN is generally not worthwhile when enteral intake is expected to be adequate within 5 to 7 days. Likely candidates for TPN include patients who are unable to ingest or absorb nutrients via the GI tract, as in short bowel syndrome, severe disease of the small bowel (for instance, inflammatory bowel disease, collagen-vascular diseases, intestinal pseudo-obstruction, or radiation enteritis), or intractable vomiting. TPN may be warranted in patients receiving high-dose chemotherapy, radiation, and bone marrow transplantation, where nutritional intake is apt to be poor for several weeks resulting from a combination of stomatitis, nausea, vomiting, diarrhea, and anorexia. It may also be useful in patients who can benefit from a period of bowel rest, including those with moderate to severe pancreatitis or with enterocutaneous fistulae. In both cases, enteral intake (which stimulates secretion of digestive enzymes) is likely to exacerbate the condition, whereas bowel rest may promote healing. In addition, some postoperative, trauma, or burn patients may need temporary TPN.[1]

***Routes for TPN.*** TPN may be delivered through either central or peripheral veins. Because it requires an indwelling catheter, central vein TPN carries an increased risk of sepsis, as well as potential insertion-related complications such as pneumothorax and hemothorax. Air embolism is also more likely with central vein TPN. However, central venous catheters provide very secure IV access and allow delivery of more hyperosmolar solutions than peripheral TPN. TPN solutions containing 25% to 35% dextrose are commonly used via central veins, and this provides an inexpensive source of calories. It is increasingly common for patients requiring multiple IV therapies and frequent blood sampling to have multilumen central venous catheters and for TPN to be infused via these catheters. Infection rates in patients receiving TPN via multilumen catheters have been reported to be as much as three times higher than those in patients with single lumen catheters.[30,32] Scrupulous aseptic technique is essential in maintaining multilumen catheters; the manipulation involved in frequent changes of intravenous (IV) fluid and blood drawing through these catheters increases the risk of catheter contamination. Also, patients requiring these catheters are likely to be very ill and immunocompromised.

Peripheral TPN is rarely associated with serious infectious or mechanical complications, but it does necessitate good peripheral venous access. Therefore, it may not be appropriate for long-term nutrition support or for patients receiving multiple IV therapies. Furthermore, peripheral veins tolerate very hyperosmolar solutions poorly, and thus peripheral solutions are limited to about 10% dextrose. Daily use of IV lipid emulsions, which are isotonic, is necessary to provide adequate calories during peripheral TPN, unless the patient is consuming substantial amounts by mouth and the TPN is being used only as a supplement.

***Summary of nursing care.*** Nursing care of the patient receiving TPN includes catheter care, administration of solutions, prevention or correction of complications, and evaluation of patient responses to IV feedings. Information regarding nursing management of TPN complications is summarized in Table 6-6. Infectious complications are of particular concern.

The indwelling central venous catheter provides an excellent nidus for infection. The nurse has a major role in preventing this complication of TPN therapy. Catheter care includes maintaining an intact dressing at the catheter insertion site and manipulating the catheter and administration tubing with aseptic technique. Dressings for TPN catheters

**Table 6-6** Nursing management of TPN complications

| Complication | Signs/symptoms | Prevention/correction |
|---|---|---|
| Catheter-related sepsis | Fever, chills, glucose intolerance, positive blood culture | Maintain an intact dressing, change if contaminated by vomitus, sputum, etc.; use aseptic technique when handling catheter, IV tubing, and TPN solutions; hang a bottle of TPN no longer than 24 hr, lipid emulsion no longer than 12-24 hr; use an in-line 0.22 μm filter with TPN to remove microorganisms; avoid drawing blood, infusing blood or blood products, piggybacking other IV solutions or medications into TPN IV tubing, or attaching manometers or tranducers via the TPN infusion line, if at all possible<br>If catheter-related sepsis is suspected, remove catheter or assist in changing the catheter over a guidewire and administer antibiotics as ordered |
| Air embolism | Dyspnea, cyanosis, apnea, tachycardia, hypotension, "millwheel" heart murmur; mortality estimated at 50% (depends on quantity of air entering) | Use Luer-Lok syringe or secure all connections well; use an in-line 0.22 μm air-eliminating filter; have patient perform Valsalva maneuver during tubing changes; if the patient is on a ventilator, change tubing quickly at end expiration; maintain occlusive dressing over catheter site for at least 24 hr after discontinuing catheter to prevent air entry through catheter tract<br>If air embolism is suspected, place patient in left lateral decubitus and Trendelenburg position (to trap air in the apex of the right ventricle, away from the outflow tract) and administer oxygen and CPR as needed; immediately notify physician, who may attempt to aspirate air from the heart |
| Pneumothorax | Chest pain, dyspnea, hypoxemia, hypotension, radiographical evidence, needle aspiration of air from pleural space | Throughly explain catheter insertion procedure to patient, because when a patient moves or breathes erratically he or she is more likely to sustain pleural damage; perform x-ray examination following insertion or insertion attempt<br>If pneumothorax is suspected, assist with needle aspiration or chest tube insertion, if necessary; chest tubes are usually used for pneumothorax >25% |
| Central venous thrombosis | Edema of neck, shoulder, and arm on same side as catheter; development of collateral circulation on chest; pain in insertion site; drainage of TPN from the insertion site; positive findings on venogram | Follow measures to prevent sepsis; repeated or traumatic catheterizations are most likely to result in thrombosis<br>If thrombosis is suspected, remove catheter and administer anticoagulants and antibiotics as ordered |
| Catheter occlusion or semiocclusion | No flow or a sluggish flow through the catheter | If infusion is stopped temporarily, flush catheter with heparinized saline.<br>If catheter appears to be occluded, attempt to aspirate the clot; if this is ineffective, physician may order thrombolytic agent such as streptokinase or urokinase instilled in the catheter |
| Hypoglycemia | Diaphoresis, shakiness, confusion, loss of consciousness | Infuse TPN within 10% of ordered rate; observe patient carefully for signs of hypoglycemia following discontinuance of TPN*<br>If hypoglycemia is suspected, administer oral carbohydrate; if the patient is unconscious or oral intake is contraindicated, the physician may order a bolus of IV dextrose |
| Hyperglycemia | Thirst, headache, lethargy, increased urinary output | Administer TPN within 10% of ordered rate; monitor blood glucose at least daily until stable; the patient may require insulin added to the TPN if hyperglycemia is persistent; sudden appearance of hyperglycemia in a patient who was previously tolerating the same glucose load may indicate onset of sepsis |

*The nurse should observe the patient especially closely for the first 1-2 hr after abrupt discontinuance of TPN (without tapering of the rate), because hypoglycemia is most probable at this time.[36]

may consist either of gauze and tape or transparent film. Usually gauze dressings are changed three times weekly, and transparent dressings are changed every 5 to 7 days. Both types are also changed whenever they become wet, soiled, or nonadherent. These types of dressings are associated with comparable rates of catheter-related sepsis,[16,31,42] but the transparent dressings usually decrease nursing time spent on dressing changes and may reduce irritation of sensitive skin.[16,42] After removal of the old dressing, the skin at the insertion site is commonly cleansed with povidone iodine, which is used because it has both antibacterial and antifungal activity. Chlorhexidine hydrochloride can be substituted for povidone iodine for patients allergic to iodine.

TPN solutions usually consist of amino acids, dextrose, electrolytes, vitamins, minerals, and trace elements. Although dextrose-amino acid solutions are commonly thought of as good growth media for microorganisms, they actually suppress the growth of most organisms usually associated with catheter-related sepsis, except yeasts.[8] However, because the many manipulations required to prepare solutions increase the possibility of contamination, TPN solutions are best used with caution. They should be prepared under laminar flow conditions in the pharmacy, with avoidance of additions on the nursing unit. Solution containers should be inspected for cracks or leaks before hanging, and solutions should be discarded within 24 hours of hanging. A 0.22 μm-line filter, which eliminates all microorganisms but not endotoxins, may be used in administration of solutions. Use of the filter, however, should not be substituted for scrupulous aseptic technique, because there is no conclusive evidence that filters decrease sepsis rates.[12]

In contrast to dextrose–amino acid solutions, IV lipid emulsions support the proliferation of many microorganisms.[5] Furthermore, lipid emulsions cannot be filtered through the 0.22 micron filters that remove most microorganisms, because some particles in the emulsions are larger than 0.22 μm. Lipid emulsions should be handled with strict asepsis, and they should be discarded within 12 to 24 hours of hanging. There is a trend toward mixing lipid emulsions with dextrose–amino acid TPN solutions. Although this saves nursing time, the nurse must be extremely careful in administering these solutions. TPN solutions containing lipids cannot be filtered through 0.22 micron filters, and they support the growth of most bacteria and *Candida albicans* better than dextrose–amino acid TPN solutions.[8]

## NUTRITIONAL MANAGEMENT BY SYSTEMS

### Nutrition in cardiovascular alterations

Diet and cardiovascular disease may interact in a variety of ways. In one situation, excessive nutrient intake, manifested by overweight or obesity and a diet rich in cholesterol and saturated fat, is a risk factor for development of arteriosclerotic heart disease. Conversely, the consequences of chronic myocardial insufficiency can include malnutrition.

**Nutritional assessment in cardiovascular alterations.** A nutritional assessment provides the nurse and other members of the health care team the information necessary to plan the patient's nutrition care and teaching. Key points of the nutritional assessment of the cardiovascular patient are summarized in Table 6-7. The major nutritional concerns relate to appropriateness of body weight, serum lipid levels, and blood pressure.

#### Nutrition intervention in cardiovascular alterations

***Myocardial infarction.*** The following guidelines will assist the nurse in providing appropriate nutritional care for the patient in the immediate post–myocardial infarction (MI) period:

1. Limit meal size for the patient with severe myocardial compromise or postprandial angina. While typical size meals are less stressful than a bed bath or shower for the patient with an uncomplicated condition, these meals increase cardiac index, stroke volume, heart rate, myocardial oxygen consumption, and whole body oxygen consumption; thus they increase cardiac work. Five to six small meals daily are less likely than three larger meals to increase myocardial work, promote ischemia, and cause angina.[44]
2. Monitor the effect of caffeine on the patient, if caffeine is included in the diet. Because caffeine is a stimulant, it might be expected to increase heart rate and myocardial oxygen demand. In the United States and in most industrial nations, coffee is the richest source of caffeine in the diet, with about 150 mg of caffeine per 180 ml (6 fluid ounces) of coffee. In comparison, the caffeine content of the same volume of tea or cola is approximately 50 mg or 20 mg, respectively. Schneider[56] found that one cup of caffeine-containing coffee had no effect on heart rate, blood pressure, myocardial oxygen consumption, and cardiac rhythm in patients convalescing from acute MI. Similarly, a double-blind study in which patients recovering from MI received 300 mg caffeine or a placebo revealed no increase in ventricular dysrhythmias after caffeine intake.[50] However, the acute MI patient should be carefully monitored during and after coffee consumption to rule out any adverse effects.
3. Avoid serving foods at temperature extremes. Very hot or very cold foods could potentially trigger vagal or other neural input and cause cardiac dysrhythmias.

***Hypertension.*** The primary nutritional intervention for hypertensive patients is to limit sodium intake, usually to no more than 2 g/day. The primary sodium source in the American diet is salt (sodium chloride) added during food processing and food preparation or at the table. One teaspoon of salt provides about 2.3 g of sodium. Most salt substitutes contain potassium chloride and may be used with the physician's approval by the patient who has no renal impairment. "Lite salt" is about half sodium chloride and half potassium chloride. It too may be used if the physician agrees, but it must be used very sparingly to achieve a sodium intake of 2 g or less daily.

Caffeine causes an acute increase in blood pressure but apparently has no sustained effect, and the incidence of hypertension is no higher among caffeine users than non-

**Table 6-7** Cardiovascular nutritional assessment

| Area of concern | Significant findings | | |
|---|---|---|---|
| | **History** | **Physical assessment** | **Laboratory data** |
| Overweight/obesity | Excessive kcal intake (consult dietitian regarding nutrition history)<br>Sedentary lifestyle | Weight >120% of desirable<br>Triceps skinfold >90th percentile* | |
| Protein-calorie malnutrition (cardiac cachexia) | Chronic cardiopulmonary disease causing:<br>Decreased food intake related to angina, respiratory embarrassment, or fatigue during eating<br>Malabsorption of nutrients (hypoxia of the gut impairs absorption;[46] in chronic congestive heart failure or cardiomyopathy, the amount of malabsorption may be significant)<br>Medications that impair appetite, e.g., digitalis, quinidine | Weight <85% of desirable<br>Triceps skinfold <10th percentile†<br>Muscle wasting<br>Loss of subcutaneous fat | Serum albumin <3.5 g/dl (or low serum transferrin or prealbumin)<br>Negative nitrogen balance<br>Creatinine excretion <17 mg/kg/day (women) or 23 mg/kg/day (men) |
| Elevated serum lipid levels | Frequent or daily use of foods high in cholesterol and saturated fat, including red meat, cold cuts, bacon or sausage, butter, cream or nondairy creamer, foods containing shortening or lard or fried in those products, eggs, organ meats, cheese, ice cream<br>Sedentary lifestyle<br>Family history of hyperlipidemia<br>Overweight or obesity | Xanthomas, or yellowish plaques deposited in the skin (uncommon) | Serum cholesterol >200 mg/dl (age 20-29), >220 (age 30-39), >240 (>40 yr)[51]<br>Low-density lipoprotein cholesterol >130 mg/dl[52] |
| Elevated blood pressure | Daily use of high-sodium foods and salt at the table<br>Consumption of >2 ounces of alcohol/day | | |

Adapted from Moore MC: Pocket guide to nutrition and diet therapy, St Louis, 1988, Mosby–Year Book, Inc.
*20 mm for men and 34 mm for women.
†6 mm for men and 14 for women.

users. Therefore restriction of the caffeine intake of hypertensive patients does not appear to be necessary.[53]

***Congestive heart failure.*** Nutrition intervention in congestive heart failure is designed to reduce fluid retained within the body and thus reduce preload.[54] Since fluid accompanies sodium, limitation of sodium is necessary in order to reduce fluid retention. Specific interventions include (1) limiting sodium intake, usually to 2 g/day or less and (2) limiting fluid intake as appropriate. The amount ordered is usually 1.5 to 2 L/day, to include both fluids in the diet and those given with medications and for other purposes. The nurse should remember that some foods that are normally served as solids are actually liquids at body temperature. These include gelatins (100% water), custard (75% water), sherbet and fruit ices (50% water), and ice cream (33% water).

***Cardiac cachexia.*** The severely malnourished cardiac patient **(cardiac cachexia)** often suffers from congestive heart failure. Therefore sodium and fluid restriction, as previously described, are appropriate. It is important to concentrate nutrients into as small a volume as possible and to serve small amounts frequently, rather than three large daily meals that may overwhelm the patient.

Because the patient is likely to tire quickly and to suffer from anorexia, tube feeding or total parenteral nutrition (TPN) may be necessary. When tube feeding is needed, formulas with 2 or more calories/ml are preferable. (Most commonly used formulas provide 1 calorie/ml.) Formulas appropriate for the fluid-restricted patient include Magnacal (Biosearch), Isocal HCN (Mead Johnson), TwoCal HN (Ross), and Nutrisource (Sandoz). During TPN, 20% lipid emulsions with 2 calories/ml provide a concentrated energy source. (The 10% emulsions, in contrast, contain only 1.1 calorie/ml.)

The nurse must monitor the fluid status of these patients carefully when they are receiving nutrition support. Body weight must be recorded daily; a consistent gain of more than 0.11 to 0.22 kg (¼ to ½ pounds) a day usually indicates fluid retention rather than gain of fat and muscle mass. The nurse must also check the patient frequently for increasing pulmonary and peripheral edema.

### Nutrition in Pulmonary Alterations

Malnutrition has extremely adverse effects on respiratory function, decreasing both surfactant production and vital capacity.[63] Moreover, individuals who lose weight lose proportionately more mass from the diaphragm than total body mass, and this further impairs ventilation.[59] Early detection and treatment of nutritional deficits seem to be especially important in patients with pulmonary alterations. Patients with acute respiratory disorders find it difficult to consume adequate oral nutrients and can rapidly become malnourished. Patients with chronic disorders and long-term weight loss have proved challenging to rehabilitate nutritionally. Goldstein and others[59] have shown that patients who do tolerate nutritional repletion demonstrate significant improvements in forced expiratory volume at 1 minute ($FEV_1$) and forced vital capacity (FVC), as well as increased sensitivity to $PaCO_2$ levels. Patients with undernutrition and end-stage chronic obstructive pulmonary disease (COPD), however, are unable to tolerate the increase in metabolic demand that occurs during refeeding. Also, they are at significant risk for development of cor pulmonale and often fail to tolerate the fluid required for delivery of enteral or parenteral nutrition support. Prevention of severe nutritional deficits, rather than correction of deficits once they have occurred, is the key to nutritional management of these patients.

**Nutritional assessment in pulmonary alterations.** Nutritional assessment is summarized in Table 6-8. The patient with respiratory compromise is especially vulnerable to the effects of fluid volume and carbohydrate excess and must be assessed continually for these complications.

**Nutrition intervention in pulmonary alterations**

***Prevent or correct undernutrition and underweight.*** The nurse and dietitian can work together to encourage oral intake in the undernourished or potentially undernourished patient who is capable of eating. Small, frequent feedings are especially important, since a very full stomach can in-

***Table 6-8*** Pulmonary nutritional assessment

| Area of concern | Significant findings: History | Significant findings: Physical assessment | Significant findings: Laboratory data |
|---|---|---|---|
| Protein-calorie malnutrition | Chronic lung disease: Poor intake of protein and calories because of:<br>Breathing difficulty from pressure of a full stomach on the diaphragm<br>Unpleasant taste in the mouth from chronic sputum production<br>Gastric irritation from bronchodilator therapy<br>Increased energy expenditure from increased work of breathing[59] | Muscle wasting<br>Loss of subcutaneous fat<br>Recent weight loss, or weight <90% of desirable<br>Triceps skinfold <10th percentile* | Serum albumin <3.5 g/dl, or low transferrin or prealbumin<br>Total lymphocyte count <1200/mm³<br>Creatinine excretion <17 mg/kg (women) or 23 mg/kg (men) |
| | Acute respiratory alterations:<br>Inadequate intake of protein and calories because of:<br>Upper airway intubation<br>Altered state of consciousness | Same as for chronic disease | Same as for chronic disease |

*6 mm for men and 14 mm for women.

*Continued.*

***Table 6-8*** Pulmonary nutritional assessment—cont'd

| Area of concern | Significant findings | | |
|---|---|---|---|
| | **History** | **Physical assessment** | **Laboratory data** |
| Protein-calorie malnutrition—cont'd | Dyspnea<br>Increased protein and calorie requirements due to increased work of breathing or acute pulmonary infections<br>Catabolism resulting from corticosteroid use | | |
| Overweight/obesity (in patients with chronic lung disease) | Decreased caloric needs resulting from decreasing metabolic rate with aging (metabolic rate declines 2%/decade after age 30) or decreased activity to compensate for impaired respiratory function | Weight >120% of desirable<br>Triceps skinfold >90th percentile† | |
| Elevated respiratory quotient (RQ)‡ | Use of glucose or other carbohydrate to provide 70% or more of nonprotein calories<br>Consumption of excess calories | Tachypnea, shortness of breath | RQ ≥1<br>Elevated $\dot{V}O_2$ and $\dot{V}CO_2$<br>Elevated $PaCO_2$ (not always present) |
| Fluid volume excess | Administration of more than 35-50 ml fluid/kg/day<br>Increased antidiuretic hormone (ADH) release resulting from stress and ventilator dependency | Dependent edema<br>Pulmonary rales<br>Bounding pulse<br>Shortness of breath | Serum sodium <135 mEq/L<br>BUN, hematocrit, and serum albumin decreased from previous values |
| Excess lipid intake | Administration of IV lipids | | Serum triglycerides >150 mg/dl<br>Low $V_A/Q$§ |

†20 mm for men and 34 mm for women.
‡RQ, or $CO_2$ produced ÷ $O_2$ consumed, is measured by indirect calorimetry, which is not available in all institutions. However, pulmonary function tests can provide some indication of RQ, as the "laboratory data" column demonstrates. Carbon dioxide production (and RQ) rises in the patient who is depending primarily on carbohydrate for fuel (e.g., the patient receiving TPN in whom dextrose is supplying almost all calories, rather than receiving a balance between dextrose and lipid calories) and especially the patient who is being overfed so that adipose tissue is being accumulated.
§The defect is not usually sufficient to alter $PaO_2$ or $PaCO_2$ except in patients with the most severe lung disease.[60]

terfere with diaphragmatic movement. Mouth care needs to be provided before meals and snacks to clear the palate of the flavors of sputum and medications. Administering bronchodilators with food can help to reduce gastric irritation.

Because of anorexia, dyspnea, and debilitation, however, many patients will require tube feeding or TPN. Some, but not all, investigators[58,61,66] have found pulmonary aspiration to be increased in patients with artificial airways who are receiving tube feedings, and it is especially important for the nurse to be alert to the risk of pulmonary aspiration. See the nursing management plan "High Risk for Aspiration," p. 476.

***Avoid excess carbohydrate administration.*** The production of carbon dioxide increases when carbohydrate is relied on as the primary energy source. This is unlikely to be significant in the patient who is eating foods. Instead, it is an iatrogenic complication of TPN in which glucose is often the predominant calorie source, or occasionally of tube feeding in a patient with a very high carbohydrate formula.[64] Excessive carbohydrate intake can raise $PaCO_2$ sufficiently to make it difficult to wean a patient from the ventilator. Patients not dependent on a ventilator may experience tachypnea or shortness of breath on a high carbohydrate regimen.

The nurse who notes an increasing $PaCO_2$ in a patient receiving carbohydrate-based TPN should discuss with the physician the possibility of providing daily lipid infusions for the patient. A regimen with approximately equal amounts of the nonprotein calories from lipid and carbohydrate is probably optimal for the patient with respiratory compromise.

***Avoid excessive serum lipid levels.*** Excessive lipid intake can impair capillary gas exchange in the lungs, although this is not usually sufficient to produce an increase in $Paco_2$ or decrease in $Pao_2$.[60] However, the patient with severe respiratory alteration may be further compromised by lipid overdose. If lipid intake is maintained at no more than 2 g/kg/day, lipid excess is rarely a problem. (Lipids are available as 20 g lipid per 100 ml of 20% lipid emulsion and 10 g/100 ml of 10% emulsion.) Serum triglycerides should be maintained less than 150 mg/dl. Higher levels may indicate inadequate clearance and a need to decrease the lipid dosage.

***Prevent fluid volume excess.*** Pulmonary edema and right heart failure, which may result from fluid volume excess, further worsen the status of the patient with respiratory compromise. Strict intake records must be maintained to allow for accurate totals of fluid intake. Usually the patient requires no more than 35 to 50 ml/kg/day of fluid. For the patient receiving nutrition support, fluid intake can be reduced by using 20% lipid emulsions as a source of calories, using tube feeding formulas providing at least 2 calories/ml (the dietitian can suggest appropriate choices), and choosing oral supplements that are low in fluid. Some examples are cottonseed oil (Lipomul, Upjohn), an oral lipid supplement providing 6 calories/ml, and powdered glucose polymers, which increase caloric intake without increasing volume. The nurse plays a valuable role in continually reassessing the patient's state of hydration and alerting other team members to changes that may dictate an increase or decrease in fluid intake.

### Nutrition in Neurological Alterations

Because neurological disorders tend to be long-term problems, they necessitate good nutritional care to prevent nutritional deficits and promote well-being.

**Nutritional assessment in neurological alterations.** Nutrition-related assessment findings vary widely in the patient with neurological alterations, depending on the type of disorder present. Some common findings are shown in Table 6-9.

**Nutrition intervention in neurological alterations**

***Prevention or correction of nutritional deficits.***

**ORAL FEEDINGS.** Patients with dysphagia or weakness often experience the greatest difficulty in swallowing foods that are dry or thin liquids such as water that are difficult to control. For these patients, the nurse and dietitian can work together to plan suitable meals and evaluate patient acceptance and tolerance. Some suggestions that may help the patient with dysphagia or weakness of the swallowing musculature include the following.*

1. Serve soft, moist foods. Tender chopped meats and poultry; casseroles; gravies and sauces over meats and vegetables; applesauce; cooked or canned fruits; ripe banana; cottage cheese; yogurt; poached, soft-cooked, or scrambled egg; mashed potatoes; cooked cereals; pudding; and custard are examples.

2. Thicken beverages with infant cereal, yogurt, or ice cream if the patient has difficulty swallowing fluids or chokes on water and other thin liquids. Alternatively, fluid can be provided by gelatin, sherbet, sorbet, fruit ices, popsicles, and ice cream. Fruit nectars may be better tolerated than juices.

3. Do not rush the patient who is eating, because this may increase the risk of pulmonary aspiration. Providing small amounts of food at frequent intervals, rather than larger amounts only at mealtimes, may help the patient feel less need to hurry. Keep suction equipment available in case aspiration does occur.

4. Place the patient in Fowler's position before feedings, if possible, to allow gravity to encourage effective swallowing.

5. Serve the main meal early in the day to the patient with myasthenia gravis, because muscle strength is greatest at that time.

**TUBE FEEDINGS OR TPN.** Patients who are unconscious or unable to eat because of severe dysphagia, weakness, ileus, or other reasons will need tube feedings or TPN. Prompt initiation of nutrition support must be a priority in the patient with neurological impairments. Needs for protein and calories are increased by infection and fever, as may occur in the patient with encephalitis and meningitis. Needs for protein, calories, zinc, and vitamin C are increased during wound healing, as in the trauma patient and the patient with decubitus ulcers.

Tube feeding can be successful in many patients with neurological impairment. Because these patients have an increased risk of certain complications, particularly pulmonary aspiration, they require especially careful nursing care, however. Patients of most concern are (1) those with an impaired gag reflex, such as some patients with cerebral vascular accident, (2) those with delayed gastric emptying, such as patients in the early period after spinal cord injury and patients with head injury treated with barbiturate coma, and (3) patients likely to experience seizures. To prevent aspiration in this high risk population refer to the nursing management plan "High Risk for Aspiration," p. 476.

Continuous tube feedings decrease absorption of oral phenytoin as much as 70%. While it might be possible to increase the phenytoin dose to compensate for the impaired absorption, this poses a danger of drug toxicity if the tube feeding is abruptly halted.[80] Current recommendations are that tube feedings not be given for 2 hours before and 2 hours after a single daily dose of phenytoin and that blood levels of phenytoin be monitored carefully in patients receiving continuous feedings.[67,80]

Hyperglycemia is a common complication in patients receiving corticosteroids. Patients treated with these drugs should have blood glucose levels monitored regularly and

*See also the nursing management plan "High Risk for Aspiration," p. 476

***Table 6-9*** Neurological nutritional assessment

| Area of concern | Significant findings: History | Significant findings: Physical assessment | Significant findings: Laboratory data |
|---|---|---|---|
| **DISORDERS OF PROTEIN AND CALORIE NUTRITURE** | | | |
| Protein-calorie malnutrition | Decreased intake because of:<br>Coma or confusion<br>Feeding/swallowing difficulties such as dribbling of food and beverages from mouth, dysphagia, weakness of muscles involved in chewing and swallowing<br>Ileus resulting from spinal cord injury or use of pentobarbital<br>Anorexia resulting from depression<br>Increased needs because of:<br>Hypermetabolism and catabolism following head injury<br>Increased needs for protein and calories to heal trauma and surgical wounds<br>Loss of protein from decubitus ulcers | Muscle wasting<br>Loss of subcutaneous fat<br>Weight <90% of desirable<br>Triceps skinfold <10th percentile*<br>Change in hair texture, loss of hair | Serum albumin <3.5 g/dl (or low transferrin or prealbumin values)<br>Negative nitrogen balance<br>Total lymphocyte count <1200/mm$^3$<br>Creatinine excretion <17 mg/kg/day (women) or <23 mg/kg/day (men) |
| Overweight/obesity | Decreased caloric needs resulting from inactivity<br>Reliance on soft or pureed foods, which are often more dense in calories than higher fiber foods<br>Increased food intake resulting from depression/boredom | Weight >120% of desirable<br>Triceps skinfold >90th percentile† | |
| **VITAMIN AND MINERAL DEFICIENCIES** | | | |
| Iron (Fe) | Poor intake of meats resulting from chewing difficulties (e.g., myasthenia gravis)<br>Loss of blood in trauma | Pallor, blue sclerae<br>Koilonychia | Microcytic anemia (low hct, hgb, MCV, MCH, MCHC)<br>Serum Fe <50 μg/ml |
| Zinc (Zn) | Poor intake of meat resulting from chewing problems<br>Increased needs for healing decubitus ulcers, trauma, or surgical wounds | Hypogeusia, dysgeusia<br>Diarrhea<br>Seborrheic dermatitis<br>Alopecia | Serum Zn <60 μg/ml |
| **FLUID ALTERATIONS** | | | |
| Fluid volume deficit | Poor intake resulting from difficulty swallowing (e.g., in cerebral vascular accident), inability to express thirst, fluid restriction in an effort to reduce intracranial edema | Poor skin turgor<br>Decreased urinary output<br>Dry, sticky mucous membranes | Serum sodium >145 mEq/L<br>Serum osmolality >300 mOsm/kg<br>Increased BUN and hct<br>Urine specific gravity >1.030 |

Adapted from Moore MC: Pocket guide to nutrition and diet therapy, St Louis, 1988, Mosby–Year Book, Inc.
hct, hematocrit; hgb, hemoglobin; MCV, mean cell volume; MCH, mean cell hemoglobin; MCHC, mean cell hemoglobin concentration; BUN, blood urea nitrogen.
*6 mm (men) or 14 mm (women).
†20 mm (men) or 34 mm (women).

may require insulin to prevent substantial loss of glucose in the urine, as well as osmotic diuresis, loss of excessive amounts of potassium, and other fluid and electrolyte disturbances.

Tube feedings may not be possible in some patients with neurological alterations. Certain patients with head injury may not tolerate tube feedings for a prolonged period of time because of vomiting and poor gastrointestinal motility. Intolerance of enteral feedings seems to be related to the severity of the injury and to increased intracranial pressure.[76] Another group of patients who are not good candidates for enteral feedings are those with frequent or uncontrolled seizures.

TPN is needed by most patients who fail to tolerate tube feedings or those who cannot be enterally fed for at least 5 to 7 days. Prompt use of TPN is especially important for patients with head injuries, because head injury causes marked catabolism,[78] even in patients who receive barbiturates, which should decrease metabolic demands.[68,72] Head-injured patients rapidly exhaust glycogen stores and begin to utilize body proteins to meet energy needs, a process that can quickly cause protein-calorie malnutrition. The catabolic response to head injury is partly a result of the corticosteroids often used in treatment.[70] However, the hypermetabolism and hypercatabolism is also caused by dramatic hormonal responses to this type of injury.[78] Levels of cortisol, epinephrine, and norepinephrine increase, with levels of norepinephrine elevating as much as seven times normal. These hormones increase the metabolic rate and caloric demands, causing mobilization of body fat and proteins to meet the increased energy needs. Furthermore, head-injured patients undergo an inflammatory response and may be febrile, creating increased needs for protein and calories. Improved survival has been observed in head-injured patients who received TPN early in the hospital course, rather than being deprived of adequate nutrition or provided with only enteral feedings for several days or weeks after injury.[77,79]

As mentioned previously, patients receiving corticosteroids are especially prone to hyperglycemia, and they must be monitored carefully for development of this complication while receiving TPN. Administering insulin, usually as an additive in the TPN, or decreasing the glucose intake and substituting increased amounts of calories from intravenous lipid emulsions will help to control blood glucose.

### Nutrition in Renal/Fluids Alterations

Providing adequate nutritional care for the patient with renal disease can be extremely challenging. While renal disturbances and their treatments can markedly increase needs for nutrients, necessary restrictions in intake of fluid, protein, phosphorus, and potassium make delivery of adequate calories, vitamins, and minerals difficult. Thorough nutrition assessment provides the basis for successful nutritional care in patients with renal disease.

**Nutritional assessment in renal/fluids alterations.** Assessment is summarized in Table 6-10.

**Nutrition intervention in renal/fluids alterations.** The goal of nutritional interventions is to administer adequate nutrients, including calories, protein, vitamins, and minerals, while avoiding excesses of fluid, protein, electrolytes, and other nutrients with potential toxicity.

***Protein.*** Evidence suggests that a low-protein diet retards the progression of renal damage. It is postulated that a high-protein intake increases glomerular flow and pressures, as the kidney attempts to excrete the urea and other nitrogenous products derived from the protein. The increase in glomerular pressures may hasten the death of the glomeruli.[84] Consequently, decreased protein intake (0.6 g/kg/day compared with the 0.8 g/kg/day recommended for the healthy person and the 1.7 g/kg/day actually consumed by the average American) is recommended for the undialyzed patient with renal failure.[92] Although uremia necessitates control of protein intake, the patient with renal failure often has many problems that actually increase protein/amino acid needs: losses in dialysis, wounds, and fistulae; use of corticosteroid drugs that exert a catabolic effect; increased endogenous secretion of catecholamines, corticosteroids, glucagon, and parathyroid hormone, all of which can cause or aggravate catabolism; and catabolic conditions such as trauma, surgery, and sepsis associated or coincident with the renal disturbances.[85,94] Therefore, protein needs may actually be increased. During hemodialysis and arteriovenous hemofiltration, amino acids are freely filtered and lost, but proteins such as albumin and immunoglobulins are not. Both proteins and amino acids are removed during peritoneal dialysis, creating a greater nutritional requirement for protein.[95] Protein needs are estimated at 1 to 1.2 or more g/kg/day for patients receiving hemodialysis or hemofiltration, and 1.2 to 1.4 or more g/kg/day for those receiving peritoneal dialysis.[90] Although these amounts are greater than the recommended daily level for healthy adults, they are probably lower than the amount found in the diet before the patient's illness, and thus most patients will perceive them as restrictions.

Controversy exists regarding the type of amino acids to be provided to the patient in renal failure. Some authorities advocate using primarily essential amino acids, those which the body cannot make, with the idea that the patient will form adequate amounts of nonessential amino acids via the process of transamination (transfer of amine groups from one carbon backbone to another). Foods containing protein of high biological value, such as eggs, milk, beef, poultry, and fish, are richer in essential amino acids than foods with lower biological value protein, such as grains, legumes, and vegetables. Therefore foods containing lower biological value protein would need to be especially restricted. Specialized essential amino acid products have been developed for nutrition support. These include Amin-Aid (Kendall McGaw) and Travasorb Renal (Travenol) for enteral feed-

***Table 6-10*** Renal nutritional assessment

| Area of concern | History | Physical assessment | Laboratory data |
|---|---|---|---|
| Protein-calorie malnutrition | Poor dietary intake because of:<br>Dietary restrictions on protein-containing foods<br>Anorexia caused by zinc deficiency (lost in dialysis or decreased in diet because of restrictions on meats, whole grains, legumes)<br>Increased protein and amino acid losses from:<br>Dialysis (hemodialysis losses ≈ 14 g/session; CAPD losses ≈ 9-12 g/day)<br>Tissue catabolism resulting from corticosteroid use<br>Proteinuria (e.g., nephrotic syndrome)<br>Increased needs for protein and calories during peritonitis and other infections | Muscle wasting<br>Loss of subcutaneous tissue<br>Weight <90% of desirable<br>Triceps skinfold <10th percentile*<br>(Loss of weight and subcutaneous fat may be masked by edema)<br>Loss of hair, change of texture | Serum albumin <3.5 g/dl or low transferrin or prealbumin levels<br>Total lymphocyte count <1200/$mm^3$<br>Negative nitrogen balance |
| Altered lipid metabolism | Nephrotic syndrome, with elevated cholesterol levels<br>Excess carbohydrate (CHO) consumption from:<br>Emphasis on CHO in the diet to replace some of the calories normally provided by protein<br>Use of glucose as an osmotic agent in dialysis | | Serum cholesterol >250 mg/dl<br>Serum triglycerides >180 mg/dl |
| Potential fluid volume excess | Oliguria or anuria<br>Patient knowledge deficit about or noncompliance with fluid restriction | Edema<br>Hypertension<br>Acute weight gain (≥1%-2% of body weight) | Hematocrit decreased from previous levels |
| **DISORDERS OF MINERALS/ELECTROLYTES** | | | |
| Phosphorus (P) excess | Oliguria or anuria | Tetany | Serum P >4.5 mg/dl<br>Calcium × P product (Ca in mg/dl × P in mg/dl) >70 |
| Zinc (Zn) deficit | Poor intake because of restriction of protein-containing foods<br>Loss in dialysis | Hypogeusia, dysgeusia<br>Alopecia<br>Seborrheic dermatitis<br>Diarrhea | Serum Zn <60 μg/ml |
| Iron (Fe) deficit | Decreased intake because of restriction of protein-containing foods<br>Loss of blood in dialysis tubing | Fatigue<br>Pallor, blue sclerae<br>Koilonychia | Hematocrit <37% (women) or 42% (men), hemoglobin <12 g/dl (women) or 14 g/dl (men), low MCV, MCH, MCHC |
| Sodium excess | Oliguria or anuria | Edema<br>Hypertension | |
| Potassium ($K^+$) excess | Oliguria or anuria | Weakness, flaccid muscles | Serum $K^+$ >5 mEq/L<br>Elevated T wave and depressed ST segment on ECG |

Adapted from Moore, MC: Pocket guide to nutrition and diet therapy, St Louis, 1988, Mosby–Year Book, Inc.
CAPD, continuous ambulatory peritoneal dialysis; MCV, mean cell volume; MCH, mean cell hemoglobin; MCHC, mean cell hemoglobin concentration.
*6 mm for men and 14 mm for women.

***Table 6-10*** Renal nutritional assessment—cont'd

| Area of concern | History | Physical assessment | Laboratory data |
|---|---|---|---|
| Aluminum (Al) excess | Use of aluminum-containing phosphate binders<br>Al contamination of TPN constituents, especially Ca and vitamins[89] | Ataxia, seizures<br>Dementia<br>Renal osteodystrophy with bone pain and deformities | Plasma Al >100 μg/L |
| **DISORDERS OF VITAMIN NUTRITURE** | | | |
| A excess | Oliguria or anuria<br>Daily administration of tube feedings, TPN, or oral supplement with vitamin A | Anorexia<br>Alopecia, dry skin<br>Hepatomegaly<br>Fatigue, irritability | Serum retinol >80 μg/dl |
| C deficit | Loss in dialysis<br>Decreased intake due to restriction of $K^+$-containing fruits and vegetables | Gingivitis<br>Petechiae, ecchymoses | Serum ascorbate <0.4 mg/dl |
| $B_6$ deficit | Failure of the diseased kidney to activate vitamin $B_6$<br>Loss in dialysis | Dermatitis<br>Ataxia<br>Irritability, seizures | Plasma pyridoxal phosphate <34 nmol (normal values not well established) |
| Folic acid | Loss in dialysis<br>Decreased intake resulting from restriction of meats, fruits, and vegetables | Glossitis (inflamed tongue)<br>Pallor | Hematocrit <37% (women) or 42% (men), elevated MCV<br>Serum folate <6 ng/ml |

ings and Aminosyn RF (Abbott), RenAmin (Travenol), and Nephramine (Kendall McGaw) for use in preparation in TPN. Reliance on these solutions may delay the need for dialysis. However, it is not clear that outcome is improved in patients receiving essential amino acid preparations, and many physicians now recommend the use of more balanced preparations, containing both essential and nonessential amino acids, in settings in which dialysis is available.[85,86] For the stressed, catabolic renal patient, provision of adequate amounts of all types of amino acids required for anabolism appears to be more important than delaying initiation of dialysis.

Some nephrologists advocate the use of ketoanalogues (carbon structures related to the amino acids, but lacking the amine group) rather than or in addition to essential amino acids. Patients can form amino acids from the ketoanalogues and circulating nitrogenous compounds. Use of ketoanalogues requires reduction of protein intake to at least 0.4 g/kg/day.[91,93] Because these compounds are relatively unpalatable, they may need to be given by tube.

***Fluid.*** Patients are usually limited to a fluid intake resulting in a gain of no more than 0.45 kg (1 pound) per day on the days between dialysis. This generally means a daily intake of 500 ml plus the volume lost in urine, diarrhea, and vomitus. With the use of continuous peritoneal dialysis, hemofiltration, or arteriovenous hemodialysis, the fluid intake can be liberalized. A liberal fluid allowance permits more adequate nutrient delivery, whether by oral, tube, or parenteral feedings. Enteral formulas providing 2 calories/ml or more, such as Nutrisource (Sandoz), TwoCal HN (Ross), Isocal HCN (Mead Johnson), and Magnacal (Biosearch), are useful in providing a concentrated source of calories for tube-fed patients who require fluid restriction. Intravenous lipids, particularly 20% emulsions, can be used to supply concentrated calories for the TPN patient.

***Calories.*** It is essential that the renal patient receive adequate amounts of calories to prevent catabolism of body tissues to meet energy needs. Catabolism not only reduces the mass of muscle and other functional body tissues but also releases nitrogen that must be excreted by the kidney. Adults with renal failure need about 35 to 45 calories/kg/day, compared with the 25 to 30 calories/kg needed by healthy adults, in order to prevent catabolism and ensure that all protein consumed is used for anabolism rather than to meet energy needs. After renal transplantation, when the patient usually receives large doses of corticosteroids, it is especially important to ensure that adequate caloric intake continue to prevent undue catabolism.[94]

High-carbohydrate foods such as hard candies, sugar, honey, jelly, jellybeans, and gumdrops are often used as a means of supplying calories to the patient with renal failure, because these foods are low in sodium and potassium, which are retained in renal failure. However, hypertriglyceridemia is found in a substantial number of patients with renal disorders. This condition is worsened by excessive intake of simple refined sugars such as sucrose (table sugar) or glucose. To help control hypertriglyceridemia, only about 35% of the patient's calories should come from carbohydrates, with the emphasis placed on complex carbohydrates (starches and fibers). Breads, pastas, and cereals can provide most of these complex carbohydrates, with some also being supplied by vegetables. (In general, bread and pasta made from white flour are preferred, because the bran portion of grains is high in phosphorus. Low-protein breads, pasta, and cereals are available for cases in which regular products would provide excessive amounts of protein.) When glucose is used as the osmotic agent in peritoneal dialysis and arteriovenous hemodialysis, approximately 70% of the glucose in the dialysate may be absorbed, and this must be considered part of the patient's carbohydrate intake.[85,90] For the tube-fed patient, enteral formulas that contain some fiber, such as Compleat (Sandoz) and Enrich (Ross), may help to control hypertriglyceridemia.

To help control hypertriglyceridemia and to provide concentrated calories in minimal fluid, fat should supply about half or more of the patient's calories. Because hypercholesterolemia is frequently found in patients with renal failure, polyunsaturated fats and oils—corn, soy, cottonseed, safflower, and sunflower—are preferred over saturated fats, which tend to raise cholesterol levels. The necessary restriction of meat, milk, and other protein foods in the diet will help to lower cholesterol and saturated fat intake. For patients who need a caloric supplement, Lipomul (Upjohn) is a palatable oral lipid supplement providing 6 calories/ml with minimal sodium and potassium. Intravenous lipids and the long-chain fats found in most enteral formulas, except those prepared from blended foods, are primarily polyunsaturated. Some formulas are rich in medium-chain triglycerides, or fats. Although these triglycerides are saturated, they do not contribute to hypercholesterolemia and thus may be used for the renal patient.

***Other nutrients.*** Table 6-11 is a summary of the recommended nutrient intake for patients with renal disorders, where recommendations are different from those for healthy adults. The recommendations for healthy adults are included to provide a basis for comparison. Certain nutrients are restricted because they are excreted by the kidney. Phosphorus is one example; its restriction appears to delay progression of renal damage.[92] Phosphorus is found primarily in meat, milk, nuts, and whole grains, so that limitation of protein intake will also help to lower phosphorus levels. The patient has no specific requirement for the fat-soluble vitamins A, E, and K because they are not removed in appreciable amounts by dialysis, and restriction prevents development of toxicity. Elevated levels of vitamin A are a common finding in dialyzed patients.[87,88] On the other hand, needs for several water-soluble vitamins and trace minerals are increased in the dialysis patient because they are small enough to pass freely through the dialysis filter. If the patient is not receiving supplements of the water-soluble vitamins listed in Table 6-11, or, if levels of trace elements are not being monitored, the nurses should consult with the physician about the need for such measures. Similarly, if the patient is receiving vitamin A–containing TPN or tube feed-

***Table 6-11*** Daily nutritional recommendations for patients with renal failure

| Nutrient | Recommended dietary allowance (RDA) for healthy persons | Daily amount in renal failure |
|---|---|---|
| Protein or amino acids (g/kg) | 0.8 | 0.6 (undialyzed)* |
| | | 1-1.2+ (hemodialysis)* |
| | | 1.2-1.4+ (peritoneal dialysis)* |
| Calories/kg | 25-30 | 35-45 |
| Electrolytes and minerals† | | |
| Sodium | Unspecified | 87-109 mEq (2-2.5 g)‡ |
| Potassium | Unspecified | 70-80 mEq (2.7-3.1 g) |
| Calcium (mg) | 800 | 1000-1500 |
| Phosphorus (mg) | 800 | 700-800 |
| Magnesium (mg) | 280-350 | 200-300 |
| Trace minerals | | |
| Iron (mg) | 10-15 | 15 mg +, as needed to prevent deficiency |
| Zinc (mg) | 12-15 | 15 mg +, as needed to prevent deficiency |
| Vitamins | | |
| C (mg) | 60 | 70-100 |
| $B_6$ (mg) | 1.6-2 | 5-10 |
| Folic acid (mg) | .18-.2 | 1 |

Adapted from Feinstein EI: Nutr Clin Prac 3:9, 1988; Kopple JD and Blumenkrantz MJ: Kidney Int (suppl) 16:S295, 1983; and Maschio G and others: Kidney Int 22:371, 1982.
*Based on estimated dry weight.
†Dosages given are representative ranges; serum levels and physical findings help to determine actual individual intake. For instance, the presence of edema and hypertension usually necessitates a reduced sodium allowance. These are enteral recommendations, and parenteral levels may be lower.
‡Levels for continuous ambulatory peritoneal dialysis (CAPD) may be higher.

ing daily, the nurse can discuss with the physician, pharmacist, and dietitian the desirability of devising nutrient solutions providing only the water-soluble vitamins.

## Nutrition in Gastrointestinal Alterations

Because the gastrointestinal (GI) tract is so inherently related to nutrition, it is not surprising that catastrophic occurrences in the GI tract—hemorrhage, perforation, infarct, or related organ failure—have acute and severe adverse effects on nutritional status.

**Nutritional assessment in gastrointestinal alterations.** Assessment is summarized in Table 6-12. The area and amount of the GI tract affected determine, to a large extent, the likelihood and degree of nutritional deficits. The ileum

***Table 6-12*** Gastrointestinal nutritional assessment

| Area of concern | History | Physical assessment | Laboratory data |
|---|---|---|---|
| Protein-calorie malnutrition | Decreased oral intake caused by:<br>Fear of symptoms—pain, cramping, diarrhea—associated with eating (e.g., peptic ulcer, dumping syndrome)<br>Alcohol abuse<br>Nausea, vomiting, anorexia<br>Increased losses because of:<br>Maldigestion or malabsorption (e.g., inadequate bile salt production, increased loss of bile salts in short bowel syndrome, diarrhea, inadequate absorptive area in short bowel syndrome)<br>GI bleeding<br>Fistula drainage<br>Increased requirements caused by:<br>Needs for healing (e.g., surgical wounds, fistulae) | Muscle wasting<br>Loss of subcutaneous fat<br>Weight <90% of desirable or recent weight loss<br>Triceps skinfold <10th percentile*<br>Hair loss or change in texture | Serum albumin <3.5 g/dl or low transferrin<br>Total lymphocyte count <1200/mm³<br>Creatinine excretion <17 mg/kg/day (women) or 23 mg/kg/day (men)<br>Negative nitrogen balance<br>Fecal fat >5 g/day or >5% of intake |
| Potential fluid volume deficit | Losses caused by severe vomiting or diarrhea (e.g., GI obstruction, short bowel syndrome) | Poor skin turgor<br>Dry, sticky mucous membranes<br>Complaint of thirst<br>Loss of ≥0.23 kg (0.5 pounds) in 24 hr | Hct >52% (men) or 47% (women)<br>BUN >20 mg/dl<br>Serum sodium >145 mEq/L<br>Serum osmolality >300 mOsm/kg<br>Urine specific gravity >1.030 |
| **DISORDERS OF MINERAL/ELECTROLYTE NUTRITURE** | | | |
| Calcium (Ca) | Increased loss because of steatorrhea (Ca forms soaps with fat in the stool and thus becomes unabsorbable) | Tingling of fingers<br>Muscular tetany and cramps<br>Carpopedal spasm<br>Convulsions | Serum Ca <8.5 mg/dl (Severe deficits only) |
| Magnesium (Mg) | Inadequate intake because of poor diet in alcoholism<br>Increased losses because of:<br>Diarrhea or steatorrhea<br>Loss of small bowel fluid (e.g., in short bowel syndrome, fistulae) | Tremor<br>Hyperactive deep reflexes<br>Convulsions | Serum Mg <1.5 mEq/L |

Adapted from Moore MC: Pocket guide to nutrition and diet therapy, St Louis, 1988, Mosby–Year Book, Inc. *Continued.*

*hct, hematocrit; BUN, blood urea nitrogen; hgb, hemoglobin; MCV, mean cell volume; MCH, mean cell hemoglobin; MCHC, mean cell hemoglobin concentration; Ca, calcium.*

**6 mm for men and 14 mm for women.*

*Table 6-12* Gastrointestinal nutritional assessment—cont'd

| Area of concern | History | Physical assessment | Laboratory data |
|---|---|---|---|
| Iron (Fe) | Blood loss<br>Impaired absorption because of decreased upper GI acidity with gastrectomy or use of antacids and cimetidine<br>Inadequate intake (e.g., restriction of protein foods in hepatic failure) | Pallor, blue sclerae<br>Fatigue<br>Koilonychia | Hct <42% (men) or 37% (women), hgb <14 g/dl (men) or 12 g/dl (women), low MCV, MCH, MCHC<br>Serum Fe <60 μg/dl |
| Zinc (Zn) | Increased losses caused by:<br>Diarrhea, steatorrhea<br>Loss of small bowel fluid<br>Diuretic use (in hepatic failure)<br>Increased urinary losses in alcoholism<br>Inadequate intake caused by:<br>Protein restriction in hepatic failure<br>Poor diet in alcoholism | Anorexia<br>Hypogeusia, dysgeusia<br>Seborrheic dermatitis | Serum Zn <60 μg/ml |
| Potassium ($K^+$) | Increased loss caused by:<br>Diarrhea<br>Diuretic use<br>Hyperaldosteronism (in hepatic failure)<br>GI suction | Muscle weakness, ileus<br>Diminished reflexes | Serum $K^+$ <3.5 mEq/L |
| **DISORDERS OF VITAMIN NUTRITURE** | | | |
| A | Increased loss in steatorrhea (vitamin A dissolves in fatty stools)<br>Impaired release of vitamin A from storage in the liver because of inadequate production of retinol-binding protein, the transport protein, in malnutrition or liver failure) | Drying of skin and cornea<br>Poor wound healing<br>Follicular hyperkeratosis (resembles gooseflesh) | Serum retinol <20 μg/dl |
| K | Impaired absorption in steatorrhea<br>Decreased production because of destruction of intestinal bacteria by antibiotic usage | Petechiae, ecchymoses<br>Prolonged bleeding | Prothrombin time >12.5 sec (not accurate in liver failure) |

is among the most nutritionally important areas. Fat and bile salt absorption occur in this area, as does absorption of fat-soluble vitamins and vitamin $B_{12}$. Patients with ileal disease or resection are likely to become malnourished as a result of significant loss of calories, as well as vitamins and minerals, in the feces. The ileocecal valve is especially critical in maintaining adequate nutrition. Not only does it slow entry of GI contents into the large bowel, allowing more time for absorption to take place in the small bowel, but it also helps prevent migration of the microorganisms from the large bowel into the small bowel. Proliferating microorganisms in the small bowel deconjugate the bile salts, impairing fat absorption. Deconjugated bile salts also irritate the intestinal mucosa and raise the osmolality within the bowel, promoting diarrhea.[100]

**Nutrition intervention in gastrointestinal alterations.** The GI tract is the preferred route for delivery of nutrients in GI disease, as it is in all other disease states. However, following damage or resection, enteral nutrition support may be inadequate or impossible, at least temporarily. Nursing care of patients receiving enteral feedings and TPN has already been described. Since bowel resection and hepatic failure are two of the most nutritionally challenging GI alterations, most of this discussion will be devoted to them.

***Short bowel syndrome (bowel resection)***

**ADMINISTRATION OF FLUIDS AND ELECTROLYTES.** Extensive

bowel resection is associated with marked gastric hypersecretion. The increase in gastric juices, coupled with the sudden loss of absorptive area, results in the loss of several liters of fluid daily, along with potassium, magnesium, and zinc. The nurse's role in management of these patients includes (1) strict intake and output records, including volume or weight of stools if they are frequent or loose, (2) ongoing assessment of the patient's state of hydration, and (3) administration of fluids and electrolytes and evaluation of the patient's response, including daily weight measurements to evaluate the adequacy of fluid replacement.

**ADMINISTRATION OF NUTRITION SUPPORT.** The major nutritional problems associated with bowel resection are loss of absorptive area, with increased fecal losses of fluids, electrolytes, fat, protein, and other nutrients; increased loss of bile salts, especially if the terminal ileum was resected, with further malabsorption of fat; and micronutrient deficiencies resulting from trapping of minerals and fat-soluble vitamins within the excreted fat. Following bowel resection, the remaining intestine undergoes marked hyperplasia, with increasing length of the remaining villi, which increases the available absorptive area. The result is improved absorption of water, electrolytes, and glucose.[98] Some patients with 70% to 80% resection of the small bowel can eventually be maintained on enteral feedings only, especially if the terminal ileum and ileocecal valve are retained, but patients with resection of more than 90% of the small bowel usually require permanent TPN.[96,100] The small bowel is estimated to be approximately 350 to 650 cm in length, depending on whether measurements are made during surgery, when the GI tract retains much of the muscle tonus, or on postmortem examination, when minimal tone is present.[100] It is difficult to estimate the amount remaining at the time of intestinal resection, and thus many patients undergo contrast radiographs when stable to determine the length of the remaining bowel. The adaptive response may take up to a year to become complete, and it does not occur without the presence of nutrients within the gut.[98] Therefore every attempt is made to introduce some enteral feedings early in the course of recovery.

Patients are supported with TPN until fecal output declines, usually to less than 1 L/day. At that point, very small amounts of enteral feedings are begun. Feedings may consist of an elemental, or predigested, diet given by tube. Fat is the most difficult nutrient to absorb, and the formula will ordinarily be very low in fat or will be high in medium-chain triglycerides (MCTs), which are more readily absorbed than the long-chain triglycerides predominating in most foods. Tube feedings should be given on a continuous basis, to promote optimal absorption. Intragastric rather than transpyloric feedings are preferable to utilize every available centimeter of intestinal surface area. Alternatively, a low-fat, high-starch diet may be given by mouth. Foods such as white rice; enriched white bread and toast; plain pasta; and peeled boiled or baked potato, without added milk, cheese, butter, margarine, or other fat are examples of those allowed initially. Low-fat meats such as chicken without skin are gradually added, and then small amounts of fruits and vegetables are introduced.[97] Lactose, or milk sugar, is often tolerated poorly by patients with bowel resection, but low-fat cottage cheese or yogurt, which are relatively low in lactose, may be tolerated. MCTs can be served in juice or used in food preparation to increase caloric intake. Patients receiving oral feedings often require much encouragement to eat, because they may associate eating with worsening of diarrhea. As more and more enteral intake is tolerated, TPN is gradually tapered. Careful records must be kept of all enteral and parenteral intake to determine when TPN can be decreased or discontinued.

**ADMINISTRATION OF MEDICATIONS.** The nurse may need to discuss with the physician the possibility of using medications to control severe, watery diarrhea. In some patients with short bowel syndrome, in whom diarrhea is prolonged or especially severe and causes anal excoriation or copious ostomy output, antidiarrheal agents such as diphenoxylate with atropine or codeine may be beneficial. Anticholinergic drugs such as glycopyrrolate can also be used to counteract the gastric hypersecretion.

***Hepatic failure.*** Hepatic failure is associated with a wide spectrum of metabolic alterations. Because the diseased liver has impaired ability to deactivate hormones, there are elevated levels of circulating glucagon, epinephrine, and cortisol. These hormones promote catabolism of body tissues. Glycogen stores are rapidly exhausted. Although release of lipids from their storage depots is accelerated, the liver has decreased ability to metabolize them for energy. Furthermore, as many as half of the patients with hepatic failure may have malabsorption of fat because of inadequate production of bile salts by the liver. Therefore body proteins are increasingly utilized for energy sources, producing rapid tissue wasting. The branched chain amino acids (BCAA), leucine, isoleucine, and valine, are especially well utilized for energy, and their levels in the blood decline. Conversely, levels of the aromatic amino acids (AAA), phenylalanine, tyrosine, and tryptophan, rise as a result of tissue catabolism and impaired ability of the liver to clear them from the blood. While hyperammonemia is a feature of hepatic failure, it probably is not the causative agent in encephalopathy; instead, AAAs appear to be the culprits. After transport across the blood-brain barrier, they can be converted to "false neurotransmitters," which compete with the normal neurotransmitters for binding sites. The net result is to impede normal neurotransmission and produce hepatic encephalopathy.[102]

**MONITORING OF FLUID AND ELECTROLYTE STATUS.** Ascites and edema occur because of decreased colloid osmotic pressure in the plasma as the diseased liver produces less albumin and other plasma proteins, increased portal pressure caused by obstruction, and renal sodium retention from secondary hyperaldosteronism. To control the fluid retention, restriction of sodium (usually 500 to 1500 mg, or 20 to 65 mEq, daily) and fluid (1500 ml or less) is generally necessary, in conjunction with administration of diuretics. Patients must be weighed daily to evaluate the success of treatment. In addition, laboratory and physical status must be closely observed for potassium deficits caused by diuretic therapy and hyperaldosteronism.

## Nutrition in Endocrine Alterations

Because of the far-reaching effects on all body systems, endocrine alterations have an impact on nutritional status in a variety of ways.

**Nutritional assessment in endocrine alterations.** The nutritional assessment process is summarized in Table 6-13. Because of the prevalence of non–insulin-dependent diabetes mellitus (NIDDM) patients among the hospitalized population, the nutritional problems most commonly noted in patients with endocrine alterations are overweight and obesity.

**Nutrition intervention in endocrine alterations**

***Underweight and malnourished patients.*** The most severely undernourished patients are usually those with pancreatitis, because of loss of pancreatic exocrine function. Pancreatic insufficiency, with inadequate release of trypsin, chymotrypsin, and pancreatic lipase and amylase, results in impaired digestion and subsequent loss of nutrients in the stool. Fat malabsorption is the most marked effect of pancreatic insufficiency. Fat lost in the stools is accompanied by calcium, zinc, and other minerals, along with the fat-soluble vitamins. Nutritional care in malabsorptive disorders is discussed more thoroughly in the section concerning nutrition in gastrointestinal alterations.

Patients with insulin-dependent diabetes mellitus (IDDM) or endocrine dysfunction caused by pancreatitis often have weight loss and malnutrition as a result of tissue catabolism, because they cannot utilize dietary carbohydrate to meet energy needs. Although patients with NIDDM are more

***Table 6-13*** Endocrine nutritional assessment

| Area of concern | History | Physical findings | Laboratory data |
|---|---|---|---|
| Underweight or protein-calorie malnutrition | Increased losses of calories in urine or feces caused by:<br>Impaired glucose metabolism and glucosuria in type I diabetes mellitus<br>Steatorrhea in pancreatitis<br>Decreased intake because of:<br>Discomfort with eating (in pancreatitis)<br>Alcoholism (often a cause of pancreatitis) | Weight less than 90% of desirable<br>Recent weight loss<br>Wasting of muscle and subcutaneous tissue<br>Triceps skinfold <10th percentile* | Urine glucose >0.5%<br>Fecal fat >5 g/24 hr or >5% of intake<br>Serum albumin <3.5 g/dl, or low transferrin or prealbumin levels<br>Total lymphocyte count <1200/mm³<br>Creatinine excretion <17 mg/kg/day (women) or 23 mg/kg/day (men) |
| Overweight | NIDDM<br>Sedentary lifestyle | Weight >120% of desirable<br>Triceps skinfold >90th percentile† | |
| Potential fluid volume deficit | Diuresis (from diabetes insipidus or osmotic diuresis of HHNK or ketoacidosis) | Poor skin turgor<br>Dry, sticky mucous membranes<br>Thirst<br>Loss of >0.23 kg (0.5 pounds) in 24 hr<br>Increased urine output | Serum glucose >250 mg/dl<br>Urine glucose >0.5%<br>Serum sodium >145 mEq/L<br>Increasing hct<br>BUN >20 mg/dl |
| Potential fluid volume excess | Fluid retention caused by SIADH | Edema (peripheral and/or pulmonary)<br>Gain of >0.23 kg (0.5 pounds) in 24 hr | Serum sodium <135 mEq/L<br>Decreasing hct |
| Potential zinc deficiency | Impaired absorption in steatorrhea<br>Increased urinary losses in diuresis, diabetes mellitus, and alcoholism<br>Poor intake in alcoholism | Hypogeusia, dysgeusia<br>Alopecia<br>Seborrheic dermatitis<br>Impaired wound healing | Serum zinc <60 μg/ml |

Adapted from Moore MC: Pocket guide to nutrition and diet therapy, St Louis, 1988, Mosby–Year Book, Inc..
Hct, hematocrit; BUN, blood urea nitrogen; SIADH, syndrome of inappropriate secretion of antidiuretic hormone; NIDDM, non-insulin–dependent diabetes mellitus.
*6 mm for men and 14 mm for women.
†20 mm for men and 34 mm for women.

likely to be overweight than underweight, they too may become malnourished as a result of chronic or acute infections, trauma, major surgery, or other illnesses. Delivery of nutrition support in these patients, especially control of blood glucose, can be challenging. Blood glucose should be monitored regularly, usually several times a day until the patient is stable. Regular insulin added to the solution is the most common method of managing hyperglycemia in the patient receiving TPN. The dosage required is almost always larger than the patient's usual subcutaneous dose, because some of the insulin adheres to glass bottles and plastic bags or administration sets. Continuous subcutaneous infusion of insulin may also be used. Hyperglycemia is also a common problem in tube-fed patients, particularly when feedings are given continuously. Twice-daily doses of intermediate-acting insulin or more frequent doses of regular insulin may be inadequate to control hyperglycemia in continuously fed patients. One solution is to administer feedings intermittently, on a "meal-type" schedule, and to administer oral hypoglycemics, regular insulin, or intermediate-acting insulin based on this schedule.[113] However, some diabetic patients require continuous feedings. For example, patients with severe gastroparesis may need transpyloric feedings because poor gastric emptying makes intragastric feedings impossible or inadequate. Transpyloric feedings must almost always be given continuously, since dumping syndrome and poor absorption often occur if feedings are given rapidly into the small bowel. For the continuously tube-fed diabetic patient, control of blood glucose may be improved either with continuous insulin infusion or by use of a formula containing fiber, if possible. Examples are Compleat (Sandoz) and Enrich (Ross). Fiber slows the absorption of the carbohydrate in the formula, producing a more delayed and sustained glycemic response.

***Overweight patients.*** Aggressive attempts at weight loss are rarely warranted among very ill patients, although weight loss in overweight patients with NIDDM improves glucose tolerance. Instead of suggesting a low-calorie diet, nurses should encourage patients to select foods providing fiber and starches (for example, dried beans and peas, whole-grain breads and cereals, pasta, fresh fruits and vegetables) rather than more refined carbohydrates (for example, white bread, fruit juice, and "instant" mashed potatoes). Diets rich in complex carbohydrates have been shown to lower insulin requirements, increase the sensitivity of the peripheral tissues to insulin, and decrease serum cholesterol levels.[108] Although results of studies of the use of high-fiber diets in an effort to promote weight loss are inconclusive,[115] it appears that reliance on bulky, high-fiber foods may help to reduce caloric intake.[107,112] Weight loss may occur because fiber delays gastric emptying and increases satiety, so the patient is satisfied with less food. Also, absorption of nutrients such as starch and fats from a high-fiber diet may be less complete than absorption from a low-fiber diet.[112,117]

Nutrition support should not be neglected simply because a patient is obese, because protein-calorie malnutrition develops even among such patients. When a patient is not expected to be able to eat for at least 5 to 7 days, or inadequate intake persists for that period of time, the nurse should consult with the physician regarding initiation of tube feedings or TPN if no steps have been taken to do so. There is no disease process that benefits from starvation, and development or progression of nutritional deficits may contribute to complications (for example, decubitus ulcers, pulmonary or urinary tract infections, and sepsis, which prolong hospitalization, increase the costs of care, and may even result in death[111,114,116]).

## REFERENCES

### Nutritional Assessment and Support


1. American Society for Parenteral and Enteral Nutrition: Guidelines for use of total parenteral nutrition in the hospitalized adult patient, J Parent Ent Nutr 10:441, 1986.
2. American Society for Parenteral and Enteral Nutrition: Standards for nutrition support: hospitalized patients, Nutr Clin Prac 3:28, 1988.
3. Brinson R, Curtis WD, and Singh M: Diarrhea in the intensive care unit: the role of hypoalbuminemia and the response to a peptide-based, chemically defined diet, J Am Coll Nutr 6:517, 1987.
4. Coale M and Robson J: Dietary management of intractable diarrhea in malnourished patients, J Am Diet Assoc 76:444, 1980.
5. Crocker KS and others: Microbial growth comparisons of five commercial parenteral lipid emulsions, J Parent Ent Nutr 8:391, 1984.
6. Crocker KS and others: Microbial growth in clinically used enteral delivery systems, Am J Infect Control 14:250, 1986.
7. Cutie AJ, Altman E, and Lenkel L: Compatibility of enteral products with commonly employed drug additives, J Parent Ent Nutr 7:186, 1983.
8. D'Angio R and others: The growth of microorganisms in total parenteral nutrition admixtures, J Parent Ent Nutr 11:394, 1987.
9. Donowitz LG and others: Alteration of normal gastric flora in critical care patients receiving antacid and cimetidine therapy, Infect Control 7:23, 1986.
10. Driver AG and LeBrun M: Iatrogenic malnutrition in patients receiving ventilatory support, JAMA 244:2195, 1980.
11. Flynn KT, Norton LC, and Fisher RL: Enteral tube feeding: indications, practices and outcomes, Image J Nurs Sch 19:16, 1987.
12. Goldman DA and Maki DG: Infection control in total parenteral nutrition, JAMA 223:1360, 1973.
13. Hiebert JM and others: Comparison of continuous vs intermittent tube feedings in adult burn patients, J Parent Ent Nutr 5:73, 1981.
14. Kagawa-Busby KS and others: Effects of diet temperature on tolerance of enteral feedings, Nurs Res 29:276, 1980.
15. Kamath SK and others: Hospital malnutrition: a 33-hospital screening study, J Am Diet Assoc 86:203, 1986.
16. Kellam B, Fraze DE, and Kanarek KS: Central line dressing material and neonatal skin integrity, Nutr Clin Prac 3:65, 1988.
17. Keohane P and others: Relation between osmolality of diet and gastrointestinal side effects in enteral nutrition, Br Med J 288:678, 1984.
18. Kittinger JW, Sandler RS, and Heizer WD: Efficacy of metoclopramide as an adjunct to duodenal placement of small-bore feeding tubes: a randomized, placebo-controlled, double-blind study, J Parent Ent Nutr 11:33, 1987.
19. Levenson R and others: Do weighted nasoenteric feeding tubes facilitate duodenal intubations? J Parent Ent Nutr 12:135, 1988.
20. Lipman TO, Kessler T, and Arabian A: Nasopulmonary intubation with feeding tubes: case reports and review of the literature, J Parent Ent Nutr 9:618, 1985.
21. Marcuard SP: Dissolution of clotted enteral feeding, J Parent Ent Nutr 11:16S, 1987.
22. Marcuard SP and Perkins AM: Clogging of feeding tubes, J Parent Ent Nutr 12:403, 1988.

23. Metheny N: Measures to test placement of nasogastric and nasointestinal feeding tubes: A review. Nurs Res 37:324-329, 1988.
24. Metheny N, Eisenberg P, and McSweeney M: Effect of feeding tube properties and three irrigants on clogging rates, Nurs Res 37:165, 1988.
25. Metheny NA, Eisenberg P, and Spies M: Aspiration pneumonia in patients fed through nasoenteral tubes, Heart Lung 15:256, 1986.
26. Metheny NA, Spies MA, and Eisenberg P: Measures to test placement of nasoenteral feeding tubes, West J Nurs Res 10:367, 1988.
27. Nicholson LJ: Declogging small-bore feeding tubes, J Parent Ent Nutr 11:594, 1987.
28. Niemiec PW and others: Gastrointestinal disorders caused by medication and electrolyte solution osmolality during enteral nutrition, J Parent Ent Nutr 7:387, 1983.
29. Payne-James JJ and others: Enteral tube design and its effect on spontaneous transpyloric passage and duration of tube usage, J Parent Ent Nutr 12:21S, 1988.
30. Pemberton LB and others: Sepsis from triple- vs single-lumen catheters during total parenteral nutrition in surgical or critically ill patients, Arch Surg 121:591, 1986.
31. Powell C and others: Op-Site dressing study: a prospective randomized study evaluating povidone iodine ointment and extension set changes with 7-day Op-Site dressings applied to total parenteral nutrition subclavian sites, J Parent Ent Nutr 9:443, 1985.
32. Powell C, Fabri PJ, and Kudsk KA: Risk of infection accompanying the use of single-lumen vs double-lumen subclavian catheters: a prospective randomized study, J Parent Ent Nutr 12:127, 1988.
33. Taylor TT: A comparison of two methods of nasogastric tube feedings, J Neurosurg Nurs 14:49, 1982.
34. Treloar DM and Stechmiller J: Pulmonary aspiration in tube-fed patients with artificial airways, Heart Lung 13:667, 1984.
35. Valentine RJ and Turner WW: Pleural complications of nasoenteric feeding tubes, J Parent Ent Nutr 9:605, 1985.
36. Wagman LD and others: The effect of acute discontinuation of total parenteral nutrition, Ann Surg 204:524, 1986.
37. Warnold I and Lundhold K: Clinical significance of preoperative nutritional status in 215 noncancer patients, Ann Surg 199:299, 1984.
38. Weinsier RL and others: Hospital malnutrition: a prospective evaluation of general medical patients during the course of hospitalization, Am J Clin Nutr 32:418, 1979.
39. Weizman Z, Schmueli A, and Deckelbaum RJ: Continuous nasogastric drip elemental feeding: alternative for prolonged parenteral nutrition in severe prolonged diarrhea, Am J Dis Child 137:253, 1983.
40. Whatley K and others: When does metoclopramide facilitate transpyloric intubation? J Parent Ent Nutr 8:679, 1984.
41. Wrobel J and Bodin T: Are serum albumin levels detrimental to enteral formulation tolerance? J Parent Ent Nutr 12:21S, 1988.
42. Young GP and others: Catheter sepsis during parenteral nutrition: the safety of long-term OpSite dressings, J Parent Ent Nutr 12:365, 1988.

## Nutrition in Cardiovascular Alterations

43. American Heart Association: Dietary guidelines for healthy American adults, Dallas, 1986, The Association.
44. Bagatell CJ and Heymsfield SB: Effect of meal size on myocardial oxygen requirements: implications for postmyocardial infarction diet, Am J Clin Nutr 39:421, 1984.
45. Kaplan NM: Non-drug treatment of hypertension, Ann Int Med 102:359, 1985.
46. Kelsen SG: The effects of undernutrition on the respiratory muscles, Clin Chest Med 7:101, 1986.
47. Kinsella JE: Food components with potential therapeutic benefits: the n-3 polyunsaturated fatty acids of fish oils, Food Technol 40:89, 1986.
48. Kromhout D, Bosscheiter ED, and deLezenne Coulander C: The inverse relation between fish consumption and 20-year mortality from coronary heart disease, N Engl J Med 312:1205, 1985.
49. Kuhn MM: Nutritional support for the shock patient, Crit Care Nurs Clin North Am 2(2):201, 1990.
50. Myers MG and others: Caffeine as a possible cause of ventricular arrhythmias during the healing phase of acute myocardial infarction, Am J Cardiol 59:1024, 1987.
51. National Cholesterol Education Program: Cholesterol treatment recommendations for adults, Bethesda, Md, 1987, National Heart, Lung, and Blood Institute.
52. National Institutes of Health Consensus Development Conference: Lowering blood cholesterol to prevent heart disease, JAMA 253:2080, 1985.
53. Nonpharmacological approaches to the control of high blood pressure: final report of the subcommittee on nonpharmacological therapy of the 1984 joint national committee on detection, evaluation, and treatment of high blood pressure, Hypertension 8:444, 1986.
54. Poindexter SM, Dear WE, and Dudrick SJ: Nutrition in congestive heart failure, Nutr Clin Prac 1:83, 1986.
55. Rock CL and Coulston AM: Weight-control approaches: a review by the California Dietetic Association, J Am Diet Assoc 88:44, 1988.
56. Schneider JR: Effects of caffeine ingestion on heart rate, blood pressure, myocardial oxygen consumption, and cardiac rhythm in acute myocardial infarction patients, Heart Lung 16:167, 1987.
57. Stevens J: Does dietary fiber affect food intake and body weight? J Am Diet Assoc 88:939, 1988.

## Nutrition in Pulmonary Alterations

58. Flynn KT, Norton LC, and Fisher RL: Enteral tube feeding: indications, practices and outcomes, Image J Nurs Sch 19:16, 1987.
59. Goldstein SA, Thomashow B, and Askanazi J: Functional changes during nutritional repletion in patients with lung disease, Clin Chest Med 7:141, 1986.
60. Hageman JR and Hunt CE: Fat emulsions and lung function, Clin Chest Med 7:69, 1986.
61. Metheney NA, Eisenberg P, and Spies M: Aspiration pneumonia in patients fed through nasoenteral tubes, Heart Lung 15:256, 1986.
62. Rothkopf MM and others: Nutritional support in respiratory failure, Nutr Clin Prac 4(5):166, 1989.
63. Sahebjami H: Nutrition and the pulmonary parenchyma, Clin Chest Med 7:111, 1986.
64. Shanbhogue RLK and others: The nutritional management of a patient on long-term mechanical ventilation, Nutr Clin Prac 2:23, 1987.
65. Taylor TT: A comparison of two methods of nasogastric tube feedings, J Neurosurg Nurs 14:49, 1982.
66. Treloar DM and Stechmiller J: Pulmonary aspiration in tube-fed patients with artificial airways, Heart Lung 13:667, 1984.

## Nutrition in Neurological Alterations

67. Bauer RC: Interference of oral phenytoin absorption by continuous nasogastric feedings, Neurology 32:570, 1982.
68. Clifton GL, Robertson CS, and Constant CF: Enteral hyperalimentation in head injury, J Neurosurg 62:186, 1985.
69. Cox SAR and others: Energy expenditure after spinal cord injury: an evaluation of stable rehabilitating patients, J Trauma 25:419, 1985.
70. Hausmann D and others: Effects of steroid on nitrogen loss and plasma amino acid profiles after head injury, J Parent Ent Nutr 11:10S, 1987.
71. Kiver KF and others: Pre- and post-pyloric enteral feeding: analysis of safety and complications, J Parent Ent Nutr 8:95, 1984.
72. Lander V and others: Enteral feeding during barbiturate coma, Nutr Clin Prac 2:56, 1987.
73. Metheney NM, Eisenberg P, and Spies M: Aspiration pneumonia in patients fed through nasoenteral tubes, Heart Lung 15:256, 1986.
74. Metheny N, Eisenberg P, and McSweeney M: Effect of feeding tube properties and three irrigants on clogging rates, Nurs Res 37:165, 1988.
75. Middaugh PA: Early nutritional management post-head injury, J Head Trauma Rehab 4(4):17, 1989.

76. Norton J and others: Intolerance to enteral feeding in brain injured patients: possible mechanisms, J Parent Ent Nutr 11:10S, 1987.
77. Ott L and others: Does nutritional support affect outcome from severe head injury: a reexamination, J Parent Ent Nutr 11:10S, 1987.
78. Ott L, Young B, and McClain C: The metabolic response to brain injury, J Parent Ent Nutr 11:488, 1987.
79. Rapp RP and others: The favorable effect of early parenteral feeding on survival in head-injured patients, J Neurosurg 58:906, 1983.
80. Saklad JJ, Graves RH, and Sharp WP: Interaction of oral phenytoin with enteral feedings, J Parent Ent Nutr 10:322, 1986.
81. Saltzberg D and others: Pulmonary aspiration during nasogastric (NG) feeding, J Parent Ent Nutr 11:20S, 1987.
82. Shizgal HM and others: Body composition in quadriplegic patients, J Parent Ent Nutr 10:364, 1986.
83. Varella LD: Nutritional support and head trauma, Crit Care Nurse 9(6):28, 1989.

### Nutrition in Renal Alterations

84. Brenner MB, Meyer TW, and Hostetter TH: Dietary protein intake and the progressive nature of kidney disease: the role of hemodynamically mediated glomerular injury in the pathogenesis of progressive glomerular sclerosis in aging, renal ablation and intrinsic renal disease, N Engl J Med 307:652, 1982.
85. Feinstein EI: Total parenteral nutritional support of patients with acute renal failure, Nutr Clin Prac 3:9, 1988.
86. Freund HR and others: The effect of different intravenous nutritional regimens on renal function during acute renal failure in the rat, J Parent Ent Nutr 11:556, 1987.
87. Gleghorn EE and others: Observations of vitamin A toxicity in three patients with renal failure receiving parenteral alimentation, Am J Clin Nutr 44:107, 1986.
88. Johnson KS, Hendricks DG, and Wyse BW: Vitamin A and vitamin E status of hemodialysis patients, Dial Transplan 12:477, 1983.
89. Koo WWK and others: Aluminum in parenteral nutrition solution—sources and possible alternatives, J Parent Ent Nutr 10:591, 1986.
90. Kopple JD and Blumenkrantz MJ: Nutritional requirements for patients undergoing continuous ambulatory peritoneal dialysis, Kidney Int 16(suppl):S295, 1983.
91. Lucas PA and others: The risks and benefits of a low protein–essential amino acid–keto acid diet, Kidney Int 29:995, 1986.
92. Maschio G and others: Effects of dietary protein and phosphorus restriction on the progression of early renal failure, Kidney Int 22:371, 1982.
93. Mitch WE and others: The effect of a ketoacid–amino acid supplement to a restricted diet on the progression of chronic renal failure, N Engl J Med 311:623, 1984.
94. Seagraves A and others: Net protein catabolic rate after kidney transplantation: impact of corticosteroid immunosuppression, J Parent Ent Nutr 10:453, 1986.
95. Twardowski ZJ and Nolph KD: Blood purification in acute renal failure, Ann Int Med 100:447, 1984.

### Nutrition in Gastrointestinal Alterations

96. American Society for Parenteral and Enteral Nutrition Board of Directors: Guidelines for the use of enteral nutrition in the adult patient, J Parent Ent Nutr 11:435, 1987.
97. Beyer PL and Frankenfield DC: Enteral nutrition in extreme short bowel, Nutr Clin Prac 2:60, 1987.
98. Bristol JB and Williamson RCN: Nutrition, operations, and intestinal adaptation, J Parent Ent Nutr 12:299, 1988.
99. Cerra FB and others: Disease-specific amino acid infusion (F080) in hepatic encephalopathy: a prospective, randomized, double-blind, controlled trial, J Parent Ent Nutr 9:288, 1985.
100. Cowan GSM Jr, Luther RW, and Sykes TR: Short bowel syndrome: causes and clinical consequences, Nutr Supp Serv 4:25, 1984.
101. Gulledge AD and others: Psychosocial issues of home parenteral and enteral nutrition, Nutr Clin Prac 2:183, 1987.
102. Hiyama DT and Fischer JE: Nutritional support in hepatic failure: current thought in practice, Nutr Clin Prac 3:96, 1988.
103. Lerebours E and others: Comparison of the effects of continuous and cyclic nocturnal parenteral nutrition on energy expenditure and protein metabolism, J Parent Ent Nutr 12:360, 1988.
104. Millikan WJ Jr and Hooks MA: Nutritional support in hepatic failure: clinical controversies, Nutr Clin Prac 3:94, 1988.
105. Wahren JJ and others: Is intravenous administration of branched chain amino acids effective in the treatment of hepatic encephalopathy? A multicenter study, Hepatology 3:475, 1983.

### Nutrition in Endocrine Alterations

106. American Diabetes Association: Nutritional recommendations and principles for individuals with diabetes mellitus, Diabetes Care 13(1): Suppl. 18, 1990.
107. Anderson JW: High fiber diets for obese diabetic men on insulin therapy: short-term and long-term effects. In Vahouny GV, editor: Dietary fiber and obesity, New York, 1985, Alan R Liss.
108. Anderson JW and others: Dietary fiber and diabetes: a comprehensive review and practical application, J Am Diet Assoc 87:1189, 1987.
109. Bogardus C and others: Effects of physical training and diet therapy on carbohydrate metabolism in patients with glucose intolerance and non–insulin dependent diabetes, Diabetes 33:311, 1984.
110. Franz MJ: Exercise and the management of diabetes mellitus, J Am Diet Assoc 87:872, 1987.
111. Holmes R and others: Serum albumin (SA): a predictor of pressure sores, J Parent Ent Nutr 11:4S, 1987.
112. Krotkiewski M: Effect of guar gum on body weight, hunger ratings and metabolism in obese subjects, Br J Nutr 52:97, 1984.
113. Phillips ML: Enteral nutrition support in diabetes mellitus, Nutr Clin Prac 2:152, 1987.
114. Reilly JJ and others: Economic impact of malnutrition: a model system for hospitalized patients, J Parent Ent Nutr 12:371, 1988.
115. Stevens J: Does dietary fiber affect food intake and body weight? J Am Diet Assoc 88:939, 1988.
116. Warnold I and Lundhold K: Clinical significance of preoperative nutritional status in 215 noncancer patients, Ann Surg 199:299, 1984.
117. Wilmhurst P and Crawley JCW: The measure of gastric transit time using 24-Na and the effects of energy content and guar gum on gastric emptying and satiety, Br J Nutr 44:1, 1980.

UNIT III

# CARDIOVASCULAR ALTERATIONS

CHAPTER 7

# Cardiovascular Assessment and Diagnosis

## CHAPTER OBJECTIVES

- *Use the technique of palpation to thoroughly assess the vascular system.*
- *Locate the cardiac auscultation areas of the precordium.*
- *Verbalize the difference between the first and second heart sounds according to anatomical cause and the auscultation areas where each sound is best heard.*
- *Define and explain the significance of physiological and paradoxical splitting of the second heart sound, ventricular and atrial gallops, and systolic and diastolic murmurs.*
- *Describe the murmurs that may occur after a myocardial infarction.*
- *Describe the difference between central and peripheral cyanosis.*
- *Describe the electrocardiographic changes that occur with hypokalemia and hyperkalemia.*
- *List important aspects of the normal chest radiograph with which the critical care nurse should be familiar.*
- *Describe proper placement of the electrodes for cardiac monitor leads II, $MCL_1$, and $MCL_6$*
- *Explain the three methods for determining cardiac rate from an electrocardiogram.*
- *Explain the important electrocardiographic findings, assessment aspects, and nursing actions for each of the dysrhythmias described in the chapter.*
- *State the expected nursing actions for elevations in the central venous pressure and the pulmonary artery pressure and the pathologies responsible for these elevations.*

## KEY TERMS

central cyanosis, p. 98
peripheral cyanosis, p. 98
jugular venous distention (JVD), p. 99
point of maximal impulse (PMI), p. 101
excitability, p. 109
automaticity, p. 109
contractility, p. 109
resting membrane potential, p. 109
depolarization, p. 111
absolute refractory period, p. 112
sinoatrial (SA) node, p. 114
atrioventricular (AV) node, p. 114
bundle of His, p. 114
Purkinje fibers, p. 114
Holter monitoring, p. 121
phonocardiography, p. 135
echocardiography, p. 135
nuclear magnetic resonance (NMR), p. 137
cardiac output (CO), p. 140
preload, p. 140
afterload, p. 142
inotropy, p. 142
pulmonary artery wedge pressure (PAWP), p. 148
left ventricular end-diastolic pressure (LVEDP), p. 148

The purpose of this chapter is to describe clinical, laboratory, and diagnostic assessment techniques that guide the practitioner in planning and implementing care for the patient with cardiovascular alterations.

Interpretation of this data, combined with the cardiovascular history, enables the critical care team to diagnose, treat, and assess the patient's response to therapeutic interventions.

## CLINICAL ASSESSMENT

### History

The patient history (see the box on p. 98) is important for providing data that contribute to the cardiovascular diagnosis and the treatment plan. The patient's presenting symptoms or complaints should direct the history-taking part of the assessment. Each symptom should be further explored with the questions detailed in Table 7-1. Other symptoms that may be indicative of cardiovascular problems are listed

### DATA COLLECTION FOR CARDIOVASCULAR HISTORY

#### COMMON CARDIOVASCULAR SYMPTOMS

Chest pains
Palpitations
Dyspnea
Cough
Nocturia
Edema
Dizziness/syncope
Claudication

#### PATIENT PROFILE

Personal habits
  Use of tea, coffee, alcohol, recreational drugs; over-the-counter drug use; smoking; exercise; and dietary habits
Lifestyle pattern
  Working, relaxing, coping
Recent life changes
  Within the past 6 months
Emotional state
  Evidence of psychological stress, worry, anxiety
Perception of illness and its meaning for the future

#### RISK FACTORS

Sex/age
Family history
Hypertension
Diabetes mellitus
Obesity
Smoking history
High serum cholesterol
Sedentary lifestyle

#### FAMILY HISTORY

Coronary artery disease
Myocardial infarction
Hypertension
Stroke
Diabetes mellitus
Lipid disorders

#### CARDIAC STUDIES IN PAST

Cardiac catheterization
Cardiac ultrasound
ECG
Exercise tolerance test
Myocardial imaging with radiographic isotopes
Percutaneous transluminal coronary angioplasty
Valvuloplasty

#### PAST MEDICAL HISTORY

Childhood
  Murmurs, cyanosis, streptococcal infections, rheumatic fever
Adult
  Heart failure, coronary artery disease, heart valve disease, mitral valve prolapse, myocardial infarction, peripheral vascular disease, diabetes mellitus, hypertension, hyperlipidemia, dysrythmias, murmurs, endocarditis, psychiatric illnesses
Allergies
  Especially to radiographic contrast agents or iodine
Surgical history
  Coronary artery bypass grafting, valve replacement, peripheral vascular bypasses or repairs

#### CURRENT MEDICATION USAGE

Digitalis
Diuretics
Potassium
Antidysrhythmics
Beta blockers
Calcium channel blockers
Nitrates
Antihypertensives
Anticoagulants

in the box above under "common cardiovascular symptoms" and should be inquired about even if the patient does not complain of them.

## Physical Examination

**Inspection.** Inspection of the cardiovascular system centers on the patient's general appearance—face, extremities, neck, thorax, and abdomen. Important aspects for inspection of the cardiovascular system are listed in the box on p. 99. Inspection for presence of cyanosis is an important component of the examination. **Central cyanosis** is a bluish discoloration of the skin, lips, circumoral area, mucous membranes, and nailbeds. It indicates a decreased oxygen saturation of the circulating hemoglobin molecule and may occur as a result of right-to-left intracardiac shunting, impaired pulmonary function, or hypoxia from any cause.[51] **Peripheral cyanosis** indicates reduction of peripheral blood flow as a result of vascular disease or decreased cardiac output and is usually seen in the nailbeds or the tip of the nose.[51]

Clubbing of the nailbeds is associated with central cyanosis as a sign of chronic oxygen deficiency. Clubbing is evaluated by assessing the angle between the nail and the nail base, which is normally less than 180 degrees. A flattened angle (equaling 180 degrees) with a springy or spongy nail base is "early" clubbing, and an angle greater than 180

***Table 7-1*** Clarification of symptoms by asking specific questions

| Determine | Typical question |
|---|---|
| Location, radiation | Where is it? Does it move or stay in one place? |
| Quality | What's it like? |
| Quantity | How severe is it? How frequent? How long does it last? |
| Chronology | When did it begin? How has it progressed? |
| Aggravating and alleviating factors | What are you doing when it occurs? What do you do to get rid of it? |
| Associated findings | Are there any other symptoms you feel at the same time? |
| Treatment sought and effect | Have you seen a doctor in the past for this same problem? What was the treatment? |

degrees with a swollen nail base is "late" clubbing.

The external jugular vein should be assessed for distention. Normally, in the upright position, the jugular veins are nondistended. **Jugular venous distention** (JVD) occurs when central venous pressure is elevated. The procedure for assessing JVD is as follows. With the patient reclined at a 30- to 45-degree angle, the examiner stands on the patient's right side and turns the patient's head slightly toward the left (Fig. 7-1). If the jugular vein is not visible, light finger pressure is applied across the sternocleidomastoid muscle, just above and parallel to the clavicle. This will fill the external jugular vein by obstructing flow. Once the location of the vein has been identified, the pressure is released and the presence of JVD is assessed. Because inhalation decreases venous pressure, JVD should be assessed at the end of exhalation. Any fullness in the vein extending more than 3 cm above the sternal angle is evidence of increased venous pressure.[51]

**Palpation.** Palpation is a technique that utilizes the sense of touch. The finger tips are sensitive to pressure, the backs of the fingers are sensitive to temperature, and the base of the fingers on the palmar side, as well as the lateral edge of the palm, are sensitive to pressure and vibrations. Palpation is done with a light touch and an unhurried, relaxed approach. The information obtained with palpation reinforces data collected with inspection. Important components for palpation of the cardiovascualr system are delineated in the box on p. 100.

## INSPECTION OF THE CARDIOVASCULAR SYSTEM

### GENERAL APPEARANCE

Weight
Nutritional status
Position of comfort
Color of skin

### FACE

Expression
Emotional state
Presence of diaphoresis
Color of lips
Color of mucous membranes
Color of conjunctiva

### EXTREMITIES

Nailbed color
Nailbed clubbing
Skin color
Skin condition
Hair distribution
Presence of edema
Presence of varicosities
Comparison of circumferences

### EXTERNAL JUGULAR VEIN

### THORAX

Skeletal deformities
Skin condition (scars, bruises, wounds)
Presence of pacemaker generator

### ABDOMEN

Skin conditions (scars, bruises, wounds)
Abdominal aortic pulsation

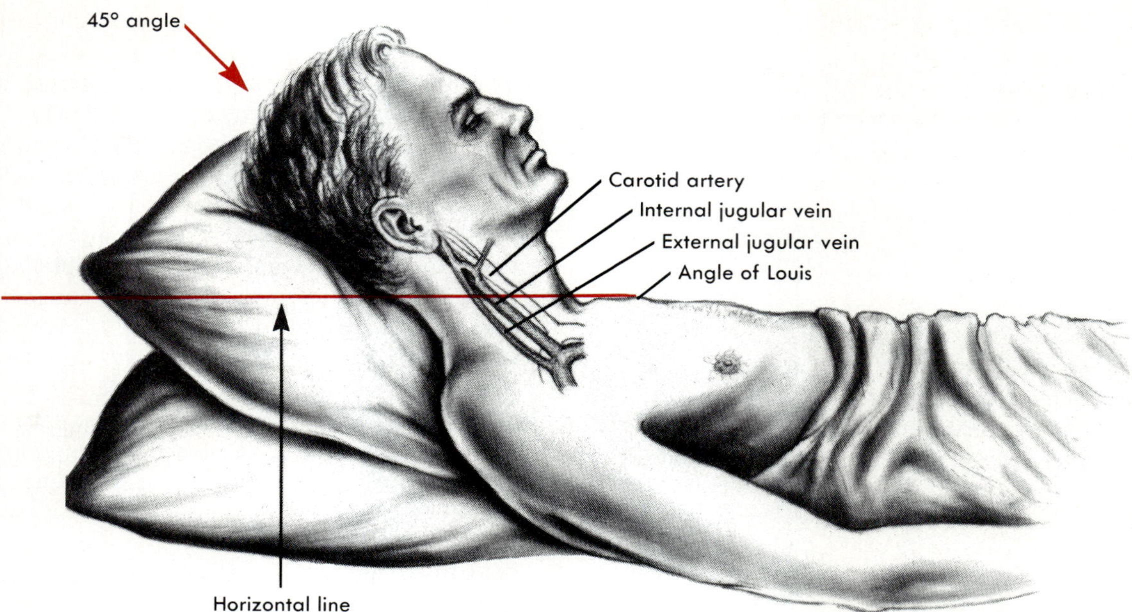


***Fig. 7-1*** Position of the internal and external jugular veins. (From Thompson JM and others: Clinical nursing, ed 2, St Louis, 1989, Mosby–Year Book, Inc.)

Examination of the major arterial areas in the extremities includes bilateral assessment for quality and consistency. The extremity pulses are assessed separately and compared bilaterally to check consistency. Pulse volume is graded on a scale of 0 to 4+.

The radial and the brachial arteries are palpated for pulse quality in the upper extremities. These same arteries are also often punctured or cannulated for arterial blood gas specimens. It is imperative to frequently assess the pulse quality when the artery is cannulated, as well as the color, temperature, and pulse quality distal to the cannulated site. Occlusion of arterial blood flow would be reflected by the absence of a pulse and/or coolness and pallor of the distal extremity. Capillary refill assessment is a maneuver done on the nailbeds to evaluate arterial circulation to the extremity. The nailbed should be compressed to produce blanching, and release of the pressure should result in a return of blood flow and nail color in less than 3 seconds. The severity of arterial insufficiency is directly proportional to the amount of time necessary to reestablish flow and color.

The lower extremity pulses are the most difficult to locate—the popliteal pulses perhaps being the most elusive. The dorsalis pedis pulses and the posterial tibial pulses may be congenitally absent, but their presence is not entirely ruled out until they are checked with the patient's extremity in the dependent position.

Edema of the lower extremities can be caused by heart, liver, or renal failure and venous insufficiency with venous stasis. The amount of edema is quantified by pressing the skin of the feet, ankles, and shins against the underlying bone. If there is an impression left in the tissue when the

## PALPATION OF THE CARDIOVASCULAR SYSTEM

### UPPER EXTREMITIES

Brachial pulses
Radial pulses
Temperature
Capillary refill

### LOWER EXTREMITIES

Popliteal pulses
Posterior tibial pulses
Dorsalis pedis pulses
Edema of feet, ankles, shins
Presence of phlebitis

### NECK

Carotid pulses

### PRECORDIUM

Apical impulse
Other chest pulsations (lifts, thrusts, heaves, thrills)

### ABDOMEN

Femoral pulses
Abdominal aortic pulse

thumb is removed, it is called "pitting edema," and the depth, if quantified, should be recorded in millimeters.

The veins of the lower extremities are assessed with palpation, specifically for thrombophlebitis. By squeezing or pressing the calves against the tibia, pain or tenderness or increased firmness or tension in the muscle may be elicited. These signs suggest phlebitis and should alert the examiner to check other parameters that may aid the diagnosis, such as comparing leg circumferences, checking for increased heat in the extremity or for unexplained fever or tachycardia. Homan's sign, in the company of the other signs, can assist the diagnosing of phlebitis.[51] To elicit Homan's sign, the patient's knee should be flexed, and the examiner should forcefully and abruptly dorsiflex the patient's foot. The sign is positive when there is reported pain in the popliteal region and the calf.

The carotid pulses are assessed by palpation for cardiac rate and rhythm. With an increased pulse pressure, such as that which occurs with hyperdynamic states such as fever, anxiety, hyperthyroidism, anemia, and exercise, the carotid pulse is large and "bounding." Aortic insufficiency can also cause a bounding pulse because of the rapid runoff of blood through the incompetent valve. If the carotid pulse is regular and alternates between bounding and weak pulse palpations with every other pulse being weak, it is called *pulsus alterans*. Pulsus alterans indicates left-sided heart failure.

If blood flow through the carotid arteries is compromised at all by arteriosclerosis or plaques, palpation could easily cause total occlusion; thus only one carotid artery at a time should be palpated. Also, they should be palpated in the lower half of the neck, well below the level of the carotid bodies, which, when stimulated, cause a decrease in heart rate.

The anterior thorax must be inspected for the apical impulse, sometimes referred to as the **point of maximal impulse** (PMI). The apical impulse occurs as the left ventricle contracts during systole and rotates forward causing the left ventricular apex to hit the chest wall. The impulse is a quick, localized (2 × 2 cm), outward movement normally located just lateral to the left midclavicular line at the fifth intercostal space in the adult patient (Fig. 7-2). The apical impulse is the only normal pulsation palpated on the chest wall, and the location, size, and character should be noted.

Once the apical impulse has been examined, the entire precordium (the chest area overlying the heart and great vessels) must be assessed for other pulsations. The terminology used to communicate palpatory findings should describe as accurately as possible the sensation the examiner feels. Generally speaking, accepted terminology refers to "thrusts" as localized and "heaves" or "lifts" as more diffuse movements. "Thrills" are vibrations that feel like a cat's purr and are associated with loud murmurs. Description of location, amplitude, duration, direction (inward or outward), distribution (localized or diffuse), and timing in the cardiac cycle (systole or diastole) are helpful for determining the cause of a pulsation.

**Percussion.** Percussion may be used in the cardiac physical assessment to outline the left cardiac border. The apical impulse, however, located by inspection and palpation, is more reliable in determining the size of the left ventricle and is more quickly assessed.

**Auscultation.** Auscultation is used for blood pressure measurement, detection of carotid and femoral bruits, and assessment of normal and abnormal heart sounds and murmurs.

***Vasculature.*** The carotid and femoral arteries should be

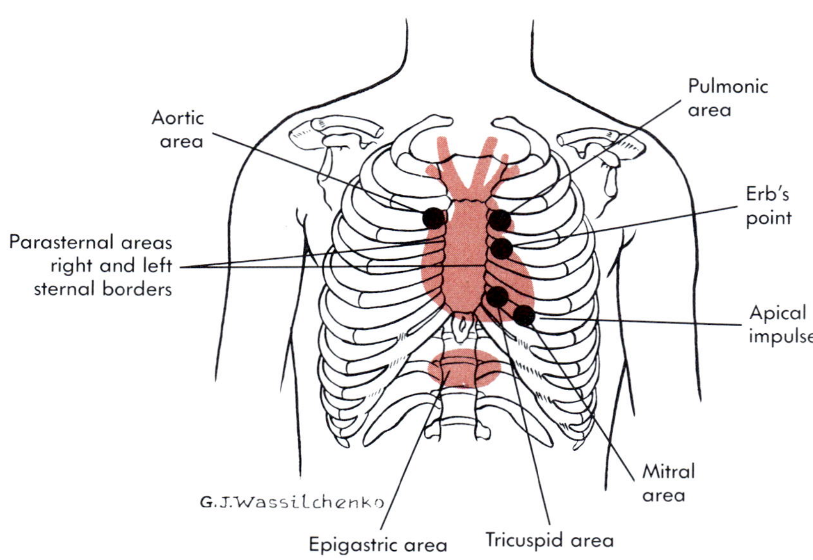


***Fig. 7-2*** Thoracic palpation and auscultation points.

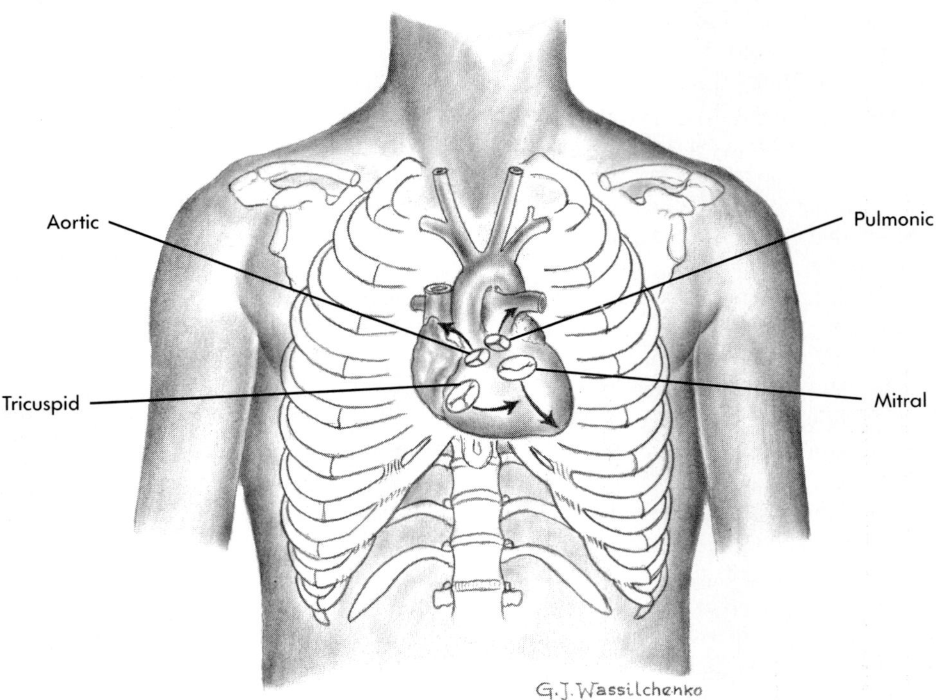


*Fig. 7-3* Transmission of heart sounds to the thorax and their relationship to the anatomical position of the heart valves.

auscultated for bruits. A bruit is an extracardiac vascular sound resulting from either (1) blood flow through a tortuous or a partially occluded vessel or (2) from increased blood flow through a normal vessel. The sound is a high-pitched "sh-sh" sound that vacillates in volume with systole and diastole. Because the diaphragm of the stethoscope is usually too big to auscultate the carotid or femoral areas comfortably, the bell, pressed firmly enough into the skin to create a seal, will act as a good substitute. Light but firm pressure is the key when using the bell of the stethoscope to create a diaphragm.

***Heart.*** Auscultation of the heart can be the most challenging part of the cardiac physical examination. Transmission of heart sounds to the thorax and their relationship to the anatomical position of the heart valves is illustrated in Fig. 7-3.

**FIRST AND SECOND HEART SOUNDS ($S_1$ AND $S_2$).** Normal heart sounds are referred to as "sound one" ($S_1$) and "sound two" ($S_2$). $S_1$ is produced by the rapid deceleration of blood flow when the atrioventricular (mitral and tricuspid) valves close at the beginning of systole. $S_2$ is heard at the end of systole when the semilunar (aortic and pulmonic) valves reach closure. The actual sounds are caused not by the valve leaflets touching each other when they close, but by the vibrations created by the abrupt interruption of retrograde blood flow against the closed, tensed valve leaflets.[106] Both sounds are high pitched and heard best with the diaphragm of the stethoscope. Each sound is loudest in an auscultation area located "downstream" from the actual valvular component of the sound (see Fig. 7-3).

Both $S_1$ and $S_2$ are split sounds because of asynchronous left and right ventricular contraction. When there are no ventricular conduction blocks, the left side of the heart contracts milliseconds before the right. The left-sided heart valves, mitral and aortic, are the first heard components of each sound and are usually the loudest. The splits are best heard in the areas overlying the quieter components, the tricuspid and pulmonic valves. The $S_2$ is more obviously split, and the audible distance between the aortic and pulmonary components is increased with inhalation. This respiratory variation is called physiological splitting and occurs because inspiration causes changes in pulmonary vascular impedence and in systemic and pulmonary venous return. All the components of the split sounds will be high pitched and best heard with the diaphragm of the stethoscope. This information should help to differentiate the normal split sound from the ventricular filling sounds that may indicate pathology.[106] See Table 7-2 for detailed characteristics of the normal heart sounds.

**THIRD AND FOURTH HEART SOUNDS ($S_3$ AND $S_4$).** The abnormal heart sounds are labeled "sound three" ($S_3$) and "sound four" ($S_4$) and are referred to as "gallops" when auscultated during tachycardia. They are ventricular filling sounds, occurring during diastole, and are low pitched. One can differentiate between right and left ventricular gallops by location. Left ventricular $S_3$ and $S_4$ are heard best with

***Table 7-2*** Characteristics of heart sounds one ($S_1$) and two ($S_2$)

| $S_1$ | $S_2$ |
|---|---|
| High pitched | High pitched |
| Loudest in mitral area (apex) | Loudest in aortic area (base) |
| Normal split <20 msec | Normal split <30 msec |
| Split heard best in tricuspid area | Split heard best in pulmonic area |
| Important to differentiate between split $S_1$ and $S_4$ | ↑ Split with inhalation<br>↓ Split with exhalation |
| Occurs immediately before carotid upstroke | |

***Table 7-3*** Characteristics of heart sounds three ($S_3$) and four ($S_4$)

| $S_3$ | $S_4$ |
|---|---|
| **PHYSIOLOGICAL CAUSES** | **PHYSIOLOGICAL CAUSES** |
| Related to diastolic motion and rapid filling of ventricles in early diastole | Related to diastolic motion and ventricular dilitation with atrial contraction in late diastole |
| Can be normal in children and young adults (<40 yr) | May occur with or without cardiac decompensation |
| **PATHOLOGICAL CAUSES** | **PATHOLOGICAL CAUSES** |
| Ventricular dysfunction with an increase in end systolic volume (MI, congestive heart failure, valvular disease, systemic or pulmonary hypertension) | Ventricular hypertrophy with a decrease in ventricular compliance (CAD, systemic hypertension, cardiomyopathy, aortic or pulmonary stenosis, ↑ in intensity with acute MI or angina) |
| Hyperdynamic states (anemia, thyrotoxicosis, mitral or tricuspid regurgitation) | Acute valvular regurgitation |
| | Hyperkinetic states (anemia, thyrotoxicosis, arteriovenous fistula) |
| **RHYTHMIC WORD ASSOCIATION** | **RHYTHMIC WORD ASSOCIATION** |
| Ken....tuck..y<br>$S_1$ $S_2$ $S_3$ | Ten...nes.....see<br>$S_4$ $S_1$ $S_2$ |
| **SYNONYMS** | **SYNONYMS** |
| Ventricular gallop<br>Protodiastolic gallop | Atrial gallop<br>Presystolic gallop |

the bell of the stethoscope positioned lightly over the apical impulse with the patient in the left lateral decubitus position, and right ventricular gallops are heard best at the left lower sternal border (LLSB). They are rhythmic (like horses cantering) and have mimetic sounds as listed in Table 7-3. The $S_3$ occurs at the beginning of diastole, and when associated with ventricular failure, has a sound similar to that of a stone dropping into water at the bottom of a well—dull and "thuddy." The $S_4$ occurs at the end of diastole when the ventricle is full and is associated with the atrial contraction (kick). It is a hollow, snappy sound, as if the noncompliant ventricle cannot accept any more volume unless it flows in hard and fast.[93]

**MURMURS.** Heart murmurs are prolonged extra sounds that occur during systole or diastole. The sounds are vibrations caused by turbulant blood flow through the cardiac chambers. Not all murmurs are caused by cardiac valvular disease. Some murmurs are caused by a high rate of blood flow through the ventricle as with fever, anemia, and exercise (high output states), and other murmurs may be caused by structural defects such as patent foramen ovale (opening in the septum between the right and left atria). Murmurs are characterized by their timing (systolic/diastolic), location and radiation, quality (blowing, grating, harsh), pitch (high or low), and intensity (loudness graded on a scale of I to VI, the higher the number, the louder the murmur). Table 7-4 describes the most common murmurs in terms of these characteristics.

When auscultating murmurs, it is again helpful to visualize the cardiac anatomy, specifically the location of the heart valves and the direction of sound transmission with valve closure and murmur. Generally the systolic valvular murmurs will radiate downstream from the valve that is narrowed (stenotic), and the diastolic valvular murmurs, indicating a backflow of blood through an incompetent valve, will be auscultated best directly over the area of the valve (see Fig. 7-3).

**MURMURS ASSOCIATED WITH MYOCARDIAL INFARCTION.** At the bedside, the nurse is often the first person to auscultate a murmur. The holosystolic or pansystolic murmurs that can occur in the acute myocardial infarction period are good examples. The auscultation of a new, high-pitched, holosystolic, blowing murmur at the cardiac apex heralds mitral valve regurgitation secondary to papillary muscle dysfunction. This murmur may be soft (I/VI or II/VI) and occur only during ischemic episodes when the papillary muscle contractility is impaired, but its presence is associated with persistent pain, heart failure, and higher mortality.[68] If the murmur is loud (V/VI or VI/VI), harsh, and radiating in all directions from the apex, the papillary muscle or chordae tendineae may have ruptured. This is an emergency situation requiring immediate medical and often surgical intervention.

Ventricular septal defect, or rupture, is another emergency situation. It creates the same type of harsh, holosystolic murmur, loudest along the left sternal border. The clinical picture associated with both the papillary muscle rupture and the ventricular septal defect is that of acute heart failure and cardiogenic shock. Immediate diagnosis and treatment is necessary to prevent deaths.

***Table 7-4*** Characteristics of some murmurs

| Defect | Pitch, intensity, quality | Location, radiation |
|---|---|---|
| **SYSTOLIC MURMURS** | | |
| Mitral regurgitation | High<br>Harsh<br>Blowing | Mitral area<br>May radiate to axilla |
| Tricuspid regurgitation | High<br>Often faint, but varies<br>Blowing | Tricuspid RLSB, apex, LLSB, epigastric areas<br>Little radiation |
| Ventricular septal defect | High<br>Loud<br>Blowing | Left sternal border |
| Aortic stenosis | → → →<br>↗ Chhhh hh ↘<br>Medium<br>Rough, harsh | Aortic area to suprasternal notch, right side of neck, apex |
| Pulmonary stenosis | Low to medium<br>Loud<br>Harsh, grinding | Pulmonic area<br>No radiation |
| **DIASTOLIC MURMURS** | | |
| Mitral stenosis | Low<br>Quiet to loud with thrill<br>Rough rumble | Mitral area<br>Usually no radiation |
| Tricuspid stenosis | Medium<br>Quiet, louder with inspiration<br>Rumble | Tricuspid area or epigastrim<br>Little radiation |
| Aortic regurgitation | High<br>Faint to medium<br>Blowing | Aortic area to LLSB and aorta<br>Erb's point |
| Pulmonic regurgitation | Medium<br>Faint<br>Blowing | Pulmonic area<br>No radiation |

RLSB, right lower sternal border; LLSB, left lower sternal border.

**PERICARDIAL FRICTION RUB.** A pericardial friction rub is a sound that can occur within the first week of a myocardial infarction and/or cardiac surgery and is secondary to pericarditis. It is a "to-and-fro," scratchy sound that corresponds with cardiac motion within the pericardial sac (that is, ventricular systole, ventricular diastole, and atrial systole), so it can be both a systolic and diastolic sound. It is high pitched and best auscultated at Erb's point (the third ICS to the left of the sternum). It is often associated with chest pain and it is important to differentiate pericarditis from myocardial ischemia. The detection of the pericardial friction rub can assist in the proper diagnosis and treatment.

## LABORATORY ASSESSMENT

Laboratory studies of blood serum are performed to assess (1) other organ systems that reflect or secondarily affect cardiac status, (2) electrolyte levels that directly affect cardiac function, (3) enzyme levels that may reflect myocardial infarction, and (4) hematological status for determination of anemia or infection that may be a cause of cardiac disease or coagulation problems.

### General Chemistry Studies

The presence of increased glucose during a fasting state may indicate diabetes mellitus, which is believed to accel-

***Table 7-5*** Potassium and calcium effects on cardiac function

| Electrolyte | Serum value | Effect on cardiac function |
|---|---|---|
| Potassium | > 5.5 mEq/L | Decreased rate of depolarization<br>Shortened repolarization<br>Depressed AV conduction<br>ECG changes: Tall, peaked T waves; widened QRS complex; prolongation of P wave and PR interval |
| | < 3.5 mEq/L | Prolonged ventricular repolarization<br>ECG changes: Prominent U wave; sudden occurrence of supraventricular and ventricular dysrhythmias |
| Calcium | > 11 mg/dl | Strengthened contractility<br>Shortened ventricular repolarization<br>ECG change: Shortened QT interval |
| | < 9 mg/dl | Prolonged repolarization<br>ECG change: prolonged QT interval |

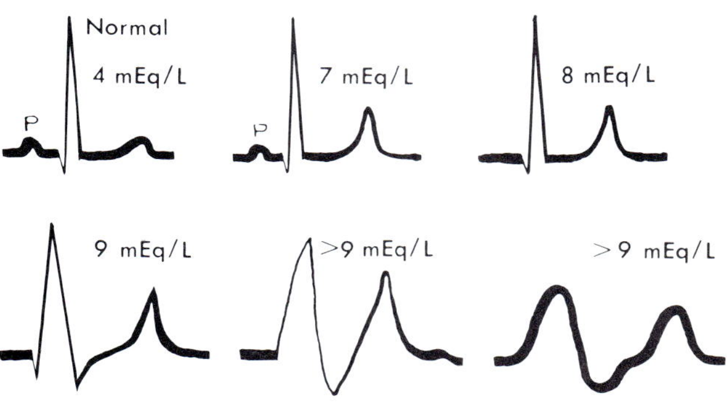


***Fig. 7-4*** Effects of hyperkalemia. The earliest electrocardiogram (ECG) change with hyperkalemia is peaking (tenting) of the T wave. With progressive increases in serum potassium, the QRS complexes widen, P waves disappear, and, finally, ventricular fibrillation develops. These changes do not necessarily occur with a specific serum potassium level. For example, some patients can have a normal ECG with a potassium level of 7 mEq/L, whereas other patients will have ventricular fibrillation at 9 mEq/L or less. (From Goldberger AL and Goldberger E: Clinical electrocardiography: a simplified approach, ed 4, St Louis, 1990, Mosby–Year Book, Inc.)

erate atherosclerosis. Renal failure, assessed by determining increased levels of urea nitrogen and creatinine, may cause electrolyte imbalances of potassium and calcium, which affect cardiac conduction and contractility. Abnormal liver function tests may alert the medical team to liver dysfunction caused by failure of the right side of the heart that is not clinically evident. Liver function indices seen on the chemistry report include alkaline phosphatase, bilirubin, aspartate aminotransferase (AST), and alanine aminotransferase (ALT).

### Potassium

During depolarization and repolarization of nerve and muscle fiber, potassium and sodium exchange occurs intracellularly and extracellularly. Thus both an excess or a deficiency of potassium can alter cardiac muscle function. If serum potassium levels rise above 10 to 14 mEq/L, depressed A-V conduction will lead to cardiac standstill or ventricular fibrillation. Coexisting low serum sodium, calcium, or pH levels potentiate the cardiac effects of hyperkalemia.

Rhythm disturbances resulting from potassium levels below 2.6 mEq/L are reversible with potassium replacement.[64] Table 7-5 summarizes the effects of potassium on cardiac function. ECG changes found in hyperkalemia and hypokalemia are illustrated in Figs. 7-4 and 7-5.

### Calcium

Maintaining a normal serum calcium level is important because of its affect on myocardial contractility and cardiac

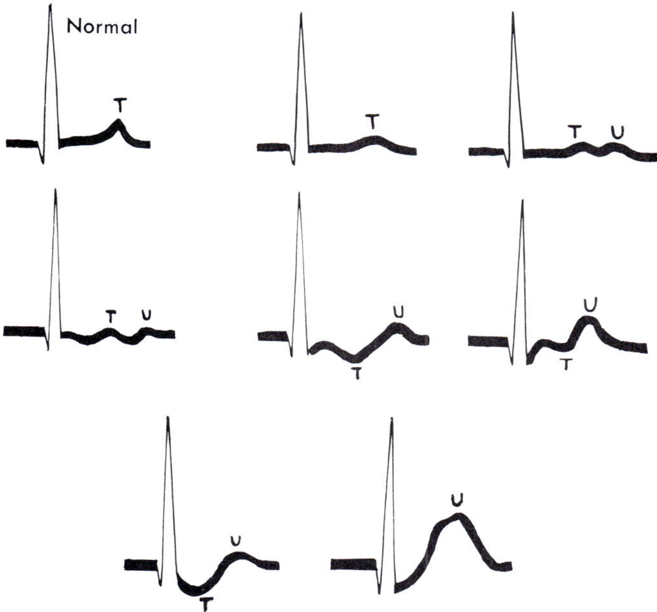


***Fig. 7-5*** Hypokalemia. Variable ECG patterns, ranging from slight T wave flattening to the appearance of prominent U waves, sometimes with ST segment depressions or T wave inversions, may be seen with hypokalemia. These patterns are not directly related to the specific level of serum potassium. (From Goldberger AL and Goldberger E: Clinical electrocardiography: a simplified approach, ed 4, St Louis, 1990, Mosby–Year Book, Inc.)

*Table 7-6* Cardiac enzyme serum levels associated with myocardial infarction

| Cardiac enzymes | Elevation (hours) | Peak (hours) | Duration (days) |
|---|---|---|---|
| Creatine phosphokinase (CPK) | 4-8 | 12-24 | 3-4 |
| Creatine phosphokinase-MB (CPK-MB) | 4-8 | 12-20 | 2-3 |
| Lactate dehydrogenase (LDH) | 12-48 | 72-144 | 8-14 |
| $LDH_1:LDH_2$ (normally <1) | 12-14 ($LDH_1:LDH_2$ >1) | 72-144 | 14 |

excitability. Effects of calcium on cardiac function are summarized in Table 7-5. Below a level of 6 mg/dl, QT prolongation is common, proportional to the amount of hypocalcemia, and reversed with infusion of calcium.[51]

### Cardiac Enzymes

Cardiac enzymes are proteins that are released from irreversibly damaged tissue cells. The enzymes released by damaged myocardial tissue include creatine phosphokinase (CPK), asparate aminotransferase (AST), and lactate dehydrogenase (LDH). Other organs, when damaged or necrotic, will emit these same enzymes. Therefore, when measured as a whole, the enzymes are not cardiac specific. Each enzyme, however, can be broken into its component parts, labeled isoenzymes, and the serum level of these cardiac-specific components will yield information of diagnostic value for cardiac disease. The typical sequence of appearance of CPK and LDH and their isoenzymes is listed in Table 7-6.

Both CPK and LDH have isoenzymes that are cardiac specific. CPK has three isoenzymes composed of varying amounts of M (muscle) and B (brain) subunits. The brain and gastrointestinal tract contain high concentrations of CPK-BB; skeletal muscle and myocardium contain CPK-MM. Myocardial cells contain the CPK-MB isoenzyme that is only minimally found in any other tissue and appears in the serum only subsequent to myocardial cell death. CPK-MB is, at present, the most specific and sensitive serum index for diagnosing myocardial infarction in patients evaluated within 24 hours of onset of chest pain.[81] It can be used to estimate infarct size.[64] Serial samples should be drawn during admission and 12 and 24 hours after admission to help establish or rule out the diagnosis of myocardial infarction.

LDH is composed of five isoenzymes ($LDH_1$, $LDH_2$, $LDH_3$, $LDH_4$, $LDH_5$), and myocardial cells contain a majority of $LDH_1$ and $LDH_2$. When myocardial infarction occurs, both the $LDH_1$ and the $LDH_2$ levels rise, and the $LDH_1:LDH_2$ ratio becomes greater than 1 (normally it is less than 1). The $LDH_1:LDH_2$ ratio can flip back and forth, making it important to collect more than one specimen over time.

It cannot be overemphasized that all of these enzymes are found in multiple other tissues and are released by these tissues in times of stress or tissue damage.[51,64,80,109] Therefore a diagnosis of myocardial infarction can be determined only after assessing the ECG changes and clinical signs and symptoms, as well as the serum enzyme levels.

### Hematological Studies

Hematological laboratory studies that are routinely ordered for the management of patients with altered cardiovascular status are listed in the box below.

## DIAGNOSTIC PROCEDURES

### Chest Radiography

**Basic principles.** Chest radiography is the oldest noninvasive method for visualizing images of the heart, yet it remains a frequently used and valuable diagnostic tool. In the critical care unit, the nurse may be the first person to view the chest radiograph of an acutely ill patient. Nurses also have an important role in influencing the quality of the film through proper positioning and instruction of the patient. For these reasons, it is vital that critical care nurses gain a basic understanding of chest x-ray techniques and interpretation as it applies to the cardiovascular system.

As x-rays travel through the chest from the emitting tube to the film plate, they are absorbed to a varying degree by the tissues through which they pass. Dense structures will appear white, since they block x-rays, whereas air-filled structures will appear dark (Table 7-7). Thoracic structures can be studied best by examining their borders. Two structures with the same density, when located next to each other, will have no visible border. If a structure is located next to

**HEMATOLOGICAL STUDIES FOR ASSESSMENT OF THE CARDIOVASCULAR PATIENT**

Red blood cell (RBC or erythrocyte) level
Hemoglobin (Hb) level
Hematocrit (Hct) level
Erythrocyte sedimentation rate (ESR)
White blood cell (WBC or leucoctye) level
Coagulation studies:
  Prothrombin time (PT)
  Partial thromboplastin time (PTT)

*Table 7-7* X-ray densities of intrathoracic structures

| Metal or bone (white) | Fluid (grey) | Air (black) |
|---|---|---|
| Ribs, clavicle, sternum, spine | Blood | Lung |
| Calcium deposits | Heart | |
| Surgical wires or clips | Veins | |
| Prosthetic valves | Arteries | |
| Pacemaker wires | Edema | |

a contrasting density (for example, vascular structures next to an air-filled lung), even subtle changes in size and shape can be seen.[15]

Ideally, the chest radiograph is taken in the x-ray department with the patient in an upright position, the film exposed during a deep, sustained inhalation, and the x-ray tube aimed horizontally 6 feet from the film. This is a posterior-anterior (PA) film, since the beam traverses the patient from posterior to anterior.

Since most patients in critical care units are too ill to go to the x-ray department, chest radiographs are routinely obtained by using portable x-ray machines, with the patient either sitting upright or lying supine, depending on the patient's clinical condition and the judgment of the nurse. In both cases, the film plate is placed behind the patient's back. Whenever possible, the upright (AP) film is preferred to the supine because it is quicker, it shows more of the lung since the diaphragm is lower, and the images are sharper and less magnified.

A deep, sustained inhalation is important. During exhalation, the lungs appear to cloud and the heart appears larger, possibly leading to an erroneous diagnosis of congestive heart failure. Alert patients will be encouraged by the radiology technician to take in a deep breath and hold it while the exposure is taken. With patients receiving mechanical ventilatory support, the exposure must be timed to coincide with maximal inhalation. Some patients will simply be unable to maintain a sustained inhalation on command, resulting in a distorted cardiac shadow and poor visualization of the lung fields. For this reason it is important to be able to compare and contrast serial chest films before determining that progress or deterioration has occurred.

**Cardiac radiographic findings.** Diagnosis from cardiac x-ray film is twofold; it involves observation of anatomical structures and observation of the pulmonary vascular bed to infer physiological data. Anatomical considerations center around evaluation of the size and shape of cardiac chambers and great vessels, as well as valve calcifications, if present. Physiological observations are related to specific x-ray findings that suggest changes in pulmonary venous pressure, pulmonary artery pressure, or changes in pulmonary blood flow.

***Enlargement of the heart and great vessels.*** There are four major factors that can cause enlargement of the heart and great vessels: pressure overload, volume overload, abnormal tissue, and poststenotic dilation.

Pressure overload, which results from obstruction of outflow, can be either a gradual process, as in chronic hypertension, or of sudden onset, such as that which occurs with a massive pulmonary emboli. Congestive heart failure is the most common example of a clinical condition that causes volume overload. Abnormal cardiac tissues resulting in heart/vessel enlargement are cardiomyopathies and thoracic aortic aneurysms. Poststenotic dilation applies only to arteries. It occurs because of turbulent flow distal to an obstruction. Clinical examples include pulmonic valve stenosis, resulting in dilation of the trunk of the pulmonary artery, and aortic valve stenosis, resulting in dilation of the middle ascending aorta.

***Assessment of chamber enlargement.*** Two basic principles apply to the assessment of cardiac enlargement through chest x-ray film: (1) in general, each chamber enlarges in a direction away from the remainder of the heart, and (2) if a particular chamber enlarges enough to come into contact with a rigid structure such as the spine or sternum, further enlargement will cause displacement and rotation of the entire heart.

***Cardiothoracic ratio.*** Estimation of the cardiothoracic ratio (often abbreviated CT ratio) is a technique used to measure overall heart size, with some limitations (Fig. 7-6). It is done with a frontal view (AP or PA). The maximal cardiac diameter is measured and compared against the maximal thoracic diameter measured to the inner border of the ribs. The CT ratio is considered abnormal if the cardiac diameter is greater than 50% of the total thoracic diameter.[15] It is most sensitive in detecting left-ventricular enlargement, since the left ventricle enlarges toward the left chest wall. It is best to compare serial films, using the CT ratio to follow the progression of enlargement.[29]

In the frontal view of the chest, the right atrium composes the border of the right side of the heart, and the left ventricle represents the border of the left side (Fig. 7-7). Enlargement of either of these chambers could be seen and localized from this view. Use of the chest radiograph to determine specific chamber enlargement is not as accurate as the estimation of overall heart size.[78] The superior vena cava forms the upper right border of the mediastinum on the frontal view. Since only the right border is defined (the left border blends in with the opacity of the rest of the mediastinal structures), the size of the superior vena cava cannot be measured accurately by chest x-ray film. The inferior vena cava is seen best in the lateral view. The posterior border is visible from where it leaves the diaphragm to where it enters the pericardial sac. The thoracic aorta lies within the mediastinum and is not clearly visible on either PA or lateral films if normal. When enlarged, the thoracic aorta rises out of the mediastinum and into contact with lung tissue, making it easier to visualize.

Pericardial effusions can sometimes be visible on a chest radiograph. A pericardial effusion will cause the entire out-

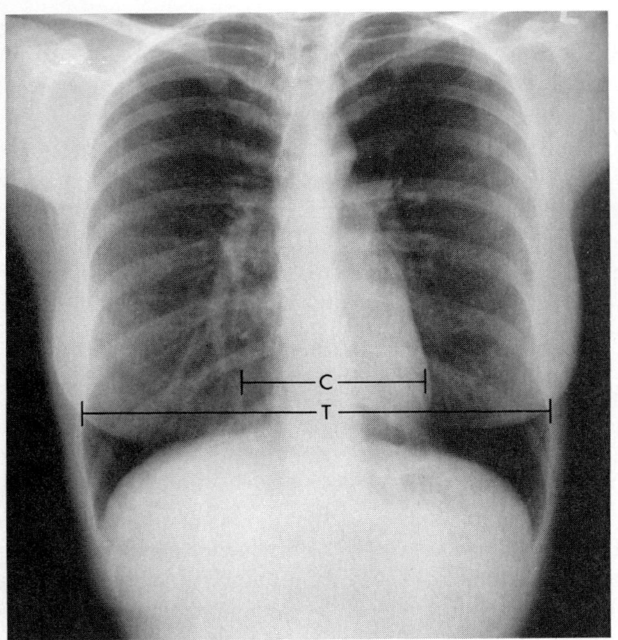


*Fig. 7-6* Cardiothoracic (CT) ratio, a technique for estimating heart size on a PA chest film. Normally the cardiac diameter is 50% or less of the thoracic diameter when measured during full inhalation. *C,* Maximal cardiac diameter; *T,* maximal thoracic diameter measured to the inside of the ribs.

line of the heart to enlarge symmetrically.[47] However, other noninvasive procedures such as echocardiography are much more specific in diagnosing and quantifying pericardial effusions.

### Pulmonary Vascular Patterns

Under normal conditions the pulmonary arteries and veins are sharply defined, with a gradual decrease in blood vessel diameter from the center of the lungs to the periphery.

Pulmonary artery hypertension exists when pulmonary artery pressures are elevated because of obstruction at the pulmonary arteriolar level. This condition is seen clinically in patients who have chronic obstructive pulmonary disease and in those who have had multiple pulmonary emboli. The major vascular change visible on chest radiograph is dilation of the main pulmonary artery and its central hilar branches. The degree of dilation of the pulmonary arteries seen on x-ray film correlates closely with the degree and duration of pressure elevation; in addition, peripheral vessels may appear decreased in size, and, if chronic, tortuosity of lobar and segmental arterial branches occurs.

Pulmonary venous hypertension actually represents high pressures throughout the pulmonary circulation, beginning in the left atrium, being transmitted backward across the pulmonary veins, pulmonary capillaries, and pulmonary arteries, and resulting in right-ventricular systolic hypertension. This entire sequence is caused by increased resistance to flow in the left side of the heart, either at the level of the mitral valve, as in mitral stenosis, or secondary to left-ventricular failure.

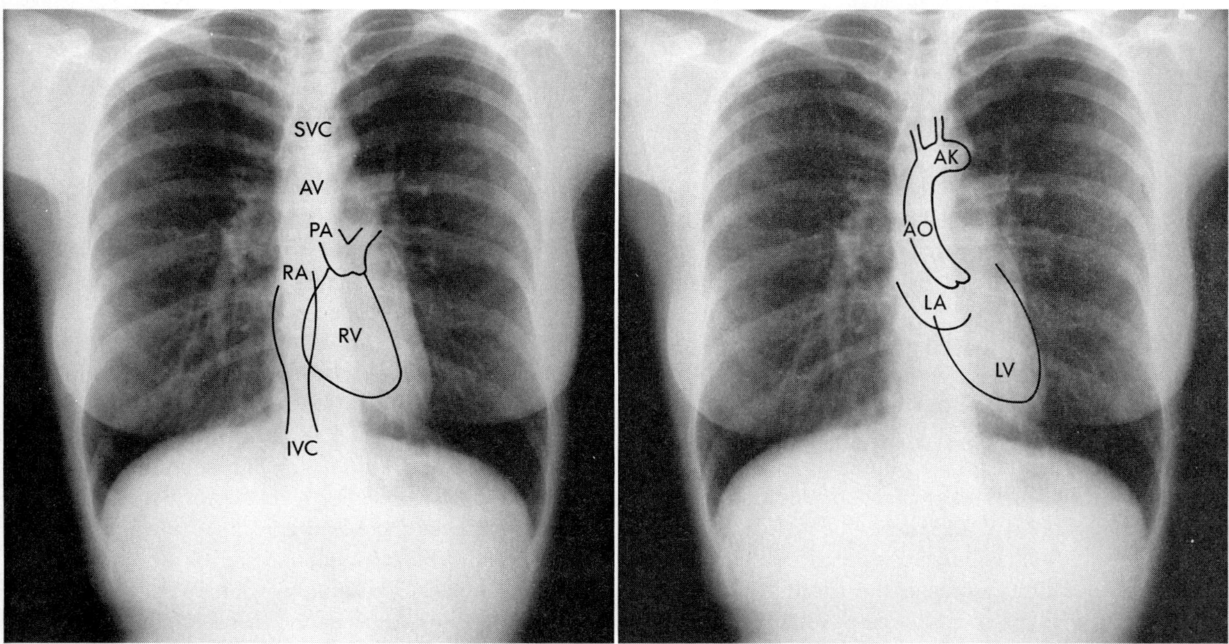


*Fig. 7-7* Location of cardiac structures on a PA chest film. *AV,* Azygos vein; *SVC,* superior vena cava; *PA,* pulmonary artery; *RA,* right atrium; *RV,* right ventricle; *IVC,* inferior vena cava; *AO,* aorta; *AK,* aortic knob; *LA,* left atrium; *LV,* left ventricle.

***Table 7-8*** Chest x-ray estimation of PAWP

| Pulmonary artery wedge pressure (mm Hg) | Chest x-ray findings |
|---|---|
| 5-10 | Normal |
| 10-15 | Equal perfusion of upper and lower lung fields |
| 15-20 | Upper lung perfusion > lower lung perfusion |
| 20-25 | Interstitial edema in lower lobes |
| 25-35 | Kerley-B lines; increased size of main pulmonary artery and hilar branches; perihilar haze |
| >35 | Diffuse perihilar infiltrates |

Pulmonary venous pressure can be measured directly by a balloon-tipped pulmonary artery catheter wedged in the pulmonary capillary bed. As pulmonary venous congestion develops, pulmonary artery wedge pressure (PAWP) can be estimated from the venous markings on the chest x-ray film (Table 7-8).[87] The *Kerley-B lines,* which occur with a PAWP of 25 to 35, are fine, straight, linear shadows that appear at right angles to the pleura and are approximately 1 to 2 cm long. They first appear in the dependent basilar area of the lung.

The chest radiograph often continues to show evidence of pulmonary edema even after treatment has been initiated and pulmonary artery pressures have returned to normal. X-ray findings and extravascular lung water usually return to normal within 2 days if the onset was acute or within 5 days if it was caused by an exacerbation of chronic heart failure.[45,107] Sometimes, coexisting conditions such as pneumonia or atelectasis render the chest radiograph less helpful in determining the extent of pulmonary edema. Although the chest x-ray film may be useful in determining the presence of overt pulmonary edema, it may not be as accurate in detecting modest changes in the amount of extravascular lung water in critically ill patients with coexisting lung disease when using films obtained by portable machines with the patient supine.[45]

### Electrocardiography

Electrocardiography is a very complex subject and necessitates a requisite understanding of the cardiac cell structure and function. This section will review the following concepts: microscopic structure of the heart, electrical and mechanical properties of the heart, the cardiac cycle, and the conduction system. In addition, a general description of dysrhythmias commonly encountered in clinical practice will be provided.

**Cardiac microscopic structure.** To understand and appreciate the unique pumping ability of the heart, attention must be given to the cardiac cell structure and function. Cardiac muscle fibers are typically found in a latticework arrangement. The fiber cells (myofibrils) divide and then rejoin and then separate again. In general, cardiac myofibrils run on a longitudinal axis, and the fibers appear striped, or striated. When viewed under an electron microscope, these striations are actually the contractile proteins (Fig. 7-8). The areas separating each myocardial cell from its neighbor are called *intercalcated discs,* which are continuous with the *sarcolemma,* or cell membrane. At the point where a longitudinal branch of the cell meets another cell branch is the tight junction (or *gap junction*), which offers much less of an impedance to electrical flow than the sarcolemma. Because of this, depolarization will occur from one cell to another with relative ease.[31] Also, the cardiac muscle is a *functional syncytium,* in which depolarization started in any cardiac cell will quickly be spread to all of the heart.

Intracellularly, each cardiac cell contains two types of contractile proteins, *actin* and *myosin*. These proteins abound in the cell in organized longitudinal arrangements. The actin filaments are connected to the Z bands on one end, leaving the other end free to interact with the myosin crossbridges. In the resting muscle cell, the actin and myosin partially overlap. The ends of the myosin filament that overlap with the actin have tiny projections. For contraction to occur, these projections interact with the actin to form crossbridges. The portion of the muscle fiber between two Z bands is called a *sarcomere*. Another extremely important intracellular structure necessary for successful contraction is the *sarcoplasmic reticulum* (SR). Calcium ions are stored in the SR and released for use following depolarization. Deep invaginations into the sarcomere are called *transverse tubules,* or T-tubules. The T-tubules are essentially an extension of the cell membrane and thus function to conduct depolarization to structures deep within the cytoplasm, such as the SR. The cardiac cells abound with *mitochondria,* which contain respiratory enzymes necessary for oxidative phosphorylation. This enables the cell to keep up with the tremendous energy requirements of the repetitive contraction.

**Electrical activity.** Electrical and mechanical properties include **excitability,** conductivity, **automaticity,** rhythmicity, **contractility,** and refractoriness. The following section will relate these concepts specifically to cardiac cells (Table 7-9).

Electrical potentials across cell membranes are present in essentially all cells of the body. Some cells, such as nerve and muscle cells, are specialized for conduction of electrical impulses along their membranes. This electrical potential, or *transmembrane potential,* refers to the relative electrical difference between the interior of a cell and that of the fluid surrounding the cell. Ionic channels are pores in cell membranes that allow passage of specific ions at specific times or signals. Transmembrane potentials and ionic channels are extremely important in myocardial cells, because they form the basis for electrical impulse conduction and muscular contraction.[85]

***Resting membrane potential.*** In a myocardial cell, the normal **resting membrane potential** (RMP) is approxi-

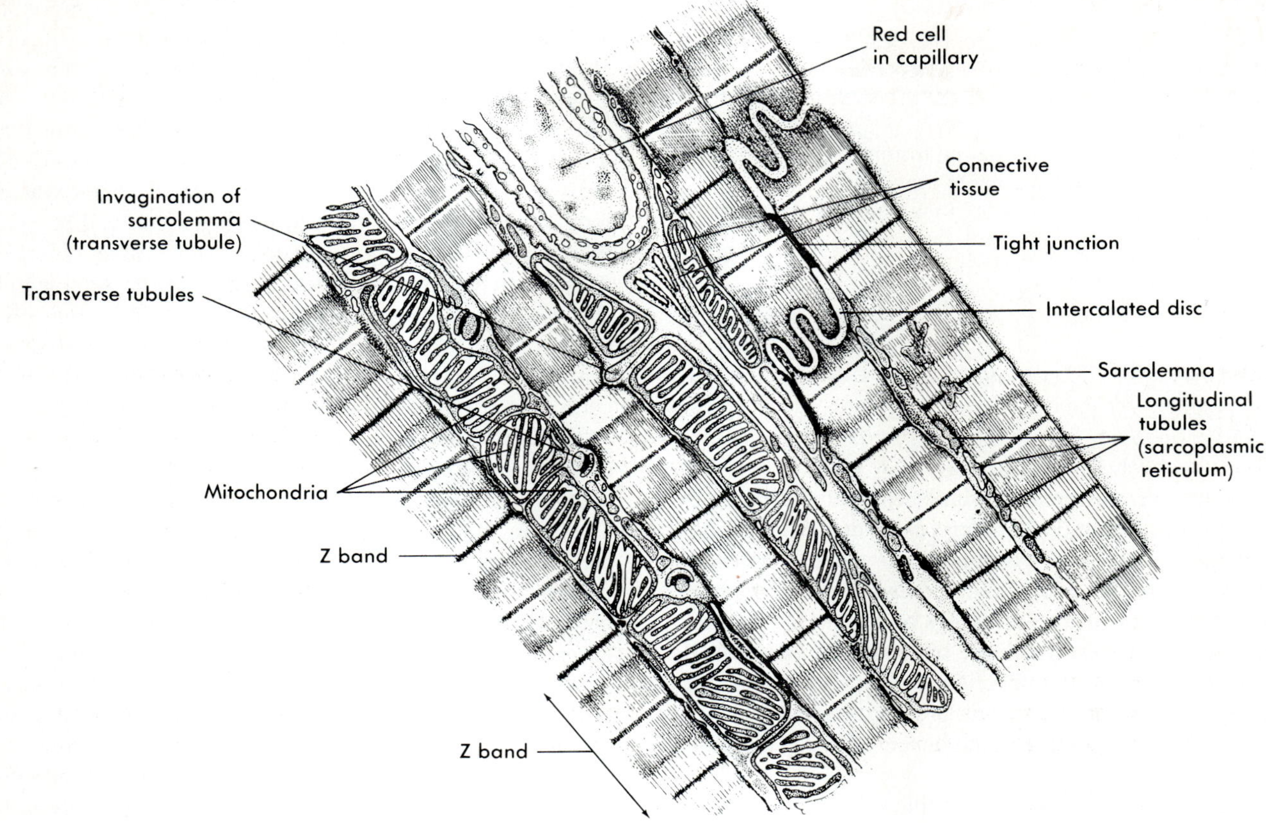


***Fig. 7-8*** Diagram of an electron micrograph of cardiac muscle showing the large numbers of mitochondria, the intercalated disks with tight junctions, the transverse tubules, and the longitudinal tubules (also known as the sarcoplasmic reticulum). (Approximately × 30,000) (From Berne RM and Levy MN: Cardiovascular physiology, ed 6, St Louis, 1991, Mosby–Year Book, Inc.)

***Table 7-9*** Definitions of terms related to cardiac tissue function

| Term | Definition |
|---|---|
| Excitability | The ability of a cell or tissue to depolarize in response to a given stimulus |
| Conductivity | The ability of cardiac cells to transmit a stimulus from cell to cell |
| Automaticity | The ability of certain cells to spontaneously depolarize ("pacemaker potential") |
| Rhythmicity | Automaticity generated at a regular rate |
| Contractility | The ability of the cardiac myofibrils to shorten in length in response to an electrical stimulus (depolarization) |
| Refractoriness | The state of a cell or tissue during repolarization when the cell or tissue either cannot depolarize regardless of the intensity of the stimulus, or requires a much greater stimulus than is normally required |

***Table 7-10*** The approximate extracellular and intracellular concentrations of $K^+$, $Na^+$, and $Ca^{++}$ in a resting myocardial cell

| Ion | Extracellular concentration (mM/L) | Intracellular concentration (mM/L) |
|---|---|---|
| $K^+$ | 4 | 135 |
| $Na^+$ | 145 | 10 |
| $Ca^{++}$ | 2 | 0.0001 |

From Berne and Levy: Cardiovascular physiology, ed 6, St Louis, 1991, Mosby–Year Book, Inc.

mately −80 to −90 mV. This means that the interior of the cell is relatively negative compared with the exterior medium when the cell is at rest. The relative negativity of the cell interior is created by an uneven distribution of positively charged ions and negatively charged ions. Hence there are relatively more of the positively charged ions outside of the cell than there are inside.

When the cell is at rest, the intracellular potassium ($K^+$) is very high, and sodium ($Na^+$) is low. Conversely, the extracellular $K^+$ is relatively low, compared with a high concentration of $Na^+$ (Table 7-10). Like $Na^+$, calcium ($Ca^{++}$) also has a much higher concentration outside the cell. These large differences in individual ion concentrations are responsible for the *chemical gradients,* that is, the tendency of a ion to move from the area of higher concentration to the area of lower concentration. However, there is also an *electrical gradient,* in which the positively charged ions will move to the area of relative negativity. For example, the chemical gradient of $K^+$ is to move out of the cell, since the intracellular concentration is so much higher than the outside medium. But, as a result of the relative negativity inside the cell, the electrical gradient will work to retain the positively charged $K^+$ ion. An important factor influencing both gradients is *membrane permeability,* or the selectivity of the membrane to ionic movements. Even at rest, there is some slight movement of ions across the cell membrane. The cell membrane is approximately 50 times more permeable to $K^+$ than it is to $Na^+$. Because $K^+$ movement out of the cell will create more negativity inside the cell, potassium is therefore the most important ion for maintaining the negative RMP.[16]

***Phases of the action potential.*** In a myocardial cell, when there is a sudden increase in the permeability of the membrane to $Na^+$, there follows a rapid sequence of events that lasts a fraction of a second. This sequence of events is termed **depolarization.** The graphic representation of depolarization is the *action potential,* or AP (Fig. 7-9). As the membrane is depolarized, $Na^+$ begins to enter the cell, thus causing the interior of the cell to become more positive. At about −65 mV, the membrane reaches *threshold,* the point at which the inward $Na^+$ current overcomes the efflux of $K^+$. With the fast $Na^+$ channels open, the inward rush of $Na^+$ is extremely rapid and briefly causes the inside of the cell to become slightly more positive than the outside of the cell. This is known as phase 0 of the AP.

When the rapid influx of $Na^+$ is terminated, a brief period of partial repolarization occurs (phase 1 of the AP). This is followed by phase 2, or the plateau. During this phase, another set of channels, the slow $Na^+$ and $Ca^{++}$ channels, open and allow the influx of $Ca^{++}$ and $Na^+$. Also during phase 2, $K^+$ tends to diffuse out of the cell, balancing the slow inward flux of $Na^+$ and $Ca^{++}$, thereby maintaining the plateau of the AP. The $Ca^{++}$ entering the cell at this phase causes cardiac contraction, which will be described later in this chapter.

Phase 3 of the AP is the final repolarization phase, and

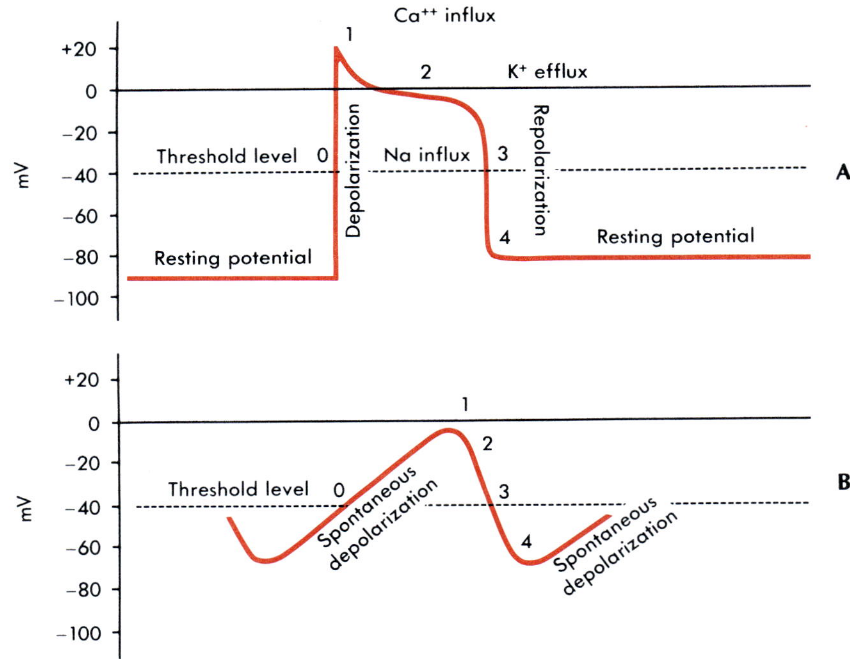


***Fig. 7-9*** Cardiac action potentials. **A,** Action potential phases 0 to 4 of a nonpacemaker cell. **B,** Action potential of a pacemaker cell. (From Thompson JM and others: Clinical nursing, ed 2, St Louis, 1989, Mosby–Year Book, Inc.)

depends upon two processes. The first is the inactivation of the slow channels, thereby preventing further influx of $Ca^{++}$ and $Na^{+}$. The other is the continued efflux of $K^{+}$ out of the cell. Both of these processes will cause the intracellular environment to become more negative, thereby reestablishing the RMP. Phase 4 of the AP is the return to RMP. The excess $Na^{+}$ that entered the cell during depolarization is now removed from the cell in exchange for $K^{+}$ by means of the $Na^{+}$ and $K^{+}$ pump. This mechanism returns the intracellular concentrations of $Na^{+}$ and $K^{+}$ to the levels prior to depolarization and is essential for normal ionic balance.[119]

***Fiber conduction and excitability.*** Propagation of an AP along a cardiac fiber occurs as a result of ionic shifts discussed previously. As a local section of the cell becomes depolarized, reaches threshold, and completely depolarizes, it affects the adjacent area of the cell and begins depolarization in that area. Thus the AP propagates down the fiber in a wavelike fashion.

The time from the beginning of depolarization until the time when the fiber can again be depolarized is called the *effective* or **absolute refractory period.** During this period, the cell cannot be depolarized regardless of the amount or intensity of the stimulus. This period lasts from the beginning of depolarization to approximately −50 mV during phase 3. Immediately following the absolute refractory period is the *relative refractory period*. At this time, the cell is not fully repolarized, but could depolarize with a strong enough stimulus (Fig. 7-10). This can be a particularly dangerous time for ectopy to occur. This period lasts from approximately −50 mV during phase 3 to when the cell returns to RMP. At phase 4, the cell is fully repolarized and is again at RMP, ready to respond to the next stimulus.

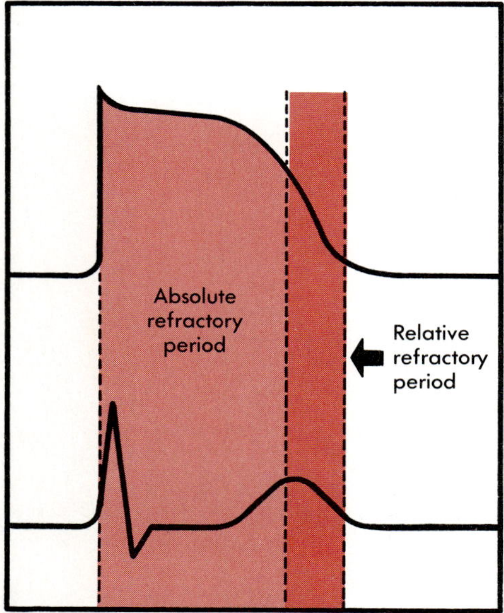


***Fig. 7-10*** Absolute and relative refractory periods correlated with the cardiac muscle's action potential and with an ECG tracing.

**Mechanical activity.** The electrical activity discussed in the previous section is the basis for mechanical contraction. As the myocardial cell is depolarized, specifically during phase 2 of the AP, some $Ca^{++}$ enters the cytoplasm through the cell membrane via special $Ca^{++}$ channels. The majority of $Ca^{++}$ enters the cytoplasm from stores in the sarcoplasmic reticulum (SR).[62] The cytoplasmic $Ca^{++}$ then binds with troponin and tropomyosin, molecules that are present on the actin filaments, resulting in contraction. Occurring throughout the myocardium, the result is myocardial contraction. Once contraction has occurred, $Ca^{++}$ is taken back up into the SR and the cytoplasmic concentration of $Ca^{++}$ falls leading to muscular relaxation. Both contraction and relaxation are active processes because they require adenosine triphosphate (ATP) and because the $Ca^{++}$ is removed from the cell by way of a $Na^{+}/Ca^{++}$ pump.[50,82,105,123]

**The cardiac cycle.** The cardiac cycle refers to one complete mechanical cycle of the heart beat, beginning with ventricular contraction and ending with ventricular relaxation.

***Ventricular systole.*** As the ventricles are depolarized, the septum and papillary muscles tense first. This provides a stable outflow tract and competent AV valves. The ventricles begin to tense (endocardium to epicardium), causing a rise in pressure. When the intraventricular presure exceeds that of the intraatrial pressure, the mitral and tricuspid valves close. This stage is known as *isovolumic contraction,* because, even though the ventricular muscle is tensing, the ventricular volume does not change. As the ventricular tension increases, the intraventricular pressures exceed those of the aorta and pulmonary arteries, causing the aortic and pulmonic valves to open. The blood ejected from the ventricles is called the *stroke volume*. Usually more than half of the total ventricular blood volume is ejected; the blood that remains in the ventricles is the *residual* or *end-systolic volume*. The *ejection fraction* is the ratio of the stroke volume ejected from the left ventricle per beat to the volume of blood in the left ventricle at the end of diastole (left ventricular end-diastolic volume). It is expressed as a percent, normal being at least greater than 50%. Both ejection fraction and LVEDV are widely used clinically as indices of contractility and cardiac function.

***Ventricular diastole.*** Following ventricular systole is ventricular diastole. The first phase is *isovolumic relaxation,* which occurs between closure of the semilunar (aortic and pulmonic) valves and the opening of the AV (mitral and tricuspid) valves. Immediately following is the rapid filling phase, in which the AV valves open and the majority of the ventricular filling occurs. The next phase is ventricular diastasis or a reduced ventricular filling period. This is passive flow of blood from the periphery and pulmonary vasculature into the ventricles. The last part of ventricular diastole, known as atrial kick, provides approximately 30% of total

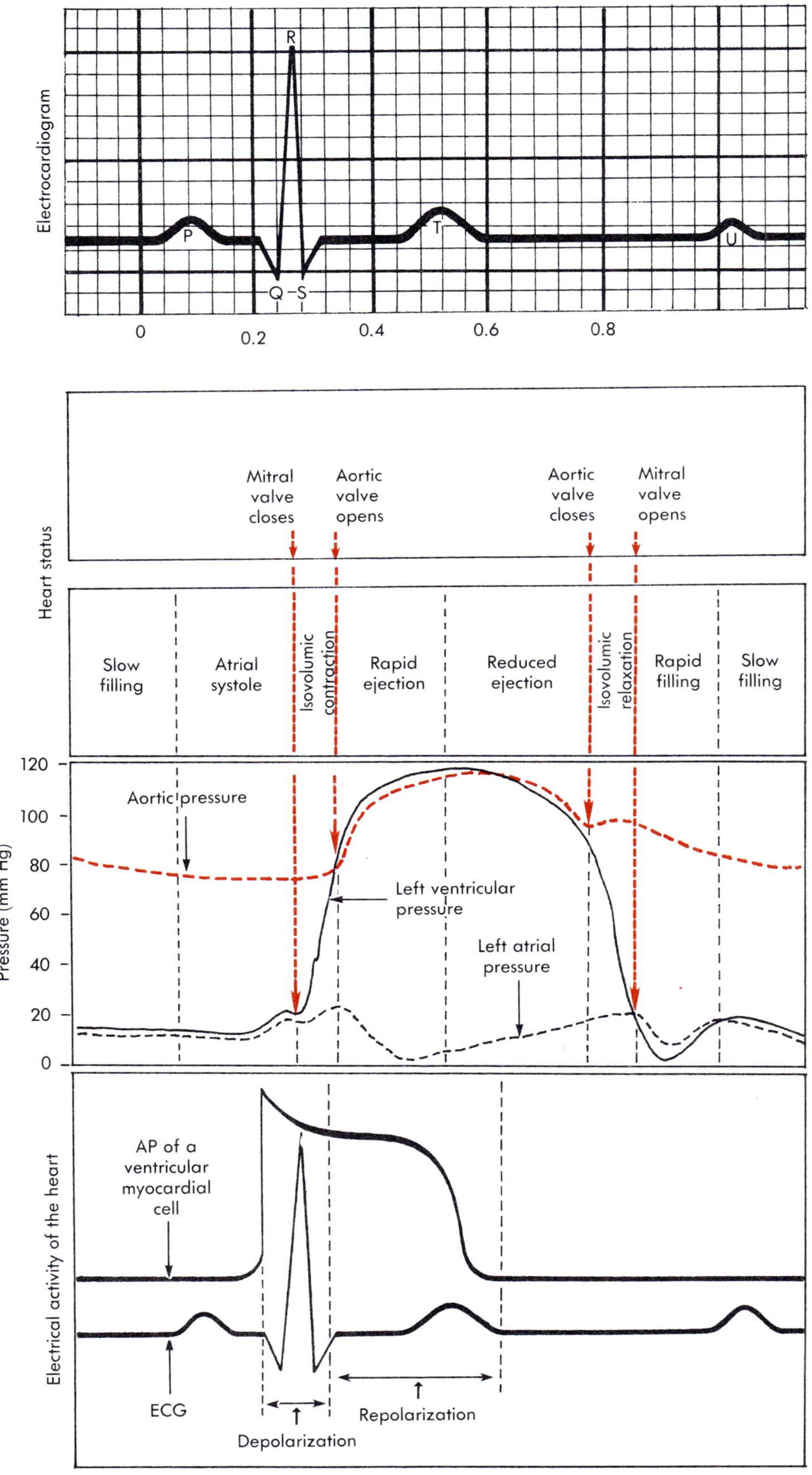


*Fig. 7-11* The cardiac cycle.

ventricular filling. With this, the cycle is complete and begins once again with systole (Fig. 7-11).

**The conduction system.** The history of the discovery of the conduction system dates back to 1845, when Purkinje wrote a classic paper describing ventricular conductive cells. Breakthroughs in electrophysiology have advanced not only clinical cardiology but also have entered the cardiac surgery arena.[99,102] This section will discuss the three main areas of impulse propagation and conduction—the SA node, the AV node, and the His/Purkinje fibers.

***Sinoatrial node.*** The **sinoatrial (SA) node** is considered the natural pacemaker of the heart because it has the highest degree of automaticity or intrinsic heart rate (Table 7-11). The node is usually a spindle-shaped structure located near the mouth of the superior vena cava, on the posterior aspect of the right atrium (Fig. 7-12). There is some normal variability in the position and shape of the node. The SA node contains basically two types of cells, the specialized pacemaker cells found in the node center and the border zone cells. Both the pacemaker cells and the border zone cells have inherent depolarization capabilities (they automatically depolarize 60 to 100 times per minute). It is the cells in the nodal center that are responsible for the actual pacemaking of the heart. The fibers in the border zone cells also have intrinsic pacemaker properties, but depolarization is depressed by the surrounding atrial tissue.[12]

Once the center nodal cells have depolarized, the impulse is conducted through the nodal border zone toward the atrium. Atrial depolarization occurs both cell to cell and also through four specialized conduction pathways that exit the SA node (Fig. 7-13, *A*). These conduction pathways are Bachman's bundle, which is directed to the left atrium, and three internodal pathways that are directed to the AV node.

***Atrioventricular node.*** The **atrioventricular (AV) node** is located posteriorly on the right side of the interatrial septum (see Fig. 7-12). Because the atria and ventricles are separated by nonconductive tissue, all electrical impulses initiated in the atria will be conducted to the ventricles solely via the AV node. Although the AV node also possesses pacemaker cells, the intrinsic rhythmicity is less than that of the SA node (Table 7-11). So, as an impulse from the SA node arrives at the AV node, the AV node will be depolarized (Fig. 7-13, *B*), resetting its own pacemaker potential. This prevents the AV node from initiating its own pacemaker impulse that would compete with the SA node.

***Table 7-11*** Intrinsic pacemaker rates of cardiac conduction tissue

| Location | Rate (beats/min) |
|---|---|
| SA node | 60-100 |
| AV node | 40-60 |
| Purkinje fibers | 15-40 |

As the depolarization impulse from the SA node arrives at the AV node, a slight conduction delay occurs through the AV node. This delay is a result of the inherent properties of the nodal structures that cause a slowing of conduction velocity. The purpose of this delay is to allow adequate time for optimal ventricular filling from atrial contraction. The AV nodal delay also functions as a protection mechanism for the ventricles. As a result of the slowed conduction velocity through the AV node, conduction is thus time dependent and hence limits the contraction frequency of the ventricles. For example, when there is an abnormal number of electrical impulses bombarding the AV node during atrial flutter or atrial fibrillation, the AV nodal delay limits the number of impulses that move through to the ventricles. Without this delay, the ventricles would receive each atrial impulse, and the heart would quickly decompensate.

Another property described in the AV node is that of retrograde (backward) conduction. This means that an electrical impulse that is initiated in or below the AV node can be conducted in a backward fashion. When this happens, the propagation time is generally longer than that of antegrade (forward) conduction. In this instance, the coordinated efforts of atria and ventricles are diminished or lost, resulting in lack of atrial kick to ventricular filling.

***Bundle of His and Purkinje fibers.*** Electrical impulses are conducted in the ventricles through the **bundle of His** and the **Purkinje fibers** (Fig. 7-13, *C*). The bundle of His fibers runs through the subendocardium down the right side of the interventricular septum. About 12 mm from the AV node, the bundle of His divides into the right and left bundle branches. The right bundle branch continues down the right side of the interventricular septum toward the right apex (see Fig. 7-12). The left bundle branch is thicker than the right and takes off from the bundle of His at almost a right angle. It then traverses the septum to the subendocardial surface of the left interventricular wall, where it divides into a thin anterior and a thick posterior branch. Functionally, when one of the left branches is blocked, it is referred to as a hemiblock. All of the bundle branches are subject to conduction defects (bundle branch blocks) and give rise to characteristic changes in the electrocardiogram.

The right bundle branch and the two divisions of the left bundle branch eventually divide into the Purkinje fibers. These divide many times, terminating in the subendocardial surface of both ventricles. The Purkinje fibers have the fastest conduction velocity of all heart tissue. Ventricular muscle depolarization follows (Fig. 7-13, *D*).

**Basic principles of electrocardiography**

***Electrocardiographic leads.*** All electrocardiographs use a system of one or more *leads*. A lead consists of three electrodes: a positive electrode, a negative electrode and a ground electrode. The function of the ground electrode is to prevent the display of background electrical interference on the ECG tracing.

The positive electrode on the skin acts as a camera. If the wave of depolarization travels toward the positive elec-

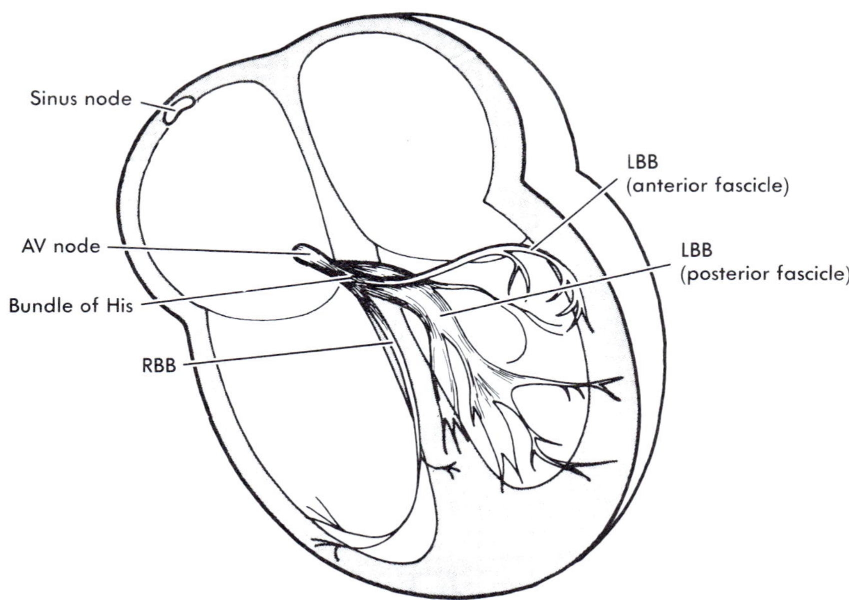


***Fig. 7-12*** Cardiac conduction system. (From Conover MB: Understanding electrocardiography: arrhythmias and the 12-lead ECG, ed 5, St Louis, 1988, Mosby–Year Book, Inc.)

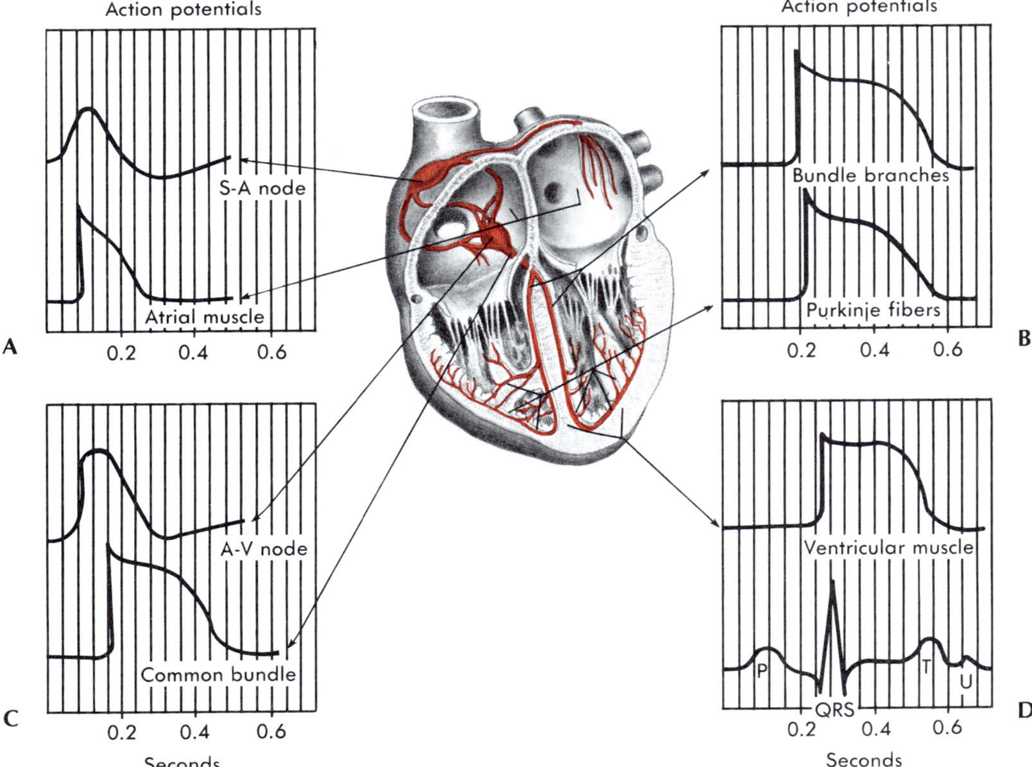


***Fig. 7-13*** Heart with normal conduction pathways and transmembrane action potentials of **A,** SA node and atrial muscle, **B,** AV node, **C,** bundle branches, and **D,** ventricular muscle. (From Thompson JM and others: Clinical nursing, ed 2, St Louis, 1989, Mosby–Year Book, Inc.)

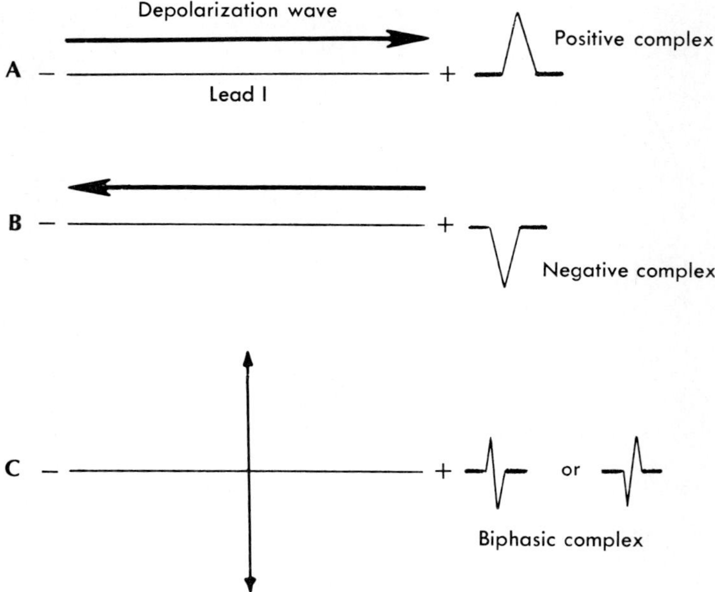


***Fig. 7-14*** Three basic laws of electrocardiography. **A,** Flow of depolarization toward the positive electrode results in a positive deflection on the ECG. **B,** Flow of depolarization away from the positive electrode results in a negative deflection on the ECG. **C,** Flow of depolarization perpendicular to the positive electrode results in a biphasic deflection on the ECG. These three basic laws apply to both the P wave and the QRS complex. (From Goldberger AL and Goldberger E: Clinical electrocardiography: a simplified approach, ed 4, St Louis, 1990, Mosby–Year Book, Inc.)

trode, an upward stroke, or *positive deflection,* is written on the ECG paper (Fig. 7-14, *A*). If the wave of depolarization travels away from the positive electrode, a downward line, or *negative deflection,* will be recorded on the ECG (Fig. 7-14, *B*). A biphasic complex occurs when depolarization moves perpendicular to the positive electrode (Fig. 7-14, *C*). The size of the muscle mass also has an effect, with the larger muscle mass having a greater influence on the tracing.

The wave of ventricular depolarization in the healthy heart travels from right to left and head to toe. The appearance of the waveforms on the ECG will vary, depending on the location of the positive electrode. The standard 12-lead ECG provides a picture of electrical activity in the heart from the 12 different positions of the positive electrodes.

A 12-lead ECG consists of six standard limb leads and six chest leads (Fig. 7-15, *A, B,* and *C*). The limb leads are obtained by placing electrodes on all four extremities. Leads I, II, and III are bipolar limb leads in that they consist of a positive and a negative electrode. The other three limb leads are labeled aVR, aVL, and aVF, representing augmented vector right, left, and foot. These unipolar leads consist only of a positive electrode, with the negative electrode calculated within the machine at roughly the center of the heart. Under these circumstances the ECG tracing would ordinarily be very small, so the machine enhances, or *augments,* it. The term *vector* refers to directional force.

The precordial chest leads are labeled "V" leads and are distributed in an arch around the left chest. They are useful for viewing electrical forces traveling from right to left or front to back but are not helpful in evaluating vertical forces in the heart. For an accurate interpretation, all 12 leads must be taken into consideration.

***Baseline distortion.*** It is important that the tracing have a flat baseline, which is that portion of the tracing that is between the various waveforms. Two forms of artifact can distort the baseline: 60-cycle interference and muscular movement. Sixty-cycle interference (Fig. 7-16, *A*) results from leakage of electrical current somewhere within the system and appears as a generalized thickening of the baseline. It can usually be resolved by ensuring that all electrical equipment at the bedside is well grounded. Occasionally, it may be necessary to unplug one piece of equipment at a time until the offending device is found. Muscular movement (Fig. 7-16, *B*) is displayed as a coarse, erratic disturbance of the baseline. In most cases, asking the patient to lie quietly while the ECG is being run is sufficient. If movement is caused by shivering or seizure activity, it is best to wait until the activity subsides before obtaining the 12-lead ECG.

***Specialized ECG paper.*** ECG paper records the speed and magnitude of electrical impulses on a grid composed of small and large boxes (Fig. 7-17). There are five small boxes in every large box. At a standard paper speed of 25

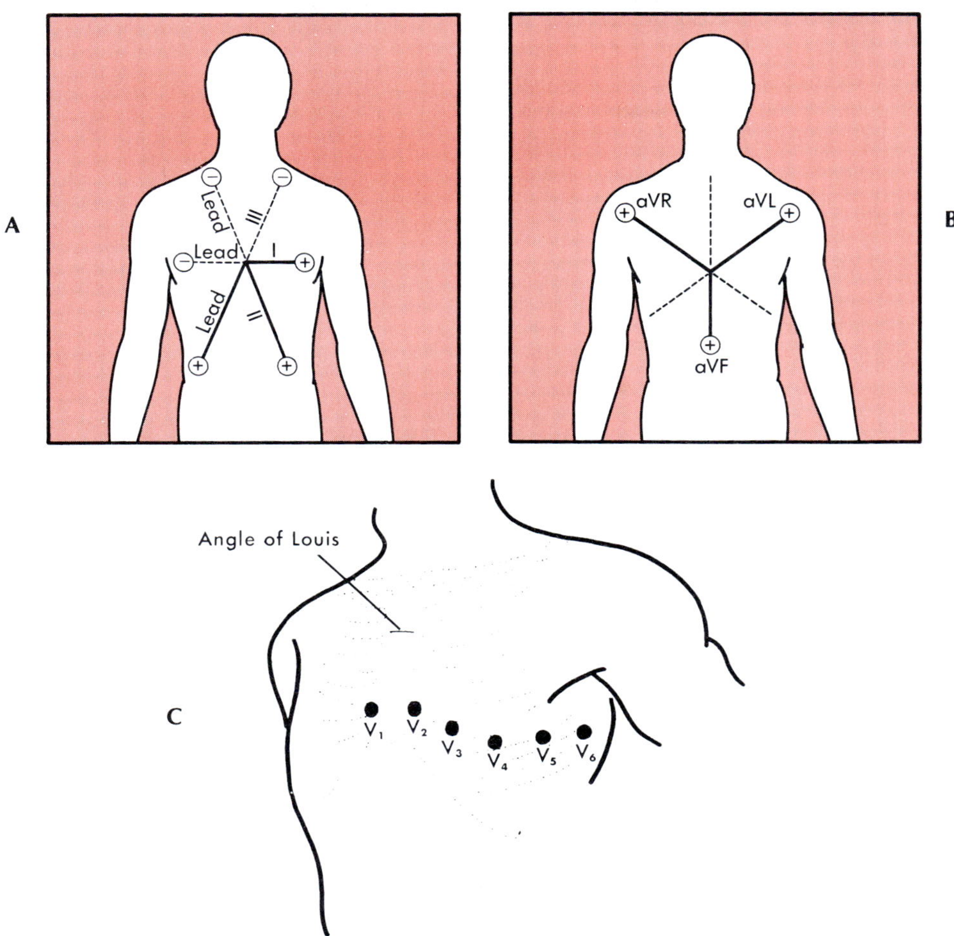


***Fig. 7-15*** **A,** Limb leads I, II, and III. Leads are actually located on the extremities. Illustrated are the angles from which these leads view the heart. **B,** Lead placement for augmented limb leads aVR, aVL, and aVF. These are unipolar leads that use the calculated center of the heart as their negative electrode. **C,** Lead placement for the chest electrodes: $V_1$, fourth intercostal space at the right sternal border; $V_2$, fourth intercostal space at the left sternal border; $V_3$, equidistant between $V_2$ and $V_4$; $V_4$, fifth intercostal space at the left midclavicular line; $V_5$, anterior axillary line and same horizontal level as $V_4$; $V_6$, midaxillary line and same horizontal level as $V_4$. (**C** from Goldberger AL and Goldberger E: Clinical electrocardiography: a simplified approach, ed 4, St Louis, 1990, Mosby–Year Book, Inc.)

mm/second, one small box (1 mm) is equivalent to 0.04 second, and one large box (5 mm) represents 0.20 second. Distances along the horizontal axis represent speed and are stated in seconds rather than in millimeters or number of boxes. The vertical axis represents magnitude or strength of force. At standard calibration, one small box equals 0.1 mV, and one large box equals 0.5 mV. It is important to look for the *standardization mark,* which is usually located at the beginning of the tracing (Fig. 7-18). The mark indicates 1 mV and at standard calibration should go up two large boxes.

***Wave forms and intervals.*** The letter Q is used to describe an *initial* negative deflection; in other words, only if the first deflection from the baseline is negative will it be labeled a Q wave. The letter R applies to any positive deflection. If there are two positive deflections in one QRS complex, the second is labeled R′ (read "R prime") and is commonly seen in lead $V_1$ in right bundle branch block. The letter S refers to any subsequent negative deflections. Any combination of these deflections can occur and is collectively called the QRS complex.

Duration of waveforms and intervals should be evaluated (Fig. 7-19). The PR interval is measured from the beginning of the P wave to the beginning of the QRS complex. Since most of this time period results from delay of the impulse in the A-V node, the PR interval is an indicator of A-V nodal function. The portion of the wave that extends from the end of the QRS to the beginning of the T wave is labeled the ST segment. Its duration is not measured. Instead, its shape and location are evaluated. The ST segment should be flat and at the same level as the isoelectric baseline. Elevation or depression is expressed in millimeters and may indicate ischemia. The QT interval is measured from the beginning of the QRS complex to the end of the T wave. The normal value of a QT interval is very dependent on heart rate.

***Cardiac monitor lead analysis.*** During continuous cardiac monitoring, adhesive pregelled electrodes are used to obtain an ECG tracing that is similar to one lead of a 12-lead ECG. At a minimum, this requires three electrodes: one positive, one negative, and one ground. In some clinical areas, five electrodes are used, either to monitor two leads simultaneously or to allow selection of several different leads at any time through a lead selector switch on the monitor. Three leads, II, $MCL_1$, and $MCL_6$, are commonly used for continuous monitoring, although others may also be used.

**LEAD II.** The positive electrode is placed on the lower left torso, the negative electrode is placed on the right shoulder, and the ground electrode is usually placed on the left shoulder (Fig. 7-20, *A*). The location of the ground is not significant. In most patients, this lead displays in a waveform

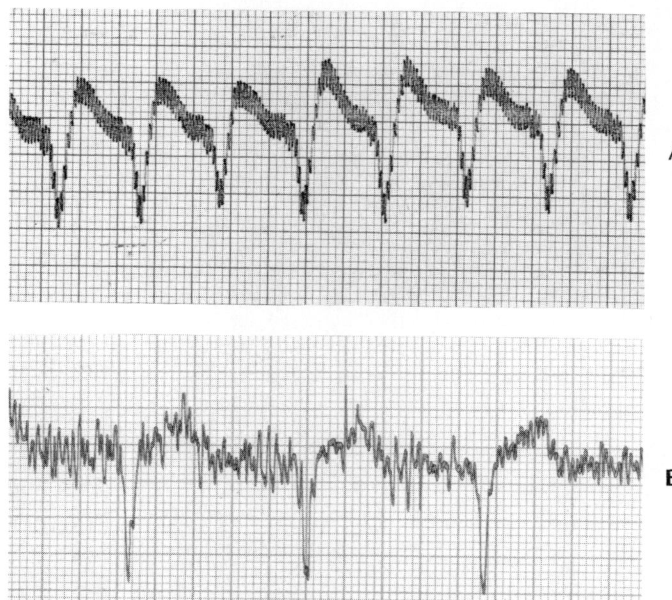


***Fig. 7-16*** **A,** Artifact—60-cycle interference. **B,** Artifact—muscular movement.

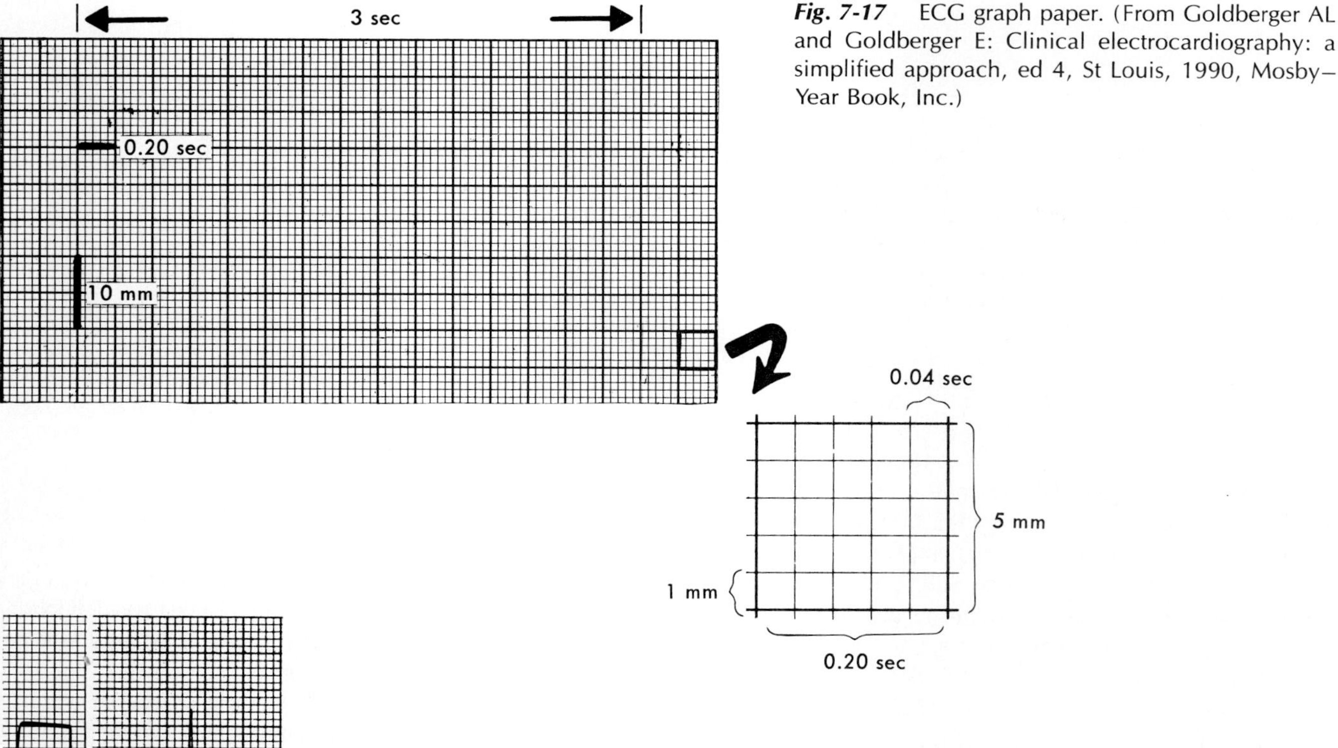


***Fig. 7-17*** ECG graph paper. (From Goldberger AL and Goldberger E: Clinical electrocardiography: a simplified approach, ed 4, St Louis, 1990, Mosby–Year Book, Inc.)

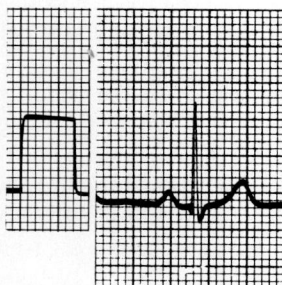

***Fig. 7-18*** Standardization mark. Before beginning the ECG, the machine must be calibrated so that the standardization mark is 10 mm tall. (From Goldberger AL and Goldberger E: Clinical electrocardiography: a simplified approach, ed 4, St Louis, 1990, Mosby–Year Book, Inc.)

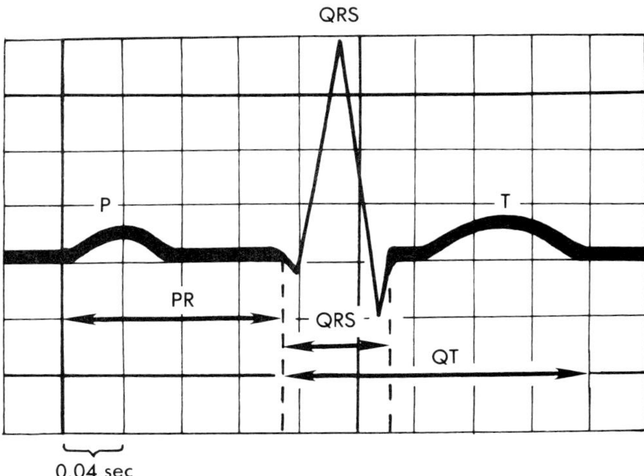


*Fig. 7-19* ECG waveforms and intervals. The P wave represents atrial depolarization. The QRS complex represents ventricular depolarization and is normally 0.10 seconds or less. The T wave represents ventricular repolarization. The PR interval represents the time between sinus node discharge and the beginning of ventricular depolarization and is between 0.12 to 0.20 seconds. The QT interval represents the time from initial depolarization of the ventricles to the end of repolarization and is normally less than one half the RR interval (measured from one QRS complex to the next). (From Conover MB: Understanding electrocardiography: arrhythmias and the 12-lead ECG, ed 5, St Louis, 1988, Mosby–Year Book, Inc.)

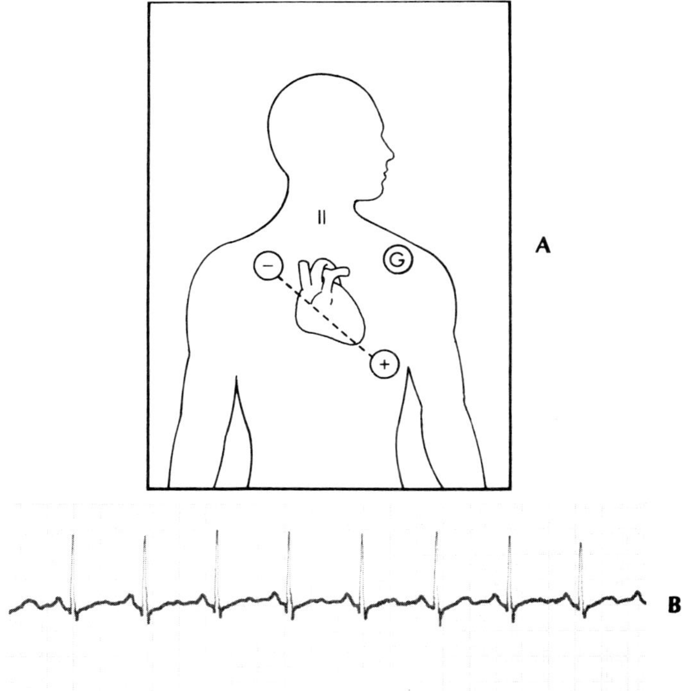


*Fig. 7-20* **A,** Electrode placement for monitoring lead II. **B,** Typical ECG tracing in lead II.

that is predominantly upright (Fig. 7-20, *B*). For this reason, it has been a popular monitoring lead. P waves are usually easy to identify in lead II.

**LEAD $MCL_1$.** "$MCL_1$" stands for "modified chest lead one." It is equivalent to a $V_1$ lead on a 12-lead ECG. The tracings are similar but not identical. In both, the positive electrode is at the fourth intercostal space just to the right of the sternum. With $MCL_1$ the ground electrode is usually placed on the right shoulder (Fig. 7-21, *A*). Since the positive electrode is to the right of the heart and most of the electrical activity in the heart is directed toward the left ventricle, the QRS complex in lead $MCL_1$ will normally be negative (Fig. 7-21, *B*). Interventricular conduction changes such as bundle branch block are easier to identify in lead $MCL_1$ than in lead II. Differentiation of wide complex tachycardia (ventricular tachycardia versus supraventricular tachycardia with aberrancy) is also clearer in $MCL_1$, making it a popular monitoring lead in cardiac patients who are at high risk for these dysrhythmias.

**LEAD $MCL_6$.** An alternative to lead $MCL_1$ is lead $MCL_6$. This is a modified $V_6$, with the positive electrode located in the $V_6$ position (left fifth intercostal space, midaxillary line). The negative electrode is placed below the left shoulder, and the ground can be placed below the right shoulder. Lead $MCL_6$ is also an adequate lead for monitoring interventricular conduction changes.

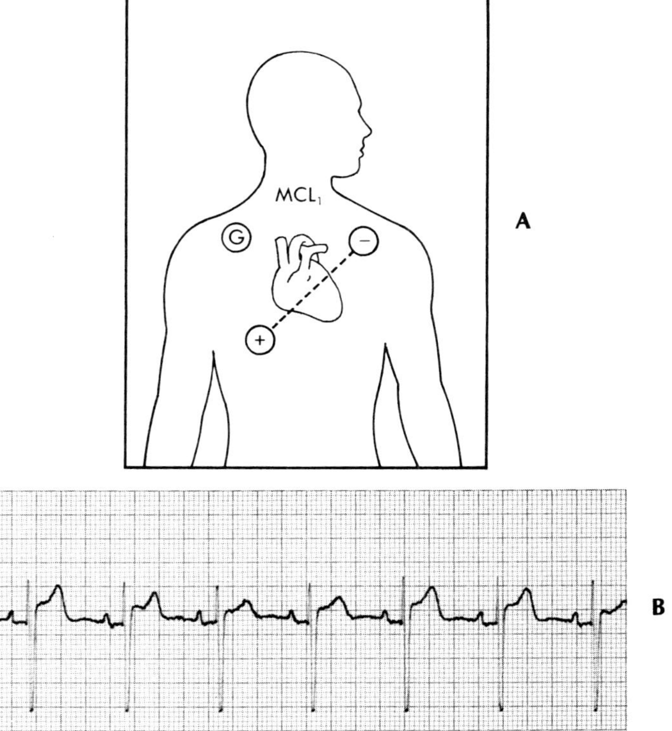


*Fig. 7-21* **A,** Electrode placement for monitoring lead $MCL_1$. **B,** Typical ECG tracing in lead $MCL_1$.

**EVALUATION OF RHYTHM STRIPS**

1. Calculate the ventricular and atrial rates.
2. Determine the rhythm.
3. Analyze the P wave.
4. Measure the PR interval.
5. Determine the QRS interval.
6. Measure the QT interval.
7. Analyze the ST segment.
8. Analyze the T wave.

**Dysrhythmia interpretation.** A dysrhythmia is any disturbance in the normal cardiac conduction pathway. Dysrhythmias can be detected on a 12-lead ECG, but very often they occur only sporadically. For this reason patients in a critical care unit are monitored continuously, using a single lead, and rhythm strips are recorded routinely, as well as any time there is a change in the patient's rhythm. A systematic approach to evaluation of a rhythm strip is introduced first in this section, followed by specific criteria for common dysrhythmias encountered in clinical practice. A summary of key points on which to evaluate rhythm strips is found in the box above.

The first thing to assess when evaluating a rhythm strip is the ventricular rate. Regardless of the dysrhythmia involved, the ventricular rate holds the key to whether or not the patient will be able to tolerate the dysrhythmia, that is, maintain adequate blood pressure, cardiac output, and mentation. If the ventricular rate is consistently >200 or <30, emergency measures must be started to correct the rate. Three methods for calculating rate are described in Fig. 7-22. In the healthy heart, the atrial rate and the ventricular rate are the same. However, in many dysrhythmias the atrial and ventricular rates are different; thus both must be calculated. The choice of method for calculating the heart rate depends on the regularity of the rhythm. If the rhythm is irregular, the first method is used. If the rhythm is regular, it is more accurate to use the second or third method. The second method can be easier to use when two consecutive R waves fall exactly on dark lines, and it provides a rapid estimate of rate. The third method is recommended when both R waves do not fall exactly on dark lines.

The term *rhythm* refers to the regularity with which the P waves or R waves occur. Calipers assist in determining rhythm. One point of the calipers is placed on the beginning of one R wave, while the other point is placed on the very next R wave. Leaving the calipers "set" at this interval, each succeeding RR interval is checked to be sure it is the same width. If the rhythm is *regular,* the RR intervals are the same, ±10%. If the rhythm is *irregular,* that is, the RR intervals are not the same, then a pattern must be sought. Discovering a pattern may aid in the interpretation of the dysrhythmia. Common patterns include grouped beats, cyclic speeding up and slowing down, or pairing of beats. If no pattern can be found, the pattern is described as *irregularly irregular* (Fig. 7-23).

The P wave should be analyzed by answering the follow-

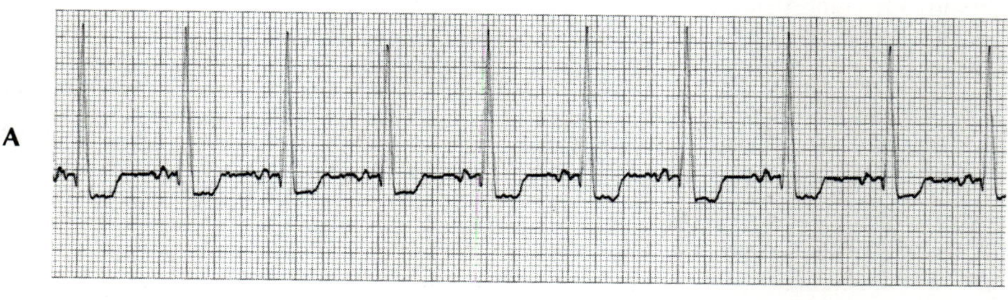


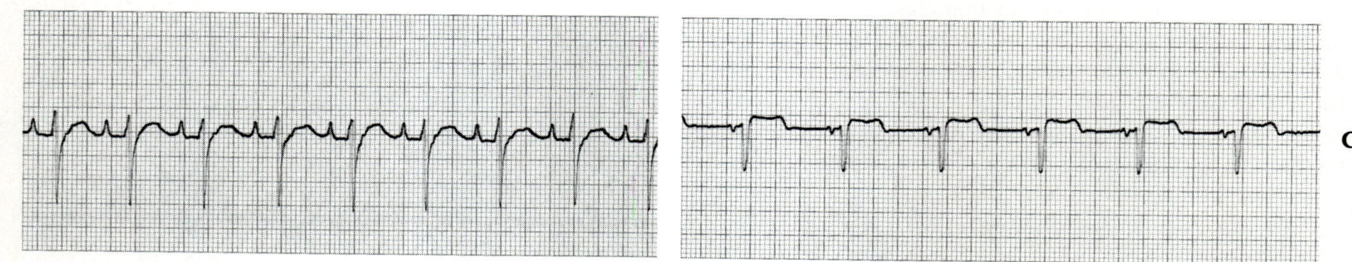


***Fig. 7-22*** Methods for calculating rate. **A,** Rate method number 1: number of RR intervals in 6 seconds multiplied by 10 (for example, 8 × 10 = 80/min). **B,** Rate method number 2: number of large boxes between QRS complexes divided into 300 (for example , 300 ÷ 3 = 100/min). **C,** Rate method number 3: number of small boxes between QRS complexes divided into 1500 (for example, 1500 ÷ 20 = 75/min).

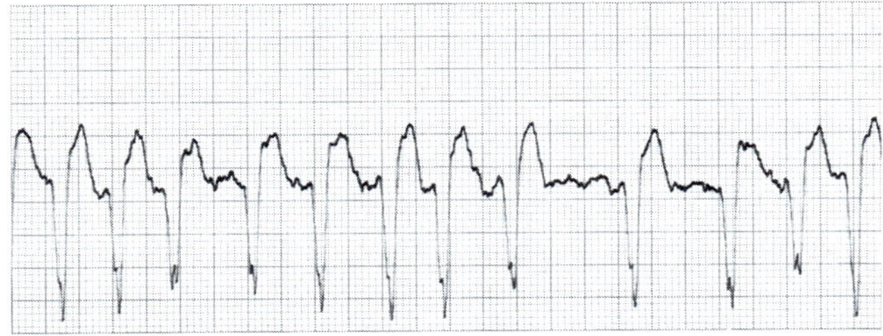

***Fig. 7-23*** Rhythm—irregularly irregular with no constant pattern.

ing questions. First, is the P wave present or absent? Second, is it related to the QRS? Sometimes there may be two, three, or four P waves in front of every QRS. If this pattern is consistent, the P wave and QRS are still related, although not on a 1:1 basis.

The duration of the PR interval is measured, and all PR intervals on the strip are checked to be sure they are the same duration as the original interval.

The entire ECG strip must be evaluated to ascertain that the QRS complexes are the same shape and width. If there is more than one QRS shape on the strip, each QRS must be measured (Fig. 7-24).

The QT interval must be measured as part of the routine analysis. The QT varies with heart rate; with heart rates of 60 to 100 beats per minute, the QT is usually 0.35 to 0.44 seconds.[111]

Determine whether the ST segment is isoelectric, depressed, or elevated. Analyze the T wave for shape, for example, round, flat, or peaked, and whether it is upright or inverted.

**Dysrhythmia recognition.** A general description of dysrhythmias commonly encountered in clinical practice is presented in Figs. 7-25 through 7-30. The figures contain a representative ECG strip, diagnostic criteria, etiologic factors, treatment, and other key points about the dysrhythmia. Discussion is organized into six areas: sinus rhythms, atrial dysrhythmias, junctional dysrhythmias, premature ventricular contractions, ventricular dysrhythmias, and AV conduction disturbances. More in-depth discussion on rhythm disturbances can be obtained through literature devoted specifically to electrocardiography and dysrhythmia interpretation.[23,41,72]

### CLINICAL USES OF HOLTER MONITORING

- Detection of supraventricular and ventricular dysrhythmias
  - In patients at high risk for asymptomatic dysrhythmias
  - For correlation of patient's symptoms with dysrhythmic occurrence
- Detection of paroxysmal heart block
- Evaluation of antidysrhythmic therapy
  - Reveals decrease in frequency and/or severity of dysrhythmias with therapy
  - Reveals increase in frequency and/or severity of dysrhythmias because of prodysrhythmic effect of some drugs
- Detection of ST segment level or shape in patients with or without suspected ischemic heart disease
- Evaluation of pacemaker function or dysfunction

Modified from Morganroth J: Ann Intern Med 102(1):73, 1985.

### Holter Monitoring

**Holter monitoring,** also known as continuous ambulatory electrocardiography, is a technique that records the electrocardiogram (ECG) of patients while they perform their usual activities. The patient wears skin electrodes and carries a box very similar to a tape recorder, either with a shoulder strap or clipped to his or her belt or pocket. Usually the monitor is left on for 24 hours and then is returned to the hospital or clinic for reading. This is a totally noninvasive procedure with no immediate adverse effects. As technology has improved, the recording devices have become even smaller so that at present a 4- × 6-inch recorder weighs less than 1 pound.

**Indications.** Holter monitors are widely used in a variety of clinical situations (see the box above). Often transient symptoms such as syncope, palpitations, or chest pain can-

*Text continued on p. 133.*

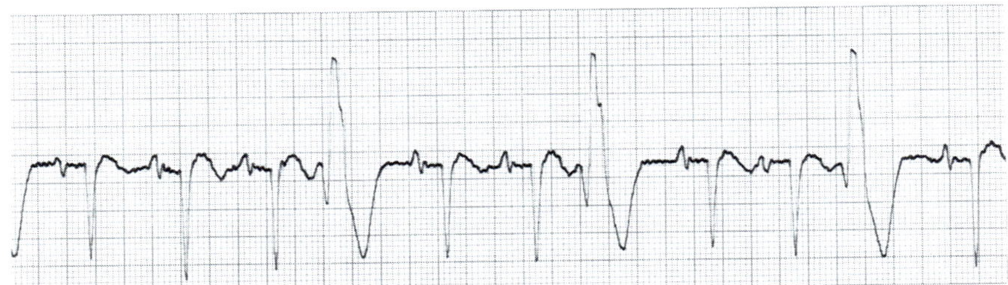

***Fig. 7-24*** QRS duration illustrating both normal and abnormal intervals. The narrow QRS complexes measure 0.08 seconds, which is normal. The wide QRS complexes measure 0.20 second and are caused by ventricular ectopy.

***Fig. 7-25*** Sinus rhythm.

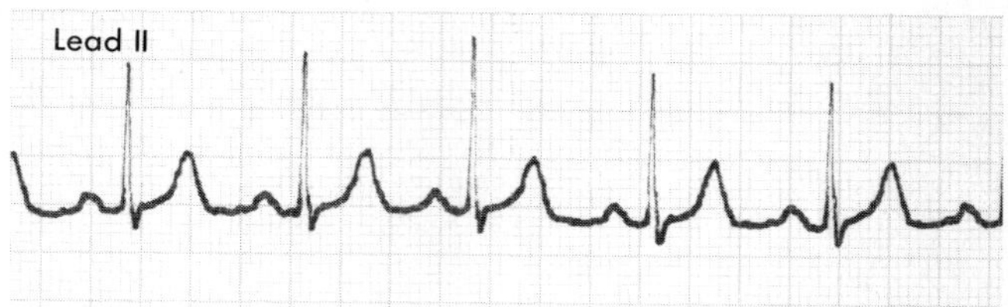


**A,** Normal sinus rhythm.

RATE: 60 to 100/min
RHYTHM: Regular

P WAVE: Present, with 1/QRS complex
PR INTERVAL: 0.12 to 0.20 sec; constant
QRS INTERVAL: 0.06 to 0.10 sec

ETIOLOGIC FACTORS: Normal conduction
TREATMENT: None necessary

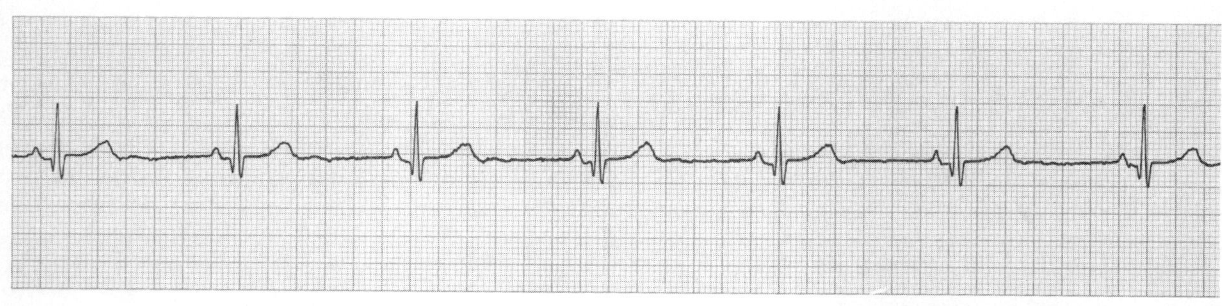

**B,** Sinus bradycardia.

RATE: Less than 60/min
RHYTHM: Regular

P WAVE: Present, with 1/QRS complex
PR INTERVAL: 0.12 to 0.20 sec; constant
QRS INTERVAL: 0.06 to 0.10 sec

ETIOLOGIC FACTORS: Athletes, vagal stimulation, increased intracranial pressure, drug therapy with digoxin or beta blockers, ischemia of the sinus node caused by acute anterior wall myocardial infarction.

TREATMENT: Not usually treated unless accompanied by symptoms of hypoperfusion (i.e., hypotension, dizziness, chest pain, changes in level of consciousness).

***Fig. 7-25, cont'd*** Sinus rhythm.

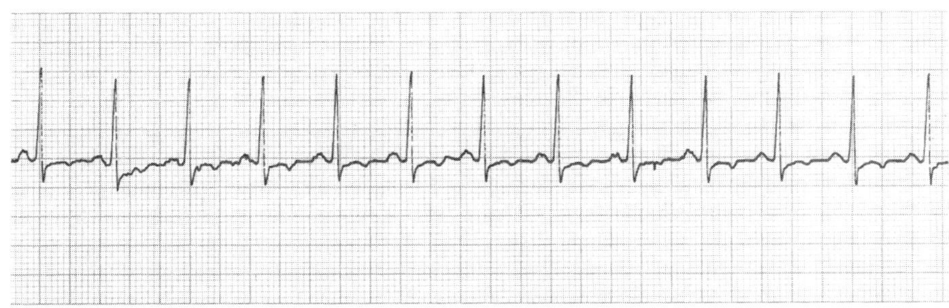

**C,** Sinus tachycardia.

RATE: Greater than 100/min
RHYTHM: Regular
P WAVE: Present, with 1/QRS complex
PR INTERVAL: 0.12 to 0.20 sec; constant
QRS INTERVAL: 0.06 to 0.10 sec

ETIOLOGIC FACTORS: Exercise, emotion, pain, fever, hemorrhage, shock, congestive heart failure, drugs (i.e., dopamine, aminophylline, hydralazine, epinepherine, and overuse of atropine).

TREATMENT: Treatment is aimed at the cause (i.e., fever, pain, and so on). Drugs such as calcium channel blockers and beta blockers are widely used.

KEY POINTS: Tachycardia is detrimental to anyone with ischemic heart disease because it decreases coronary blood supply by decreasing diastole, which is when the majority of coronary artery perfusion occurs. At the same time, tachycardia will increase the myocardial oxygen demand and the work of the heart. Cardiac output is the product of stroke volume multiplied by heart rate. If stroke volume is reduced as a result of myocardial damage, the only way that the heart can compensate is by increasing heart rate. Therefore caution should be taken in the administration of drugs to slow the heart rate, because slowing of the sinus node may cause severe and relatively immediate heart failure due to an inadequate cardiac output.

Rates of greater than 150/min should be closely examined for a triggering focus other than the sinus node (i.e., atrial flutter may be difficult to diagnose due to the high ventricular rate).

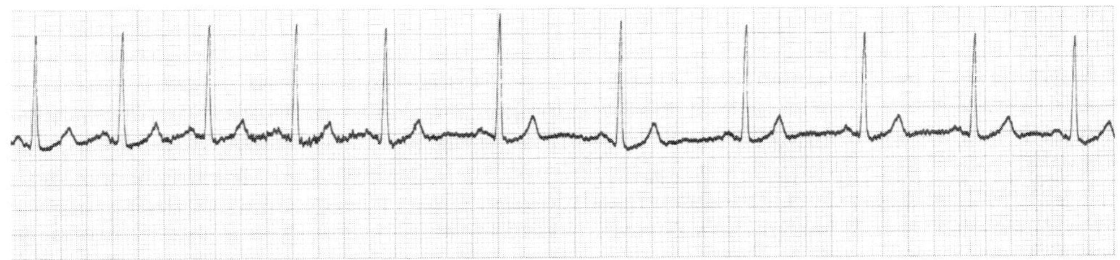

**D,** Sinus arrhythmia.

RATE: 60 to 100
RHYTHM: Irregular; respiratory variation
P WAVE: present, with 1/QRS complex
PR INTERVAL: 0.12 to 0.20 sec; constant
QRS INTERVAL: 0.06 to 0.10 sec

ETIOLOGIC FACTORS: Irregularity coincides with respiratory pattern (i.e., heart rate increases with inspiration and decreases with exhalation); frequently occurs in children.

TREATMENT: None necessary.

***Fig. 7-26*** Atrial dysrhythmias.

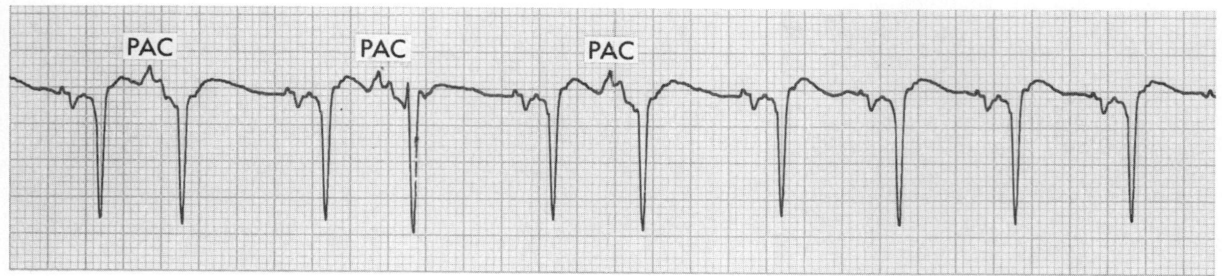


**A,** Premature atrial contraction (PAC).

RATE: Determined by underlying rhythm
RHYTHM: Variable

P WAVE: Present; different contour and configuration than others or may be buried in the preceeding T wave
PR INTERVAL: 0.12 to 0.20 sec or prolonged
QRS INTERVAL: 0.06 to 0.10 sec

ETIOLOGIC FACTORS: Can occur normally, accentuated by emotional disturbances, caffeine, nicotine, and digitalis; mitral valve prolapse and congestive heart failure may also cause PACs.
TREATMENT: None, if infrequent. If more frequent and patient is symptomatic, treat the cause (i.e., omit the irritants such as caffeine, reduce emotional distress, modify digitalis dosages, treat congestive heart failure. If pharmacologic therapy is necessary, procainamide or quinidine can be used).
KEY POINTS: Whenever an unexpected pause occurs in a rhythm, the T wave preceding the pause should be examined very carefully and compared with other T waves on the same strip. Look for distortions that may reveal a hidden, early P wave.

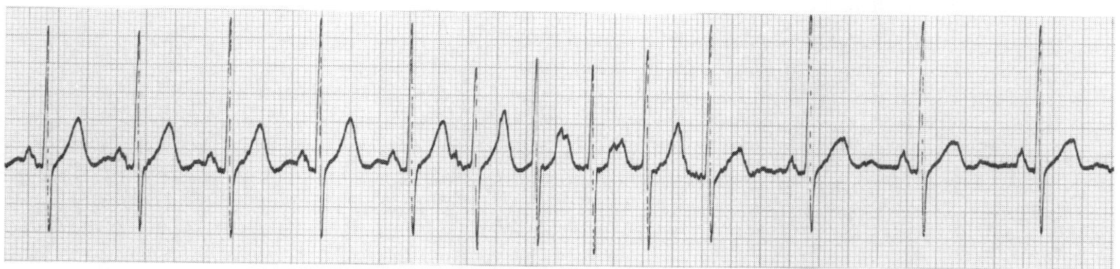

**B,** Paroxysmal atrial tachycardia (PAT).

RATE: Atrial: 150 to 250/min
Ventricular: Same as atrial or less if not all p waves are conducted
RHYTHM: Regular

P WAVE: Present; abnormally shaped
PR INTERVAL: 0.12 to 0.20 sec or prolonged
QRS INTERVAL: 0.06 to 0.10 sec

ETIOLOGIC FACTORS: Same as those for premature atrial contractions.
TREATMENT: PAT usually responds rapidly to medical management such as direct or indirect vagal maneuvers, intravenous calcium channel–blocking agents, or electrical cardioversion.
KEY POINTS: PAT refers to the sudden interruption of sinus rhythm by an ectopic focus that fires rapidly, and the condition starts and ends abruptly. PAT is significant clinically, especially if it is sustained for any length of time, because it occurs at such a rapid rate. If untreated, congestive heart failure, angina, or myocardial infarction may occur as a direct result of the rapid rate.

***Fig. 7-26, cont'd*** Atrial dysrhythmias.

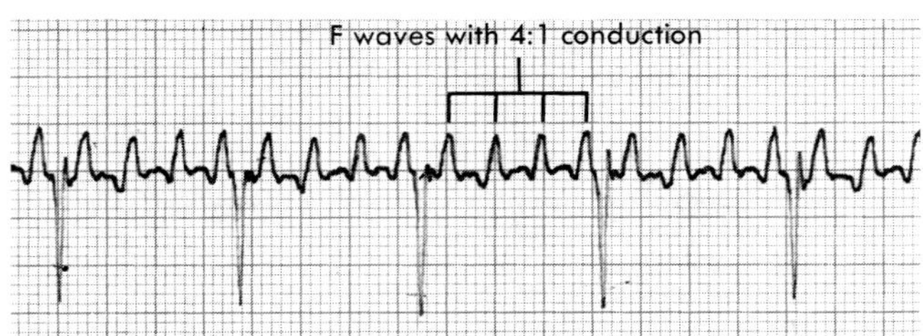


**C,** Atrial flutter (AF).

RATE: Atrial: 250 to 350/min
Ventricular: Half of atrial or less

RHYTHM: Atrial: Regular
Ventricular: May or may not be regular

P WAVE: Flutter (F) waves

PR INTERVAL: Conduction ratio: flutter waves per QRS

QRS INTERVAL: 0.06 to 0.10 sec

ETIOLOGIC FACTORS: Ischemic heart disease, coronary artery disease, cor plumonale, mitral or tricuspid valvular disease.

TREATMENT: Vagal maneuvers are useful to better visualize the flutter waves but rarely terminates AF. The main forms of therapy include cardioversion; drug therapy (i.e., digitalis, verapimil, quindine); and overdrive pacing.

KEY POINTS: AF is believed to be caused by a steady circular pathway through which the wave of depolarization is continually passing. At this high rate, P waves are lost and a "saw-tooth" pattern occurs with characteristic "F waves." The AV node does not allow all of the impulses to be conducted to the ventricles, so both atrial rates and ventricular rates must be calculated. In describing AF, the PR interval is no longer used. Instead, the conduction ratio is described to designate the number of flutter waves per QRS (i.e., 2:1, 3:1, 4:1). Once the impulse has passed through the AV node, conduction through the ventricles remains unaltered; thus a normal QRS complex appears.

The major key to the clinical significance of AF is the ventricular response rate. With an atrial rate of 300 and conduction ratio of 4:1, the ventricular rate is 75. However, if the ratio is 2:1, the ventricular response rate is 150, which may lead to angina, congestive heart failure, or other signs of cardiac decompensation.

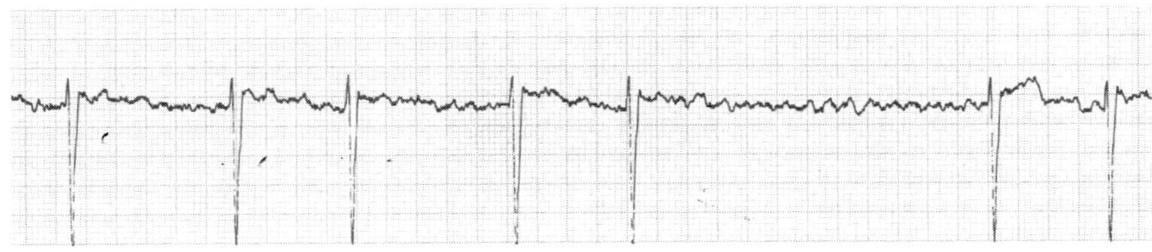

**D,** Atrial fibrilation (A Fib)

RATE: Atrial: Greater than 350/min (unable to count since no P waves can be identified)
Ventricular: 60 to 100 (controlled); greater than 100 (uncontrolled)

RHYTHM: Irregularly irregular

P WAVE: Fibrallatory (f) waves

PR INTERVAL: Absent

QRS INTERVAL: 0.06 to 0.10 sec

ETIOLOGIC FACTORS: Coronary artery disease, hypertension, mitral valve disease, thyrotoxicosis, acute MI, chronic obstructive lung disease, congestive heart failure, pericarditis.

TREATMENT: Drug therapy with digitalis, calcium channel blockers, beta blockers; cardioversion.

KEY POINTS: A Fib consists of numerous sites in the atria firing spontaneously, resulting in a quivering of the atrial muscle with no effective contraction. The ECG is characterized by an uneven baseline, an absence of P waves with f waves appearing instead. The AV node acts as a filter and allows only a portion of the impulses to reach the ventricles.

Cardioversion is more often successful when A Fib has been present for only a short time. If A Fib has been present for more than a few days, there is the threat of precipitating emboli since blood may pool in the walls of the atria and form thrombus. For this reason, anticoagulation therapy is often initiated several days or weeks before elective cardioversion.

***Fig. 7-27*** Junctional dysrhythmias.

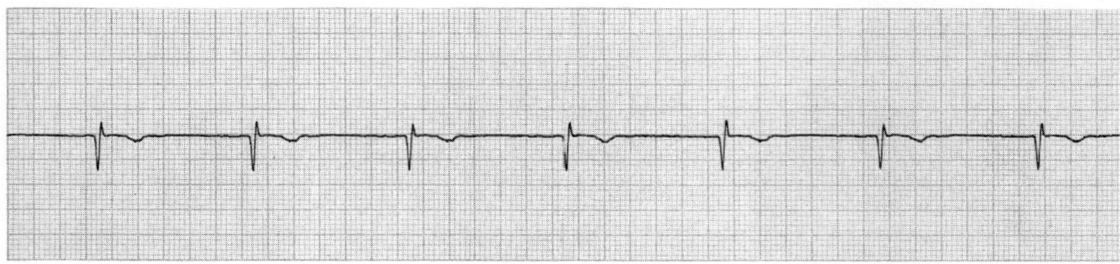

**A,** Junctional escape rhythm.

RATE: 40 to 60/min
RHYTHM: Regular
P WAVE: May be present or absent; inverted in lead II
PR INTERVAL: Less than 0.12 sec
QRS INTERVAL: 0.06-0.10 sec

ETIOLOGIC FACTORS: Conditions effecting the SA node, such as sinus bradycardia, and conditions in which AV automaticity is enhanced (i.e., digitalis toxicity, acute anterior wall MI, or rheumatic fever).

TREATMENT: Treatment of condition effecting the SA or AV node; drug therapy (i.e., atropine); pacemaker.

KEY POINTS: The condition is usually well tolerated. When the sinus node fails to fire, the junctional impulses are able to spontaneously depolarize and pace the heart. It is a protective mechanism to prevent asystole in the event of SA node failure.

After an ectopic impulse arises in the junction, it spreads in two directions at once. The upward spread through the atria causes an inverted P wave. The normal downward spread of depolarization through the ventricles results in a normal QRS. Sometimes the atria and the ventricles depolarize simultaneously, in which case the P wave is not visible.

If only a single ectopic impulse generates in the junction, it is simply called a "premature junctional contraction." On ECG, the rhythm will be normal from the sinus node except for one early QRS complex of normal shape and duration. If a P wave can be found, it will closely precede or follow the QRS and will be inverted in lead II.

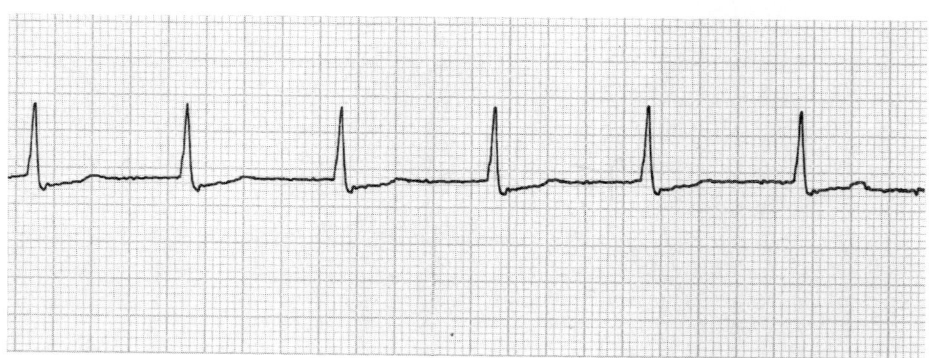

**B,** Accelerated junctional rhythm.

RATE: 60 to 100min
RHYTHM: Regular
P WAVE: May be present or absent; inverted in lead II
PR INTERVAL: Less than 0.12 sec
QRS INTERVAL: 0.06 to 0.10 sec

ETIOLOGIC FACTORS: Digitalis toxicity, inferior wall MI, myocarditis.

TREATMENT: Withold digitalis if toxicity is present; treat causes.

KEY POINTS: *Accelerated* refers to the situation of a junctional rate that is greater than normal for the junction, but less than that considered for tachycardia. This condition is usually well tolerated since it is within the normal range for heart rate.

*Junctional tachycardia* occurs when the junctional rate is greater than 100 and may not be as well tolerated by the patient due to the higher rate.

***Fig. 7-28*** Premature ventricular contraction (PVC).

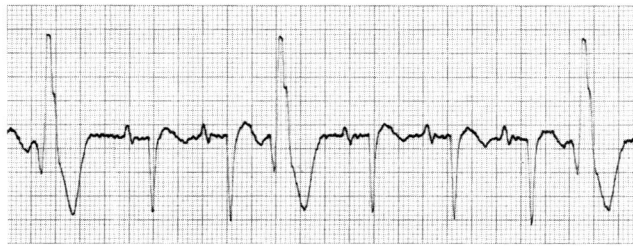

**A,** Unifocal PVCs.

QRS: Prolonged and greater than 0.12 sec; it is the width of the QRS, not the height, that is important in diagnosing ventricular ectopy.
ETIOLOGIC FACTORS: A PVC originates in a ventricular cell that has become abnormally permeable to sodium, usually as the result of damage. PVCs are commonly encountered in conditions such as ischemia, acute MI, cardiomyopathies, ventricular anurysms, hypokalemia, hypoxemia, acidosis, digitalis toxicity, and heart failure.
TREATMENT: Not all PVCs require treatment. When immediate therapy is indicated, lidocaine is the drug of choice and is administered by a bolus followed by a continuous infusion. Procainamide or bretylium can be given intravenously when lidocaine fails. Numerous oral antidysrhythmic agents can be administered for long-term control (i.e., quinidine, procainamide, mexiletine, propranolol, verapimil, amiodarone, and others). If digitalis toxicity is present, the digitalis is discontinued. Hypokalemia is treated with potassium replacement. Oxygen is administered and acidosisis reversed.
KEY POINTS: A single ectopic impulse originating in the ventricles is called a PVC. Some PVCs are very small in height but remain wider than 0.12 sec. If in doubt, a different lead should be evaluated. The shape of the QRS will vary, depending on the location of the ectopic focus. If all of the ventricular ectopic beats look the same in that particular lead, they are called *unifocal PVCs.*

PVCs can develop concurrently with any supraventricular dysrhythmia. Therefore when describing the condition, the underlying rhythm is described first (i.e., "sinus bradycardia with frequent unifocal PVCs").

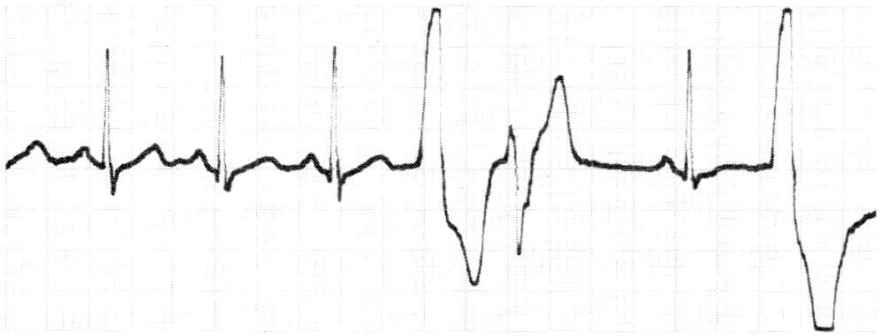

**B,** Multifocal PVCs.

KEY POINTS: Ventricular ectopics of various shapes in the same lead are called *multifocal PVCs.* Multifocal ventricular ectopics are more serious than unifocal because they indicate a greater area of irritable myocardial tissue and are more likely to deteriorate into a more serious condition, such as ventricular tachycardia or fibrillation.

***Fig. 7-28, cont'd*** Premature ventricular contraction (PVC).

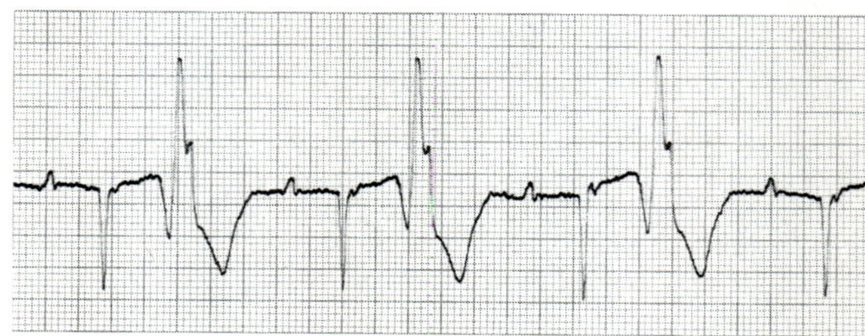

**C,** Ventricular bigeminy.

KEY POINTS: When a PVC follows each normal beat, *ventricular bigeminy* is present. If a PVC follows every third beat, it is called *ventricular trigeminy*.

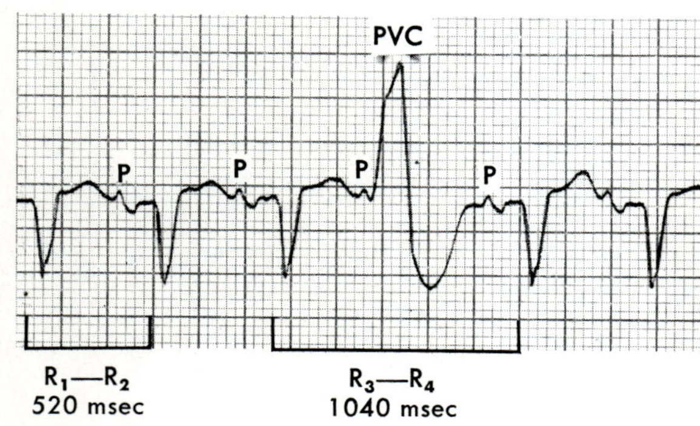


**D,** PVC with fully compensatory pause.

KEY POINTS: Some PVCs cause a fully compensatory pause—the interval between the two sinus beats that surround the PVC ($R_3$ and $R_4$ in this case) is exactly two times the normal interval between sinus beats ($R_1$ and $R_2$). Notice that the P waves come on time except that the third P wave is interrupted by the PVC and therefore does not conduct normally through the A-V junction. The next (fourth) P wave also comes on time. The fact that the sinus node continues to pace despite the PVC results in the fully compensatory pause. (From Goldberger AL and Goldberger E: Clinical electrocardiography: a simplified approach, ed 4, St Louis, 1990, Mosby–Year Book, Inc.)

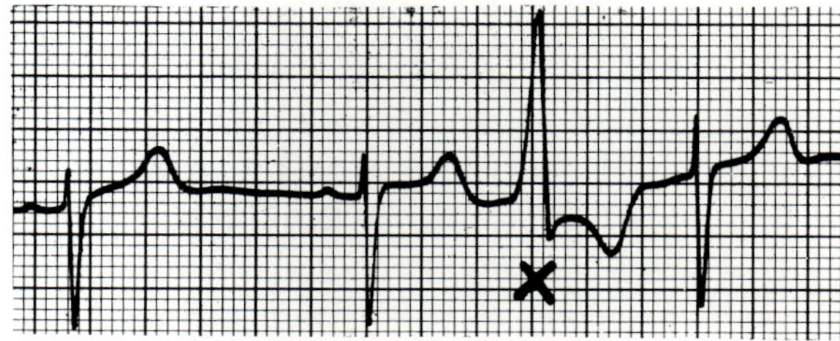


**E,** Interpolated PVC.

KEY POINTS: Sometimes a PVC *(X)* will fall between two normal QRS complexes without disturbing the rhythm. This is called an interpolated PVC. Note that the RR interval between sinus beats remains unchanged. (From Goldberger AL and Goldberger E: Clinical electrocardiography: a simplified approach, ed 4, St Louis, 1990, Mosby–Year Book, Inc.)

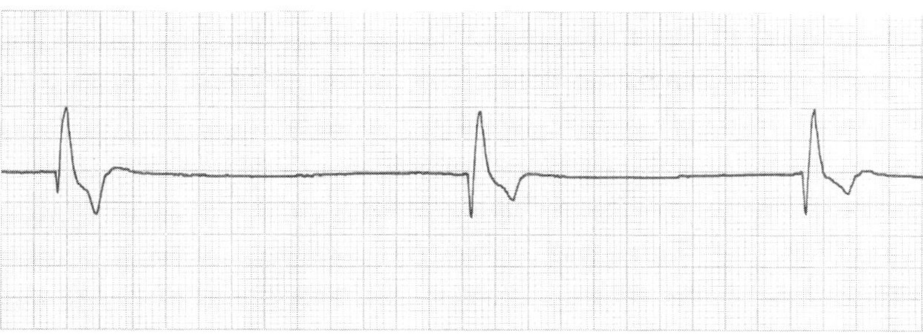

**A,** Idioventricular rhythm.

RATE: 20 to 40/min
RHYTHM: Usually regular
P WAVE: Absent or retrograde
PR INTERVAL: None
QRS INTERVAL: Greater than 0.12 sec

ETIOLOGIC FACTORS: Acute MI, digitalis toxicity.
TREATMENT: Atropine, pacemaker, CPR, epinepherine.
KEY POINTS: When both the sinus node and the AV node fail to function, an idioventricular pacemaker takes over control as a protective mechanism. Treatment is aimed at increasing the effective heart rate rather than abolishing the ventricular beats.

An *accelerated idioventricular* rhythm occurs when the ventricular rate is greater than 40 but less than 100 per minute. Although relatively benign, this rhythm must be closely observed for any increase in rate or hemodynamic deterioration. Usually, it is not treated if well tolerated.

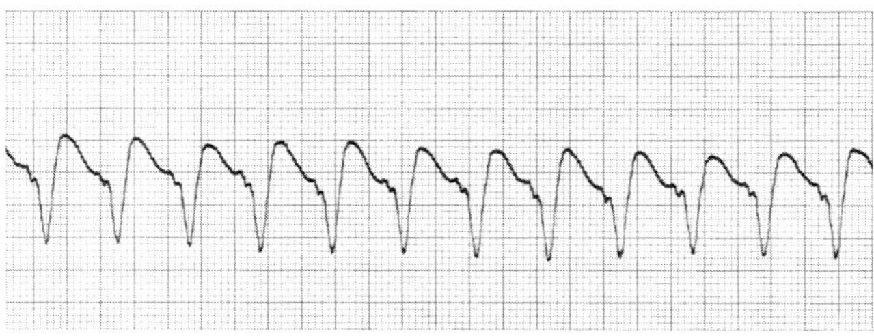

**B,** Ventricular tachycardia (V tach).

RATE: Greater than 100/min
RHYTHM: Usually regular
P WAVE: Absent or retrograde
PR interval: None
QRS INTERVAL: Greater than 0.12 sec

ETIOLOGIC FACTORS: Myocardial ischemia, acute MI, digitalis toxicity, electrolyte disturbances, adverse reaction to antidysrhythmic drugs, chronic severe heart disease (i.e., cardiomyopathy or ventricular aneurysm).
TREATMENT: Intravenous drug therapy (i.e., lidocaine, procainamide, bretylium); cardioversion; if hypokalemic, administer potassium intravenously; if hypoxemic, administer oxygen.
KEY POINTS: More than 3 PVCs in a row is considered V tach; however, it is helpful to state how many beats of V tach occurred if the run was short (e.g., less than 20 beats).

Some types of PVCs have been associated with future development of V tach or ventricular fibrillation. They have been called *warning, complex,* or *malignant* ectopy: frequent PVCs, multifocal PVCs, three or more beats of V tach in a row. In addition, the *R-on-T phenomenon,* in which the PVC occurs during the relative refractory period, can lead to ventricular fibrillation.

In most cases the sinus node is not affected, and it will continue to depolarize the atria; P waves can sometimes be seen on ECG but are not related to the QRS.

V tach is a serious dysrhythmia and must be treated quickly. Its rapid rate alone makes the dysrhythmia poorly tolerated. The cardiac output will fall, leading to loss of consciousness. If V tach is not terminated quickly, ventricular fibrillation and death may result.

***Fig. 7-29, cont'd*** Ventricular dysrhythmias.

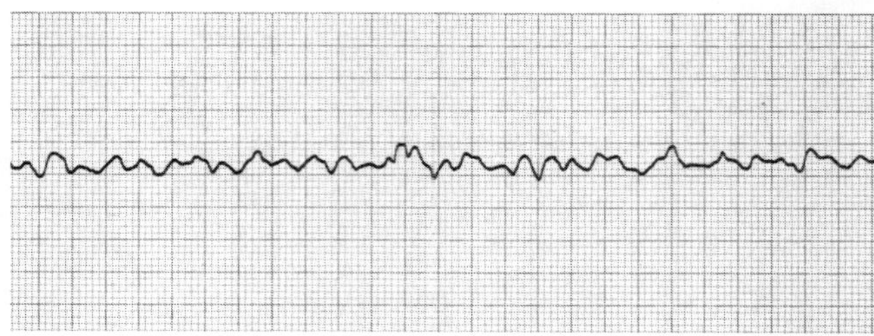

**C,** Ventricular fibrillation (V fib).

RATE: Undeterminable
RHYTHM: Irregular
P WAVE: Absent
PR INTERVAL: Absent
QRS INTERVAL: Absent

ETIOLOGIC FACTORS: Acute MI, R-on-T phenomenon, digitalis toxicity, chronic severe heart disease, dying heart.
TREATMENT: Precordial thump; rapid defibrillation with countershock; initiation of CPR.
KEY POINTS: V fib is the result of rapid discharge of impulses from multiple foci in the ventricles, resulting in ventricles that are unable to respond completely and effectively. The ventricles merely quiver, and there is no forward flow of blood and no palpable blood pressure or audible apical heart tones. Clinically, V fib is indistinguishable from asytole. On the ECG, V fib appears as a course wavy baseline.

***Fig. 7-30*** Atrioventricular conduction disturbances.

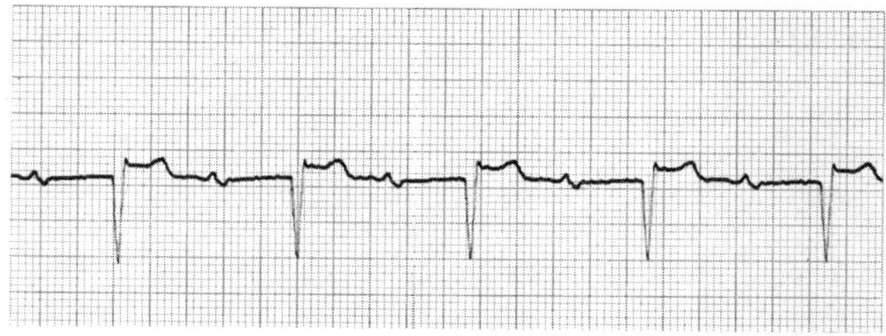

**A,** First-degree AV block.

RATE: Determined by sinus rate
RHYTHM: Regular
P WAVE: 1 P wave/QRS
PR INTERVAL: Greater than 0.20 sec and constant
QRS INTERVAL: 0.06 to 0.10 sec

ETIOLOGIC FACTORS: May occur in both normal and diseased hearts; drugs (i.e., digitalis, beta blockers, calcium channel blockers); cardiac surgery; myocarditis; calcification of the AV node due to aging.
TREATMENT: None necessary.
KEY POINTS: First-degree heart block is not clinically significant by itself. In the presence of acute MI, it may be a forerunner of more severe conduction disturbances and requires close monitoring.

***Fig. 7-30, cont'd*** Atrioventricular conduction disturbances.

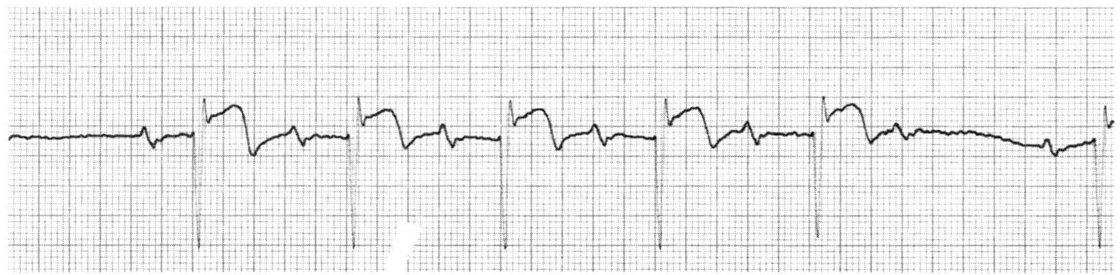

**B,** Second-degree AV block, Mobitz type I (Wenckebach).

RATE: Normal or slow

RHYTHM: Irregular

P WAVE: Intermittently not conducted, yielding more P waves than QRS complexes

PR INTERVAL: Increases with each consecutively conducted P wave

QRS INTERVAL: 0.06 to 0.10 sec

ETIOLOGIC FACTORS: Ischemia, acute inferior MI, digitalis toxicity.

TREATMENT: Close observation; temporary transvenous pacemaker.

KEY POINTS: The AV conduction time progressively lengthens until a P wave is not conducted. Mobitz I is caused by an abnormally long relative refractory period. The rate of conduction depends on the moment of the impulse arrival: the earlier the impulse arrives in the AV node, the longer it takes to conduct; the later it arrives, the shorter the conduction time. The actual anatomical site of the block is at the level of the AV node itself.

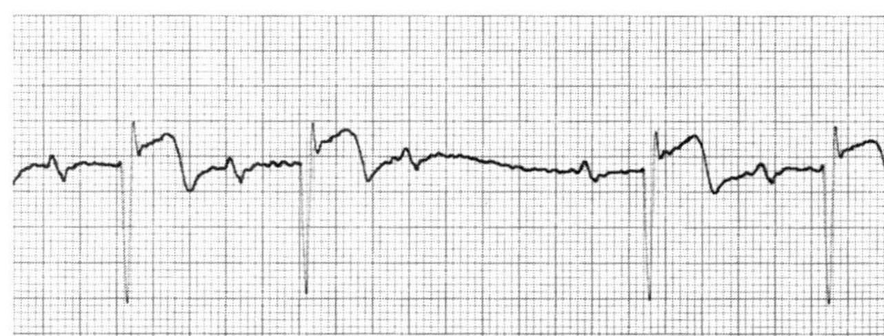

**C,** Second-degree AV block, Mobitz type II.

RATE: Usually slow

RHYTHM: Irregular

P WAVE: Intermittently not conducted, yielding more P waves than QRS complexes

PR INTERVAL: Constant

QRS INTERVAL: May be normal, but usually coexists with bundle branch block (greater than 0.12 sec)

ETIOLOGIC FACTORS: Acute anterior wall MI.

TREATMENT: Close observation; drug therapy (i.e., atropine, isoproteranol, epinepherine); temporary transvenous pacemaker; external pacemaker.

KEY POINTS: Mobitz type II block occurs in the presence of a long absolute refractory period with virtually no relative refractory period. Usually, the block is below the AV node, either in the His bundle or in both bundle branches. Most often, it occurs when one bundle branch is blocked and the other is ischemic. It is clinically more ominous than Mobitz I block, and often progresses to complete AV block.

***Fig. 7-30, cont'd*** Atrioventricular conduction disturbances.

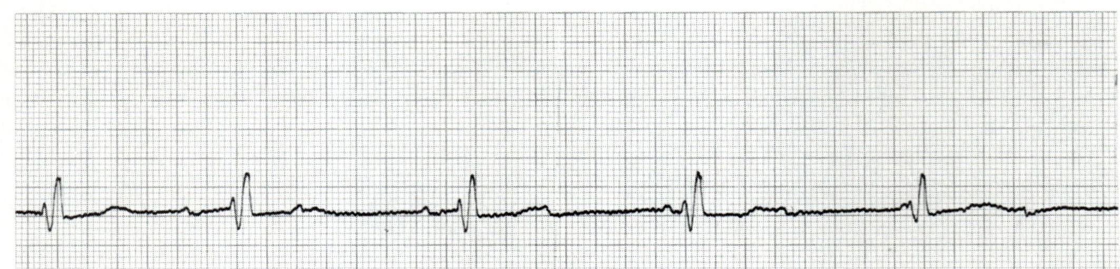

**D,** Third-degree AV block (complete heart block).

RATE: Less than 60/min, depending on escape pacemaker
RHYTHM: Regular

P WAVE: P waves are independent and not related to the QRS complexes
PR INTERVAL: Varies randomly
QRS INTERVAL: 0.06 to 0.10 sec if junctional escape pacemaker activates the vertricles; greater than 0.12 sec if ventricular escape pacemaker activates the ventricles

ETIOLOGIC FACTORS: Acute inferior wall MI, cardiac surgery, digitalis toxicity, myocarditis.
TREATMENT: Temporary transvenous pacemaker; external pacemaker; IV atropine; IV epinepherine; isoproteronol drip as last resort, if hemodynamically unstable.
KEY POINTS: Third-degree heart block is a condition in which no atrial impulses can conduct through the AV node to cause ventricular deplorization. The opportunity for conduction is optimal, yet none occurs. It is hoped that a junctional or ventricular focus will depolarize spontaneously at its intrinsic rate of 20 to 60 beats/min, and ventricular contraction will continue. If not, asystole occurs; there is no pulse and death will result if treatment is not initiated.

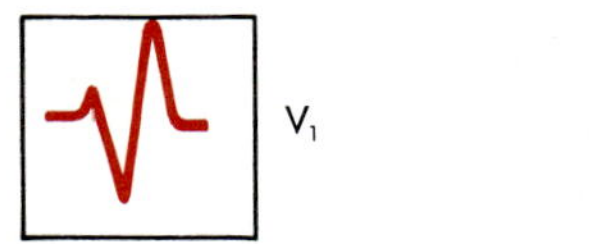


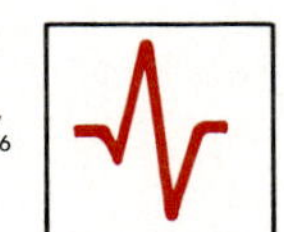


**E,** Right bundle branch block (RBBB).

ETIOLOGIC FACTORS: CAD, right ventricular hypertrophy, premature supraventricular beats that are aberrantly conducted.
TREATMENT: None necessary unless accompanied by incomplete left bundle branch block and first-degree AV block. This is called *trifascicular block* and may not require a pacemaker.
KEY POINTS: RBBB occurs when there is a complete interruption of conduction through the right bundle branch. In a complete RBBB, the QRS will always be greater than 0.12 sec.

The chest leads are the most useful in identifying bundle branch blocks, specifically $V_1$ and $V_6$, since they are located on either side of the heart. A RBBB exists if the final forces of the QRS are upright in $V_1$ and negative in $V_6$.

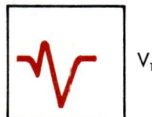

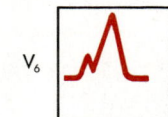

**F,** Left bundle branch block (LBBB).

ETIOLOGIC FACTORS: Ischemia, rheumatic heart disease, hypertension, valvular heart disease.
TREATMENT: None, unless accompanied by first-degree AV block, in which case a pacemaker may be inserted.
KEY POINTS: LBBB occurs when there is a complete interruption of conduction through the left bundle branch. In a complete LBBB, the QRS will always be greater than 0.12 sec.

Since a normal QRS complex is not recorded, ECG changes associated with MI may be difficult to ascertain.

On ECG, the final forces of the QRS will be negative in $V_1$ and upright in $V_6$.

not be reproduced in the clinical or hospital setting, but through use of a Holter monitor designed to be worn in the patient's usual environment, documentation of dysrhythmias or ST segment changes can be correlated with symptoms. Patients with cardiac disease may be asymptomatic yet can have significant ventricular ectopy, which places them at a higher risk for sudden death. Holter monitors are useful in identifying these high-risk patients, quantifying the frequency of the dysrhythmias, and evaluating the response to antidysrhythmic agents once treatment has begun.

**Procedure.** All Holter monitors record at least two leads, primarily to minimize inaccurate interpretation caused by artifact. Usually five electrodes are placed. Two of them are positive electrodes, corresponding approximately to the $V_1$ and $V_5$ positions on a standard 12-lead ECG. There are also two negative electrodes and one ground. Occasionally, additional electrodes are used to improve diagnostic capabilities. For example, a separate lead can be used to detect pacemaker spikes if the patient is being monitored for pacemaker dysfunction.[36] The skin electrodes are disposable, pregelled, and self-adhering. They should be kept dry—not because of any electrical danger, but to prevent their falling off before the recording is completed. If skin irritation or hypersensitivity occurs, it can usually be relieved with hydrocortisone cream. The recorder is battery powered and can use either a reel-to-reel or cassette magnetic tape. Reel-to-reel tapes have fewer technical problems and can provide a clearer recording, but cassette tapes are smaller and more convenient for the patient.

Many variations of Holter monitors exist, but at present they can be divided into three basic recording modes.[75] The first and most common is the continuous recording mode. In this mode the tape saves all of the ECG tracings for a given period of time, usually 8 to 24 hours. The tape can correlate time with the tracing and display the time that an event occurred when the tape is decoded. Most also have an event marker, which the patient can press to indicate the onset of symptoms or another event that may be important. The patient is asked to keep a diary of his or her activities, symptoms, and any medications that are taken.

When the tape is returned to the hospital or clinic for reading, a technician places it in a machine that displays the tracing for review. The tracing is run at a faster speed than normal, or it would take 24 hours to read a 24-hour recording, and the cost would be prohibitive. Printed reports are also generated as the tape is read. Real-time printouts, at normal speed, can be run when any significant dysrhythmias are noted. A trend plot of heart rate, ST segment level, or number of ectopics can also be printed. Most decoding machines count ectopics automatically, but it is up to the operator to validate that the decoder is really counting ectopy and not artifact.

A second type of recording mode is the intermittent, or patient-activated, recording mode. In this mode, when the patient is having symptoms, he or she presses a button to initiate the recording manually. Some of the newer devices can transmit this recording telephonically to a diagnostic center. Advantages of this mode center around the ability to leave the recorder on the patient for longer periods of time. Patients with infrequent symptoms do not benefit from a 24-hour continuous recording if the symptoms do not occur during that time.[52] With the intermittent recorder mode, the device can be worn for up to 96 hours, and the patient can trigger active recording at the appropriate times.

Real-time analytical or event recording is the most recent recording mode development. A built-in computer analyzes the ECG as it is recorded and stores only abnormal patterns. The device weighs approximately twice as much as a standard Holter monitor because of the built-in computer. It also costs three to five times more, but this cost is offset by the decrease in man-hours needed for interpretation. This recording mode is very useful because the recorder can be used over a longer period of time (since the entire tracing is not stored) and interpretation is immediately available from the computer without needing an operator to decode it.

**Summary of nursing care.** Many patients' symptoms do not occur every day and may be missed during a random 24-hour recording. Often symptoms tend to occur in association with specific activities. The nurse should inquire about the types of activities that tend to provoke symptoms for a specific patient and encourage the patient to pursue those activities while wearing the monitor. In general, the patient should be encouraged to be as active as possible. Keeping an accurate diary of activities is important, since it allows correlation of an identified dysrhythmia with a specific activity or symptom. The only activities that are restricted while wearing a Holter monitor are those that would get the chest electrodes or monitor wet, such as swimming and taking a shower or tub bath. Sponge baths are permitted as long as the chest electrodes are avoided.

### Exercise Electrocardiography

Exercise places unique demands on the cardiovascular system. Systemic oxygen consumption increases markedly, requiring the heart to increase cardiac output to meet these demands. Myocardial contractility increases, resulting in greater stroke volume and systolic blood pressure. Heart rate is also increased as a result of circulating catecholamines. Normally, as heart rate and stroke volume rise, cardiac output is increased dramatically, and the tissue needs for oxygen are met. This enhanced myocardial performance is not without its price. Even at rest, the heart muscle extracts 70% of the oxygen available in the circulating blood.[19] When the myocardial demand for oxygen increases during exercise, coronary blood flow must increase to maintain an adequate oxygen supply. In patients with coronary artery disease, coronary blood flow is not able to increase sufficiently to provide the high metabolic needs of the myocardium during exercise, and ischemia will result.

**Indications.** Exercise tolerance testing, or stress testing, is clinically useful in several settings. It helps evaluate the presence, absence, or severity of coronary artery disease, both in patients with known coronary heart disease, as well as in those initially seen with chest pain of unclear origin. Stress testing can evaluate the functional capacity of patients with or without heart disease and can be done serially to evaluate the effectiveness of medical or surgical therapy.

**Procedure.** Originally exercise tests were conducted using a two-step platform that the patient climbed up and down repeatedly. This is called a Master's two-step exercise test and is still used in a few places because the cost of the equipment is minimal. The vast majority of exercise tests in the United States, however, are now performed using a treadmill on which both speed and slope can be varied. A number of protocols have been developed using a treadmill. All reach virtually the same end point, but they vary the speed with which they approach that end point. Two popular ones are the Bruce protocol, in which both grade and speed are varied every 3 minutes, and the Balke protocol, in which speed remains constant and grade is gradually increased every minute.

The exercise test can be performed on an outpatient or inpatient basis. In either case, a physician must be present to supervise the test directly. It would be ideal always to conduct the exercise test in the morning after an overnight fast. Logistically, however, exercise tests must be performed throughout the day. Patients are advised to eat a light meal no closer than 3 hours before the test is scheduled. They should dress comfortably in light clothing and wear comfortable shoes for brisk walking or running.

A 12-lead ECG is recorded at rest before beginning the exercise protocol, and another 12-lead ECG is usually recorded on completion of the test. Various lead positions are used during the testing, depending on the number of leads that the equipment is able to monitor. Additional leads improve the accuracy of the test, since ischemia may be missed if there is not a lead monitoring that particular portion of the myocardial wall. Most facilities currently use three leads, usually II, $V_3$, and $V_5$. Lead II will detect ischemic changes in the inferior wall, lead $V_3$ will show ischemia in the anterior wall, and lead $V_5$ will reveal ischemia in the lateral wall. Skin preparation for electrode placement is of vital importance, since the recording will be meaningless if an electrode falls off during exercise. A blood pressure cuff is also placed on one arm to measure the blood pressure response to exercise.

Regardless of the protocol used, the electrocardiogram (ECG) is printed at 1-minute intervals, as well as during any symptoms, visible ECG changes, or dysrhythmias. Blood pressure is also measured and recorded every minute.

The treadmill test is terminated whenever the patient requests that it be stopped, if symptoms such as chest pain, dyspnea, dizziness, or fatigue occur, if there are significant ECG changes or dysrhythmias, or if there is significant hypotension or hypertension. Blood pressure is expected to rise during exercise, but a systolic blood pressure >220 mm Hg or a diastolic blood pressure >110 mm Hg is considered high enough to stop the test.[19] If none of the above situations occur, the test is stopped when a desirable level, based on the patient's heart rate, is reached. A maximal stress test is one in which the predicted maximal heart rate for that patient is reached. A goal of 85% to 90% of the predicted maximal heart rate is set for a submaximal test, and in most patients this level of exercise is sufficient to unmask any significant coronary artery disease.

A low-level stress test is sometimes performed before discharge from the hospital on patients who have suffered an acute myocardial infarction. In this case the heart rate is raised only to 120 or 130 beats per minute. Current results indicate that ST segment depression or elevation that occurs during the predischarge low-level stress test is a reliable indicator of additional myocardium at risk. However, exercise-induced angina or abnormal blood pressure responses to exercise often do not appear during a low-level stress test, so a "normal" predischarge stress test must be followed later by a test closer to maximal level.[46]

**Interpretation of results.** Considerable controversy exists about interpretation criteria for a positive exercise ECG test. ST-segment depression, either horizontal or downsloping, of 1 mm or more during or after exercise is the most diagnostic of coronary artery disease. Criteria that are

***Table 7-12*** Criteria for positive exercise ECG test

| Definitely positive | Strongly suggestive |
|---|---|
| Horizontal ST-segment depression of 1 mm or more during or after exercise | Horizontal or downsloping ST-segment depression of <1 mm during or after exercise |
| Downsloping ST-segment depression of 1 mm or more during or after exercise | Upsloping ST-segment depression of 2 mm or more beyond 0.08 sec from J point during or after exercise |
| | Horizontal or upsloping ST-segment elevation of 1 mm or more during or after exercise |
| | ST-segment sagging 1 mm or more during or after exercise |
| | Hypotension |
| | Inverted U wave |
| | Frequent premature ventricular contractions (PVCs), multifocal PVCs, grouped PVCs, ventricular tachycardia provoked by mild exercise (70% or less of maximal heart rate) |
| | Exercise-induced typical angina $S_3$, $S_4$, or heart murmur |

strongly suggestive of a positive exercise ECG test are listed in Table 7-12.

**Summary of nursing care.** It is important for the nurse to teach the patient before the procedure. Many fears about the procedure and the patient's ability to tolerate the test can be allayed. In addition to describing the procedure itself, the nurse should instruct the patient to fast for 3 hours before the test, refrain from smoking for at least 2 hours before the test, and wear comfortable shoes and loose-fitting clothes. The patient should be reassured that his or her heart will be monitored closely during the test and a physician will be standing by. Although the patient will be encouraged to continue as long as possible, the test will be stopped at the patient's request for symptoms such as fatigue, shortness of breath, or leg cramps. The patient should also be told that the diagnostic value of the test is based on the maximal heart rate achieved, not on the length of time that he or she is able to remain on the treadmill.

After the exercise test is completed, the patient will be assisted into a supine position. The ECG, pulse rate, and blood pressure will be monitored for at least 10 more minutes to detect dysrhythmias or signs of ischemia. The patient should be instructed to rest for the next 30 to 60 minutes after release from the exercise laboratory. Hot showers should be avoided for 3 to 4 hours to prevent development of orthostatic hypotension.

The nurse performing the test must be certain that emergency medications and a defibrillator are available in the test area and should be familiar with their use.

### Phonocardiography

**Indications.** A sound recording, or phonocardiogram, permits accurate timing of sounds and events and can reveal information about underlying hemodynamic events that is not obtainable through the physical examination alone. For example, the width of an $S_2$ split can be used as an index of severity in pulmonic stenosis.[114] The phonocardiogram can point out abnormalities of valve function or wall structure (such as idiopathic hypertrophic subaortic stenosis).

Another advantage of a phonocardiogram over simple auscultation is that it provides a permanent, objective record of events. Subsequent comparisons can be made to evaluate progression of valvular dysfunction or to measure the degree of improvement after therapeutic interventions.

**Phonocardiography** can be combined with echocardiography to yield more information than either technique alone. The echocardiogram provides a time-frame reference for the phonocardiogram, allowing identification of sound components by their relationship to certain defined valvular motions. At the same time, the phonocardiogram provides reference points for the echocardiogram, which improves the timing of certain phases of the cardiac cycle.

**Procedure.** Phonocardiography is the graphic display on paper of the sounds that occur in the heart and great vessels. The sounds are recorded from a transducer placed on the surface of the chest wall. The recording corresponds to the sounds heard during cardiac auscultation with a stethoscope.

**Summary of nursing care.** Patient teaching is important in relieving anxiety and eliciting cooperation. A quiet environment is desirable for proper recording of a phonocardiogram, since the equipment is very sensitive to sound waves. Several small microphones are placed on the patient's chest. In males, small areas of the chest may need to be shaved to improve skin contact with the microphones. The procedure is not uncomfortable and is usually completed in less than 20 minutes. When combined with echocardiography, which is often the case, the entire procedure may take as long as 45 minutes to 1 hour.

### Echocardiography

**Indications. Echocardiography** is used to detect cardiac abnormalities such as mitral valve stenosis and regurgitation, prolapse of mitral valve leaflets, aortic stenosis and insufficiency, idiopathic hypertrophic subaortic stenosis, atrial septal defects, and pericardial effusions. Recent developments also allow detection of wall-motion abnormalities, estimation of ejection fraction and pulmonary artery pressures, and identification of intracardiac myomas.

**Procedure.** Echocardiography uses waves of ultrasound to obtain and display images of cardiac structures. While the test is performed, the patient is in either a supine, left-lateral, or semi-Fowler's position. Which position is used depends on the patient's clinical condition and on which position provides the best view of the structures examined. A transducer is placed on the skin, with lubricant between the transducer and the skin to improve contact and reduce artifact. The transducer is usually placed in the third or fourth intercostal space to the left of the sternum, since at that point the pericardium is in direct contact with the chest wall and the ultrasonic waves are not obstructed by either air or bone. Other positions are sometimes used if the standard location does not provide adequate visualization of the cardiac structures.

Ultrasound is reflected best at interfaces between tissues that have different densities. In the heart these are the blood, cardiac valves, myocardium, and pericardium. Since all these structures differ in density, their borders can be seen on the echocardiogram.

In one type of echocardiography, a thin beam of ultrasound is directed through the heart (Fig. 7-31). Each interface is represented by a dot, and when recorded over time (like an ECG), each dot becomes a line on an oscilloscope. A strip-chart recording can be made of this tracing as the heart beats. Since this is a recording of heart motion over time, this technique is called an *M-mode* (motion-mode) echocardiogram. The M-mode echocardiogram is particularly useful for measuring cardiac wall thickness and chamber size, evaluating valve motion, and assessing contractile motion of certain portions of the heart wall. It provides a good view of the anterior interventricular septum, the left-ventricular posterior wall from the base to the midportion, the aortic and mitral valves, and the left atrium.

**A**

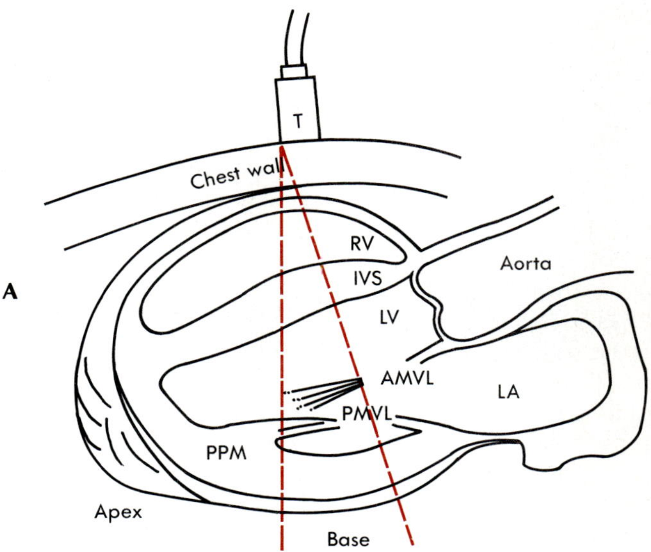


**B**

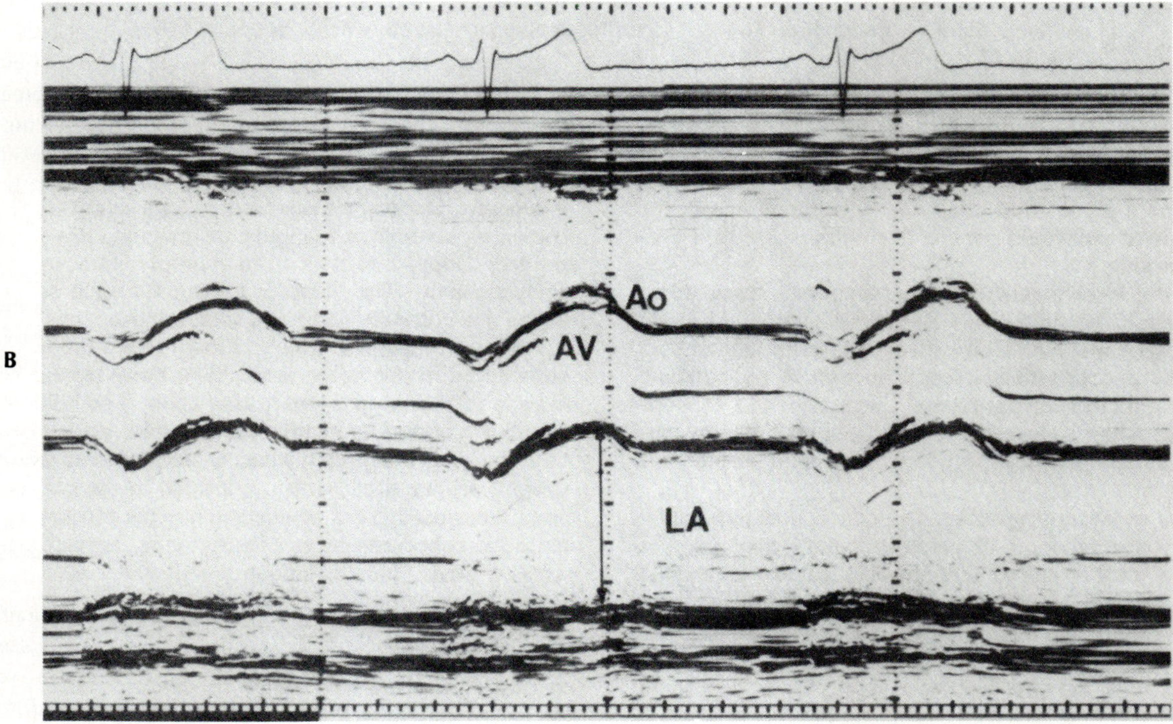


***Fig. 7-31*** **A,** Schematic presentation of cardiac structures transversed by two echo beams. *RV,* right ventricle; *LV,* left ventricle; *IVS,* interventricular septum; *En,* endocardium; *Pe,* pericardium; *Ch,* chordae. *AMLV,* anterior mitral valve leaflet; *PMVL,* posterior mitral valve leaflet; *PPM,* posterior papillary muscle; *LA,* left atrium; *T,* transducer. **B,** Normal, M-mode echocardiogram at the level of the aorta *(Ao),* aortic valve *(AV)* leaflets, and left atrium *(LA).* (**B** from Kinney M and others: Comprehensive cardiac care, ed 7, St Louis, 1991, Mosby–Year Book, Inc.)

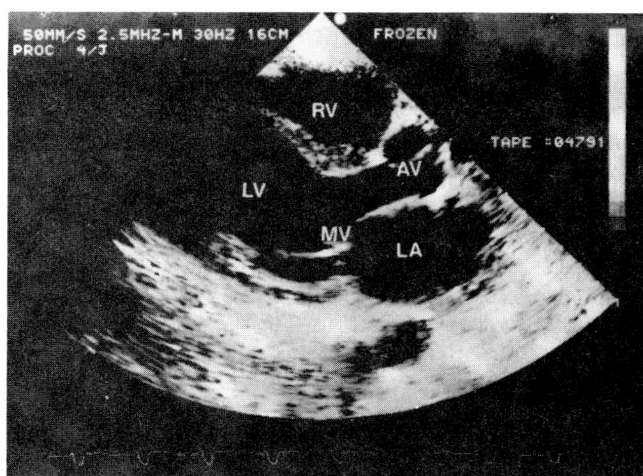


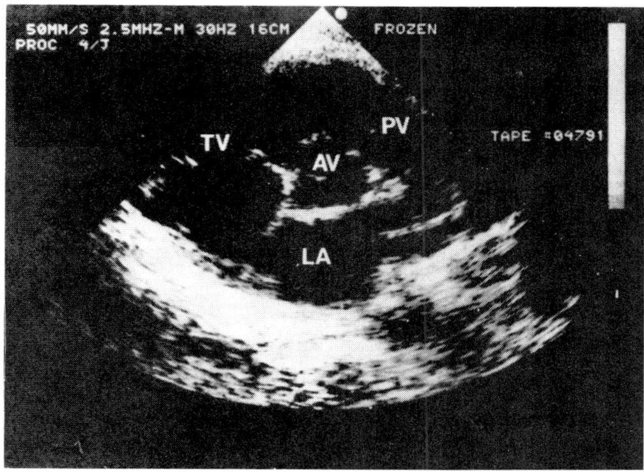


***Fig. 7-32*** 2-D echocardiogram. Note that several sections of the heart can be viewed at one time, and it is easier to see the relationship of the chambers to one another. Abbreviations are as in Figure 7-31, plus *RA,* right atrium; *TV,* tricuspid valve; *LV,* left ventricle. (From Kinney M and others: Comprehensive cardiac care, ed 7, St Louis, 1991, Mosby–Year Book, Inc.)

The *two-dimensional (2-D) echocardiogram* uses numerous crystals in the transducer to create a cross-sectional imaging plane. Sections of the heart are then viewed from a number of different angles (Fig. 7-32). The picture is displayed on an oscilloscope, and photographs are taken to serve as a permanent record. Since there are no timing markers built into this technique, it is less accurate in measuring stroke volume when the rhythm is irregular and in detecting constrictive pericarditis and tamponade.[75] In many other ways it is superior to the M-mode echocardiogram. The 2-D echocardiogram provides better quantification of valvular stenosis and a greater ability to detect ventricular aneurysms. Because a whole "slice" of the heart is seen at once, the location of various structures in relationship to the rest of the heart is better appreciated, and the size of dyskinetic wall segments can be determined.

*Doppler echocardiography* provides a special kind of echocardiogram that assesses blood flow. It uses a pulsed or continuous wave of ultrasound that records frequency shifts of reflected sound waves, showing velocity and direction of blood flow relative to the transducer. Doppler echocardiography is especially useful in patients with valvular heart disease. Both regurgitation and stenosis can be detected and estimates made of their severity. When multiple valves are involved, the Doppler technique can clarify the extent of damage to the individual valves. Prosthetic valve function can also be evaluated, along with congenital anomalies, especially shunts and atresias, measurement of volume flow, and assessment of cardiac output.

**Summary of nursing care.** The echocardiograph can be brought to the bedside if necessary, but whenever possible the patient should be transported to the echocardiography laboratory. The room will be somewhat dark to improve the visual clarity of the images displayed on the screen. Lubricant is placed on the patient's chest, and a transducer is placed in various positions to visualize cardiac and valvular structures. The procedure is not uncomfortable, but it may be tiresome for certain patients because of the length of the procedure, which is usually 30 to 60 minutes.

### Nuclear Magnetic Resonance

**Nuclear magnetic resonance** (NMR) is a noninvasive imaging technique that can obtain specific biochemical information from body tissue without the use of ionizing radiation. The procedure does not present any known hazard to living cells. In many respects, the image created is superior to both x-ray film and ultrasonography because bone does not interfere with magnetic resonance imaging.

**Indications.** Currently, cardiac magnetic resonance imaging can provide information about tissue integrity, wall-motion abnormalities and aneurysms, ejection fraction,[118] cardiac output, and patency of proximal coronary arteries.[89] The drawbacks to magnetic resonance imaging outweigh its advantages for most patients (Table 7-13), and it is currently not competitive with echocardiography and angiography.

**Procedure.** The method by which NMR scanning is performed is quite complex, but the basic concept is fairly simple. Certain atoms within molecules act as tiny bar magnets with north and south poles. The nuclei spin around this axis like a spinning top. Under normal conditions these small atomic magnets are arranged at random. If a patient is placed within a strong magnetic field, many of the nuclei line up in the same direction as the magnetic force. When a radio frequency wave is sent, some of the nuclei absorb this en-

**Table 7-13** Advantages and limitations of cardiac nuclear magnetic resonance imaging

| Advantages | Limitations |
|---|---|
| Entirely noninvasive | Time-consuming |
| Does not involve ionizing radiation | Accurate gating limited to patients in normal sinus rhythm |
| Provides images in multiple planes with uniformly good resolution | Not widely available |
| | Expensive |
| Provides information about tissue characterization and blood flow | Cannot be used on critically ill patients because of access and equipment problems |

From Stratemeier E and others: Ejection fraction determination by MR imaging: comparison with LV angiography, Radiology 158:775, 1986.

**Table 7-14** Metallic implants in nuclear magnetic resonance imaging

| Safe | Unsafe |
|---|---|
| Metallic orthopedic devices | Cardiac pacemaker |
| Surgical wires | Other electrical stimulating devices |
| Surgical clips | Aneurysm clips |
| Skin staples | Unknown types of metal implants in potentially dangerous areas of the body |
| Central nervous system shunting devices | |
| Tantalum mesh | |

From Laakman R and others: Imaging in patients with metallic implants, Radiology 157:711, 1985.

ergy, causing them to fall out of alignment and wobble like a gyroscope that is winding down. This "wobbling" out of alignment is termed *resonance*.

Each type of atom has its own unique resonance and relaxation pattern. The easiest one to record at present is the hydrogen ion, although other atoms such as phosphorus, sodium, and carbon are also being studied. Since there are two hydrogen ions per molecule of water, magnetic resonance imaging is especially sensitive to changes in tissue water content. Myocardial ischemic injury results in predictable increases in regional myocardial water content,[21] allowing differentiation between normal and ischemic tissue. Infarction leading to myocardial scarring will result in tissue with a decreased water content, which can be identified on a magnetic resonance scan as an area of decreased signal intensity.

Magnetic resonance imaging works well for structures that have little or no motion such as the brain. Cardiac applications have been limited because of the constant motion of the heart. In an attempt to overcome this limitation, various gating or slicing techniques have been used in attempts to time the images at exact phases of the cardiac cycle. The gating can be timed from the R wave of the ECG or from the arterial pulse tracing.[89] Either method is satisfactory as long as the patient is in normal sinus rhythm. With any irregularity of the rhythm, the gating technique becomes much less helpful.

**Summary of nursing care.** Magnetic resonance imaging is actually a very safe procedure. The main hazard is related to the presence of other metal substances in the environment. Since the magnetism used is approximately 40,000 times stronger than the magnetic field of the earth, metal objects such as intravenous (IV) poles or oxygen tanks can become projectiles if they come close enough to the magnet's pull. To avoid this, adequate security around the scanner is important, and many facilities use a metal detector to screen for metal objects on all people entering the area. Safe and unsafe metallic implants in nuclear magnetic resonance imaging are listed in Table 7-14.

### Radionuclide Study: Thallium Scan

**Indications.** The purpose of a thallium scan is to determine whether there is a perfusion defect in cardiac muscle.[6] It was developed as an adjunct to the exercise electrocardiogram (ECG) stress test. A thallium scan is indicated for the patient with chest pain and known or suspected coronary artery disease and for the patient with a left bundle branch block (LBBB) or a permanent pacemaker in whom an ECG stress test may be difficult to interpret.

A thallium scan combines the techniques of both cardiology and radiology. In cardiology coronary artery anatomy is important because regional myocardial blood supply is from specific coronary arteries and any blockage of an artery can lead to a discrete myocardial perfusion defect, meaning that the blood supply to this area is either decreased or absent. Although coronary arteriography will define the anatomy of the coronary arteries, it does not show whether the arteries perfuse the cardiac muscle. The radiology component involves the use of thallium 201 and a specialized perfusion scanning camera. Thallium 201 is a low-energy radioactive isotope. It is an analogue of potassium and acts like potassium when injected into the bloodstream. Because thallium is similar to potassium, it is absorbed from the bloodstream by cardiac muscle cells as part of the sodium-potassium adenosine triphosphatase (ATPase) pump. Thallium uptake is dependent on two factors: (1) the patency of the coronary arteries and (2) the amount of healthy myocardium with a functional sodium-potassium ATPase pump. If an area of myocardium is infarcted (dead), it will not take up thallium. Once thallium has been injected, a specialized scintillation camera and computer system can detect the areas of thallium concentration (uptake).

**Procedure.** Before the thallium scan the patient should have the procedure fully explained, including a description of the equipment since it may be overwhelming to some patients. The patient is usually fasting because a thallium scan involves vigorous exercise. He or she should have a patent intravenous line inserted before the test. The thallium test takes place in a specialized laboratory that contains ECG monitoring equipment, cardiovascular exercise equipment (treadmill or stationary bicycle), and an Anger gamma scintillation camera. Once in the laboratory the patient is asked to exercise vigorously for up to 1 minute or longer or until angina or fatigue develops. At this point the thallium is injected into the bloodstream. After the injection the patient is asked to exercise vigorously for another minute to stress the heart and circulate the thallium.

As soon as possible after exercise (within 10 minutes), the patient is asked to lie on the examination table for the first perfusion scan by the scintillation camera. The camera examines the heart from three angles, anterior, left anterior oblique, and left lateral oblique, to increase accuracy. On the camera screen the heart image looks like a circle with a hole. The myocardium appears, but the fluid-filled center does not. If no perfusion defect is seen, the test is complete for that patient. If a perfusion defect is noted, the patient will be asked to return for a repeat scan in 4 hours. A perfusion defect present 4 hours later means the area is infarcted. If the perfusion defect has taken up thallium since the first test (redistribution), the area is ischemic.

Occasionally, a patient who cannot tolerate a thallium/ECG stress test will have a pharmacological thallium test. In this case the patient is given dipyridamole (Persantine) to increase coronary artery blood flow, and the thallium test is then performed.

### Cardiac Catheterization and Coronary Arteriography

**Indications.** Cardiac catheterization and coronary arteriography are routine diagnostic procedures for patients with known or suspected heart disease. Clinical indications for cardiac catheterization include myocardial ischemia, unstable angina, evolving myocardial infarction, congestive heart failure with a history that suggests coronary artery disease or valvular disease, and congenital heart disease. Cardiac catheterization is used both to confirm physical findings and to provide a baseline for medical or surgical therapy.

**Procedure.** Before the catheterization the patient will meet with the cardiologist to discuss the purpose, benefit, and risks of the study. For many patients, cardiac catheterization is the first major procedure after a diagnosis of possible cardiac disease. The patient is often very anxious and has many questions. It is important that both nursing and medical staff fully answer patients' questions about the catheterization experience.

The morning of the procedure the patient fasts except for ingesting prescribed cardiac medications. Light premedication is given before the patient goes to the catheterization laboratory. If there is a history of allergy, an antihistamine or corticosteroid may be administered to prevent an anaphylactic reaction to the radiopaque contrast. Throughout the cardiac catheterization the patient remains awake and alert. He or she is positioned on a hard table with a C- or U-shaped camera arm overhead or to the side. This arm can be moved to view the heart from several different angles. Cardiac catheterization catheters, available in a variety of designs and sizes, are placed in the groin area after the patient receives a local anesthetic. The choice of catheters is based on the cardiologist's experience and the diagnostic study required. The femoral artery is used to catheterize the left side of the heart, including the coronary arteries. The femoral vein is used to pass catheters to the right side of the heart.

During catheterization of the left side of the heart, hemodynamic pressure measurements are taken in the aortic root, the left ventricle, and the left atrium. Radiopaque contrast (dye) is used to visualize the left side of the heart (angiogram) and the coronary arteries (arteriogram). Catheterization of the right side of the heart is performed using a thermodilution pulmonary artery catheter. Information obtained includes hemodynamic pressure measurements in the right atrium, right ventricle, pulmonary artery, and pulmonary capillary wedge and measurement of cardiac output, calculated hemodynamic values, oxygen saturations, and an angiogram of the right heart chambers using radiopaque contrast.

During the study the patient receives heparin systemically to reduce the risk of emboli. Many patients also receive nitroglycerin to control chest pain, particularly when the coronary arteries are full of contrast material during the coronary arteriographic procedure. At this time the patient may also experience bradycardia or hypotension. To move the contrast dye more quickly and minimize the vagal effect on heart rate and blood pressure, the patient may be asked to cough. If the bradycardia persists, atropine or, occasionally, a transvenous pacemaker may be used. If hypotension continues, intravenous (IV) fluids are administered as a bolus.

At the end of the study the heparin effect is reversed with protamine sulfate. The catheters are then removed, and pressure is placed on the groin area until bleeding has stopped. After catheterization the patient remains flat for 6 hours. Nursing care involves care of the groin site, which is checked frequently for evidence of bleeding or hematoma. Pedal and posterior tibial pulses are assessed every 15 minutes for the first hour after the catheterization and every 30 minutes to 1 hour thereafter. The patient is encouraged to drink large amounts of clear liquids, and the IV fluid rate is increased to 100 ml/hour. The additional fluid is given for rehydration because the radiopaque contrast acts as an osmotic diuretic. Patients who have an elevated blood urea nitrogen (BUN) or creatinine before catheterization are at risk for renal failure from the dye. For these patients the quantity of contrast material is consciously limited to preserve kidney function. After the catheterization the cardiologist will meet with the patient and family to discuss the findings and plan of care.

**Table 7-15** Hemodynamic pressures and normal values

| Hemodynamic pressure or value | Abbreviation | Normal range |
|---|---|---|
| Mean arterial pressure | MAP | 70-90 mm Hg |
| Central venous pressure | CVP | 2-4 mm Hg<br>3-8 cm water ($H_2O$) |
| Left atrial pressure | LAP | 5-10 mm Hg |
| Pulmonary artery pressure (systolic, diastolic, mean) | PAP, PA systolic (PAS), PA diastolic (PAD), PAP mean ($PAP_M$) | PAS 20-30 mm Hg<br>PAD 5-10 mm Hg<br>$PAP_M$ 10-15 mm Hg |
| Pulmonary capillary wedge pressure or pulmonary artery wedge pressure | PCW or PCWP or PAWP | 5-12 mm Hg |
| Cardiac output | CO | 4-6 L/min (at rest) |
| Cardiac index | CI | 2.5-4.0 L/min/$m^2$ |
| Stroke volume | SV | 60-70 ml |
| Stroke volume index | SI | 40-50 ml/$m^2$ |
| Systemic vascular resistance | SVR | 10-18 units or 800-1400 dynes/sec/$cm^{-5}$ |
| Systemic vascular resistance index | SVRI | 2000-2400 dynes/sec/$cm^{-5}/m^2$ |
| Pulmonary vascular resistance | PVR | 1.2-3.0 units or 100-250 dynes/sec/$cm^{-5}$ |
| Pulmonary vascular resistance index | PVRI | 225-315 dynes/sec/$cm^{-5}/m^2$ |
| Left cardiac work index | LCWI | 3.4-4.2 kg-m/$m^2$ |
| Left ventricular stroke work index | LVSWI | 50-62 g-m/$m^2$ |
| Right cardiac work index | RCWI | 0.54-0.66 kg-m/$m^2$ |
| Right ventricular stroke work index | RVSWI | 7.9-9.7 g-m/$m^2$ |

### Bedside Hemodynamic Monitoring

Invasive hemodynamic monitoring has become one of the major skill areas necessary for the critical care nurse. Using invasive catheters and sophisticated monitors, the nurse evaluates a patient's cardiac function, circulating blood volume, and physiological response to treatment.

Knowledge of hemodynamic monitoring will assist the clinician in developing decision-making skills to move beyond recording vital signs to interpretation and analysis of that information to formulate a nursing plan of care appropriate for the individual patient. Table 7-15 lists hemodynamic pressures and normal values.

**Indications for hemodynamic monitoring.** The range of medical diagnoses for which hemodynamic monitoring can be used consists of pathophysiological processes that alter one of the four mechanisms that support normal cardiovascular function: preload, afterload, heart rate, and contractility (Table 7-16). A brief review of these four concepts will be given before discussion of hemodynamic monitoring.

**Determination of cardiac output. Cardiac output** (CO) is defined as the volume of blood ejected from the heart over 1 minute. Therefore the determinants of CO are heart rate (HR) in beats per minute and stroke volume (SV) in milliliters per beat. The equation is as follows:

$$CO = HR \times SV$$

CO is normally expressed in liters per minute (L/min). The normal CO in the human adult is approximately 4 to 6 L/min. Cardiac index (CI) is the CO divided by the individual's estimated body surface area, expressed in square meters ($m^2$). The normal range for CI is 2.5 to 4.5 L/min/$m^2$. Changes in either the SV or HR can change the CO. However, all three parameters must be individually assessed. For example, for a person with an HR of 72 and SV of 70 ml,

$$CO = 72 \text{ (beats/min)} \times 70 \text{ (ml/beat)} = 5.040 \text{ L/min}$$

If, however, the parameters change to an HR of 140 and SV of 40 ml,

$$CO = 140 \text{ (beats/min)} \times 40 \text{ (ml/beat)} = 5.600 \text{ L/min}$$

Clearly, although the latter CO is greater, it does not reflect improved cardiac status. Rather, it could mean that cardiac decompensation is imminent. The determinants of cardiac output are illustrated in Fig. 7-33.

***Preload.*** The concept of **preload** was introduced by Frank Starling who found that as he increased the volume infused into a denervated heart, the cardiac output increased. And as the volume increased, so did the CO, until it reached a point at which further infusion actually caused the CO to decrease. This is now known as Starling's law of the heart, and it is graphically described as the Starling curve.[43]

With the advent of critical care units and sophisticated monitoring, the Starling principle gained great significance in clinical practice. For example, after a myocardial infarction (MI), the ability of the left ventricle to pump may be

***Table 7-16*** Medical diagnoses and pathological processes altering normal cardiovascular function

| Medical diagnosis | Pathophysiology | Impact on hemodynamic function |
|---|---|---|
| Acute myocardial infarction | Acute heart muscle damage | Decreased contractility<br>Increased preload<br>Decreased or increased heart rate |
| Aortic or mitral valve disease<br>Cardiomyopathy (dilated) | Chronic heart muscle damage | Decreased contractility<br>Increased preload<br>Decreased or increased heart rate |
| Cardiac tamponade<br>Trauma<br>Aortic dissection into the pericardium<br>After open heart surgery<br>Effusion (pericardial)<br>Cardiomyopathy (restrictive) | Decreased venous return and compression of heart chambers | Decreased preload<br>Decreased contractility<br>Equalization of intracardiac pressures |
| Hypothermia after cardiopulmonary bypass/open heart sugery<br>Septic shock (late)<br>Coarctation of the aorta | Increased left-ventricular workload with increased systemic vascular resistance | Increased afterload |
| Aortic stenosis<br>Cardiomyopathy (hypertrophic) | Increased left-ventricular workload with normal systemic vascular resistance | Increased contractility<br>Normal systemic vascular resistance |
| Idiopathic pulmonary hypertension<br>Chronic obstructive pulmonary disease<br>Congenital heart disease (with right-to-left shunt) | Increased right-ventricular workload | Increased pulmonary vascular resistance |
| Bleeding<br>Traumatic injury<br>After surgery<br>Coagulopathy<br>Internal bleeding (occult)<br>Dehydration | Decreased circulating blood volume | Decreased preload<br>Increased heart rate<br>Increased afterload |
| Bradycardia<br>Third-degree heart block<br>Idioventricular rhythm<br>Myocardial infarction | | Decreased heart rate |
| Tachycardia<br>Paroxysmal atrial tachycardia<br>Ventricular tachycardia | Decreased diastolic filling time with decreased stroke volume | Increased heart rate<br>Decreased preload |
| Ventricular tachycardia<br>Ventricular fibrillation<br>Asystole | Loss of heart rhythm | Cardiac arrest |
| Rewarming after open heart surgery<br>Septic shock (early)<br>Use of inotropic/vasodilator therapy | Vasodilation | Decreased afterload<br>Decreased preload<br>Increased heart rate |
| Congestive heart failure<br>Cardiogenic pulmonary edema<br>Failure of right side of heart, causing pedal edema, ascites | Increased intravascular and extravascular fluid<br>Pulmonary and systemic edema | Increased preload<br>Decreased contractility |
| Noncardiogenic pulmonary edema or acute respiratory distress syndrome (ARDS) | Increased intravascular and extravascular fluid<br>Pulmonary edema | Normal preload and contractility |

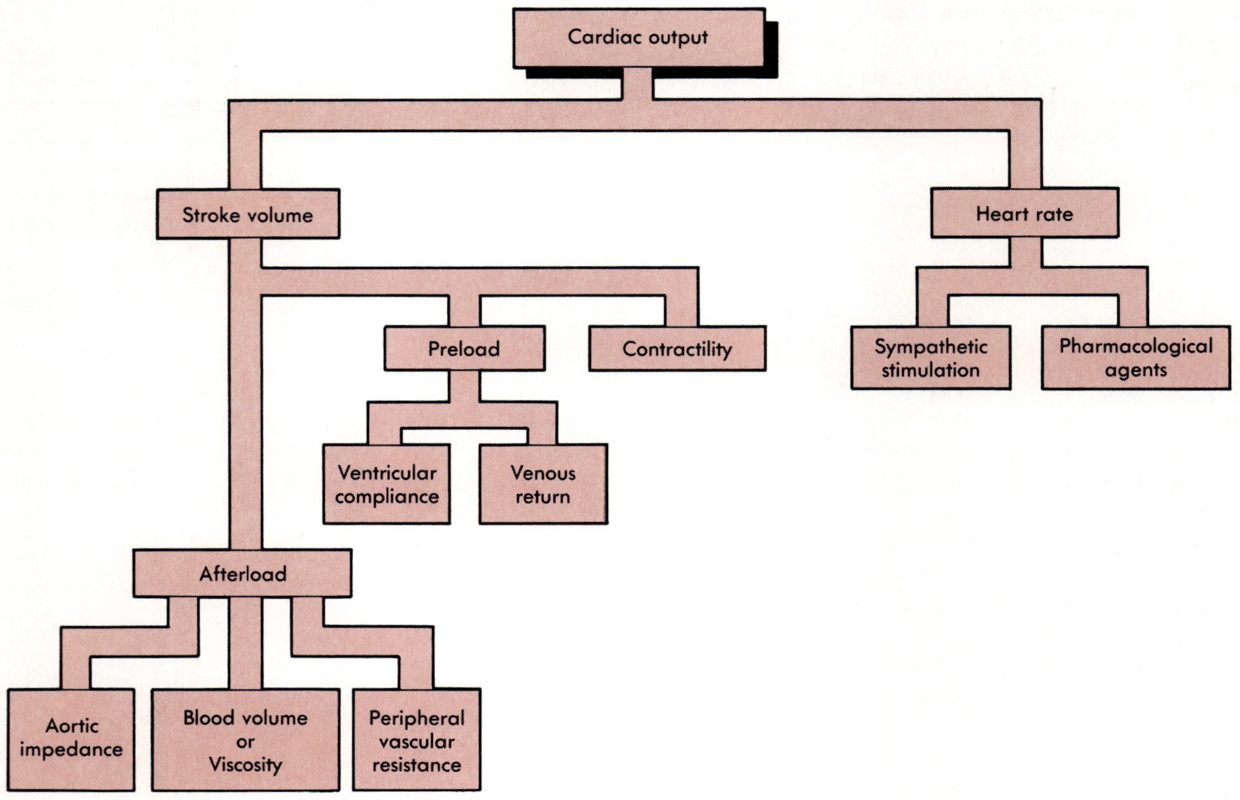


***Fig. 7-33*** Determinants of cardiac output.

impaired. It is desirable to optimize the contractility of the remaining viable heart muscle by "stretching" it with added volume. But if the intravascular volume exceeds the stretch limit, cardiac output will diminish.

Preload, then, is a function of the volume of blood presented to the left ventricle and also the compliance (the ability of the ventricle to stretch) of the ventricles at the end of diastole. It has been described as left ventricular end-diastolic pressure (LVEDP). Factors affecting the volume aspect include venous return, total blood volume, and atrial kick. Factors affecting the compliance of the ventricles are the stiffness and thickness of the muscular wall. Preload is best measured hemodynamically as the pulmonary artery wedge pressure.[43]

***Afterload.*** **Afterload** can be defined as the ventricular wall tension or stress during systolic ejection. An increase in afterload usually means an increase in the work of the heart. Afterload is increased by factors that oppose ejection. Examples of increased afterload would include aortic impedance (high diastolic aortic pressure, aortic stenosis), septal hypertrophy (obstruction in the outflow tract), vasoconstriction (increased systemic vascular resistance), and increased blood volume or viscosity. Therapeutic management to decrease afterload is done to decrease the work of the heart, thereby decreasing the myocardial oxygen demand.[43]

An increase in afterload can evoke a type of autoregulation in which the ventricle adapts to changes in filling pressure without a continued increase in resting fiber length (the Anrep effect). For example, when peripheral vascular resistance increases abruptly during vasoconstriction, ventricular diastolic pressure rises temporarily until the ventricle reaches a new equilibrium level of pressure.

***Contractility.*** Contractility refers to the heart's contractile force. It is also referred to as **inotropy** (literally, *ino* = strength and *tropy* = enhancing), which can be positive (stronger contraction) or negative (weaker contraction). As previously discussed, contractility can be increased by the Starling mechanism and by the sympathetic nervous system. It can be greatly affected by pharmacological agents, particularly those which mimic the sympathetic nervous system (sympathomimetic, adrenergics).[82]

Contractility may also be altered by a variety of other physiological phenomena. One such mechanism is the staircase or treppe phenomenon, which occurs when cardiac muscle contractions rapidly follow a period of normal rate. During this tachycardia, the force of contraction progressively increases until a new steady state is reached. In addition, situations that cause an increase in the cytoplasmic $Ca^{++}$ may result in positive inotropy. An example of this is the drug digoxin. Digoxin inhibits the $Na^+/K^+$ pump, which causes a slight rise in the intracellular $Na^+$. This rise in turn slows the $Na^+/Ca^{++}$ pump that is responsible for removing the cytoplasmic $Ca^{++}$ during diastole. The impaired $Na^+/Ca^{++}$ pump causes a slight increase in cytoplasmic $Ca^{++}$, which is the basis for the increased inotropic properties of digoxin.[16,116,119]

**Hemodynamic monitoring overview.** A hemodynamic monitoring system has three component parts: (1) the invasive catheter and tubing attached to the patient, (2) the transducer, which receives the physiologic signal from the catheter and converts it into electrical energy, and (3) the amplifier/recorder, which increases the volume of the electrical signal and displays it on an oscilloscope and on a digital scale read in millimeters of mercury (mm Hg).

Although many different catheters are inserted to monitor hemodynamic pressures, all catheters are connected to similar equipment, which consists of a bag of 0.9% normal saline solution with 1 or 2 units of heparin per milliliter of the solution, a 300 mm Hg pressure infusion cuff, intravenous (IV) tubing, three-way stopcocks, and an in-line flush device for both continuous and manual fluid infusion. The IV setup is designed to maintain catheter patency and to connect the invasive catheter to the transducer to avoid damping (flattening) of the waveform and resulting in inaccurate pressure readings. There are several types of transducers in clinical use, all of which provide the same information. The transducer may be fully disposable or reusable with a disposable sterile dome.

To ensure accurate hemodynamic pressure readings, two baseline measurements are necessary: (1) calibration of the system to atmospheric pressure, and (2) use of the phlebostatic axis for transducer height placement. To calibrate the equipment, the three-way stopcock nearest to the transducer is turned simultaneously to open the transducer to air (atmospheric pressure) and to close it to the patient and the flush system. The monitor is adjusted so that "0" is displayed, which equals atmospheric pressure. Then, using the monitor, the upper scale limit is calibrated while the system remains open to air. Standard scale limits for that monitor system are used. Finally, the stopcock is returned to its original position to visualize the waveform and hemodynamic pressures.

The phlebostatic axis is a physical reference point on the chest that is used as a baseline for consistent transducer height placement. To obtain the axis, a theoretical line is drawn from the fourth intercostal space where it joins the sternum to a midaxillary line on the side of the chest. This point approximates the level of the atria. If the transducer air-reference stopcock is level with this reference point, accurate hemodynamic pressure measurements can be obtained for most patients if the head of the bed is positioned up to 45 degrees.[64] If several clinicians will be taking measurements, the reference point can be marked on the side of the patient's chest to ensure accurate measurements.

**Intraarterial blood pressure monitoring**

***Indications.*** Intraarterial blood pressure monitoring is indicated for any major medical or surgical condition that compromises cardiac output or fluid volume status as described in Table 7-15. The system is designed for continuous measurement of three blood pressure parameters—systole, diastole, and mean arterial blood pressure (MAP). In addition, the direct arterial access is helpful in the management of patients with acute respiratory failure who require frequent arterial blood gas (ABG) measurements.

***Catheters.*** The size of the catheter used is proportionate to the diameter of the cannulated artery. In small arteries such as the radial or dorsalis pedis a 20-gauge, 3.8- to 5.1-cm, nontapered Teflon catheter is most often used. If the larger femoral or axillary arteries are used, a 19- or 20-gauge, 16-cm, Teflon catheter is used. Teflon catheters are preferred because of their lower risk of causing thrombosis.[27]

***Insertion.*** Several major peripheral arteries are suitable for receiving a cannula and for long-term hemodynamic monitoring. The most frequently used site is the radial artery. If this artery is not available, the dorsalis pedis, femoral, axillary, or brachial arteries may be used. The major advantage of the radial artery is that collateral circulation to the hand is provided by the ulnar artery and palmar arch in most of the population; thus there are other avenues of circulation if the radial artery becomes blocked after catheter placement.

The catheter insertion is usually percutaneous, although the technique varies with vessel size. Cannulas are most frequently inserted in the smaller arteries, using a "catheter-over-needle" unit in which the needle is used as a temporary guide for catheter placement. With this method, once the unit has been inserted into the artery, the needle is withdrawn, leaving the supple plastic cannula in place. Insertion of a cannula into a larger artery usually necessitates use of the Seldinger technique. This procedure involves (1) entry into the artery, using a needle, (2) passage of a supple guidewire through the needle into the artery, (3) removal of the needle, (4) passage of the catheter over the guidewire, and (5) removal of the guidewire, leaving the cannula in the artery. If a cannula cannot be inserted into the artery using percutaneous methods, an arterial cutdown may be performed. This procedure involves a skin incision to expose the artery directly.

***Summary of nursing care.*** Intraarterial blood pressure monitoring is designed for continuous assessment of arterial perfusion to the major organ systems of the body. Mean arterial pressure (MAP) is the clinical parameter most frequently used to assess perfusion because MAP represents perfusion pressure throughout the cardiac cycle. Because one third of the cardiac cycle is spent in systole and two thirds in diastole, the MAP calculation must reflect the greater amount of time spent in diastole.

A MAP greater than 60 mm Hg is necessary to perfuse the coronary arteries, brain, and kidneys. A MAP between 70 and 90 mm Hg is ideal. Systolic and diastolic pressures are monitored in conjunction with the MAP as further guide to the accuracy of perfusion. Should cardiac output decrease, the body will compensate by constricting peripheral vessels to maintain the blood pressure. In this situation the MAP may remain constant, but the pulse pressure (differ-

***Table 7-17*** Nursing measures to ensure patient safety and to troubleshoot problems with hemodynamic monitoring equipment

| Problem | Prevention | Troubleshooting |
|---|---|---|
| Damping of waveform | Provide continuous infusion of solution containing heparin through an in-line flush device (1 unit of heparin for each millimeter of flush solution). | Before insertion, completely flush the line and/or catheter. In a line attached to a patient, back flush through the system to clear bubbles from tubing or transducer. |
| Clot formation at end of catheter | Provide continuous infusion of solution containing heparin through an in-line flush device (1 unit of heparin for each millimeter of flush solution). | If a clot in the catheter is suspected because of a damped waveform or resistance to forward flush of the system, gently aspirate the line using a small syringe inserted into the proximal stopcock. Then flush the line again once the clot is removed and inspect the waveform. It should return to a normal pattern. |
| Hemorrhage | Use Luer-lock (screw) connections in line setup. Close and cap stopcocks when not in use. | Once a blood leak is recognized, tighten all connections, flush the line, and estimate blood loss. |
| | Ensure that the catheter is either sutured or securely taped in position. | If the catheter has been inadvertently removed, put pressure on the cannulation site. When bleeding has stopped, apply a sterile dressing, estimate blood loss, and inform the physician. If the patient is restless, an armboard may protect lines inserted in the arm. |
| Air emboli | Ensure that all air bubbles are purged from a new line setup before attachment to an indwelling catheter. | Since it is impossible to get the air back once it has been introduced into the bloodstream, prevention is the best cure. |
| | Ensure that the drip chamber from the bag of flush solution is more than half full before using the in-line fast-flush system. | If any air bubbles are noted, they must be vented through the in-line stopcocks, and the drip chamber must be filled. |
| | Some sources recommend removing all air from the bag of flush solution before assembling the system. | The left atrial pressure (LAP) line setup is the only system that includes an air filter specifically to prevent air emboli. |
| Normal waveform with *low* digital pressures | Ensure that the system is calibrated to atmospheric pressure. | Recalibrate the equipment if transducer drift has occurred. |
| | Ensure that the transducer is placed at the level of the phlebostatic axis. | Reposition the transducer at the level of the phlebostatic axis. Misplacement can occur if the patient moves from the bed to the chair or if the bed is placed in a Trendelenburg position. |
| Normal waveform with *high* digital pressure | Ensure that the system is calibrated to atmospheric pressure. | Recalibrate the equipment if transducer drift has occurred. |
| | Ensure that the transducer is placed at the level of the phlebostatic axis. | Reposition the transducer at the level of the phlebostatic axis. This situation can occur if the head of the bed was raised and the transducer was not repositioned. Some centers require attachment of the transducer to the patient's chest to avoid this problem. |
| Loss of waveform | Always have the hemodynamic waveform monitored so that changes or loss can be quickly noted. | Check the line setup to ensure that all stopcocks are turned in the correct position and that there is not a kink in the tubing. Sometimes the catheter migrates against a vessel wall, and having the patient change position will restore the waveform. |
| Infection | Change the bag of flush solution every 24 hours. Change the line setup and the disposable transducer every 72 hours. Change the catheter insertion site dressing every 24 hours, and inspect the cannulation site for signs of infections. Apply antiseptic ointment and a sterile dressing to the catheter site. | If local infection occurs, the catheter must be placed elsewhere by the physician, and the new insertion site must be dressed using antiseptic ointment and a sterile dressing. Sterile equipment must always be used, disposable equipment must not be reused, and nondisposable transducers must be sterilized after each patient usage. Hands should be washed before handling monitoring setup or dressings. |

ence between systolic and diastolic pressures) will narrow.

The nurse caring for the patient with an arterial line must be able to assess whether a low MAP, or narrowed perfusion pressure, represents decreased arterial perfusion or equipment malfunction. Assessment of the arterial waveform on the oscilloscope in combination with clinical assessment will yield the answer. If there are air bubbles, clots, or kinks in the system, the waveform will become damped or flattened, and the troubleshooting methods described in Table 7-17 can be implemented. If the line is unreliable or becomes dislodged, a cuff pressure can be used as a reserve system. There are slight differences between cuff and arterial pressures, but in the normovolemic patient differences of 5 to 10 mm Hg do not affect clinical management. If the patient has a low cardiac output or is in shock, the cuff pressure will be unreliable because of vasoconstriction, and an arterial line should be inserted.

***Arterial pressure waveform interpretation.*** The arterial pressure waveform represents the ejection phase of left-ventricular systole. As the aortic valve opens, blood is ejected from the left ventricle and is recorded as an increase of pressure in the arterial system. The highest point recorded is called systole. Following peak ejection (systole) there is a decrease in force and a drop of pressure. A notch (the dicrotic notch) may be visible on the downstroke of this arterial waveform, representing closure of the aortic valve. The dicrotic notch signifies the beginning of diastole. The remainder of the downstroke represents diastolic runoff of blood flow into the arterial tree. The lowest point recorded is called diastole. A normal arterial pressure tracing is described in Figure 7-34. Note that the arterial pressure tracing always follows the initiating QRS.

A low arterial blood pressure waveform is shown in Fig. 7-35. In this case the digital readout correlated well with the patient's own cuff pressure, confirming that the patient was hypotensive. This arterial waveform is more rounded, without a dicrotic notch, when compared with the normal waveform in Fig. 7-34. A damped (flattened) arterial waveform is shown in Fig. 7-36. In this case the patient's cuff pressure was significantly higher than the digital readout, thus representing a problem with equipment. A damped waveform occurs when communication from the artery to the tranducer is interrupted and produces false values on the monitor and oscilloscope. Damping may be caused by a clot at the end of the catheter, by kinks in the catheter or tubing, or by air bubbles in the system. Troubleshooting techniques (see Table 7-17) are used to find the origin of the problem and to remove the cause of damping. If there is any doubt about the accuracy of the arterial waveform, a cuff blood pressure reading should be taken. As part of the routine nursing assessment, a cuff blood pressure should be taken every shift and correlated with the intraarterial pressure.

### Central venous pressure monitoring

***Indications.*** Central venous pressure (CVP) monitoring is indicated whenever a patient has an alteration in fluid volume (see Table 7-15). The CVP can be used as a guide in fluid volume replacement in hypovolemia and to assess the impact of diuresis after diuretic administration in the case of fluid overload. Additionally, when a major intravenous (IV) line is required for volume replacement, a central venous line is a good choice because large volumes of fluid can be easily delivered.

***Catheters.*** Since many patients are awake and alert when

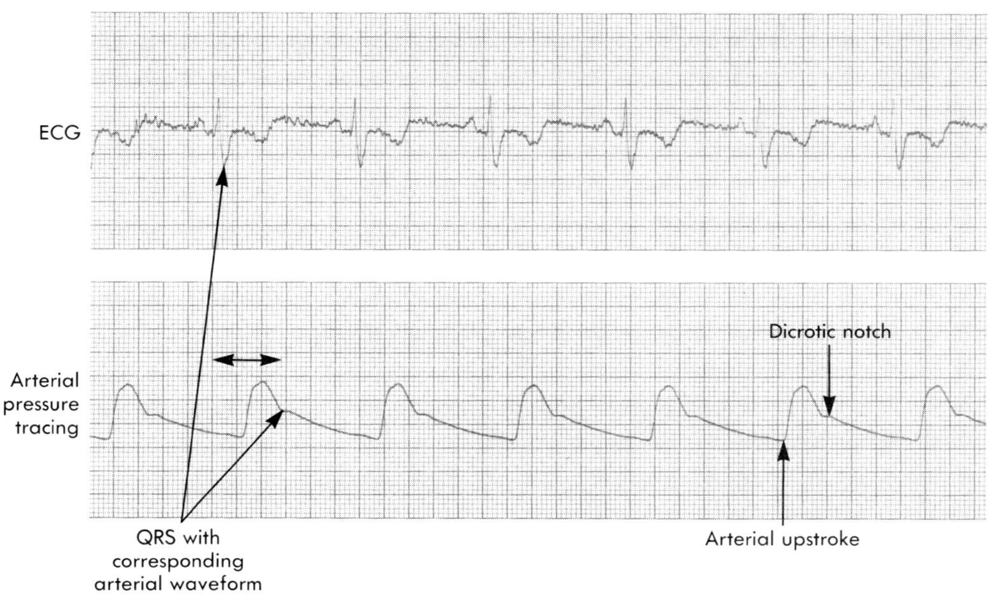


***Fig. 7-34*** Simultaneous ECG and arterial pressure tracing.

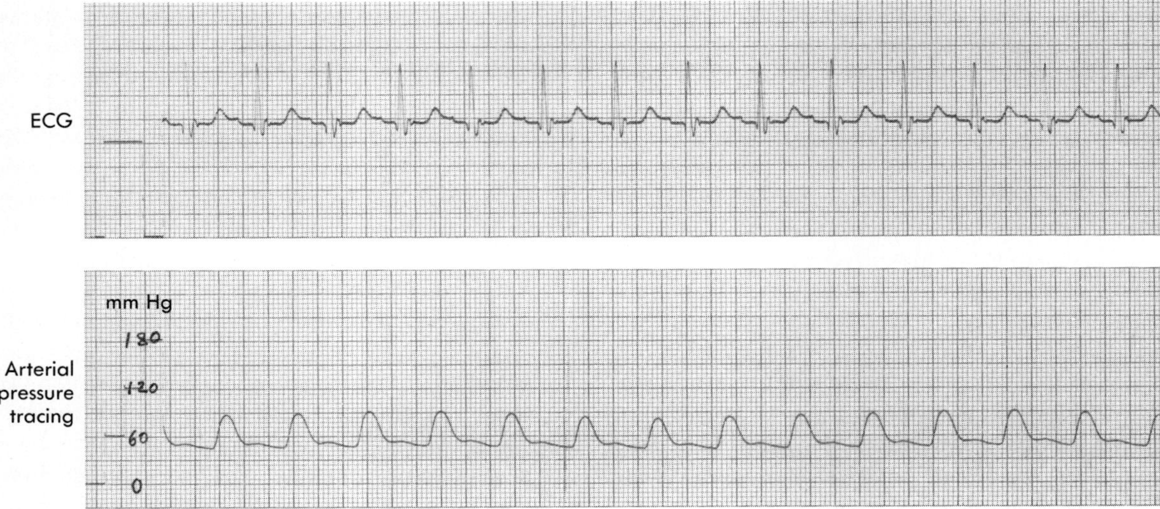


*Fig. 7-35* Simultaneous ECG and arterial pressure tracing showing a low arterial pressure waveform.

a CVP catheter is inserted, a brief explanation about the procedure will minimize patient anxiety and gain cooperation during the insertion. This cooperation is important because it is a sterile procedure and because the supine or Trendelenburg position may not be comfortable for many patients.

CVP catheters are available as single-, double-, or triple-lumen infusion catheters, depending on the specific needs of the patient. The catheters are designed for placement by percutaneous injection after skin preparation and administration of a local anesthetic. The standard CVP kit contains sterile towels, a needle introducer, syringe, guidewire, and catheter.

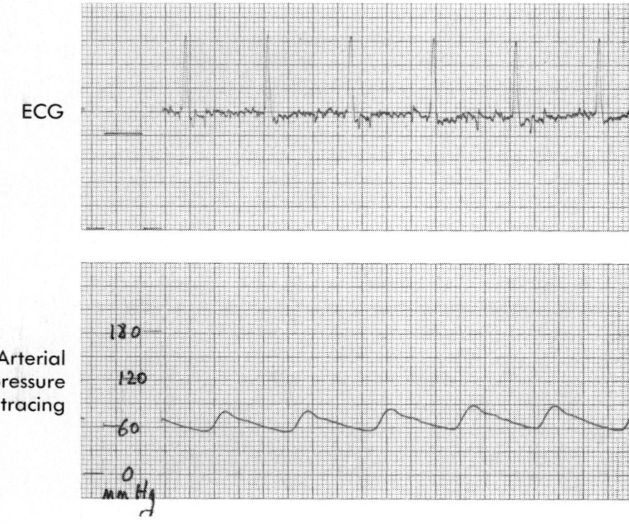


*Fig. 7-36* Simultaneous ECG and arterial pressure tracing showing a damped arterial pressure waveform.

***Insertion.*** The large veins of the upper thorax (subclavian or internal jugular) are most frequently used for percutaneous CVP line insertion. During insertion the patient may be placed in a Trendelenburg position. Placing the head in a dependent position causes the internal jugular veins in the neck to become more prominent, facilitating line placement. To minimize the risk of air embolus during the procedure, the patient may be asked to hold his or her breath any time the needle or catheter is open to air.

The Seldinger technique is the preferred method of placement in which the vein is located by using a needle and syringe. A guidewire is passed through the needle, the needle is removed, and the catheter is passed over the guidewire. Once the catheter is correctly placed at the level of the right atrium, the guidewire is removed. Finally, an IV setup is attached, and the catheter is sutured in place.

After cannulation of the internal jugular or subclavian vein, a chest radiograph should be obtained to verify placement of the catheter and the absence of an iatrogenic pneumothorax. Other suitable insertion sites include the femoral and antecubital fossae veins. In the rare case that it is not possible to insert a CVP catheter percutaneously, a surgical cutdown may be performed.

***Summary of nursing care.*** The CVP is used to measure the filling pressures of the right side of the heart. During diastole when the tricuspid valve is open and blood is flowing from the right atrium to the right ventricle, the CVP will accurately reflect right ventricular end diastolic pressure (RVEDP). The normal CVP is 2 to 5 mm Hg (3 to 8 cm $H_2O$).

The CVP is used in combination with the mean arterial pressure (MAP) and other clinical parameters to assess hemodynamic stability. In the hypovolemic patient, the CVP will fall before there is a significant fall in MAP because peripheral vasoconstriction will keep the MAP normal. Thus the CVP is an excellent early warning system for the patient who is bleeding, vasodilating, receiving diuretics, or rewarming after cardiac surgery. The CVP, however, is not a reliable indicator of left-ventricular dysfunction. Left-ventricular dysfunction, which can occur after an acute myocardial infarction, will increase filling pressures on the left side of the heart. The CVP, since it measures RVEDP, will remain normal until the increase in pressure from the left side is reflected back through the pulmonary vasculature to the right ventricle. In this situation a pulmonary artery catheter that measures pressures on the left side is the monitoring method of choice.

To take CVP measurements the clinician has a choice of two methods—either a mercury (mm Hg) system, using a transducer and a monitor, or a water (cm $H_2O$) manometer system. To achieve accurate CVP measurements the phlebostatic axis should be used as a reference point on the body, and the transducer or water manometer zero should be level with this point. If the phlebostatic axis is used and the transducer or water manometer are correctly aligned, any head-of-bed position up to 45 degrees may be accurately used for CVP readings. Elevating the head of bed is especially helpful for the patient with respiratory or cardiac problems who will not tolerate a flat position.

The risk of air embolus, although uncommon, is always present for the patient with a central venous line in place. Air can enter during insertion through a disconnected or broken catheter or along the path of a removed CVP catheter. This is more likely if the patient is in an upright position because air can be pulled into the venous system with the increase in negative intrathoracic pressure during inhalation. If a large volume of air (200 to 300 cc) is infused rapidly, it may become trapped in the right-ventricular outflow tract, stopping blood flow from the right side of the heart to the lungs. The patient may experience respiratory distress and cardiovascular collapse. Treatment involves administering 100% oxygen and placing the patient on the left side with the head downward (left-lateral Trendelenburg position). This position displaces the air from the right-ventricular outflow tract to the apex of the heart where it can be either reabsorbed or aspirated. Precautions to prevent an air embolism in a CVP line include using only Luer-lock connections, avoiding long loops of IV tubing, and using screw caps on three-way stopcocks.

***CVP waveform interpretation.*** The right-atrial (CVP) waveform has three positive deflections, called a, c, and v waves, that correspond to specific atrial events in the cardiac cycle (Fig. 7-37). The a wave reflects atrial contraction and follows the P wave seen on the electrocardiogram (ECG).

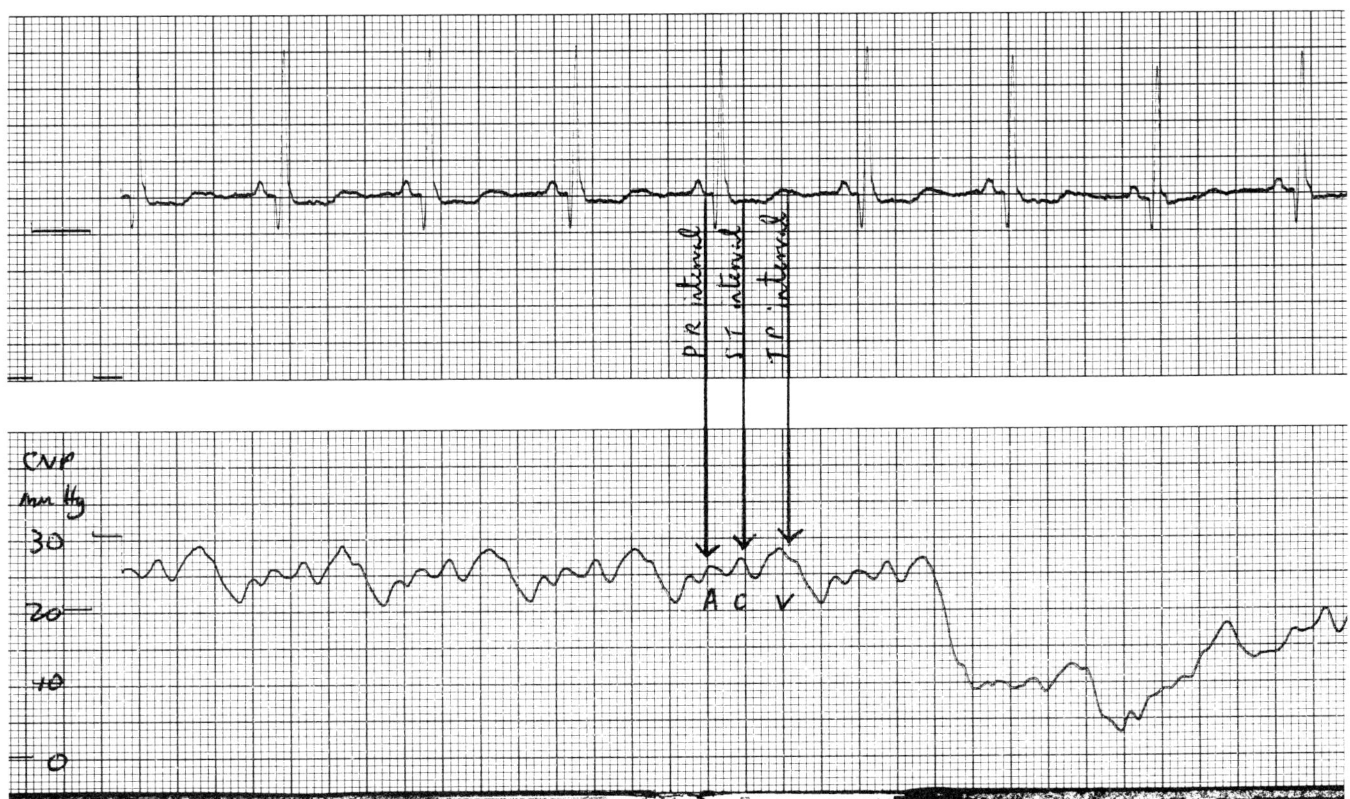


*Fig. 7-37* Simultaneous ECG and CVP tracing.

The downslope of this wave is called the x descent and represents atrial relaxation. The c wave reflects the closure of the tricuspid valve as it moves toward the right atrium in early ventricular contraction. The c wave is small and not always visible but corresponds to the QRS-T interval on the ECG. The v wave represents atrial filling and pressure increase against the closed tricuspid valve in early diastole. The downslope of the v wave is named the y descent and represents the fall in pressure as the tricuspid valve opens and blood flows from the right atrium to the right ventricle.

Certain heart rhythms can change the normal CVP waveform. In atrial fibrillation the CVP waveform has no recognizable pattern because of the disorganization of the atria. Pathological conditions such as advanced right-ventricular failure or tricuspid valve insufficiency allow backflow of blood from the right ventricle to the right atrium during ventricular contraction, producing large v waves on the right-atrial waveform.

**Left-atrial pressure monitoring**

***Indications.*** Left atrial pressure (LAP) monitoring is used in selected cases after major cardiac surgery. Until the advent of the pulmonary artery catheter in the 1970s, LAP monitoring was used to assess hemodynamics on the left side of the heart. Today it is not used for routine monitoring. However, it has been found clinically effective in the postoperative management of the cardiac surgery patient who has significant pulmonary hypertension. In this case, inotropic drugs are infused directly into the left side of the heart, while vasodilator drugs are infused into the right heart through a right-atrial catheter.[28] This technique optimizes pulmonary vasodilation and minimizes the vasoconstrictive effect of inotropic drugs on the hypertensive pulmonary bed. In addition, accurate left atrial pressures can be obtained.

***Insertion.*** The LAP catheter is inserted into the left atrium during open heart surgery. The single-lumen catheter exits through the chest wall and is attached to a routine hemodynamic monitoring setup that contains an in-line air filter.

***Summary of nursing care.*** The placement of the LAP catheter directly into the left atrium places the patient at particular risk for air or tissue emboli. Nursing care is planned to reduce these equipment-related risks. An in-line air filter is added to the flush system that contains heparin to reduce the risk of air emboli. If the waveform becomes damped, noninvasive methods of troubleshooting such as repositioning the patient are performed. The catheter is not manually flushed since to do so may increase the risk of emboli resulting from clot formation at the tip of the catheter. Some sources recommend gentle aspiration of the LAP catheter. If there is no blood return, the catheter should be removed. Pericardial tamponade is a potential complication of LAP catheter removal. Therefore mediastinal chest tubes should be left in position until after the catheter is discontinued. Because of these risks, the LAP catheter is rarely left in place for more than 48 hours.

***LAP waveform interpretation.*** The LAP waveform consists of two positive deflections, which are termed the a and

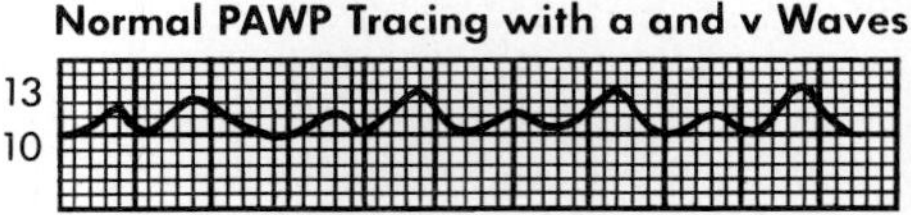


***Fig. 7-38*** Left atrial pressure tracing.

v waves (Fig. 7-38). The a wave represents atrial contraction, and the v wave represents filling of the left atrium against a closed mitral valve. Normal LAP pressure ranges from 5 to 10 mm Hg and is elevated with mitral valve disease or severe heart failure on the left side.

**Pulmonary artery pressure monitoring**

***Indications.*** When specific hemodynamic and intracardiac data are required for diagnostic and treatment purposes, a thermodilution pulmonary artery (PA) catheter may be inserted. This catheter is used for diagnosis and evaluation of heart disease, shock states, and medical conditions that cause an alteration in cardiac output or fluid volume (see Table 7-16). In addition, the PA catheter is used to evaluate patient response to treatment as described in Table 7-18.

A significant advantage of the PA catheter over the previously described methods of monitoring is that it simultaneously assesses several hemodynamic parameters, including pulmonary artery systolic and diastolic pressures, the pulmonary artery mean pressure, and the **pulmonary artery wedge pressure** (PAWP).

Although the PA catheter is inserted into the right side of the heart, it is used to measure pressures on the left side of the heart through the pulmonary artery wedge pressure (PAWP) and the pulmonary artery diastolic (PAD) pressure. This is possible because during ventricular diastole when the mitral valve is open, there is a clear pathway between the tip of the catheter and the left ventricle. In the absence of pulmonary hypertension, the pressure along this pathway (from catheter tip to left ventricle) is equal; thus the pressure that registers on the cathether tip is identical to the pressure registered within the left ventricle. The pressure recorded in the left ventricle is called **left ventricular end-diastolic pressure** (LVEDP).

Measurement and interpretation of LVEDP allow the clinician to make accurate judgments about a patient's cardiac status and fluid volume status. Diastole is the filling stage of the cardiac cycle so that the volume that has filled the left ventricle by end diastole represents the amount of blood available for ejection during systole. This left-ventricular volume is known as the preload. Although it is not possible to measure preload volume at the bedside, the pressure created by this volume can be measured using the PA catheter. Preload is equal to LVEDP as measured by the PAWP or left atrial pressure (LAP).

A significant relationship exists between LVEDP and myocardial dysfunction. As a general rule, the higher the LVEDP, the greater is the degree of myocardial dysfunction because the compromised ventricle is unable to eject all of

*Table 7-18* Pulmonary artery catheters: selected indications for use and response to treatment

| Diagnostic indications* | Possible cause | Hemodynamic profile† | Treatment and expected response |
|---|---|---|---|
| Hypovolemic shock | Trauma<br>Surgery<br>Bleeding<br>Burns<br>Excessive diuresis | Low CO<br>Low CI<br>High SVR<br>Low PAP<br>Low PAWP | *Treatment:* Fluid challenge<br>*Expected hemodynamic response:*<br>Decreased heart rate (HR)<br>Increased BP<br>Increased PAP<br>Increased PAWP, CVP<br>Increased CO, CI<br>Decreased SVR |
| Early septic shock | Sepsis | High CO<br>High CI<br>Low SVR<br>Low PAP<br>Low PAWP<br>Low CVP | *Treatment:*<br>Intravenous (IV) fluid to maintain hemodynamic function<br>Peripheral vasoconstricting agent (alpha) to increase SVR<br>Antibiotics and laboratory cultures to find site of infection<br>*Expected hemodynamic response:*<br>Decreased HR<br>Increased BP<br>Increased PAP<br>Increased PAWP, CVP<br>Increased CO, CI<br>Increased SVR |
| Advanced septic shock *or* multisystem failure shock | Sepsis<br>Multisystem failure | Low CO<br>Low CI<br>High SVR<br>High or low PAP<br>High or low PAWP<br>High or low CVP | *Treatment:*<br>Vasodilators to decrease SVR<br>Antibiotics<br>Support of body systems as necessary (e.g., mechanical ventilation or hemodialysis)<br>*Expected hemodynamic response:*<br>Decreased HR<br>Increased BP<br>Normal PAP, PAWP, CVP<br>Decreased SVR, PVR<br>Increased CO, CI |
| Cardiogenic shock | Left-ventricular pump failure caused by acute myocardial infarction, severe mitral or aortic valve disease | Low CO<br>Low CI<br>High SVR<br>High PAP<br>High PAWP<br>High CVP<br>Low SI<br>Low LCWI<br>Low LVSWI | *Treatment:*<br>Inotropic drugs to increase left-ventricular contractility<br>Vasodilators or intra-aortic balloon pump (IABP) to decrease afterload<br>Diuretics to decrease preload<br>Optimization of heart rate and control of dysrhythmias<br>*Expected hemodynamic response:*<br>Decreased HR<br>Increased BP<br>Decreased PAP<br>Decreased PAWP<br>Decreased CVP<br>Decreased SVR<br>Decreased PVR<br>Increased CO, CI<br>Increased SI<br>Increased LCWI<br>Increased LVSWI |

*Patients undergoing major vascular or cardiac surgery may also have a PA catheter in situ to follow the trend of CO/CI, SVR/PVR, and fluid status during the first 24 hours after surgery.
†See Table 7-15 for normal values of hemodynamic parameters listed in this table.

*Continued.*

**Table 7-18** Pulmonary artery catheters: selected indications for use and response to treatment—cont'd

| Diagnostic indications* | Possible cause | Hemodynamic profile† | Treatment and expected response |
|---|---|---|---|
| Acute respiratory distress syndrome (ARDS) *or* noncardiogenic pulmonary edema | Trauma<br>Sepsis<br>Shock<br>Inhaled toxins (smoke, chemicals, 100% oxygen)<br>Aspiration of gastric contents<br>Metabolic disorders | Normal CO<br>Normal CI<br>Normal SVR<br>Normal PAWP<br>High PAP<br>High PVR<br>Low RCWI<br>Low RVSWI | *Treatment:*<br>Eliminate cause of ARDS<br>Support pulmonary function as necessary<br>*Expected hemodynamic response:*<br>Decreased HR<br>Normal BP<br>Decreased PAP<br>Decreased PVR<br>Increased RCWI<br>Increased RVSWI<br>Normal CO, CI<br>Normal SVR |

the preload blood volume. A normal left-ventricular ejection fraction (EF) is 70%. The greater the degree of myocardial dysfunction, the lower is the EF and the higher the preload and LVEDP.

LVEDP can be measured by two methods using a PA catheter. The most accurate is to use the PAWP. When the small latex balloon is inflated and lodged in a pulmonary capillary, it occludes the vessel and blocks the pulmonary arterial pulsations. Thus the only pressure the catheter tip measures is the left atrial pressure, which is a reflection of LVEDP, because the mitral valve is open during diastole but closed during systole; thus the PA catheter does not record left-ventricular systolic pressures. The second method is to use the pulmonary artery diastolic (PAD) pressure, because during diastole the PAD is equal to mean PAWP and LVEDP. However, if the patient has lung disease that has elevated the PA pressures independently from the cardiac pressures, the PAD will not accurately reflect function of the left side of the heart. With pulmonary disease the PAD may be significantly higher than the PAWP. In failure of the left side of the heart, both the PAWP and the PAD pressure will be elevated and equal.

***Catheters.*** The traditional PA catheter has four lumens for measurement of central venous pressure (CVP), PA pressures, PAWP, and cardiac output (Fig. 7-39, *A*). Catheters may have additional lumens, which can be used for intravenous (IV) infusion (Fig. 7-39, *B*) to measure continuous mixed venous oxygen saturation ($Svo_2$)[121] (Fig. 7-39, *C*), or to pace the heart using transvenous pacing electrodes (Fig. 7-39, *D* and *E*).

The PA catheter is 110 cm in length. The most frequently used size is No. 7 French, although 5 and 7.5 French sizes are available. Each of the four lumens exits into the heart at a different point along the catheter length (see Fig. 7-39, *D*). The proximal (CVP) lumen is situated in the right atrium and is used for IV infusion, CVP measurement, withdrawal of venous blood samples, and injection of fluid for cardiac output determinations. The distal (PA) lumen is located at the end of the PA catheter and is situated in the pulmonary artery. It is used to record PA pressures and can be used for withdrawal of blood samples to measure $Svo_2$. The third lumen opens into a latex balloon at the end of the catheter that can be inflated with 0.8 to 1.5 cc of air. The balloon is inflated during catheter insertion once the catheter reaches the right atrium to assist in forward flow of the catheter and to minimize right-ventricular ectopy from the catheter tip. It is also inflated to obtain PAWP measurements when the PA catheter is correctly positioned in the pulmonary artery. The fourth lumen is a thermistor used to measure changes in blood temperature. It is located 4 cm from the catheter tip and is used to measure thermodilution cardiac output. The connector end of the lumen is attached directly to the cardiac output computer.

If continuous $Svo_2$ will be measured, the catheter will have an additional fiberoptic lumen that exits at the tip of the catheter. If cardiac pacing will be used, two PA catheter methods are available. One type of catheter has three atrial (A) and two ventricular (V) pacing electrodes attached to the catheter so that when it is properly positioned, the patient can be connected to a pacemaker and A-V paced. The other catheter method uses a specific transvenous pacing wire that passes down an additional catheter lumen and exits in the right ventricle if ventricular pacing is required.

***Insertion.*** If a PA catheter is to be inserted into a patient who is awake, some brief explanations about the procedure are very helpful to ensure that the patient understands what is going to happen. The insertion techniques used for placement of a PA catheter are very similar to those described in the section on CVP line insertion. In addition, because the PA catheter will be positioned within the heart chambers and pulmonary artery on the right side of the heart, catheter passage is monitored, using either fluoroscopy or waveform analysis on the bedside monitor.

Before inserting the catheter into the vein, the physician, using sterile technique, will test the balloon for inflation and will flush the catheter with normal saline solution to

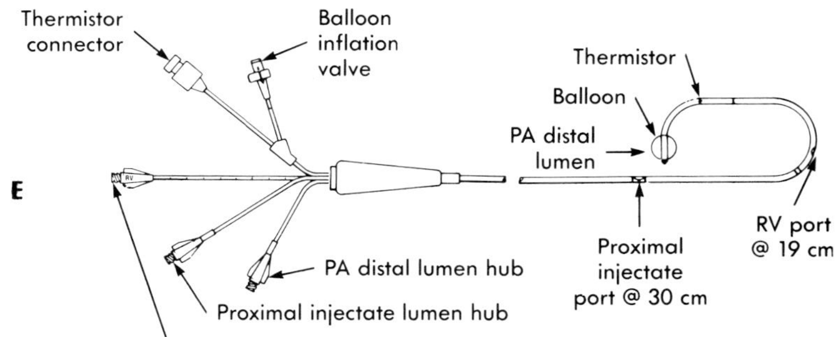

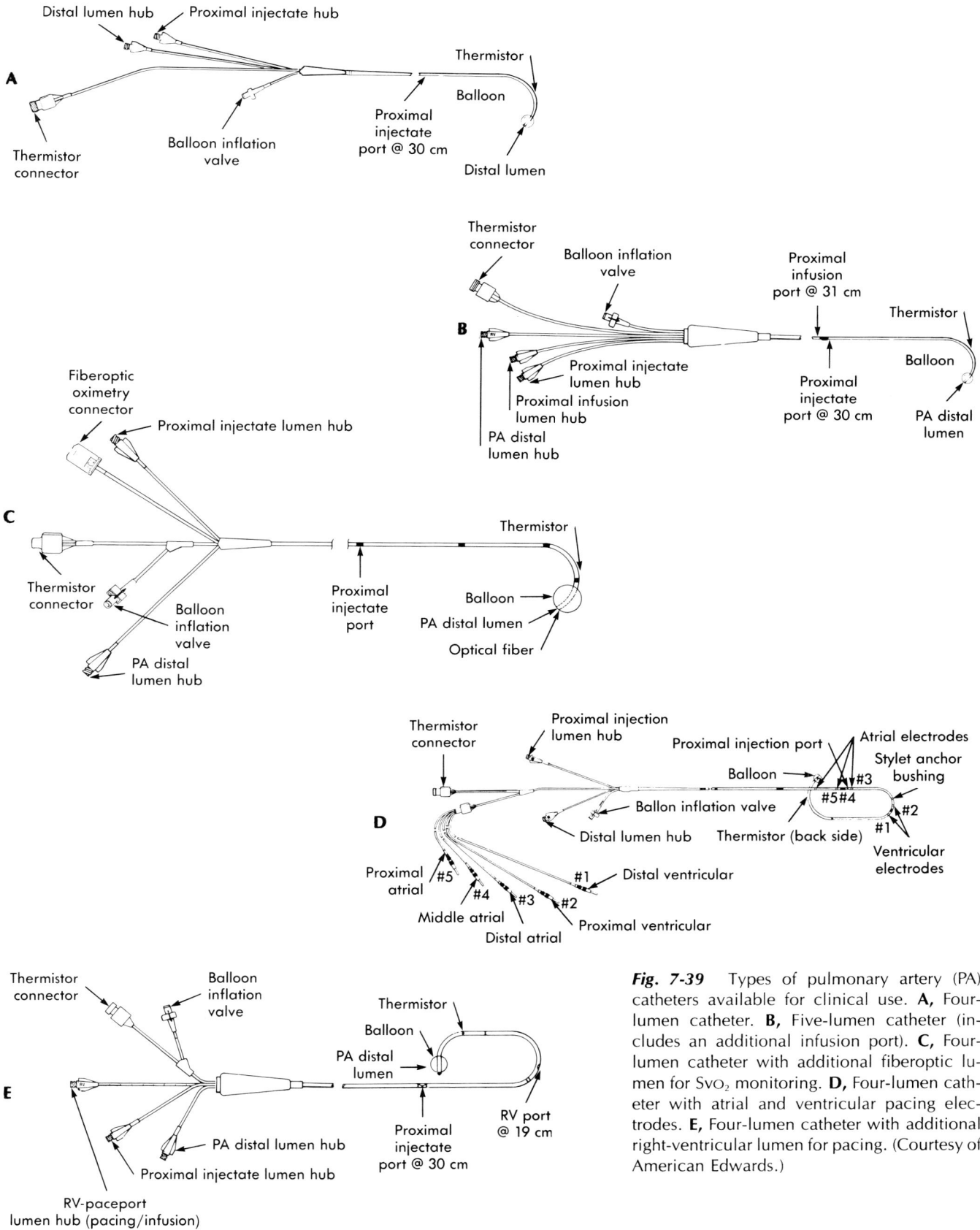


***Fig. 7-39*** Types of pulmonary artery (PA) catheters available for clinical use. **A,** Four-lumen catheter. **B,** Five-lumen catheter (includes an additional infusion port). **C,** Four-lumen catheter with additional fiberoptic lumen for $SvO_2$ monitoring. **D,** Four-lumen catheter with atrial and ventricular pacing electrodes. **E,** Four-lumen catheter with additional right-ventricular lumen for pacing. (Courtesy of American Edwards.)

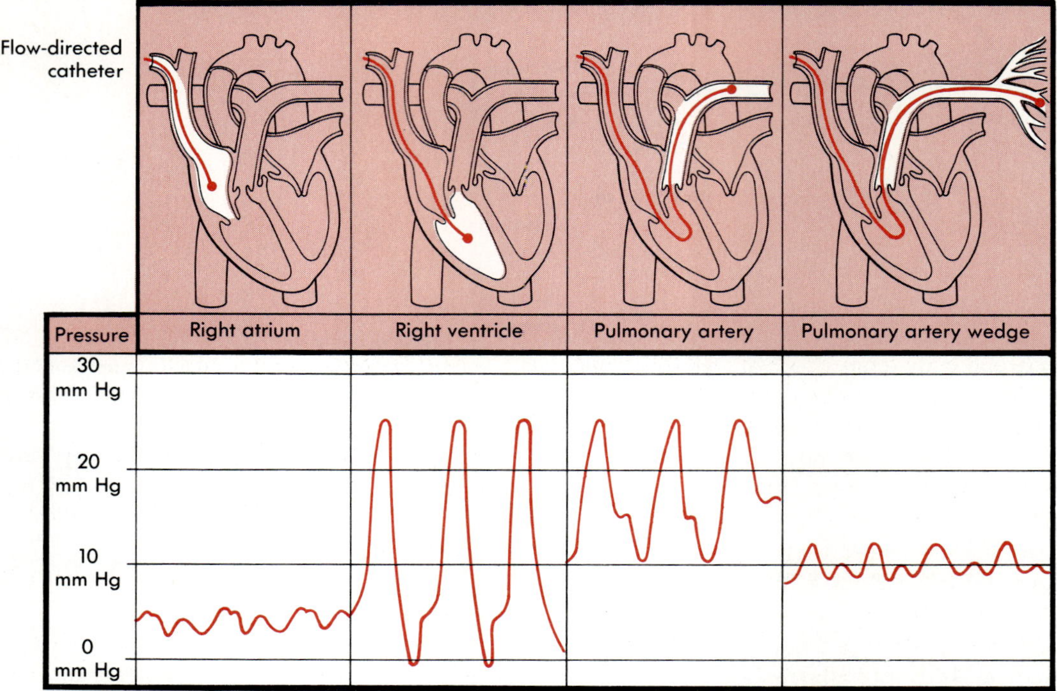


***Fig. 7-40*** PA catheter insertion with corresponding waveforms.

remove any air. The PA catheter is then attached to the bedside hemodynamic line setup and monitor so that the waveforms can be visualized while the catheter is advanced through the right side of the heart (Fig. 7-40).

***PA waveform interpretation.*** During insertion as the PA catheter is advanced into the right atrium, a right-atrial waveform should be visible on the monitor, with recognizable a, c, and v waves (see Fig. 7-40). The normal mean pressure in the right atrium is 2 to 5 mm Hg. Before passage through the tricuspid valve, the balloon at the tip of the catheter is inflated for two reasons: first, it cushions the pointed tip of the PA catheter so that if the tip comes into contact with the right ventricular wall, it will cause less myocardial irritability and consequently fewer ventricular dysrhythmias; second, inflation of the balloon assists the catheter to float with the flow of blood from the right ventricle into the pulmonary artery. The right-ventricular waveform has a saw-toothed pattern and is pulsatile, with distinct systolic and diastolic pressures. Normal right-ventricular pressures are 20-30/0-5 mm Hg. Even with the balloon inflated, it is not uncommon for ventricular ectopy to occur at this time. All patients who have a PA catheter inserted must have simultaneous electrocardiographic monitoring, with defibrillator and emergency resuscitation equipment nearby.

As the catheter enters the pulmonary artery, the waveform again changes. The diastolic pressure rises. Normal PA systolic and diastolic pressures are 20-30/10 mm Hg. A dicrotic notch, visible on the downslope of the waveform, represents closure of the pulmonic valve.

While the balloon remains inflated, the catheter is advanced into the wedge position. Here, the waveform decreases in size and is nonpulsatile, reflective of a normal left-atrial tracing with a and v wave deflections. This is described as a wedge tracing because the balloon is "wedged" into a small pulmonary vessel (see Fig. 7-40). The balloon occludes the pulmonary vessel so that the PA lumen is only exposed to left atrial pressure and is protected from the pulsatile influence of a normal PA tracing. When the balloon is deflated, the catheter should spontaneously float back into the pulmonary artery. When the balloon is reinflated, the wedge tracing should be visible. The PAWP ranges from 4 to 12 mm Hg.

**CARDIAC OUTPUT.** The PA catheter measures cardiac output (CO), using the thermodilution method. This technique can be performed at the bedside and results in CO calculated in liters per minute. A known amount (5 or 10 ml) of iced or room temperature normal saline solution is injected into the proximal lumen of the catheter. The injectant exits into the right atrium and travels with the flow of blood past the thermistor (temperature sensor) at the distal end of the catheter. The thermodilution CO method uses the indicator-dilution principle, in which a known temperature is the indicator, and it, in turn, is based on the principle that the change in temperature over time is inversely proportional to blood flow.[55] Blood flow can be diagrammatically represented as a CO curve, on which temperature is plotted against time. Many of the most recent hemodynamic monitors display this CO curve, which must then be interpreted to determine whether the CO injection is valid. The normal curve has a smooth upstroke, with a rounded peak and a gradually tapering downslope. If the curve has an uneven pattern, it may indicate faulty injection technique, and the CO measurement should be repeated. Patient movement or coughing will also alter the CO.

Generally, three cardiac outputs that are within a 10% mean range are obtained and are averaged to calculate CO. To ensure accurate readings, the difference between injectant temperature and body temperature must be at least 10° to 12° C, and the injectant must be delivered within 4 seconds, with minimal handling of the syringe to prevent warming of the solution.[67] The injectant should always be delivered at the same point in the respiratory cycle; usually end exhalation is used.[63,67] Reliable CO measurements can be obtained with the head of bed elevated up to 20 degrees, with the patient in the supine or lateral position.[63,67]

**CALCULATED HEMODYNAMIC PROFILES.** For the patient with a thermodilution PA catheter in place, additional hemodynamic information can be calculated using routine vital signs, cardiac output, and body surface area. Hemodynamic pressures and normal values are listed in Table 7-15.

***Summary of nursing care.*** When caring for a patient with a PA catheter, the PA tracing must be continuously monitored. A significant component of the nursing assessment involves evaluation of the PA waveform to ensure that the catheter has not migrated forward into the wedge position since a segment of lung can be infarcted if the catheter occludes an arteriole for a prolonged period. Other factors that affect PA measurement include head-of-bed position and lateral body position relative to transducer height placement, respiratory variation, and positive end-expiratory pressure (PEEP).[63] If the transducer is placed at the level of the phlebostatic axis, a head-of-bed position up to 45 degrees is appropriate for most patients in the supine position.[63] In the lateral position the fourth intercostal space and midsternum are suggested as the reference level.[63]

All PA and PAWP tracings are subject to respiratory interference, especially if the patient is on a positive pressure volume-cycled ventilator. During inhalation the ventilator "pushes up" the PA tracing to produce an artificially high reading (Fig. 7-41, *A*). During spontaneous respiration, negative intrathoracic pressure "pulls down" the waveform and can produce an erroneously low measurement (Fig. 7-41, *B*). To minimize the impact of respiratory variation, the PAD should be read at end exhalation, which is the most stable point in the respiratory cycle. If the digital number fluctuates with respiration, a paper readout can be obtained to verify true PAD.

If PEEP greater than 10 cm $H_2O$ is used, PAWP and PA pressure will be artificially elevated. Because of this impact of PEEP, patients were taken off the ventilator to record PA pressure measurements in the past. However, today it is believed that since patients remain on PEEP for treatment, they may remain on it during measurement of PA pressures. In this situation the trend of PA readings is more important than one individual measurement.

Use of PA catheters is not entirely risk free. Potential complications include ventricular dysrhythmias, rupture of a pulmonary artery, endocarditis, pulmonary artery thrombosis, embolus, or hemorrhage.[98]

#### Continuous monitoring of mixed venous oxygen saturation

***Indications.*** Continuous monitoring of mixed venous oxygen saturation ($S\bar{v}O_2$) is indicated for the patient who has the potential to develop an imbalance between oxygen supply and metabolic tissue demand. This includes the patient in a shock state and the patient with severe respiratory compromise such as adult respiratory distress syndrome (ARDS). Continuous $S\bar{v}O_2$ monitoring measures the balance achieved between arterial oxygen supply ($SaO_2$) and oxygen demand at the tissue level by sampling desaturated venous mixed blood from the pulmonary artery ($S\bar{v}O_2$).[121] It is called mixed venous blood because it is a mixture of all of the venous blood saturations from many body tissues. Under normal conditions the cardiopulmonary system achieves a balance between oxygen supply and demand. The four factors that contribute to this balance include cardiac output (CO), hemoglobin (Hb), arterial oxygen saturation ($SaO_2$), and tissue metabolism ($\dot{V}O_2$). Three of these factors (CO, Hb, and $SaO_2$) contribute to the *supply* of oxygen to the tissues. Tissue metabolism determines the quantity of oxygen extracted at tissue level or oxygen consumption, and creates the *demand* for oxygen.[35]

***Catheters.*** In 1981 a fiberoptic pulmonary artery catheter was designed that continuously monitored $S\bar{v}O_2$. The catheter contains the traditional four lumens plus a lumen containing optical fibers. The fiberoptics are attached to an optical module that is connected by a cable to a small bedside computer (Fig. 7-42). The optical module transmits a narrow band–width light. The light travels down one optical fiber, is reflected off the hemoglobin in the blood, and returns to the optical module through the second fiberoptic. The $S\bar{v}O_2$ signal is averaged every 5 seconds and is recorded on a continuous display or printout.[121]

The catheter is calibrated before insertion into the patient by using a standard color reference system, which comes as part of the catheter package. Insertion technique and insertion sites are identical to those used for placement of a conventional pulmonary artery catheter. Waveform analysis and/or $S\bar{v}O_2$ can be used for accurate placement. Once the catheter is inserted, recalibration is unnecessary unless the catheter becomes disconnected from the optical module. To calibrate when the catheter is inserted in a patient, a mixed venous blood sample must be withdrawn from the pulmonary artery lumen and sent to the laboratory for analysis of oxygen saturation ($S\bar{v}O_2$). To obtain accurate results, the laboratory should use a "reflectance" technique similar to the principle used by the fiberoptic catheter.

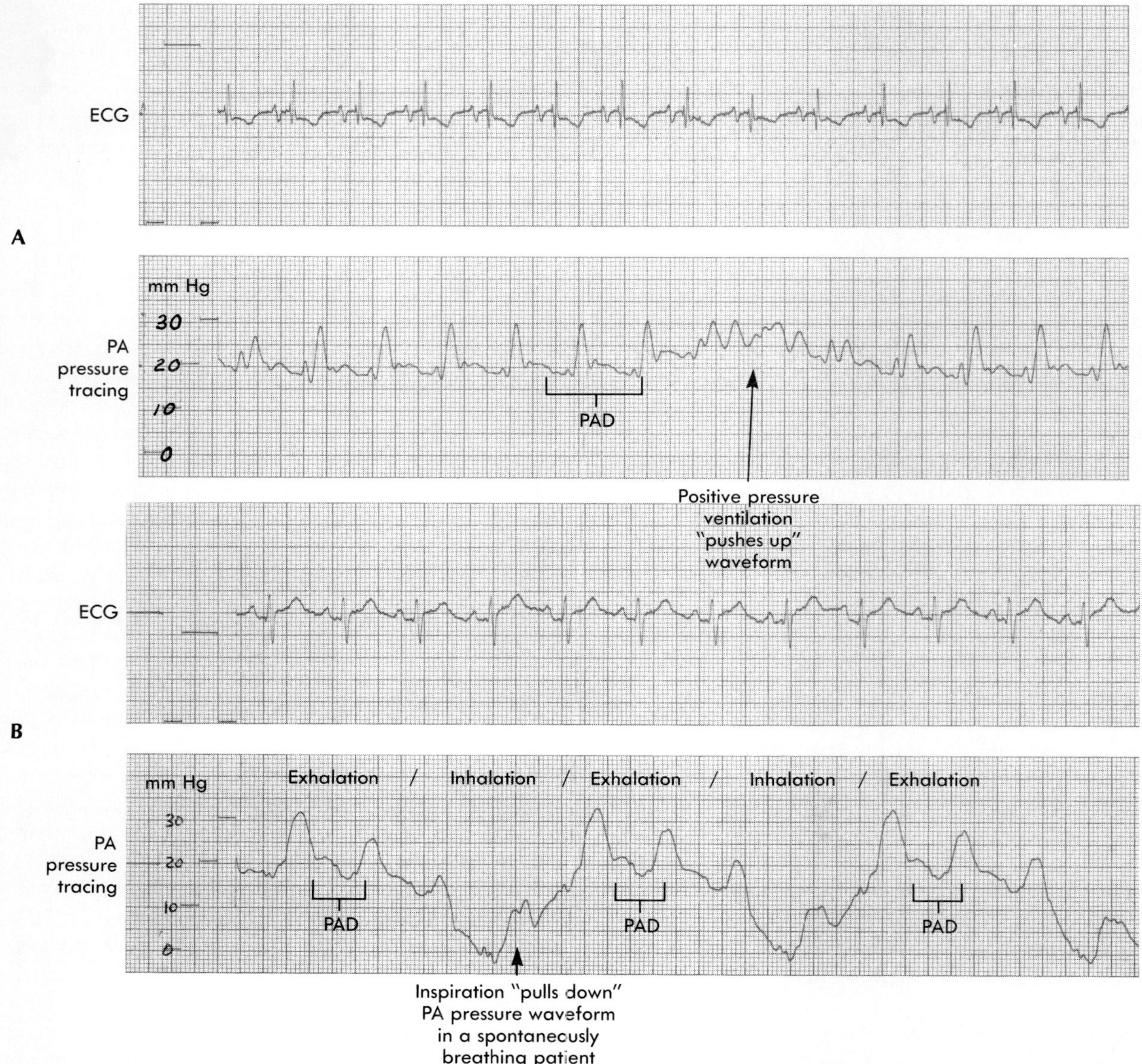


***Fig. 7-41*** PA waveforms that demonstrate the impact of ventilation on PA pressure readings. For accuracy, PA pressures should be read at end exhalation. **A,** Positive pressure ventilation: the increase in intrathoracic pressure during inhalation "pushes up" the PA pressure waveform, creating a false high reading. **B,** Spontaneous breathing: the decrease in intrathoracic pressure during normal inhalation "pulls down" the PA waveform, creating a false low reading.

***Summary of nursing care.*** $Svo_2$ monitoring provides a continuous assessment of the balance between oxygen supply and oxygen demand for an individual patient. Nursing assessment includes evaluation of the $Svo_2$ value and evaluation of the four factors ($Sao_2$, CO, Hb, and $Vo_2$) that maintain the oxygen supply–demand balance.

Normal $Svo_2$ is 75%. For most critically ill patients, an $Svo_2$ value between 60% and 80% is evidence of adequate balance between oxygen supply and demand. If the $Svo_2$ value changes by more than 10% and this change is maintained for more than 10 minutes, the nurse should determine which of the four factors is affecting $Svo_2$.

**ASSESSMENT OF ARTERIAL OXYGEN SATURATION.** The change in $Svo_2$ may be caused by a change in $Sao_2$. If the $Sao_2$ is increased because supplemental oxygen is being given, the $Svo_2$ will also rise. If the $Sao_2$ is decreased, $Svo_2$ will fall. Decreased $Sao_2$ can be caused by any action or disease that reduces oxygen supply, including ARDS, endotracheal suctioning, removing a patient from the ventilator, or removal of an oxygen mask. Figure 7-43 shows a

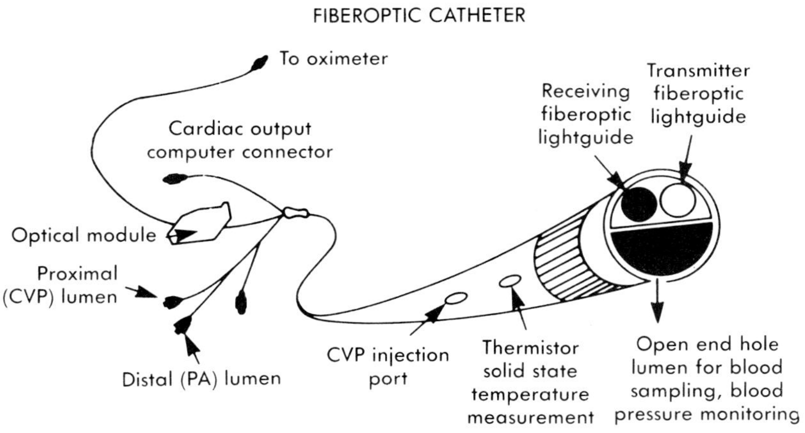

FIBEROPTIC CATHETER

To oximeter
Cardiac output computer connector
Optical module
Proximal (CVP) lumen
Distal (PA) lumen
CVP injection port
Thermistor solid state temperature measurement
Receiving fiberoptic lightguide
Transmitter fiberoptic lightguide
Open end hole lumen for blood sampling, blood pressure monitoring

***Fig. 7-42*** Oximetric fiberoptic PA catheter and optical module. (Courtesy Abbott Critical Care and Control Systems, Mountain View, Calif.)

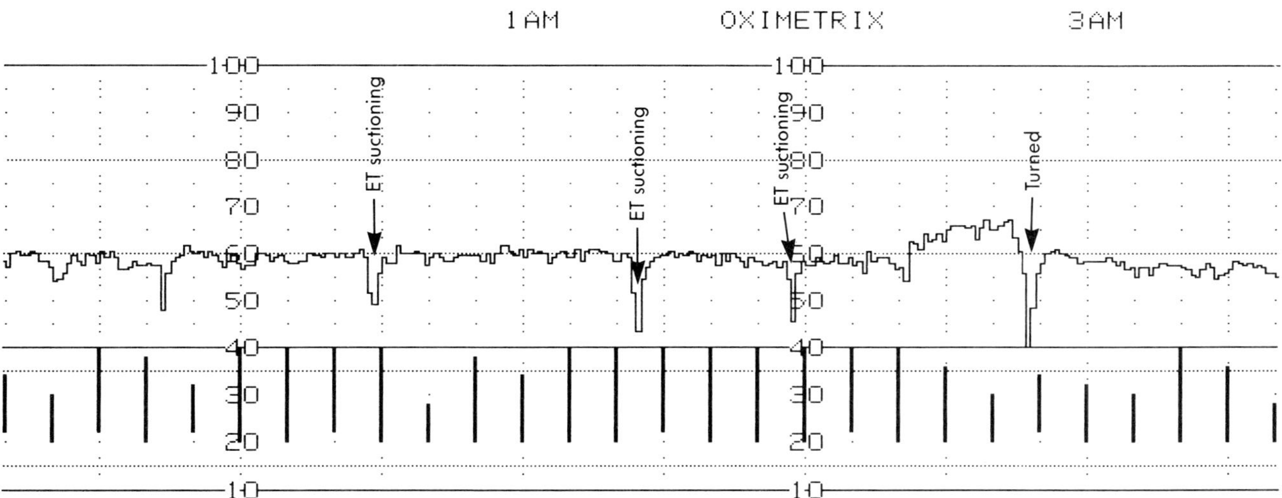


***Fig. 7-43*** Fall in $Svo_2$ during endotracheal suctioning.

fall in $Svo_2$ after suctioning in a patient with ARDS. Transient decreases in $Svo_2$ related to a nursing action such as endotracheal suctioning are not usually a cause for concern. Some patients may be slow to resaturate up to the presuction level of $Svo_2$. In this case an appropriate nursing intervention is to wait until $Svo_2$ has again returned to baseline before initiating other nursing activities.

**ASSESSMENT OF CARDIAC OUTPUT.** A change in $Svo_2$ may also be caused by an alteration in cardiac output (CO). Four hemodynamic factors affect CO—preload, afterload, heart rate, and contractility. Changes in one or more of these individual factors will affect CO.

**ASSESSMENT OF HEMOGLOBIN.** If the hemoglobin level falls as a result of bleeding or red cell destruction, the body maintains oxygen transport by increasing cardiac output and using oxygen reserves in the venous blood return. Therefore the body is able to compensate efficiently for anemia. In the healthy person hemoglobin must be extremely low before $Svo_2$ falls. However, in an anemic patient with a compromised cardiovascular system who is unable to adequately increase cardiac output, $Svo_2$ will decline as venous oxygen reserves are consumed by the body.

**ASSESSMENT OF OXYGEN CONSUMPTION.** Oxygen consumption ($\dot{V}o_2$) describes the amount of oxygen the body tissues consume for normal function in 1 minute. If the body's metabolic demands increase because of exercise or increased metabolic rate, the body will increase cardiac output to augment oxygen supply and will also use reserve oxygen in the venous system.

For the normal individual the combination of increased

**Table 7-19** Clinical interpretation of $Svo_2$ measurements

| $Svo_2$ measurement | Physiological basis for change in $Svo_2$ | Clinical diagnosis and rationale |
|---|---|---|
| High $Svo_2$ (80%-95%) | Increased oxygen supply | Patient receiving more oxygen than required by clinical condition |
| | Decreased oxygen demand | Anesthesia, which causes sedation and decreased muscle movement<br>Hypothermia, which lowers metabolic demand (e.g., with cardiopulmonary bypass)<br>Sepsis caused by decreased ability of tissues to use oxygen at a cellular level |
| Normal $Svo_2$ (60%-80%) | Normal oxygen supply and metabolic demand | Balanced oxygen supply and demand |
| Low $Svo_2$ (less than 60%) | Decreased oxygen supply caused by | |
| | Low hemoglobin (Hb) | Anemia or bleeding with compromised cardiopulmonary system |
| | Low arterial saturation ($Sao_2$) | Hypoxemia resulting from decreased oxygen supply or lung disease |
| | Low cardiac output | Cardiogenic shock caused by left-ventricular pump failure |
| | Increased oxygen consumption ($Vo_2$) | Metabolic demand exceeds oxygen supply in conditions that increase muscle movement and increase metabolic rate, including physiological states such as shivering, seizures, and hyperthermia and nursing interventions such as obtaining bed-scale weight and turning |

CO and utilization of considerable venous oxygen reserve provides adequate compensation for increased metabolic needs. However, for the critically ill patient with either cardiac or respiratory dysfunction, an increase in activity leading to increased oxygen consumption may overwhelm the cardiopulmonary system and oxygen reserves.

Simple patient movements such as getting out of bed or being weighed on a bed scale can also decrease $Svo_2$, especially if the patient has cardiopulmonary dysfunction. In compromised patients it may take several minutes for resaturation (rise in $Svo_2$) to occur. In this situation the appropriate nursing action is to observe the patient clinically in conjunction with monitoring $Svo_2$ and to postpone additional maneuvers until the $Svo_2$ has returned to baseline.

**ASSESSMENT OF $Svo_2$.** Clinical interpretation of $Svo_2$ measurements is summarized in Table 7-19.

It is helpful to assess the cause of decreased $Svo_2$ in a logical sequence that reflects knowledge of the meaning of the $Svo_2$ value: (1) to assess whether decreased $Svo_2$ is caused by decreased oxygen supply, verify the effectiveness of the ventilator or oxygen mask or check arterial oxygen saturation ($Sao_2$) by transcutaneous oximetry or from arterial blood gas values, (2) to assess cardiac function, perform a CO measurement, (3) to assess hemogobin (Hb), draw a blood sample for laboratory analysis, and (4) to assess whether decreased $Svo_2$ is the result of a recent patient movement ($Vo_2$) or a nursing action, clinically assess the patient.

If $Svo_2$ falls below 40%, the balance of oxygen supply and demand may not be adequate to meet tissue needs at the cellular level. The cells change from an aerobic to anaerobic mode of metabolism, which results in the production of lactic acid and is representative of a shock state in which cellular injury or cell death may result. At this point every attempt should be made to determine the cause of the low $Svo_2$ and to correct the oxygen supply–oxygen demand imbalance.

## REFERENCES


1. Allwork S: The applied anatomy of the arterial blood supply to the heart in man, J Anat 153:1, 1987.
2. Annoni G, Chirillo R, and Swannie D: Prognostic value of mitochondrial aspartate aminotransferase in acute myocardial infarctions, Clin Biochem 19(4):235, 1986.
3. Ashton J and Cassidy S: Reflex depression of cardiovascular function during lung inflation, J Appl Physiol 58(1):137, 1985.
4. Beattie S, Billiard S, and Meinhardt S: The use of cardiac catheterization data to design nursing care plans, Crit Care Nurs 10(6):43, 1990.
5. Benner P: From novice to expert, Menlo Park, Calif, 1984, Addison-Wesley Publishing Co.
6. Bentley LJ: Radionuclide imaging techniques in the diagnosis and treatment of coronary heart disease, Focus Crit Care 14(6):27, 1987.
7. Berman D, Rozanski A, and Knoebel S: The detection of silent ischemia: cautions and precautions, Circulation 75(1):101, 1987.
8. Bhandari A and Sheinman M: The long QT syndrome, Mod Conc Cardiovasc Dis 54(9):45, 1985.
9. Biondi J, Schulman D, and Matthay R: Effects of mechanical ventilation on right and left ventricular function, Clin Chest Med 9(1):55, 1988.
10. Blaine E: Emergence of a new cardiovascular control system: atrial natriuretic factor, Clin Exp Hypertens 7(5-6):835, 1985.

11. Blaine E: Role of atriopeptin in blood pressure regulation, Am J Med Sci 295(4):293, 1988.
12. Bonke F and others: Impulse propagation from the SA-node to the ventricles, Experientia 43:1044, 1987.
13. Bruce R and others: ST segment elevation with exercise: a marker for poor ventricular function and poor prognosis, Circulation 77 (4):897, 1988.
14. Bumann R and Speltz M: Decreased cardiac output: a nursing diagnosis, Dimens Crit Care Nurs 8(1):6, 1989.
15. Canobbio M: Chest x-ray film interpretation, Focus Crit Care 11(2):18, 1984.
16. Carmeliet E and others: Potassium currents in cardiac cells, Experientia 43:1175, 1987.
17. Chapleau M, Hajduczok G, and Abboud F: Mechanisms of resetting of arterial baroreceptors: an overview, Am J Med Sci 295(4):327, 1988.
18. Charette A: Bridging the gap between hemodynamics and monitoring, Crit Care Nurs Clin North Am 1(3):539, 1989.
19. Chung E: Manual of exercise ECG testing, New York, 1986, Yorke Medical Books.
20. Caccio J: Measurements of hemodynamics in side-lying positions: a review of the literature, Focus Crit Care 17(3):250, 1990.
21. Come P: Diagnostic cardiology: noninvasive imaging techniques, Philadelphia, 1985, JB Lippincott Co.
22. Conner R: The Wenckebach phenomenon, Heart Lung 16(5):506, 1987.
23. Conover M: Pocket guide to electrocardiography, St Louis, 1990, Mosby–Year Book, Inc.
24. Cowan M and others: Comparative accuracy of computerized spatial vectorcardiography and standard electrocardiography for detection of myocardial infarction, J Electrocardiol 18(2):111, 1985.
25. Cranefield P: The conduction of the cardiac impulse 1951-1986, Experientia 43:1040, 1987.
26. Daily EK and Schroeder J: Techniques in bedside hemodynamic monitoring, St Louis, 1989, Mosby–Year Book, Inc.
27. Daily EK and Tilkian AG: Hemodynamic monitoring. In Tilkian AG and Daily EK, editors: Cardiovascular procedures, St Louis, 1986, Mosby–Year Book, Inc.
28. D'Ambra MN and others: Prostaglandin E, J Thorac Cardiovasc Surg 89(4): 567, 1985.
29. Davis J and others: A comparison of objective measurements on the chest roentgenogram as screening tests for right or left ventricular hypertrophy, Am J Cardiol 58(7):658, 1986.
30. deBold AJ and others: A rapid and potent natriuretic response to intravenous injection of atrial myocardial extract in rats, Life Sci 28:89, 1981.
31. Deleze J: Cell-to-cell communication in the heart: structure-function correlations, Experientia 43:1068, 1987.
32. DiLucente L: Mimics of coronary artery disease on the electrocardiogram, Crit Care Nurse 10(6):31, 1990.
33. Dunn F: Hypertensive heart disease in the patient with normal electrocardiogram and chest radiograph, J Cardiovasc Pharmacol (suppl 6):5870, 1984.
34. Enger E: Pulmonary wide pressure: when it's valid, when it's not, Crit Care Nurs Clin North Am 1(3):603, 1989.
35. Fahey PJ: Continuous measurement of blood oxygen saturation in the high risk patient, Mountain View, Calif, 1985, Oximetric, Inc.
36. Famularo M and Kennedy H: Ambulatory electrocardiography to assess pacemaker function, Am Heart J 104:1086, 1982.
37. Forrester JS and others: Filling pressures in the right and left sides of the heart in acute myocardial infarction, N Engl J Med 285(4):190, 1971.
38. Francis G: Neurohumoral mechanisms involved in congestive heart failure, Am J Cardiol 55(2):15A, 1985.
39. Franey M and Bergstrom D: Clinical management using direct and derived parameters, Crit Care Nurs Clin North Am 1(3):547, 1989.
40. Gardner P: Cardiac output, theory, technique, and troubleshooting, Crit Care Nurs Clin North Am 1(3):577, 1989.
41. Goldberger AL and Goldberger E: Clinical electrocardiography: a simplified approach, ed 4, St Louis, 1990, Mosby–Year Book, Inc.
42. Greene A and Shoukas A: Changes in canine cardiac function and venous return curves by the carotid baroreflex, Am J Physiol 251(part 2):H283, 1986.
43. Greenway C and Lautt W: Blood volume, the venous system, preload, and cardiac output, Can J Physiol Pharmacol 64(4):383, 1986.
44. Groom L, Elliott M, and Frisch S: Injectate temperature: effects on thermodilution CO measurements, Crit Care Nurs 10(5):112, 1990.
45. Halperin B and others: Evaluation of the portable chest roentgenogram for quantitating extravascular lung water in critically ill adults, Chest 88(5):649, 1985.
46. Handler C and Sowton E: Stress testing predischarge and 6 weeks after myocardial infarction to compare submaximal and maximal exercise predischarge and to assess the reproducibility of induced abnormalities, Int J Cardiol 9(2):173, 1985.
47. Heinsimer J and others: Supine cross-table lateral chest roentgenogram for the detection of pericardial effusion, JAMA 257(23):3266, 1987.
48. Hindman N and others: Relation between electrocardiographic and enzymatic methods of estimating acute myocardial infarct size, Am J Cardiol 58(1):31, 1986.
49. Hoffman I: Clinical vectorcardiography in adults, Am Heart J 100:239, 1980.
50. Horackova M: Transmembrane calcium transport and the activation of cardiac contraction, Can J Physiol Pharmacol 62:874, 1984.
51. Hurst J, editor-in-chief: The heart, arteries, and veins, ed 6, New York, 1986, McGraw-Hill Book Co.
52. Hysing J and Grendahl H: Ambulatory 24-hour ECG in patients with a history of syncope: a retrospective follow-up study over 2 years, Eur Heart J 6(2):120, 1985.
53. Jacob J and others: Studies on neural and humoral contributions to arterial pressure lability, Am J Med Sci 295(4):341, 1988.
54. Julius S: The blood pressure seeking properties of the central nervous system, J Hypertens 6(3):177, 1988.
55. Kadota LT: Theory and application of thermodilution cardiac output measurement: a review, Heart Lung 14(6):605, 1985.
56. Kitzman DW: Age-related changes in normal human hearts during the first 10 decades of life. Part II (maturity): a quantitative anatomic study of 765 specimens from subjects 20 to 99 years old, Mayo Clin Proc 63:137, 1988.
57. Kligfield P and others: Evaluation of coronary artery disease by an improved method of exercise electrocardiography: the ST segment/heart rate slope, Am Heart J 112(3):589, 1986.
58. Klocke FJ and others: Coronary pressure-flow relationships, Circ Res 56:310, 1985.
59. Kloner R and Parisi A: Acute myocardial infarction: diagnostic and prognostic applications of two-dimensional echocardiography, Circulation 75(3):521, 1987.
60. Kowey P: The calamity of cardioversion of conscious patients, Am J Cardiol 61(13):1106, 1988.
61. Laakman R and others: Magnetic resonance imaging in patients with metallic implants, Radiology 157:711, 1985.
62. Langer G: The role of calcium at the sarcolemma in the control of myocardial contractility, Can J Physiol Pharmacol 65:627, 1987.
63. Laurent-Bopp D and Gardner PE: Clinical nursing research in cardiac care. In Kern L, editor: Cardiac critical care nursing, Rockville, Maryland, 1988, Aspen Publishers, Inc.
64. Lee TH and Goldman L: Serum enzyme assays in the diagnosis of acute myocardial infarction, Ann Intern Med 105(2):221, 1986.
65. Leonard JJ and others: Examination of the heart. Part four. Auscultation, Dallas, 1974, American Heart Association.
66. Levy MN: Cardiac sympathetic-parasympathetic interactions, Fed Proc 43:2596, 1984.
67. Loveys BJ and Woods SL: Current recommendations for thermodilution cardiac output measures, Prog Cardiovasc Nurs 1(1):242, 1986.
68. Maisel AS and others: The murmur of papillary muscle dysfunction

in acute myocardial infarction: clinical features and prognostic implications, Am Heart J 112(4):705, 1986.

69. Maki DG and others: Prospective study of replacing administration sets for intravenous therapy at 48- vs. 72-hour intervals, JAMA 258(13):1777, 1987.
70. Malasanos L and others: Health assessment, ed 4, St Louis, 1990, Mosby–Year Book, Inc.
71. Marriott HJL: AV block: an overdue overhaul, Emerg Med 13(6):85, 1981.
72. Marriott HJL: Practical electrocardiography, Baltimore, 1988, Williams & Wilkins.
73. Masters S: Complications of pulmonary artery catheters, Crit Care Nurse 9(9):82, 1989.
74. Missri J: Clinical Doppler echocardiography, New York, 1986, Yorke Medical Books.
75. Morganroth J: Ambulatory holter electrocardiography: choice of technologies and clinical uses, Ann Intern Med 102(1):73, 1985.
76. Morganroth J, Parisi A, and Pohost G: Noninvasive cardiac imaging, St Louis, 1983, Mosby–Year Book, Inc.
77. Murphy M and others: Reevaluation of ECG criteria for left, right and combined cardiac ventricular hypertrophy, Am J Cardiol 53:1140, 1984.
78. Murphy M and others: The reliability of the routine chest roentgenogram for determination of heart size based on specific ventricular chamber evaluation at post-mortem, Invest Radiol 20(1):21, 1985.
79. Musewe N and others: Validation of Doppler-derived pulmonary arterial pressure in patients with ductus arteriosus under different hemodynamic states, Circulation 76(5):1081, 1987.
80. Ng RHB and others: Increased activity of creatine kinase isoenzyme MB in a theophylline-intoxicated patient, Clin Chem 31(10):741, 1985.
81. Niblock AE and others: Changes in mass and catalytic activity concentrations of aspartate aminotransferase isoenzymes in serum after a myocardial infarction, Clin Chem 32(3):496, 1986.
82. Noble D: Experimental and theoretical work on excitation and excitation-contraction coupling in the heart, Experientia 43:1146, 1987.
83. Noll ML and Fountain R: Effect of backrest position on mixed venous oxygen saturation in patients with mechanical ventilation after coronary artery bypass graft, Heart Lung 19(3):243, 1990.
84. Pandian N, Skorton D, and Kerber R: Role of echocardiography in myocardial ischemia and infarction, Mod Conc Cardiovasc Dis 53(4):19, 1984.
85. Pelzer D and Trautwein W: Currents through ionic channels in multicellular cardiac tissue and single heart cells, Experientia 43:1153, 1987.
86. Phipps WJ and others: Medical-surgical nursing: concepts and clinical practice, ed 4, St Louis, 1991, Mosby–Year Book, Inc.
87. Pistolesi M and others: The chest roentgenogram in pulmonary edema, Clin Chest Med 6(3):315, 1985.
88. Platia E: Management of cardiac arrhythmias: the nonpharmacologic approach, Philadelphia, 1987, JB Lippincott Co.
89. Pohost G and Canby R: Nuclear magnetic resonance imaging: current applications and future prospects, Circulation 75(1):88, 1987.
90. Pollard D and Seliger E: An implementation of bedside physiological calculations, Waltham, GA, 1985, Hewlett Packard.
91. Presti C and others: Digital two-dimensional echocardiographic imaging of the proximal left anterior descending coronary artery, Am J Cardiol 60(6):1254, 1987.
92. Quaal S: Hemodynamic monitoring: a review of the literature, Applied Nurs Research 1:58, 1988.
93. Reddy PS, Salerni R, and Shaver JA: Normal and abnormal heart sounds in cardiac diagnosis. Part II. Diastolic sounds, Curr Prob Cardiol 10(4):1, 1985.
94. Reis D and Ledoux J: Some central neural mechanisms governing resting and behaviorally coupled control of blood pressure, Circulation 76(suppl I):2, 1987.
95. Reuter J: Calcium channel modulation by beta-adrenergic neurotransmitters in the heart, Experientia 43:1173, 1987.
96. Richards K: Doppler echocardiography in the diagnosis and quantification of valvular disease, Mod Conc Cardiovasc Dis 56(8):43, 1987.
97. Roberts R: Recognition, pathogenesis and management of non-Q-wave infarction, Mod Conc Cardiovasc Dis 56(4):17, 1987.
98. Robin ED: The cult of the Swan-Ganz catheter, Ann Intern Med 103:445, 1985.
99. Rosen M: The links between basic and clinical cardiac electrophysiology, Circulation 77(2):251, 1988.
100. Schriner D: Using hemodynamic waveforms to assess cardiopulmonary pathologies, Crit Care Nurs Clin North Am 1(3):563, 1989.
101. Sclarovsky S and others: Unstable angina: the significance of ST segment elevation of depression in patients without evidence of increased myocardial oxygen demand, Am Heart J 112(3):459, 1986.
102. Sealy W: Morphology of the conduction system and arrhythmia surgery, PACE 11:362, 1988.
103. Seidel HM and others: Mosby's guide to physical examination, ed 2, St Louis, 1991, Mosby–Year Book, Inc.
104. Sevilla D and others: Anatomic validation of electrocardiographic estimation of the size of acute or healed myocardial infarcts, Am J Cardiol 65:1301, 1990.
105. Shamoo AE and Ambudkar IS: Regulation of calcium transport in cardiac cells, Can J Physiol Pharmacol 62:9, 1984.
106. Shaver JA, Salerni R, and Reddy PS: Normal and abnormal heart sounds in cardiac diagnosis. Part I. Systolic sounds, Curr Prob Cardiol 10(3):1, 1985.
107. Slutsky R and Brown J: Chest radiographs in congestive heart failure: response to therapy in acute and chronic heart disease, Radiology 154(3):557, 1985.
108. Spodick D: Left axis deviation and left anterior fascicular block, Am J Cardiol 61(1):869, 1988.
109. Staubli M and others: Creatine kinase and creatine kinase MB in endurance runners and in patients with myocardial infarction, Eur J Applied Physiol 54(1):40, 1985.
110. Steger K, Remy J, and Krueger S: Drug-induced torsade des pointes: case report and implications for the critical care staff, Heart Lung 15(2):200, 1986.
111. Stillwell S and Randall E: Pocket guide to cardiovascular care, St Louis, 1990, Mosby–Year Book, Inc.
112. Stodieck L and Luttges M: Relationships between the ECG and phonocardiogram: potential for improved heart monitoring, Biomed Sci Instrum 20:47, 1984.
113. Stratemeier E and others: Ejection fraction determination by magnetic resonance imaging: comparison with left ventricular angiography, Radiology 158:775, 1986.
114. Tavel M: Clinical phonocardiography and external pulse recording, St Louis, 1985, Mosby–Year Book, Inc.
115. Thompson JM and others: Clinical nursing, ed 2, St Louis, 1989, Mosby–Year Book, Inc.
116. Tsien R, Hess P, and Nilius B: Cardiac calcium currents at the level of single channels, Experientia 43:1169, 1987.
117. Urban N: Hemodynamic clinical profiles, Clin Issues Crit Care Nurs 1(1):119, 1990.
118. Van Rossum A and others: Evaluation of magnetic resonance imaging for determination of left ventricular ejection fraction and comparison with angiography, Am J Cardiol 62(9):628, 1988.
119. Vassalle M: Contribution of the $Na^+/K^+$-pump to the membrane potential, Experientia 43:1135, 1987.
120. Weidmann S: Cardiac cellular electrophysiology: past and present, Experientia 43:133, 1987.
121. White KM: Completing the hemodynamic picture $Svo_2$, Heart Lung 114(3):272, 1985.
122. Willette R and others: Cardiovascular control by cholinergic mechanisms in the rostral ventrolateral medulla, J Pharmacol Exp Ther 231(2):457, 1984.
123. Winegrad S: Regulation of cardiac contractile proteins, Circ Res 55:565, 1984.

CHAPTER 8

# Cardiovascular Disorders

## CHAPTER OBJECTIVES

- *Describe the epidemiology and pathophysiology associated with coronary artery disease.*
- *Identify and describe the pathological significance of nonmodifiable, minor modifiable, and major modifiable risk factors for the development of coronary artery disease.*
- *List the electrocardiographic, hemodynamic, and physiological changes associated with myocardial infarction.*
- *List important aspects of the diagnosis and treatment of patients with congestive heart failure, cardiogenic shock, endocarditis, cardiomyopathy, valvular heart disease, hypovolemic shock, hypertensive crisis, and peripheral vascular disease.*
- *List important aspects in the nursing assessment and care of patients with myocardial infarction, congestive heart failure, cardiogenic shock, endocarditis, cardiomyopathy, valvular heart disease, hypovolemic shock, hypertensive crisis, and peripheral vascular disease.*

## KEY TERMS

coronary artery disease (CAD), p. 159
nonmodifiable risk factors, p. 160
modifiable risk factors, p. 160
low density lipoproteins (LDL), p. 160
high density lipoproteins (HDL), p. 160
atherosclerosis, p. 161
angina pectoris, p. 162
unstable angina, p. 162
Prinzmetal's angina, p. 162
myocardial infarction, p. 164
ventricular aneurysm, p. 171
ventricular septal defect, p. 171
papillary muscle rupture, p. 172
pericarditis, p. 172
congestive heart failure, p. 174
pulmonary edema, p. 175
cardiogenic shock, p. 179
hypovolemic shock, p. 179
hypertensive crisis, p. 181
cardiomyopathies, p. 182
endocarditis, p. 183
valvular heart disease, p. 184
peripheral vascular disease, p. 186
aortic dissection, p. 188
thrombophlebitis, p. 188

## CORONARY ARTERY DISEASE

### Description

**Coronary artery disease (CAD)** is an insidious, progressive disease of the coronary arteries that results in their narrowing or complete occlusion. There are multiple causes for coronary artery narrowing: atherosclerosis, thrombosis, spasm, coronary dissection, and aneurysm formation. Atherosclerosis is the most prevalent and affects the medium-sized arteries perfusing the heart, brain, kidneys, and extremities and the large arteries branching off the aorta. Atherosclerotic lesions may take different forms, depending on their anatomical location; the individual's age, genetic makeup, and physiological status; and the number of risk factors the individual manifests.

CAD has a long latent period. Fatty streaks appear within the aorta shortly after birth, but most individuals are not symptomatic until late middle age when they have coronary artery lesions that are greater than 75% (that is, 75% of the vessel lumen is occluded by atherosclerotic plaque).

### Etiology

Epidemiological and actuarial data collected during the past 40 years have demonstrated an association between specific risk factors and the development of CAD. One of the most important epidemiological studies is the Framingham Heart Study,[21,52] which began in 1948 and continues today with a second generation of subjects. As a result of this study and others like it, specific lifestyle habits have been identified that are associated with an increased prob-

**CARDIAC RISK FACTORS**

| NONMODIFIABLE | MODIFIABLE |
|---|---|
| | **Major** |
| Age | Elevated serum lipids |
| Sex | Hypertension |
| Family history | Cigarette smoking |
| Race | Impaired glucose tolerance |
| | Diet high in saturated fat, cholesterol, and calories |
| | **Minor** |
| | Sedentary lifestyle |
| | Psychological stress |
| | Personality type |

ability of developing CAD. These lifestyle habits are referred to as coronary risk factors.[13,45,123] Several tools have been developed to assist the clinician in quickly and accurately identifying patients and populations at risk.[10]

**Risk factors.** The risk factors for development of CAD are age, sex, race, elevated serum cholesterol, elevated blood pressure, cigarette smoking, abnormal glucose tolerance, sedentary lifestyle, stress, and type A behavior pattern. These factors are further delineated into nonmodifiable and major and minor modifiable factors (see the box above).

***Nonmodifiable risk factors.*** CAD occurs approximately 10 years later in women than it does in men. After menopause, rates become the same for both sexes. Family history is another significant risk factor. An individual has a positive family history if a close blood relative has had a myocardial infarction or stroke before age 60 years. Since 1968, nonwhite populations of both sexes have had higher CAD mortality rates than white populations.[110]

***Major modifiable risk factors***

**ELEVATED SERUM LIPIDS.** Hyperlipidemia is a leading factor responsible for severe atherosclerosis. Cholesterol, triglycerides, and free fatty acids are all plasma lipids that are carried in the blood. Cholesterol is a steroid that is obtained endogenously by synthesis, especially in the liver, and exogenously from a diet high in saturated fats.

Serum cholesterol levels below 200 mg/dl are associated with minimal risk of CAD, whereas levels >270 mg/dl carry a fourfold increase in the risk.[110] Cholesterol and triglycerides are transported in the blood by lipoprotein complexes, of which there are four major classes. These classes are distinguished by their protein density or by the percent of protein they carry.

High density implies a high protein content, whereas low density indicates a low protein content. The first of these lipoproteins, chylomicrons, are composed primarily of triglycerides. The second, very low density lipoproteins (VLDL), also known as B-lipoprotein, transport mainly triglycerides. The third, **low density lipoproteins (LDL)** are B-lipoproteins, which are metabolized from VLDL and carry 60% to 75% of the total plasma cholesterol. The fourth, **high density lipoproteins (HDL),** are composed of 50% protein, 25% phospholipid, 20% cholesterol, and 5% triglyceride. High density lipoproteins apparently clear cholesterol from the tissues and transport it to the liver. Children and premenopausal women often have an elevated HDL concentration, and both groups are considered low coronary risks. High density lipoprotein levels are thought to increase in response to increasing one's activity level and especially in response to aerobic exercises, weight loss, and cessation of cigarette smoking.[38]

**HYPERTENSION.** In the context of CAD, hypertension is the elevation of either systolic or diastolic pressure. Elevated systolic pressure is more predictive of risk, with levels consistently above 160 mm Hg of definite concern. The risk for developing CAD in the presence of hypertension is proportional to the degree of blood pressure elevation. Hypertension is thought a risk factor because it causes damage to the vessel's endothelium and disrupts the antithrombogenic and permeability barrier. Hypertension has a profound effect on the CAD risk profile in populations with elevated cholesterol levels (>160 mg/dl).

**CIGARETTE SMOKING.** Several studies have indicated that the risk of developing CAD is directly proportional to the number of cigarettes smoked per day.[38] Cigarette smoking unfavorably alters lipid levels, decreasing HDL levels and increasing LDL levels and triglyceride levels. Smoking results in cardiac electrical instability within cell membranes and impairs oxygen transport and use while increasing myocardial oxygen demand. Smoking is also thought to alter intimal endothelial permeability and to foster platelet agglutination. Fortunately, after cessation the coronary risk falls rapidly, with a decrease of approximately 50% within 1 year.[10,13]

**DIABETES MELLITUS.** Women with diabetes mellitus are at greater risk for developing CAD than men with diabetes mellitus. The mechanism of how diabetes effects the coronary arteries is not well understood. However, it may alter platelet function or increase red blood cell adhesion. There is also a positive association between diabetes and hypertension, hypertriglyceridemia, and low levels of HDL. Diabetics also tend to be more susceptible to both macrovascular and microvascular disease.

**OBESITY.** Obesity apparently affects the coronary artery risk profile by enhancing an individual's susceptibility to developing other risk factors such as hypertension, impaired glucose tolerance, and hyperlipidemia, with increased LDL and decreased HDL levels. Obesity is also often associated with a sedentary lifestyle.

**ORAL CONTRACEPTIVES.** Oral contraceptives increase a woman's risk, especially after age 35, because oral contraceptives (1) alter blood coagulation, (2) alter platelet function, (3) alter fibinolytic activity, and (4) may inversely affect the integrity of vascular endothelium. This risk becomes significantly greater if the woman also smokes.

### *Minor modifiable risk factors*

**SEDENTARY LIFESTYLE.** Evidence continues to accumulate that a sedentary lifestyle has an effect on the risk of developing CAD. A sedentary lifestyle is also associated with lower HDL levels, higher LDL levels, hypertension, obesity, increased glucose intolerance, and elevated triglycerides.[79]

**STRESS AND PERSONALITY.** Type A personality was identified by Rosenman and Friedman[13,52] as associated with increased coronary risk. How stress or behavior influence the development of CAD is not well understood, but stress is associated with increased circulating catecholamines, which may precipitate hypertension, alteration in platelet function, increased fatty acid mobilization, and a resultant elevation of free fatty acids.[10]

## Pathophysiology of CAD

Normal arterial walls are composed of three cellular layers: the intima, the innermost layer; the media, the middle layer; and the adventitia, the outermost layer. The intima is the most susceptible to trauma; hence, most primary lesions occur there, whereas the lesions that occur in the media are associated with more severe disease.

Three key elements that result in luminal narrowing or occlusions have been identified. They include the following[45]:

1. Smooth muscle proliferation
2. Formation of a connective tissue matrix composed of collagen, elastic fibers, and proteoglycans
3. Accumulation of lipids

**Stages of plaque development.** Three stages of atherosclerotic plaque development have been identified (Fig. 8-1).[13,23,45] The first stage, *fatty streaks,* consists of broad-based lesions composed of lipid-laden macrophages and smooth muscle cells. The second stage, the *fibrous plaque phase,* is usually identified by the occurrence of "classic" atherosclerotic plaques. The third stage, the *advanced (complicated) lesion phase,* consists of lesions usually seen with advancing age. The fibrous plaque undergoes several changes: (1) it becomes vascularized, (2) the core becomes calcified, and (3) the surface may desegregate and ulcerate, possibly resulting in (4) hemorrhage and thromboembolic episodes. Furthermore, the media may develop aneurysmal changes resulting from the decrease in smooth muscle cells.

**Hemodynamic effect.** The major hemodynamic effect of CAD is the disturbance in the delicate balance between myocardial oxygen supply and demand. **Atherosclerosis** alters the normal coronary artery's response to increased demand in two ways: (1) lesions that result in vessel-lumen occlusion of 75% or more restrict flow under resting conditions, and (2) the vessels become stiff and lose the ability to dilate. The result is decreased driving pressure beyond the site of the lesion and less oxygenated blood available to the myocardial cells perfused by that vessel.[60] As a result, the myocardium is forced to shift from aerobic metabolism to anaerobic metabolism, the consequences of which are (1) less efficient energy production, (2) lactic acid buildup, (3) intracellular hypokalemia, (4) intracellular acidosis, (5) intracellular hypernatremia, and (6) interference with the release of calcium from its storage sites in the sarcoplasmic reticulum.[13,45,60]

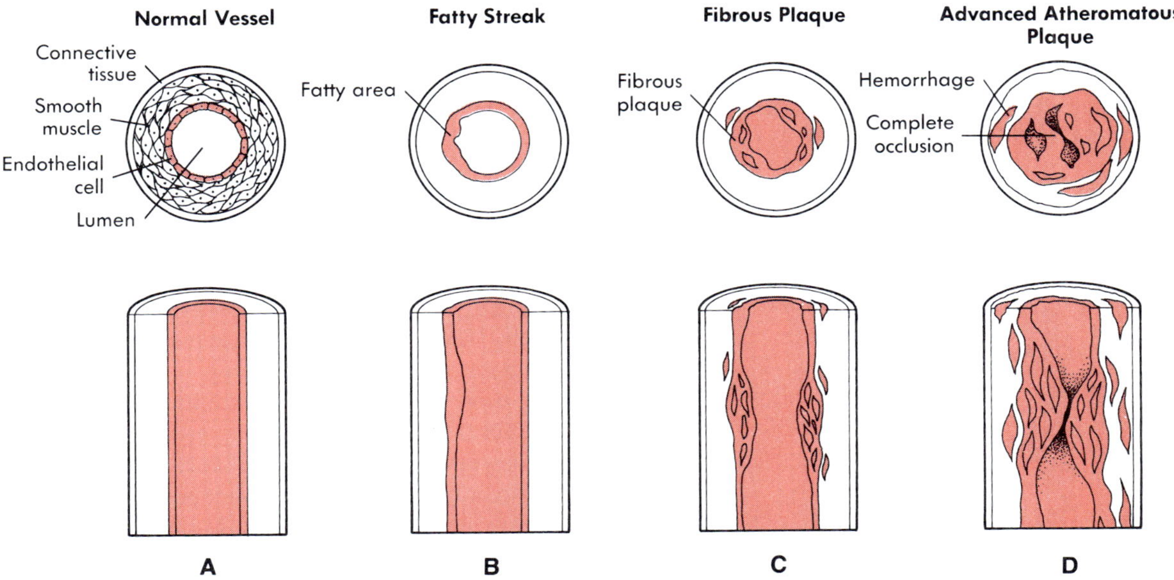


***Fig. 8-1*** The progression of atherosclerosis shown in both the longitudinal and the cross-sectional views. **A,** Normal vessel. **B,** First stage, fatty streaks. **C,** Second stage, fibrous plaque development. **D,** Third stage, advanced (complicated) lesions.

The end result of atherosclerosis is left-ventricular dysfunction. This impaired left-ventricular function results in decreased fiber stretch and contractility, decreased stroke volume, increased left-ventricular end diastolic volume (LVEDV), and increased left-ventricular end diastolic pressure (LVEDP). Further, the impairment of the calcium mechanism causes incomplete ventricular relaxation. This, in combination with poor ventricular emptying, may increase the LVEDP even more. Tissue hypoxia or ischemia is the final stage of this process.

### Angina

**Angina** is the sensory response to a transient lack of oxygen in the myocardium. It is not a disease but rather a symptom of CAD. Angina has many characteristics (see the box below), but the word itself was intended to describe a sensation of strangling in the breast, accompanied by anxiety or a fear of death.[13]

Anginal pain may occur anywhere in the chest, neck, arms, or back, but the most common location is the retrosternal region. The pain frequently radiates to the left arm but may also radiate to both arms, the mandible, and/or the neck (Fig. 8-2). Levine's sign, a clenched fist placed over the sternum, is frequently demonstrated when patients indicate the location of their discomfort.[13]

Angina is classified as stable, unstable, and variant.

*Stable angina* usually begins gradually and reaches maximal intensity during a matter of minutes before dissipating. It may be precipitated by activity, tachycardia, systemic hypertension, thyrotoxicosis, sympathomimetic drugs, systemic illness, or anemia. Correction of the precipitating event or the administration of vasodilators will usually result in the termination of the angina.[100]

Stable angina may be subdivided into *fixed threshold angina* or *varied threshold angina*. Fixed threshold angina is that which is predictable and caused by the same precipitating factors. It is usually the result of fixed lesions, with little acute vasoconstriction involved. Varied threshold angina is unpredictable. Patients may be able to walk two blocks pain free some days, whereas on other days they may need to stop after only one block.[17]

**Unstable angina** is defined as a change in a previously established stable pattern or a new onset of severe angina. It is usually more intense than stable angina and is often described as pain rather than discomfort. Unstable angina can also be referred to as *preinfarction* or *crescendo angina*, *acute coronary insufficiency*, or *intermediate coronary syndrome*. It may be precipitated by the same events associated with stable angina or by (1) acceleration of atherosclerosis in multiple vessels, (2) left main coronary disease, (3) increase in localized platelet agglutination, (4) acute or chronic thrombosis, (5) plaque hemorrhage or fissure, or (6) acute vasoconstriction.[17,24]

Unstable angina may occur after a myocardial infarction as the result of mechanical problems such as left-ventricular aneurysm, mitral regurgitation secondary to ruptured papillary muscles, ventricular septal defect, or global left-ventricular failure.[19] It is usually more intense, persists longer (up to 30 minutes), and may awaken patients from sleep.[13] The symptoms of unstable angina may only be partially relieved by rest or nitrates.

*Variant*, or **Prinzmetal's, angina** is defined as a reversible focal reduction in coronary artery diameter, leading to myocardial ischemia in the absence of preceding increases in myocardial oxygen consumption. Variant angina frequently occurs at rest and can also be cyclical, occurring at the same time everyday. It is usually associated with ST segment elevation and occasionally with transient abnormal Q waves.[13] Smoking tobacco and ingestion of alcohol and cocaine may also precipitate spasm.

Treatment of variant angina is aimed at decreasing the

#### CHARACTERISTICS OF ANGINA PECTORIS

**LOCATION**

Beneath sternum, radiating to neck and jaw
Upper chest
Beneath sternum, radiating down left arm
Epigastric
Epigastric, radiating to neck, jaw, and arms
Neck and jaw
Left shoulder, inner aspect of both arms
Intrascapular

**DURATION**

0.5 to 30 minutes

**QUALITY**

Sensation of pressure or heavy weight on the chest
Feeling of tightness, like a vise
Visceral quality (deep, heavy, squeezing, aching)
Burning sensation
Shortness of breath, with feeling of suffocation
Most severe pain ever experienced

**RADIATION**

Medial aspect of left arm
Jaw
Left shoulder
Right arm

**PRECIPITATING FACTORS**

Exertion/exercise
Cold weather
Exercising after a large, heavy meal
Walking against the wind
Emotional upset
Fright, anger
Coitus

**NITROGLYCERIN RELIEF**

Usually within 45 seconds to 5 minutes of administration

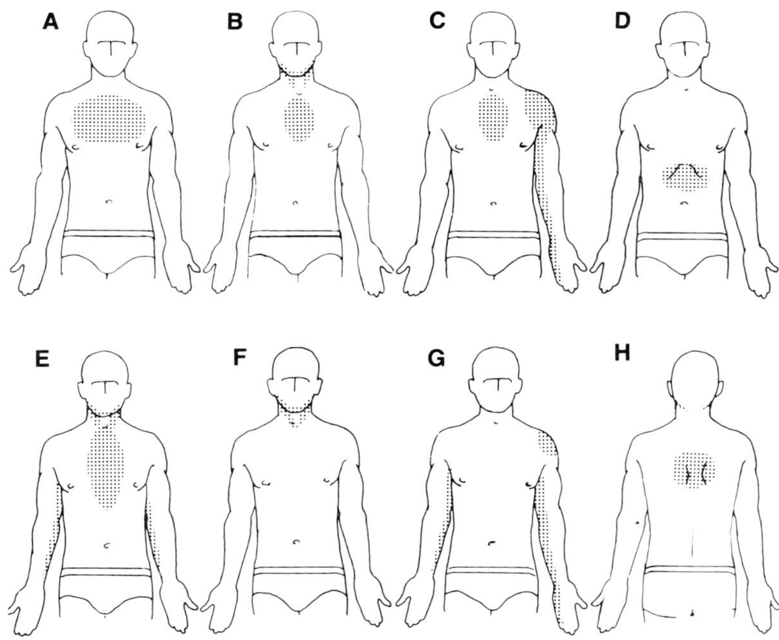


***Fig. 8-2*** Common sites for anginal pain. **A,** Upper chest. **B,** Beneath sternum radiating to neck and jaw. **C,** Beneath sternum radiating down left arm. **D,** Epigastric. **E,** Epigastric radiating to neck, jaw, and arms. **F,** Neck and jaw. **G,** Left shoulder. **H,** Intrascapular. (From Phipps WJ and others: Medical-surgical nursing: concepts and clinical practice, ed 4, St Louis, 1991, Mosby–Year Book, Inc.)

incidence of spasm and thereby reducing the risk of infarction or sudden death. Drugs of choice for the treatment of spasm are vasodilators such as nitroglycerin (either sublingual, paste, patch, or spray), isosorbide dinitrate, or calcium channel blockers such as nifedipine and diltiazem. If a patient has a fixed atherosclerotic lesion, coronary artery bypass surgery may be indicated. Percutaneous transluminal coronary angioplasty (PTCA) may be performed with selected patients as long as extreme care is taken not to induce spasm.

## Treatment of CAD

The major goals of medical therapy for CAD are to increase coronary perfusion and decrease myocardial work. Medical management will depend on the frequency, severity, duration, and hemodynamic consequences of the angina. Pharmacological therapy may include nitrates, beta adrenergic blockers, and calcium channel antagonists. CAD risk factors such as hypertension or hyperlipidemia should be aggressively treated. A low-sodium, low-cholesterol diet may be recommended. Activity will be restricted until episodes of angina are controlled. If pain persists despite maximal pharmacological therapy and rest, an intraaortic balloon may be inserted to increase coronary artery perfusion pressure and reduce afterload.

Tachycardias will usually be treated with digoxin, calcium blockers, beta blockers, or antidysrhythmics. Hypertension will be treated with diuretics or afterload reducers. Anemia may be treated with blood transfusions or iron supplements. Coronary spasm may be treated with nitrates and/or calcium blockers.

The change from stable to unstable angina represents a serious problem. The patient is usually admitted to a hospital, and bed rest is prescribed. It is important that any identified precipitating problems be treated. If the anginal pain continues, cardiac catheterization, intraaortic balloon support, thrombolic therapy, PTCA, or surgery may be indicated.

## Summary of Nursing Care

Nursing diagnoses and management of CAD and angina are summarized in the box on p. 164. Nursing care of the patient admitted with angina focuses on continuous assessment and documentation of episodes of chest pain and on providing an environment that will help alleviate fear and anxiety and provide rest and security.

On admission, cardiac monitoring should be instituted, a 12-lead ECG obtained, and any ongoing pain controlled. Complaints of chest pain must be evaluated quickly. Chest pain in the patient with known or suspected coronary disease may represent myocardial ischemia, which must be treated while it is still reversible. Assessment parameters should include the factors[103] listed in the box on p. 164.

**Nursing Diagnosis and Management**
***Coronary artery disease/angina***

- Acute Pain related to transmission and perception of noxious stimuli secondary to myocardial ischemia, p. 485
- Activity Intolerance related to myocardial tissue perfusion alterations, p. 464
- Anxiety related to threat to biological, psychological, and/or social integrity, p. 448
- Knowledge Deficit: ________ (Specify) related to lack of previous exposure to information, p. 441
- Body Image Disturbance related to actual change in body function, p. 443
- Altered Sexuality Patterns related to fear of death during coitus, secondary to myocardial infarction, p. 453

## MYOCARDIAL INFARCTION

### Description

**Myocardial infarction** is the term used to describe irreversible cellular loss and myocardial necrosis secondary to an abrupt decrease or total cessation of coronary blood flow to a specific area of the myocardium. Infarction is more prevalent in the left ventricle, and occlusions are most likely to cause myocardial necrosis when occurring in vessels that have not developed collateral flow. Infarction also occurs with more frequency in individuals with multivessel occlusions.

### Etiology

Atherosclerosis is responsible for the majority of myocardial infarctions because it causes luminal narrowing and reduced blood flow, resulting in decreased oxygen delivery to the myocardium. The three mechanisms that are primarily responsible for the reduction in oxygen delivery to the myocardium are (1) coronary artery thrombosis, (2) plaque fissure or hemorrhage, and (3) coronary artery spasm.

Coronary artery thrombi are now thought present in almost all acute occlusions. These thrombi, usually composed of platelets, fibrin, erythrocytes, and leukocytes, may be superimposed on a plaque or may align adjacent to a plaque. They release thromboxane A2, serotonin, and thrombin, all vasoconstricting substances that compound the vessel narrowing and set up a vicious cycle of recurrent occlusion.[38]

Scientists have not determined the cause of thrombus formation, but plaque fissure and/or hemorrhage are thought predisposing events.[13,23,45,69] Coronary artery thrombosis has been associated with rupture or cracks of the plaques and release of the plaque material into the vascular lumen. Plaque rupture can induce thrombosis by (1) forming a platelet plug, (2) releasing tissue thromboplastin from the plaque material activating the clotting cascade, and (3) obstructing the vessel lumen with plaque components.

The role of coronary artery spasm in partial or complete coronary artery occlusion remains a mystery. Direct evidence has shown vasospasm is present, but it is not known whether this results from hyperactive smooth muscle or whether it is a secondary response related to a plaque rupture and the release of vasoactive substances.

### Pathophysiology

**Coronary blood supply.** The coronary circulation consists of those vessels which supply the heart structures with oxygenated blood (coronary arteries) and then return the blood to the general circulation (Coronary veins). The right and left coronary arteries arise at the base of the aorta immediately after the aortic valve. After leaving the base of the aorta, the coronary arteries traverse along the outside of the heart in the natural grooves (sulci). To perfuse the thick heart muscle, branches from these main arteries arise at acute angles, penetrating the muscular wall and eventually feeding the endocardium.

The *right coronary artery* (RCA) serves the right atrium and the right ventricle in most people. In over half the population, it also is the usual blood supply for the SA and AV nodes. The *left coronary artery* (also referred to as the "widow maker," because occlusion of this main vessel usually results in immediate death) divides into two large arteries, the *left anterior descending* (LAD) and the *circum-*

**CHEST PAIN ASSESSMENT FACTORS**

- Onset (either sudden or gradual)
- Precipitating factors (did visitors come or leave; was the patient up moving around?)
- Location (was it substernal; was it located in same area as previous pain?)
- Radiation (did it radiate to the jaw, neck, arm, or shoulder?)
- Quality (was it similar to previous anginal pain; was it less or worse?)
- Intensity (on a scale of 1 to 10, where would the patient rate it?)
- Duration (did it last seconds or minutes; how soon after onset did the patient call for help?)
- Relieving factors (what made it better—changing position, nitroglycerin, oxygen, the presence of the nurse?)
- Aggravating factors (did the environment, telephone calls, waiting for help worsen the pain?)
- Associated symptoms (was the pain accompanied by nausea, vomiting, diaphoresis, or dyspnea?)
- Emotional response (how did the patient feel about the pain; was he or she anxious, fearful, angry?)

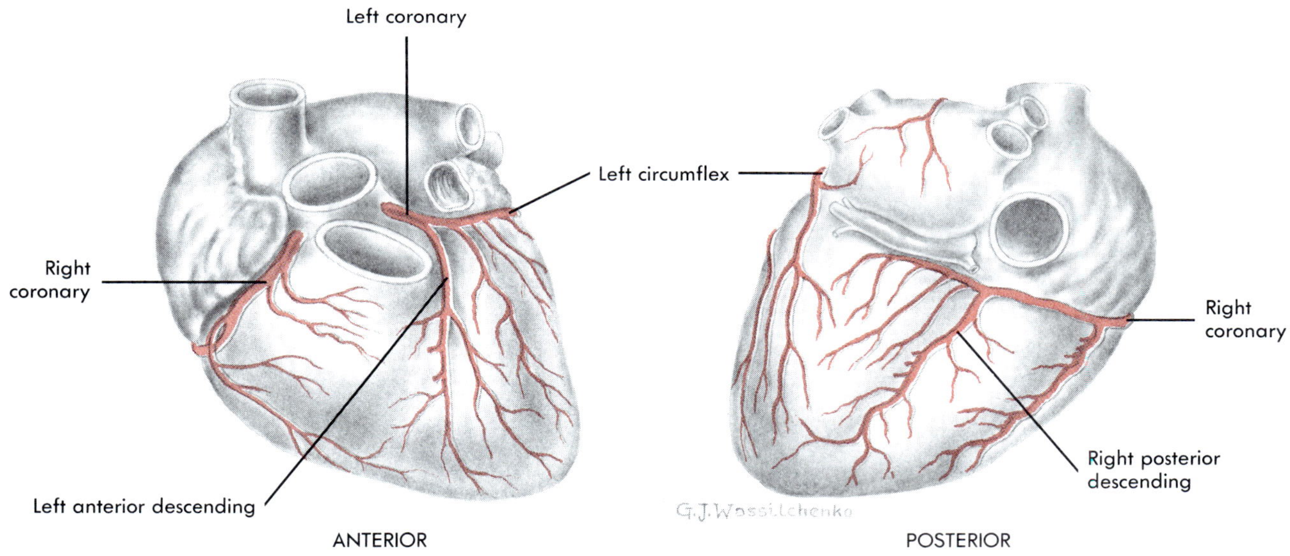


***Fig. 8-3*** Anterior and posterior views of the coronary artery circulation.

*flex*. These vessels serve the left atria and most of the left ventricle (Fig. 8-3). There is a huge spectrum of variation in the disposition of coronary arteries. The *dominant coronary artery* is that artery which traverses the posterior interventricular sulcus and supplies the posterior part of the ventricular septum and often part of the posterolateral wall of the left ventricle.[45]

After blood passes through the coronary capillaries, the majority of it is returned to the right atrium via the coronary veins, exiting via the coronary sinus. In addition, the *thebesian vessels* are small veins that connect capillary beds directly with the cardiac chambers and also communicate with cardiac veins and other thebesian veins. However, some of the blood returns directly to the chambers via vascular communications of irregular endothelium-lined sinuses within the muscular structure. These veins that drain into the left ventricle would therefore add unoxygenated blood to the freshly oxygenated blood.

Several clinical situations merit a brief discussion here. During ventricular contraction, there is no blood flow to the cardiac tissue. Coronary artery circulation is highest during early diastole, after the aortic valve has closed. During an episode of tachycardia, diastolic time is greatly diminished, hence coronary perfusion time is diminished. This offers a possible explanation for compromised coronary blood flow during times of rapid heart rate. Conversely, during bradycardia, there is prolonged diastole. However, coronary inflow may also be compromised as a result of the lack of adequate pressure and aortic recoil in late diastole to perfuse the myocardium.[45]

**Zones of infarction, ischemia, and injury.** The area of cellular death and muscle necrosis in the myocardium is known as the *zone of infarction* (Fig. 8-4). On the electrocardiogram evidence of this zone is seen by pathological Q or QS waves, which reflect a lack of depolarization from the cardiac surface involved in the myocardial infarction (Fig. 8-5, *D*). As healing takes place, the cells in this area are replaced by scar tissue.

The infarcted zone is surrounded by injured but still potentially viable tissue in an area known as the *zone of injury* (see Fig. 8-4). Cells in this area do not fully repolarize because of the deficient blood supply. This is recorded as elevation of the ST segment (Fig. 8-5, *C*).

The outer region, as illustrated in Figure 8-4, is the *zone of ischemia* and is composed of viable cells. Repolarization in this zone is impaired but is eventually restored to normal. Repolarization of the cells in this area is manifested as T wave inversion (Fig. 8-5, *B*). This region also is the apparent site of many of the dysrhythmias associated with an infarction because of the impaired repolarization.

During the first 6 weeks after an infarction, the myocardium itself undergoes many changes. Approximately 6 hours after the infarction, the muscle becomes distended, pale, and cyanotic. Over the next 2 days the myocardium becomes reddish purple, and an exudate may form on the epicardium. Leukocyte scavenger cells begin to infiltrate the muscle and carry away the necrotic debris, thereby thinning the necrotic wall. Approximately 3 to 4 weeks after the infarction, scar tissue begins to form, and the affected wall becomes whiter and thicker.[13]

***Classification of infarctions.*** Myocardial infarctions are frequently classified according to their location on the myocardial surface and the muscle layers affected. A *transmural infarction* involves all three muscle layers—the endocardium, the myocardium, and the epicardium (Fig. 8-6). Transmural infarctions, because they result in full-thickness necrosis, have a higher incidence of left-ventricular dysfunction.

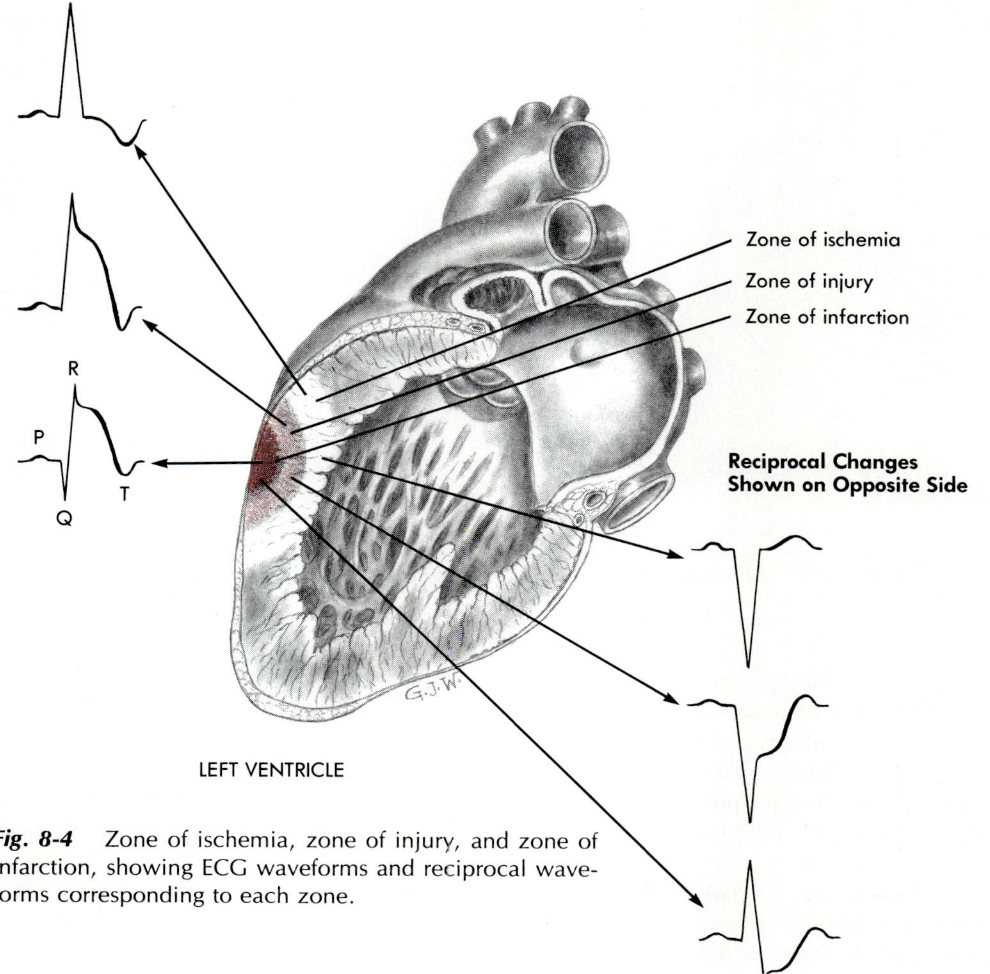


***Fig. 8-4*** Zone of ischemia, zone of injury, and zone of infarction, showing ECG waveforms and reciprocal waveforms corresponding to each zone.

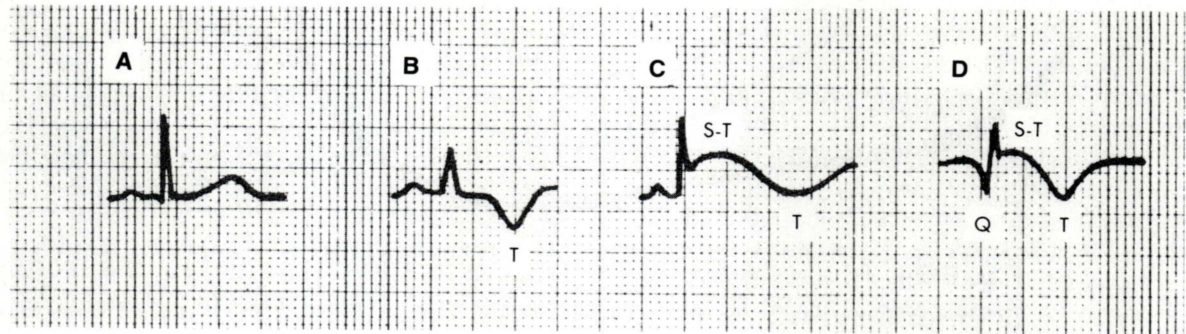


***Fig. 8-5*** ECG changes indicative of ischemia, injury, and infarction (necrosis) of the myocardium. **A,** Normal ECG. **B,** Ischemia indicated by inversion of the T wave. **C,** Ischemia and current of injury indicated by T wave inversion and ST segment elevation. The ST segment may be elevated above or depressed below the baseline, depending on whether the tracing is from a lead facing toward or away from the infarcted area and depending on whether epicardial or endocardial injury occurs. Epicardial injury causes ST elevation in leads facing the epicardium. **D,** Ischemia, injury and myocardial necrosis. The Q wave indicates necrosis of the myocardium. (From Kinney M and others: Comprehensive cardiac care: a text for nurses, physicians, and other health practitioners, ed 7, St Louis, 1991, Mosby–Year Book, Inc.)

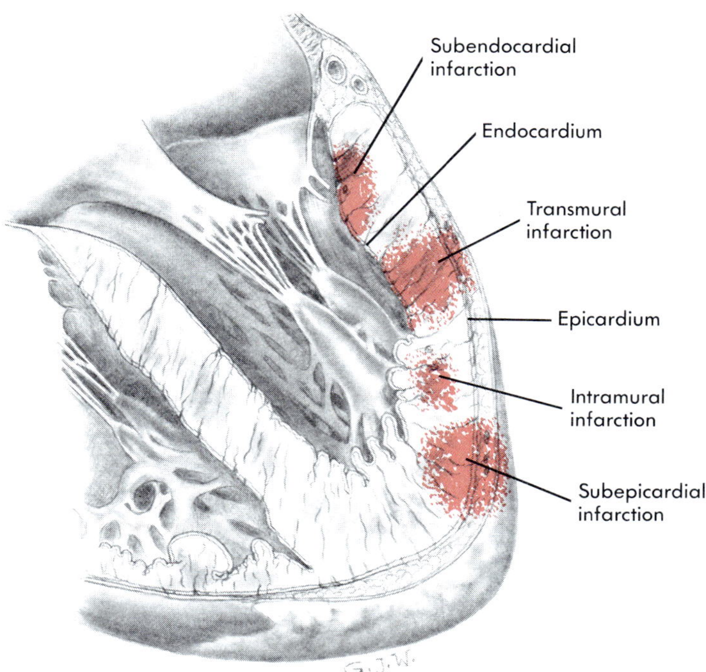


***Fig. 8-6*** Location of infarctions in the ventricular wall.

*Nontransmural infarctions* are classified as either subendocardial, involving the endocardium and the myocardium, or subepicardial, involving the myocardium and the epicardium (see Fig. 8-6). Because the endocardium has a much higher oxygen need than the epicardium, subendocardial infarctions are the more common of the nontransmural infarctions.

***Location of infarctions.*** The location and extent of a myocardial infarction is dependent on (1) the site and severity of coronary artery narrowing, (2) the presence, site, and severity of coronary artery spasm, (3) the size of the vascular bed perfused by compromised vessels, (4) the extent of collateral vessels, and (5) the oxygen needs of the poorly perfused myocardium.[45]

The location of infarction can be determined by correlating the electrocardiographic (ECG) leads with Q waves and the ST segment–T wave abnormalities. Infarction most commonly occurs in the left ventricle and the interventricular septum; however, close to 25% of all patients who sustain an inferior myocardial infarction have some right ventricular damage.[115] Although rare, atrial infarcts have also been reported.

When examining an ECG, it is essential that groups of leads, rather than one lead at a time, be evaluated. Correlating a group of leads that display ECG change with the area of the heart reflected by the leads allows (1) identification of the location of the infarction and (2) anticipation of potential electrical or mechanical complications. Remembering that the right coronary artery (RCA) perfuses the SA node, the proximal bundle of His, and the AV node and that an inferior wall infarction results from RCA occlusion will make one alert to the conduction disturbances that are possible with an inferior wall myocardial infarction. Changes in the leads overlooking the anterior wall will alert the observer to the possibility of mechanical problems or pump failure.

The three ECG manifestations used to diagnose infarction and to pinpoint the area of damaged ventricle are inverted T waves, indicative of myocardial ischemia; ST segment elevation, indicative of myocardial injury; and pathological Q waves, indicative of cell death or infarction. Location of ECG changes during myocardial infarction is summarized in Table 8-1, and timing of the ECG changes is listed in Table 8-2.

Because the anterior surface is so large, it is often subdivided into anteroseptal, true anterior, and anterior-lateral sections. *Anteroseptal infarctions* and *true anterior infarctions* (Fig. 8-7) usually result from occlusion of the left anterior descending (LAD) artery. *Anteriorlateral infarction* occurs as a result of occlusion of the circumflex coronary artery. *Inferior (diaphragmatic) infarctions* (Fig. 8-8) occur with occlusion of the right coronary artery. *Posterior infarctions* (Fig. 8-9) occur with occlusion of the circumflex branch of the left coronary artery. The location of an infarction may be very indicative of overall outcome. Anterior and anteroseptal infarctions, which result from occlusion of the LAD, are the least favorable types because of the serious left-ventricular dysfunction that results. Anterior wall infarctions are associated with twice the mortality of inferior wall infarctions.[16]

***Table 8-1*** Location of ECG changes during myocardial infarction

| Location of MI | Leads involved |
|---|---|
| Inferior | II, III, $aV_F$ |
| Lateral | I, $aV_L$ |
| Anterior | $V_2$-$V_4$ |
| Septal | $V_1$, $V_2$ |
| Apical | $V_5$, $V_6$ |
| Posterior | $V_1$, $V_2$ (reciprocal changes) |

***Table 8-2*** Timing of ECG changes during myocardial infarction

| Timing | Change |
|---|---|
| Immediate | ST segment elevation in leads over the area of infarction |
| Within a few hours | Giant upright T waves |
| Several hours to 2 weeks | ST segment normalizes; T waves invert symmetrically |
| Several hours to days; usually remain for life | Q waves or reduced R-wave voltage |

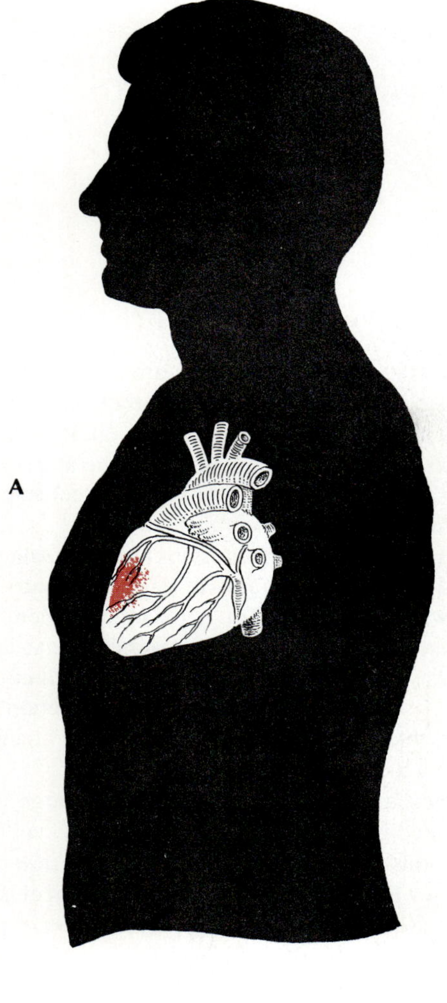


***Fig. 8-7*** **A,** Position of an anterior wall infarction. **B,** Anterior wall infarction. Note the QS complexes in leads $V_1$ and $V_2$, indicating anteroseptal infarction. There is also a characteristic notching (*arrow,* $V_2$) of the QS complex, often seen in infarctions. In addition, note the diffuse ischemic T wave inversions in leads $aV_L$ and $V_2$ to $V_5$, indicating generalized anterior wall ischemia. (**B** from Goldberger AL and Goldberger E: Clinical electrocardiography: a simplified approach, ed 4, St Louis, 1990, Mosby–Year Book, Inc.)

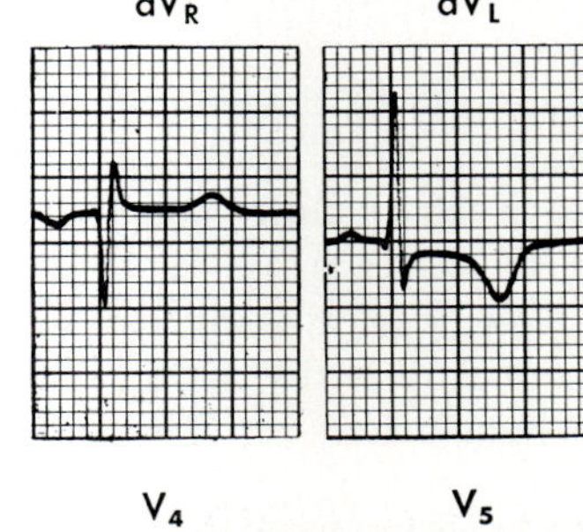


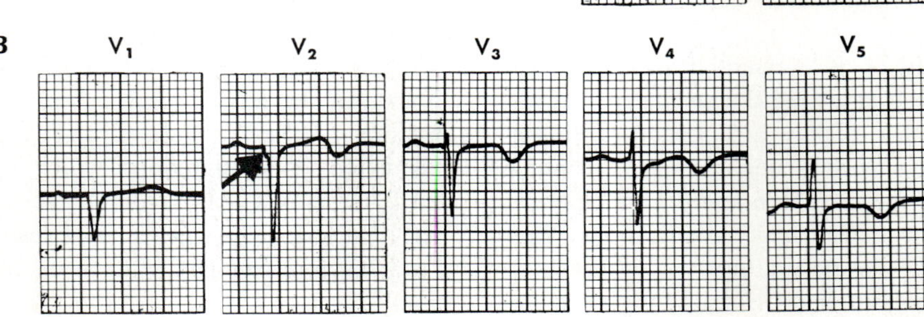

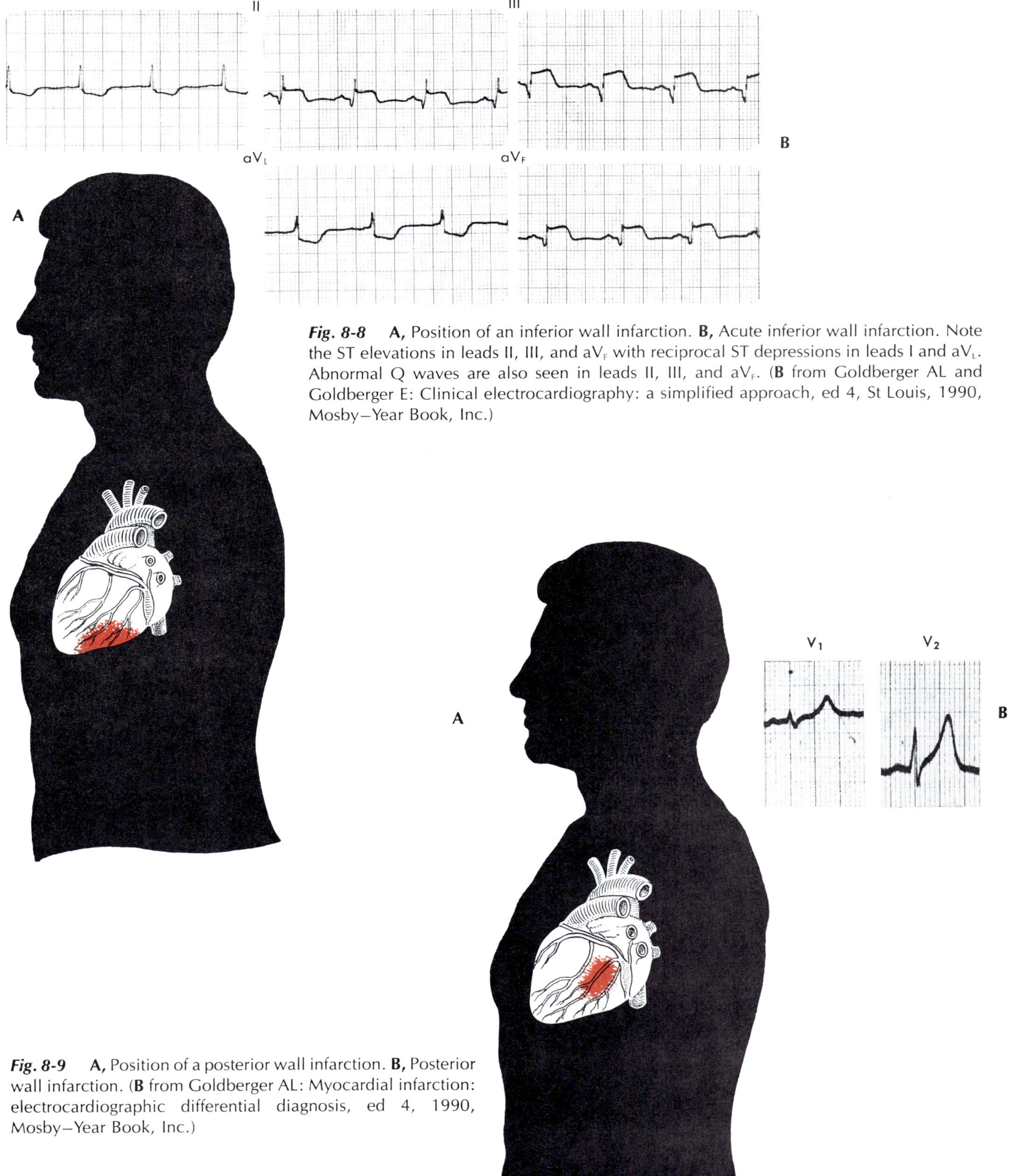


***Fig. 8-8*** **A,** Position of an inferior wall infarction. **B,** Acute inferior wall infarction. Note the ST elevations in leads II, III, and aV$_F$ with reciprocal ST depressions in leads I and aV$_L$. Abnormal Q waves are also seen in leads II, III, and aV$_F$. (**B** from Goldberger AL and Goldberger E: Clinical electrocardiography: a simplified approach, ed 4, St Louis, 1990, Mosby–Year Book, Inc.)

***Fig. 8-9*** **A,** Position of a posterior wall infarction. **B,** Posterior wall infarction. (**B** from Goldberger AL: Myocardial infarction: electrocardiographic differential diagnosis, ed 4, 1990, Mosby–Year Book, Inc.)

### Assessment and Diagnosis

The definitive diagnosis of myocardial infarction is based on the patient's clinical signs and symptoms, electrocardiographic changes discussed in the previous section, and enzyme levels.

**Clinical manifestations.** The most common clinical manifestation of infarction is prolonged severe chest pain, which is frequently associated with nausea, vomiting, and diaphoresis. This pain generally lasts 30 minutes or more and is usually located in the substernal or left precordial area. Unlike angina, which is often described as a discomfort, the pain of infarction may be described as the most severe pain the individual has ever experienced. Descriptors used are "a heaviness," "like an elephant sitting on my chest," or a "viselike tightness." The pain may radiate to the back, the neck, the jaw, or the left arm, particularly down its ulnar aspect. Neither rest nor nitrates relieve the pain. Other commonly occurring clinical manifestations of infarction may include tachycardia or bradycardia; tachypnea; diminished heart sounds, especially $S_1$; presence of $S_3$ and $S_4$; pulmonary crackles; restlessness; and anxiety.

**Enzyme manifestations.** A complete discussion of the relationship of enzymes to diagnosis of myocardial infarction was presented in Chapter 7. The reader is referred to that chapter for review.

### Complications of Myocardial Infarction

Unfortunately, many patients will have complications occurring either early or late in their postinfarction course (see the following box). These complications may result from pumping or electrical dysfunctions. Pumping complications include congestive heart failure (CHF), pulmonary edema, and cardiogenic shock. Electrical dysfunctions include bradycardia, bundle branch blocks, and varying degrees of heart block.[47,93]

**Dysrhythmias.** Close to 95% of all patients who experience a myocardial infarction will have dysrhythmias.[96] There are many potential causes such as those included in the box above, but ischemia of the pacemaker cells is the most common cause.

#### COMPLICATIONS OF MYOCARDIAL INFARCTION

Dysrhythmias
Ventricular aneurysms
Ventricular septal defect
Papillary muscle rupture
Pericarditis
Cardiac rupture
Sudden death
Congestive heart failure
Pulmonary edema
Cardiogenic shock

#### CAUSES OF DYSRHYTHMIAS IN MYOCARDIAL INFARCTION

Tissue ischemia
Hypoxemia
Autonomic nervous system influences
Metabolic derangements
  Acid-base imbalances
Hemodynamic abnormalities
Drugs (especially digoxin toxicity)
Electrolyte imbalances (e.g., hypokalemia)
Fiber stretch
  Chamber dilation
  Cardiomyopathy

*Sinus bradycardia* (heart rate $< 60$) occurs in approximately 40% of all patients who sustain an acute myocardial infarction and is more prevalent with an inferior wall infarction[105] and most frequently seen in the immediate postinfarction period.

*Sinus tachycardia* (heart rate $>100$) most often occurs with anterior wall myocardial infarctions. Tachycardia must be corrected, not only because it greatly increases myocardial oxygen consumption, but because it shortens diastolic filling time, thereby decreasing stroke volume, systemic perfusion, and coronary artery filling.

*Premature atrial contractions* (PACs) occur in almost one half of all patients who sustain acute infarction.[13] PACs are most commonly caused by cell irritability resulting from distention of the left atrium secondary to increased left-ventricular end diastolic pressure and volume.

*Atrial fibrillation* is a commonly seen atrial dysrhythmia associated with myocardial infarction and is more prevalent with an anterior wall infarction. It may occur spontaneously or be preceded by PACs or atrial flutter. With atrial fibrillation there is loss of atrial contraction, hence a loss of atrial kick and the extra stroke volume it carries, which may result in decreased cardiac output.

Within the first few hours after a myocardial infarction, almost all patients will have *premature ventricular contractions* (PVCs).[84] PVCs are usually controlled well by administering oxygen to reduce tissue hypoxia, correcting any acid-base imbalance, and administering intravenous lidocaine or other antidysrhythmic drugs.

PVCs and ventricular tachycardia occurring early (within the first few hours) in the postinfarction course are usually transient. However, when these same dysrhythmias occur late in the course, they tend to be associated with high hospital mortality, because they are usually related to the cumulative loss of myocardium.[84,115]

*AV heart block* most frequently follows an inferior wall myocardial infarction. Because the right coronary artery perfuses the AV node in 90% of the population, occlusion

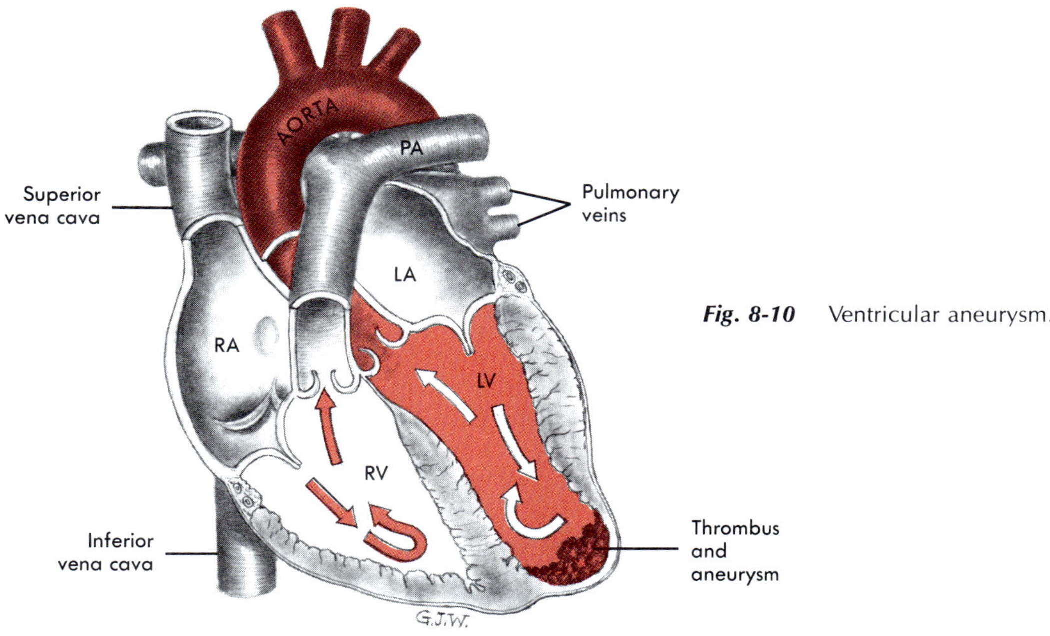


***Fig. 8-10*** Ventricular aneurysm.

of it leads to ischemia and infarction of the cells of the AV node.

The major goals of therapy for any dysrhythmia are treatment of the underlying cause and preservation of cardiac output and tissue perfusion. Medications must be used with caution, particularly those which increase the cardiac workload or depress myocardial function.

**Ventricular aneurysm.** A **ventricular aneurysm** (Fig. 8-10) is a noncontractile, thinned left-ventricular wall, which results in a reduction of the stroke volume. It occurs in approximately 12% to 15% of patients who survive acute transmural infarction.[93] A ventricular aneurysm most frequently occurs in the apical area and may develop within hours, or it may develop and enlarge over a period of weeks. The most common complications of a ventricular aneurysm are congestive heart failure, ventricular tachycardias, and embolism. Treatment is usually directed towards management of these complications.

The prognosis depends on the size of the aneurysm, overall left-ventricular function, and the severity of coexisting coronary artery disease. Rupture of the aneurysm is very rare and usually only occurs if there is reinfarction of the border of the aneurysm.

**Ventricular septal defect.** When rupture of the ventricular septal wall (Fig. 8-11) occurs, it usually does so within the first week after the infarction.[13] This complication affects approximately 1% to 3% of the patients who sustain acute infarctions and is the result of severe multivessel disease, with a lack of blood flow to the septum.[13] The rupture is often followed by congestive heart failure and shock, the seriousness of which is dependent on the size of the defect.

Rupture of the septum is manifested by severe chest pain, syncope, hypotension, and sudden hemodynamic deterioration caused by shunting of blood from the left ventricle into the right ventricle through the septal opening. A new holosystolic murmur (accompanied by a thrill) can be auscultated and is best heard along the left sternal border. A definitive diagnosis of a **ventricular septal defect** (VSD) can be made at the bedside by using the pulmonary artery catheter. Blood samples drawn from both the distal pul-

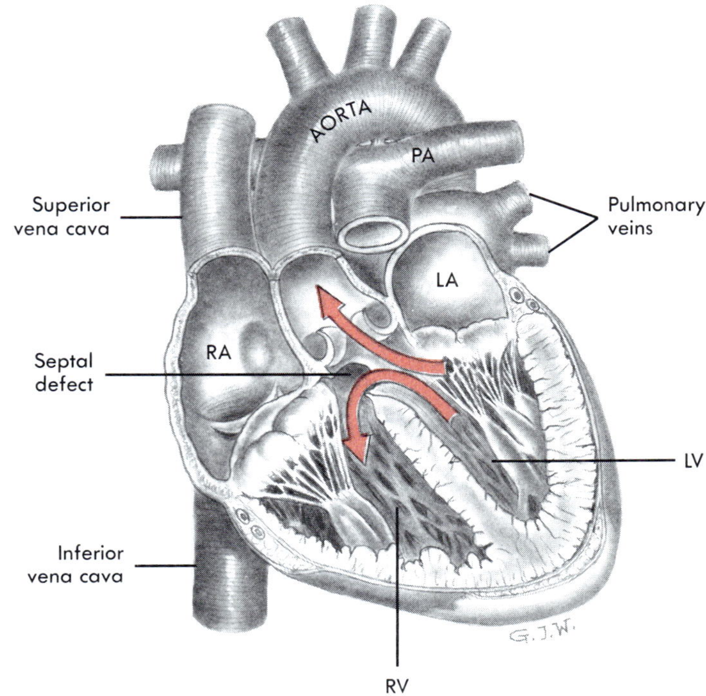


***Fig. 8-11*** Ventricular septal defect.

monary artery (PA) port and proximal central venous pressure (CVP) port will show an increase in oxygen saturation in the right ventricle (sampled from the CVP port) with a VSD. Normally, oxygen saturation in the right ventricle is 75%; with a VSD the saturation level will be increased to approximately 85%.

Since rupture of the septum is a medical and surgical emergency, patients must first be stabilized with vasodilators and an intraaortic balloon pump to decrease afterload and then have surgical closure of the defect. The surgical approach is usually through the left ventricle and frequently through the infarction itself. The septum is patched with a knitted Dacron velour patch lined, if possible, with pericardium to make it immediately leakproof.[59] If pericardium is not used, there may be residual shunting until platelets and fibrin agglutinate along the patch to seal it.

**Papillary muscle rupture. Papillary muscle rupture** can occur when the myocardial infarction involves the area around the mitral valve. Infarction of the papillary muscles results in their inability to effect a mitral valve seal; consequently, blood is forced through the weakened mitral valve back into the lower-pressured left atrium during ventricular systole.

The rupture may be partial or complete. Complete rupture is catastrophic and precipitates severe acute mitral regurgitation, shock, and death. Partial rupture (Fig. 8-12) will also result in mitral regurgitation, but usually the condition can be stabilized with the intraaortic balloon pump and vasodilators before surgery, during which a mitral valve replacement will take place.

**Pericarditis. Pericarditis** is inflammation of the pericardial sac that occurs after acute myocardial infarction when the damage extends into the epicardial surface of the heart (as in transmural infarction). The damaged epicardium then becomes rough and tends to irritate and inflame the pericardium lying adjacent to it, precipitating the development of pericarditis.

Pain is the most common symptom of pericarditis, whereas the presence of a pericardial friction rub is the most common sign and is considered a clinical hallmark. Although the friction rub may not be audible at all times, it is best heard at the sternal border during inhalation and is described as a grating, scraping, or leathery scratching. Friction rubs often change from one examination to the next, thus complicating documentation. However, pericardial pain is aggravated by deep ventilations, change of position, swallowing, and coughing. Aspirin, indomethacin, and the nonsteroidal antiinflammatory drugs, dexamethasone or methylprednisolone, are administered to treat the inflammation.

**Cardiac rupture.** Fifteen percent of deaths following myocardial infarction can be attributed to cardiac rupture,[93] which often occurs in older patients who have systemic hypertension during the acute phase of their infarctions. Rupture frequently occurs around the fifth postinfarction day when leukocyte scavenger cells are removing necrotic debris, thinning the myocardial wall.

The onset is usually sudden. Bleeding into the pericardial sac results in tamponade, cardiogenic shock, electromechanical dissociation, and death. Survival is rare, and emer-

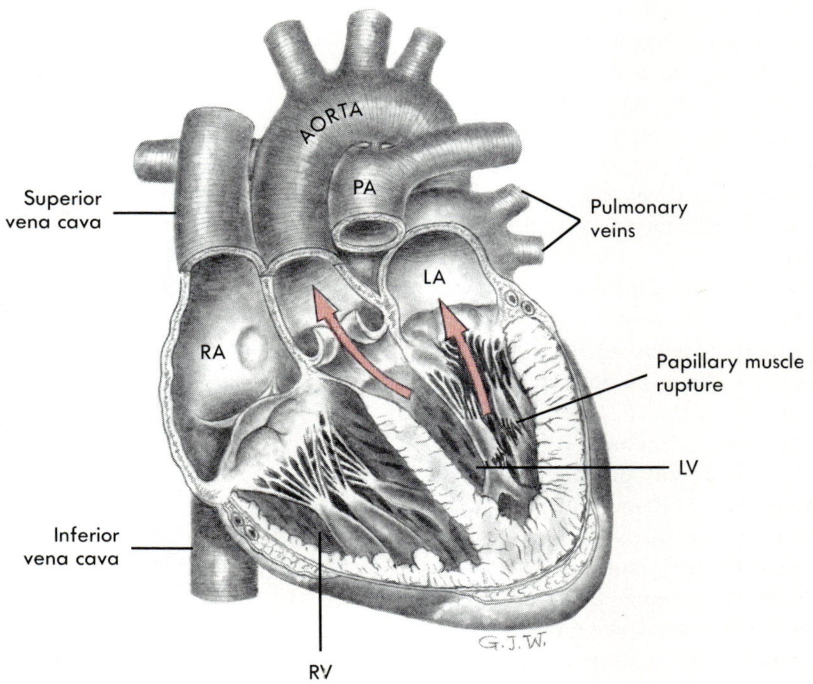


***Fig. 8-12*** Papillary muscle rupture.

gency pericardiocentesis is required to relieve the tamponade until a surgical repair can be attempted.

**Sudden death.** Death that occurs within 2 hours of onset of symptoms is classified as sudden. More than 1000 people per day in the United States are classified as having sudden death.[89] The majority are men aged 20 to 60 years. Many have had no prior symptoms of cardiac disease, although on autopsy nearly all have extensive multivessel coronary artery disease.[89]

The most common cause of sudden death is ventricular fibrillation. Precipitating factors include left-ventricular dysfunction, with an ejection fraction less than 30%, clinical diagnosis of congestive heart failure, and residual myocardial ischemia. Two major therapeutic goals for the prevention of sudden death are the identification and treatment of high-risk patients. Survivors are usually placed on antidysrhythmics and overdrive pacing or, in some cases, may have an internal defibrillator unit implanted.

### Treatment of Myocardial Infarction

The three principal goals of medical management for myocardial infarction are relief of pain, control of lethal dysrhythmias, and preservation of the myocardium.

The first 6 hours following the onset of chest pain constitute the crucial period for salvage of the myocardium. During this period it may be possible to achieve reperfusion of the infarcting myocardium with either intravenous or intracoronary thrombolysis, thrombolysis with percutaneous transluminal coronary angioplasty (PTCA), emergency PTCA, or emergency coronary artery bypass surgery (these therapies are discussed in Chapter 9).

Pain control is a priority since continued pain is a sign of ongoing ischemia, which places additional risk on noninfarcted myocardial tissue. Morphine remains the analgesic of choice, since it decreases anxiety, restlessness, autonomic nervous system activity, and preload, thereby decreasing myocardial oxygen demands.

Intravenous nitrates, beta-blocking agents, and calcium-channel antagonists may be instituted to reduce myocardial oxygen demand by decreasing both preload and afterload or by direct effect on the coronary circulation. Beta-blocking agents may reduce infarct size by decreasing sympathetic tone, thus decreasing afterload.

Oxygen is used for a minimum of 24 to 48 hours postinfarction to treat tissue hypoxia, which may be caused by left-ventricular failure. Because ventricular dysrhythmias are most prevalent in the early postinfarction period, the patient is monitored for heart rate and rhythm. Many times a pulmonary artery catheter is inserted, which allows correlation of chamber pressures to heart rate, blood pressure, urine output, and cardiac output. Stool softeners are used to decrease the risk of constipation from analgesics and bed rest and to decrease the risk of straining. For the first 24 hours the patient may be placed on a liquid or soft diet to decrease the risk of aspiration should cardiac arrest occur during this time.

Anticoagulants are sometimes used to decrease the incidence of embolic complications from deep-vein thrombosis and left-ventricular thrombi, especially while bed rest is prescribed for the patient. Antiplatelet agents may also be started to decrease release from platelets of thromboxane A2, which causes vasoconstriction and platelet aggregation. This therapy may be continued for an indefinite period of

#### Nursing Diagnosis and Management
***Myocardial infarction and complications***

- Acute Pain related to transmission and perception of noxious stimuli secondary to myocardial ischemia, p. 485
- Decreased Cardiac Output related to relative excess of preload and afterload secondary to impaired ventricular contractility, p. 457
- Decreased Cardiac Output related to supraventricular tachycardia, p. 456
- Decreased Cardiac Output related to ventricular tachycardia, p. 460
- Decreased Cardiac Output related to atrioventricular (AV) heart block, p. 458
- Activity Intolerance related to decreased cardiac output and/or myocardial tissue perfusion alterations, p. 464
- Sleep Pattern Disturbance related to fragmented sleep and/or circadian desynchronization, p. 455
- Sensory-Perceptual Alterations related to sensory overload, sensory deprivation, and sleep pattern disturbance, p. 489
- Anxiety related to threat to biological, psychological, and/or social integrity, p. 448
- Ineffective Individual Coping related to situational crisis and personal vulnerability, p. 447
- Powerlessness related to illness-related regimen, p. 445
- Altered Role Performance related to physical incapacity to resume usual or valued role, p. 444
- Body Image Disturbance related to actual change in body function, p. 443
- Sexual Dysfunction related to activity intolerance secondary to myocardial infarction, p. 450
- Altered Sexuality Patterns related to fear of death during coitus secondary to myocardial infarction, p. 453
- Altered Health Maintenance related to lack of perceived threat to health, p. 439
- Knowledge Deficit: Activity Restrictions, Fluid Restrictions, Medication, Reportable Symptoms related to lack of previous exposure to information, p. 441.

time since recent studies have documented the beneficial antiplatelet effect of prophylactic aspirin.[54]

Diagnostic studies that assess left-ventricular function (such as echocardiography and angiography) and studies that assess electrical function (such as 24-hour Holter monitoring and exercise stress testing) are all important in the decision-making process for risk assessment and both short-term and long-term management of the patient with acute myocardial infarction.

### Summary of Nursing Care

The focus of the plan of care for the patient with a myocardial infarction must include (1) the recognition and treatment of potentially life-threatening complications, (2) the manipulation of the critical care environment so that it is therapeutic, and (3) the identification of the psychosocial impact of the infarction on the patient. The box on p. 173 lists nursing diagnoses and management for the patient with myocardial infarction.

A considerable portion of time will be spent monitoring the patient for dysrhythmias and conduction defects and assessing vital signs for indications of shock, breath sounds for signs of pulmonary congestion, and heart sounds for abnormalities such as an $S_3$ or an $S_4$ or a murmur.

Medications must be administered as prescribed, followed by assessment for side effects or toxic responses. If the patient develops chest pain or dysrhythmias, it is important to record the onset in relation to the medication schedule. If dysrhythmias continue, it is important to assess for non-cardiac causes such as fever, anxiety, tissue hypoxia, position of the pulmonary wedge catheter, and acid-base or electrolyte disturbances.

During the time bed rest is prescribed for the patient, it is important that he or she is in an upright or semi-Fowler's position to foster better lung expansion, and to decrease venous return, lower preload, and decrease cardiac work.

The nurse needs to control the critical care unit's environment to decrease noise, diminish sensory overload, and allow adequate rest periods.

## CONGESTIVE HEART FAILURE

The most common cause of in-hospital mortality for patients with cardiac disease is **congestive heart failure** (CHF).[104] CHF is responsible for one third of the deaths of patients with an acute myocardial infarction. The heart failure rate is higher in men than in women for all age groups.

### Description

*Heart failure* is a pathophysiological state in which an abnormality of cardiac function is responsible for the failure of the heart to pump blood at a volume commensurate with venous return and/or with the requirements of the metabolizing tissues.[13,61,106] Impaired cardiac function results in failure to empty the venous system and reduces delivery of blood to the pulmonary and arterial circulation—hence, heart failure.

*Congestive heart failure* (CHF) is circulatory overload secondary to heart failure and fluid overload secondary to activation of compensatory mechanisms.[80] In this section all references to heart failure relate to CHF.

**Failure of right side of heart.** Failure of the right side of the heart is defined as ineffective right-ventricular contractile function. Pure failure of the right side of the heart may result from an acute condition such as a pulmonary embolus or a right-ventricular infarction, but it is most commonly caused by failure of the left side of the heart or the backing up of blood behind the left ventricle. Its common manifestations are weakness, peripheral or sacral edema, jugular venous distention, hepatomegaly, jaundice, liver tenderness, and elevated central venous pressure. If peripheral perfusion is greatly compromised, cyanosis may be present. Gastrointestinal symptoms include anorexia, nausea, and a feeling of fullness.[68]

**Failure of left side of heart.** Failure of the left side of the heart is defined as a disturbance of the contractile function of the left ventricle, resulting in pulmonary congestion and edema and/or decreased cardiac output. It most frequently occurs in patients with left-ventricular infarctions, hypertension, and aortic and/or mitral valve disease. Over a period of time with progression of the disease state, the fluid accumulation behind the dysfunctional left ventricle will produce dysfunction of the right ventricle, resulting in failure of the right side of the heart and its manifestations.

**Acute versus chronic heart failure.** Acute versus chronic failure refers to the rapidity with which the syndrome develops, the presence and activation of compensatory mechanisms, and the presence or absence of fluid accumulation in the interstitial space. Any condition that results in a sudden drop in cardiac output will also result in the manifestations of acute heart failure. Chronic failure results when more gradual ventricular dysfunction occurs, allowing the development of compensatory mechanisms such as ventricular hypertrophy; thus the manifestations of failure will not be sudden. Chronic failure may be abruptly exacerbated by the onset of dysrhythmias or by acute ischemia, causing the individual to display the manifestations of acute failure. In summary, acute heart failure has a sudden onset, with no compensatory mechanisms. Chronic failure has a progressive onset, with symptoms that may be suppressed by medication, diet, and low activity level. However, the chronic state can be exacerbated to acute failure by sudden illness or by cessation of medications.

**Low-ventricular versus high-ventricular output failure.** Low ventricular output failure is defined as a low-ventricular output state that can be caused by infarction, hypotension, cardiomyopathy, or hemorrhage. Classic signs and symptoms are those of decreased peripheral perfusion such as weak or diminished pulses; cool, pale extremities; and peripheral cyanosis. High-ventricular output failure occurs in conditions that increase the cardiac output such as thyrotoxicosis, anemia, and pregnancy. Peripherally, the pulse is strong, and the extremities are warm and pink.[13]

**PRECIPITATING CAUSES OF CHF**

Reduction or cessation of medication
Dysrhythmias
Systemic infection
Pulmonary embolism
Physical, environmental, and emotional stress
Pericarditis, myocarditis, and endocarditis
High-ventricular output states
Development of serious systemic illness
Administration of a cardiac depressant or salt-retaining drug
Development of a second form of heart disease

## Etiology

The elderly, men, the hypertensive, individuals with coronary artery disease, smokers, diabetics, and individuals with elevated cholesterol levels have been identified by the Framingham study as having high CHF risk profiles.[13,80,87,94,104] Many precipitating causes of CHF are listed in the box above.

## Pathophysiology

When the heart begins to fail and the cardiac output is no longer sufficient to meet the metabolic needs of the tissues, three major compensatory mechanisms are activated: the adrenergic system, the renin-angiotensin-aldosterone system, and the development of ventricular hypertrophy. These compensatory mechanisms maintain adequate perfusion pressure and enhance cardiac output by the manipulation of one or more of five factors: (1) heart rate, (2) stroke volume, (3) preload, (4) contractility, and (5) afterload.

The adrenergic compensatory mechanism is a result of increased sympathetic activity, which stimulates the release of catecholamines and increases the levels of circulating catecholamines, especially epinephrine.[31,33] The increase in circulating catecholamines results in peripheral vasoconstriction, which leads to shunting of blood from nonvital organs such as the kidneys and skin to vital organs such as the heart and brain.[31,33] This, in turn, increases venous return, which increases preload.

Activation of the renin-angiotensin-aldosterone system results in constriction of the renal arterioles, decreasing the glomerular filtration rate and increasing the reabsorption of sodium from the proximal and distal tubules, which promotes fluid retention. Severe heart failure will increase the antidiuretic hormone level, enhancing the retention of water.

The final compensatory mechanism is the increase in ventricular wall thickness known as ventricular hypertrophy. Myocardial hypertrophy increases the force of contraction. Therefore hypertrophy helps the ventricle overcome an increase in afterload.

In summary, the compensatory mechanisms may sustain cardiac function, especially at rest, but over a period of time may worsen the degree of failure as the retention of sodium and water leads to overdistention of the ventricles and a consequent decrease in the force of ventricular contraction. Tachycardia may eventually become a negative factor because it increases myocardial oxygen demand while shortening coronary artery perfusion. This imbalance can lead to myocardial ischemia, which may decrease ventricular contraction, reduce ventricular filling, and necessitate a higher filling pressure.

## Assessment and Diagnosis

The clinical manifestations of CHF result from tissue hypoperfusion and organ congestion.[116] Symptoms can be cardiac or noncardiac in origin. Signs and symptoms are frequently described according to the form of failure. Failure of the right side of the heart manifests as systemic venous congestion and peripheral edema, whereas failure of the left side results in pulmonary venous congestion and pulmonary edema (Table 8-3).

The severity of signs and symptoms progresses as heart failure worsens. Initially signs and symptoms appear only with exertion, but eventually occur at rest.

Dyspnea, which is labored breathing and is frequently described by patients as shortness of breath, results from pulmonary vascular congestion and decreased lung compliance. Dyspnea may then progress to orthopnea (difficulty breathing when supine) because of an increase in venous return (preload) that occurs in the supine position. Paroxysmal nocturnal dyspnea is a severe form of orthopnea in which the patient awakens from sleep gasping for air. Other respiratory symptoms include cardiac asthma (dyspnea with wheezing), a nonproductive cough, and pulmonary crackles progressing to the gurgling sounds of pulmonary edema.

**Pulmonary edema. Pulmonary edema** (Fig. 8-13) inhibits gas exchange by impairing the diffusion pathway between the alveolus and the capillary. Pulmonary edema is caused by increased left-atrial and left-ventricular pressure and results in an excessive accumulation of serous or serosanguineous fluid in the interstitial spaces and alveoli of the lungs. The most common causes are left-ventricular failure resulting from acute myocardial infarction, acute myocardial ischemia, tight mitral stenosis, or rupture of chordae tendineae and severe aortic regurgitation or aortic stenosis.[38]

With acute onset, patients are often extremely breathless and anxious. They expectorate pink, frothy liquid, causing them to feel as if they are drowning. They may sit bolt upright, gasp for breath, or thrash about. The respiratory rate is elevated, and the use of accessory muscles of ventilation becomes apparent by observation of nasal flaring and bulging neck muscles. Respirations are characterized by loud inspiratory and expiratory gurgling sounds. Diaphoresis is profuse, and the skin is usually cold, ashen, and cyanotic, reflecting low cardiac output, increased sympa-

***Table 8-3*** Signs and symptoms of failure of right and left sides of heart

| Left-ventricular failure | | Right-ventricular failure | |
|---|---|---|---|
| **Signs** | **Symptoms** | **Signs** | **Symptoms** |
| Tachypnea | Fatigue | Peripheral edema | Weakness |
| Tachycardia | Dyspnea | Hepatomegaly | Anorexia |
| Cough | Orthopnea | Splenomegaly | Indigestion |
| Bibasilar crackles | Paroxysmal noctural dyspnea | Hepatojugular reflux | Weight gain |
| Gallop rhythms ($S_3$ and $S_4$) | Nocturia | Ascites | Mental changes |
| Increased pulmonary artery pressures | | Jugular venous distention | |
| Hemoptysis | | Increased central venous pressure | |
| Cyanosis | | Pulmonary hypertension | |
| Pulmonary edema | | | |

thetic stimulation, peripheral vasoconstriction, and desaturation of arterial blood.

Arterial blood gas values may be variable. In the early stage of pulmonary edema, respiratory alkalosis may be present because of hyperventilation. However, as the pulmonary edema progresses and as gas exchange becomes impaired, respiratory acidosis and hypoxemia will ensue. Laboratory studies may also document elevated liver function, bilirubin, liver enzymes, serum glutamic-oxaloacetic transaminase (SGOT), and serum glutamic-pyruvic transaminase (SGPT). Elevated blood urea nitrogen (BUN) and creatinine levels reflect renal hypoperfusion. Urine output will be low, and urine will be concentrated, with low urine sodium and high urine osmolarity levels because of dilutional hyponatremia. The serum potassium level may vary, depending on the overall state of renal function and aggressiveness of diuresis.

The chest radiograph usually confirms an enlarged cardiac silhouette, pulmonary venous congestion, and interstitial edema. The interstitial edema markings or chest radiograph are frequently referred to as Kerley-B lines.[119]

## Treatment

The goals of management of heart failure are threefold: (1) to identify and correct precipitating causes, (2) to relieve symptoms, and (3) to enhance cardiac performance.

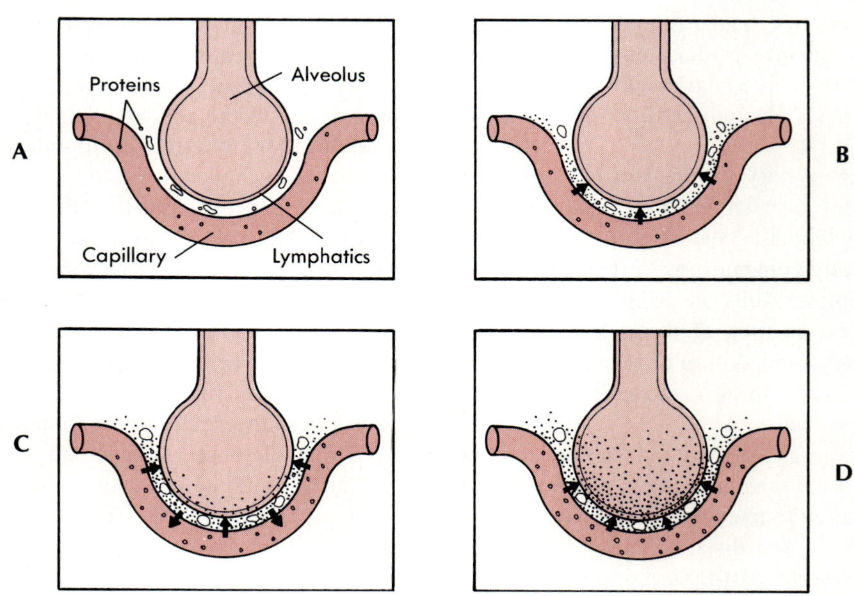


***Fig. 8-13*** As pulmonary edema progresses, it inhibits oxygen and carbon dioxide exchange at the alveolar capillary interface. **A,** Normal relationship. **B,** Increased pulmonary capillary hydrostatic pressure causes fluid to move from the vascular space into the pulmonary interstitial space. **C,** Lymphatic flow increases in an attempt to pull fluid back into the vascular or lymphatic space. **D,** Failure of lymphatic flow and worsening of left heart failure results in further movement of fluid into the interstitial space and into the alveoli.

In the acute phase the patient will usually have a pulmonary artery catheter in place so that left-ventricular function can be followed closely. Diuretics are administered to decrease preload. The intraaortic balloon pump and vasodilators such as sodium nitroprusside and intravenous nitroglycerin may be required to decrease afterload. Digitalis and positive inotropic agents such as dopamine or dobutamine may be administered to increase ventricular contractility. If the patient develops pulmonary edema, morphine and diuretics will be used to remove excess fluid, to facilitate peripheral dilation, and to decrease anxiety.

Hemodialysis or continuous arterial-venous hemofiltration with or without dialysis may be required to control sodium and water retention.

### Summary of Nursing Care

The focus of the plan of care for a patient with CHF must include interventions that will decrease cardiac work, optimize cardiac function, and promote emotional and physical rest. Refer to boxes on this page.

#### Nursing Diagnosis and Management

***Acute congestive heart failure and pulmonary edema***

- Impaired Gas Exchange related to ventilation-perfusion inequality secondary to pulmonary vascular congestion, p. 474
- Decreased Cardiac Output related to relative excess of preload and afterload secondary to impaired ventricular contractility, p. 457
- Activity Intolerance related to decreased cardiac output, p. 464
- High Risk for Impaired Skin Integrity risk factors: reduced mobility, poor subcutaneous tissue support (peripheral and sacral edema), p. 499
- High Risk for Infection risk factors: invasive monitoring devices, p. 465
- Sensory-Perceptual Alterations related to sensory overload, sensory deprivation, and sleep pattern disturbance, p. 489
- Anxiety related to threat to biological, psychological, and/or social integrity, p. 448
- Ineffective Individual Coping related to situational crisis and personal vulnerability, p. 447
- Sleep Pattern Disturbance related to circadian desynchronization, p. 455
- Knowledge Deficit: Medications, Fluid Restrictions, Activity Restrictions, Diet, Reportable Symptoms related to lack of previous exposure to information, p. 441

During periods of breathlessness, activity must be restricted; bed rest is usually prescribed for the patient, who is positioned with the head of the bed elevated to allow maximal lung expansion. The legs may be placed in a dependent position to encourage venous pooling, thereby decreasing venous return.

Breath sounds should be auscultated frequently to determine adequacy of respiratory effort and to assess for onset or worsening of congestion, and oxygen is administered to relieve dyspnea. If the patient is not hypotensive, morphine may be administered to decrease hyperventilation and anxiety. If the patient's ventilatory status worsens, the nurse must be prepared for endotracheal intubation and mechanical ventilation.

Patients in CHF require aggressive pharmacological therapy, and the patient's hemodynamic response to these agents, as well as to diuretic therapy and fluid restrictions, must be closely monitored.

The ECG must be evaluated for any dysrhythmias that may be present or may develop as a result of drug toxicity or electrolyte imbalance. Patients in heart failure are prone to digoxin toxicity secondary to decreased renal perfusion, as well as to electrolyte (most frequently, sodium and potassium) imbalances.

#### Nursing Diagnosis and Management

***Chronic congestive heart failure***

- Impaired Gas Exchange related to ventilation-perfusion inequality secondary to pulmonary vascular congestion, p. 474
- Decreased Cardiac Output related to relative excess of preload and afterload secondary to impaired ventricular contractility, p. 457
- Activity Intolerance related to decreased cardiac output, p. 464
- Activity Intolerance related to postural hypotension secondary to prolonged immobility, vasodilator therapy, p. 463
- High Risk for Impaired Skin Integrity risk factors: reduced mobility, poor subcutaneous tissue support (peripheral and sacral edema), p. 499
- Anxiety related to threat to biological, psychological, and/or social integrity, p. 448
- Sleep Pattern Disturbance related to fragmented sleep secondary to paroxysmal nocturnal dyspnea, p. 455
- Noncompliance: Medications, Fluid Restrictions, Activity Restrictions, Diet related to knowledge deficit and/or lack of resources, p. 440
- Altered Health Maintenance related to lack of perceived threat to health, p. 439

The patient in heart failure may be prone to skin breakdown resulting from immobility, bed rest, inadequate nutrition, edema, and decreased perfusion to the skin and subcutaneous tissue. Frequent position changes and padding of dependent areas and bony prominences may be helpful. Patients in failure frequently experience decreased appetite; therefore small, frequent meals may be more appropriate than the standard three large meals.

Another major nursing function is to maintain an environment that fosters physical and emotional rest. The nurse needs to assess the patient's understanding of conservation of energy in planning activities and to collaborate with the patient in organizing the day's schedule. Rest periods must be carefully planned and adhered to, while independence within the patient's activity prescription is fostered.

## CARDIOGENIC SHOCK

### Description

Whenever there is loss of more than 40% of functional myocardium, a clinical syndrome manifested by decreased perfusion, hypotension, decreased or absent urine output, obtundation, sweating, pallor, and tachycardia occurs. Close to 20% of patients sustaining an anterior myocardial infarction will develop this syndrome—**cardiogenic shock.**[41,52]

### Etiology

The most common cause of cardiogenic shock is extensive left-ventricular dysfunction resulting from an acute myocardial infarction with or without associated complications. Examples of complications that may result in cardiogenic shock include papillary muscle rupture, left-ventricular free wall rupture, acute ventricular septal defect (VSD), end stage cardiomyopathy, severe valvular dysfunction, myocardial contusion, cardiac tamponade, left-atrial myxoma, and thrombus and/or a massive pulmonary embolus.

### Stages of Cardiogenic Shock

Four stages of cardiogenic shock have been identified (Table 8-4). The first, the initial stage, is identified when the cardiac output begins to decrease in the absence of clinical symptoms. The second stage, the compensatory stage, is a period wherein the cardiac output is decreased and early clinical signs and symptoms are evident. Stage III is the progressive stage. If the shock state is not reversed by this time, the compensatory mechanisms become debil-

***Table 8-4*** Stages of shock

| Stage | Definition | Signs and symptoms |
|---|---|---|
| Initial | Cardiac output decreased in absence of symptoms | Decreased cardiac output |
| Compensatory | Attempt by body's compensatory mechanisms, mediated by the sympathetic nervous system, to increase cardiac output | Sinus tachycardia<br>Elevated pulmonary artery wedge pressure readings; PAW >18-20 mm Hg<br>Cool palm, clammy skin<br>Decreased urinary output, usually <20 ml/hr<br>Decreased urinary sodium; increased urinary osmolarity<br>Rapid, deep ventilations; respiratory alkalosis<br>Altered level of consciousness<br>Decreased bowel sounds<br>Hyperglycemia<br>Hypernatemia |
| Progressive | Compensatory mechanisms no longer helpful but now perpetuate shock cycle | Severe peripheral vasoconstriction<br>Decreased oxygen delivery to cells<br>Anaerobic metabolism<br>Metabolic acidosis<br>Sinus tachycardia, weak pulse<br>Chest pain, palpitations<br>Nausea, vomiting, anorexia<br>Rapid, shallow ventilations<br>Elevated pulmonary artery pressure readings |
| Refractory | Irreversible stage; signs and symptoms not changed by therapy | Cardiac failure (severely decreased cardiac output)<br>Elevated pulmonary artery pressure readings<br>Acidosis<br>Alterations in blood clotting<br>Inadequate cerebral perfusion<br>Cardiac and respiratory arrest<br>Death |

**CLINICAL MANIFESTATIONS OF CARDIOGENIC SHOCK**

**HEMODYNAMICS**

- Systolic blood pressure >90 mm Hg (in a previously hypertensive patient, there will be a 30-60 mm Hg decrease)
- Tachycardia
- Elevated PA pressures

**RENAL**

- Progressive oliguria unresponsive to diuretics

**RESPIRATORY**

- Rapid, shallow respirations
- Crackles and rhonchi on auscultation

**GASTROINTESTINAL**

- Decreased to absent bowel sounds

**NEUROLOGICAL**

- Moderate to severe obtundation

**SKIN**

- Cool, pale, diaphoretic
- Mottled and cyanotic in later stages

**HEMATOLOGICAL**

- Abnormalaties in clotting

itating. Stage IV is the refractory stage. At this point the shock state is irreversible to any form of therapy.

### Assessment and Diagnosis

Cardiogenic shock is a multisystem disease. The cardiac injury tends to be progressive and interrelated so that decreasing function adversely affects the other body systems.[8] Clinical manifestations depend on the severity of the shock state and the patient's underlying medical status. Furthermore, some clinical manifestations are related to decreased tissue perfusion and/or to the effect of the compensatory mechanisms. Clinical manifestations are listed in the box above.

### Treatment

Therapies are directed toward reducing infarct size, improving coronary and systemic perfusion, decreasing myocardial oxygen consumption, controlling heart rate, and increasing ventricular contractility. These goals may be accomplished by using venovasodilators to decrease preload and arterial vasodilators to decrease afterload. The intraaortic balloon pump is used for afterload reduction, whereas positive inotropic agents are used to increase ventricular contractility. Care must be taken to maintain an adequate perfusion pressure when using vasodilators. Inotropic agents must be used cautiously so that myocardial $\dot{V}O_2$ is not increased excessively. Pulmonary artery wedge pressures (PAWPs) or pulmonary artery diastolic pressures (PADPs) should be used to guide the administration of pharmacological agents.

Oxygenation must be supported to keep the $PaO_2$ above 80 mm Hg. If ventilatory failure ensures (arterial partial pressure of carbon dioxide [$PaCO_2$] above 50 mm Hg in a previously normocapnic patient), endotracheal intubation and mechanical ventilation will be necessary.

### Summary of Nursing Care

The focus of nursing care for the patient in cardiogenic shock is the continuous assessment of tissue and organ perfusion.

Patients experiencing cardiogenic shock will have an arterial line, pulmonary artery catheter, urinary drainage catheter, and, frequently, an intraaortic balloon pump. Oxygen is administered, and arterial blood gas values are closely monitored. Respiratory assessment for pulmonary congestion is performed hourly or more often to assess the need for ventilatory support. Patients in cardiogenic shock are sometimes confused and restless. Safety precautions must be taken to protect them, as well as to maintain the security of invasive catheters and tubes.

It is important to maintain the patient in a positive nitrogen balance; most often, this is accomplished with hyperalimentation or tube feedings. If the patient is receiving parenteral intake, bowel sounds must be auscultated every shift because shock may precipitate intestinal ischemia. Care must also be taken to see that the patient does not aspirate.

The skin integrity of patients in shock may be compromised secondary to their low perfusion state, and interventions must be directed toward maintenance of skin integrity. A list of nursing diagnoses related to cardiogenic shock is found in the box on p. 180.

## HYPOVOLEMIC SHOCK

### Description

**Hypovolemic shock** is the most commonly occurring of the shock states. It results from reduction of the circulating blood volume, leading to an inability of the circulation to meet the body's metabolic needs.

### Etiology

Hypovolemic shock may result from either direct or indirect volume loss. Direct volume losses result from hemorrhage, severe diarrhea and/or vomiting, massive diuresis, and loss of plasma from skin lesions or burns.[74]

Indirect volume loss frequently results from sequestering of fluids into another body space because of an alteration in capillary permeability or a fall in colloidal osmotic pressure. Indirect loss frequently occurs with cirrhosis, hemorrhagic pancreatitis, long-bone fracture, severe sodium depletion, ruptured spleen, addisonian crisis, or hypopituitarism.

**Nursing Diagnosis and Management**

***Cardiogenic shock***

- Decreased Cardiac Output related to relative excess of preload and afterload secondary to impaired ventricular contractility, p. 457
- High Risk for Altered Peripheral Tissue Perfusion risk factor: vasopressor therapy, p. 462
- High Risk for Infection risk factor: invasive monitoring devices, p. 465
- High Risk for Aspiration risk factors: endotracheal tube, situation hindering elevation of upper body, reduced level of consciousness, p. 476
- Ineffective Airway Clearance related to impaired cough secondary to loss of glottic closure with cuffed endotracheal tube, p. 468
- Sleep Pattern Disturbance related to circadian desynchronization, p. 455
- Sensory-Perceptual Alterations related to sensory overload, sensory deprivation, sleep pattern disturbance, p. 489
- Body Image Disturbance related to functional dependence on life-sustaining technology, p. 443
- Anxiety related to biological, psychological, and/or social integrity, p. 448

### Pathophysiology

The loss of intravascular volume leads to decreased venous return (preload), decreased cardiac filling pressures, decreased stroke volume, decreased cardiac output, and ultimately, decreased tissue perfusion. Once this spiral begins and the body's compensatory mechanisms, mediated by the sympathetic nervous system, are activated, vasoconstriction occurs, the renin-aldosterone system is activated, and antidiuretic hormone is secreted.

Hypovolemic shock may be classified as mild, moderate, or severe, depending on the estimated fluid loss.[8]

### Assessment and Diagnosis

The clinical manifestations of shock depend on the severity of fluid loss. Mild shock is defined as a volume loss of approximately 10% to 25% or 500 to 1200 ml of fluid. In this stage the patient may be hypotensive and slightly tachycardic.

Moderate hypovolemic shock results from a fluid loss of approximately 25% to 35% or 1200 to 1800 ml of fluid. At this time a marked decrease in blood pressure and cardiac output follow. Clinical manifestations include severe arterial vasoconstriction; diminished blood flow to the kidneys, gastrointestinal tract, and liver; development of a rapid, thready pulse; diaphoresis; decreased urine output; and increasing anxiety and restlessness.

A fluid loss of 35% to 50% or 1800 to 2500 ml results in severe shock causing the patient to be severely hypotensive, with marked peripheral vasoconstriction, marked diaphoresis, obtundation, and anuria.

### Treatment

The major goal of therapy is to restore and maintain tissue perfusion and to correct the underlying physiological abnormality. This is accomplished by replacing intravascular volume with either a crystalloid (for example, Ringer's lactate or other balanced electrolyte solution) or a colloid (that is, blood or blood components) solution or a combination of both. Initially, the lost volume is replaced quickly through one to three large peripheral intravenous catheters until the shock state is corrected or there is evidence of fluid overload. Autotransfusion, the collection and administration of the patient's own blood, may be used for trauma injuries. A Pneumatic Anti-Shock Garment (PASG) may also be used for a patient in profound shock as a means of increasing venous return, and vasopressors may be used to maintain perfusion pressure as the fluid resuscitation continues.

### Summary of Nursing Care

The focus of nursing care for the patient in hypovolemic shock is to assess overall perfusion status, administer fluids as ordered, assess pulmonary and renal status, and observe for signs or symptoms of fluid overload (see the box below).

**Nursing Diagnosis and Management**

***Hypovolemic shock***

- Fluid Volume Deficit related to active blood loss, p. 495
- High Risk for Altered Peripheral Tissue Perfusion risk factor: vasopressor therapy, p. 462
- High Risk for Infection risk factor: invasive monitoring devices, p. 465
- High Risk for Aspiration risk factors: endotracheal tube, situation hindering elevation of upper body, reduced level of consciousness, p. 476
- Ineffective Airway Clearance related to impaired cough secondary to loss of glottic closure with cuffed endotracheal tube, p. 468
- Sleep Pattern Disturbance related to circadian desynchronization, p. 455
- Sensory-Perceptual Alterations related to sensory overload, sensory deprivation, sleep pattern disturbance, p. 489

Patients in shock may have pulmonary artery catheters, central venous catheters, and/or arterial lines in place, depending on the severity and the cause of the shock and their preshock medical history. The patient in shock requires frequent documentation of hemodynamic response to therapy and assessment of renal status, pulmonary function, and mentation.

Patients are positioned with their legs elevated, trunk flat, and head and shoulders elevated higher than the chest to increase venous return.[74]

## HYPERTENSIVE CRISIS

### Description/Etiology

**Hypertensive crisis** represents a clinical situation in which hypertension is associated with irreversible vital organ damage or a threat to life over a short period of time. The critical factor in hypertensive crisis is the accelerated rise of the blood pressure, which results in complications occurring over a period of hours or days rather than days to weeks.[73] A diastolic pressure greater than 130 mm Hg is usually labeled as severe hypertension.

The overall incidence of hypertensive crisis is less than 1% of known hypertensives. It is usually precipitated by the conditions listed in the box below, left.

### Pathophysiology

The exact mechanism of hypertensive crisis is not known, but it is characterized by fibrinoid necrosis of the arterioles.

### Assessment and Diagnosis

Hypertensive crisis is manifested by CNS compromise (headache, papilledema, coma), cardiovascular compromise (angina, myocardial infarction), acute renal failure, and a history consistent with catecholamine excess.

### Treatment

Hypertensive crisis necessitates admitting the patient to a critical care unit where antihypertensive therapy can be administered parenterally and blood pressure monitored continuously using an arterial line. Frequently used medications include furosemide, sodium nitroprusside, diazoxide, trimethaphan camsylate, and labetalol.

Clonidine administered in hourly doses of 0.1 to 0.2 mg lowers severe hypertension. Other parenteral drugs that apparently are effective during crisis are guanabenz, minoxidil, oral nifedipine, and captopril. A loop diuretic and beta blocker are usually used concurrently to prevent reflex tachycardia and fluid retention, both of which may increase the blood pressure.[62,73]

### Summary of Nursing Care

The focus of nursing care for the patient with hypertensive crisis is to return the blood pressure to the desired range and then to identify the factors that resulted in this life-threatening condition (see the box at left).

During the acute phase the patient must be closely observed for signs and symptoms of cardiac or neurological compromise such as cardiovascular collapse, ischemia, dysrhythmias, mental confusion, stupor, seizures, or coma.

Antihypertensives should be administered as ordered and the blood pressure closely monitored. If potent vasodilators such as nitroprusside are being used, they should be infused

#### CONDITIONS PRECIPITATING HYPERTENSIVE CRISIS

**CARDIOVASCULAR COMPROMISE**

- Unstable angina
- Myocardial infarction
- Aortic dissection
- Severe hypertension
- Pheochromocytoma (very rare)
- Aortic aneursmectomy
- Carotid endarterectomy
- Coronary artery bypass grafting

**CENTRAL NERVOUS SYSTEM COMPROMISE**

- Increased intracranial pressure
- Malignant hypertension (any cause)
- Hypertensive encephalopathy (any cause)
- Cerebrovascular accident
- Brain tumor
- Brain trauma
- Eclampsia

**ACUTE RENAL FAILURE**

- Malignant hypertension
- Vasculitis
- Scleroderma
- Glomerulonephritis

**HISTORY CONSISTENT WITH CATECHOLAMINE EXCESS**

- Pheochromocytoma
- MAOI in combination with certain drugs and foods
- Clonidine and guanabenz withdrawal

From McRae RP and Liebson PR: Med Clin North Am 70(4):749, 1986.

#### Nursing Diagnosis and Management
*Hypertensive crisis*

- Anxiety related to threat to biological, psychological, and/or social integrity, p. 448
- Altered Cerebral Tissue Perfusion related to increased intracranial pressure secondary to hemorrhage, p. 480

through an infusion pump, and an arterial line should be placed in the patient.

While obtaining the health history, the nurse needs to identify risk factors and also clarify any misconceptions the patient may have regarding hypertension and its treatment.

## CARDIOMYOPATHY

### Description

**Cardiomyopathies** are diseases of the heart muscle and are classified as primary or secondary. Primary, or *idiopathic, cardiomyopathy* is defined as heart muscle disease of unknown cause, although both viral infections and autoimmunity are suspected causes.[55] Treatment of idiopathic cardiomyopathy is not curative but is directed toward controlling symptoms. Treatment includes a decrease in activity; restriction of sodium intake; administration of diuretics, positive inotropic agents, vasodilators, and antidysrhythmics; and administration of oxygen during periods of acute exacerbations of heart failure; ultimately, cardiac transplantation may be the patient's only hope for survival.

*Secondary cardiomyopathy* is defined as heart muscle disease secondary to some other systemic disease such as coronary artery disease, valvular disease, or severe hypertension.[1,45]

### Categories of Cardiomyopathies

Cardiomyopathies are further classified into three main categories based on abnormalities of structure and function. These categories include hypertrophic, restrictive, and congestive cardiomyopathy.

**Hypertrophic cardiomyopathy.** Hypertrophic cardiomyopathy is a genetically transmitted autosomal dominant trait, which frequently appears in relatives who may be asymptomatic. It is characterized by left-ventricular hypertrophy and bizarre cellular hypertrophy of the upper-ventricular septum, which may or may not result in outflow tract obstruction. Frequently, septal hypertrophy pulls the papillary muscle out of alignment, resulting in altered function of the anterior leaflet of the mitral valve and mitral regurgitation. The myocardial muscle becomes stiff and less compliant, resulting in increased resistance to blood entering the left atrium and an increase in diastolic filling pressures.

The most common symptom is exertional dyspnea related to elevated left-ventricular diastolic pressure and increased wall stiffness, resulting in a decreased cardiac output. Syncope or "graying out" spells are also common because of the inability to increase the cardiac output with exertion.

Treatment is aimed at relaxing the ventricle and decreasing obstruction of the outflow tract. Most frequently used therapies are beta blockers and calcium channel blockers.[51,66] It must be clearly stated in the patient's record that positive inotropic drugs should not be administered because of their propensity to increase ventricular contractility, thereby increasing outflow tract obstruction.

**Congestive cardiomyopathy.** Congestive (dilated) cardiomyopathy is characterized by grossly dilated ventricles without muscle hypertrophy. The muscle fibers contract poorly, resulting in global left-ventricular dysfunction, low cardiac output, atrial and ventricular dysrhythmias, pooling of blood, leading to embolic episodes, and eventually refractory congestive heart failure and premature death.

**Restrictive cardiomyopathy.** Restrictive cardiomyopathy is the least common form of cardiomyopathy and is characterized by abnormal diastolic function. This cardiomyopathy results in ventricular-wall rigidity as a direct conseqeunce of wall fibrosis. The overall effect is to obstruct ventricular filling. Restrictive cardiomyopathy may be misdiagnosed as constrictive pericarditis.

Heart failure, low cardiac output, dyspnea, orthopnea, and liver engorgement are the most common signs and symptoms of restrictive cardiomyopathy. Treatment is directed toward the improvement of pump function, the removal of excess fluid, and administration of a low sodium diet.

### Summary of Nursing Care

Many of the nursing interventions for the patient with cardiomyopathy are similar to those for the patient with congestive heart failure. Refer to the box below.

Nursing interventions should also be directed at maintaining the patient's current level of conditioning and toward collaborating with the physical therapist to maintain and, hopefully, improve the patient's functional level. Activity plans need to reflect energy conservation; therefore activities should be clustered and include frequent rest periods.

#### Nursing Diagnosis and Management
*Cardiomyopathy*

- Decreased Cardiac Output related to relative excess of preload and afterload secondary to impaired ventricular contractility, p. 457
- Activity Intolerance related to knowledge deficit of energy-saving techniques, p. 463
- Activity Intolerance related to decreased cardiac output, p. 464
- Anxiety related to threat to biological, psychological, and/or social integrity, p. 448
- Powerlessness related to illness-related regimen and physical deterioration despite compliance, p. 445
- Powerlessness related to physical deterioration despite compliance, p. 445
- Hopelessness related to perceptions of failing or deteriorating physical condition, p. 446
- Sensory-perceptual alterations related to sensory overload, sensory deprivation, and sleep pattern disturbance, p. 489

The patient's understanding of his or her illness and his or her coping mechanisms and support systems must be assessed. Patients and families need to know what support services are available.

## ENDOCARDITIS

### Description/Etiology

Infection by a microorganism of a platelet-fibrin vegetation on the endothelial surface of the heart results in infective **endocarditis.** It is a relatively uncommon disorder, which is seen more frequently in men than women. Major predisposing factors are listed in the box below.

The development of endocarditis is dependent on two factors: (1) there must be a susceptible lesion in the vascular endothelium, and (2) there must be an organism to establish an infection.[5] The source of the organism may be unknown, or it may be traced to any type of invasive procedure. Streptococci and staphylococci account for approximately 90% of all endocarditis.

Endocarditis begins after the onset of bacteremia and the colonization of thrombotic vegetation.[4] The bacteria is then encased in a platelet and fibrin shell, which protects it from destruction by phagocytic neutrophils, leading to a zone of localized agranulocytosis. It is because of this extensive protective mechanism and its ability to restrict the body's normal response to infection that antibiotic therapy must be so intensive and extensive.[25,76]

### Pathophysiology

The disease may be classified as acute and subacute. Acute infection develops on normal valves, progresses rapidly, causes severe destruction, and may be fatal if the patient is not treated. Subacute infection occurs on damaged heart valves and progresses much more slowly, and the outcome is usually positive with treatment. Survival may be possible even without treatment. The term subacute *bacterial* endocarditis (SBE) is not always accurate because, although most infections are bacterial, some are caused by yeast or fungus. It is much more useful to classify the disease according to causative microorganism.[76]

#### PREDISPOSING FACTORS IN ENDOCARDITIS

Rheumatic heart disease
Congenital heart disease
Mitral valve prolapse
Marfan's syndrome
Idiopathic hypertropic subaortic stenosis
Peripheral arteriovenous fistulas
Indwelling intravenous or intraarterial catheters
Cardiac and prosthetic valve surgery
Prosthetic aortic grafts
Degenerative heart disease
Alcoholism
Chronic hemodialysis
Intravenous drug abuse
Syphilitic aortic disease
Immunosuppression
Severe burns

#### SIGNS AND SYMPTOMS OF ENDOCARDITIS

Fever
Splenomegaly
Hematuria
Petechiae
Cardiac murmurs
Easy fatigability
Osler nodes (small raised tender areas most commonly found in pads of fingers and toes)
Splenic hemorrhages
Roth's spots (round or oval spots consisting of coagulated fibrin; seen in the retina and leads to hemorrhage)

### Assessment and Diagnosis

See the box above for the signs and symptoms of endocarditis. A positive blood culture is usually necessary for a definitive diagnosis.

### Treatment

Treatment requires prolonged parenteral therapy with adequate doses of bactericidal antibiotics.[25,53,58] An increasing number of patients are being discharged home to continue their parenteral therapy. Home patients should be followed closely to assess for acute valvular incompetence or acute onset of prosthetic valve dehiscence with accompanying cardiac failure, which will require emergency cardiac surgery.[53,117,120]

### Summary of Nursing Care

The focus of nursing care for patients with infective endocarditis is resolution of infection, prevention of or early identification of complications, and preventive teaching (see the box on p. 184).

Endocarditis requires a long course, usually 6 weeks, of intravenous antibiotics. During this time the patient must be continuously assessed for any signs of worsening or recurrence of the infection. The nurse must be alert for signs and symptoms of heart failure secondary to worsening valve dysfunction. Therefore the cardiovascular assessment should include the auscultation of heart sounds for the presence of or change in cardiac murmur.

A patient with infective endocarditis is also at risk for embolic events, either cerebral or pulmonary. Therefore level of consciousness, any visual changes, or headache should be documented. Any shortness of breath or chest pain with hemoptysis must also be reported.

As the patient recovers, he or she needs to know what

**Nursing Diagnosis and Management**
***Endocarditis***

- Activity Intolerance related to decreased cardiac output secondary to valvular dysfunction, p. 464
- High Risk for Infection risk factor: invasive lines, p. 465
- Knowledge Deficit: Home Intravenous Medication Regimen related to lack of previous exposure to information, p. 441
- Altered Health Maintenance related to lack of perceived threat to health, p. 439

signs and symptoms to report to the physician, how to take an oral temperature, activities that place him or her at risk for recurrence, and the necessity of letting other health care providers (for example, dentist, podiatrist) know of the history of endocarditis. Before discharge from the hospital, the patient should obtain a Medic Alert bracelet or emergency identification card.

## VALVULAR HEART DISEASE
### Description/Etiology

**Valvular heart disease** is a cardiac dysfunction produced by structural and/or functional abnormalities of single or multiple cardiac valves. The result is alteration in blood flow across the valve.

There are two types of lesions, *stenotic* and *regurgitant*. Valvular stenosis results in impeded flow across the valve, and valvular regurgitation results in bidirectional flow of blood across the valve. Valvular dysfunction affects overall cardiac function by increasing pressure work with stenotic lesions and by increasing volume work with regurgitant lesions. In an attempt to compensate for these dysfunctions, the myocardium will either dilate to accommodate an increased volume or hypertrophy to increase contractility to maintain forward flow.[107]

Valvular heart disease is caused by conditions such as rheumatic fever, infective endocarditis, inborn defects of connective tissue, dysfunction or ruptures of the papillary muscles, and congenital malformations.[117]

**Mitral valve dysfunction.** *Mitral valve stenosis* (Table 8-5) is a progressive narrowing of the mitral valve orifice from 4 to 6 cm to less than 1.5 cm. This narrowing is usually the result of acute rheumatic valvulitis, which results in diffuse leaflet thickening or fibrotic thickening of the margins of closure. The diffuse leaflet fibrosis and fusion of one or both commissures contributes to reduced leaflet mobility. The chordae tendineae may also be thickened, shortened, and fused, further contributing to the stenotic mitral orifice. As a result, the mitral valve is no longer able to open and close passively in response to chamber pressure changes; therefore blood flow across the valve is impeded. Symptoms do not usually appear until the valve orifice is narrowed to 1.5 cm.[107]

*Mitral valve regurgitation* (see Table 8-5) can be secondary to rheumatic disease or it can be caused by endocarditis, papillary muscle dysfunction, or a number of other causes. In mitral valve regurgitation the valve annulus, leaflets, commissures, chordae tendineae, and papillary muscles may all be dysfunctional, or the dysfunction may be isolated to just one component of the valve. The primary effects of mitral valve regurgitation result in thickening and retraction of a portion of the leaflet. Mitral valve regurgitation results in retrograde flow of blood into the left atrium with each ventricular contraction. The left atrium dilates to accommodate this additional volume, whereas the left ventricle hypertrophies as it tries to maintain forward flow and an adequate stroke volume.

**Aortic valve dysfunction.** *Aortic valve stenosis* (see Table 8-5) can occur secondary to aging, calcification of a congential bicuspid valve, or rheumatic valvulitis. Irrespective of its cause, the effect is to impede ejection of blood from the left ventricle into the aorta, resulting in increased left-ventricular systolic pressure, left-ventricular hypertrophy, and eventually, at end-stage disease, left-ventricular dilation. Additionally, when the increase in volume and pressure is communicated back to the atrial and pulmonary vasculature, the result is an increase in left-atrial pressure and volume, pulmonary venous pressure, and pulmonary congestion.

*Aortic valve regurgitation* (see Table 8-5) can occur secondary to rheumatic fever, systemic hypertension, Marfan's syndrome, syphilis, rheumatoid arthritis, or discrete subaortic stenosis. Aortic valve regurgitation results in reflux of blood back into the left ventricle during ventricular diastole.

**Tricuspid valve dysfunction.** *Tricuspid valve stenosis* (see Table 8-5) is rarely an isolated lesion and usually occurs in conjunction with mitral and/or aortic disease. Its origin is most often rheumatic fever. Tricuspid valve stenosis increases the pressure work of the usually low-pressure right atrium, resulting in right-atrial hypertrophy. *Tricuspid valve regurgitation* (see Table 8-5) usually occurs secondary to advanced failure of the left side of the heart or severe pulmonary hypertension.

**Pulmonary valve dysfunction.** *Pulmonary valve disease* is most often related to congenital anomalies and produces failure of the right side of the heart. If untreated, it can result in severe irreversible pulmonary vascular changes.

**Mixed valvular lesions.** Many people will have mixed lesions, that is, an element of both stenosis and regurgitation. Mixed lesions can accentuate a condition the way aortic stenosis and aortic regurgitation do when they both increase left-ventricular volume and pressure and thereby multiply the degree of left-ventricular work. On the other hand, mitral valve stenosis and aortic valve stenosis protect the left ventricle from the strain produced by aortic valve stenosis alone.

***Table 8-5*** Valvular dysfunction

| Pathophysiology | Signs/symptoms | Diagnosis |
|---|---|---|
| **MITRAL VALVE STENOSIS** | | |
| Left atrium must generate more pressure to propel blood beyond the lesion<br>Rise in left-atrial pressure and volume reflected retrograde into pulmonary vessels<br>Right-ventricular hypertrophy<br>Right-ventricular failure | Dyspnea on exertion<br>Fatigue and weakness<br>Pronounced respiratory symptoms—orthopnea, paroxysmal nocturnal dyspnea<br>Mild hemoptysis with bronchial capillary rupture<br>Susceptibility to pulmonary infections | Chest radiograph—pulmonary congestion, redistribution of blood flow to upper lobes<br>Electrocardiogram (ECG)—atrial fibrillation and other atrial dysrhythmias<br>Auscultation—diastolic murmur, accentuated $S_1$, opening snap<br>Catherization—elevated pressure, gradient across valve; increased left-atrial pressure, pulmonary artery wedge, pulmonary artery pressure; low cardiac output |
| **MITRAL VALVE REGURGITATION** | | |
| Left-ventricular dilation and hypertrophy<br>Left-atrial dilation and hypertrophy | Weakness and fatigue<br>Exertional dyspnea<br>Palpitations<br>Severe symptoms precipitated by left-ventricular failure, with consequent low output and pulmonary congestion | Chest radiograph—left-atrial and left-ventricular enlargement, variable pulmonary congestion<br>ECG—P-mitrale, left-ventricular hypertrophy, atrial fibrillation<br>Auscultation—murmur throughout systole<br>Catherization—opacification of left-atrium during left-ventricular injection, V waves, increased left-atrial and left-ventricular pressures<br>Variable elevations of pulmonary pressures |
| **AORTIC VALVE STENOSIS** | | |
| Left-ventricular hypertrophy<br>Progressive failure of ventricular emptying<br>Pulmonary congestion<br>Failure of right side of heart, with systemic venous congestion<br>Sudden death | Exertional dyspnea<br>Exercise intolerance<br>Syncope<br>Angina<br>Congestive heart failure (left-ventricular failure) | Chest radiograph—poststenotic aortic dilation, calcification<br>ECG—left-ventricular hypertrophy<br>Auscultation—systolic ejection murmur<br>Catherization—significant pressure gradient, increased left ventricular end diastolic pressure |
| **AORTIC VALVE REGURGITATION** | | |
| Increased volume load imposed on left ventricle<br>Left-ventricular dilation and hypertrophy | Fatigue<br>Dyspnea on exertion<br>Palpitations | Chest radiograph—boot-shaped elongation of cardiac apex<br>ECG—left-ventricular hypertrophy<br>Auscultation—diastolic murmur<br>Catherization—opacification of left ventricle during aortic injection<br>Peripheral signs—hyperdynamic myocardial action and low peripheral reistance |
| **TRICUSPID VALVE STENOSIS** | | |
| Right atrium must generate higher pressure to eject blood beyond the lesion<br>Right-atrial dilation<br>Systemic venous engorgement<br>Increased venous pressures | Venous distention<br>Peripheral edema<br>Ascites<br>Hepatic engorgement<br>Anorexia | Chest radiograph—right-atrial enlargement<br>ECG—right-atrial enlargement (P pulmonale)<br>Auscultation—diastolic murmur<br>Catherization—elevated right-atrial pressure with large a waves; pressure gradient across the tripcuspid valve |

*Continued.*

*Table 8-5* Valvular dysfunction—cont'd

| Pathophysiology | Signs/symptoms | Diagnosis |
|---|---|---|
| Right-ventricular hypertrophy and dilation | Decreased cardiac output<br>Neck vein distention<br>Hepatic engorgement<br>Ascites<br>Edema<br>Pleural effusions | Chest radiograph—right-atrial and ventricular enlargement<br>ECG—right-ventricular hypertrophy and right-atrial enlargement, atrial fibrillation<br>Auscultation—murmur throughout systole<br>Catheterization—elevated right-atrial pressure and V waves |

Mitral valve stenosis, by decreasing forward flow from the left atrium to the left ventricle, reduces the residual volume in the left ventricle because of the aortic valve stenosis.[34,51]

### Pathophysiology/Diagnosis

Pathophysiology, clinical signs and symptoms, and diagnostic criteria for valvular dysfunction are listed in Table 8-5.

### Summary of Nursing Care

The focus of care for the patient with valvular heart disease is to assess the patient's functional activity level and fluid volume status and to monitor for signs of heart failure, syncope, or anginal pain (refer to the box below).

## PERIPHERAL VASCULAR DISEASE

Atherosclerosis is the most common cause of **peripheral vascular disease**. Alterations can occur in either the venous or arterial systems, with most occurring in the vessels of the lower extremities. Risk factors associated with peripheral vascular disease are the same as those for coronary artery disease.

> **Nursing Diagnosis and Management**
> ***Valvular heart disease***
>
> - Decreased Cardiac Output related to relative excess of preload and afterload, p. 457
> - Activity Intolerance related to decreased cardiac output, p. 464
> - Activity Intolerance related to postural hypotension secondary to prolonged immobility, vasodilator therapy, p. 463
> - High Risk for Altered Peripheral Tissue Perfusion risk factor: vasopressor therapy, p. 462
> - Body Image Disturbance related to actual change in body function, p. 443

### Arterial Disease

**Occlusive arterial disease.** There are two major causes of occlusive arterial disease. The first is *arteriosclerosis obliterans*, a consequence of atherosclerosis. These lesions tend to occur at the origin or bifurcations of a vessel. The aortoiliac vessels, femoropopliteal vessels, and popliteal-tibial vessels are the most common sites for atherogenesis.

The second major cause of occlusive arterial disease is *thromboangiitis obliterans* (Buerger's disease), an occlusion caused by inflammation and thrombosis. Thrombi may originate in the left side of the heart as a consequence of atrial fibrillation or mitral stenosis. Thrombogenesis also occurs at the site of artherosclerotic plaque. Arterial occlusion obstructs blood flow to the distal extremity.

***Assessment and diagnosis.*** Signs and symptoms of occlusive arterial disease are listed in the box on p. 187. Acute occlusions usually are initially seen with sudden onset of severe pain, loss of pulses, collapse of superficial veins, coldness and pallor, and impaired motor and sensory function.

***Treatment.*** Medical therapy is geared toward controlling or eliminating risk factors, providing good foot care, and suggesting alterations in lifestyle to promote rest and pain relief. Therapy may also include the use of anticoagulants, vasodilators, or antiplatelet drugs. If the above-listed therapies do not produce positive results, the patient may be a candidate for angioplasty.

Surgical therapy may be required if symptoms become disabling or threaten limb viability. Surgical procedures and the purpose of each include the following: (1) arterial reconstruction—to restore unimpeded flow and to redirect blood flow around the site of occlusion, (2) endarterectomy—to remove discrete plaque, and (3) lumbar sympathectomy—to decrease sympathetic tone and increase peripheral vasodilation. Severe occlusions may necessitate limb or partial limb amputation.

### SIGNS AND SYMPTOMS OF OCCLUSIVE ARTERIAL DISEASE

**INTERMITTENT CLAUDICATION (CRAMPING, ACHING PAIN DURING AMBULATION)**

- Pain is relieved by rest; as disease progresses, pain also occurs during rest.
- Relief is obtained by placing the extremity in a dependent position.
- Site of the pain is indicative of the location of the lesion.
- Arterial pulses may be diminished, transiently present (vessel spasm), or absent distal to the site of occlusion.

**CHANGES IN SKIN COLOR**

- With extremity elevation, the limb becomes pale.
- With dependency of the extremity, there is a rubor or purplish discoloration.

**ATROPHIC TISSUE CHANGES**

- Nails thicken, and skin becomes dry.
- Hair loss occurs on the lower leg, dorsum of the feet, and toes.
- Temperature gradient is usually present as a line of demarcation.
- There is wasting of muscle, as well as soft skin tissue.
- Ulcerations and gangrene set in as the disease progresses.

### Nursing Diagnosis and Management
***Peripheral vascular disease***

- Altered Peripheral Tissue Perfusion related to compromised arterial flow and knowledge deficit secondary to arterial occlusive disease, p. 462
- Acute Pain related to transmission and perception of noxious stimuli secondary to tissue ischemia, p. 485
- Anxiety related to threat to biological, psychological, and/or social integrity, p. 448
- Powerlessness related to physical deterioration despite compliance, p. 445
- Hopelessness related to perceptions of failing or deteriorating physical condition, p. 446

***Summary of nursing care.*** The focus of nursing care for the patient with arterial insufficiency is to increase the arterial blood supply, decrease venous pooling, promote vasodilation, maintain tissue integrity, treat tissue hypoxia, and provide patient teaching. Refer to the box above, right for specific nursing diagnoses and management.

**Aneurysmal arterial disease.** An aneurysm is a localized dilation of the arterial wall that results in an alteration in vessel shape and blood flow. Figure 8-14 displays the four types of aneurysms. Causes of aneurysms are listed in the box on p. 188.

Medial degeneration is the most common pathology of aneurysm formation. Medial degeneration occurs as a normal part of the aging process and as a complication of Marfan's syndrome. The ascending aorta and the aortic arch are the sites of the greatest hemodynamic stress and are also the most frequent sites of arterial dissection. Extensive medial degeneration frequently occurs in hypertensive patients and is a major contributing factor to aneurysmal risk.

***Assessment and diagnosis.*** For many years a person may be asymptomatic or the aneurysm may be detected during routine abdominal examination as a palpable, pulsatile mass located in the umbilical region of the abdomen to the left of midline. A thoracic aneurysm may be identified on a routine chest x-ray film. Cardiovascular symptoms include

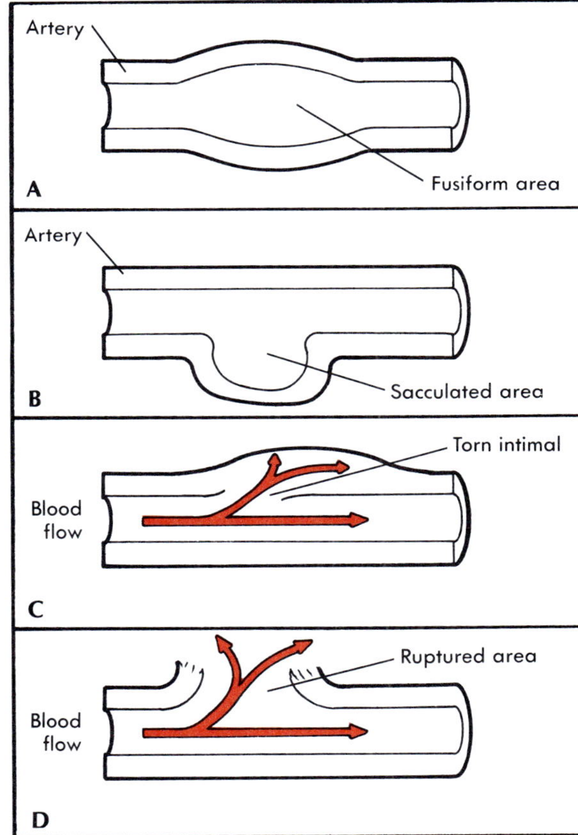


***Fig. 8-14*** Four basic types of aneurysms. **A,** Fusiform aneurysm, in which an entire segment of an artery is dilated, thus taking on a spindle or bulbous shape. Fusiform aneurysms occur most often in the abdominal aorta secondary to atherosclerosis. **B,** Sacculated aneurysm, which involves only one side of an artery and is usually located in the ascending aorta. **C,** Dissecting aneurysm, which occurs because of a tear in the intima, resulting in the shunting of blood between the intima and media of a vessel. **D,** Pseudoaneurysm, which results from a ruptured artery.

**CAUSES OF ANEURYSM**

Hypertension
Atherosclerotic changes in the thoracic and abdominal aorta
Blunt trauma (deceleration injury)
Cystic medical necrosis (Marfan's syndrome)
Pregnancy
Iatrogenic injury or dissection

**INDICATIONS FOR ANEURYSM SURGERY**

Aneurysm greater than 5 cm
Aneurysm progressively increasing in size
Impending rupture
Symptoms resulting from cerebral or coronary ischemia
Pericardial tamponade
Uncontrollable pain
Aortic insufficiency

severe hypertension, acute neurological deficits, fleeting peripheral pulses, and a new murmur indicative of aortic insufficiency.

***Treatment.*** An aneurysm less than 4 cm in size can be managed medically with frequent monitoring of blood pressure and ultrasound testing to document any changes in size of the aneurysm. The patient will be encouraged to lose weight if obesity is a factor, and blood pressure will be carefully monitored and hypertension treated to decrease hemodynamic stress on the site. An aneurysm greater than 6 cm is usually treated surgically (see box above, right).

**Aortic dissection.** An **aortic dissection** occurs when there is separation of the vascular layers by a column of blood. This creates a false lumen, which communicates with the true lumen through a tear in the intima. This separation extends along the length of the vessel rather than coursing around the circumference.

***Assessment and diagnosis.*** Signs and symptoms of dissection are listed in the box below, right. The location of the dissection may be established by the site of pain. A distal dissection is usually accompanied by chest pain, which radiates to the back, abdomen, or legs. Central chest pain is indicative of an ascending dissection.[24]

***Treatment.*** Medical management involves controlling hypertension and pain. Progression of the dissection is evaluated by the patient's report of worsening or new pain.

Surgical procedures include resection of the affected areas, followed by graft placement, repair or replacement of the aortic valve, and restoration of blood flow to major branches of the aorta.

***Summary of nursing care.*** The focus of nursing care for the patient with an aortic dissection is to maintain the blood pressure within prescribed parameters, stabilize the patient hemodynamically, and control the pain. Since analgesics can mask the pain of further dissection, they are administered judiciously.

### Venous Disease

Venous disease occurs when there is alteration in the integrity of veins, resulting in decreased venous return or thrombosis.

**Thrombolic venous disease.** The most common form of venous disease is usually manifested as thrombophlebitis.

**Thrombophlebitis** is the formation of a thrombus, accompanied by inflammation, pain, tenderness, and redness at the site. The incidence is greatest in the lower-extremity vessels, especially the saphenous, femoral, and popliteal veins. Thrombophlebitis can occur in either deep or superficial vessels and in upper- or lower-extremity vessels.

Stasis of blood, endothelial injury, and hypercoagulability of blood are referred to as Virchow's triad. Usually two of the three conditions must be present for thrombosis to occur.

***Superficial thromboses.*** Superficial thromboses are characterized by cordlike veins that are readily palpable. The area surrounding the affected vessel will often be tender to palpation, erythematous, and warm. The most common cause of superficial thromboses of the arms is intravenous therapy.

**TREATMENT.** Patients with superficial thromboses do not usually require anticoagulation therapy, and bed rest may be prescribed until the extremity is less tender and ambulation can be considered. Warm compresses may be used,

**SIGNS AND SYMPTOMS OF AORTIC DISSECTION**

- Sudden onset of intense, severe, tearing pain, which may be localized initially in the chest, abdomen, or back. As dissection extends, pain radiates to the back or distally toward the lower extremities.
- New murmur of aortic regurgitation if the dissection moves retrograde, extending to the aortic valve. Coronary arteries may be at risk and lead to myocardial infarction. Signs of shock develop quickly with this type of lesion.
- Severe hypertension
- Loss of peripheral pulses
- Acute neurological deficits, i.e., syncope, altered LOC, varying levels of paralysis and paresthesia, CVA
- Gastrointestinal symptoms, i.e., acute abdominal pain, melena, hyperactive bowel sounds
- Renal symptoms, i.e., oliguria, hematuria

along with elastic stockings. Superficial thromboses are usually not precursors of more serious conditions.

***Deep vein thrombophlebitis.*** Obstruction of blood flow can occur within a deep vessel of the pelvis or lower extremity. This markedly increases the patient's risk of pulmonary embolism and long-term disability resulting from chronic venous insufficiency.

Development of deep-vein thrombosis may be very insidious. It occurs as a result of edema, causes of which include increased intravascular volume and increased intravascular pooling of blood. Pain is described as an aching or throbbing sensation, which worsens with ambulation. A positive Homan's sign, which is pain on dorsiflexion of the foot, heightens the suspicion of a deep vein thrombosis. Other manifestations include increased tissue turgor with swelling, increased skin temperature, dilation of superficial veins, and mottling and cyanosis caused by stagnant flow.

**TREATMENT.** Major therapeutic emphasis is placed on prophylaxis. The patient is confined to bed rest, along with elevation of the limb, anticoagulation therapy, and local applications of moist heat. Analgesics are prescribed to reduce discomfort. Most patients will be managed medically with anticoagulants, but those at high risk for pulmonary embolism (that is, cancer patients, patients with bleeding disorders, or patients who have a spinal cord injury, or who are comatose) may require surgical intervention. Possible procedures include venous thrombectomy, femoral vein interruption, inferior vena cava interruption, insertion of filtering devices, thrombolytic therapy, angioplasty, and laser treatment.

**Chronic venous insufficiency.** Chronic venous insufficiency is produced by extensive deep vein thrombosis with resultant venous valve insufficiency. It is usually precipitated by chronic venous stasis and elevation of venous pressures, resulting in stretching and weakening of the valves. Over a period of time, this condition may lead to the development of stasis ulcers.

**Summary of nursing care.** The focus of care for the patient with venous disease is to increase blood flow and to prevent complications from deep vein thrombosis or anticoagulant therapy. Range-of-motion exercises should be performed with the unaffected leg. The patient should be instructed to avoid use of the knee gatch because elevation of the knee impedes venous return. Calf and/or thigh measurements should be obtained daily.

The patient with a deep vein thrombosis should be closely monitored for signs of pulmonary embolism, and the patient should be instructed to report immediately any chest pain, dyspnea, or tachypnea. Once the patient is ambulatory, he or she should be encouraged to walk but not to sit or stand for long periods of time. When sitting in a chair, low elevation of the affected extremity should be maintained.

Anticoagulant therapy should be monitored by obtaining daily coagulation values. Bleeding should be treated promptly. Stools should be checked for occult blood. Mechanical trauma should be avoided (for example, the patient should use an electric razor, soft toothbrush, and unobstructed walkway).

## REFERENCES


1. Abelmann WH: Classification and natural history of primary myocardial disease, Prog Cardiovasc Dis 27(2):73, 1984.
2. Anderson UK: Mitral valve prolapse: a diagnosis for primary nursing intervention, J Cardiovasc Nurs 1(3):41, 1987.
3. Barzilai B and others: Prognostic significance of mitral regurgitation in acute myocardial infarction, Am J Cardiol 65(18):1169, 1990.
4. Bayless R and others: Incidence, mortality and prevention of infective endocarditis, J R Coll Physicians Lond 20(1):12, 1986.
5. Benditt E: The origin of atherosclerosis, Sci Am 236:74, 1977.
6. Benditt EP and Benditt JM: Evidence for a monoclonal origin of human atherosclerotic plaques, Proc Natl Acad Sci 70:1753, 1973.
7. Bigger JT and others: Prognosis after recovery from acute myocardial infarction, Annu Rev Med 35:127, 1984.
8. Billhardt RA and Rosenbush SW: Cardiogenic and hypovolemic shock, Med Clin North Am 70(4):853, 1986.
9. Black L, Coombs V, and Townsend S: Reperfusion and reperfusion injury in acute myocardial infarction, Heart Lung 19(3):274, 1990.
10. Blessey R: Epidemiology, risk factors, and pathophysiology of ischemic heart disease, Phys Ther 65(12):1796, 1985.
11. Bondestam E and others: Pain assessment by patients and nurses in the early phase of acute MI, J Adv Nurs 12(6):677, 1987.
12. Bondy B: An overview of arterial disease, J Cardiovasc Nurs 1(2):1, 1987.
13. Braunwald E, editor: Heart disease, ed 3, Philadelphia, 1988, WB Saunders Co.
14. Bressack MA and Raffin TA: Importance of venous return, venous resistance and mean circulatory pressure in the physiology and management of shock, Chest 92(5):906, 1987.
15. Burke LE: Nursing grand rounds: risk-factor modification in the prevention of coronary heart disease, J Cardiovasc Nurs 1(4):67, 1987.
16. Bush DE and Healy B: Management of a patient recovering from myocardial infarction: a decision tree, Adv Intern Med 31:469, 1986.
17. Cohn JM: Management of acute myocardial infarction, Am J Med 77:67, 1984.
18. Condini MA: Management of acute myocardial infarction, Med Clin North Am 70(4):769, 1986.
19. Conti CR: Unstable angina before and after infarction: thoughts on pathogenesis and therapeutic strategies, Heart Lung 15(4):361, 1986.
20. Cox JL and others: Laser-assisted angioplasty treating peripheral vascular disease, AORN J 46(5):835, 1987.
21. Dawber TR and others: Epidemiological approaches to heart disease: the Framingham study, Am J Public Health 41:279, 1951.
22. Deans KW and Hartshorn JC: Cardiovascular pharmacology: nitrates in the treatment of coronary artery disease, J Cardiovasc Nurs 1(1):81, 1986.
23. DeWood MA and others: Prevalence of total coronary occlusion during the early hours of transmural MI, N Engl J Med 303:897, 1980.
24. Dixon MB: Acute aortic dissection, J Cardiovasc Nurs 1(2):24, 1987.
25. Donabedian H and Freimer EH: Pathogenesis and treatment of endocarditis, Am J Med 78(6A):127, 1985.
26. Doyle JE: Treatment modalities in peripheral vascular disease, Nurs Clin North Am 21(2):241, 1986.
27. Eberts A: Advances in the pharmacologic management of angina pectoris, J Cardiovasc Nurs 1(1):15, 1986.
28. Epstein SE and Palmeri ST: Mechanisms contributing to precipitation of unstable angina and acute myocardial infarction: implications regarding therapy, Am J Cardiol 54(10):1245, 1984.
29. Ferguson RK and others: Clinical applications of angiotensin-converting enzyme inhibitors, Am J Med 77(4):690, 1984.
30. Fozzard HA and Makielski JC: The electrophysiology of acute myocardial ischemia, Annu Rev Med 36:275, 1985.

31. Francis GS: Neurohumoral mechanisms involved in congestive heart failure, Am J Cardiol 55(2):15A, 1985.
32. Francis GS and Archer SL: Diagnosis and management of acute congestive heart failure in the intensive care unit, J Inten Care Med 4(2):84, 1989.
33. Francis GS and Cohn JN: The autonomic nervous system in congestive heart failure, Annu Rev Med 37:235, 1986.
34. Gillum RF and others: Decline in coronary heart disease mortality. Old questions and new facts, Am J Med 76(6):1055, 1984.
35. Glueck CJ: Role of risk factor management in progression and regression of coronary and femoral artery atherosclerosis, Am J Cardiol 57(14):35G, 1986.
36. Goldberg RJ and others: The role of anticoagulant therapy in acute myocardial infarction, Am Heart J 108(5):1387, 1984.
37. Goldberg RJ and others: Long-term anticoagulant therapy after acute myocardial infarction, Am Heart J 109(3):616, 1985.
38. Goldman L and Cook EF: The decline in ischemic heart disease mortality rates. An analysis of the comparative effects of medical interventions and changes in lifestyle, Ann Intern Med 101(6):825, 1984.
39. Guido B and Mocogni F: Hypercholesterolemia as a cardiovascular risk factor: nursing implications, Crit Care Nurs Q 12(2):73, 1989.
40. Haas G and Leier C: Invasive cardiovascular testing in chronic congestive heart failure, Crit Care Med 18(1):51, 1990.
41. Handler CE: Cardiogenic shock, Postgrad Med J 61(718):705, 1985.
42. Hansson L and Lundin S: Hypertension and coronary heart disease: cause and consequence or associated diseases? Am J Med 76(2A):41, 1984.
43. Herman J: Nursing assessment and nursing diagnosis in patients with peripheral vascular disease, Nurs Clin North Am 21(2):219, 1986.
44. Hjalmarson A: Early intervention with a beta-blocking drug after acute myocardial infarction, Am J Cardiol 54(11):11E, 1984.
45. Hurst W, editor: The heart, ed 6, New York, 1986, McGraw-Hill Book Co.
46. Irwin S: Clinical manifestations and assessment of ischemic heart disease, Phys Ther 65(12):1806, 1985.
47. Jaffe AS: Complications of acute myocardial infarction, Cardiovasc Clin 2(1):79, 1984.
48. Jarzemsky P: Nursing care of the patient with dilated cardiomyopathy, Crit Care Nurs 6(2):10, 1986.
49. Jeffries PR and Whelan SK: Cardiogenic shock: current management, Crit Care Nurs 11(1):48, 1988.
50. Johnson J: Valvular heart disease in the elderly, J Cardiovasc Nurs 1(2):72, 1987.
51. Josephson MA and Singh BN: Use of calcium antagonists in ventricular dysfunction, Am J Cardiol 55(3):81B, 1985.
52. Kannel WB and others: A general cardiovascular risk profile: the Framingham study, Am J Cardiol 38:46, 1976.
53. Kaye D: Prophylaxis for infective endocarditis: an update, Ann Intern Med 104(3):419, 1986.
54. Kelly DT: Clinical decisions in patients following myocardial infarction, Curr Probl Cardiol 10(11):1, 1985.
55. Kereiakes DJ and Parmley WW: Myocarditis and cardiomyopathy, Am Heart J 108(5):1318, 1984.
56. Kern LS: Advances in the surgical treatment of coronary artery disease, J Cardiovasc Nurs 1(1):1, 1986.
57. King K and Harkness JL: Infective endocarditis in the 1980s. Part 1. Etiology and diagnosis, Med J Aust 144(10):536, 1986.
58. King K and Harkness JL: Infective endocarditis in the 1980s. Part 2. Treatment and management, Med J Aust 144(11):588, 1986.
59. Kirklin JW and Barratt-Boyes BG: Cardiac surgery, New York, 1986, John Wiley & Sons, Inc.
60. Kjekshus JK: The coronary circulation in normal and ischemic hearts, Scand J Clin Lab Invest 173:9, 1984.
61. Klamerus KJ: Current concepts in clinical therapeutics: congestive heart failure, Clin Pharm 5(6):481, 1986.
62. Kochar MS and Woods KD: Hypertension control for nurses and other health professionals, ed 2, New York, 1985, Springer-Verlag Publishing Co.
63. Lanoue AS, Snyder BA, and Galan KM: Percutaneous transluminal coronary angioplasty: nonoperative treatment of coronary artery disease, J Cardiovasc Nurs 1(1):30, 1986.
64. Levy RI: Changing perspectives in the prevention of coronary artery disease, Am J Cardiol 57(14):17G, 1986.
65. Lewis VC: Monitoring the patient with acute myocardial infarction, Nurs Clin North Am 22(1):15, 1987.
66. Mancini DM and others: Inotropic drugs for the treatment of heart failure, J Clin Pharmacol 25(7):540, 1985.
67. Mancini DM and others: Intravenous use of amrinone for the treatment of the failing heart, Am J Cardiol 56(3):8B, 1985.
68. Mancini DM and others: Central and peripheral components of cardiac failure, Am J Med 80(2B):2, 1986.
69. Maseri A and others: Pathophysiology of coronary occlusion in acute infarction, Circulation 73(2):233, 1986.
70. Massie B: Updated diagnosis and management of congestive heart failure, Geriatrics 41(3):30, 1986.
71. Mayberry-Toth B and Landron S: Complications associated with acute myocardial infarction, Crit Care Nurs Q 12(2):49, 1989.
72. McKool K: Facilitating smoking cessation, J Cardiovas Nurs 1(4):28, 1987.
73. McRae RP and Liebson PR: Hypertensive crisis, Med Clin North Am 70(4):749, 1986.
74. Meyers KA and Hickey MK: Nursing management of hypovolemic shock, Crit Care Nurs 11(1):57, 1988.
75. Nowakowski JF: Use of cardiac enzymes in the evaluation of acute chest pain, Ann Emerg Med 15(3):354, 1986.
76. Oikawa JH and Kaye D: Endocarditis: epidemiology, pathophysiology, management, and prophylaxis, Cardiovasc Clin 16(2):335, 1986.
77. Opie LH: Drugs and the heart four years on, Lancet 1(8375):496, 1984.
78. Owens-Jones S and Hopp L: Viral myocarditis, Focus Crit Care 15(1):25, 1988.
79. Paffenbarger RS and others: Physical activity as an index of heart attack risk in college alumni, Am J Epidemiol 108:161, 1978.
80. Parmley WW: Pathophysiology of congestive heart failure, Am J Cardiol 55:9A, 1985.
81. Pearle DL: Nifedipine in acute myocardial infarction, Am J Cardiol 54(11):21E, 1984.
82. Perret C: Acute heart failure in myocardial infarction: principles of treatment, Crit Care Med 18(1):526, 1990.
83. Pitt B: Evaluation of the patient with congestive heart failure and ventricular arrhythmias, Am J Cardiol 57(3):19B, 1986.
84. Pratt CM and others: The clinical significance of ventricular arrhythmias after myocardial infarction, Cardiol Clin 2(1):3, 1984.
85. Quaal SJ: Thrombolytic therapy: an overview, J Cardiovasc Nurs 1(1):45, 1986.
86. Rafalowski M: Cardiac valve replacement: the homograft, Focus Crit Care 17(2):111, 1990.
87. Remme WJ: Congestive heart failure—pathophysiology and medical treatment, J Cardiovasc Pharmacol 8(suppl 1):36, 1986.
88. Renlund DG and Gerstenblith G: Angina: current approaches to diagnosis, drug therapy, and surgical referral, Geriatrics 41(1):35, 1986.
89. Rosenthal ME and others: Sudden cardiac death following acute myocardial infarction, Am Heart J 109(4):865, 1985.
90. Ross R and Glomset J: Atherosclerosis and the arterial smooth muscle cell, Science 180:1332, 1973.
91. Ross R and Glomset JA: The pathogenesis of atherosclerosis, Part I, N Engl J Med 295(7):369, 1976.
92. Ross R and Glomset JA: The pathogenesis of atherosclerosis, Part II, N Engl J Med 295(8):420, 1976.

93. Rude RE: Acute myocardial infarction and its complications, Cardiol Clin 2(2):163, 1984.
94. Ruggie N: Congestive heart failure, Med Clin North Am 70(4):829, 1986.
95. Ryan P: Strategies for motivating life-style change, J Cardiovasc Nurs 1(4):54, 1987.
96. Sasyniuk BI: Symposium on the management of ventricular dysrhythmias. Concept of reentry versus automaticity, Am J Cardiol 54(2):1A, 1984.
97. Schakenbach LH: Physiologic dynamics of acquired valvular heart disease, J Cardiovasc Nurs 1(3):1, 1987.
98. Schroeder JS: Combination therapy with isosorbide dinitrate: current status and the future, Am Heart J 110(1):284, 1985.
99. Scrima DA: Infective endocarditis: nursing considerations, Crit Care Nurse 7(2):47, 1987.
100. Silverman KJ and Grossman W: Angina pectoris. Natural history and strategies for evaluation and management, N Engl J Med 310(26):1712, 1984.
101. Smilack JD and Horn VP: Acute infective endocarditis, Cardiol Clin 2(2):201, 1984.
102. Smith A: Physiology, diagnosis, and life-style modifications for hyperlipidemia, J Cardiovasc Nurs 1(4):15, 1987.
103. Smith CE: Assessing chest pain, Nursing 88 18(5):52, May 1988.
104. Smith WM: Epidemiology of congestive heart failure, Am J Cardiol 55:3A, 1985.
105. Sobel BE: Early intervention in acute myocardial infarction: one center's perspective, Am J Cardiol 54(11):2E, 1984.
106. Srebro J and Karliner JS: Congestive heart failure, Curr Probl Cardiol 23(6):301, 1986.
107. Stapleton JF: Natural history of chronic valvular disease, Cardiovasc Clin 16(2):105, 1986.
108. Streff MM: Exercise in the prevention of coronary artery disease, J Cardiovasc Nurs 1(4):42, 1987.
109. Stuart EM and others: Nonpharmacologic treatment of hypertension: a multiple-risk-factor approach, J Cardiovasc Nurs 1(4):1, 1987.
110. Superko HR and others: Coronary heart disease and risk factor modification. Is there a threshold? Am J Med 78(5):826, 1985.
111. Sutton FJ: Vasodilator therapy, Am J Med 80(2B):54, 1986.
112. Turk M: Acute pericarditis in the post–myocardial infarction patient, Crit Care Nurse Q 12(3):34, 1989.
113. Turner J: Nursing interventions in patients with peripheral vascular disease, Nurs Clin North Am 21(2):233, 1986.
114. Tyroler HA: Cholesterol and cardiovascular disease. An overview of Lipid Research Clinics (LRC) epidemiologic studies as background for the LRC Coronary Primary Prevention Trial, Am J Cardiol 54(5):14C, 1984.
115. Wagner GS: Arrhythmias in acute myocardial infarction, Med Clin North Am 68(4):1001, 1984.
116. Wagner MM: Pathophysiology related to peripheral vascular disease, Nurs Clin North Am 21(2):195, 1986.
117. Waller BF: Rheumatic and nonrheumatic conditions producing valvular heart disease, Cardiovasc Clin 16(2):3, 1986.
118. Warbinek E and others: Peripheral arterial occlusive disease: nursing assessment and standard care plans, Part 2, Cardiovasc Nurse 22(2):6, 1986.
119. Weber KT and others: Advances in the evaluation and management of chronic cardiac failure, Chest 85(2):253, 1984.
120. Weinstein L: Life-threatening complications of infective endocarditis and their management, Arch Intern Med 146(5):953, 1986.
121. Wenger NK: Coronary disease in women, Annu Rev Med 36:285, 1985.
122. Whalen K: Level of nursing care required by the unstable angina patient, Crit Care Med 18(5):505, 1990.
123. Wilhelmsen L: Risk factors for coronary heart disease in perspective. European intervention trials, Am J Med 76(2A):37, 1984.

CHAPTER 9

# Cardiovascular Therapeutic Management

## CHAPTER OBJECTIVES

- *Discuss the prevention, identification, and management of pacemaker malfunction.*
- *Describe the immediate postoperative medical and nursing management of the adult cardiac surgical patient.*
- *Summarize the nursing interventions pertinent to the patient undergoing percutaneous transluminal coronary angioplasty.*
- *Describe the role of the critical care nurse during and following the administration of thrombolytic therapy.*
- *Identify the major nursing implications related to the administration of antidysrhythmic and vasoactive drug therapy.*

## KEY TERMS

asynchronous pacemaker, p. 195
synchronous pacemaker, p. 195
AV sequential pacemaker, p. 195
pacing artifact, p. 199
electromagnetic interference (EMI), p. 199
runaway pacemaker, p. 199
cardiopulmonary bypass (CPB), p. 203
percutaneous transluminal coronary angioplasty (PTCA), p. 205
streptokinase (SK), p. 207
urokinase (UK), p. 208
tissue plasminogen activator (t-PA), p. 208
anisoylated plasminogen streptokinase activator complex (APSAC), p. 208
intraaortic balloon pump (IABP), p. 209
ventricular assist device (VAD), p. 212

## TEMPORARY PACEMAKERS

Pacemakers are electronic devices that can be used to initiate the heartbeat when the heart's intrinsic electrical system is unable to effectively generate a rate adequate to support cardiac output. Pacemakers can be used temporarily, either supportively or prophylactically, until the condition responsible for the rate or conduction disturbance (actual or potential) has resolved. Pacemakers can also be used on a permanent basis if the patient's condition persists despite adequate therapy. The use of temporary pacemakers as a diagnostic tool is also gaining in popularity.[23,47]

### Indications

The clinical indications for instituting temporary pacemaker therapy are similar regardless of the cause of the rhythm disturbance necessitating the placement of a pacemaker (see the box below). Such causes range from drug toxicities and electrolyte imbalances to sequelae related to acute myocardial infarction or cardiac surgery.

Dysrhythmias that are unresponsive to drug therapy and result in compromised hemodynamic status are a definite indication for pacemaker therapy. The goal of therapy in the case of bradydysrhythmia is to increase the ventricular

**INDICATIONS FOR TEMPORARY PACING**

- Bradydysrhythmias
  - Sinus bradycardia and arrest
  - Sick sinus syndrome
  - Heart blocks
- Tachydysrhythmias
  - Supraventricular
  - Ventricular
- Permanent pacemaker failure
- Support of cardiac output
  - Status following cardiac surgery
- Diagnostic studies
  - Electrophysiology studies (EPSs)
  - Atrial electrogram (AEG)

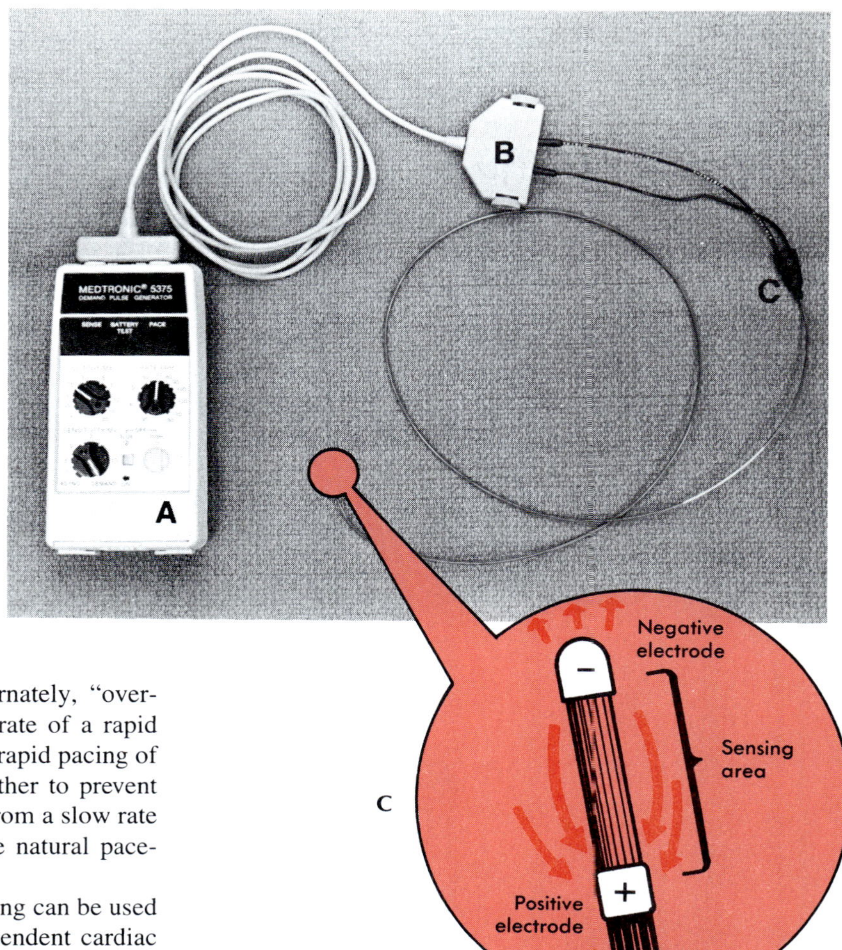


***Fig. 9-1*** The components of a temporary bipolar transvenous pacing system. **A,** External pulse generator. **B,** Bridging cable. **C,** Pacing lead. (Adapted from Persons CB: Critical care procedures and protocols: a nursing approach, Philadelphia, 1987, JB Lippincott Co.)

rate and thus enhance cardiac output. Alternately, "overdrive" pacing can be used to decrease the rate of a rapid supraventricular or ventricular rhythm. This rapid pacing of the heart, or overdrive pacing, functions either to prevent the "breakthrough" ectopics that can result from a slow rate or "capture" an ectopic focus and allow the natural pacemaker to regain control.

Following cardiac surgery, temporary pacing can be used to improve a transiently depressed, rate-dependent cardiac output. In addition, conduction disturbances that can occur following valvular surgery can be managed effectively with temporary pacing.[81]

Several diagnostic uses for temporary pacing have evolved over the past several years. Electrophysiology studies (EPS) use special pacing electrodes to induce dysrhythmias in patients with recurrent symptomatic dysrhythmias.[47,52] This allows the physician to closely evaluate the particular dysrhythmia and determine appropriate therapy.

The atrial electrogram (AEG) is simply an amplified recording of atrial activity that can be obtained through the use of atrial pacing wires and a standard electrocardiogram (ECG) machine.[23] It is often used after cardiac surgery to facilitate the diagnosis of supraventricular dysrhythmias in patients with temporary atrial epicardial electrodes already in place.[73]

### The Pacemaker System

A pacemaker system is a simple electrical circuit consisting of a pulse generator and a pacing lead (an insulated electrical wire) with either one or two electrodes. The pulse generator is designed to generate an electrical current that travels through the pacing lead and exits through an electrode (exposed portion of the wire) that is in direct contact with the heart. This electrical current initiates a myocardial depolarization. The current then seeks to return by one of several ways to the pulse generator to complete the circuit.

The power source for a temporary external pulse generator is the standard alkaline or mercury battery. Implanted permanent pacemaker batteries are now either nuclear powered or, as is more often the case, long-lived lithium cells.

The pacing lead used for temporary pacing may be bipolar or unipolar. The bipolar lead used in transvenous pacing has two electrodes in close proximity. The distal, or negative, electrode is at the tip of the pacing lead and is in direct contact with the heart. Approximately 1 cm above the negative electrode is a positive electrode. The negative electrode is attached to the negative terminal, and the positive electrode is attached to the positive terminal of the pulse generator, either directly or via a bridging cable (Fig. 9-1).

The bipolar epicardial lead system used for temporary pacing following cardiac surgical procedures has two separate insulated wires (one negative and one positive electrode) loosely secured with sutures to the cardiac chamber to be paced and attached to the pulse generator as just described.[30]

Sensing antenna area

Unipolar

Pulse generator

Metal case acts as positive terminal

Negative electrode

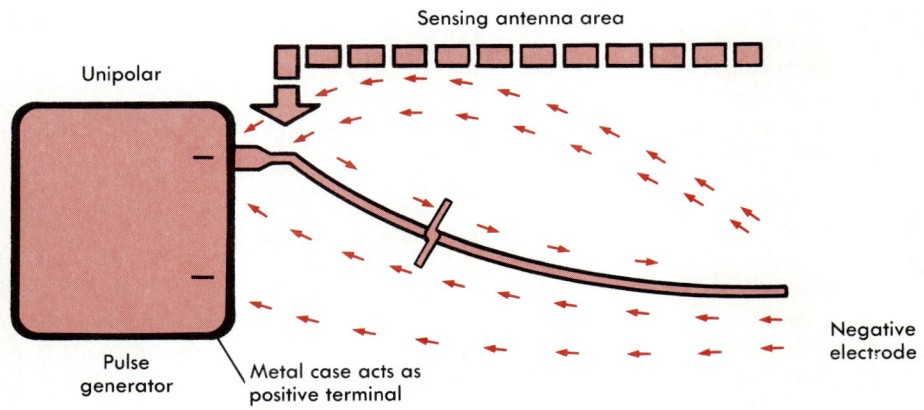

***Fig. 9-2*** The components of a permanent unipolar transvenous pacing system.

A

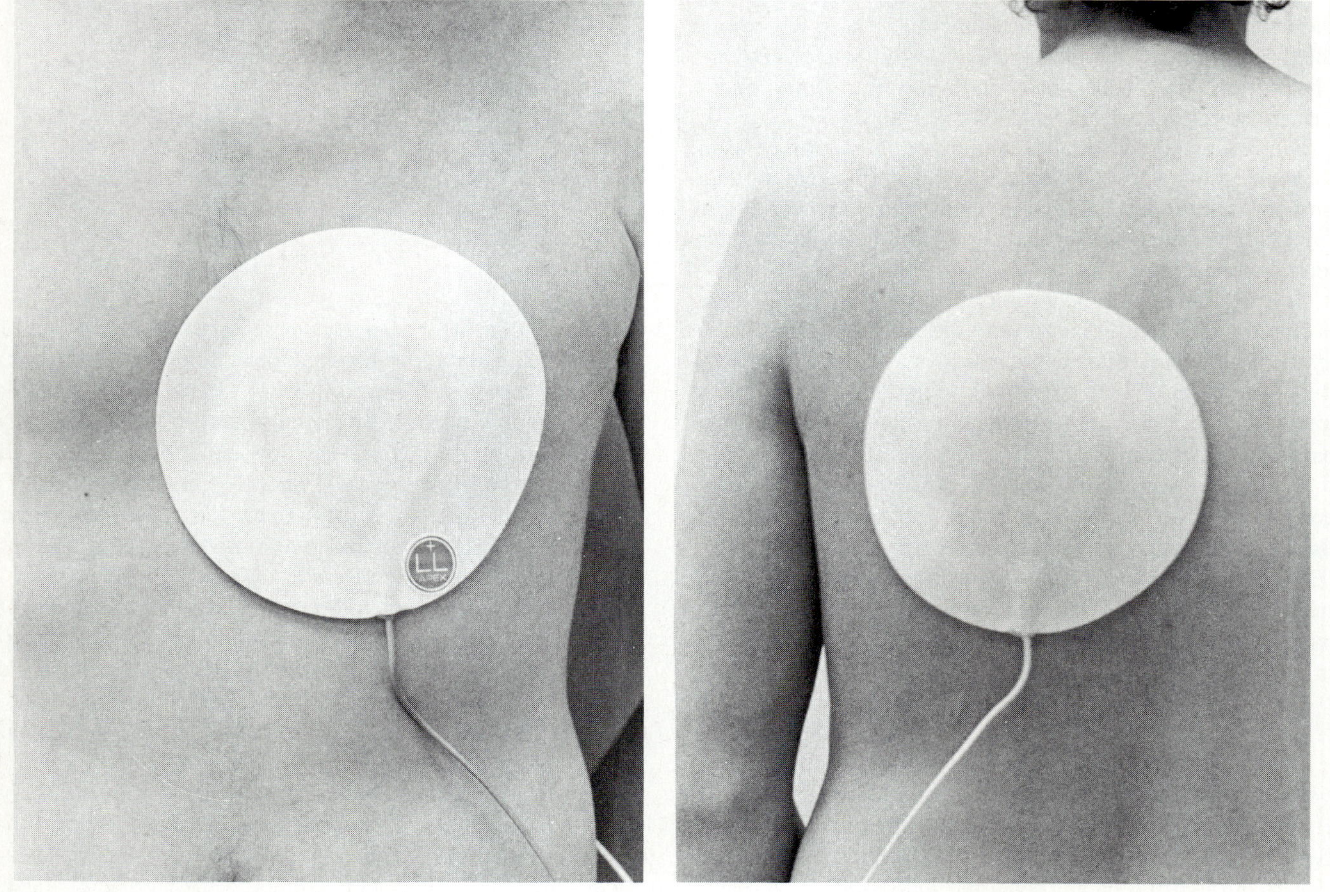

B

***Fig. 9-3*** Placement of transcutaneous pacing electrodes. (From Persons CB: Critical care procedures and protocols: a nursing approach, Philadelphia, 1987, JB Lippincott Co.)

In both cases, the current will flow from the negative terminal of the pulse generator down the pacing lead to the negative electrode and into the heart. The current is then picked up by the positive electrode and flows back up the lead to the positive terminal of the pulse generator.

A unipolar pacing system has only one electrode (a negative electrode) making contact with the heart. In the case of a permanent pacemaker, the positive electrode can be created by the metallic casing of the subcutaneously implanted pulse generator (Fig. 9-2). Or as is the case with a unipolar epicardial lead system, the positive electrode can be formed by a piece of surgical steel wire sewn into the subcutaneous tissue of the chest.[30]

Because the unipolar pacing system has a wide sensing area as a result of the relatively large distance between the negative and positive electrodes, it has better sensing capabilities than a bipolar system. However, this makes the unipolar system more susceptible to electromagnetic interference (EMI) or stray electrical impulses from the heart itself or from the critical care environment such as intravenous infusion pumps that can adversely affect pacemaker function.[40]

### Pacing Routes

Several routes are available for temporary cardiac pacing. Permanent pacing is usually accomplished transvenously, although in situations in which a thoracotomy is otherwise indicated, such as cardiac surgery, the physician may elect to insert permanent epicardial pacing wires.

Transcutaneous cardiac pacing is enjoying a revival of sorts, after having been abandoned many years ago because of the painful muscle contractions and soft tissue burns it caused.[56] Transcutaneous cardiac pacing involves the use of two skin electrodes, one placed anteriorly and the other posteriorly on the chest, connected to an external pulse generator (Fig. 9-3). It is a rapid, noninvasive procedure that nurses can perform in the emergency setting and has been gaining in popularity since improved technology has helped to minimize the problems associated with it.

Transthoracic pacing is also an emergency procedure that involves the insertion of a pacing wire into the ventricle through a needle inserted through the chest wall. However, this is an invasive procedure associated with serious complications such as pneumothorax and cardiac tamponade.[2]

The insertion of temporary epicardial pacing wires has become a routine procedure during most cardiac surgical cases. Ventricular, and in many cases atrial, pacing wires are loosely sewn to the epicardium. The terminal pins of these wires are pulled through the skin before closing the chest. If both chambers have pacing wires attached, the atrial wires exit subcostally to the right of the sternum and the ventricular wires exit in the same region but to the left of the sternum.[30] These wires can be removed by gentle traction at the skin surface with minimal risk of bleeding.

Temporary transvenous endocardial pacing is accomplished by advancing a pacing electrode wire through a vein, often the subclavian or internal jugular, into the right atrium or right ventricle. Insertion can be facilitated either through direct visualization with fluoroscopy or by the use of the standard electrocardiogram. Electrode placement can be accomplished electrocardiographically by attaching the distal electrode of the pacing catheter to the V lead of a properly grounded ECG machine via an alligator clamp. With the limb leads attached and the lead selector switch set on V, the distal electrode serves as an exploring electrode that will display various intracardiac ECG patterns verifying proper advancement and placement of the electrode.

### Pacemaker Classification Code

In the 1960s, pacemaker terminology was limited to "fixed-rate" and "demand" pacing, followed by the introduction of "AV sequential" pacing in the early 1970s. Although these terms are still useful today for understanding pacemaker function (see the box below), the continued expansion of functional capabilities of pulse generators made it necessary to develop a more precise classification system. Therefore, in 1974, the Inter-Society Commission for Heart Disease (ICHD) adopted a three-letter code for describing the various pacing modalities available. The code was updated in 1981 by adding two more letters to include increased programming characteristics and antitachycardia functions.[55] (See Table 9-1 for revised five-letter code.)

However, this revised code is already becoming obsolete with the development of newer devices that are rate-responsive or that combine pacing and shocking capabilities.[7,14] The code is based on three categories, each represented by a letter. The first letter refers to the cardiac chamber that is paced. The second letter designates which chamber is sensed, while the third letter indicates the response to the sensed event. For example, a VVI pacemaker will pace the ventricle if the pacemaker fails to sense an

#### PACEMAKER TERMINOLOGY

**FIXED-RATE (ASYNCHRONOUS)**

Delivers a pacing stimulus at a set (fixed) rate regardless of the occurrence of spontaneous myocardial depolarizations.

**DEMAND (SYNCHRONOUS)**

Delivers a pacing stimulus only when the heart's intrinsic pacemaker fails to function at a predetermined rate; the pacing stimulus will either be inhibited or triggered into the QRS complex when the intrinsic pacemaker functions.

**AV SEQUENTIAL (DUAL-CHAMBER PACING)**

Delivers a pacing stimulus to both the atrium and ventricle in proper sequence with sufficient AV delay to permit adequate ventricular filling.

***Table 9-1*** ICHD classification code

| Chamber(s) paced | Chamber(s) sensed | Mode of response | Programmable functions | Antitachycardia function |
|---|---|---|---|---|
| V—ventricle | V—ventricle | T—triggered | P—programmable (rate and output) | B—bursts |
| A—atrium | A—atrium | I—inhibited | M—multiprogrammable | N—normal rate competition |
| D—double (both A and V) | D—double | D—double (ventricular inhibited; atrial triggered) | C—communicating | S—scanning |
| | O—none | O—none<br>R—reverse | O—none | E—external control<br>O—none |

From Parsonnet V, Furman S, and Smyth N: PACE 4:401, 1981.

intrinsic ventricular depolarization. However, sensing of a spontaneous ventricular depolarization will inhibit ventricular pacing. (See Table 9-2 for description of all types of pacemakers.)

### Pacemaker Settings

The controls on all external temporary pulse generators are similar, and their function should be thoroughly understood so that pacing can be initiated quickly in an emergency situation and troubleshooting can be facilitated should problems with the pacemaker arise.

**Rate.** The rate control (Fig. 9-4) regulates the number of impulses that can be delivered to the heart per minute. The rate setting will vary depending on the physiological needs of the patient, but in general will be maintained between 60 and 80 beats/min. Pacing rates for overdrive

***Table 9-2*** Descriptions of pulse generators

| Pulse generator | Description |
|---|---|
| AOO | Atrial fixed rate<br>Atrial pacing, no sensing |
| VOO | Ventricular fixed rate<br>Ventricular pacing, no sensing |
| DOO | AV sequential fixed rate<br>Atrial and ventricular pacing, no sensing |
| VVI | Ventricular demand<br>Ventricular pacing, ventricular sensing, inhibited response to sensing |
| VVT | Ventricular demand<br>Ventricular pacing, ventricular sensing, triggered response to sensing |
| AAI | Atrial demand<br>Atrial pacing, atrial sensing, inhibited response to sensing |
| AAT | Atrial demand<br>Atrial pacing, atrial sensing, triggered response to sensing |
| VAT | AV synchronous<br>Ventricular pacing, atrial sensing, triggered response to sensing (The ventricular pacing stimulus will fire at a set time following sensing of a spontaneous atrial depolarization.) |
| DVI | AV sequential<br>Atrial and ventricular pacing, ventricular sensing, inhibited response to sensing (Both atrial and ventricular pacing is inhibited if spontaneous ventricular depolarization is sensed; if no spontaneous ventricular activity is sensed, then the atrial and ventricle will be paced sequentially.) |
| VDD | Atrial synchronous, ventricular inhibited<br>Ventricular pacing, atrial and ventricular sensing, inhibited response to sensing in the ventricle and triggered response to sensing in the atrium |
| DDD | Universal<br>Both chambers are sensed and paced, inhibited response to sensing in the ventricle and triggered response to sensing in the atria |

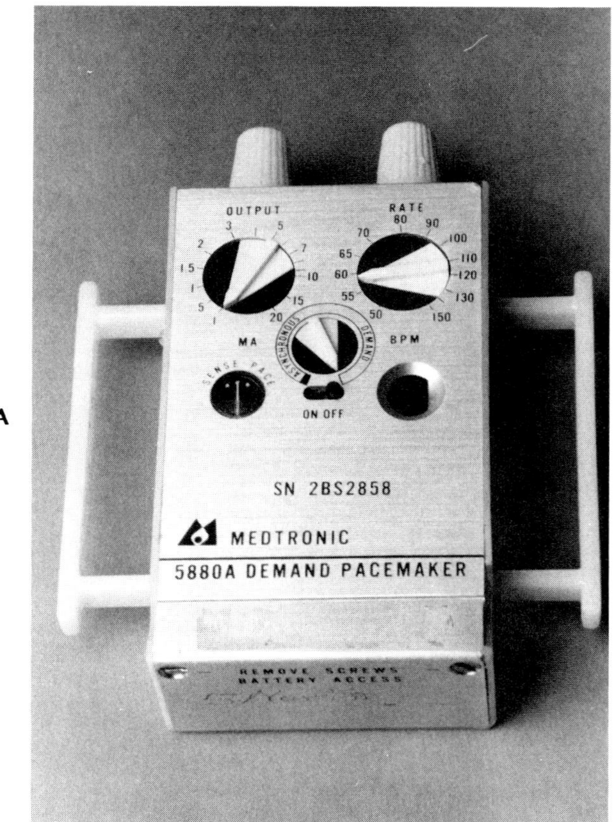


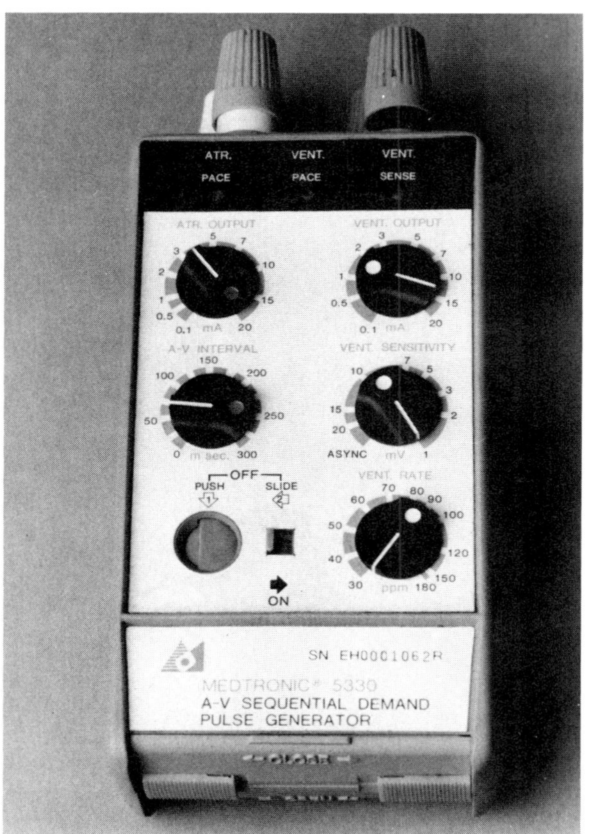


***Fig. 9-4*** External demand pulse generator **(A)** and AV sequential pulse generator **(B)**.

suppression of tachydysrhythmias may greatly exceed these values. If the pacemaker is operating in the AV sequential mode, the ventricular rate control will also regulate the atrial rate.

**Output.** The output dial regulates the amount of electrical current (measured in milliamperers or mA) that is delivered to the heart to initiate depolarization. The point at which depolarization occurs is termed *threshold* and is indicated by a myocardial response to the pacing stimulus (capture). Threshold can be determined by gradually decreasing the output from 20 mA until 1 : 1 capture is lost. The output setting is then slowly increased until 1 : 1 capture is reestablished; this threshold to pace should be less than 1.0 mA with a properly positioned pacing electrode. However, the output should be set two to three times higher than threshold, since thresholds tend to fluctuate. There will be separate output controls for both the atrium and the ventricle when an AV sequential pulse generator is utilized.

**Sensitivity.** The sensitivity control regulates the ability of the pacemaker to detect the heart's intrinsic electrical activity. If the sensitivity is turned all the way up, that is, a setting of 1 mV millivolts (mV), the pacemaker is maximally sensitive and will be able to respond to even low-amplitude electrical signals coming from the heart. On the other hand, turning the sensitivity all the way down (adjusting the dial to a setting of 20 mV or to area labeled "async") will result in the inability of the pacemaker to sense any intrinsic electrical activity and cause the pacemaker to function at a fixed rate. The sensitivity control is usually set at 6 mV. There is a sense indicator (often a light) on the pulse generator that will signal each time intrinsic cardiac electrical activity is sensed. A pulse generator may be designed to sense atrial or ventricular activity or both. The pacemaker's sensing ability is evaluated by observing for a change in pacing rhythm in response to spontaneous depolarizations. (See the section on pacemaker malfunctions for sensing problems.)

**AV interval.** The AV interval control (only available on AV sequential pacers) regulates the time interval between the atrial and ventricular pacing stimuli. Proper adjustment of this interval to between 150 to 250 msec preserves AV synchrony in order to maximize ventricular stroke volume and enhance cardiac output.

**On/off.** Finally, an on/off switch is provided with a safety feature that prevents the accidental termination of pacing.

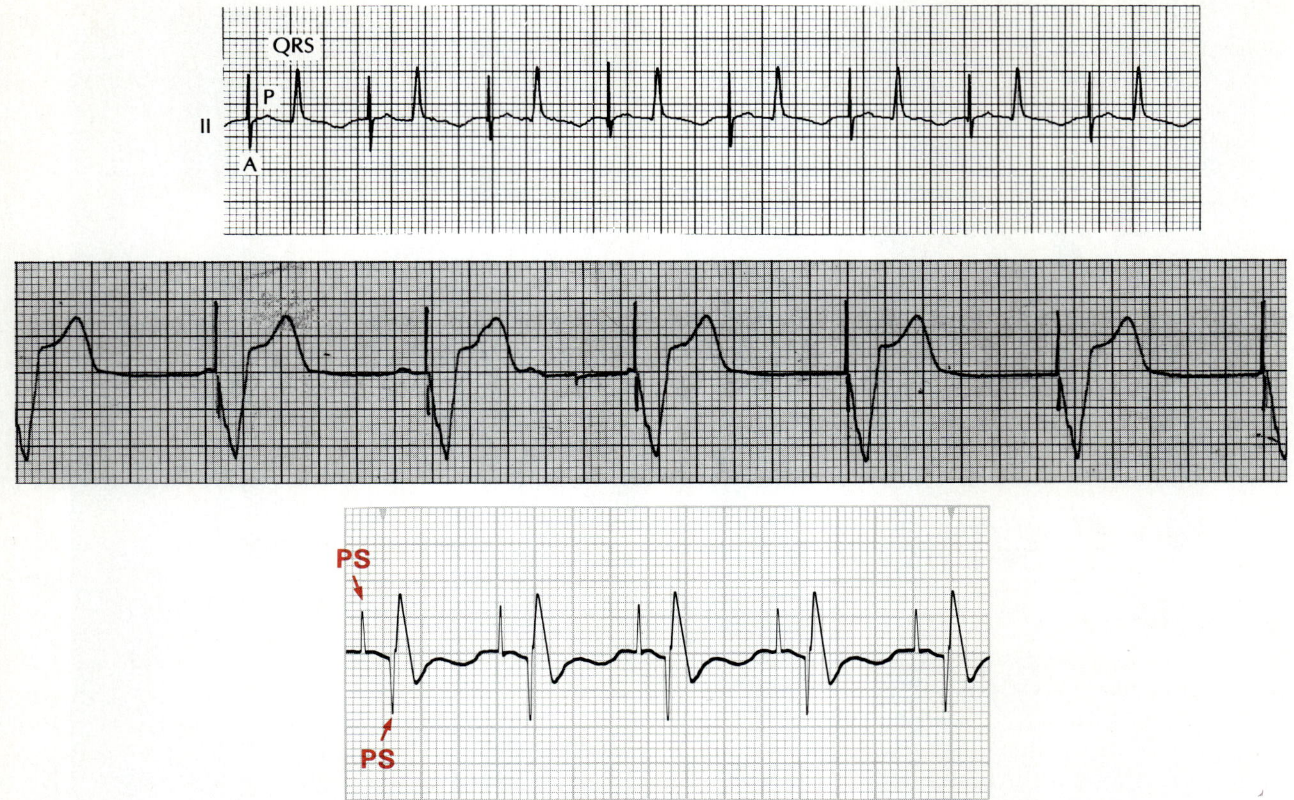


***Fig. 9-5*** **A,** Atrial pacing. **B,** Ventricular pacing. **C,** Dual chamber pacing. (**A** from Goldberger AL and Goldberger E: Clinical electrocardiography: a simplified approach, ed 4, St Louis, 1990, Mosby–Year Book, Inc. **B** from Conover MB: Understanding electrocardiography: arrhythmias and the 12-lead ECG, ed 5, St Louis, 1988, Mosby–Year Book, Inc. **C** from Huszar R: Basic dysrhythmias, ed 2, St Louis, 1991, Mosby–Year Book, Inc.)

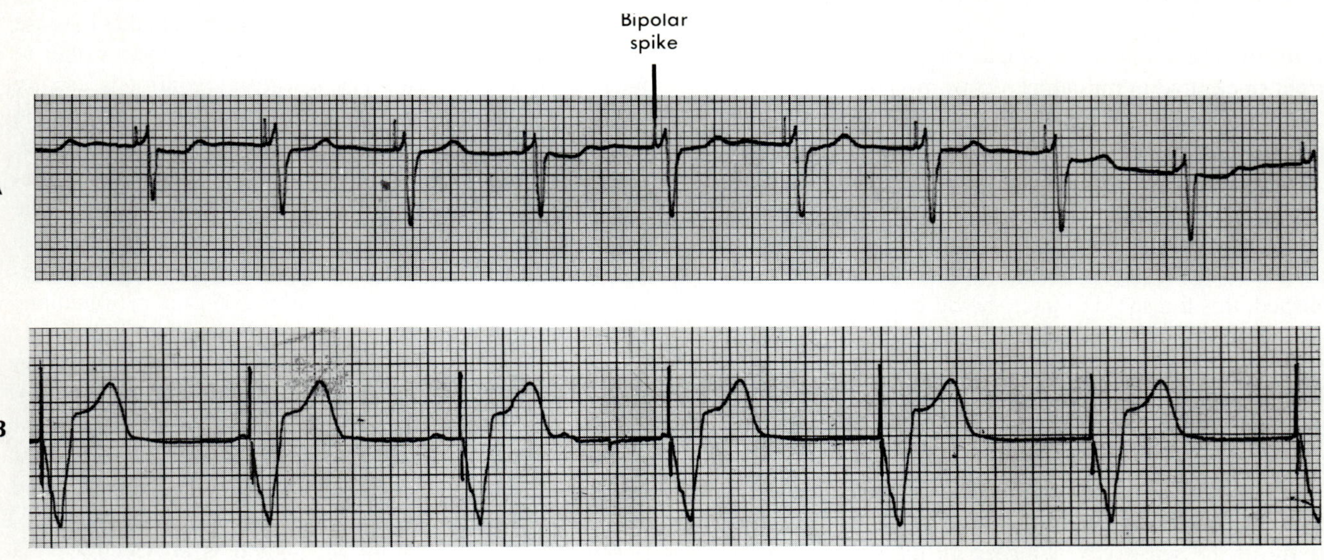


***Fig. 9-6*** **A,** Bipolar pacing artifact. **B,** Unipolar pacing artifact. (From Conover MB: Understanding electrocardiography, ed 5, St Louis, 1988, Mosby–Year Book, Inc.)

## Pacing Artifacts

All patients with temporary pacemakers should have continuous ECG monitoring. The **pacing artifact** is the spike that is seen on the ECG tracing as the pacing stimulus is delivered to the heart. A P wave should be visible following the pacing artifact if the atrium is being paced (Fig. 9-5, *A*). Similarly, a QRS complex should follow a ventricular pacing artifact (Fig. 9-5, *B*). A pacing artifact will precede both the P wave and the QRS complex with dual chamber pacing (Fig. 9-5, *C*).

Not all paced beats look alike. For example, the artifact produced by a unipolar pacing electrode is larger than that produced by a bipolar lead (Fig. 9-6). Furthermore, the QRS complex of paced beats will appear different, depending on the location of the pacing electrode. If the pacing electrode is positioned in the right ventricle, an LBBB pattern will be displayed on the ECG. On the other hand, an RBBB pattern will be visible if the pacing stimulus originates from the left ventricle.

## Pacemaker Malfunctions

The majority of pacemaker malfunctions can be broken down into abnormalities of either pacing or sensing.

Problems with pacing can involve the failure of the pacemaker to deliver the following: the pacing stimulus, a pacing stimulus that depolarizes the heart, or the correct number of pacing stimuli per minute.

Failure of the pacemaker to deliver the pacing stimulus will result in the disappearance of the pacing artifact, even though the patient's intrinsic rate is less than the set rate on the pacer (Fig. 9-7). This can occur either intermittently or continuously and can be attributed to failure of the pulse generator or its battery, a loose connection between the various components of the pacemaker system, broken lead wires, or stimulus inhibition as a result of **electromagnetic interference (EMI).** Tightening connections, replacing the batteries or the pulse generator itself, or removing the source of EMI may restore pacemaker function.

If the pacing stimulus fires but fails to initiate a myocardial depolarization, a pacing artifact will be present but will not be followed by the expected P wave or QRS complex, depending on the chamber being paced (Fig. 9-8). This "loss of capture" can most often be attributed to either displacement of the pacing electrode or to an increase in threshold (electrical stimulus necessary to elicit a myocardial depolarization) as a result of drugs, metabolic disorders, electrolyte imbalances, and fibrosis or myocardial ischemia at the site of electrode placement.[54] Repositioning the patient to the left side or increasing the output (mA) may elicit capture.

Pacing can also occur at inappropriate rates. For example, impending battery failure can result in a gradual decrease in paced rate or "rate drift." Another phenomenon, commonly referred to as **runaway pacemaker,** will result in firing of the pacemaker stimulus at rates greater than the set rate. This malfunction is universally caused by failure of the pulse generator's circuitry necessitating replacement.

Sensing abnormalities include both failure to sense and oversensing. Failure to sense is the inability of the pacemaker to sense spontaneous myocardial depolarizations. This will result in competition between paced complexes and the heart's intrinsic rhythm. This malfunction can be demonstrated on the ECG by pacing artifacts that follow too closely behind spontaneous QRS complexes (Fig. 9-9). "R on T" phenomenon is a real danger with this type of pacer aberration; therefore the nurse must act quickly to determine the cause. Often the cause can be attributed to inadequate wave amplitude (or height of the P or R wave). If this is the case, the situation can be promptly remedied by increasing the sensitivity (moving the sensitivity dial toward its lowest setting). Other possible causes include lead displacement or fracture, pulse generator failure, or EMI-precipitated asynchronous pacing.

Oversensing results from the inappropriate sensing of extraneous electrical signals leading to unnecessary triggering or inhibiting of stimulus output, depending on the pacer mode. The source of these electrical signals can range from the presence of tall, peaked T waves to EMI in the critical care environment. Since the majority of temporary pulse generators currently in use today are ventricular inhibited, oversensing will result in unexplained pauses in the ECG tracing as the extraneous signals are sensed and inhibit ventricular pacing. Often, simply moving the sensitivity dial toward 20 mV will stop the pauses.

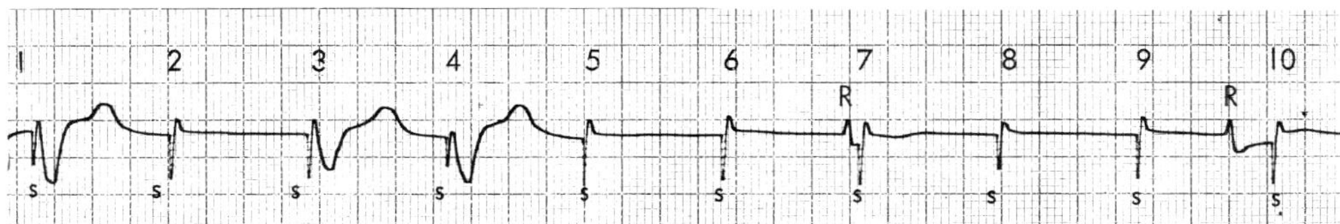


***Fig. 9-7*** Pacemaker malfunction: failure to pace. Notice that beats *1, 3,* and *4* show the pacemaker spikes *(s)* and normally paced QRS complexes and T waves. The remaining beats show only pacemaker spikes. *R* represents the patient's slow spontaneous QRS complexes. (From Goldberger E: Treatment of cardiac emergencies, ed 5, St Louis, 1990, Mosby–Year Book, Inc.)

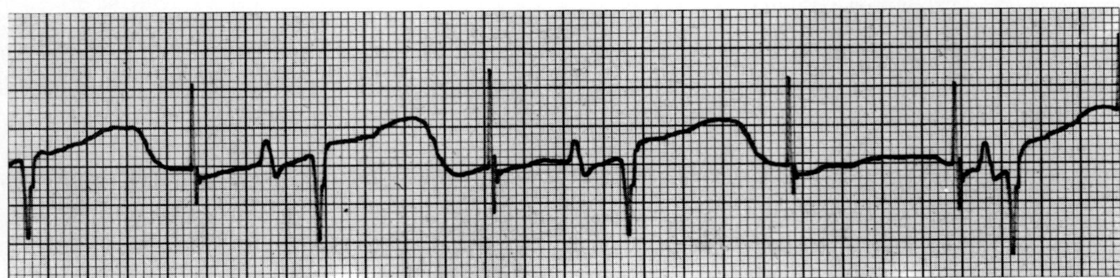

***Fig. 9-8*** Failure to capture. (From Conover MB: Understanding electrocardiography, ed 5, St Louis, 1988, Mosby–Year Book, Inc.)

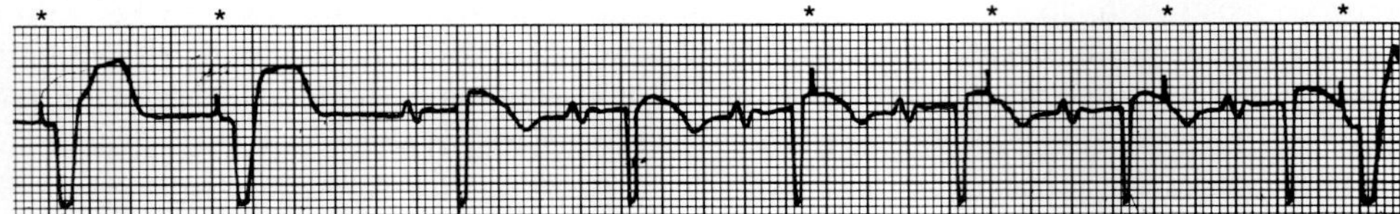

***Fig. 9-9*** Pacemaker malfunction: failure to sense. Notice that after the first two paced beats there is a series of sinus beats with first-degree AV block. Failure of the pacemaker unit to sense these intrinsic QRS complexes leads to inappropriate pacemaker spikes (*), which fall on T waves. Three of these spikes do not capture the ventricle because they occur during the refractory period of the cardiac cycle. (From Conover MH: Understanding electrocardiography, ed 5, St Louis, 1988, Mosby–Year Book, Inc.)

## Summary of Nursing Care

There are a myriad of nursing responsibilities associated with the care of a patient who has a temporary pacemaker, but four major areas should be emphasized: surveillance for complications, protection against microshock, prevention of pacemaker malfunction, and patient teaching. A summary of potential nursing diagnoses related to temporary pacemakers is found in the box on p. 201.

Infection at the lead insertion site is one complication associated with pacemakers. The site(s) should be carefully inspected for purulent drainage, erythema, or edema, and the patient should be monitored for signs of systemic infection. Although most infections remain localized, endocarditis can occur in patients with endocardial pacing leads. A less frequent complication associated with transvenous pacing is myocardial perforation, which can result in rhythmic hiccoughs or cardiac tamponade.

Because the pacing electrode is in intimate contact with the heart, special care must be taken while handling the external components of the pacing system to avoid conducting stray electrical current from other equipment. Even a small amount of stray current could precipitate a lethal tachycardia. The possibility of "microshock" can be minimized by wearing rubber gloves when handling the pacing wires and by properly insulating terminal pins of pacing wires when they are not in use. The latter can be accomplished either by using caps provided by the manufacturer or improvising with a needle cover or section of disposable rubber glove. The wires should then be taped securely to the patient's chest to avoid accidental electrode displacement. Additional safety measures include using a nonelectric or a properly grounded electric bed, keeping all electrical equipment away from the bed, and permitting the use of only rechargeable electric razors.[63]

Continuous ECG monitoring is essential to facilitate prompt recognition of and appropriate intervention for pacemaker malfunction. But there is much the nurse can do to prevent pacing abnormalities.

As previously mentioned, the temporary pacing lead and bridging cable should be properly secured to the body with tape to prevent the accidental displacement of the electrode, which can result in failure to pace or sense. The external pulse generator can be secured to the patient's waist with a strap or placed in a telemetry bag for the mobile patient. For the patient on bed rest, suspending the pulse generator with twill tape from an IV pole mounted overhead on the ceiling will not only prevent tension on the lead while moving the patient (given adequate length of bridging cable) but will also alleviate the possibility of accidental dropping of the pulse generator.

The nurse should be aware of all sources of EMI which, within the critical care environment, could interfere with the pacemaker's function. Sources of EMI in the clinical area include electrocautery, defibrillation current, radiation therapy, magnetic resonance imaging devices, and transcutaneous electrical nerve stimulation (TENS) units.[63] In

**Nursing Diagnosis and Management**

***Temporary pacemakers***

Decreased Cardiac Output risk factor atrioventricular heart block, p. 458

High Risk for Infection risk factor: invasive monitoring devices, p. 465

Knowledge Deficit: Position Restrictions related to lack of previous exposure to information, p. 441

Body Image Disturbance related to functional dependence on life-sustaining technology, p. 443

Self-Esteem Disturbance related to feelings of guilt over physical deterioration, p. 442

Powerlessness related to health care environment or illness-related regimen, p. 445

Anxiety related to threat to biological, psychological, and/or social integrity, p. 448

most cases, if EMI is suspected of precipitating pacemaker malfunction, converting to the asynchronous mode (fixed-rate) will maintain pacing until the cause of the EMI can be removed. If the patient requires defibrillation, the pulse generator should be temporarily turned off during delivery of the shock to prevent possible damage to the pacemaker circuitry.

Finally, the nurse should inspect for loose connections between lead and pulse generator on a regular basis. In addition, there should always be replacement batteries and pulse generators available on the unit. Although the battery has an anticipated life span of 1 month, it is probably sound practice to change the battery if the pacemaker has been operating continually for several days. The pulse generator should always be labeled with the date that the battery was replaced.

Patient teaching for the client with a temporary pacemaker should emphasize the same areas of prevention that the nurse must address in her or his care. The patient should be instructed not to handle any exposed portion of the lead wire and to notify the nurse should the dressing over the insertion site become soiled or dislodged. The patient should also be advised not to use any electric devices brought in from home that could interfere with pacemaker functioning. Furthermore, patients with temporary transvenous pacemakers need to be taught to restrict movement of the affected extremity to prevent lead displacement.

## CARDIAC SURGERY

The nursing care of the cardiac surgical patient is a demanding yet exciting job requiring the talents of an experienced team of critical care nurses. The following discussion introduces basic cardiac surgical techniques and principles of cardiopulmonary bypass and highlights the key points about postoperative care of the adult patient who requires either valve replacement or coronary revascularization.

### Coronary Artery Bypass Surgery

Myocardial revascularization involves the use of a conduit or channel designed to bypass an occluded coronary artery. Currently, the two most successful conduits are the saphenous vein graft (SVG) and the internal mammary artery (IMA) graft.[38] SVG involves the anastomosis of an excised portion of the saphenous vein proximally to the aorta and distally to the coronary artery below the obstruction (Fig. 9-10). The IMA, which remains attached to its origin at the subclavian artery, is swung down and anastomosed distally to the coronary artery (Fig. 9-11). Although only recently introduced, the IMA graft is gaining in popularity because it has demonstrated both short-term and long-term patency rates superior to those of the SVG.[45]

### Valvular Surgery

Valvular disease results in various hemodynamic dysfunctions that can usually be managed medically so long as the patient remains asymptomatic. There is reluctance to surgically intervene early in the course of the disease because of the surgical risks and long-term complications associated with prosthetic valve replacement. However, this must be weighed against the possibility of irreversible deterioration in left ventricular function that may develop during the compensated asymptomatic phase.

There are two categories of prosthetic valves: mechanical and biological or tissue valves. Mechanical valves are made from combinations of metal alloys, pyrolite carbon, and dacron (Fig. 9-12). Their construction renders them highly durable, but all patients will require anticoagulation to reduce the incidence of thromboembolism. The biological or tissue valves, usually constructed from animal or human cardiac tissue, offer the patient freedom from therapeutic anticoagulation as a result of their low thrombogenicity (Fig. 9-13). However, their durability is limited by their tendency toward early calcification. (See the box on p. 202 for a description of various valvular prostheses.)

The choice of a valvular prosthesis depends on many factors. For example, because mechanical valves are more durable, they may be chosen over a tissue valve for a young person who has a relatively long life span ahead. Similarly, a bioprosthesis may be chosen for an older patient (older than 65 years of age), because although the valve has a reduced longevity, the patient has a decreased life expectancy. For patients with medical contraindications to anticoagulation or patients whose past compliance with drug therapy has been questionable, a tissue valve should be selected. Technical considerations such as the size of the annulus (or anatomic ring in which the valve sits) can also influence the choice of valve (a bioprosthesis may be too big for a small aortic root).[8]

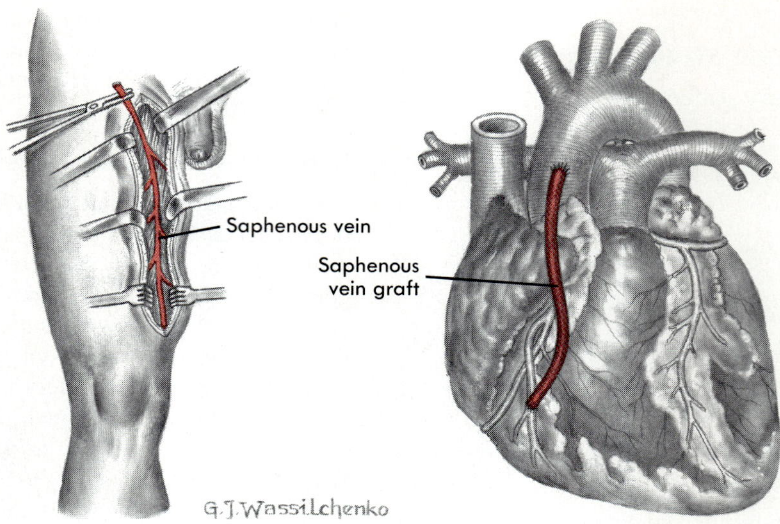


***Fig. 9-10*** Saphenous vein graft.

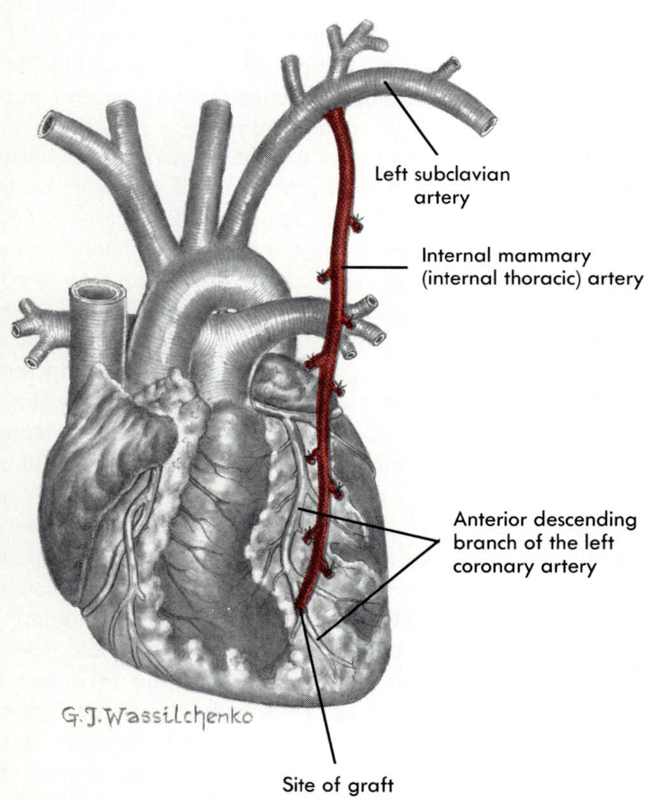


***Fig. 9-11*** Internal mammary vein graft.

## CLASSIFICATION OF PROSTHETIC CARDIAC VALVES

### MECHANICAL VALVES

Tilting-disk: a free-floating lens-shaped disk mounted onto a circular sewing ring
- Bjork-Shiley
- Omniscience (Lillehei-Kaster)
- Medtronic-Hall (Hall-Kaster)

Caged-ball: a ball moves freely within a three- or four-sided metallic cage mounted on a circular sewing ring
- Starr-Edwards

Bileaflet: two semicircular leaflets, mounted on a circular sewing ring, that open centrally
- St. Jude Medical

### BIOLOGICAL TISSUE VALVES (BIOPROSTHESES)

Porcine heterograft: a porcine aortic valve mounted on a semiflexible stent and preserved with glutaraldehyde
- Hancock
- Carpentier-Edwards

Bovine pericardial heterograft: bovine pericardium fashioned into three identical cusps that are then mounted on a cloth-covered frame
- Ionescu-Shiley

Homograft: a human heart valve (aortic or pulmonic) harvested from a donated heart and cryopreserved; may or may not be mounted on a support ring

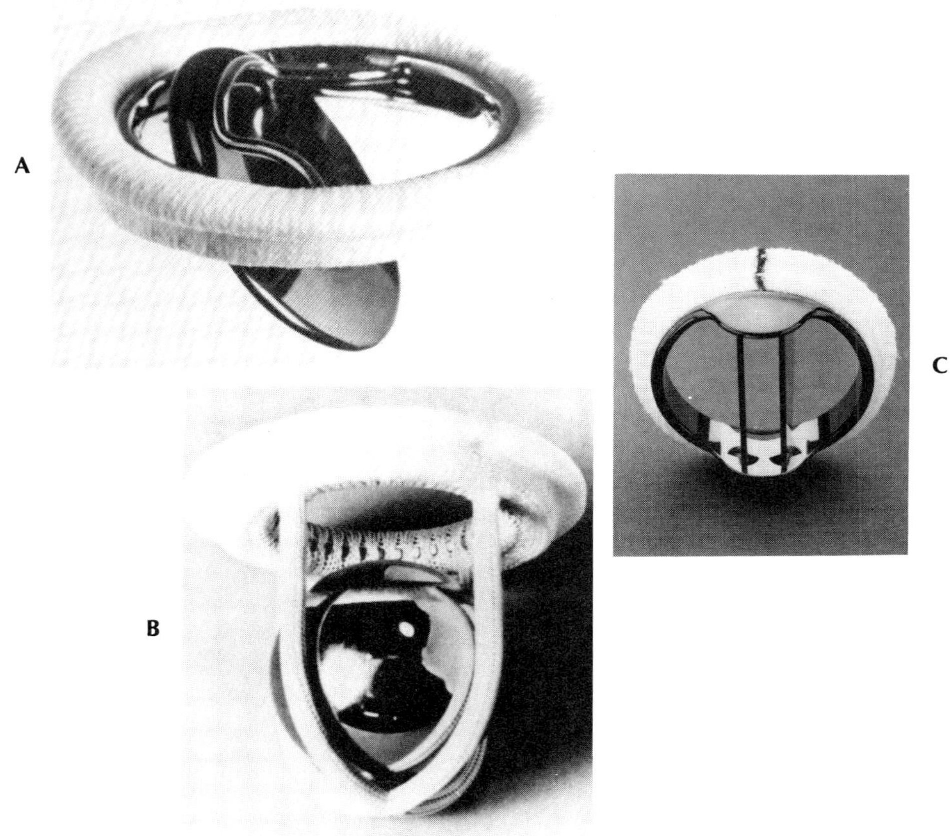


***Fig. 9-12*** **A,** The Bjork-Shiley tilting disc valve with pyrolytic-carbon disc, stellite cage, and Teflon cloth sewing ring. The valve opens to 60 degrees. **B,** Starr-Edwards caged-ball valve model 6320 with completely cloth-covered stellite cage and hollow stellite ball with specific gravity close to that of blood. **C,** The St. Jude medical heart valve, a mechanical central flow disc. (**A** and **B** from Eagle K and others: The practice of cardiology, ed 2, Boston, 1989, Little Brown & Co. **C** courtesy St. Jude Medical, Inc., St. Paul, Minn.)

## Cardiopulmonary Bypass

**Cardiopulmonary bypass (CPB)** is a mechanical means of circulating and oxygenating a patient's blood while diverting most of the circulation from the heart and lungs during cardiac surgical procedures.[83] The extracorporeal circuit consists of cannulas that drain off venous blood, an oxygenator that oxygenates the blood by one of several methods, and a pump head that pumps the arterialized blood back to the aorta through a single cannula. The patient is systemically heparinized before initiation of bypass to prevent clotting within the bypass circuit.

Systemic hypothermia during bypass can reduce tissue oxygen requirements to 50% of normal, which affords the major organs additional protection from ischemic injury.[83] Lowering the body temperature to about 28° C (82.4° F) is accomplished through a heat exchanger incorporated into the pump. The blood is warmed back up to normal body temperature before bypass is discontinued.

The technique of hemodilution is also used to enhance tissue oxygenation by improving blood flow through the systemic and pulmonary microcirculation during bypass. Hemodilution refers to the dilution of autologous (patient's own) blood with the isotonic crystalloid solution used to prime the pump. Capillary perfusion is enhanced by hemodilution, because the reduced viscosity (stickiness) of the blood decreases both resistance to flow through the capillaries and the possibility of microthrombi formation. At the completion of CPB, the large quantities of "pump blood" that remain in the bypass circuit can be collected and used for initial postoperative volume replacement.

## Postoperative Management

Postoperative management of the cardiovascular surgery patient is focused on six areas: cardiovascular support, control of bleeding, pulmonary care, control of neurological complications, prevention of infection, and renal involvement (refer to the box on p. 204).

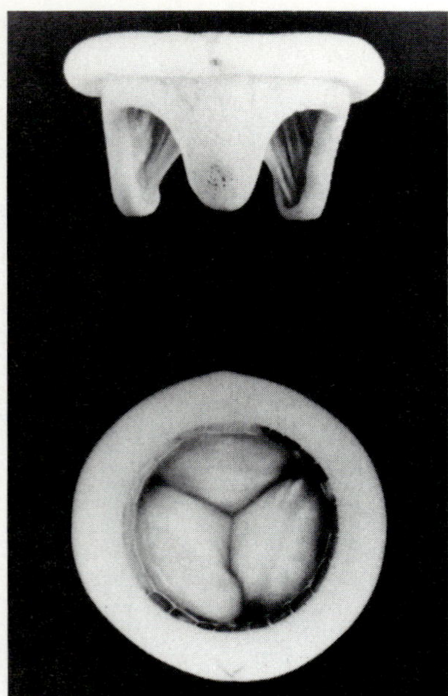

***Fig. 9-13*** Hancock II porcine aortic valve is chemically treated to retard calcification. The flexible Delrin stent and sewing ring are covered in Dacron cloth. (From Eagle K and others: The practice of cardiology, ed 2, Boston, 1989, Little Brown & Co.)

### Summary of Nursing Care

Nursing diagnoses and mangement for the post–open heart surgery patient are summarized in the box on p. 205.

Hypothermia can contribute to depressed myocardial contractility in the cardiac surgical patient. While hyperthermia blankets are used to warm the patient, care should be taken to remove the blankets promptly when the temperature reaches 98.4° F to prevent subsequent excessive temperature elevations.[59]

Chest tube stripping, done to maintain patency of the tubes, is controversial because the high negative pressure generated by routine methods of stripping is believed to result in tissue damage that can contribute to bleeding.[32] However, this risk must be carefully weighed against the very real danger of cardiac tamponade if blood is not effectively drained from around the heart. Therefore chest tube stripping is frequently advocated in instances of postoperative bleeding. However, the technique of milking the chest tubes may be advisable for routine postoperative care because this technique generates less negative pressure and decreases the risk of bleeding.[32]

Patients and family members need to be reassured that postcardiotomy psychosis is a temporary phenomenon that will resolve quickly. Meanwhile, every effort should be made to keep the patient informed of all that is going on in the surroundings so that unfamiliar sights, sounds, and smells are not overwhelming and confusing. Painful stimuli should be kept to a minimum, and meaningful stimuli such as touching should be encouraged. Nursing care should be organized to maximize optimal sleep patterns.

#### POSTOPERATIVE MANAGEMENT OF THE CARDIOVASCULAR SURGERY PATIENT

**CARDIOVASCULAR SUPPORT**

Treatment of low cardiac output resulting from preexisting heart disease, prolonged pump time, and/or inadequate myocardial protection:

1. Regulate heart rate via temporary pacing or drug therapy.
2. Enhance preload via administration of volume, i.e., colloid or PRBCs.
3. Decrease afterload via vasodilator therapy.
4. Enhance contractility via positive inotropic support.
5. Institute intraaortic balloon pumping if unresponsive to drug therapy.

**CONTROL OF BLEEDING**

Treatment of bleeding from the mediastinal tubes caused by inadequate hemostasis, disruption of suture lines, or coagulapathy associated with CPB:

1. Administer clotting factors, i.e., fresh-frozen plasma, platelets.
2. Administer protamine.
3. Replace blood loss.
4. Prophylactic use of positive end-expiratory pressure.
5. Rewarm patient.

**PULMONARY CARE**

Atelectasis and pleural effusions may be eliminated or diminished by intubation for at least 1 night after surgery; patients with underlying pulmonary disease may require longer periods of ventilatory support.

**CONTROL OF NEUROLOGICAL COMPLICATIONS**

Transient neurological dysfunction attributed to decreased cerebral perfusion and cerebral microemboli related to the pump run; postcardiotomy psychosis will be treated according to the severity of the dysfunction.

**PREVENTION OF INFECTION**

Persistent elevations above 101° F should be investigated and treated accordingly.

**RENAL INVOLVEMENT**

Low urine output (less than 25-30 ml/hr) and "pink-tinged" urine, which may be the result of homolysis during CPB, may be treated with furosemide (Lasix).

### Recent Advances in Cardiac Surgery

Malignant ventricular dysrhythmias, the major culprit in sudden cardiac death, can now be managed surgically when drug therapy has been unsuccessful or has produced intol-

## Nursing Diagnosis and Management

***Status post–open heart surgery***


Decreased Cardiac Output related to hemopericardium secondary to open heart surgery, p. 458

Decreased Cardiac Output related to supraventricular tachycardia, p. 456

Decreased Cardiac Output related to atrioventricular heart block, p. 458

Decreased Cardiac Output related to ventricular tachycardia, p. 460

Decreased Cardiac Output related to decreased preload secondary to mechanical ventilation with or without PEEP, p. 457

Decreased Cardiac Output related to relative excess of preload and afterload secondary to impaired ventricular contractility, p. 457

Fluid Volume Deficit related to active blood loss, p. 495

High Risk for Altered Peripheral Tissue Perfusion risk factor: vasopressor therapy, p. 462

High Risk for Aspiration risk factors: endotracheal tube, gastrointestinal tube, depressed cough and gag reflexes secondary to anesthesia, decreased gasrointestinal motility secondary to an anesthesia, situation hindering elevation of upper body, p. 476

Ineffective Airway Clearance related to impaired cough secondary to loss of glottic closure with cuffed endotracheal tube, p. 468

Ineffective Airway Clearance related to thoracic pain, p. 469

Ineffective Breathing Pattern related to thoracic pain, p. 472

Acute Pain related to transmission and perception of noxious stimuli secondary to leg and/or sternotomy incision, p. 485

High Risk for Infection risk factor: invasive monitoring devices, p. 465

Activity Intolerance related to postural hypotension secondary to immobility, narcotics, vasodilator therapy, p. 463

Sensory-Perceptual Alterations related to sensory overload, sensory deprivation, sleep pattern disturbance, p. 489

Sleep Pattern Disturbance related to circadian desynchronization, p. 455

Knowledge Deficit: Postoperative Exercise Regimen, Fluid Restrictions, Medication, Wound Care, Reportable Symptoms related to lack of previous exposure to information, p. 441

Body Image Disturbance related to actual change in body structure, function, and appearance, p. 443

Altered Sexuality Patterns related to fear of death during coitus secondary to myocardial infarction, p. 453


erable side effects.[28] The origin of the dysrhythmia is first located with specialized pacing electrodes during the open chest procedure (referred to as intraoperative endocardial mapping). The offending area of endocardium is then either excised or eliminated by cryosurgery. If the ventricular tachydysrhythmia is not amenable to surgical ablation, an automatic implantable cardioverter-defibrillator (AICD) can be implanted. The AICD is a pulse generator capable of identifying and terminating life-threatening ventricular dysrhythmias by countershocking the heart with electrodes that have been surgically placed.[48] The immediate postoperative care is very similar to that given any cardiac surgery patient. Currently a new device is being tested clinically that incorporates bradycardia backup and antitachycardia pacing capabilities.

Coronary endarterectomy is currently enjoying a modest revival as an adjunct to bypass procedures in patients with diffuse or small vessel disease.[38] Laser technology has paved the way for investigation into intraoperative coronary laser recanalization. The introduction of heart transplantation has generated much excitement and anticipation for patients who suffer from otherwise untreatable heart disease.

Although future trends in the surgical management of cardiac disease are difficult to predict, the critical care nurse must continue to be prepared to meet the challenge of providing a high level of nursing care at the bedside. A solid knowledge base and keen assessment skills are prerequisite for the accurate anticipation of problems and prompt intervention necessary to stabilize the patient and prevent the occurrence of life-threatening complications.

## PERCUTANEOUS TRANSLUMINAL CORONARY ANGIOPLASTY

**Percutaneous transluminal coronary angioplasty (PTCA)** involves the use of a balloon-tipped catheter that when advanced through an atherosclerotic coronary lesion (atheroma) can be intermittently inflated for the purpose of dilating the stenotic area and improving blood flow through it (Fig. 9-14). The mechanism of dilation was originally thought to be plaque compression that resulted in the im-

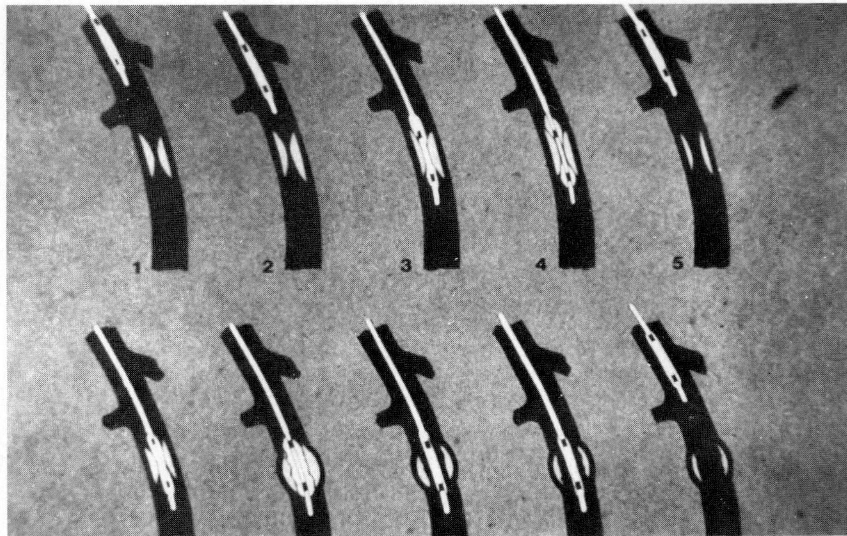


***Fig. 9-14*** Balloon compression of an atherosclerotic lesion. (From Kinney M and others: Comprehensive cardiac care, ed 7, St Louis, 1991, Mosby—Year Book, Inc.)

mediate expression of plaque contents or its redistribution within the vessel wall. However, it is now believed that the stretching of the vessel wall as a result of high balloon inflation pressures results in fracture of the plaque that enlarges the vessel lumen.[82] PTCA provides an alternative to both traditional medical management of atherosclerotic heart disease and coronary artery bypass surgery, as well as a valuable adjunct to thrombolytic therapy in terms of reducing a severe stenosis that persists following thrombolysis.[85] Indications for PTCA are summarized in the box on p. 207.

### Procedure

PTCA is performed in the cardiac catheterization laboratory by means of fluoroscopy. Introducer sheaths are commonly inserted percutaneously into the femoral artery and vein. The venous sheath can be used to perform a right heart catheterization with a Swan-Ganz catheter and/or to insert a pacing catheter.

The patient is systemically heparinized to prevent clots from forming on or in any of the catheters. A special guiding catheter designed to engage the coronary ostia is inserted through the arterial sheath and advanced in retrograde manner through the aorta. Nitroglycerin or calcium channel blockers may be given at this time to prevent coronary artery spasm and maximize coronary vasodilation during the procedure. A guidewire is then advanced down the coronary artery and negotiated across the occluding atheroma. The balloon catheter is advanced over this guidewire and positioned across the lesion. The balloon is inflated and deflated repetitively (each inflation not to exceed 90 seconds) until evidence of dilation is demonstrated on angiogram.[43]

The patient is transferred to the coronary care unit for overnight care and observation. The introducer sheaths are left in place for several reasons. First, the intravenous infusion of heparin is continued for 6 to 24 hours following PTCA to prevent clot formation on the roughened endothelium at the site of dilation.[43,82] Therefore removal of the sheaths during this time would predispose to bleeding. Second, it allows for rapid vascular access should redilation become necessary. However, the arterial sheath must be attached to a continuous heparinized saline flush, and intravenous fluids must be infused through the venous sheath to maintain luminal patency. If the patient's postangioplasty course is uneventful, the sheaths are usually removed within 24 hours.

### Complications

As stated earlier, serious complications can result from angioplasty that will necessitate emergency CABG surgery. These complications include persistent coronary artery spasm, myocardial infarction, and acute coronary occlusion.[16] Other complications that can occur in the period immediately after angioplasty include bleeding and hematoma formation at the site of vascular cannulation, compromised blood flow to the involved extremity, allergic reaction to radiopaque contrast dye, dysrhythmias, and vasovagal response (hypotension, bradycardia, and diaphoresis) during manipulation or removal of introducer sheaths. Restenosis can occur up to 6 months after angioplasty; however, this late complication is typically amenable to repeat angioplasty. The mechanism involved in restenosis may be related to platelet deposition and thrombus formation.[43] For this reason, patients are started on a regimen of antiplatelet drugs, for example, a combination of aspirin and dipyridamole.

Coronary atherectomy, laser angioplasty, and placement

**INDICATIONS FOR PTCA**

Multiple vessel disease
Characteristics of the lesion
  Concentric*/eccentric
  Noncalcified*/calcified
  Proximal*/distal
  Partial*/total occlusions
  Discrete*/diffuse
Angina
  Chronic stable
  Angina after CABG
  Recent onset/postinfarct unstable
  With MI alone/with thrombolytic therapy
Aysmptomatic with positive treadmill test
Must be a candidate for CABG
Partial occlusions of SV or IMA grafts

*Higher probability of success

of coronary stent prosthesis are new interventional technologies developed to address the problems of acute closure and restenosis associated with PTCA.[78] *Atherectomy* is the excision and removal of the atherosclerotic plaque by cutting, shaving, or grinding with specialized coronary catheters to achieve a more controlled mechanism of injury which, it is hoped, is less prone to complications. Laser plaque ablation in coronary arteries is currently in clinical trials.[70] During *laser balloon angioplasty,* heat and pressure are applied simultaneously to the coronary wall to create a less thrombogenic surface and to "weld" together the fractured intimal segment. Another major coronary technology that has recently evolved is the *coronary stent prosthesis.* This is a self-expanding stent that is introduced into the cornary artery over a guidewire in a region that has been previously dilated with PTCA to prevent acute closure and restenosis.[66]

### Summary of Nursing Care

The nursing care of the patient following angioplasty focuses on accurate assessment and prompt intervention. The nurse is in the unique position at the bedside to continuously monitor for signs of potential problems and take quick and appropriate action to minimize the deleterious effects of complications related to angioplasty.

It is essential that the nurse assess the patient for recurrent angina. Angina during angioplasty is an expected occurrence at the time of balloon inflation. It is a result of the temporary interruption of blood flow through the involved artery. However, it should subside with deflation or removal of the balloon and/or the administration of nitroglycerin. Angina following PTCA may be a result of transient coronary vasospasm or it may herald a more serious complication. In any case, the nurse must act quickly to assess for signs and symptoms of myocardial ischemia and initiate appropriate interventions as indicated.

Bleeding or hematoma at the sheath insertion site may occur while the sheath is in place or after its removal as a result of the effects of heparin. The nurse must monitor for bleeding or swelling at the puncture site as well as frequently assess for adequacy of circulation to the involved extremity. The nurse should also assess the patient for back pains, which might indicate retroperitoneal bleeding from oozing puncture sites. The patient should be instructed to keep the involved leg straight and not to elevate the head of the bed any more than 45 degrees while the sheath is in place (to prevent dislodgement) and for several hours after its removal (to prevent bleeding). Use of an eggcrate mattress may help alleviate the lower back pain experienced by many patients while immobile after undergoing PTCA.[6] Following sheath removal, direct pressure should be applied to the puncture site for 15 to 30 minutes; a sandbag may be ordered if the former is inadequate for hemostasis. Patients are usually allowed to resume ambulation 6 to 8 hours later, depending on institutional protocol.

Typically, patients undergoing elective angioplasty are hospitalized for only a few days. Because PTCA is only a palliative procedure, these patients need education in risk factor modification. Because of abbreviated hospital stay, the nurse often has insufficient time to do more than identify the offending risk factors and initiate basic instruction. Patients should be referred to local cardiac rehabilitation centers for more extensive teaching and follow-up to facilitate understanding and compliance with the therapeutic regimen.

Another teaching need that must be addressed is the patient's knowledge deficit related to discharge medications. It is essential that the patient clearly understand the rationale for therapy as well as potential side effects of each drug.

## THROMBOLYTIC THERAPY

Thrombolytic therapy offers a promising new approach for the patient experiencing acute myocardial infarction (AMI). Before the introduction of streptokinase as a thrombolytic agent, the medical management of AMI focused on decreasing myocardial oxygen demands in an effort to minimize myocardial necrosis and thus preserve ventricular function. Recently, however, efforts to limit the size of infarction have been directed toward the timely reperfusion of the jeopardized myocardium. The use of thrombolytic therapy to accomplish this is predicated on the prevailing theory that the terminal event in the majority of transmural infarctions is a fresh thrombus superimposed on a high-grade coronary lesion.[57] The administration of a thrombolytic agent will result in the lysis of the acute thrombus, thus recanalizing the obstructed coronary artery and restoring blood flow to the affected myocardium.

### Thrombolytic Agents

**Streptokinase. Streptokinase (SK)** is a thrombolytic agent derived from beta-hemolytic streptococci, which, when combined with plasminogen, catalyzes the conversion of plasminogen to plasmin, the enzyme responsible for clot dissolution in the body.[67] SK can be administered either intravenously or by an intracoronary approach necessitating cardiac catheterization. The efficacy of both routes has been established, and both have been used in clinical practice.[77] However, because of the significant lag time between onset of symptoms and the initiation of intracoronary SK, the intracoronary route is now considered obsolete.[11,77,85]

The three major problems associated with the use of SK are its systemic lytic effects coupled with a long half-life, its potential antigenic effects if readministered, and hypotension. Because the anticoagulant action of streptokinase is indiscriminate (non-clot specific) and prolonged (half-life 10 to 18 minutes), bleeding is a common complication that should be carefully monitored for during the 12 hours immediately following administration.[85] In addition, because streptokinase is a bacterial protein, it is strongly antigenic and can produce a variety of allergic reactions, including anaphylaxis, especially when administered to a patient who has either received SK therapy previously or had a recent streptococcal infection.

**Urokinase. Urokinase (UK)** is an enzymatic protein secreted by the parenchyma of the human kidney. Its thrombolytic effect results from the direct activation of plasminogen to form plasmin. This differs from streptokinase, which must first form a complex with plasminogen to activate plasmin to dissolve the clot.[67] UK is also non-clot-specific (activates circulating, non-clot-bound plasminogen as well as clot-bound plasminogen) but has a shorter half-life than SK.[85] Although a systemic lytic state may also be produced, its administration is associated with fewer bleeding complications.[60] Because urokinase is produced by the kidney, it is nonantigenic and thus well suited for use if subsequent thrombolytic therapy is indicated. However, it is currently difficult and expensive to produce and only approved for intracoronary administration in the treatment of AMI, precluding extensive clinical use.

**Tissue plasminogen activator.** A promising advance in thrombolytic therapy was the introduction of **tissue plasminogen activator (t-PA).**[67] Marketed under the name Activase, t-PA is a naturally occurring enzyme (thus nonantigenic) that is clot specific and has a very short half-life (3 to 5 minutes).[42] It converts plasminogen to plasmin after binding to the fibrin-containing clot. This clot specificity results in an increased concentration and activity of plasmin at the site of the clot where it is needed.[11] It was hoped that this characteristic of t-PA would prevent the induction of a systemic lytic state that occurs with SK therapy. However, the results of recent studies comparing the adverse effects of SK and t-PA show similar incidences of bleeding following administration.[75] Nonetheless, the intravenous administration of t-PA appears to be superior to intravenous streptokinase in terms of efficacy (recanalization of the affected coronary artery).[42]

**Anisoylated plasminogen streptokinase activator complex (APSAC). Anisoylated plasminogen streptokinase activator complex (APSAC, Eminase)** is the newest thrombolytic agent approved by the FDA (February, 1990) for use in the treatment of acute myocardial infarction. Often referred to as a second generation streptokinase, it has certain advantages over SK specifically related to duration of action, ease of administration, and fibrin selectivity.[41,65] Compared with SK, the duration of action has been quadrupled and the time of administration has been reduced from 60 minutes to 2 to 5 minutes.[65] In addition, it is administered in an inactive form resistant to neutralization by plasmin inactivators. So although it is a non–clot specific agent, there is enhanced binding to fibrin clots before activation due to its unique molecular structure.[41] Disadvantages include the induction of allergic reactions and hypotension similar to those seen with the use of SK. However, there is evidence to suggest the lytic state produced by APSAC and the other non–clot specific agents (UK, SK) may account for the reduced tendency for rethrombosis sometimes seen after thrombolytic therapy.[64]APSAC is a promising therapeutic alternative which, along with SK and tPA, is well suited for thrombolytic therapy.

## Eligibility Criteria

Certain criteria have been developed, based on research findings, to determine the patient population that would most likely benefit from the administration of thrombolytic therapy. In general, patients with recent onset of chest pain (less than 6 hours' duration) may be selected to receive thrombolytic therapy. Research suggests that the earlier the treatment is instituted, the higher the likelihood of successful reperfusion.[37] However, a recent study demonstrated a reduction in mortality rate even when thrombolytic therapy was begun between 6 to 24 hours after onset of chest pain.[33]

Patients with persistent ST segment elevation despite sublingual nitroglycerin or nifedipine, indicative of impending transmural infarction, are considered candidates for therapy. Patients with abnormal Q waves should not be excluded from therapy, because it is not necessarily evidence of a completed infarction.

Other common criteria for the use of thrombolytic therapy are included in the box below.

### SELECTION CRITERIA

- Less than 6 hours from onset of chest pain
- ST segment elevation on ECG
- Ischemic chest pain of 30 minutes' duration
- Chest pain unresponsive to sublingual nitroglycerine or nifedipine
- Less than 76 years of age
- No conditions that might predispose to hemorrhage

### Evidence of Reperfusion

Several phenomenon can be observed following the reperfusion of an artery that has been completely occluded by a thrombus. Initially, there is an abrupt cessation of ischemic chest pain as blood flow is restored. Another reliable indicator of reperfusion is the appearance of various "reperfusion" dysrhythmias. Accelerated idioventricular rhythm (AIVR) is the most common reperfusion dysrhythmia, but premature ventricular contractions, bradycardias, heart block, ventricular tachycardia, and, rarely, ventricular fibrillation may also occur.[72] The reason for the occurrence of these dysrhythmias remains unclear. However, vigilant monitoring of the patient's ECG is essential because a stable condition may rapidly deteriorate when recanalization occurs, and dysrhythmias should be treated appropriately.

Another noninvasive marker of recanalization is the rapid resolution of the previously elevated S-T segments indicating restoration of blood flow to previously ischemic myocardial tissue. For this reason, a monitoring lead should be chosen that clearly demonstrates ST elevation before the initiation of therapy.[12]

The serum concentration of creatine kinase (formerly creatine phosphokinase) rises rapidly and markedly following reperfusion of the ischemic myocardium.[11] This phenomenon is termed "washout," because it is thought to be a result of the rapid readmission into the circulation of creatine kinase, an enzyme released by damaged myocardial cells, following restoration of blood flow to previously unperfused areas of the heart.

Recognition of these noninvasive markers of recanalization is essential for documenting the patient's response to thrombolytic therapy.

### Administration

**Streptokinase.** Intravenous streptokinase, although not as effective in terms of recanalization as intracoronary streptokinase, has the advantage of being more practical in that it can be administered more rapidly following the onset of symptoms.[60] Therefore SK is now routinely administered intravenously (even though this route of administration has not yet been approved by the Food and Drug Administration). The recommended dosage is 1,500,000 IU of streptokinase administered intravenously over 30 to 60 minutes to achieve clot lysis. The patient is then heparinized to prevent early rethrombosis.

**Tissue plasminogen activator.** Tissue plasminogen activator was approved specifically for intravenous administration. The total dose of t-PA is 100 mg, 60 mg of which is administered over 1 hour to rapidly recanalize the infarct-related coronary artery. The remaining 40 mg is given over the following 2 hours; after that a heparin drip to maintain patency of the recanalized artery and prevent rethrombosis is given.

**APSAC.** Since it is inactive on administration, APSAC can be given rapidly as a bolus injection. The recommended dose is 30 mg injected intravenously over 2 to 5 minutes. Because the half-life of APSAC is markedly increased (90 to 105 minutes), concomitant heparin therapy if employed should begin 4 to 6 hours after administration to decrease risk of bleeding associated with the prolonged fibrinolytic activity.[64]

### Summary of Nursing Care

The most common complication related to thrombolysis is bleeding, not only as a result of the thrombolytic therapy itself but also because the patients routinely receive anticoagulation therapy for several days to minimize the possibility of rethrombosis. Therefore the nurse must continually monitor for signs and symptoms of bleeding. Mild gingival bleeding and oozing around venipuncture sites is common and therefore not to be considered worrisome.[53] Should serious bleeding occur, such as intracranial or internal bleeding, all fibrinolytic and heparin therapy should be discontinued, and appropriate volume expanders and/or coagulation factors should be administered.

In addition to accurate assessment of the patient for the evidence of bleeding, the nurse should also intervene appropriately to prevent possible bleeding episodes. The nurse should avoid nonessential handling of the patient, keep injections to a minimum, and remember to keep additional pressure on injection, venipuncture, and particularly arterial puncture sites. Antacids can be given prophylactically, especially if the patient complains of gastric discomfort. The patient should be cautioned against vigorous toothbrushing and told to refrain from using straight-edge razors.

## MECHANICAL CIRCULATORY ASSIST DEVICES

### Intraaortic Balloon Pump

**The intraaortic balloon pump (IABP)** is currently the most widely employed temporary mechanical circulatory assist device used to support failing circulation[10,21] (see the box below). Its therapeutic effects are based on the hemodynamic principles of diastolic augmentation and afterload reduction.

#### COMMON INDICATIONS FOR THE USE OF IABP

Left ventricular failure after cardiac surgery
Unstable angina refractory to medications
Recurrent angina following AMI
Complications of AMI
- Cardiogenic shock
- Papillary muscle dysfunction/rupture with mitral regurgitation
- Ventricular septal defect
- Refractory ventricular dysrhythmias

The most commonly used intraaortic balloon consists of a single sausage-shaped polyurethane balloon that is wrapped around the distal end of a vascular catheter and positioned in the descending thoracic aorta just distal to the take-off of the left subclavian artery. The second generation of intraaortic balloon catheters is more flexible and can be wrapped to a smaller diameter than their predecessors and therefore can be inserted into the femoral artery percutaneously rather than surgically.[10] When attached to a bedside pumping console and properly synchronized to the patient's ECG pattern, the intraaortic balloon will inflate during diastole and deflate just before systole.

Initially, as the balloon is inflated in diastole concurrent with aortic valve closure, the blood in the aortic arch above the level of the balloon will be displaced retrograde (backward) toward the aortic root, augmenting diastolic coronary arterial blood flow and increasing myocardial oxygen supply (Fig. 9-15, *A*). The blood volume in the aorta below the level of the balloon will be propelled forward toward the peripheral vascular system, which may enhance renal perfusion. Subsequently, the deflation of the balloon just before the opening of the aortic valve creates a potential space or vacuum toward which blood will flow unimpeded during systole (Fig. 9-15, *B*). This decreased resistance to left ventricular ejection, or decreased afterload, will facilitate ventricular emptying and reduce myocardial oxygen demands. The overall physiological effect of IABP therapy is an improvement in the balance between myocardial oxygen supply and demand.[36] Contraindications to balloon pumping include aortic aneurysm, aortic valve insufficiency, and severe peripheral vascular disease.

Although the actual management of the pumping console and its timing functions are usually delegated to specially trained personnel on the unit, there are several important nursing responsibilities related to the care of the patient on the intraaortic balloon pump.

The ECG and arterial pressure tracing should be constantly monitored to verify the timing and effect of balloon counterpulsations (Fig. 9-16). Dysrhythmias can adversely affect the timing of balloon inflation and deflation, thus rhythm disturbances must be detected and treated promptly.[10] In addition, balloon deflation can be accidentally triggered by pacemaker spikes that are mistaken for R waves. The resulting early deflation is not dangerous, but, since it limits effective afterload reduction, an ECG lead that minimizes the pacing spike should be selected. Mean arterial pressure should be maintained at about 80 mm Hg with adequate pumping.

A major complication of IABP is ischemia of the involved limb secondary to occlusion of the femoral artery either by the catheter itself or by emboli from thrombus formation on the balloon. Consequently, the presence and quality of peripheral pulses distal to the catheter insertion site should be frequently assessed along with color, temperature, and cap-

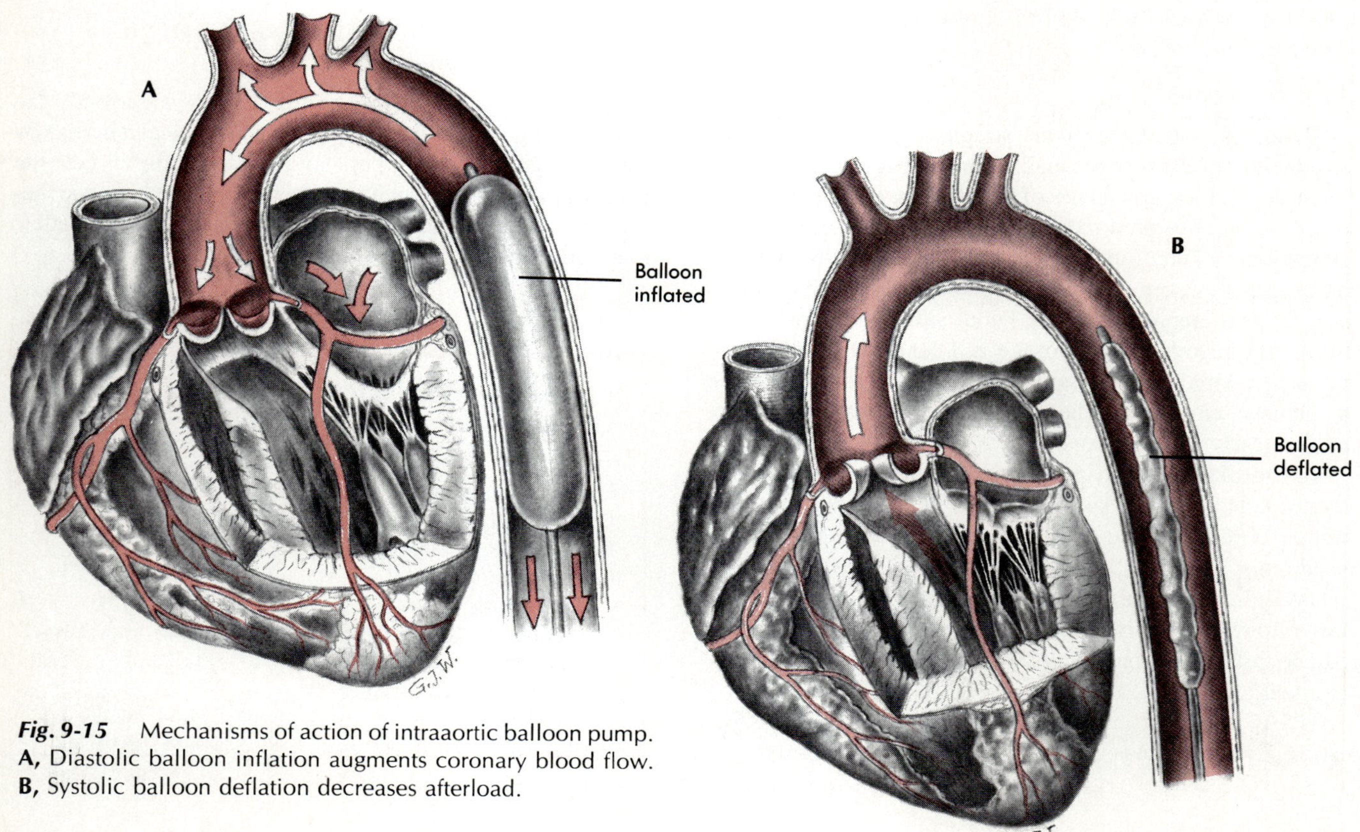


***Fig. 9-15*** Mechanisms of action of intraaortic balloon pump. **A,** Diastolic balloon inflation augments coronary blood flow. **B,** Systolic balloon deflation decreases afterload.

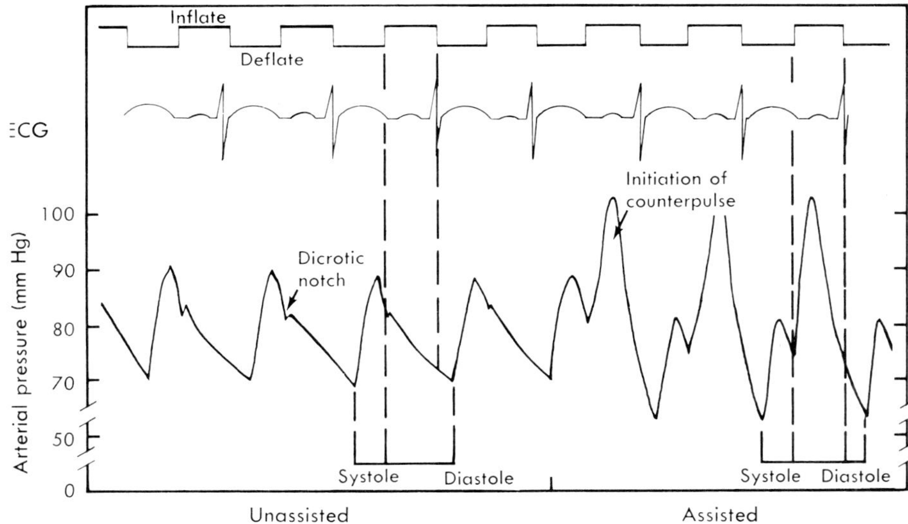


***Fig. 9-16*** Timing and effect of counterpulsation sequence by the ECG and arterial pressure waveform. With initiation of counterpulsation, diastolic pressure is heightened and systolic and end-diastolic pressures are lowered. (From Daily EK and Schroeder JS: Techniques in bedside hemodynamic monitoring, ed 4, St Louis, 1989, Mosby—Year Book, Inc.)

illary refill of the involved extremity. Other vascular complications of IABP include acute aortic dissection and the development of pseudoaneurysms.[27]

In addition, the balloon catheter may migrate proximally, occluding the left subclavian artery or distally compromising renal circulation. Therefore careful assessment of the left radial pulse and urinary output is essential. Measures to avoid accidental displacement of the balloon catheter include keeping the patient on complete bedrest with the head of the bed elevated no more than 30 degrees and preventing any flexion of the involved hip.

The patient should be log rolled from side to side every 2 hours to maintain skin integrity and to prevent pulmonary atelectasis. The presence of the balloon pump should never be a deterrent to appropriate pulmonary toilet. Thrombocytopenia may occur as a result of mechanical destruction of the platelets by the pumping action of the balloon. Therefore platelet counts should be closely monitored, and the patient watched for evidence of bleeding. Since the groin insertion site is at high risk for contamination, a daily regimen of aseptic dressing changes with betadine should be adhered to closely.

Finally, the psychological needs of the patient must not be overlooked. Sleep deprivation is not at all uncommon, partly a result of the continuous nursing care requirements of the patient but also related to the noise level in the unit, including the sounds made by the balloon pumping device. In addition, these patients universally experience anxiety related to fear of not recovering and loss of control because of forced immobility.

Weaning from the balloon pump should be considered when the patient has been hemodynamically stable with no or only minimal pharmacological support. The weaning procedure consists of slowly decreasing the pumping frequency from every beat down to every eighth beat as tolerated.[36] The IABP should remain at this minimal pumping ratio (or in a flutter mode) until its removal, to prevent thrombus formation on the balloon surface.

### External Counterpulsation

External counterpulsation (ECP) is a noninvasive method of diastolic augmentation in which the lower extremities are used as the pumping chambers. The system consists of two tapered, rigid cylinders that enclose the legs from ankle to thigh[69] (Fig. 9-17). Between the leg and the rigid outer housing is a water-filled bag that obliterates the remaining space to form an airtight seal. Water is then pumped in and out of the bag in synchrony with the ECG to apply alternating positive and negative pressure to veins and arteries within the legs. During diastole, inflation of the bag forces both venous and arterial blood back toward the heart, increasing preload and coronary filling, respectively. Negative pressure can be generated during systolic deflation to produce a vacuum effect similar to that seen with IABP that decreases afterload.

Compromised lower extremity circulation is the major complication associated with ECP. Patients will frequently complain of pain, muscular cramping, and numbness and tingling in the lower extremities that in some cases may necessitate discontinuance of therapy. Prolonged periods of pumping should be interrupted for brief periods when possible to provide skin care and passive range of motion.

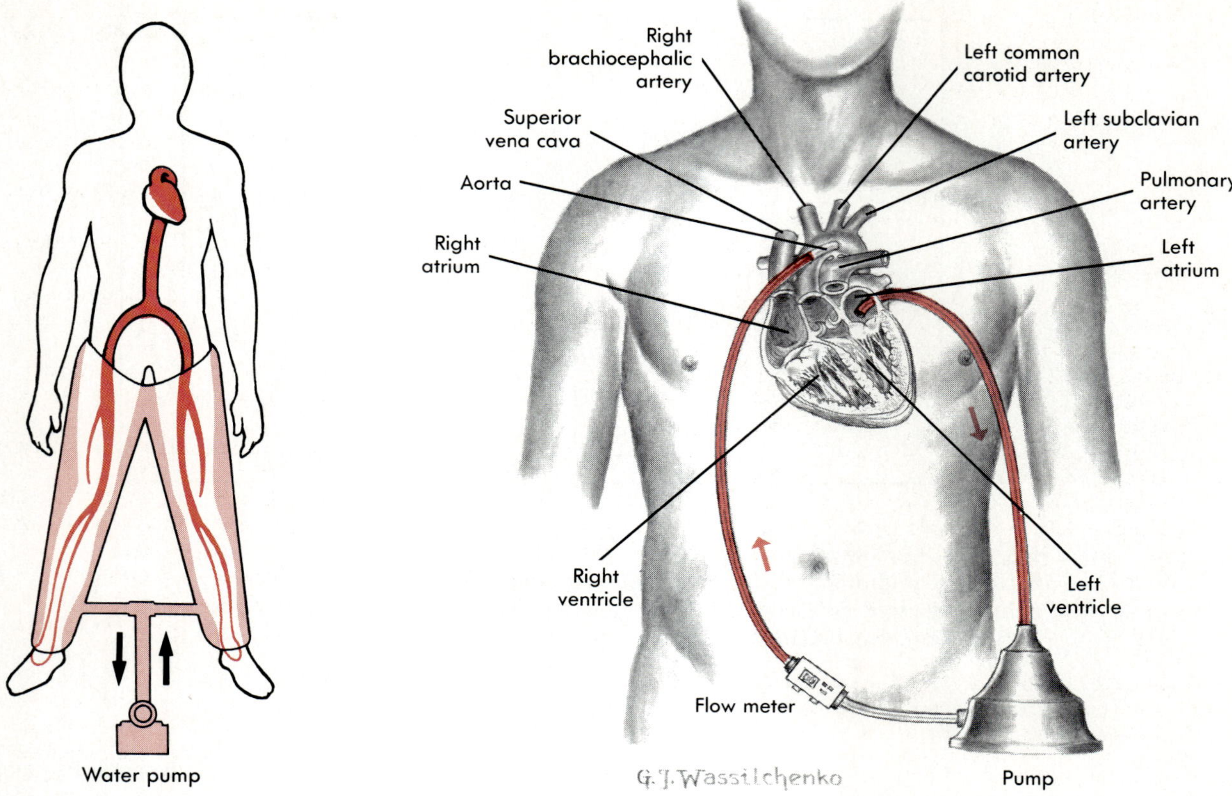


***Fig. 9-17*** External counterpulsation (ECP).

***Fig. 9-18*** Left ventricular assist device (L-VAD).

Indications for ECP are similar to those for IABP, with the obvious exceptions of patients who have undergone coronary revascularization with saphenous vein grafts.

## Ventricular Assist Devices

The **ventricular assist device (VAD)** is indicated for patients who, despite aggressive medical therapy, cannot be weaned from cardiopulmonary bypass because of persistent ventricular failure with cardiogenic shock.[49] VAD application in refractory cardiogenic shock following AMI and in patients whose condition is deteriorating while awaiting cardiac transplantation is currently being studied.[35]

The basic premise underlying the use of VAD following an acute myocardial infarction or after cardiac surgery is that myocardial function will improve if the heart is given time to rest and recover. This is accomplished by diverting a moderate amount of systemic blood flow (25% to 50%) around the failing ventricle by means of an extracorporeal pump.[9]

The left ventricular assist device (L-VAD) is used most commonly because LV failure occurs more frequently than RV failure.[9] Surgically placed cannulas in the left atrium and aorta are attached to an external pump device by connecting tubing (Fig. 9-18). Both cannulae exit the skin either through the sternal incision or through separate chest incisions.[49] Blood is diverted from the left atrium via the atrial cannula into the pumping device, which then pumps the blood out to the systemic circulation by way of the aortic cannula.

Weaning proceeds after several days by gradually decreasing flow rates to allow the patient's ventricle to contribute more to total blood flow. Patients on the VAD are routinely anticoagulated to prevent clotting in the extracorporeal circuit. These patients are also extraordinarily prone to infection because of the multiple portals of entry (invasive lines and, in some cases, open sternal incision); every precaution must be taken to prevent unnecessary exposure to organisms, and the patient should be closely monitored for signs and symptoms of infection.[9]

### REFERENCES

1. American Heart Association: Standards for cardiopulmonary resuscitation and emergency cardiac care, JAMA 255:2905, 1986.
2. American Heart Association: Textbook of advanced cardiac life support, Dallas, 1987, The Association.
3. Banasik JL and Tyler ML: The effect of prophylactic positive end-expiratory pressure on mediastinal bleeding after coronary revascularization surgery, Heart Lung 15:43, 1986.
4. Barr S: Inocor, Crit Care Nurs 5:64, 1985.
5. Bassan MM, Oded S, and Eliakim A: Improved prognosis during long-term treatment with beta-blockers after myocardial infarction: analysis of randomized trials and pooling of results, Heart Lung 13:164, 1984.

6. Beattie MS and Geden E: Reducing pain and discomfort following percutaneous transluminal coronary angioplasty, Dimens Crit Care Nurs 9(3):150, 1990.
7. Bernstein AD and others: The NASPE/BPEG generic pacemaker code for antibradyarrhythmia and adaptive-rate pacing and antitachyarrhythmia devices, PACE 10:794, 1987.
8. Bonchek LI: Basis for selecting a valve prosthesis, Cardiovasc Clin 17:107, 1987.
9. Brannon PHB and Towner SB: Ventricular failure: new therapy using the mechanical assist device, Crit Care Nurs 6:70, 1986.
10. Bregman D and Kaskel P: Advances in percutaneous intraaortic balloon pumping, Crit Care Clin 2:221, 1986.
11. Brewer CC and Markis JE: Streptokinase and tissue plasminogen activator in acute myocardial infarction, Heart Lung 15:552, 1986.
12. Briones TL: Tissue-plasminogen activator: nursing implications, Dimens Crit Care Nurs 8(4):203, 1989.
13. Catalano JT: Antiarrhythmic medications classified by their autonomic properties, Crit Care Nurse 6:44, 1986.
14. Catalano JT: Dual-chamber pacemaker rhythm, Crit Care Nurs 10(3):67, 1990.
15. Collen D and others: Coronary thrombolysis with recombinant human tissue-type plasminogen activator: a prospective, randomized placebo-controlled trial, Circulation 70:1012, 1984.
16. Cowley MJ and others: Acute coronary events associated with percutaneous transluminal coronary angioplasty, Am J Cardiol 53:12C, 1984.
17. DeAngelis R: Amiodarone, Crit Care Nurse 6:12, 1986.
18. Dorros G and others: Percutaneous transluminal coronary angioplasty in patients with prior coronary artery bypass grafting, J Thorac Cardiovasc Surg 87:17, 1984.
19. Earp JK: Thermal gradients and shivering following open heart surgery, Dimens Crit Care Nurs 8(5): 267, 1989.
20. Eberts MA: Advances in the pharmacologic management of angina pectoris, J Cardiovasc Nurs 1:15, 1986.
21. Fenton M: Intra-aortic balloon pump therapy, Crit Care Nurse 5:54, 1985.
22. Finkelmeier BA and O'Mara SR: Temporary pacing in the cardiac surgical patient, Crit Care Nurse 4:108, 1984.
23. Finkelmeier BA and Salinger MH: The atrial electrogram: its diagnostic use following cardiac surgery, Crit Care Nurse 4:42, 1984.
24. Fox J: Laser coronary angioplasty, J Cardiovasc Nurs 1:57, 1986.
25. Gallo JA and Todd BA: Mediastinitis after cardiac surgery, Crit Care Nurs 10(6):64, 1990.
26. Gershan JA and Jirika MK: Percutaneous transluminal coronary angioplasty: implications for nursing, Focus Crit Care 11:28, 1984.
27. Goran SF: Vascular complications of the patient undergoing intra-aortic balloon pumping, Crit Care Nurs Clinics N Amer 1(3):459, 1989.
28. Grosso MA, Brown JM, and Harken AH: Surgical treatment of cardiac arrhythmias, Prim Cardiol 14:51, 1989.
29. Gurevich I: Infectious complications after open heart surgery, Heart Lung 13:472, 1984.
30. Haywood DL: Temporary A-V sequential pacing using an epicardial lead system, Crit Care Nurse 5:21, 1985.
31. Huang SK and Marcus FI: Antiarrhythmic drug therapy of ventricular arrhythmias, Current Probl Cardiol 11:1, 1986.
32. Isaacson JJ, George LT, and Brewer MJ: The effect of chest tube manipulation on mediastinal drainage, Heart Lung 15:601, 1986.
33. ISIS-2 Collaborative Group: Randomized trial of intravenous streptokinase, oral aspirin, both or neither among 17,187 cases of suspected acute myocardial infarction, Lancet 2:349, 1988.
34. Jansen KJ and McFadden PM: Postoperative nursing management in patients undergoing myocardial revascularization with internal mammary artery bypass, Heart Lung 15:48, 1986.
35. Jorge E, Pae WE, and Pierce WS: Left heart and biventricular bypass, Crit Care Clin 2:267, 1986.
36. Jorge E and Pierce WS: Mechanical support or replacement of the heart, Cardiovasc Clin 17:361, 1987.
37. Kennedy JW and others: Acute myocardial infarction treated with intracoronary streptokinase: a report of the society for cardiac angiography, Am J Cardiol 55:871, 1985.
38. Kern LS: Advances in the surgical treatment of coronary artery disease, J Cardiovasc Nurs 1:1, 1986.
39. Kienzle MG and others: Antiarrhythmic drug therapy for sustained ventricular tachycardia, Heart Lung 13:614, 1984.
40. Killip T: Coronary bypass surgery—where we stand today, Drug Therap 14:71, 1984.
41. Kleuen MR: Comparison of thrombolytic agents: mechanism of action, efficacy, and safety, Heart Lung 17(6):750, 1988.
42. Kline EM: Recombinant tissue-type plasminogen activator in acute myocardial infarction: role of the critical care nurse, Heart Lung 16:779, 1987.
43. Lanoue AS, Snyder BA, and Galen KM: Percutaneous transluminal coronary angioplasty: nonoperative treatment of coronary artery disease, J Cardiovasc Nurs 1:30, 1986.
44. Lasater MG: Torsades des pointes etiology and treatment, Focus Crit Care 13:17, 1986.
45. Loop FD and others: Influence of the internal-mammary-artery graft on 10 year survival and other cardiac events, N Engl J Med 314:1, 1986.
46. Meier B and Gruentzig A: Learning curve for PTCA: skills, technology on patient selection, Am J Cardiol 53:65C, 1984.
47. Mercer ME: The electrophysiology study: a nursing concern, Crit Care Nurse 7:58, 1987.
48. Moser SA, Crawford D, and Thomas A: Caring for patients with implantable cardioverter defibrillators, Crit Care Nurs 8(2):52, 1988.
49. Mulford E: Nursing perspectives for the patient receiving post-operative ventricular assistance in the critical care unit, Heart Lung 16:246, 1987.
50. Mullet K: State of the art in neurostimulation, PACE 10:162, 1987.
51. Murdock DK and others: Pacemaker malfunction: fact or artifact?, Heart Lung 15:150, 1986.
52. Nieminski KE, Kay RH, and Rubin DA: Current concepts and management of the sick sinus syndrome, Heart Lung 13:675, 1984.
53. Ong YC and Wescott BL: Intravenous fibrolytic therapy in a community hospital, Focus Crit Care 5:30, 1986.
54. Parker MM and Lemberg L: Pacemaker update 1984. Part I. Introduction to electrocardiographic analysis of pacing function and site, Heart Lung 13:315, 1984.
55. Parsonnet V, Furman S, and Smyth N: A revised code for pacemaker identification, PACE 4:401, 1981.
56. Persons CB: Transcutaneous pacing—meeting the challenge, Focus Crit Care 14:13, 1987.
57. Quaal SJ: Thrombolytic therapy: an overview, J Cardiovasc Nurs 1:45, 1986.
58. Quinless FW, Cassese M, and Atherton N: The effect of selected preoperative, intraoperative, and postoperative variables on the development of postpericardiotomy psychosis in patients undergoing open heart surgery, Heart Lung 14:334, 1985.
59. Rafalowski MM: Relationship of core temperature at time of blanket removal to subsequent core temperature in patients immediately after coronary artery bypass, Heart Lung 16:9, 1987.
60. Relman AS: Intravenous thrombolysis in acute myocardial infarction, N Engl J Med 312:915, 1985.
61. Rice V: Shock management. Part II. Pharmacologic intervention, Crit Care Nurse 5:42, 1985.
62. Rotmensch HH, Vlasses PH, and Ferguson RK: Prophylactic use of beta-adrenergic blockage in survivors of myocardial infarction, Heart Lung 13:366, 1984.
63. Sager DP: Current facts on pacemaker electromagnetic interference and their application to clinical care, Heart Lung 16:211, 1987.
64. Sherry S: Pharmacology of anistreplase, Clin Card 13:v3, 1990.
65. Sherry S: Unresolved clinical pharmacologic questions in thrombolytic therapy for acute myocardial infarction, J Am Coll Cardiol 12(2):519, 1988.

66. Sigwart U, Puel J, and Mirkovitch V: Intravascular stents to prevent occlusion and restenosis after transluminal angioplasty, N Engl J Med 316(2):701, 1987.
67. Sipperly ME: Thrombolytic therapy update, Crit Care Nurs 5:30, 1985.
68. Smith A: Amiodarone: clinical considerations, Focus Crit Care 11:30, 1984.
69. Soroff HS, Hui J, and Giron F: Current status of external counter-pulsation, Crit Care Clin 2:277, 1986.
70. Spears JR and others: Percutaneous coronary laser balloon angioplasty: preliminary results of a multicenter trial, J Am Coll Cardiol 13(2):61A, 1989.
71. Steger KE, Remy J, and Krueger S: Drug-induced torsades des pointes: case report and implications for critical care staff, Heart Lung 15:200, 1986.
72. Strauss E and Rudy EB: Tissue-plasminogen activator: a new drug for reperfusion therapy, Crit Care Nurse 6:30, 1986.
73. Sulzbach LM: The use of temporary atrial wire electrodes to record atrial electrograms in patients who had cardiac surgery, Heart Lung 14:540, 1985.
74. Taylor T: Monitoring left atrial pressure in the open-heart surgical patient, Crit Care Nurse 6:62, 1986.
75. Thielbar S: Antiarrhythmic drug therapy: an overview, Crit Care Q 7:21, 1984.
76. TIMI Study Group: The thrombolysis in myocardial infarction (TIMI) trials: phase I finding, N Engl J Med 312:932, 1985.
77. Topol EJ: Clinical use of streptokinase and urokinase therapy for acute myocardial infarction, Heart Lung 16:760, 1987.
78. Topol EJ: Emerging strategies for failed percutaneous transluminal coronary angioplasty, Am J Cardiol 63(3):249, 1989.
79. Touloukian JE: Calcium channel blocking agents: physiologic basis of nursing interventions, Heart Lung 14:342, 1985.
80. Varah N, Smith J, and Baugh RF: Heparin monitoring in the coronary care unit after percutaneous transluminal coronary angioplasty, Heart Lung 19(3):265, 1990.
81. Vitello-Cicciu JM and others: Profile of patients requiring the use of epicardial pacing wires after coronary artery bypass surgery, Heart Lung 16:301, 1987.
82. Vlietstra RE and Holmes DR: Percutaneous transluminal coronary angioplasty, J Cardiac Surg 3:56, 1988.
83. Weiland AP and Walker WE: Physiologic principles and clinical sequelae of cardiopulmonary bypass, Heart Lung 15:34, 1986.
84. Wescott BL: Tissue plasminogen activator: a new advancement in fibrinolytic therapy, Focus Crit Care 13:22, 1986.
85. Zwerner PL and Gore JM: Thrombolytic therapy in acute myocardial infarction, J Intens Care Med 1:302, 1986.

UNIT IV

# PULMONARY ALTERATIONS

CHAPTER 10

# Pulmonary Assessment and Diagnostic Procedures

## CHAPTER OBJECTIVES

- *Perform a nursing assessment of the pulmonary system on a critically ill patient and correctly interpret the results.*
- *Identify and state where normal lung sounds are auscultated on the thorax.*
- *Name the three types of adventitious lung sounds and explain the pathophysiology of each.*
- *Identify abnormal arterial blood gases and initiate nursing actions that will assist in correcting the abnormalities.*
- *Identify the parameters that must be evaluated to assess total oxygenation of arterial blood.*
- *List the indications and nursing care for patients having a bronchoscopy or thoracentesis.*

## KEY TERMS

Henderson-Hasselbalch equation, p. 223
oxygen saturation, p. 224
oxygen content, p. 224
oxygen transportation, p. 224
oxyhemoglobin dissociation curve, p. 225
2,3-diphosphoglycerate (2,3-DPG), p. 226
dead space, p. 233
ventilation-perfusion scanning, p. 234

## CLINICAL ASSESSMENT

As with assessment of any body system, examination of the patient's respiratory status must be a systematic process of garnering clues leading to a diagnosis. This process can be of brief duration (for example, determining breathlessness) or can involve a detailed history and examination, depending on the nature and immediacy of the patient's situation. Whatever the setting, the nurse should develop and practice a sequential pattern of assessment to avoid omitting portions of the examination. Since the thorax is arranged symmetrically, it is necessary to compare areas of the left thorax to areas of the right thorax in an effort to observe significant differences. For example, the left apex of the lung should be compared with the right apex of the lung, as opposed to the lower lung field on the same or opposite side.

Proper assessment includes an investigation into the chronology of symptoms (history), physical signs (physical examination), and findings (laboratory diagnostic tests). Evaluation of data uncovered using these three components will generally yield a reliable determination of the patient's condition.

### History

The history of the illness is considered extremely important in determining the patient's condition. Throughout the interview, the patient's chief complaint is evaluated in an attempt to reveal the underlying cause(s). The nurse seeks to expose key signs and symptoms that can determine causation and lead to proper intervention. Table 10-1 reviews the key symptoms associated with respiratory disease.

During the discussion of symptoms, it is important to note the absence of a symptom from a usual cluster or grouping. For example, cough is generally associated with pulmonary infection; absence of any cough would be noted as a significant negative in symptoms of this disorder and could help refine the list of possible causes.

#### Symptoms

***Shortness of breath.*** Shortness of breath is probably one of the most frequent complaints that prompts patients to

**Table 10-1** Key symptoms in respiratory disease

| Symptoms | Possible causes |
|---|---|
| Dyspnea/shortness of breath, breathlessness, inability to catch breath, smothering tightness in chest, dyspnea on exertion, orthopnea | Airway obstruction; e.g., foreign body, bronchitis, mucus, asthma, chronic obstructive pulmonary disease (COPD), atelectasis, tumors, pneumothorax<br>Altered function, e.g., congestive heart failure (CHF), pulmonary embolism, pulmonary contusion, acute blood loss, anemia, splinting, chest wall deformity<br>Hyperventilation syndrome |
| Chest pain accentuated by breathing, coughing, sneezing, laughing; usually sharp, knifelike burning quality to pain | Inflammation or trauma of ribs, muscles, nerves, and pleurae; pleurisy, rib fracture, costochondritis, intercostal myositis |
| Cough with or without sputum production | Exacerbation of COPD, pneumonia, interstitial lung disease, aspiration lung disorders, CHF, pulmonary embolism, noncardiogenic pulmonary edema, chronic irritation of respiratory mucosa |

seek assistance. It is a common symptom of respiratory and cardiac disease and, since shortness of breath is a subjective complaint, its severity can be difficult to assess. One method that seems to provide quantitative data is having the patient rate shortness of breath using the Visual Analog Scale (VAS) or the Modified Borg Scale (see the box below).[3,18,44]

The VAS consists of a horizontal line with "not at all breathless" to "very breathless" at either end of the continuum. The patient is asked to locate his or her sensation of breathlessness on this line. Changes in severity or improvement can then be plotted along the continuum during the course of therapy. The Modified Borg Scale has a vertical continuum on which the patient is asked to quantify shortness of breath. Shortenss of breath may be acute or chronic in onset, or it may be associated with activity and position. Orthopnea is the term used to describe shortness of breath that is only relieved by assuming an upright position.

***Cough.*** Cough is a frequent complaint, although it is nonspecific as an indicator of pulmonary disease. Like other nonspecific complaints, cough requires careful investigation by the interviewer. One should inquire about the onset, frequency, precipitating events, and whether the cough is productive. If the cough is productive, visualization of sputum is desirable, and the patient should be asked to quantify sputum production. The investigator should also inquire about the presence or absence of hemoptysis. Table 10-2 lists abnormal sputum characteristics and their likely causes.

***Chest pain.*** Chest pain is one of the most frequently seen presenting symptoms. When not associated with trauma, chest pain may be accompanied by a heightened emotional state because of the association of chest pain with heart attack. Since there may not be physical signs associated with pain, careful questioning about the pain is essential.

Using the PQRST mnemonic can assist the practitioner in compiling a complete description of the pain complaint, allowing significant reduction in possible causes. *P* stands for provocative-palliative factors of pain; *Q* refers to quality of pain; *R* relates to region of pain and radiation to other areas; *S* refers to a description of the severity of pain; and *T* refers to the temporal characteristics of pain[7] (see the box on p. 219).

Along with the current history, the nurse should know the patient's past medical nursing history. Awareness of other disease conditions has significant bearing on planning patient care, because morbidity and mortality are affected by associated disease states.

## METHODS TO RATE SHORTNESS OF BREATH

### MODIFIED BORG SCALE

Circle the number that best matches your shortness of breath

| | |
|---|---|
| 0 | None at all |
| 0.5 | Very, very slight (just noticeable) |
| 1 | Very slight |
| 2 | Slight |
| 3 | Moderate |
| 4 | Somewhat severe |
| 5 | Severe |
| 6 | |
| 7 | Very severe |
| 8 | |
| 9 | Very, very severe (almost maximal) |
| 10 | Maximal |

### DYSPNEA VISUAL ANALOGUE SCALE

Mark the line at the point that best describes your breathing.

No difficulty breathing ———————— Extreme difficulty breathing

From Lush M and others: Heart Lung 17(5):528, 1988.

***Table 10-2*** Sputum characteristics seen in various respiratory disorders

| Appearance | Likely cause |
|---|---|
| Bloody gelatinous sputum (currant-jelly sputum) | *Klebsiella pneumoniae* |
| Rusty sputum (prune-juice sputum) | Pneumococcal pneumonias |
| Thick, greenish sputum with blood streaking it | *Klebsiella pneumoniae* |
| Stringy mucoid sputum | Asthmatic attack |
| Frothy sputum | Pulmonary edema |
| Purulent sputum of yellow, green, gray nature | Pneumonias |

### Physical Examination

Once the history has been obtained, the nurse should begin the physical examination (the search for key signs), which will move her or him further toward a diagnosis.

**Inspection.** Much can be gleaned about the respiratory status during inspection, and the nurse should focus on (1) general signs of respiratory disease, (2) chest wall movement and deformity, (3) ventilatory pattern, and (4) discharges of sputum, pus, or hemoptysis.

General signs associated with respiratory problems are numerous. Clubbing of the fingers is a significant sign of cardiopulmonary disease.[39] The mechanism responsible for clubbing is not known, but it is often associated with a chronic decrease in oxygen supply to the body tissues.[39] Clubbing includes loss of angulation at the nail plate, change in the curvature of the nail, and floating of the nail root (Fig. 10-1).[7,25]

Central cyanosis may be associated with hypoxic pulmonary disease and is seen as a blue color of the skin and mucous membranes. Cyanosis occurs when large amounts of unsaturated hemoglobin are present in the capillaries (>5 g/dl blood).[7,21,39]

Although central cyanosis is evidence of hypoxemia, it is an insensitive assessment parameter because cyanosis is not detected by the human eye until oxyhemoglobin saturation falls below 80%.[24] Inspection of lips, ears, and molar regions helps to differentiate central from local peripheral cyanosis. Other general findings may include various lesions such as petechiae, Osler nodes, and erythema multiforme, which can be associated with staphylococcal pneumonias.[5] Osler nodes are tender reddish bumps on the hands that develop as embolic lesions of the bacteria, and erythema multiforme is an associated skin lesion characterized by redness.

Chest wall movement and symmetry should be carefully observed. Whenever possible, observation of the thorax and chest wall movement should be accomplished with the patient in a sitting position. Since sitting is not feasible for many critically ill patients, the nurse must adjust for the variation of chest wall movements created by the patient's position. The shape of the chest should be assessed for structural deformities such as kyphosis, scoliosis, or pectus excavatum. Any scars should be noted, as should all surgical incisions. The presence of other iatrogenic features such as chest tubes, central venous lines, artificial airways, and/or nasogastric tubes must be noted since they may affect assessment findings.

Breathing should be observed for the effort it necessitates. Normal, quiet breathing is relatively effortless, whereas difficult breathing can range from mild to extreme dyspnea. Extreme dyspnea is exemplified by the breathing of a patient suffering an exacerbation of chronic obstructive pulmonary

#### DESCRIBING PAIN USING THE PQRST APPROACH

**PROVOCATIVE-PALLIATIVE**

Document factors that aggravate or alleviate pain. Distinguish if pain is increased or unchanged during ventilation. Pain associated with movement can often be localized to displaced tissues. Assess whether pain is affected by position or inactivity.

**QUALITY**

Pain is usually described as (1) burning, (2) pricking or sharp, and (3) deep or aching. Superficial pain is often associated with burning, pricking, and sharp characteristics and is localized. Throbbing or cramping may be described. Deep pain is usually longer in duration and is associated with pressure and aching.

**REGION-RADIATION**

Ask the patient to indicate the area of pain; with superficial pain, the patient can often identify the exact spot. Any radiation of pain should be determined. Radiation is usually associated with deep, visceral pain.

**SEVERITY**

Pain's severity defies precise measurement; use a pain-rating scale for quantification of patient's pain (0 equals pain free, 10 equals worst pain imaginable). Studies show pain rated <7 on a 0 to 10 scale usually responds to nonnarcotic drugs and/or nursing measures that increase naturally occurring endorphins. Pain rated as >7 on a 0 to 10 scale usually requires narcotic drug intervention and cannot be relieved by nursing measures alone. Intense pain is usually associated with other signs such as tachycardia, diaphoresis, facial grimacing, posturing, splinting, and/or nausea and vomiting.[21,28,29]

**TEMPORAL**

These characteristics of pain give information about onset and duration of pain. Assess whether pain is acute or chronic, periodic in occurrence, and brief or extended in duration.

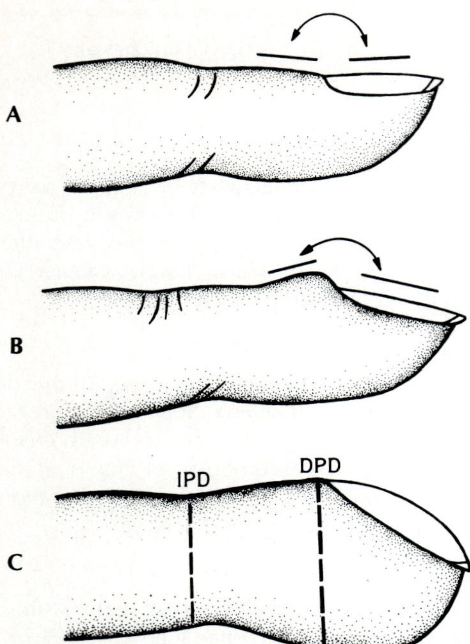


*Fig. 10-1* **A,** Normal digit configuration. **B,** Mild digital clubbing with increased hyponychial angle. **C,** Severe digital clubbing; depth of finger at base of nail *(DPD)* is greater than depth of interpharyngeal joint *(IPD)* with clubbing. (From Scanlan CL and others: Egan's fundamentals of respiratory care, ed 5, St Louis, 1990, Mosby–Year Book, Inc.)

disease (COPD) who sits in high-Fowler's position and leans forward, using neck and chest accessory muscles to inhale and pursed-lip breathing to exhale. Gasps for air may make the distress readily apparent. Lesser degrees of dyspnea are reflected by the same factors—patient position, active effort to breathe, use of the accessory muscles of ventilation, presence of intercostal retraction, unequal movement of chest and thoracic wall, flaring of nares, or pausing midsentence to take a breath.

Inspection would not be complete without determining the patient's breathing pattern, since several types of irregular breathing patterns may occur in certain disease states. Table 10-3 outlines irregular breathing patterns. The depth of inhalation should also be grossly determined during observation of the respiratory cycle. Kussmaul respiration (air hunger) is a deep, regular, sighing breathing that may be associated with a slow or fast rate. It occurs in response to metabolic acidosis, peritonitis, severe hemorrhage, and pneumonia. Noting noisy breathing, especially stridulous breathing, which is the high-pitched whistling or crowing sound associated with glottic narrowing, gives additional clues. Stridulous breathing may presage complete airway obstruction and requires immediate intervention.

**Palpation.** Palpation of the chest wall should reveal areas of tenderness and lumps or bony deformities. Tracheal position should be assessed by placing the fingers on the middle of the top of the manubrium and moving upward. The trachea should be located in the midline. Deviations to either side may indicate a pneumothorax, a large pleural effusion, or severe atelectasis.

Vibratory palpation (tactile fremitus) involves using the examiner's hands to evaluate air vibration. As the patient speaks, the palmar surface of each hand is held firmly against the patient's chest to assess the chest wall vibrations that occur during speech. Alterations within the lung or pleura change the ease with which vibrations are transmitted to the chest wall. Pleural effusions decrease the vibrations, whereas consolidation of lung tissue increases the vibrations.

Respiratory excursion is measured by placing the hands on either side of the posterior thorax while the patient breathes. Excursion should be evaluated in the upper, middle, and lower posterior thorax. Evaluation of posterior excursion is facilitated by placing the thumbs together on the spinal column with fingers reaching around each side of the chest wall. Noting movement of thumbs away from each other allows estimation of respiratory excursion and determination of symmetry. Asymmetrical movement of the chest

***Table 10-3*** Irregular breathing patterns

| Pattern | Defining characteristics | Possible causes |
|---|---|---|
| Cheyne-Stokes respiration | A pattern of breathing characterized by shallow ventilations, which increase in depth, reach a peak, and decline. A period of apnea occurs as the ventilations decline, after which the pattern is repeated. | Normal variation in children and in elderly people; left cardiac failure, aortic valvular problems, low diastolic pressure, increased cerebral pressure, brain injury, morphine and its derivatives, barbiturates |
| Biot's breathing | Uncommon variant of Cheyne-Stokes respiration. Periods of apnea irregularly interrupt breaths of equal depth. | Meningitis |
| Painful breathing | Normal breathing interrupted by pain and splinting. | Pleurisy, inflamed and traumatized muscle, fractured ribs or cartilages, subphrenic inflammation |
| Sighing respirations | Normal rhythm periodically interrupted by deep sighing. | Psychoneurosis, physiological sighing |

***Table 10-4*** Characteristics of normal breath sounds

| Sound | Characteristics | Findings |
|---|---|---|
| Vesicular | Heard over most of lung field; low pitch; soft and short exhalation and long inhalation | |
| Bronchovesicular | Heard over main bronchus area and over upper right posterior lung field; medium pitch; exhalation equals inhalation | |
| Bronchial | Heard only over trachea; high pitch; loud and long exhalation | |

Modified from Thompson JM and others: Mosby's manual of clinical nursing, ed 2, St Louis, 1989, Mosby–Year Book, Inc.

can occur in pneumothorax, pneumonia, splinting, or other disorders that interfere with lung inflation.

**Percussion.** The density of organs and tissues is evaluated by percussion. When struck, different tissues emit characteristic sounds described as resonant, tympanic, dull, or flat, depending on the pitch and timbre. These sounds defy verbal description and are best distinguished by the examiner through practice. The sound emitted by air-filled lung is referred to as resonance, percussion of the stomach yields tympany, the heart sounds dull, and muscle sounds flat when percussed. The sound emitted when percussing over a pneumothorax is termed hyperresonance. In the acute care setting, percussion of lung fields is infrequently used after the initial baseline assessment has been completed. During percussion, as with other maneuvers, like areas of the lungs should be compared; that is, percussion of the posterior left apex should be compared with the posterior right apex, using a back-and-forth movement. Both anterior and posterior chest fields should be percussed.

**Auscultation.** Listening over the lung fields with a stethoscope permits the nurse to evaluate air movement and the presence of adventitious sounds. Air movement creates turbulence as it flows through the branching network of airways.

***Normal breath sounds.*** Because of the variation in airway size encountered, *normal breath sounds* change as airway size changes. Air movement heard over large airways such as the trachea or mainstem bronchi is referred to as bronchial breath sounds. Other breath sounds include vesicular and bronchovesicular sounds. Table 10-4 reviews the characteristics of these normal breath sounds.

***Voice sounds.*** Besides listening to breath sounds, the nurse should assess voice sounds. Voice sounds are particularly useful in detecting consolidation. The two types of voice sounds assessed are whispered pectoriloquy and bronchophony. In healthy lungs, whispered and spoken words will not be clearly heard during auscultation. An increase in the loudness and distinctiveness of whispered or spoken words indicates pathology (Table 10-5).

Egophony is a form of bronchophony. It is also referred to as an "e" to "a" change. If the lung is compressed such as with a pleural effusion, the letter "e" will be heard as "a" when spoken by the patient.

***Adventitious sounds.*** Although a multitude of names exist for extra or adventitious sounds heard in the lung, the Joint Committee on Pulmonary Nomenclature has recommended use of the terms "crackles and wheezes."[15]

*Crackles* is used to describe the sounds previously called *rales*. Once thought caused by air passing through fluid-filled airways, acoustical studies show that these sounds are caused by pressure variations in the airways and reflect the

***Table 10-5*** Voice sounds, normal and abnormal results

| Voice sounds | Results |
|---|---|
| Bronchophony: using diaphragm of stethoscope, listen to posterior chest as patient says "ninety-nine" | Normal response: muffled "nin-nin" sound heard<br>Abnormal response: clear, loud "ninety-nine" response heard because the lung tissue is consolidated |
| Whispered pectoriloquy: using stethoscope, listen to posterior chest as patient whispers "one, two, three" or "ninety-nine" | Normal response: muffled sounds heard<br>Abnormal response: clear "one, two, three" or "ninety-nine" heard because of lung consolidation |
| Egophony: using stethoscope, listen to posterior chest as the patient says "e-e-e" | Normal response: muffled "e-e-e" sound heard<br>Abnormal response: sound of e changes to an "a-a-a" sound, referred to as "e" to "a" change, because of consolidation |

From Thompson JM and others: Mosby's manual of clinical nursing, ed 2, St Louis, 1989, Mosby–Year Book, Inc.

**Table 10-6** Causes and characteristics of adventitious sounds

| Sound | Causes | Characteristics |
|---|---|---|
| Crackles | Pressure variations in airways | Discontinuous and categorized as early or late inspiratory |
| Early inspiratory crackles | Same as above | Low pitched and few in number; vary in loudness and not abolished by cough or deep breathing; frequently audible at mouth, as well as over lung fields |
| Late inspiratory crackles | Same as above | Numerous, gravity dependent, and affected by position changes; may be abolished or decreased by deep breathing or coughing; heard only over lung fields |
| Wheezes | Bronchial wall oscillations and opening and closing of airways | Continuous sounds heard during inhalation and/or exhalation; musical or snoring in character |
| Friction rubs | Rubbing together of inflamed and roughened pleural surfaces | Creaking or grating quality during inhalation and exhalation; heard best in lower anteriolateral chest (area of greatest thoracic expansion); not affected by coughing; disappears when patient pauses in breathing |

opening of collapsed alveoli in the lung. *Wheezes* are associated with bronchial wall oscillations and the airways' opening and closing. Table 10-6 outlines adventitious sounds.

Other adventitious sounds that can be heard are pleural friction rub and mediastinal emphysema (Hammans' sign). Pleural friction rub is a grating, rough sound caused by inflammation within the pleura. The sound corresponds to ventilation and disappears with breath holding[3,25]; thus it can be differentiated from pericardial friction rub, which does not vary with ventilation. Mediastinal emphysema is caused by air in the mediastinum and sounds like high-pitched crunching and crackling heard around the mediastinum.[4]

When listening for adventitious sounds, it is necessary to eliminate any outside source of sounds (for example, the sound of the bubbling of water from ventilator tubing, which can be transmitted to a patient's chest during auscultation) that could be transmitted to the lung. Before auscultation, listening to the environmental sounds created by equipment supporting the patient can help the nurse identify potential sources of random sounds that could be confused during the auscultory process.

## LABORATORY ASSESSMENT

### Arterial Blood Gas Analysis

Interpretation of arterial blood gas levels can be difficult, especially if one is under pressure to do it quickly and accurately as is so often the case in critical care. One way that the nurse can help to ensure accuracy when analyzing arterial blood gas levels is by following the same steps of interpretation each time.

A specific method to be used each time blood gas values must be interpreted is presented here. Understanding this method and the normal blood gas values will greatly assist in successful interpretation.

**Step 1: Look at the $Pa_{O_2}$ and answer the question, "Does the $Pa_{O_2}$ show hypoxemia?"** The $Pa_{O_2}$ is a measure of the partial pressure of oxygen dissolved in arterial blood plasma, with *P* standing for "partial pressure" and *a* standing for "arterial." Sometimes $Pa_{O_2}$ is shortened to $P_{O_2}$. It is reported in millimeters of mercury (mm Hg).

The normal range for $Pa_{O_2}$ on room air breathed at sea level is 80 to 100 mm Hg. However, the normal range is age-dependent in two groups: persons aged 60 years and older and infants. The normal level for infants breathing room air is 40 to 70 mm Hg.[41] The normal level for persons 60 years of age and older decreases with age as changes occur in the ventilation-perfusion ratio in the aging lung.[8,31] The correct $Pa_{O_2}$ for older persons can be ascertained by subtracting 1 mm Hg for every year that a person is over 60 years of age from 80 mm Hg (the lowest normal value). Using this formula, it will be found that a 65-year-old individual can have a $Pa_{O_2}$ as low as 75 mm Hg and still be within the normal range. (Formula: 5 years over 60 years of age; 80 mm Hg − 5 mm Hg = 75 mm Hg.) In the same way, an acceptable range for an 80-year-old person would begin at 60 mm Hg. (Formula: 20 years over the age of 60; 80 mm Hg − 20 mm Hg = 60 mm Hg.) At any age, a $Pa_{O_2}$ less than 40 mm Hg represents a life-threatening situation that requires immediate action. If the $Pa_{O_2}$ is less than the predicted lowest value, it shows *hypoxemia,* which means that a lower than normal amount of oxygen is dissolved in plasma. That is why the question "Does the $Pa_{O_2}$ show hypoxemia?" is asked.

**Step 2: Look at the pH level and answer the question, "Is the pH on the acid or alkaline side of 7.40?"** The pH is the hydrogen ion concentration of plasma. The normal range is 7.35 to 7.45 with the mean being 7.40. If the pH is less than 7.40, it is on the acid side of the mean. Less than 7.35 is called *acidemia,* and the overall condition is called *acidosis*.

If the pH is greater than 7.40, it is on the alkaline side of the mean. Greater than 7.45 is called *alkalemia,* and the overall condition is called *alkalosis*. Calculation of the pH is accomplished by using the partial pressure of carbon dioxide ($Paco_2$) and the plasma bicarbonate level ($HCO_3$). The formula used is the **Henderson-Hasselbalch equation** (see the box below).

**Step 3: Look at the $Paco_2$ and answer the question, "Does the $Paco_2$ show respiratory acidosis, alkalosis, or normalcy?"** The $Paco_2$ is a measure of the partial pressure of carbon dioxide dissolved in arterial blood plasma, and it is reported in mm Hg. It is the acid-base component that reflects the effectiveness of ventilation in relation to the metabolic rate. In other words, the $Paco_2$ value indicates whether the patient can ventilate well enough to rid his or her body of the carbon dioxide produced as a consequence of metabolism. When the patient cannot ventilate well enough, the $Paco_2$ will rise.

A buildup of carbon dioxide in the body is a serious health matter; thus the importance of accurate assessment of the $Paco_2$ level cannot be overemphasized. The normal range for the $Paco_2$ is 35 to 45 mm Hg. This range does not change as a person ages. A $Paco_2$ greater than 45 mm Hg defines *respiratory acidosis,* which results from alveolar hypoventilation or ventilation-perfusion inequality. Another way of stating this is to say that respiratory acidosis occurs because the patient's ventilation is not effective in removing the carbon dioxide produced by metabolism.

Ventilatory failure is diagnosed whenever the $Paco_2$ level rises above 50 mm Hg. Acute ventilatory failure occurs when the $Paco_2$ level is above 50 mm Hg with a pH below normal, usually less than 7.30.[8,41] It is referred to as acute because the pH is abnormal, thereby not allowing enough time for the body to compensate by returning the pH to normal. The student of respiratory nursing should remember ventilatory failure occurs because the patient is not breathing or *ventilating* effectively. It will be of little or no help to administer oxygen without also improving ventilation. These patients need assistance to *ventilate,* not necessarily to *oxygenate*.

Interventions that will assist the patient in ventilation include elevating the patient's chest to ease diaphragmatic descent; teaching the patient deep-breathing exercises; encouraging the patient to expectorate mucus, or if this is not possible, suctioning the mucus; and when vital capacity and tidal volume fall severely low while $Paco_2$ continues to climb, providing mechanical ventilation.

A $Paco_2$ value that is less than 35 mm Hg defines *respiratory alkalosis,* which is caused by alveolar hyperventilation.[24] Hyperventilation can result from pain, fever, chills, anxiety, overvigorous mechanical ventilation, sepsis, or as a compensatory mechanism to metabolic acidosis.

Although respiratory alkalosis does not produce the life-threatening situation of respiratory acidosis, it must not be overlooked because the alkalemia decreases cerebral blood flow and can result in cardiac, cerebral, and neuromuscular irritability.[22,24] Interventions are usually aimed at correcting the underlying cause of the alkalemia.

**Step 4: Look at the $HCO_3^-$ level and answer the question, "Does the $HCO_3$ show metabolic acidosis, alkalosis, or normalcy?"** The bicarbonate ($HCO_3$) is the "base" component of acid-base blood gas analysis and reflects kidney or metabolic function. The bicarbonate is reduced or increased in the plasma by renal mechanisms. The normal range is 22 to 26 mEq/L. A bicarbonate level of less than 22 mEq/L defines *metabolic acidosis,* which can result from ketoacidosis, lactic acidosis, renal failure, or diarrhea. A bicarbonate level that is greater than 26 mEq/L defines *metabolic alkalosis,* which can result from fluid loss from the upper GI tract (vomiting or nasogastric suction), diuretic therapy, severe hypokalemia, alkali administration, or corticosteroid therapy.

**Step 5: Look back at the pH level and answer the question, "Does the pH show a compensated or an uncompensated condition?"** If the pH level is abnormal, that is, less than 7.35 or greater than 7.45, the $Paco_2$, the $HCO_3$, or both will also be abnormal. This is an uncompensated condition, because there has not been enough time for the body to return the pH to its normal range. Two examples of uncompensated arterial blood gases follow:

1. $Pao_2$: 90 mm Hg
   pH: 7.25
   $Pco_2$: 50 mm Hg
   $HCO_3$: 22 mEq/L
   This is diagnosed as *uncompensated respiratory acidosis.*
2. $Pao_2$: 90 mm Hg
   pH: 7.25
   $Pco_2$: 40 mm Hg
   $HCO_3$: 17 mEq/L

### THE HENDERSON-HASSELBALCH EQUATION FOR BLOOD pH

The blood pH depends on the ratio of bicarbonate to dissolved carbon dioxide. As long as the ratio is 20:1, the pH will be 7.4.

$$pH = pK^* + \log \frac{base}{acid}$$

$$pH = pK + \log \frac{HCO_3^-}{CO_2}$$

$$pH = 6.1 + \log \frac{24 \text{ mEq/L}}{40 \times .03 \text{ mEq/L}}$$

$$pH = 6.1 + \log 20$$

$$pH = 6.1 + 1.3$$

$$pH = 7.4$$

*pK is the pH at which the substance is half dissociated and half undissociated—value here is 6.1; $HCO_3$ normal is 24 mEq/L; $CO_2$ normal for arterial blood is 40 mm Hg and must be converted to mEq/L to be used in this equation. Therefore the 40 mm Hg is multiplied by .03 to convert to mEq/L.

This is diagnosed as *uncompensated metabolic acidosis*.

If the pH is within normal limits and both the $Paco_2$ and the $HCO_3$ are abnormal, the condition is *compensated* because there has been enough time for the body to restore the pH to within its normal range. Two examples of compensated arterial blood gases follow:

1. $Pao_2$: 90 mm Hg
   pH: 7.37
   $Pco_2$: 60 mm Hg
   $HCO_3$: 38 mEq/L
   This is diagnosed as *compensated respiratory acidosis with metabolic alkalosis*. The acidosis is considered the main disorder and the alkalosis the compensating disorder, because the pH is on the acid side of 7.40.
2. $Pao_2$: 90 mm Hg
   pH: 7.42
   $Pco_2$: 48 mm Hg
   $HCO_3$: 35 mEq/L
   This is diagnosed as *compensated metabolic alkalosis with respiratory acidosis*. The alkalosis is considered the main disorder and the acidosis the compensating disorder, because the pH is on the alkaline side of 7.40.

This method of blood gas interpretation is reviewed in the box below.

### STEPS FOR INTERPRETATION OF BLOOD GAS LEVELS

**STEP 1**

Look at the $Pao_2$ level and answer the question, *"Does the $Pao_2$ level show hypoxemia?"*

**STEP 2**

Look at the pH level and answer the question, *"Is the pH level on the acid or alkaline side of 7.40?"*

**STEP 3**

Look at the $Paco_2$ level and answer the question, *"Does the $Paco_2$ level show respiratory acidosis, alkalosis, or normalcy?"*

**STEP 4**

Look at the $Hco_3$ level and answer the question, *"Does the $Hco_3$ show metabolic acidosis, alkalosis, or normalcy?"*

**STEP 5**

Look back at the pH level and answer the question, *"Does the pH show a compensated or an uncompensated condition?"*

## Other Considerations When Interpreting Arterial Blood Gases

**Oxygen saturation ($Sao_2$). Oxygen saturation** is a measure of the amount of oxygen bound to hemoglobin compared to hemoglobin's maximum capability for binding oxygen.[4,46] It is reported as a percentage or as a decimal with the normal being greater than 96% (.96) on room air. The $Sao_2$ level cannot reach 100% (on room air) because of the normal physiological shunting of venous blood into the arterial system via the bronchial, thebesian, and other minor systems within the lungs and heart. However, when supplemental oxygen is administered, the $Sao_2$ level may approach 100% so closely that it is reported as 100%.

Proper evaluation of the $Sao_2$ level is vital. For example, an $Sao_2$ of 97% means that 97% of the available hemoglobin is bound with oxygen. The word *available* is essential to evaluating the $Sao_2$ level, because the hemoglobin level is not always within normal limits and oxygen can only bind with what is available. A 97% saturation level associated with 10 grams of hemoglobin does not deliver as much oxygen to the tissues as does a 97% saturation associated with 15 grams of hemoglobin. Thus assessing only the $Sao_2$ level and finding it within normal limits should not lead one to believe that the patient's oxygenation status is normal. The hemoglobin level must also be evaluated before a decision on oxygenation status can be made.

**Oxygen content. Oxygen content** ($Cao_2$ or $O_2Ct$) is a measure of the total amount of oxygen carried in the blood including the amount dissolved in plasma, measured by the $Pao_2$, and the amount bound to the hemoglobin molecule, measured by the $Sao_2$. $Cao_2$ is reported in milliliters (ml) of oxygen carried per 100 ml of blood. The normal value is 18 to 20 ml of oxygen carried per 100 ml of blood; this can also be stated as 18 to 20 vol%.

To calculate the oxygen content, the $Pao_2$, the $Sao_2$, and the hemoglobin level are used; therefore a change in any of these factors will change the $Cao_2$. For instance, a low hemoglobin concentration will yield a low $Cao_2$.

The value of assessing the $Cao_2$ is best illustrated by the example in Table 10-7. Here, the arterial blood gas parameters that are most commonly used to evaluate oxygenation status ($Pao_2$ and $Sao_2$) are both normal. Assessing only the $Pao_2$ and the $Sao_2$ would lead to the false belief that, in Patient B, oxygenation status is normal. However, it can be seen by looking at the hemoglobin and the $Cao_2$ that the oxygenation of Patient B's blood is far from normal.

Table 10-7 illustrates two essential facts of oxygenation assessment: (1) checking the $Pao_2$ and the $Sao_2$ are not enough and (2) a patient may not be *hypoxemic* but may be *hypoxic*. Hypoxemia versus hypoxia is discussed in more detail in Chapter 11. By assessing oxygen content, one is assessing **oxygen transportation** in the blood.

**Oxygen transport within the blood.** Approximately 1000 ml of oxygen is transported to the cells each minute.[31] Oxygen is transported to the tissue cells by the blood in two ways. It is either *dissolved in plasma ($Pao_2$)* or *bound to*

***Table 10-7*** Assessing oxygenation status

| Patient | $Pa_{O_2}$ level (mm Hg) | $Sa_{O_2}$ level (%) | Hb level (gm%) | $Ca_{O_2}$ level (vol%) |
|---|---|---|---|---|
| A | 100 | 97 | 15 | 19.8 |
| B | 100 | 97 | 10 | 13.3 |

*hemoglobin molecules ($Sa_{O_2}$).* Most of the oxygen is transported by hemoglobin, with the portion of oxygen dissolved in plasma equal to approximately 3% of the total oxygen within the blood. However, whereas only a small portion of the total amount of oxygen carried by the blood is dissolved in plasma, it is this dissolved portion that is significant to cellular oxygenation. The pressure exerted by the oxygen dissolved in plasma is important because this oxygen diffuses across the capillary membrane into the cells first and serves as the vehicle for the unloading of the oxygen from the hemoglobin molecule. As molecules of dissolved oxygen leave the plasma and diffuse into the cells, other molecules of oxygen move off the hemoglobin molecule, dissolve into the plasma, and, in turn, diffuse into the cells. For this procedure to begin, the $Pa_{O_2}$ must be greater than the oxygen level within the cell.

***Oxyhemoglobin dissociation curve.*** The relationship between dissolved oxygen and hemoglobin-bound oxygen is illustrated graphically as the **oxyhemoglobin dissociation curve** (Fig. 10-2). The sigmoid shape of the oxyhemoglobin dissociation curve illustrates several essential points about the relationship between the two ways oxygen is carried. The *steep lower portion* of the curve, at $Pa_{O_2}$ levels of 10 to 50 mm Hg, shows that the peripheral tissues can withdraw large amounts of oxygen from the hemoglobin molecule with only a small change in $Pa_{O_2}$, thus preserving the gradient for the continued unloading of hemoglobin.

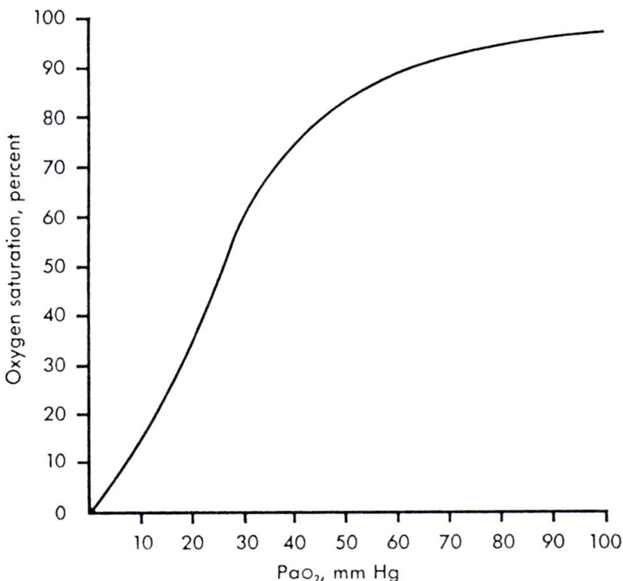


***Fig. 10-2*** Oxyhemoglobin dissociation curve.

***Table 10-8*** Predictable relationship of $Pa_{O_2}$ and $Sa_{O_2}$ on the normal oxyhemoglobin dissociation curve

| $Pa_{O_2}$ (mm Hg) | $Sa_{O_2}$ (%) |
|---|---|
| 100 | 98 |
| 90 | 97 |
| 80 | 95 |
| 70 | 93 |
| 60 | 89 |
| 50 | 84 |
| 40 | 75 |
| 30 | 57 |
| 20 | 35 |
| 10 | 14 |

The area at $Pa_{O_2}$ levels of 60 to 100 mm Hg is called the *flat upper portion* of the curve. This portion shows that the saturation of hemoglobin remains high even as the $Pa_{O_2}$ declines. For example, in a healthy person, a $Pa_{O_2}$ of 60 mm Hg yields a saturation of 89%, whereas a $Pa_{O_2}$ of 100 mm Hg yields a saturation of 98%. The great drop in $Pa_{O_2}$ (from 100 to 60 mm Hg) causes only a small drop in oxygen saturation (from 98% to 89%). For this reason, many patients with chronic lung disease manage quite well with a $Pa_{O_2}$ as low as 55 or 60 mm Hg since that level (1) provides sufficient loading of hemoglobin with oxygen and (2) provides a $Pa_{O_2}$ gradient sufficient for the unloading of hemoglobin.

The ability of human beings to live comfortably at high altitudes is based on the unique relationship between dissolved oxygen and hemoglobin-bound oxygen, illustrated by assessing the flat upper portion of the curve. At high altitudes, because of the decreased barometric pressure, the $Pa_{O_2}$ will fall. There exists a wide range in which the $Pa_{O_2}$ can fall, yet loading of the hemoglobin molecule remains quite sufficient.

***Shifting of the oxyhemoglobin dissociation curve.*** Under normal circumstances, hemoglobin has a steady and predictable affinity for oxygen. The combination of oxygen and hemoglobin based on this affinity is responsible for the position of the oxyhemoglobin dissociation curve wherein a given $Pa_{O_2}$ will yield a predictable oxygen saturation. Table 10-8 illustrates this predictable relationship between the $Pa_{O_2}$ and $Sa_{O_2}$.

Occasionally, particularly in critically ill individuals, events will occur that alter the affinity hemoglobin has for oxygen. Anytime this affinity is altered, the position of the oxyhemoglobin dissociation curve will shift (Fig. 10-3). Shifts in the position of the curve mean there is a change in the way oxygen is taken up by the hemoglobin molecule

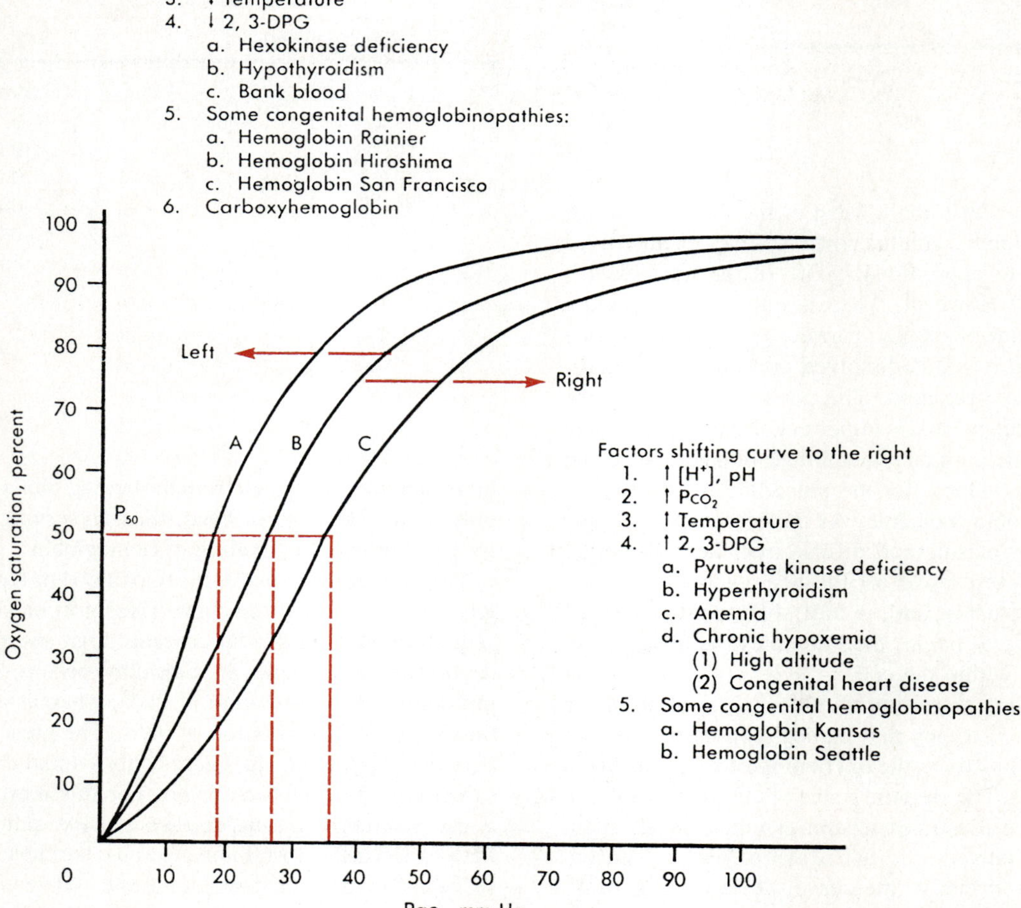


***Fig. 10-3*** Curve B is the standard oxyhemoglobin dissociation curve. Curve A shows the curve shifted to the left because of hemoglobin's increased affinity for oxygen. Curve C shows the curve shifted to the right because of hemoglobin's decreased affinity for oxygen. Factors responsible for shifting the curve are listed adjacent to curves A and C. (From Kinney MR and others: AACN's clinical reference for critical care nursing, St Louis, 1988, Mosby–Year Book, Inc.)

in the alveolar level, as well as a change in the way oxygen is delivered at the tissue level.

***Clinical implications of a shifted curve.*** When the curve is shifted to the right (Fig. 10-3, *curve C),* there is a lower oxygen saturation for any given $PaO_2$; in other words, hemoglobin has less affinity for oxygen. Although the saturation is lower than expected, a right shift enhances oxygen delivery at the tissue level because hemoglobin unloads more readily. Factors that cause this change in oxygen-hemoglobin affinity and thus shift the curve include fever, increased $PaCO_2$, acidosis, and an increase in **2,3-diphosphoglycerate (2,3-DPG)** (see the box on p. 227).

When the curve is shifted to the left (Fig. 10-3, *curve A*), quite the reverse occurs; there is a higher arterial saturation for any given $PaO_2$ because hemoglobin has an increased affinity for oxygen. Although the saturation is higher, oxygen delivery to the tissues is impaired because hemoglobin does not unload as easily. Factors that contribute to the effect include hypothermia, alkalemia, decreased $PaCO_2$, and decreased 2,3-DPG.

To assess whether the curve is shifted to the left or to the right, the $PaO_2$ at the 50% saturation level ($P_{50}$) must be assessed. Fig. 10-3 shows that when the curve is in its normal position, a $P_{50}$ is associated with a $PaO_2$ of 26.6 mm Hg. If, when looking at the $P_{50}$, the $PaO_2$ is higher, the curve is shifted to the right (Fig. 10-3, *curve C*). On the other hand, if, when looking at the $P_{50}$, the $PaO_2$ is less than 26.6 mm Hg, the curve is shifted to the left (Fig. 10-3, *curve A*).

When working in a clinical situation in which a $P_{50}$ is not

## WHAT IS 2,3-DPG?

2,3-Diphosphoglycerate (2,3-DPG), an organic phosphate found primarily in red blood cells, has the ability to alter the affinity of hemoglobin for oxygen. When the level of 2,3-DPG increases within the red blood cells, hemoglobin's affinity for oxygen is decreased (a shift in the oxyhemoglobin curve to the right), thus making more oxygen available to the tissues. Increased synthesis of 2,3-DPG apparently is an important component of the adaptive responses in healthy persons to an acute need for more tissue oxygen. Tissue hypoxia acts as the stimulus for production of 2,3-DPG, and increased amounts have been found in patients with anemia, right-to-left shunts, and congestive heart failure and in persons residing at high altitudes.[33]

A decrease in the amount of 2,3-DPG is detrimental to tissue oxygenation because this decrease causes hemoglobin's affinity for oxygen to increase (a shift in the oxyhemoglobin curve to the left). Situations resulting in decreased 2,3-DPG levels include hypophosphatemia, septic shock, and the use of banked blood.[39] Blood preserved with acid citrate dextrose loses most of its red cell 2,3-DPG within several days. Blood preserved with citrate phosphate dextrose maintains its 2,3-DPG levels for several weeks. Transfusion of blood with low 2,3-DPG will not be beneficial for tissue oxygenation until the 2,3-DPG level is restored, which may take 18 to 24 hours.[4,39]

available, one need only remember the above clinical situations that are responsible for left and for right shift of the curve.

**Expected $Pa_{O_2}$.** When a patient is put on supplemental oxygen, his or her $Pa_{O_2}$ level is expected to rise. Knowing the level to which the $Pa_{O_2}$ *should* rise in normal subjects on a given $FI_{O_2}$ and comparing that to the level in which the $Pa_{O_2}$ actually *does* rise in patients with pulmonary disease has value, because it illustrates how well the lung is functioning.

Calculating the expected $Pa_{O_2}$ is accomplished by multiplying the $FI_{O_2}$ value by 5.[41] Thus the expected $Pa_{O_2}$ on an $FI_{O_2}$ of 30% should be at least 150 mm Hg (30 × 5), whereas the expected $Pa_{O_2}$ on an $FI_{O_2}$ of 50% should be 250 mm Hg (50 × 5). These expected $Pa_{O_2}$ values represent the oxygen level achievable with healthy lungs. Pulmonary disease can radically decrease the expected $Pa_{O_2}$ level. Table 10-9 illustrates three examples of what can occur when the expected $Pa_{O_2}$ level does not reach normal.

Patient A shows a normal expected $Pa_{O_2}$ level; thus it is assumed that his or her lungs are performing normally. The fact that the expected $Pa_{O_2}$ level is reached means he or she may not require supplemental oxygen. Patient B does not reach the expected $Pa_{O_2}$ level, but at least he or she is not hypoxemic; supplemental oxygen, administered at an $FI_{O_2}$ of .50, allows the $Pa_{O_2}$ level to be above 80 mm Hg. However, because the expected $Pa_{O_2}$ level is not achieved, an assumption should be made that removal of oxygen will result in hypoxemia.[41] Therefore in situations like this, nursing care must include education of the patient, his or her family, and all caregivers about the importance of the oxygen remaining in place. Patient C does not reach the expected $Pa_{O_2}$ level, and he or she is hypoxemic; he or she needs more help. This may include emphasis on coughing or suctioning of mucus to remove a possible source of ventilation-perfusion inequality, repositioning to allow for better lung inflation and for better matching of ventilation with perfusion, and increasing the $FI_{O_2}$ or applying positive end-expiratory pressure (PEEP) if the patient is mechanically ventilated.

**Table 10-9** The expected $Pa_{O_2}$ versus the actual $Pa_{O_2}$

| Patient* | $FI_{O_2}$ level (%) | Expected $Pa_{O_2}$ level (mm Hg) | Actual $Pa_{O_2}$ level (mm Hg) |
|---|---|---|---|
| A | 30 | 150 | 160 |
| B | 50 | 250 | 85 |
| C | 50 | 250 | 60 |

*Patients are all under 60 years of age.

It is impossible to apply the "$FI_{O_2}$ value × 5" rule to achieve the expected $Pa_{O_2}$ value when the patient is on a system that delivers oxygen by liters per minute. For these situations, Table 10-10 shows the $FI_{O_2}$ levels that correspond to various oxygen delivery systems.

**Body temperature.** Body temperature will alter the normal affinity that exists between oxygen and hemoglobin. For this reason, either the patient's temperature must be taken when the arterial blood gases are drawn, or the computer that measures and records the blood gas levels must also measure the blood temperature.

Fever will decrease the normal affinity that exists between oxygen and hemoglobin, which results in a decrease in oxyhemoglobin but an increase in the oxygen dissolved in plasma. In the presence of fever, less oxygen will bind to hemoglobin, but because of its lessened affinity for hemoglobin, the oxygen will unload more readily at the tissue level.

Hypothermia will increase the normal affinity that exists between oxygen and hemoglobin, resulting in more oxyhemoglobin and a lower $Pa_{O_2}$ for any given saturation. Oxygen will less readily unload at the tissue level. This physiology is illustrated by a leftward shift of the oxyhemoglobin dissociation curve.

A general rule is that fever helps the unloading of oxygen at the tissue level (within limits), whereas hypothermia interferes with the unloading of hemoglobin.

**Base excess and base deficit.** Base excess and base deficit reflect the nonrespiratory contribution to acid-base

**Table 10-10** Guidelines for estimating $FIO_2$ with low-flow oxygen devices

| 100% $O_2$ flow rate (L) | $FIO_2$ (%) |
|---|---|
| **NASAL CANNULA OR CATHETER** | |
| 1 | 24 |
| 2 | 28 |
| 3 | 32 |
| 4 | 36 |
| 5 | 40 |
| 6 | 44 |
| **OXYGEN MASK** | |
| 5-6 | 40 |
| 6-7 | 50 |
| 7-8 | 60 |
| **MASK WITH RESERVOIR BAG** | |
| 6 | 60 |
| 7 | 70 |
| 8 | 80 |
| 9 | 90 |
| 10 | 99+ |

Note: Normal ventilatory pattern assumed.
From Shapiro BA, Harrison, RA, and Walton JR: Clinical application of blood gases, St Louis, 1989, Mosby–Year Book, Inc.

balance and are reported in milliequivalents per liter above or below the normal range of −2 mEq/L to +2 mEq/L. A negative base level is reported as a *base deficit*, which correlates with metabolic acidosis, whereas a positive base level is reported as a *base excess*, which correlates with metabolic alkalosis.

**Alveolar–arterial oxygen tension difference.** The alveolar–arterial oxygen tension difference [$(A\text{-}a)DO_2$] is also written as $P(A\text{-}a)O_2$ and referred to as the A-a gradient. It measures the difference between the oxygen tension within the alveoli (A) and the artery (a) and provides information on the efficiency of the transfer of oxygen into the blood at the alveolar-capillary level. Serial determinations of the A-a gradient provide clinically useful data on lung function and are useful guides to therapy.[34]

The normal gradient for persons under 61 years of age is 10 mm Hg (measured while breathing room air). However, the normal gradient elevates in at least two instances not related to acute lung pathology. First, age elevates the gradient, because the lungs develop ventilation-perfusion (V/Q) inequalities as a normal part of aging, thereby resulting in less efficient oxygen exchange; in one study, persons aged 61 to 75 years had an average A-a gradient of 16 mm Hg.[33] Second, the use of supplemental oxygen will elevate the gradient at least up to an $FIO_2$ of 60%.[26] Changes in $PaCO_2$ will not affect the A-a gradient.

Recently, the clinical usefulness of the A-a gradient has been questioned, particularly because of its variability when calculated on levels of oxygen above room air[40] and because of the need to calculate the $PAO_2$.[17] An elevated A-a gradient can result from V/Q inequalities, from shunt abnormality (Qs/Qt), or from diffusion limitations.

**The arterial/alveolar oxygen tension ratio.** The relationship between the $PaO_2$ and the $PAO_2$ can also be expressed as a ratio, $PaO_2/PAO_2$. Like the A-a gradient, the arterial/alveolar oxygen tension ratio ($PaO_2/PAO_2$) also requires the calculation of the alveolar $PO_2$. Unlike the A-a gradient, the $PaO_2/PAO_2$ remains relatively stable when the $FIO_2$ changes as long as the underlying lung condition is stable.[17,35]

The normal $PaO_2/PAO_2$ ratio is 0.75 to 0.90 for any $FIO_2$. A ratio of less than 0.75 indicates V/Q inequality, shunt, or diffusion limitation.

**The $PaO_2/FIO_2$ ratio.** The oxygen ratio, $PaO_2/FIO_2$, is easier to calculate than the A-a gradient or the $PaO_2/PAO_2$, because it does not require use of the alveolar gas equation in its calculation. However, it has the disadvantage of being affected by changes in the $PaCO_2$, and there is much controversy over its usefulness as a predictor of pulmonary dysfunction.[26,27] Specifically, some studies have shown it to be an insensitive indicator of changes in shunt.[17,42]

**Arterial-mixed venous oxygen content difference.** When both arterial blood samples and pulmonary arterial blood samples are available, the arterial-mixed venous oxygen content difference ($A\text{-}VDO_2$) can be calculated. The $A\text{-}VDO_2$ represents an assessment of the cardiac output in relation to metabolic needs and is useful in determining oxygen extraction and whether cardiac output is sufficient enough to meet the body's metabolic needs.

In healthy persons, the $A\text{-}VDO_2$ is 5.0 vol% with the normal range being 4.5 to 6.0 vol%.[42] Critically ill patients with adequate cardiovascular function can maintain an $A\text{-}VDO_2$ of 2.5-4.5 vol%, whereas critically ill patients with inadequate cardiovascular reserves may show an $A\text{-}VDO_2$ greater than 6.0 vol%.

### Blood Studies

Blood studies usually involve obtaining the patient's complete blood cell count (CBC), electrolytes, and general chemistry profile. Other studies are added depending on the patient's history and physical condition. Isoenzymes of creatine phosphokinase (CPK) are appropriate in chest injury when myocardial damage is questioned.

The CBC and white blood cell count (WBC) differential are general screening tests. Increased WBCs with a shift to the left (high numbers of immature neutrophils) suggest bacterial as opposed to viral infections[11,32,37] and, therefore, assist in delineating treatment of pneumonia, especially in situations where sputum analysis, for one reason or another, has not been achieved. Elevated eosinophils (more than 500/$mm^3$) accompany asthma and certain allergic lung conditions. Lung disease is often associated with polycythemia because of chronic tissue hypoxia. Polycythemia will develop even if tissue hypoxia is only present during part of the 24-hour period, such as at night when decreased ventilation and oxygen intake cause oxygen desaturation of the hemoglobin molecule.[32] The presence of anemia may explain tachypnea and persistent tissue hypoxia despite normal $Po_2$ and $O_2$ saturations.

Evaluation of electrolytes can yield important information about the patient's overall condition, and the effects of therapy or the need for therapy. Sodium levels can shed light on the fluid status of the patient, which becomes crucial in the patient critically ill with pulmonary disease. Evaluation of sodium levels in urine and blood may identify the syndrome of inappropriate secretion of antidiuretic hormone (SIADH), which can occur in ventilator-supported patients or patients receiving frequent intermittent positive-pressure breathing (IPPB) treatments.[19]

Maintaining a normal potassium level is important in treating acid-base abnormalities. The body cannot fully correct an alkalosis that occurs along with hypokalemia, because potassium is the exchange ion in the kidney that allows for retention of hydrogen ion ($H^+$) and thus lowers pH.[13] The opposite is true in acidosis associated with hyperkalemia.

Recently the role of phosphate in adequate diaphragmatic contractility has surfaced. Phosphate levels should be evaluated in patients with acute respiratory failure to determine if hypophosphatemia is contributing to poor venitilatory dynamics.[1]

An analysis of serum enzymes may be helpful in identifying patients who may have experienced pulmonary infarction. Because enzymes are present in many body tissues, more definite radiological tests are usually performed to confirm pulmonary injury.

### Sputum Studies

Sputum should always be carefully evaluated. The most difficult aspect of sputum examination is proper collection of the specimen. When the patient has difficulty producing sputum, inducing sputum with heated, nebulized saline may help to loosen secretions for expectoration. Chest physiotherapy combined with nebulization will improve the success rate. Collection of a sputum specimen is best done in the morning, because secretions have a greater volume caused by nighttime pooling.[34] The presence of an effective, forceful cough is helpful; however, many critically ill patients are unable to cough effectively and thus sputum collection by other means, such as transtracheal aspiration, is required.

**Transtracheal aspiration.** Transtracheal aspiration (TTA) in nonintubated patients is preferred over nasotracheal or bronchial washings. In this technique, a catheter is introduced by cricoid stick into the trachea. This eliminates contamination of sputum by resident flora of mouth and pharynx. The TTA maneuver should be performed by an experienced physician, because major complications can occur.[11,37] Massive intraairway hemorrhage is possible, dysrhythmias can occur, and subcutaneous emphysema can develop.

**Endotracheal/tracheal specimen collection.** Many critically ill patients will have endotracheal or tracheal tubes already in place. Collecting sputum specimens from these patients requires special attention to technique. Deep specimens should be obtained to avoid resident upper airway flora that may have migrated down the tube. This colonization of the lower airways with upper airway flora can occur within 24 hours of intubation of tracheostomy.[32,48]

**Other methods of specimen collection.** Proper specimen retrieval may require more invasive measures, such as the use of a fiberoptic bronchoscopy in association with a sheath-protected catheter specimen, a transbronchial biopsy and bronchoalveolar lavage, a transthoracic needle aspiration of lung, or an open lung biopsy.

The fiberoptic bronchoscopy is the most frequent invasive procedure used in the diagnosis of pulmonary infections. It is versatile with respect to options (that is, it can be used for simple specimen collection, biopsy, lavage, or all three) and has few side-effects. Bleeding occurs in up to 7% of patients, and hypoxemia can be associated with the procedure.[43]

Although transthoracic needle aspiration can be selectively guided by fluoroscopy, complications are frequent and significant. Hemoptysis occurs in 3% to 10% of patients, and pneumothorax occurs in 20% to 30%.[2,43]

Open biopsy offers the best opportunity for the investigation of pulmonary infection. Theoretically, by locating the proper area for specimen collection and biopsy, ineffective results should be eliminated. However, one study showed that only 70% of the cases of open biopsy yielded identification of the causative organism.[12] The mortality rate is around 5%, which poses a major disadvantage to this approach. Critically ill patients may not be able to tolerate such a procedure, and all other methods of diagnosis are generally employed first.

Once a sputum specimen is obtained, a Gram's stain followed by a culture and sensitivity (C&S) should be performed. A Gram's stain allows for cellular quantification and evaluation of the value of the specimen.

## DIAGNOSTIC PROCEDURES

### Bronchoscopy

**Indications.** Bronchoscopy is a relatively safe procedure that is most often used as a diagnostic tool (see the box "Indications for Bronchoscopy" on p. 230). Therapeutic uses include the removal of foreign bodies, removal of obstructing secretions, and resection of small, benign growths from the airway.

**Procedure.** Bronchoscopy can be performed with a rigid or flexible scope. Table 10-11 outlines the indications and disadvantages of both apparatuses. Some operators use one type of scope to supplement the capabilities of the other type, although the flexible fiberoptic scope has become the instrument of choice in most situations.

Before the bronchoscopy, a complete patient history and examination, including a chest x-ray examination, should

## INDICATIONS FOR BRONCHOSCOPY

Persistent, unexplained cough
Hemoptysis of unknown origin
Aspiration of gastric contents, foreign body, mucus
Bronchial obstruction
Pleural effusion of unknown origin
Suspected pulmonary tumor
Tissue biopsy
Retrieval of cellular elements and secretions for culture and cytology
Bronchial lavage
Staging of lung tumors
Evaluation of inhalation injury
Suspected lung cancer
Interstitial or alveolar infiltrates of unknown origin
Lung infections
Atelectasis
Guide patient intubation in neck injury

be performed. Preoperative evaluation of the patient should also include clotting studies (PT, PTT, and platelet count) and evaluation of the arterial blood gas levels. When the platelet count is less than 50,000, platelet transfusions before and during the procedure should be given.[10] Hypoxemic patients (less than 70 mm Hg $Pa_{O_2}$) need supplemental oxygen during the procedure. The patient should have nothing by mouth for 4 to 6 hours before the bronchoscopy to reduce the risk of aspiration.[19]

Although topical anesthesia can be used alone, it is generally supplemented by systemic anesthesia or analgesia. Diazepam (Valium) and midazolam HCl (Versed) are two agents frequently administered intravenously during the procedure. Preoperative medications for a diagnostic bronchoscopy may include atropine and intramuscular codeine. The atropine lessens the vasovagal response and reduces the secretions, whereas codeine decreases the cough reflex. When a bronchoscopy is performed therapeutically to remove secretions, medications other than analgesics are avoided because intratracheal topical anesthetics tend to decrease cough and impair secretion clearance.

The bronchoscopy should not be performed within a few days of other operative procedures because of increased secretions that result from local irritation. By the same token, after a bronchoscopy, patients often experience an increased cough and throat discomfort. A small amount of blood may be present in the sputum and a slight fever, should it occur, is usually self-limiting.

**Summary of nursing care.** The nursing care of patients undergoing therapeutic or diagnostic bronchoscopy involves (1) preparation of the patient psychologically and physically for the procedure and (2) monitoring the patient's responses to the procedure and assessing the patient after the bronchoscopy.

Many of the bronchoscopies performed on the critically ill patient are carried out to remove secretions interfering with proper aeration. Anxiety is often present because of the concomitant tissue hypoxia, the artificial airway, and possible ventilator support. The patient may fear the insertion of the bronchoscope because he or she assumes that it will interfere with breathing and therefore lead to suffocation. The nurse must reassure the patient that proper ventilation will occur.

The nonintubated patient undergoing a bronchoscopy should receive nothing by mouth both before the procedure and until the gag reflex returns afterwards. Periodical assessment of the gag reflex should be performed.

During the procedure, the nurse should monitor the patient's vital signs and oxygenation and inform the physician of changes. If specimen retrieval is performed during the bronchoscopy, the nurse may need to assist in preparing the specimen for transport to the laboratory.

Following the procedure, the patient must be observed for the development of complications, degree of oxygenation, and return of the cough and gag reflexes.

*Table 10-11* Comparison of rigid and flexible bronchoscope

| Indications | Disadvantages |
|---|---|
| **RIGID BRONCHOSCOPE** | |
| Evaluate large lung hemorrhage (>200 cc)<br>Removal of foreign body<br>Surgical excision of tracheal or main bronchial lesions<br>Biopsy of vascular tumor | Limited visualization of distal airways<br>Cannot be used with mechanically ventilated patients<br>Limited in patients with cervical problems<br>Less patient comfort, especially with local anesthesia |
| **FLEXIBLE BRONCHOSCOPE** | |
| Applied in full variety of diagnostic and therapeutic situations | View may be inferior in quality and easily obscured<br>May be difficult to control massive hemorrhage<br>May necessitate several withdrawals and reinsertions during procedure<br>Size can limit removal of foreign bodies and secretions |

When a tissue biopsy is performed, some hemoptysis may occur immediately after the bronchoscopy. Frank bleeding is not usual and may mean hemorrhage is occurring.

In the nonintubated patient, equipment for emergency airway management should be available to treat tracheal edema, which may result from the procedure. The patient may complain of a sore throat and hoarseness, but these side effects are generally self-limiting.

### Thoracentesis

**Indications.** Thoracentesis is a simple, usually uncomplicated procedure for the removal of fluid (pleural effusion) from the pleural space. It is most frequently used as a diagnostic measure, although in rare circumstances it may be performed therapeutically as in the case of pleural effusion drainage.

Most pleural effusions are self-limiting, and unless the cause is unknown or therapy for the patient may be altered by the results, thoracentesis is unwarranted. When a pleural effusion persists despite treatment of the primary cause, thoracentesis should be considered.

**Procedure.** The patient should be in a sitting position with legs over the side of the bed and hands and arms supported on a padded overbed table. If the patient's condition precludes sitting, the side-lying position with back flush with the edge of the bed can be used. The patient should be cautioned not to move or cough during the procedure.

During the thoracentesis, the site of the needle insertion is usually determined by previous chest x-ray examination results, CT scan, or chest percussion. A local anesthetic is used to minimize patient discomfort during insertion of the thoracentesis needle. Most institutions now have disposable thoracentesis trays, which contain all the equipment required for the procedure.

**Relative contraindications.** No absolute contraindications to thoracentesis exist, although there are risks that generally contraindicate the procedure in all but emergency situations. Factors that heighten the risk of thoracentesis include unstable hemodynamics, coagulation defects, mechanically ventilated patients, the presence of an intraaortic balloon pump,[38] or patients who are uncooperative. In most clinical situations, diagnostic thoracentesis can be delayed until these risk factors are eliminated.

**Complications.** Complications associated with thoracentesis include pain, pneumothorax, and reexpansion pulmonary edema. The risk of pain or pneumothorax is significantly reduced when the thoracentesis is performed by an experienced clinician. Reexpansion pulmonary edema can occur when a large amount of effusion fluid is removed from the pleural space.[26,36,38] Removal of the fluid increases the negative intrapleural pressure which, when the lung does not reexpand to fill the space, can lead to edema. The patient can experience severe coughing and shortness of breath. The onset of these symptoms is an indication to discontinue the thoracentesis.

**Summary of nursing care.** Nursing care of patients undergoing thoracentesis is directed at (1) preparing the patient both psychologically and physically, and (2) monitoring the patient's condition during and following the procedure. In critical care patients, performing a thoracentesis may be more problematic because of the patient's being confused and less alert or resulting from an unstable hemodynamic state or positioning limitations imposed by the patient's condition. The nurse must adjust her or his plans and responses based on the presence of complicating patient situations.

A thorough explanation should be given to patients about what will be done to them and expected from them during the thoracentesis procedure. Patient cooperation and understanding increases the safety and ease of the procedure. Supplemental oxygen should be provided, and proper positioning of the patient accomplished. Baseline vital signs should be taken, and provisions made for ongoing monitoring of these parameters.

When possible, oxygenation should be monitored by oximetry or other instantaneous measuring devices. Removal of a large pleural effusion is often accompanied by a reduction in the $PaO_2$, which can continue up to 24 hours after the procedure. Administering supplemental oxygen can lessen the hypoxemia. The removal of effusion fluid can also result in reexpansion pulmonary edema, which can be evidenced by increasing dyspnea and coughing and decreasing oxygen saturation.[38]

After the thoracentesis, a chest x-ray examination should be performed to rule out accidental pneumothorax, which is a potential complication.[36] The patient's vital signs should be checked every 15 minutes until stable, and the nurse should periodically assess lung sounds and oxygen saturation. The patient should be encouraged to lie with the uninvolved lung facing down, because research shows this position to improve oxygenation. Bleeding is a possibility, and the nurse should evaluate the patient for any signs and symptoms of hemorrhage.

### Pulmonary Function Tests

Pulmonary function tests are designed to quantify respiratory function. They are utilized in five primary ways (see the box "Uses of Pulmonary Function Tests"). Pulmonary

#### USES OF PULMONARY FUNCTION TESTS

- Initial evaluation of patients with a complaint of breathlessness
- Initial evaluation of patients with known respiratory disease
- Document course of patients with respiratory disease
- Preoperative evaluation of patients with respiratory complication
- Screening for subclinical disease

**Table 10-12** Pulmonary volumes and capacities relevant to critical care

| Volume capacity | Definition | Relevance |
|---|---|---|
| Tidal volume ($V_T$) | Volume of air exhaled after normal inhalation; estimated at 500 cc or 6 to 8 cc/kg, while off ventilator, or 10 to 15 cc/kg while on ventilator | Used to assess weaning from mechanical ventilation<br>Must be significantly greater than dead space |
| Dead space volume ($V_D$) | Inhaled air that does not take part in gas exchange<br>Normal, 150 cc (see the box "Types of Dead Space") | An excessive amount will alter normal arterial blood gas levels |
| Minute ventilation ($\dot{V}_E$) | Volume of air inhaled per minute—$V_T \times$ RR*<br>Normal, 4 to 8 L/min (adult) | Must be high enough to prevent accumulation of carbon dioxide ($PaCO_2$)<br>Used to assess weaning from mechanical ventilation |
| Minute alveolar ventilation ($\dot{V}_A$) | Volume of air reaching alveoli per minute—($V_T - V_D$) $\times$ RR | Same as $V_E$<br>Not routinely measured |
| Vital capacity (VC) | Volume of air exhaled after the deepest inhalation<br>Normal, 3 to 5 L | Essential to weaning<br>Usually must be >1 L or 10 to 15 cc/kg for successful weaning from mechanical ventilation |
| Functional residual capacity (FRC) | Volume of air in lung after normal exhalation<br>Normal, 2500 cc | Keeps the lung minimally inflated, decreasing the work of breathing<br>Provides gas exchange between breaths |

*RR, Respiratory rate.

function testing can seldom result in identification of a specific disease. Interpretations must be based on general and specific patterns of dysfunction that suggest a number of different specific disease.[6] Variations in the normal pulmonary function occur with age, gender, and body size.

**Spirometry.** Spirometry, the simplest pulmonary function testing technique, can be performed at the bedside, as well as in the pulmonary laboratory. It is used to measure such pulmonary volumes and capacities as tidal volume, vital capacity, and minute ventilation. Table 10-12 reviews those volumes and capacities that are of value in critical care nursing. Spirometry cannot measure residual volume or functional residual capacity. If these parameters are essential, the gas dilution technique or body plethysmography must be used.

Dynamic pulmonary function tests are designed to evaluate the function of the respiratory muscles, the thorax, and the lungs.[47] Ventilation is accomplished by overcoming inertia and resistance to air flow. Timed breathing studies reflect the ease of ventilation and include forced vital ca-

**Table 10-13** Dynamic pulmonary function tests

| Test | Description | Abnormal value |
|---|---|---|
| Forced vital capacity (FVC) | The maximal amount of gas a patient can exhale into a spirometer as forcefully and as quickly as possible | Flow reduced with obstructive pulmonary disease because of early airway closure caused by forced exhalation |
| Forced expiratory flow in 1 and 3 seconds ($FEV_1$ and $FEV_3$) | The maximal amount of gas a patient can exhale into a spirometer during 1 and 3 seconds of a forced exhalation | Flow reduced in obstructive disease because of early airway closure caused by forced exhalation |
| Forced expiratory flow at midpoint of vital capacity (FEF 25%-75%) | The measure of the average flow rate during the middle 50% of exhalation; also a good measure of small or distal airway function | Reduced in obstructive airway disease and is considered a good indicator of early changes indicating obstructive lung disease |
| Maximal voluntary ventilation (MVV) | The maximal amount of gas that a patient can move in 1 minute. Test usually occurs in a 10-15 second period, with L/min value calculated | Value reduced in moderate to severe obstructive airway disease |

**TYPES OF DEAD SPACE**

*Anatomical dead space* is defined as the area from mouth and nose to terminal bronchioles and is usually estimated at approximately 150 cc. A more specific method of assessing the volume of anatomical dead space uses the following formula: 1 cc of dead space per pound or 2 cc of dead space per kilogram of *ideal* body weight. Anatomical dead space is so termed because it is a component of normal pulmonary anatomy and, under normal conditions, is the only lung area in which dead space exists.

*Alveolar dead space* is pathological and occurs when a gas exchange area is no longer normally perfused. One pathology that produces alveolar dead space is pulmonary embolism. In this circumstance, the embolism decreases blood flow to the lung area distal to it, but the area may still receive ventilation. The result is an area of ventilation with no perfusion, that is, dead space. Normally, there is no measurable alveolar dead space within the lung. Other pathologic conditions that can lead to alveolar dead space include hypotension from decreased cardiac output or hemorrhage. In this case, a redistribution of blood flow and volume favors the dependent parts of the lungs, causing decreased perfusion in many well-ventilated alveoli in the upper lung areas. Positive pressure mechanical ventilation may cause alveolar dead space because the positive pressure can restrict blood flow through some pulmonary capillaries.

*Physiologic dead space* refers to the combination of anatomic and alveolar dead space. Since there is normally no alveolar dead space, physiologic dead space should equal anatomical dead space in healthy lungs.

pacity, forced expiratory flow at midpoint of vital capacity, forced expiratory flow at 1 and 3 seconds, and maximal voluntary ventilation. Table 10-13 defines these tests.

**Lung disorders and pulmonary function tests.** Pulmonary function testing allows separation of lung disorders into the two categories: restrictive and obstructive. *Restrictive disorders* can be intrinsic (within the lungs) or extrinsic (outside the lungs). An example of an intrinsic disorder is pulmonary fibrosis or interstitial lung disease, whereas kyphoscoliosis is an example of extrinsic disorder. Regardless of the cause, restrictive disorders limit lung expansion and therefore reflect diminished volumes and capacities. Restrictive disorders may have little or no effect on air flow in and out of the lungs; therefore timed studies may be normal[8,26] (see Table 10-13).

*Obstructive disorders* affect air flow; consequently, timed ventilatory values will be decreased in relationship to normal values. Volume and capacity measurements in individuals with obstructive disorders may be normal or increased (Table 10-14). As air flow out of the lung is impeded, air trapping occurs and lung overinflation results. This process tends to progress as the disease worsens. In obstructive disorders, the vital capacity reduction results from air trapping and increased residual lung volume, which compromises the vital capacity.[47]

Because critically ill patients may not be able to actively cooperate in pulmonary function studies, complete batteries are infrequently performed and results must be considered in relation to the total picture. The constraints involved with mechanical ventilation or artificial airways preclude accurate pulmonary function studies. Nevertheless, some parameters that provide information about the static and dynamic properties of the lung can be gathered.

If the patient is being mechanically ventilated, the results of some of these pulmonary function tests may be readily available for interpretation. When using this data to assess a patient's status, evaluation of the trend is more important than evaluation of an isolated finding.

In patients on IMV/SIMV ventilation, parameters that can reflect changes in the patient's condition include increasing respiratory rate, decreasing tidal volume, and increased resistance as seen by changes in pressure needed to ventilate. This can reflect airway obstruction, the need for secretion clearance, and respiratory muscle fatigue.

### Ventilation-Perfusion Scanning

**Indications.** The major goal of the lungs is to provide adequate gas exchange between people and their environment. Intimate contact between the alveolar-capillary mem-

***Table 10-14*** Pulmonary function findings in lung disorders

| Test | Predominantly reversible air flow obstruction (asthma) | Predominantly irreversible air flow obstruction | Interstitial lung disease (restrictive disease) | Emphysema (obstructive disease) |
|---|---|---|---|---|
| $FEV_1$ | ↓↓ | ↓↓ | ↓ | ↓↓ |
| FVC | ↓ | ↓ | ↓↓ | ↓ |
| $FEV_1$/FVC% | ↓ | ↓ | N or ↑ | ↓ |
| TLC | N or ↑ | N or ↑ | ↓ | ↑↑ |
| RV | ↑ | ↑ | ↓ | ↑↑ |
| $DL_{CO}$ | N or ↑ | ↓ | N or ↓ | ↓↓ |

↑, increased; ↑↑, greatly increased; ↓, decreased; ↓↓, greatly decreased; N, normal; $FEV_1$, forced expiratory volume in 1 second; FVC, forced vital capacity; RV, residual volume; TLC, total lung capacity; $D_{LCO}$, the diffusing capacity of carbon monoxide.

## DIAGNOSTIC USES OF VENTILATION-PERFUSION SCANNING

**Perfusion abnormalities**

Vasculitis
Arteriovenous fistula
Pulmonary hypertension
Tumors of hilum
Bullous emphysema
Diffuse interstitial fibrosis
Pulmonary infarction
Conditions creating regional lung hypoxia

**Ventilation abnormalities**

Chronic obstructive pulmonary disease
Bronchiectasis
Cystic fibrosis
Airway obstruction
Pneumonia
Pulmonary infarction
Severe pulmonary edema

**Evaluation of function before lung resection surgery**

brane is provided by millions of alveoli with billions of capillaries draped around them in a sheetlike fashion. With ideal matching of ventilation (air) and perfusion (blood), each alveolar-capillary unit would receive an equal amount of air and an equal amount of blood simultaneously. This would result in a ventilation-perfusion (V/Q) ratio of 1.0.[9,14] The ideal, however, never exists even in normal lungs, because of physiological and anatomic shunting of blood. In normal subjects, mismatching of V/Q relationships is not detrimental, but illnesses or diseases that substantially alter V/Q ratios can result in serious impairment of gas exchange. **Ventilation-perfusion scanning** is indicated where a serious alteration of the normal V/Q relationship is suspected. (See the box "Diagnostic Uses of Ventilation-Perfusion Scanning.")

**Procedure.** V/Q scans are one method to evaluate the relationship of air distribution and blood flow in lungs. The V/Q scan involves the use of radioisotopes, most commonly xenon or technetium, which are administered by inhalation and intravenous techniques.

Scintillation cameras record the gamma radiation images produced by the isotope as it is breathed or perfused into the lung. When an obstruction of the isotope's flow into an area of the lung occurs, the diminished radioactivity will be reflected in the camera image of that zone. Newer portable cameras have been developed that allow bedside V/Q studies to be performed on critically ill patients who are too unstable to be moved to the nuclear medicine departments.

Perfusion scans are usually obtained by injecting a radioactive nucleotide, often technetium ($^{99m}$Tc) intravenously. These particles are 50 to 1,000 times larger than other radioactive colloids and are trapped in the vascular bed as they pass through the lungs. A scintiograph camera measures the concentrations and reflects it on a cathode tube. Areas of the lung receiving more perfusion will show a more dense collection than will a less perfused lung tissue. Pulmonary emboli alter the normal perfusion pattern, hence the resulting concentration of radioactivity.

Ventilation scans may be achieved by having the patient inhale a radioactive gas. The distribution of gas in the lungs is then documented both by the concentration of radioactivity displayed on the scanner and by the time that it takes to clear the gas from the lungs. Ventilation disturbances occur in bronchitis, pneumonia, and obstructive processes.

### REFERENCES

1. Aubier M and others: Effect of hypophosphatemia on diaphragmatic contractility in patients with acute respiratory failure, N Engl J Med 4:313, 1985.
2. Baum G and Wolinsky E: Textbook of pulmonary disease, ed 3, Boston. 1983, Little, Brown & Co.
3. Burdon J and others: The perception of breathlessness in asthma, Am Rev Respir Dis 126:825, 1982.
4. Burton GG and Hodgkin JE: Respiratory care: guide to clinical practice, Philadelphia, 1984, JB Lippincott Co.
5. Chase RA and Gordon J: Overwhelming pneumonia, MCN 70(4):945, 1986.
6. Clausen JL: Clinical interpretation of pulmonary function tests, Resp Care 34(7):638, 1989.
7. DeGowan E and DeGowan R: Bedside diagnostic examination, London, 1976, McMillan Inc.
8. Fishman AP: Pulmonary diseases and disorders, ed 2, New York, 1988, McGraw-Hill Book Co.
9. Freeman L and Johnson P: Clinical radionuclide imaging, vols 1 and 2, ed 3, Orlando, Fla, 1984, Grune & Stratton, Inc.
10. Glenn W and others: Thoracic and cardiovascular surgery, ed 4, Norwalk, Conn, 1983, Appleton-Century-Crofts.
11. Griffith D and Wallace R: Bacterial pneumonia in the adult: diagnosis and therapy, Hosp Med 24:188, 1988.
12. Guenter C and Welch M: Pulmonary medicine, ed 2, Philadelphia, 1983, WB Saunders Co.
13. Guyton A: Textbook of medical physiology, Philadelphia, 1986, WB Saunders Co.
14. Harbert J and DaRocha AF: Textbook of nuclear medicine, ed 2, Philadelphia, 1984, Lea & Febiger.
15. Harper R: A guide to respiratory care, Philadelphia, 1981, JB Lippincott Co.
16. Hess D: Noninvasive monitoring in respiratory care—present, past, and future: an overview, Resp Care 35(6):482, 1990.
17. Hess D and Maxwell C: Which is the best index of oxygenation—P $(A\text{-}a)O_2$, $PaO_2/PAO_2$, or $PaO_2/FiO_2$, Resp Care 30(11):961, 1985.
18. Jansen-Bjerklie S and others: The sensation of pulmonary dyspnea, Nurs Res 35(3):25, 1986.
19. Kaye W: Invasive therapeutic techniques, Heart Lung 12(3):122, 1983.

20. Kinney MR, Packa DR, and Dunbar SB: AACN'S clinical reference for critical care nursing, St Louis, 1988, Mosby–Year Book, Inc.
21. Lane G and Pierce A: When persistence pays off, Nursing 82, 12:44, 1982.
22. Luce JM, Tyler ML, and Pierson DJ: Intensive respiratory care, Philadelphia, 1984, WB Saunders Co.
23. Lush M and others: Dyspnea in the ventilator-assisted patient, Heart Lung 17(5):528, 1988.
24. MacIntyre N: Respiratory monitoring without machinery, Resp Care 35(6):546, 1990.
25. Malasanos L and others: Health assessment, ed 4, St Louis, 1989, Mosby–Year Book, Inc.
26. Martin L: Pulmonary physiology in clinical practice: the essentials for patient care and evaluation, St Louis, 1987, Mosby—Year Book, Inc.
27. Maxwell C, Hess D, and Shefet D: Use of the arterial/alveolar tension ratio to predict the inspired oxygen concentration needed for a desired arterial oxygen tension, Respir Care 29(11):1135, 1984.
28. McCaffery M: Relieve your patient's pain fast and effectively with oral analgesics, Nursing 80, 10(11):58, 1980.
29. McCaffery M: Relieving pain with non-invasive techniques, Nursing 80, 10(12):54, 1980.
30. McCaffery M: Understanding your patient's pain, Nursing 80, 10(9):26, 1980.
31. McCance KL and Huether SE: Pathophysiology: the biologic basis for disease in adults and children, St Louis, 1990, Mosby–Year Book, Inc.
32. McDonnell K, Fahey P, and Segal M: Respiratory intensive care, New York, 1987, Little, Brown & Co.
33. Murray JF: The normal lung, Philadelphia, 1986, WB Saunders Co.
34. Murray JF and Nadel JA: Textbook of respiratory medicine, Philadelphia, 1988, WB Saunders Co.
35. Peris LV and others: Clinical use of the arterial/alveolar oxygen tension ratio, Crit Care Med 11(11):888, 1983.
36. Prosperi A, Mitchell T, and Govi J: Thoracentesis for pleural effusions, Fam Pract Recertification 8(5):29, 1986.
37. Raju L and Kahn F: Pneumonia and the elderly, Geriatrics 43(10):51, 1988.
38. Sahn S: Pleural effusions: diagnosis and management, Hosp Med 24(8):77, 1988.
39. Scanlan CL, Spearman CB, and Sheldon RL: Egan's fundamentals of respiratory care, St Louis, 1990, Mosby–Year Book, Inc.
40. Shapiro BA: Respiratory critical care: state of the art—controversies—new horizons, vol 8, Chicago, 1988, Respiratory Care Seminars, Inc.
41. Shapiro BA, Harrison RA, and Walton JR: Clinical application of blood gases, Chicago, 1982, Mosby–Year Book, Inc.
42. Shapiro BA and others: Clinical application of respiratory care, Chicago, 1985, Mosby–Year Book, Inc.
43. Sheldon RL: Flexible fiberoptic bronchoscopy, Prim Care 12(2):299, 1985.
44. Stark R and Chatterjee M: A new exercise test for clinical dyspnea, Pract Cardiology 9(6):86, 1983.
45. Washington JA: Maximizing diagnostic yield from sputum examination, J Resp Dis 7:81, 1981.
46. Welch JP, DeCasere R, and Hess D: Pulse oximetry: instrumentation and clinical applications, Resp Care 35(6):584, 1990.
47. Williams D and Cugell D: Pulmonary function tests: indications and interpretation, Hosp Med 24(5):23, 1988.
48. Wu WH and Huang S: Tracheal intubation, Consultant 26:34, 1986.

CHAPTER 11

# Pulmonary Disorders

## CHAPTER OBJECTIVES

- *Differentiate between hypoxemia and tissue hypoxia according to cause, symptoms, and treatment.*
- *Discuss important aspects of the nursing care that will prevent and/or treat atelectasis.*
- *Identify and describe the two major problems faced by patients with obstructive pulmonary disorders.*
- *Discuss important aspects of nursing care for the patient with a restrictive lung defect.*
- *Briefly describe important aspects of the care of patients with pneumonia, aspiration lung disorder, respiratory failure, and adult respiratory distress syndrome (ARDS).*

## KEY TERMS

hypoxemia, p. 236
alveolar hypoventilation, p. 236
ventilation-perfusion (V/Q) inequality, p. 237
tissue hypoxia, p. 237
methemoglobin, p. 238
obstruction of ventilation, p. 240
pursed-lip breathing, p. 242
controlled cough technique, p. 243
restriction of ventilation, p. 244
atelectasis, p. 245

## HYPOXEMIA

**Hypoxemia** is a word used to define a lower than normal amount of oxygen dissolved in plasma (see the box at right.) Thus, when the $PaO_2$ is less than predicted for the patient's age, hypoxemia is diagnosed. The causes of hypoxemia are listed in Table 11-1 and include alveolar hypoventilation, pulmonary shunting, and ventilation-perfusion (V/Q) inequalities. Most authorities now agree that diffusion impairment is not an etiological category of hypoxemia. Conditions once listed as causes of the hypoxemia related to diffusion impairment have been shown to mediate hypoxemia by one of the other three routes. Diffusion impairment is much more likely to result in hypoxemia during exercise or at high altitude, particularly in patients with chronic pulmonary disease.[64] Exercise-induced desaturation of hemoglobin and hypoxemia can occur because of disease that either increases the diffusion pathway across the alveolar-capillary membrane (for example, adult respiratory distress syndrome) or because of a decrease in the volume of the pulmonary-capillary bed (for example, emphysema).

### Cause

**Alveolar hypoventilation. Alveolar hypoventilation** occurs when the amount of oxygen being brought into the alveoli is insufficient to meet metabolic needs. The hypoxemia caused by alveolar hypoventilation is often associated with an elevated $PaCO_2$[98] and commonly results from disorders outside the lungs. Table 11-2 reviews some of these disorders. This type of hypoxemia is usually corrected by administration of supplemental oxygen and, in some cases, depending on the cause, assistance with ventilation.

**Shunt.** Shunt occurs when blood reaches the arterial system without passing through ventilated regions of the lungs. Shunts can occur as a result of congenital heart defects or pulmonary arteriovenous fistulas. A shunt can also occur because a portion of a lung is not ventilated as the result of either alveolar collapse (for example, atelectasis), alveolar consolidation (for example, pneumonia), or excessive mucus accumulation (for example, chronic bronchitis).

When a patient with a shunt is given 100% oxygen to breathe, the $PaO_2$ will fail to rise to the level seen in normal

> **RELATED DEFINITIONS**
>
> **HYPOXEMIA**
>
> A $PaO_2$ less than predicted for the patient's age.
>
> **ARTERIAL HYPOXIA**
>
> A decreased amount of oxygen in the plasma; the same as hypoxemia; this term may have been responsible for the incorrect assumption that hypoxemia and hypoxia are one and the same.
>
> **TISSUE HYPOXIA**
>
> A lower than normal amount of oxygen delivered to the tissues.

***Table 11-1*** Causes of hypoxemia

| Etiological category | Medical disorder |
|---|---|
| Alveolar hypoventilation | CNS depression, disease of the medulla and spinal cord, Guillain-Barré syndrome, myasthenia gravis, muscular dystrophy, restriction to chest wall expansion, obesity |
| Shunt | Pulmonary edema, pneumonia, adult respiratory distress syndrome, atelectasis |
| V/Q inequality | Asthma, chronic bronchitis, chronic obstructive pulmonary disease, pneumonia, atelectasis |

subjects or to the expected $PaO_2$. Indeed, with pure shunt and no accompanying ventilation-perfusion inequality, the $PaO_2$ will not rise at all upon the administration of oxygen. This happens because when a shunt occurs there is no ventilation to the affected area of the lung and no inspired air reaches that region; therefore no amount of supplemental oxygen will reach the affected region. Only shunts behave in this way. The hypoxemia mediated by alveolar hypoventilation and ventilation-perfusion inequality will show some or complete correction with administration of 100% oxygen.[98]

The shunt can be calculated with the resulting figure showing the percentage of total blood flow that is not exposed to ventilated alveoli. The calculation is:

$$\frac{Qs}{Qt} = \frac{Cco_2 - CaO_2}{Cco_2 - C\bar{v}O_2}$$

Total blood flow is designated Qt; shunt flow is Qs. The oxygen content in the pulmonary capillary (c) is derived by assuming that the capillary $Po_2$ is equal to the alveolar $Po_2$. Normally, only 2% to 5% of the cardiac output should be made up of shunted blood. In severe cases of oxygen failure, as much as 40% of the cardiac output may be shunted.[57] In most cases, the higher the Qs/Qt, the more ominous is the pulmonary pathology.

**Ventilation-perfusion inequalities. Ventilation-perfusion (V/Q) inequality** occurs when ventilation and blood flow are mismatched in various regions of the lung. In the normal lung, there is always some ventilation-perfusion inequality, since not all alveoli are completely ventilated and completely perfused. The ventilation-perfusion inequality referred to in this discussion and in pulmonary pathology means that there is an *abnormal and excessive* amount of ventilation and perfusion inequality. While with shunt, blood passes through alveoli that are *unventilated,* in many causes of V/Q inequality, blood passes through alveoli that are *underventilated*. In other words, although some air

***Table 11-2*** Causes of alveolar hypoventilation

| Disorder | Cause |
|---|---|
| Depressed respiratory center activity | Drugs, neurological disease |
| Reduced chest expansion | Pain, surgical incision, fatigue, chest wall deformity, poor patient positioning, or failure to frequently reposition patient |
| Restriction to lung expansion | Pulmonary fibrosis, pneumothorax, pleural effusion |

passes into these alveoli, it is not the normal amount. Because of this, supplemental oxygen is usually helpful in correcting the hypoxemia resulting from V/Q inequality. V/Q inequality is the most common cause of hypoxemia and is responsible for most, if not all, of the hypoxemia of chronic obstructive pulmonary disease (COPD), interstitial lung disease, and pulmonary embolism.[98]

### Symptoms

Until hypoxemia proceeds to tissue hypoxia (in most cases a $PaO_2$ of <50 mm Hg), there are no symptoms other than the low $PaO_2$. Any clinician new to pulmonary care is advised to become familiar with the causes of hypoxemia in order to anticipate hypoxemia. Many times, the progression from hypoxemia to tissue hypoxia is rapid.

### Treatment

Treatment of hypoxemia depends on its severity. Mild hypoxemia may not require oxygen therapy, whereas severe hypoxemia will always necessitate some period of oxygenation. Further, severe hypoxemia as a result of massive ventilation-perfusion inequality or pulmonary shunt may not respond to oxygen alone and may require mechanical ventilation with positive end expiratory pressure (PEEP). The box on p. 238 presents essential information for the evaluation of hypoxemia. In all cases of hypoxemia, the cause must be sought and treatment instituted against it, since hypoxemia is a *symptom* of a disorder, not a cause of a disorder. Nursing diagnosis and management are listed in the box on p. 238.

## TISSUE HYPOXIA

**Tissue hypoxia** denotes a lower than normal amount of oxygen being delivered to the tissue cells. (See the box on p. 236). Causes of tissue hypoxia include: (1) hypoxemia, (2) abnormal hemoglobin, (3) low cardiac output, (4) increased oxygen requirements, and (5) toxic substance preventing normal $O_2$ utilization.

### Causes of Tissue Hypoxia

**Hypoxemia.** A $PaO_2$ of less than 50 mm Hg can produce tissue hypoxia. Some patients with chronic pulmonary disease and persons who reside at high altitudes maintain a

## EVALUATION OF HYPOXEMIA

### DEFINING HYPOXEMIA

Patient under 60 years old breathing room air

| | |
|---|---|
| Mild hypoxemia | $PaO_2 < 80$ mm Hg |
| Moderate hypoxemia | $PaO_2 < 60$ mm Hg |
| Severe hypoxemia | $PaO_2 < 40$ mm Hg |

For each year patient over 60 years, subtract 1 mm Hg to determine lower limits of normal for patient's age

### DETERMINING HYPOXEMIA

Look at the $PaO_2$ to answer the question, "Does the $PaO_2$ show hypoxemia?" Less than predicted for age means hypoxemia

### EVALUATING OXYGEN THERAPY TO CORRECT HYPOXEMIA

| | |
|---|---|
| Corrected hypoxemia | $PaO_2 \geq$ predicted for patient's age |
| Uncorrected hypoxemia | $PaO_2 <$ predicted for patient's age |
| Overcorrected hypoxemia | $PaO_2 > 100$ mm Hg |

Modifed from Shapiro BA, Harrison RA, and Walton JR: Clinical application of blood gases, ed 4, St Louis, 1989, Mosby–Year Book, Inc.

## Nursing Diagnosis and Management

***Hypoxemia***

- Impaired Gas Exchange related to alveolar hypoventilation secondary to (specify), p. 475
- Impaired Gas Exchange related to ventilation-perfusion inequality secondary to (specify), p. 474

$PaO_2$ as low as 55 mm Hg without tissue hypoxia because of compensatory mechanisms, such as increased cardiac output and polycythemia. In these cases, the elevated cardiac output and red blood cell count allow for a greater oxygen-carrying capacity of the blood. In most cases, however, severe acute hypoxemia will result in tissue hypoxia.

**Abnormal hemoglobin.** The effect that abnormal hemoglobin has on its oxygen-carrying capacity is significant. Hemoglobin carries approximately 97% of the total amount of oxygen held within the bloodstream. This great carrying capacity is dependent on hemoglobin's being normal in amount and molecular structure. Normal adult hemoglobin is labeled hemoglobin A (Hb A). Abnormal hemoglobins do exist, and situations occur in which normal hemoglobin becomes abnormal. Most hemoglobin abnormalities affect the oxygen-carrying capability of this molecule. Methemoglobin and carboxyhemoglobin are abnormalities of hemoglobin that are sometimes present in the critically ill patient.

***Methemoglobin.*** Certain drugs (Table 11-3), particularly nitrates and sulfonamides, will change normal hemoglobin into methemoglobin (metHb). **Methemoglobin** occurs when the iron atoms within the Hb A molecule are oxidized from the ferrous state to the ferric state.[3] Methemoglobin does not carry oxygen, and, in high enough levels, will cause tissue hypoxia. It will also cause cyanosis because metHb darkens the color of the oxidized hemoglobin. Normally, approximately 1.5% of hemoglobin is in this oxidized state; an amount greater than 1.5% defines a state of methemoglobinemia.[57] Mild methemoglobinemia (metHb <30%) is treated with supplemental oxygen and removal of the offending drug. More severe cases can be treated with methylene blue, which acts as a reducing agent that converts the ferric state back to the ferrous state and returns the metHb to Hb A.

***Carboxyhemoglobin.*** Carboxyhemoglobin (HbCO) occurs when carbon monoxide (CO) combines with Hb A. HbCO exposure can be lethal because the carbon monoxide molecule uses the same binding site on the Hb molecule that oxygen uses. However, carbon monoxide's affinity for Hb is approximately 220 times that of oxygen; thus, when in competition with oxygen for the Hb binding site, carbon monoxide will always bind before oxygen can.[77] Unfortunately, the body cannot use carbon monoxide for metabolism; hence, when enough Hb becomes bound with carbon monoxide and not oxygen, tissue hypoxia will result. Normal HbCO levels are less than 2%, but levels of only 10% can lead to symptoms, whereas levels of 20% or more are indicative of cellular hypoxia. Table 11-4 shows the clinical effects of carbon monoxide poisoning.

Exposure to heavy automobile traffic or to cigarette smoke

***Table 11-3*** Some drugs implicated in causing methemoglobinemia

| Generic name | Use |
|---|---|
| Dapsone | Skin protectant |
| Benzocaine | Local anesthetic |
| Metoclopramide | Gastric stasis |
| Nitroglycerin | Angina |
| Phenazopyridine | Urinary tract analgesic |
| Prilocaine | Local anesthetic |
| Primaquine | Malaria prophylaxis and treatment |
| Trimethoprim | Urinary antibacterial |
| Amyl nitrite | Rarely used clinically; often used by drug abusers |

From Martin L: Pulmonary physiology in clinical practice: the essentials for patient care and evaluation, St Louis, 1987, Mosby–Year Book, Inc.

***Table 11-4*** Correlation of symptoms and signs with carbon monoxide level

| Percent of carbon monoxide in inspired air | Percent of HbCO in blood | Signs and symptoms |
|---|---|---|
| 0.007 | 10 | Common in cigarette smokers; dyspnea during vigorous exertion; occasional tightness in forehead; dilation of cutaneous blood vessels |
| 0.012 | 20 | Dyspnea during moderate exertion; occasional throbbing headache in temples |
| 0.022 | 30 | Severe headache; irritability; easy fatigability; disturbed judgment; possible dizziness and possible dimness of vision |
| 0.035-0.052 | 40-50 | Headache; confusion; fainting on exertion |
| 0.080-0.122 | 60-70 | Unconsciousness; intermittent convulsions; respiratory failure; death if exposure prolonged |
| 0.195 | 80 | Fatal |

From Martin L: Pulmonary physiology in clinical practice: the essentials for patient care and evaluation, St Louis, 1987, Mosby–Year Book, Inc; modified from Winter PM and Miller JN: JAMA 236:1503, 1976, Copyright 1976, American Medical Association.

can raise HbCO from its normal level up to 10%. Patients with preexisting chronic hypoxemia have decreased exercise tolerance at levels of 4% or more HbCO.[57] At levels of 5% to 8% HbCO, healthy coronary arteries will dilate to bring more blood to the myocardium to compensate for the decreased oxygen content. In persons with fixed coronary artery obstruction, dilation may not be possible, leading to compromise of cardiac oxygenation. There is also evidence that HbCO leads to a decrease in the threshold for ventricular fibrillation, possibly relating to the sudden death of smokers with coronary disease.[57]

Treatment of HbCO includes removing the source of the carbon monoxide poisoning and administering oxygen. The half-life of HbCO when an individual is breathing room air is approximately 4 to 6 hours. With administration of 100% oxygen, the half-life can be shortened to 1 hour.[59] Patients with severe poisoning may require endotracheal intubation followed by administration of 100% oxygen. Hyperbaric oxygen therapy, although not always available or practical, is highly effective. Hyperbaric therapy can dissolve enough oxygen in plasma (6 ml/100 ml plasma when breathing 100% oxygen at 3 atm) to sustain life, even if HbCO is 100%[57]

***Deoxygenated (reduced) hemoglobin.*** "Deoxygenated hemoglobin" (previously known as reduced hemoglobin) refers to the amount of hemoglobin not saturated with oxygen and means that the oxygen binding site is empty. Therefore some portion of the hemoglobin content is desaturated.

Deoxygenated hemoglobin results for various reasons, including low quantity of oxygen in the atmosphere, hypoventilation, and acute or chronic pulmonary disease. When 5 g or more of hemoglobin per 100 ml of blood are desaturated, cyanosis will be present because the color of desaturated blood is darker than the color of staturated blood. Venous blood is desaturated, hence its dark color when compared to arterial blood.

Correction of tissue hypoxia related to abnormal hemoglobin must be directed at returning the hemoglobin to a normal structure at normal levels. Supplemental oxygen can be administered to raise the $PaO_2$ in hopes of providing some added oxygen to the tissues. Oxygen therapy is particularly helpful in correcting the hypoxia resulting from carboxyhemoglobin.

**Low cardiac output.** A low cardiac output can result in tissue hypoxia because of failure of the heart to perfuse enough blood through the systemic circulation to meet the body's metabolic needs. This can follow myocardial infarction(s), cardiac dysrhythmias, heart failure, hypovolemic shock, cardiogenic shock, and other acute and chronic diseases of the cardiovascular system. Interventions to correct tissue hypoxia resulting from low cardiac output should be directed toward that system, assuming oxygenation via the pulmonary system is normal.

**Increased oxygen requirements.** Increased oxygen requirements occur in obese persons, patients with fever, and particularly in burn patients.

**Toxic substance tissue hypoxia.** This form of hypoxia is rare. An example potentially seen in critical care is the toxicity that occurs with cyanide poisoning. Cyanide prevents the use of oxygen by the cellular enzyme cytochrome oxidase. Dissolved oxygen ($PaO_2$) is unaffected; hence this is an example of tissue hypoxia occurring without hypoxemia. Patients with cyanide poisoning will not respond to oxygen therapy but must be given the antidote containing sodium nitrite, which combines with the cyanide, thus freeing cytochrome oxidase. Administration of sodium thiosulfate further degrades the cyanide. A byproduct of this antidote is methemoglobin, which can then be reduced by administration of methylene blue.[52]

### Symptoms

Symptoms of tissue hypoxia are best organized into systems, as presented in Table 11-5. Tachycardia and tachypnea are normal body compensatory mechanisms triggered to

***Table 11-5*** Symptoms of tissue hypoxia

| System | Symptoms |
|---|---|
| | polycythemia |
| Respiratory | Tachypnea, dyspnea, cyanosis, hypoxemia |
| Renal | Low urine output |
| Neurological | Headache, anxiety, agitation, confusion, weakness, double vision, impaired judgment, weakness, drowsiness, coma |

correct the hypoxia. Other symptoms such as dysrhythmias, confusion, double vision, and drowsiness are manifestations of hypoxia of specific body cells.

### Treatment

The specific treatment of each cause of hypoxia was discussed in the previous sections. In general, tissue hypoxia is treated by identifying and treating the cause, such as abnormal hemoglobin, hypoxemia, or low cardiac output. Regardless of the cause, the tissue oxygen delivery must be brought back to normal by the administration of supplemental oxygen and, when the patient is not effectively ventilating, by mechanical ventilation. If the presence of mucus is suspected, it must be cleared via effective cough, suctioning, intermittent positive pressure breathing, chest physiotherapy, or, as a last resort, bronchoscopy. Nursing diagnoses and management of tissue hypoxia are listed in the box at right.

**Nursing Diagnosis and Management**
***Tissue hypoxia***

- High Risk for Altered Peripheral Tissue Perfusion related to compromised arterial flow, p. 462
- High Risk for Altered Peripheral Tissue Perfusion risk factor: vasopressor therapy, p. 462
- High Risk for Altered Peripheral Tissue Perfusion risk factor: orthopedic injury or manipulation of an extremity, p. 462
- High Risk for Impaired Skin Integrity risk factor: altered circulation, p. 499
- Activity Intolerance related to decreased cardiac output and/or myocardial tissue perfusion alterations, p. 464

## OBSTRUCTIVE AND RESTRICTIVE LUNG DISORDERS

Pulmonary diseases are often categorized by the manner in which they alter a patient's breathing pattern. Two patterns predominate: diseases that result in obstruction of ventilation and those that result in restriction of ventilation. The following discussion will explain how these disorders affect the lower airways, resulting in the diseases often seen in critical care.

### Obstruction of Ventilation

Obstruction of ventilation means that airflow during exhalation, particularly during forced exhalation, is abnormally slow. This is usually a result of airway narrowing and/or airway collapse. Some of the diseases that are associated with this pattern of ventilation and are often seen in the critical care unit include asthma, chronic bronchitis, emphysema, and chronic obstructive pulmonary disease (COPD). Cystic fibrosis and bronchiectasis are also obstructive diseases but are not commonly seen in adult critical care.

For the most part, diseases that have an obstructive component are chronic in nature, such as bronchial asthma, chronic bronchitis, bronchiectasis, and emphysema. Acute bronchitis is an exception.

Airway narrowing or airway collapse can result from several factors. One factor is mucus within the airways, which, if it is in a large volume such as occurs in chronic bronchitis or bronchiectasis and is not expectorated, will result in obstruction to normal airflow.

Another factor involved in airway narrowing is edema of the lung tissue surrounding the bronchioles, which can compress these airways. This can occur in left-sided heart failure and pulmonary edema.

Finally, when the obstruction is caused by airway collapse, it is most often associated with emphysema, because this disease process weakens the respiratory bronchioles so that they remain open during inhalation but collapse as a result of the forces produced during exhalation.

**Obstruction of ventilation** is diagnosed when pulmonary function tests such as the forced vital capacity (FVC) and the forced expiratory volume measured over one second ($FEV_1$) show excessively prolonged exhalation.

**Major symptoms of obstructive disorders.** Two main problems associated with airway obstruction are difficulty breathing and excessive mucus production with or without cough. These are problems related to the pathophysiological process of obstructive airway disease and are treated by medical interventions such as bronchodilators, expectorants, or mechanical ventilation. However, both difficulty breathing and excessive mucus production lead to other patient problems that need to be resolved and that, in many situations, are evaluated for and resolvable by nursing care.

**Difficulty breathing.** How does obstruction of ventilation affect a patient's breathing? This question can be answered if the reader will perform the short experiment outlined in the box on p. 241.

## SIMULATING DIFFICULTY BREATHING

Imagine yourself in the position of the patient with difficulty breathing caused by an obstructive airway disease. To help with this, place a straw in your mouth and breathe through it with your nose pinched shut. Make a tight seal so that you cannot draw in air around the straw. You have just simulated airway narrowing; hence obstruction of ventilation. You are probably noticing that breathing is more difficult through the straw. Perhaps you are breathing much harder than normal because the work of drawing air in and pushing it through the small lumen of the straw is much more difficult than it is to draw it through your mouth and nose. The work of breathing has increased; it can be tiring. Wouldn't it be nice to have a straw with a bigger lumen? It would make breathing easier and would be like taking a bronchodilator.

Patients with chronic airway obstruction live with breathing difficulty constantly, and it impairs not only their physical wellness but also their emotional and social wellness. They alter their lifestyles to fit their breathing patterns, often decreasing or stopping activities they enjoy but can no longer tolerate. While a chest infection may not present a serious problem to a healthy person, it can and often does mean hospitalization to someone with obstructive lung dysfunction.

***Summary of nursing care.*** Refer to the box below for nursing diagnoses and management of obstructive lung dysfunction.

There are two breathing techniques which, when taught and used every day, are helpful to patients with difficulty breathing.

***Pursed-lip and diaphragmatic breathing.*** Pursed-lip and diaphragmatic breathing are techniques that can help improve the control of ventilation and prolong pulmonary emptying time.[14] The objectives of these breathing techniques include (1) promoting greater use of the diaphragm while decreasing use of the chest and neck accessory muscles of ventilation, (2) allowing the patient to suppress the

## Nursing Diagnosis and Management

### *Obstructive lung dysfunction*

- Ineffective Airway Clearance related to excessive secretions, p. 466
- Ineffective Airway Clearance related to knowledge deficit of controlled cough and hydration techniques, p. 468
- Ineffective Breathing Pattern related to chronic airflow limitations, p. 470
- Impaired Gas Exchange related to ventilation-perfusion inequality secondary to chronic obstructive lung dysfunction, p. 474
- Impaired Gas Exchange related to alveolar hypoventilation secondary to (specify), p. 475
- Activity Intolerance related to knowledge deficit of energy-saving techniques, p. 463
- Altered Nutrition: Less Than Body Protein-Calorie Requirements related to lack of exogenous nutrients and increased metabolic demand. (See also discussion of metabolic results from carbohydrate overfeeding, Chapter 6.)
- High Risk for Infection risk factors: protein-calorie malnourishment, steroid therapy, p. 465
- Sleep Pattern Disturbance related to fragmented sleep and/or circadian desynchronization, p. 455
- Sensory-Perceptual Alterations related to sensory overload, sensory deprivation, sleep pattern disturbance, p. 489
- High Risk for Impaired Skin Integrity risk factors: reduced mobility, protein-calorie malnourishment, steroid therapy, p. 499
- Sexual Dysfunction related to activity intolerance secondary to chronic lung disease, p. 451
- Altered Health Maintenance related to lack of perceived threat to health, p. 439
- Noncompliance: Energy-Saving Techniques, Breathing Techniques (Diaphragmatic, Pursed Lip), Hydration, Avoidance of Environmental Pollutants (Smoking), Medication Regimen, Muscle Toning Exercises related to lack of resources, p. 440
- Body Image Disturbance related to actual change in body structure, function, and appearance, p. 443
- Self-Esteem Disturbance related to feelings of guilt over physical deterioration, p. 442
- Altered Role Performance related to physical incapacity to resume usual or valued role, p. 444
- Powerlessness related to health care environment or illness-related regimen, p. 445
- Hopelessness related to perceptions of deteriorating physical condition, p. 446
- Anxiety related to threat to biological, psychological, and/or social integrity, p. 448

## PURSED-LIP BREATHING

- With mouth closed, inhale through nose.
- Exhale through mouth with lips "pursed" (lips in a whistling or kissing position).
- Make exhalation at least twice as long as inhalation (2 seconds in, 4 seconds out).

### RATIONALE

Explain to the patient that this maneuver keeps airways open longer during exhalation and evacuates trapped air. The procedure for pursed-lip breathing can be used, along with diaphragmatic breathing, during episodes of shortness of breath.

## DIAPHRAGMATIC BREATHING

Have the patient place two fingers just below the xiphoid process and push in with his or her fingers while sniffing gently. Explain that the movement felt at the fingertips is the diaphragm moving as he or she sniffs and that this muscle requires exercise so that it can increase the efficiency of breathing.

### TECHNIQUE

- Place one hand on chest, one hand on abdomen.
- Inhale, pushing abdominal hand outward.
- Exhale slowly (through pursed lips), allowing abdominal hand to fall inward.
- Chest hand should remain still.

### RATIONALE

Explain that this maneuver saves energy because the diaphragm uses oxygen more efficiently than the accessory muscles and that this technique retrains the diaphragm to assume the work of breathing. Diaphragmatic breathing is useful in terminating episodes of acute shortness of breath but should also be incorporated into a regular routine of muscle retraining.

tendency for hurried, gasping ventilations, (3) improving the effectiveness of alveolar ventilation by increasing tidal volume, prolonging pulmonary emptying time, and improving the relationship between ventilation and perfusion within the lungs and possibly, (4) improving the strength and endurance of the inspiratory muscles.

**Pursed-lip breathing** is an expiratory maneuver often adopted by dyspneic patients in an effort to control their dyspnea. This maneuver stimulates positive end-expiratory pressure (PEEP), prevents premature airway collapse, and is believed to provide internal stability of the airways during exhalation.[46]

The pursed-lip breathing technique is easily learned (see box, "Pursed Lip Breathing"). However, patients with severe shortness of breath, depending on its cause, may not benefit from instruction of this technique until their condition improves enough to allow a learning experience.

Diaphragmatic breathing (see box, "Diaphragmatic Breathing") is a method through which the patient tones his or her diaphragm. It may be particularly helpful to the patient with emphysema or to the patient with an emphysemic component to another obstructive pulmonary disease.

***Excessive mucus with or without cough.*** In addition to difficulty breathing as a result of airway narrowing, many patients with obstructive lung disease have chronic, excessive mucus production, which further complicates breathing and can lead to chronic cough. Cough is reported by patients with chronic bronchitis as their single most debilitating health problem.[98]

Regarding mucus production, two important issues should be identified. The first is that some obstructive dysfunctions are *not* accompanied by mucus production. Emphysema in its pure form, without accompanying bronchitis or an acute chest infection, is an obstructive disease that is not complicated by mucus production. Second, when a patient develops an acute chest infection superimposed on chronic obstructive lung disease, the amount of mucus normally produced will increase.

It is impossible to discuss mucus production without including cough. Patients with excessive production of mucus should be encouraged to cough, because it is a lack of an effective cough combined with excessive mucus production that results in ventilatory and respiratory failure. Therefore the teaching and assessment of effective cough are imperative, since the only other means to remove mucus is by nasopharyngeal suctioning or bronchoscopy.

***Summary of nursing care***

**TEACHING AN EFFECTIVE COUGH TECHNIQUE.** Coughing is sometimes necessary, even in a healthy individual, for the removal of mucus from the tracheobronchial tree. To be effective, however, the cough must be a composite of several distinct and necessary phases, which are listed in Table 11-6. Effective coughing depends on (1) a deep inhalation, (2) strong contraction of the muscles of exhalation, in particular the abdominal muscles, (3) a functioning glottis, and (4) airways that remain open during the terminal exhalatory phase of the cough. Abnormal functioning of any of the above mechanisms will decrease the effectiveness of coughing. Inability to take a deep breath, weak abdominal muscles, unwillingness to use the abdominal muscles because of pain or poor positioning, and chronic diffuse small airway collapse such as can occur with COPD can significantly reduce cough effectiveness. A reduction of cough effectiveness in the presence of mucus production will lead to ineffective airway clearance.

Patients with excessive mucus production often exhaust themselves coughing in an inefficient manner. Teaching a

***Table 11-6*** Factors that interfere with production of an effective cough

| Components of a normal cough | Factors that interfere with normal coughing | Nursing action |
|---|---|---|
| Inhalation to near-total lung capacity | General weakness<br>Inability to take a deep breath<br>Positioning that impairs the deep breath | Consider teaching huff or quad coughing*<br>Position for effective cough |
| Closure of the glottis | Bypass of the glottis by artificial airway | — |
| Contraction of the abdominal muscles | Weak abdominal muscles<br>Painful use of muscles<br>Positioning that impairs use of the abdominal muscles | Huff cough<br>Analgesics<br>Position for effective cough |
| Sudden opening of the glottis with explosive exhalation | Inability to exhale with force<br>Diffuse small airway collapse on exhalation<br>Bypass of the glottis by artificial airway | Quad coughing<br>Huff coughing |

*Huff and quad cough techniques are discussed on p. 243.

**controlled cough technique** that results in the effective production of mucus can be instrumental in assisting the patient to control this aspect of his or her illness. Cough instruction is useful in conjunction with all respiratory therapy modalities and with patients who have had abdominal or thoracic surgery.[84] However, only those patients who have documented mucus or who are strongly suspected of having retained mucus should be encouraged to cough. Coughing causes airway irritation and fatigue[36]; further, it promotes airway and alveolar collapse, particularly in the absence of secretions.[5]

The reader should be aware that the cough procedure presented here is not a scientifically studied technique but is one that has been received quite successfully by patients, respiratory therapists, and nurses in both the acute and rehabilitative settings.[63] This technique involves the steps listed in the box on p. 244.

There may be patients who cannot follow the controlled cough technique. Other types of coughing that successfully remove mucus such as huff or quad coughing can be encouraged.

*Huff coughing* is a series of coughs produced with the glottis held open while saying the word, "huff." The sharp sound of a cough should not be produced with a huff cough, but the sound should be that of forced exhalation.[93] Huff coughing may be helpful for COPD patients who have significant airway collapse on forced exhalation, because huff coughing is associated with higher flow rates in these patients than in the normal closed-glottis approach to coughing. Furthermore, huff coughing may assist in moving secretions from the smaller airways into the main-stem bronchi or trachea where the controlled cough technique can be used for effective expectoration.

*Quad coughing* is helpful in patients who have flaccid or weakened abdominal musculature. The most obvious example is the patient with paralysis or weakness caused by neuromuscular disorders. Quad coughing calls for the nurse to push upward and inward on the abdomen, toward the diaphragm, while the patient exhales.

**PROPER PATIENT POSITIONING.** The most effective position for coughing is upright and flexed forward at the waist. Lying supine or even in a semi-Fowler's position does not allow total lung inflation, diaphragmatic descent, or intercostal muscle action and thus decreases the efficiency of the cough.[52] Additionally, patients who have abdominal incisions may experience less incisional pain when coughing while drawing their knees up toward the chest[52] and/or by splinting the incision against a pillow. The feet should be supported rather than allowed to dangle; in this way the support can be used as a brace against which to generate greater abdominal muscle tension, producing a stronger cough. The brace will also help prevent muscular strain of the lower back.[14]

When a head-up position is contraindicated, the side-lying position with knees bent is preferable to the supine recumbent position.[14,36]

**EFFECTIVE HYDRATION AND AIRWAY HUMIDIFICATION.** Shapiro and associates[84] consider adequate systemic hydration as the second most important factor in mobilizing secretions from the airways (an effective cough is first.) Hydration decreases mucus viscosity and enhances mucociliary effectiveness and cough.[93] In the nonintubated patient, hydration can be accomplished systematically with oral or intravenous fluids. Sources recommended that 1½ to 3 L of decaffeniated fluid per day are necessary to prevent thick mucus and to facilitate cough.[36,63] However, although almost all authorities on pulmonary disease agree that adequate systemic hydration is necessary to mobilize secretions, there is no evidence that overhydration will further assist in mucus mobilization.[37] Cardiovascular and renal function should be considered before hyration orders are implemented; further, patients with COPD who are also hypercapnic tend to retain fluid even in the absence of cardiac decompensation.[37]

**CHEST PHYSIOTHERAPY.** Chest physiotherapy (CPT) is the

## CONTROLLED COUGH TECHNIQUE

1. *Maximal inhalation*—an effective cough is contingent on filling the lungs and airways distal to the mucus so that the succeeding forced exhalation will propel the mucus up to the airways. Maximal inhalation also increases airway caliber; as a result, it is more likely that the air will pass distal to partially obstructing mucus or foreign matter.[93]
2. *Hold breath 2 seconds*—this step permits the patient to prepare for exhalation and allows distribution of the inhaled air to the lung's periphery.[84]
3. *Cough twice*—the first cough will loosen mucus, the second will propel the mucus. Further coughing may use excessive oxygen and energy at a time when the lung volume has already been expelled with the first two coughs, and the effort is thus wasted.
4. *Pause*—just long enough to regain control.
5. *Inhale by sniffing*—sniffing is recommended, because a deep inhalation through the mouth may drive loose mucus back down into the airways.
6. *Rest.*

From Moser KM and others: Shortness of breath: a guide to better living and breathing, St Louis, 1983, Mosby–Year Book, Inc.

general title for a group of airway clearance therapies consisting of bronchial drainage, chest percussion, and chest vibration. Effective coughing is an essential aspect of each of these techniques. Although CPT may be initally ordered by a physician, thereby placing it in the category of medical interventions, it is often performed or supervised by the nurse, moving it into the category of a collaborative intervention. In cases of suspected ineffective airway clearance for which coughing alone is insufficent in removing secretions, CPT must be considered. It is often a nursing responsibility to evaluate the need for CPT and to inform the physician that an order should be written.

### Restriction of Ventilation

**Restriction of ventilation** means that the expansion of the lung is limited (restricted). To the patient, it means that he or she is unable to take a full, deep breath. This abnormal pattern of ventilation can be either acute or chronic and is caused by pathological conditions that fit into one of four groups: (1) lung parenchymal dysfunctions, (2) pleural membrane dysfunctions, (3) chest wall dysfunctions, and (4) neuromuscular impairment. Table 11-7 lists causes that fall into each of the four groups of restrictive dysfunction. It should be noted that a number of the acute pathological conditions such as atelectasis, pneumothorax, and pleural effusion often occur in patients who do not have primary pulmonary disease.

**Table 11-7** Restrictive lung dysfunction

| Group classification | Diseases |
|---|---|
| Lung parenchymal dysfunction | Sarcoidosis, atelectasis, diffuse interstitial fibrosis |
| Pleural membrane dysfunction | Pneumothorax, pleural effusion, pleuritis |
| Chest wall dysfunctions | Kyphoscoliosis, rib fractures/trauma, tight chest strapping, chest or upper abdominal incision, abdominal distention obesity |
| Neuromuscular disorders | Polio, Guillain-Barré syndrome, muscular dystrophy, myasthenia gravis, amotrophic lateral sclerosis |

Even though the causes in Table 11-7 have differences such as pathophysiology and chronicity, they each have one common feature. Each restricts lung expansion resulting in the predictable ventilatory pattern of restrictive lung dysfunction—that of a smaller, fixed tidal volume (Vt) associated with a more rapid ventilatory rate as a compensatory mechanism to maintain minute ventilation ($\dot{V}E$). Persons with restrictive pulmonary disease, whether acute or chronic, will demonstrate this pattern of breathing regardless of the disease responsible for pulmonary restriction. The severity of the disease plus the patient's relative health will both affect the degree to which the restriction to ventilation is manifested.

What are the consequences of this altered ventilatory pattern? One consequence may be activity limitations. The patient with restrictive disease cannot effectively increase tidal volume during stress, such as when moving about in bed, ambulating, or coughing. As the patient's metabolic rate increases in these situations, a greater minute ventilation becomes necessary. With a relatively fixed tidal volume, minute ventilation can increase only through an increased ventilatory rate. However, the patient with a restrictive ventilatory pattern may already be breathing more rapidly than most persons—thus a further increase in ventilatory rate can be difficult, if not exhausting. Any exertion on the part of the patient requires a precise nursing assessment, evaluating the patient's ability to tolerate the exertion.

Another consequence of restrictive disease is an increase in the work of breathing. This occurs because many of the diseases that result in the restrictive breathing pattern also reduce lung compliance and impede lung inflation. Some of these diseases include diffuse interstitial lung fibrosis, atelectasis, pleural effusion, sarcoidosis, and pneumothorax. The increased work of breathing and the altered ventilatory pattern (low Vt–high rate) can seriously interfere with recovery of the critically ill patient.

**Summary of nursing care.** The most important consideration when caring for a patient with a restrictive pulmonary dysfunction is evaluation of the activity level the patient can tolerate. Nursing care should be planned so that the patient's activity level does not put excessive stress on his or her breathing pattern. Assessment of a tolerable activity level is very individual. One patient may become exhausted after turning in bed or having had a portable chest x-ray taken, whereas another patient may easily tolerate sitting at the bedside. When the resting ventilatory rate is significantly elevated, for example, as high as 28 per minute or more, the patient can be so exhausted maintaining this rate that further activity is not possible. At other times, however, with other patients, a rate of 28 per minute may be tolerable even if the activity level is increased. In any situation in which there is an elevated ventilatory rate, the assessment of a patient's tolerance of activity must be made, and generous rest periods should be spaced between activities.

It is most important that critical care nurses understand that restrictive dysfunctions do not necessarily need to involve the pulmonary system and that they are, many times, acute rather than chronic. A review of Table 11-7 reveals that upper abdominal surgery, abdominal distention, tight abdominal strapping, and obesity can alter lung inflation without direct involvement of the pulmonary system. These conditions impede diaphragmatic descent and intercostal muscle action, impairing both inhalation and exhalation. Pulmonary conditions that might not be considered serious, such as kyphoscoliosis and rib fractures, can actually present a severe pulmonary restriction when coupled with other problems for which the patient may have been admitted to the critical care unit.

Impaired inhalation, in particular, is a serious problem because it is a risk factor for development of atelectasis. Abdominal distention and tight strapping of the abdomen, most often seen by the use of an abdominal binder, hinder diaphragmatic descent and the normal outward abdominal movement occurring during inhalation; hence, patients tend toward a shallow, monotonous breathing pattern. This situation can be made worse if the abdominal binder works its way to the upper abdomen or lower chest, as sometimes is the case with bedridden patients. Because the potential pulmonary problems (atelectasis, pneumonia) outweigh the need for the binder, many surgeons no longer order them. However, in those situations in which one is used, it must be repositioned whenever it is found to have slipped up toward the chest or rib cage, and nursing care should include the interventions listed in the next section that can assist in preventing atelectasis.

Kyphoscoliosis can impair intercostal rib action, thus chest and lung expansion. This chest deformity compresses the underlying lung tissue so that it may not be ventilated well enough to contribute to gas exchange. When a patient with kyphoscoliosis is admitted to the critical care unit, the chest deformity itself can be a serious enough ventilatory limitation to put him or her at risk for development of atelectasis or pneumonia, particularly because both bed rest and acute critical illness will put additional stress or limitation on the ventilatory pattern. Vigilance is necessary in the assessment of breath sounds, ventilatory rate, blood gases, and changes in activity tolerance, as well as in the application of the nursing interventions that prevent atelectasis.

Rib fractures can present the same risk as kyphoscoliosis. In this case however, pain medication may be ordered and should be provided at a level that will allow full lung inhalation without the dosage being so high as to unnecessarily prolong sleep or naps when ventilations decrease in rate and depth.

Probably the most frequently seen restrictive dysfunction resulting from hospitalization is atelectasis. Because of this and because it is so responsive to nursing interventions, it will be discussed next, under its own heading. Restrictive dysfunctions that are not frequently seen in critical care, such as those related to neuromuscular disorders and some that fall under lung parenchymal dysfunction (sarcoidosis, DIF), will not be discussed in this text. The reader is referred to a medical-surgical nursing text or a pulmonary text for these discussions. Further though, the reader is reminded that *any* disease or dysfunction that presents a restriction to ventilation should be treated with the previous nursing care section in mind. Refer to the box below for nursing diagnoses and management of restrictive lung dysfunction.

## ATELECTASIS

### Description

Pulmonary **atelectasis** is collapse of lung tissue. This should not be confused with pneumothorax. While there is alveolar collapse in both conditions, the cause of the collapse is very different. Atelectasis occurs because alveoli become underinflated or uninflated. Pneumothorax occurs because air enters the pleural space. In most cases, pneumothorax

**Nursing Diagnosis and Management**

***Restrictive lung dysfunction***

- Ineffective Breathing Pattern related to modifiable chest wall restrictions secondary to pneumothorax or pleural effusion, p. 470
- Ineffective Breathing Pattern related to unmodifiable chest wall restrictions secondary to kyphoscoliosis or obesity, p. 473
- Activity Intolerance related to knowledge deficit of energy-saving techniques, p. 463
- Body Image Disturbance related to actual change in body structure, function, and appearance, p. 443
- Powerlessness related to physical deterioration despite compliance, p. 445
- Sexual Dysfunction related to activity intolerance secondary to chronic lung disease, p. 451

is not preventable. Atelectasis, however, in most cases is preventable by appropriate nursing interventions, as will be elucidated in the following discussion.

### Cause and Pathophysiology

Atelectasis can be the result of a variety of abnormalities including: localized airway obstruction, a ventilatory pattern of shallow monotonous breathing, patient positioning that impairs adequate lung expansion, a change in the distending forces within the lung, negative airway pressure, and a deficiency of surfactant.

**Localized airway obstruction.** Local airway obstruction has long been considered a pathogenesis of atelectasis, with the offending agent believed to be an abnormal accumulation of mucus in the airways. Atelectasis then develops because the mucus completely or partially blocks the entry of fresh air into the distal lung areas. Lack of new ventilation to these areas promotes the absorption of what air is available until collapse results. This is sometimes termed absorption atelectasis, which is further discussed in the box at right. The development of atelectasis through this process is somewhat attenuated by the Pores of Kohn and the Canals of Lambert that can provide collateral air circulation to blocked airways. However, the mucus accumulation can be diffuse enough to block even these collateral pathways. Diseases associated with the development of atelectasis through this means are those notable for producing mucus, such as cystic fibrosis, chronic bronchitis, COPD, and bronchectasis. Further, any acute pulmonary disease, such as a pneumonia, superimposed on these chronic diseases further increases mucus and heightens the risk for development of atelectasis.

**Shallow, monotonous breathing pattern.** A shallow, monotonous breathing pattern has also long been considered a cause of atelectasis. Changes in ventilation that result from this breathing pattern include decreased lung volume, decreased compliance ("stiff" lungs), and pulmonary shunting.[5,80] The breathing pattern is found most commonly in patients who have had upper abdominal surgery, but it occurs to some extent following all surgeries and appears to result because the recumbent position in which most patients are placed during surgery reduces lung inflation.[21] Position is not the only surgical factor that can increase the risk for atelectasis caused by shallow, monotonous breathing. General anesthesia is known to alter normal lung mechanics and promote development of atelectasis through reduction in lung and chest wall compliance and through reduction in diaphragmatic action.[23,80] Recently, it has been reported that general anesthesia alone, regardless of the surgery, can result in 24 hours of impaired diaphragmatic activity.[94] However, the likelihood of pulmonary complications resulting from anesthesia and surgery is more a function of the type and duration of the surgery[51] and of the postoperative care.

Surgery of the upper abdomen and thorax heightens the risk of atelectasis because total lung capacity, FRC, and vital capacity can be decreased for as long as 5 to 7 days.[88] The incidence of clinically important atelectasis increases as the incision approaches the diaphragm; thus upper abdominal surgery carries a higher risk of ventilatory impairment than does lower abdominal surgery.[80]

The potential for the development of atelectasis after surgery is compounded by the tendency of patients to breathe lower tidal volumes at higher respiratory rates because this is the easiest, most pain-free pattern. Additionally, both pain and the analgesics used for pain relief disrupt the normal sighing pattern thought to open underventilated alveoli and enhance the spread of surfactant.

The shallow, monotonous breathing pattern is also found in patients who have not had surgery but whose illnesses require bed rest or prevent normal lung expansion such as will occur with chest or abdominal wall trauma. Additionally, any trauma or disease that might interfere with the normal functioning of the respiratory control centers of the central nervous system should be viewed as presenting a risk for the development of atelectasis.

**Patient positioning.** To the extent that position impairs

#### ABSORPTION ATELECTASIS

According to Shapiro[82]: "Absorption atelectasis is the most common type of acute lung collapse and is usually caused by retained secretions." Secretions that obstruct bronchi or bronchioles prevent air from entering the alveoli distal to the obstruction. This lack of fresh air with which to inflate the alveoli after each exhalation results in deflation of the alveoli and atelectasis. Collapse is not complete, however, because alveoli will remain inflated with nitrogen from the atmosphere, since nitrogen does not diffuse into the pulmonary capillary.

Absorption atelectasis can also result from the administration of an oxygen concentration that is both too high and administered over too long a period of time. Normally, alveoli are held open because they are filled by atmospheric gas largely composed of nitrogen that remains within the alveoli after all of the oxygen has diffused into the pulmonary capillary. When a concentration of oxygen above the normal atmospheric level of 21% is administered, some of the nitrogen is "washed out" or replaced by oxygen. The higher the concentration of oxygen, the greater the amount of nitrogen washed out. When nitrogen is replaced by oxygen, alveoli do not remain well inflated since all of the oxygen diffuses into the pulmonary capillary, leaving alveoli empty. Thus the higher the concentration of oxygen administered, the less well inflated will be the alveoli. This is referred to as "nitrogen wash out absorption atelectasis." Because of this pathology, it is not recommended that oxygen be administered at an $FIO_2$ above 40% to 50%.

The risk of absorption atelectasis is compounded when patients breathe at a minimal tidal volume as a result of sedation, surgical pain, or central nervous system dysfunction.[77]

normal lung inflation, atelectasis can develop as a result of improper patient positioning. In particular, any position that interferes with diaphragmatic descent or chest wall expansion can restrict lung inflation to the degree that atelectasis becomes a risk. Because of this, clinical assessment of the pulmonary system must include the evaluation of the effectiveness of ventilation in patients who cannot readily change position or who are reluctant to change position as a result of pain or decreased movement capability. Lung inflation is best achieved with the chest at least semi-upright, such as in semi-Fowler's position with the thorax elevated from waist level and in an even right to left position.

**Decreased distending forces.** The lung remains inflated as a result of the normal distending pressures that exist because of the opposing forces exerted by the natural recoil of the lung and by negative intrapleural pressure. When a pulmonary dysfunction occurs that interferes with the action of these two forces, normal lung inflation is interrupted, and the risk of developing atelectasis is increased. The loss of the normal inflation forces alone does not necessarily result in atelectasis. However, the patient is put in a position of increased risk. These disorders include pneumothorax, pleural effusion, chest wall/rib disorders, impairment of normal diaphragmatic functioning, and bullae formation resulting from emphysema.

### Assessment for Atelectasis

Symptoms resulting from atelectasis develop in proportion to the underlying respiratory impairment, the extent of the atelectasis, and the abruptness of onset. Atelectasis that develops slowly in a segment or lobe of an otherwise well-compensated patient generally causes few symptoms.[56] However, a patient who develops atelectasis and who may have an ongoing acute or chronic disease may exhibit severe symptoms.

Physical signs of atelectasis vary depending on how large an area is affected and on the patency of the airways that lead into the atelectatic area. Crackles, bronchial breath sounds, and egophony may be present if the airways are open, whereas decreased breath sounds will be found when the airways are occluded.[56] Crackles can be auscultated on the periphery of the atelectatic area, while decreased to absent breath sounds may be heard directly over the area. Large amounts of atelectatic lung tissue can produce a tracheal deviation toward the affected side, a dull percussion finding instead of the normal resonance, and decreased chest excursion on the affected side.

Arterial blood gas levels may or may not be altered by atelectasis. When they are altered, the $Pa_{O_2}$ usually shows hypoxemia. This results because blood passing through the atelectatic area does not come into contact with oxygen and proceeds to the left side of the heart in its venous concentration. There it mixes with normally oxygenated blood that has come from ventilated (nonatelectatic) lung areas. The resultant mixture shows a reduction in both $Pa_{O_2}$ and $Sa_{O_2}$ and is a consequence of what is known as right-to-left pulmonary shunting. Hypoxemia is relatively uncommon when all cases of atelectasis are considered, and it occurs most often in acute atelectasis when one or more lobes are involved.[41]

Fever may be present but has not been shown to be a reliable indicator of atelectasis.[41,73] Fever that does accompany atelectasis is most likely related to lung infection distal to the obstructed airway.[41]

Atelectasis is most often first noticed on chest radiograph by abnormalities such as displacement of lobar fissures[56] (which occurs as a result of loss of lung volume), opacity of an area, obliteration of known borders such as one of the cardiac borders,[41] or elevation of the diaphragm on the affected side. It remains one of the many dysfunctions in which the diagnosis is best confirmed by chest x-ray examination.

### Prevention

Prevention is not a usual heading under the discussion of diseases/disorders found in most critical care texts; however, atelectasis is one of the few dysfunctions in the hospitalized patient that can be prevented so easily that this discussion seems vital and will thus be included here. Very simply, atelectasis can, in many instances, be prevented with delivery of inspiratory volumes that will adequately ventilate the lung on a regular basis, such as several times every hour. Adequate ventilation can be assumed if auscultation of the lung during ventilation reveals breath sounds throughout all lung fields (discounting any previous pathology), especially at the lung bases.

There are many methods that can be used to achieve adequate ventilation, including incentive spirometry, intermittent positive pressure breathing (IPPB), mechanical ventilation, and repeated coaching by a nurse or respiratory therapist. Regardless of the method used, adequate lung ventilation must result or the efforts will be ineffective. The principle on which all prevention and treatment of atelectasis is based is that of providing regular, adequate inflation of the lung.

At this point, the reader should be assisted to understand those interventions that have not been shown to be effective in preventing atelectasis, so that ineffective interventions can be avoided in practice. *It is impossible for alveoli to inflate during exhalation; therefore forced coughing (in the absence of secretions), tracheal irritation that induces coughing, and blowing into devices have not been shown to be effective in preventing or treating atelectasis.* According to Bartlett[5]: "While it may be common practice to encourage patients to cough, it is uncomfortable and has no rational basis." Unless a patient has mucus in the airways (evaluated on chest auscultation) or is spontaneously coughing, he or she should not be encouraged to do so regardless of the much taught postoperative nursing care routine of cough-turn–deep breathe (CTDB). The only benefit that can be attributed to expiratory maneuvers may be the inhalation that occurs before coughing or use of the exhaling device.[5]

### Treatment

Once atelectasis has been diagnosed, treatment should ensue with vigor because any amount of alveolar collapse increases the work of breathing by decreasing lung compliance. This means patients must work harder to achieve lung inflation, and, if they are too weak to do so alone, they will require assistance or the atelectasis will worsen. Medical interventions include use of incentive spirometry, IPPB, mechanical ventilation if respiratory failure occurs, chest physiotherapy (CPT), administration of bronchodilators and/or mucolytics, oxygen for hypoxemia, and antibiotics when pneumonia is suspected. Atelectasis is often associated with pneumonia because it reduces both blood and lymph flow in the atelectatic area, thus hindering two major defense systems for preventing infection.[84]

Use of incentive spirometry was discussed in the section on prevention of atelectasis. The same recommendations for use apply when it is prescribed as a treatment for atelectasis.

IPPB is used more often as a treatment for atelectasis than it is as a prevention. It must be used correctly to be effective. This means that during the inhalation period of IPPB, air flow should be auscultated throughout all lung fields to ascertain the adequacy of ventilation. One of the major limitations of IPPB use occurs because patients are not supervised during the treatment. Many patients, as a result of the discomfort associated with chest inflation, stop air flow out of the machine before full lung inflation is achieved, thus negating the effectiveness of the treatment. IPPB treatments require supervision by a nurse or therapist who can instruct the patient about the depth of breath necessary to achieve maximal effect. Mechanical ventilation is used when atelectasis is associated with ventilatory failure.

CPT, the percussion and clapping of the thorax, involves positioning the atelectatic lung areas for favorable drainage followed by low-frequency (clapping) or high-frequency (vibration) percussion against the chest wall to jar secretions loose.[41] CPT is often used in conjunction with bronchodilator and mucolytic therapy.

Hypoxemia associated with atelectasis requires oxygen therapy and vigorous means of lung inflation. However, the fraction of inspired oxygen concentration ($FIO_2$) chosen should be high enough only to return the patient's $PaO_2$ to within normal limits for his or her age, because excessive amounts of oxygen are unnecessary and can be detrimental to surfactant production (see box, "Absorption Atlectasis"). Some authorities suggest that the $FIO_2$ be kept at a level that maintains the $PaO_2$ at 60 to 80 mm Hg, as that level will prevent tissue hypoxia at the lowest $FIO_2$.[65] Others feel the $PaO_2$ should be restored back to its nonhypoxemia level.

### Summary of Nursing Care

Nursing diagnoses and management of atelectasis are listed in the box above.

Nursing interventions can be extremely instumental in preventing atelectasis, and their focal points should be *teaching the patient proper ventilatory techniques and confirming maximal lung ventilation*.

#### Nursing Diagnosis and Management
*Atelectasis*

- Ineffective Breathing Pattern related to abdominal or thoracic pain, p. 472
- Ineffective Breathing Pattern related to modifiable chest wall restrictions secondary to pneumothorax or pleural effusion, p. 470
- Ineffective Airway Clearance related to excessive secretions, p. 466
- Impaired Gas Exchange related to alveolar hypoventilation secondary to (specify), p. 475
- Impaired Gas Exchange related to ventilation-perfusion inequality secondary to (specify), p. 474

Maximal deep inhalations held for approximately 3 seconds or longer (without the patient inadvertently initiating the Valsalva maneuver, prevented by keeping an open glottis) should be incorporated into the care plans for any patient at risk for developing atelectasis. Both the duration and the depth of inflation, which should be at least twice the tidal volume, are important in preventing as well as treating alveolar collapse.[56] The chest should be auscultated during inflation to ensure that all dependent parts of the lung are well ventilated and to help the patient understand the depth of breath necessary for optimum effect. In this way, when a nurse is not present for chest auscultation, the patient will know what depth yields adequate ventilation. Incentive spirometry is not necessary to prevent atelectasis, if the patient can be relied on to follow through with his or her own sustained maximal ventilations.

When an incentive spirometer is ordered, correct use is mandatory; this includes at least ten deep, effective breaths taken per hour. Ten breaths has been recommended, because research has shown it to be the average number of deep breaths (sighs) taken per hour by normal, healthy persons.[56] An hourly regimen of deep breathing is recommended because studies have indicated that some alveoli remain open for only 1 hour after the onset of hypoventilation; thus hourly hyperventilation is manadatory.[84] Close supervision of patient compliance with the prescribed regimen is recommended, as is the auscultation for breath sounds during the patient's maximum inhalations.

Many patients are reluctant to use the incentive spirometer or perform deep breathing because of associated discomfort or pain. Care must be taken to assess the level of analgesic necessary to relieve pain yet allow maximal lung inflation without oversedation so that the breathing pattern reverts to one of shallow, monotonous ventilations.

Frequent repositioning (a minimum of every 2 hours while the patient is awake) is essential because it most often results in a change in ventilatory pattern to that of deeper, more frequent ventilations. Although patients in the critical care unit are not often ambulated, those in the step-down units are, and early ambulation is essential in restoring lung function, providing several points are kept in mind.

When sitting at the bedside or ambulating, patients must be encouraged to keep the thorax in straight alignment while they breathe deeply. This position best accommodates diaphragmatic descent and intercostal muscle action, thus the breathing benefits. Also, the sitting or standing position provides enhanced ventilation to areas of the lung that are dependent in the supine position, thus accommodating maximal inflation and, in some instances, gas exchange.[66]

Adequate fluid intake is essential, in particular if the nursing assessment of a patient reveals him or her to be at increased risk for mucus production such as those patients with previous mucus history and those with an underlying mucus-producing disease (such as chronic bronchitis, pneumonia, or bronchiectasis). Collaboration with the physician and/or a nutritionist may be necessary to establish a fluid intake that will allow mobilization of secretions without causing fluid volume overload. Many patients with mucus history maintain the fluid intake at one and one half or more quarts of decaffeinated beverage per day. For patients who are not on oral intake, 24-hour intake by other means must be given at a level that allows mobilization of secretions. Whenever tenacious mucus is suctioned or expectorated, inadequate fluid intake should be suspected. Additionally, those patients with an artificial airway require humidification to that airway so that pulmonary secretions remain mobile. Collaboration with a respiratory therapist may be necessary if insufficient humidification is suspected.

Patient teaching cannot be overlooked in the prevention of atelectasis. All of the above interventions require patient cooperation and thus should be incorporated into a patient teaching plan. Preoperative teaching is most effective and should include as many of the above nursing interventions as time will allow, including practice with an incentive spirometer if postoperative orders will include its use.

Preventive interventions should also be used for treatment interventions as they achieve the same result—maximal lung inflation. However, once atelectasis has developed, more vigilance is needed on the part of patient, nurse, and respiratory therapist in performing the interventions. Because atelectasis, depending on its extent, can increase the work of breathing, significant encouragement may be necessary when the patient is performing maximal lung inflations. Also, the assessment of the length of time a patient is able to spend on lung inflation corresponding with the length of rest necessary to recover will assist in the development of a daily care plan that best accommodates patient care.

Once this dysfunction has been diagnosed, careful assessment of lung sounds, breathing pattern, presence of fever, and patient ability to withstand the current nursing and medical interventions is necessary to establish whether the atelectasis is being resolved or is progressing.

## PNEUMONIA

### Description

Once the leading cause of human death, pneumonia continues to be a major health problem. Despite antibiotics, it is still the most frequent cause of infectious mortality and remains the fifth leading cause of death in the United States.[19,29] Nosocomial pneumonias account for 15% of hospital-acquired infections, with the majority of cases occurring in critical care units or similar areas.[19,29] The morbidity and mortality associated with such cases is 20% to 50%.[19,29]

### Cause

Pneumonia is caused when virulent organisms are able to multiply in the lower respiratory system. Host defenses are multiple and bacteria must overcome these defenses to colonize the lower respiratory tract. The host mechanisms that maintain sterility below the glottis include aerodynamic energy, mucociliary action, antibody secretion, phagocytic activity, and the lymphatic response.[6,34] Table 11-8 outlines some pneumonias encountered by the practitioner in the critical care patient population.

### Pathophysiology

Development of acute pneumonia implies (1) a break in host defenses, (2) a particularly virulent organism, or (3) an overwhelming inoculation event. Bacterial invasion of the lower respiratory tract can occur by inhalation, aspiration, migration from adjacent sites, or, less commonly, hematogenous seeding.[16] The most common method appears to be that of microaspiration of bacteria colonized in the upper airway.[31]

Infection results in pulmonary inflammation with or without significant exudates. Ventilation-perfusion inequality and hypoxemia occur as lung consolidation progresses. Untreated pneumonia can result in respiratory failure and septicemia. Mortality increases with associated disease states, such as diabetes, malnutrition, immunosuppression or chronic obstructive lung disorders, and patient age.

### Assessment and Diagnosis

Dyspnea is the primary symptom experienced in diffuse pneumonia. Coughing and wheezing with sputum production may be present. Often the patient complains of fever or chills, although this may be less frequent in the elderly and immunosuppressed population.[31] Pleuritic pain may be a prominent feature. Generally, the onset will be acute with the patient feeling quite unwell in a brief period of time. However, in the hospitalized patient the onset can also be insidious.

In critically ill patients, many of whom have multiple-system problems and various invasive monitoring devices in place, the cause of an infection that presents an indolent course can be easily obscured.

Assessment reveals hyperpnea or tachypnea, possibly associated with crackles and wheezes over the area of involvement. Chest x-ray evaluation may show infiltrates,

***Table 11-8*** Characteristics of common pneumonias

| Parameter | *Pseudomonas aeruginosa* | Staphylococcal pneumonia | Streptococcal pneumonia | *Hemophilus influenzae* | Mycoplasmal pneumonia |
|---|---|---|---|---|---|
| Classic signs and symptoms | Fever, especially in morning, chills, severe dyspnea, copious purulent sputum | Sudden or insidious onset, sustained fever and pleuritic pain, productive cough, shaking chills, dyspnea, cyanosis, tachypnea, pleural effusion, rapid development of respiratory failure | Abrupt onset, fever, cough, chest pain, afternoon-evening temperature, diaphoresis, rusty sputum, chills, myalgias; consolidation with egophony, bronchophony, bronchial breathing; chest dull to percussion, crackles, wheezes auscultated | Cough, sputum production, fever, chills, dyspnea, pleuritic chest pain, increasing respiratory insufficiency | Gradual onset with sore throat, pounding headache, myalgias; dry persistent hacking cough, fatigue, low-grade fever, scant sputum/or none; crackles appear later in disease, dull to percussion, wheezes, pleural friction, rub; acute 80% cough, temperature > 101°, erythema multiforme, bullous myringitis |
| X-ray findings | Diffuse bronchopneumonia, typically bilateral; nodular infiltrates; small pleural effusions | Consolidation in segments or lobes; patchy bilateral infiltrates, pleural fluid common; when hematogenous route, large confluent, bilateral infiltrates seen | Dense homogenous shadows involving all of one or more lobes | Variable ranges from patchy infiltrates to dense consolidation effusion common | Patchy perihilar, lobar, or diffuse infiltrates; 50% infiltrates multilobar; significant effusion rare, if present, reconsider diagnosis |
| Therapy | Gentamicin, tebramycin, amikacin | Oxacillin, penicillinase-resistant semisynthetic penicillin, cephalosporin, clindamycin, tobramycin, gentamycin as last resort | Penicillin, if resistant to erythromycin, vancomycin; if allergy to penicillin, then tetracyclines, lincomycin, cephalosporins, chloramphenical | Second-generation cephalosporins, then ampicillin, if sensitive; trimethoprimsulfamethoxazole; after hospital discharge, ampicillin or cefaclor, chloramphenicol | Erythromycin, tetracycline |
| Preventive measures | Proper sterilization and use of disposable respiratory therapy devices, suction apparatus, proper hand washing | | Polyvalent pneumococcal vaccine for high-risk people | Vaccine for encapsulated hemophilus influenza type B; usual infection in critical care unit involves encapsulated forms | Erythromycin for high-risk contacts in family setting, tetracyclines |

PMNs, polymorphonuclear leukocytes.

depending on the length of illness and absence of other lung problems. An elevated leukocyte count with a shift to the left is seen in bacterial pneumonias. A normal or decreased white blood cell count in the presence of pneumonia suggests an overwhelming infection and a poor prognosis. Sputum cultures and blood cultures should be obtained to completely assess the patient's condition.

Invasive tests such as a thoracentesis for pleural fluids, transtracheal aspiration, bronchoscopy, and open biopsy are further diagnostic measures that can be used in cases in which attempts to identify the pathogen have been otherwise ineffective.

### Treatment

Treatment of pneumonia should include specific antibiotic therapy, support of respiratory function, support of nutrition, treatment of associated medical problems and complications, and proper fluid and electrolyte management. Special attention should be aimed at preventing the spread of infection, along with prompt recognition and treatment.

Although bacteria-specific therapy is the goal, this may not always be possible because of difficulties in identifying the organism and the seriousness of the patient's condition. The time involved obtaining bacterial specimens should be balanced against the need to begin some treatment based on patient condition.

Selection of the antibiotic should reflect clinical efficacy, microbiological activity, antibiotic penetration, metabolism, and side effects. With increasing awareness of the need to control cost of medical care, expense of an antibiotic can become a factor in selection. Recent literature has focused on the ability of antibiotics to penetrate the blood bronchus barrier as a criterion for successful treatment of pneumonia in some populations. Generally, this becomes a concern in people with chronically damaged or hypersecreting bronchial systems who may be significant in number in critical care settings. Some of the new cephalosporins show better penetration in research studies.[48]

Stopping antibiotic therapy is generally indicated when the patient has been afebrile for several days with a previously abnormal (elevated or depressed) white blood cell count close to or at normal levels. Reexamination of the sputum should demonstrate freedom from bacteria. X-ray infiltrates can persist for extended periods after the pneumonia has resolved and should not be considered a reason to continue drug therapy.[47,59]

Patients in critical care units, being sicker and with multiple problems, may require a longer course of antibiotic therapy. Gram-negative pneumonias, *Legionella*, and staphylococcal pneumonia may require treatment for up to 3 weeks.[59]

### Summary of Nursing Care

Refer to the box above for nursing diagnoses and management of pneumonia. Nursing care of patients with pneumonia requires a multifaceted approach: (1) safe and timely administration of antibiotic therapy, (2) monitoring and support of the patient's ventilatory efforts, and (3) prevention of further contamination by other organisms from infected patients to other critically ill patients.

The nurse has a major role in assisting with antibiotic therapy, as planned and prescribed by the physician. Often, if not always, the nurse is responsible for collecting the sputum specimens on which therapy will be based. The nurse also monitors the patient's response to antibiotic therapy by continually evaluating the patient's status. Changes in vital signs, sputum production, and sputum characteristics will generally be noticed initially by the nurse through routine patient monitoring.

Throughout the course of the pneumonia, the critical care nurse monitors and supports the patient's ventilatory function. Lung sounds are assessed at least every 4 hours, along with other vital signs (temperature, pulse, respiratory rate, and blood pressure). Efforts to support airway clearance and ventilation are directed by nursing. This will include various measures of pulmonary toilet, depending on the patient's individual condition and proper patient positioning to facilitate lung expansion. Recent research shows coached deep breathing with coughing to be more effective in raising sputum in acute pneumonias than does postural drainage and vibration techniques.[43]

Frequent changes of the patient's position should be implemented to maximize ventilation and perfusion in different

### Nursing Diagnosis and Management
***Pneumonia***

- Impaired Gas Exchange related to ventilation-perfusion inequality secondary to alveolar infiltrates, p. 474
- Impaired Gas Exchange related to ventilation-perfusion inequality secondary to (specify), p. 474
- Impaired Gas Exchange related to alveolar hypoventilation secondary to (specify), p. 475
- Ineffective Airway Clearance related to excessive secretions, p. 466
- Acute Pain related to transmission and perception of noxious stimuli secondary to pneumonia, p. 485
- Altered Nutrition: Less Than Body Protein-Calorie Requirements related to lack of exogenous nutrients and increased metabolic demand. (See also discussion of metabolic results from carbohydrate overfeeding, Chapter 6.)
- Powerlessness related to health care environment or illness-related regimen, p. 445
- Anxiety related to threat to biological, psychological, and/or social integrity, p. 448

areas of the lungs. When unilateral pneumonia exists, positioning the patient on the unaffected side (with the good lung down) can improve ventilation-perfusion matching.[66,94]

Prevention should also be directed at eradicating pathogens from the environment and interrupting the spread of organisms from person to person. Significant progress has been made in removing contaminants from the patient environment through proper disinfection of respiratory equipment and increased use of disposable supplies. Other possible environmental sources of pathogens include suctioning equipment and indwelling lines. Proper aseptic care must be directed at the management of these invasive tools. Proper hand-washing technique is the single most important measure available to prevent spread of bacteria from person to person.[42]

## ASPIRATION LUNG DISORDER

### Description

Aspiration pneumonia, a special type of pneumonia that may be seen in critical care units, is a major cause of morbidity and mortality. Aspiration has been recorded in as many as 38% of critically ill, intubated patients receiving feeding through small-bore nasogastric tubes, despite maintenance of the integrity of cuffed tracheal tubes.[17,60] Many of the risk factors leading to aspiration are present in critical care patients (see the box below).

### Cause

The presence of abnormal substances in the airways and alveoli as a result of aspiration is misleadingly called aspiration pneumonia. The title is misleading because the aspiration of toxic substances into the lung may or may not involve bacterial infection. Aspiration lung disorder would be a more meaningful title, because injury to the lung can result from chemical, mechanical, and/or bacterial characteristics of the aspirate.

**RISK FACTORS ASSOCIATED WITH ASPIRATION**

- Impaired consciousness
- Compromised glottal closure
- Compromised cough reflex
- Ileus or gastric dilation
- Nasogastric feeding tubes (large or small bore)
- Artificial airways
- Disorders affecting pharyngeal and/or esophageal motility
- Tracheoesophageal fistulas
- General anesthesia
- Cardiopulmonary resuscitation
- Improper patient positioning during tube feeding
- Esophageal strictures

### Pathophysiology

Characteristics of the aspirated material are crucial to the ultimate effects on lung tissue. Generally, an aspirate with a low pH spreading throughout the lung fields may quickly result in adult respiratory distress syndrome. As seen in animal studies, the "critical pH" of less than 2.5 is thought to cause severe chemical lung injury.[17,34] The coupling of a low pH and virulent pathogens may quickly overwhelm normal defenses of the lung. Aspiration of material from the oropharynx carries resident flora to the sterile lower respiratory tract. Elderly and hospitalized patients show a prevalence of gram-negative bacteria in the oropharynx, which increases the likelihood of gram-negative pneumonias associated with aspiration.[17,27,34,87]

Recognition of the aspiration event plays a role in outcome. Aspiration of significant amounts can be readily noticed with respiratory distress, dyspnea, wheezing, and coughing. However, aspiration of smaller amounts (silent aspiration) can occur without recognition, especially in patients with altered levels of consciousness.

Aspiration of particulate matter may have an immediate life-threatening result if large particles mechanically block the major airways. In less dramatic situations, small particles cause small segmental atelectasis by occluding bronchioles. The presence of foreign matter causes an inflammatory response in the lung, though not the dramatic fluid shift seen in acid aspiration.

Bacterial inoculation by aspiration usually follows an indolent course. Bacteria invade the lung, resulting in a clinical picture that can range from patchy bronchopneumonia to empyema and purulent lung abscesses. Anaerobic organisms predominate in community aspirations, whereas gram-negative aerobic organisms are seen in the majority of aspirations occurring in hospitalized patients.[99]

### Assessment and Diagnosis

When aspiration of a significant volume or repeated aspiration of smaller volumes occurs, the patient will develop increasing dyspnea, fever, tachypnea, and cyanosis.[17] If the cough reflex is intact, increased coughing occurs. Intubated patients may require more frequent suctioning, and aspirated material may be present in secretions. Auscultation of the lung fields demonstrates decreased breath sounds in the affected area with associated wheezes. Arterial blood gases reflect hypoxemia, and an increased $FIO_2$ is needed to maintain satisfactory oxygenation.[17] If bacterial infection becomes established, the white blood cell count may become elevated. A normal or decreased white blood cell count in the setting of infection suggests overwhelming host invasion and a poor prognosis.

Chest x-ray changes appear 12 to 24 hours after the initial aspiration. The validity of the chest x-ray in diagnosing aspiration lung disorder is related to the prior status of the patient. Patients with underlying lung involvement, as commonly seen in critical care units, may already have significant pulmonary infiltrates present on chest x-ray evaluation, clouding the interpretation. In massive aspiration, diffuse bilateral infiltrates suggest pulmonary edema is present, whereas lesser aspirations show atelectasis in the early period.[17] Later chest films show large, fluffy infiltrates.

Because of the acute vertical descent of the right mainstem bronchus, the right lung is more often the site of involvement in aspirations. The lower right and left lobes and the right middle lobe are common sites of aspiration[17] involvement with occurrences being 60%, 42%, and 32%, respectively.[34] The patient position at the time of aspiration affects the distribution pattern of the aspirate in the lungs. Patients at risk for aspiration are best kept in a head-down position, or at least supine and lateral.

### Treatment

Management includes emergency treatment and follow-up treatment. When aspiration is witnessed, emergency treatment should be instituted to secure the airway and minimize pulmonary damage. The patient should be placed in slight (6 to 8 inches head-down) Trendelburg's position and turned to right lateral decubitus position to aid drainage and avoid involvement of other lung areas.[17,59] Oropharyngeal suctioning should immediately follow. Direct visualization by bronchoscopy is indicated when large particulate aspirate blocks airways. Bronchial and pulmonary lavage is not recommended, because studies have demonstrated that this practice disseminates aspirate in lungs and increases damage.[17,59]

Following airway clearance, attention should be given to hemodynamic support, arterial blood gas monitoring, and respiratory support. Hemodynamic changes result from fluid shifts occurring in massive aspirations causing noncardiogenic pulmonary edema. Transudation of large amounts of cellular and colloidal fluids causes a disarray of pulmonary defenses and cellular injury. Arterial blood gas analysis should be obtained immediately and sequentially throughout the patient course to direct oxygen therapy. Inability to correct hypoxemia, despite supplemental oxygen, is an indication that aggressive treatment is needed. Positive end expiratory pressure (PEEP) ventilation may help maintain acceptable oxygenation with lower concentrations of inspired oxygen. However, at the same time that PEEP provides for a lower $FIO_2$, it can also decrease cardiac output, thus lowering tissue oxygenation; therefore the lowest level of PEEP needed for satisfactory oxygenation should be used.[11]

Other medical intervention involves drug therapy. Bronchodilators may be useful in situations associated with bronchospasm. Benefits of steroidal drugs remain unclear; they are frequently used in aspiration, even though current studies do not support the use of steroids.[22,96] Osmotic agents such as albumin should not be utilized as the albumin extravasates into the lung, further decreasing gas exchange at the alveolus.[17,59,71] Antibiotics should be instituted according to positive Gram's stain or culture results. When anaerobic contamination is present, Levison[48] noted a greater response to clindamycin than to penicillin. In hospital-acquired aspiration pneumonia, a broad-spectrum antibiotic such as a cephalosporin has been shown to improve patient outcome. When *Pseudomonas* is present, an aminoglycoside or betalactamase penicillin should be administered.[17]

Recent studies regarding the efficiency of administering prophylactic $H^2$ blockers to lessen gastric acidity in preoperative patients have been performed.[17] Results have shown that lessening of the acid level of gastric secretions minimizes lung injury when aspiration occurs.[9] Alteration of gastric pH in other at-risk patients may be warranted. The use of oral antacids has been efficacious in increasing the gastric pH of gastric secretions, but nonparticulate antacids such as sodium citrate appear to be preferred in high-risk patients, such as patients in the critical care unit. Metoclopramide hydrochloride, a dopamine antagonist, has been shown to decrease gastric volume and increase upper gastrointestinal motility and gastric sphincter tone.[59] It may therefore be advantageous when given preoperatively.

### Summary of Nursing Care

Refer to the box below for nursing diagnoses and management of aspiration lung disorder. During the course of caring for the critically ill patient, the nurse must implement measures for preventing aspiration lung disorder. If the aspiration event occurred before the patient's admission to the critical care unit, the nurse must direct interventions toward (1) maintaining the airway and supporting respiratory function, (2) early recognition and treatment of complications of aspiration lung disorder, and (3) preventing further aspiration events.

In at-risk patients, nursing interventions should be directed at preventing aspiration. Decisions regarding patient positioning should reflect consideration of the potential for

#### Nursing Diagnosis and Management
***Aspiration lung disorder***

- Impaired Gas Exchange related to ventilation-perfusion inequality secondary to aspiration, p. 474
- High Risk for Aspiration risk factors: reduced level of consciousness, depressed cough and gag reflexes, presence of tracheostomy or endotracheal tube, gastrointestinal tube, enteral tube feedings, decreased gastrointestinal motility, impaired swallowing, facial/oral/neck surgery or trauma, situations hindering evaluation of upper body, p. 476
- Sensory-Perceptual Alterations related to sensory overload, sensory deprivation, sleep pattern disturbance, p. 489
- Anxiety related to threat to biological, psychological, and social integrity, p. 448

aspiration. Unless contraindicated, the unconscious patient should be placed on the side in a slight Trendelburg's position to promote drainage and discourage aspiration. Placement of nasogastric (NG) tubes for gastric decompression requires careful consideration, because NG tubes paradoxically increase the risk of aspiration and have been frequently shown to empty the stomach incompletely.[59] Patients receiving continuous or intermittent tube feeding should be maintained in at least a 30-degree head elevation. If a recumbent or head down position is necessary, feedings should be interrupted every 30 minutes to 1 hour before assuming a flat position. When head elevation is contraindicated, the right lateral decubitus position is preferred, because it aids passage of gastric contents through the pylorus.[60] Also, in this situation the choice of the type of feeding tube takes on added importance.

Tube feeding into the stomach should be avoided in all unconscious patients or patients with an absent or compromised cough reflex. These patients should receive feeding into the intestine by means of a small-bore weighted tube, since these tubes are associated with a lower incidence of aspiration than the larger bore tubes. Frequent checking of tube location, as well as checking for gastric retention of the feeding, is necessary to prevent aspiration. The standard technique used to check retention may be difficult in small-bore, pliable catheters, because drawing back can collapse the lumen. Therefore abdominal girths should be monitored on a serial basis.

Monitoring nasogastric tube placement regularly is a necessary nursing task. Placement of any tube should be initially verified by x-ray examination or whenever the possibility of dislodgement is suspected. There have been several reports about small-bore tubes being inadvertently placed or dislodged into the respiratory tract.[60]

Glucose oxidase reagent strips can be used to check for glucose in tracheobronchial secretions of tube-fed patients, since normal sputum is free from detectable glucose. Small amounts of blood in the secretions can create a false-positive test, and this should be considered when oxidase strips are used.

## RESPIRATORY FAILURE

### Description

Respiratory failure is commonly seen in critical care patients as a primary disorder or as a complication of other system failures or traumatic injuries. Respiratory failure is generally accepted as being present when the $PaO_2$ is $<50$ mm Hg, and/or the $PaCO_2$ is $>50$ mm Hg at an $FIO_2$ of 21%.[4,9,55] When hypoxemia without associated hypercapnia is present (type I), respiratory failure is said to exist. Type II respiratory failure (also called ventilatory failure) exists when the patient is both hypoxemic and hypercapnic. Some conditions deteriorate from type I to type II respiratory failure in the course of the disease or when intervention is delayed or unsuccessful.

### Cause

As the boxes below indicate, many causative agents or conditions can lead to respiratory failure. When disease and disability result in an insufficient exchange of air and gas in relation to the amount needed to maintain metabolism, respiratory failure exists.

#### TYPE I RESPIRATORY FAILURE (HYPOXEMIA WITHOUT HYPERCAPNIA)

Chronic bronchitis and emphysema
Pneumonia
Pulmonary edema
Pulmonary fibrosis
Bronchial asthma
Atelectasis
Aspiration (acid-bile)
Adult respiratory distress syndrome (ARDS)
Bronchiectasis
Smoke inhalation
Pulmonary embolism
Cardiogenic shock
Cyanotic congenital heart disease
Pulmonary arteriovenous fistulas
Kyphoscoliosis
Massive obesity
Postoperative
Crushed chest injury
Fat embolism

#### TYPE II RESPIRATORY FAILURE (VENTILATORY FAILURE, HYPOXEMIA WITH HYPERCAPNIA)

Acute exacerbations of chronic pulmonary diseases
Chronic bronchitis and emphysema
Bronchial asthma
Crushed chest injury
Drug overdose (narcotic, sedative, and so on)
Central alveolar hypoventilation syndrome
Obstructive sleep apnea syndrome
Myasthenia gravis
Tetanus
Polyneuropathies, myopathies
Cervical cord injuries
Head injuries
Poliomyelitis
Hypothermia
Hypertrophy of the tonsils and adenoids
Near-drowning
Curariform drugs
Barbiturate poisoning

### Pathophysiology

Respiratory failure can be acute or chronic, depending on the speed of onset and duration of the illness. It can result from changes in the functioning of the components of the respiratory system such as the airways, the alveoli, or the alveolar-capillary membrane. Changes in how these components function in relation to the whole can result in hypoventilation, impeded diffusion, ventilation-perfusion mismatch, and increased pulmonary shunting. Combinations of these abnormalities are frequently seen in patients with respiratory failure. Type I hypoxemic respiratory failure results from V/Q mismatch, shunt, or diffusion abnormalities. Type II respiratory failure results from the same conditions that cause type I failure and includes hypoventilation. Treatments directed at improving oxygenation or breathing are necessary to correct the hypercapnia, hypoxemia, and subsequent acidosis.

### Assessment and Diagnosis

Diagnosing and following the course of respiratory failure is best accomplished by blood gas analysis. Clinical symptoms displayed by the patients are not reliable in predicting the degree of hypoxemia or hypercapnia. Blood gas analysis confirms the level of $Paco_2$, $Pao_2$, and blood pH.

### Treatment

In type I failure, aggressive treatment of hypoxemia using a high $FIo_2$ is necessary, because severe hypoxemia ($Pao_2$ <40 mm Hg) is rapidly fatal. Although the absolute level of hypoxemia varies in each individual, most treatment approaches aim to keep the oxygen saturation at 90% or above. Correcting hypoxemia by increasing the $FIo_2$ is effective in treating V/Q inequalities and diffusion impairments. When shunt exists (blood flowing through a nonventilated alveoli), increasing the $FIo_2$ of inspired air alone is ineffective. In these situations, alveolar ventilation, hence $Pao_2$, may be increased by constant positive airway pressure (CPAP) or PEEP in addition to mechanical ventilation.

In type I patients, the mixed venous $Po_2$ ($Pvo_2$) is an assessment parameter that reflects tissue oxygenation and cardiac output more accurately than arterial blood gas analysis.[25] Mixed venous $O_2$ monitoring requires a pulmonary artery catheter. The recent development of a catheter with fiberoptic bundles has allowed for constant monitoring of the $Pvo_2$ as opposed to intermittent sampling. Along with the importance of providing adequate oxygen, prolonged administration of a high $FIo_2$ should be avoided, because this results in oxygen toxicity and aggravates low V/Q ratios. When faced with a $Pao_2$<50 mm Hg, despite an $FIo_2$ of 50%, significant intrapulmonary shunt exists.[55] ARDS is a common example of this respiratory failure.

Ventilatory support in type I respiratory failure should be considered when (1) inadequate oxygenation continues despite $FIo_2$ increases, (2) retention of $CO_2$ occurs leading to increased $Paco_2$, mental depression, or increased fatigue, and (3) secretion control becomes difficult.[4,55]

Type II respiratory failure, associated with hypoventilation, requires methodology aimed at improving ventilatory dynamics. Intervention may require lowering the $FIo_2$ in patients who chronically retain carbon dioxide and thus are dependent on the hypoxic respiratory drive. Other interventions in type II respiratory failure include narcoleptic drugs, reversal of drug overdose, or mechanical ventilation if the respiratory failure results from neurological or muscle disorders of ventilatory muscle fatigue.

One of the most frequent situations leading to type II respiratory failure is acute exacerbation of chronic obstructive pulmonary disease as a result of a new pulmonary infectious process.[55] Acute deterioration in a chronic setting can be detected by the presence of acidosis in a previously compensated patient. Therapy is aimed at treating the pulmonary infection, relieving the hypoxemia, stimulating the respiratory drive, and, if necessary, providing mechanically assisted ventilation. Each approach must be evaluated on the basis of the individual patient situation.

Treating hypoxemia is a primary aim, because hypoxemia gives rise to systemic complications and, if untreated, will result in death. In most situations, conservative treatment of hypoxemia has proved more satisfactory than aggressive therapy involving intubation and assisted ventilation.[55] Low levels of $FIo_2$ are warranted to avoid depressing any hypoxic respiratory drive that might exist in patients with chronic $CO_2$ retention.

The process of ventilation is driven by many forces. One of the predominant chemical factors stimulating ventilation is the level of hydrogen ions ($H^+$) circulating in the medulla and the brain. In normal states, small increases in hydrogen ion concentration result in increasing the ventilatory drive (rate and depth of inspiration), which in turn increases the removal of $CO_2$ (an $H^+$ precursor) from the lungs. However, if the CO (and subsequently the $H^+$ level) climbs slowly over time (as in COPD), the chemoreceptors in the medulla become less and less responsive to hydrogen ion concentration. When this occurs, low tissue oxygen levels (hypoxemia) stimulate ventilation. Giving the patient too much supplemental $FIo_2$ can abolish the hypoxic drive and result in apnea. Generally, oxygen should be titrated to produce a $Pao_2$ of 50 to 60 mm Hg.[4,49]

Even careful administration of oxygen has the potential for decreasing the hypoxic drive to ventilate in patients who chronically retain carbon dioxide. As previously mentioned, clinical signs of hypercapnia and hypoxia are not reliable in reflecting the degree of abnormality. Arterial blood gases should be utilized. Frequency of sampling warrants arterial catheterization that will also allow for continuous monitoring of the blood pressure.

Methods frequently chosen to deliver lower oxygen concentrations include Venturi masks or nasal prongs at 1 to 3 L/min. Patient compliance with oxygen therapy is often better with nasal prong use than with face mask use because of perceived comfort by the patient. When the face mask is used to treat hypoxemia, the patient will often complain that the mask compromises breathing, talking, and eating and may even remove the mask. Nasal prongs allow patients to be active while continuing to receive oxygen, therefore providing a more consistent level of oxygenation.

Bronchodilation can improve air flow in patients and lessen hypoxemia. Although theophylline preparations are commonly chosen, beta blockers have proved effective, especially when delivered by nebulized inhalation. Two drugs that may be used are ipratropium bromide and salbutamol.[55]

When the patient has $CO_2$ narcosis from respiratory depression as a result of drugs or oxygen, doxapram is helpful. Doxapram has been administered in a continuous drip in an attempt to increase patients' levels of alertness and improve their ability to participate in bronchial hygiene activities.[55] Respiratory stimulants such as nikethamide offered no improvement in the course of respiratory failure. Almitrine is a newer respiratory stimulant that may have advantages not seen in other drugs. Specifically, almitrine stimulates the carotid and aortic bodies to increase ventilation. Studies in France show improvement in $Pa_{O_2}$ and decrease in the $Pa_{CO_2}$ when almitrine was given in a continuous intravenous drip.[49] (Oral forms of the drug are also available.)

When conservative measures fail to reverse the elevated $Pa_{CO_2}$ and improve oxygenation, mechanical ventilation may be necessary. Complications of mechanical ventilation such as barotrauma can occur, and difficulty in weaning the patient from a mechanical ventilator is a real possibility. Mechanical ventilation in COPD patients should be brief and instituted for short-term problems that can be aggressively reversed. Since conservative management (without mechanical ventilation) in COPD patients is as successful as the use of mechanical ventilation and carries fewer risks of complications, it should be tried first.

### Summary of Nursing Care

Nursing diagnoses and management of respiratory failure are summarized in the box below. Respiratory failure can result from a myriad of precipitating events with varying treatment approaches. Nursing care will be directed by the specific cause of the respiratory failure, although some common interventions are utilized. The nurse has a significant role in (1) monitoring the patient's course, (2) supporting and improving the ventilatory dynamics, (3) maintaining a patent airway and aiding secretion clearance, and (4) proper administration of drugs, including oxygen.

Monitoring the course of an illness is a major nursing responsibility. Since the nurse provides care on a continuous basis, changes in the patient's status are initially recognized and evaluated by the nurse caregiver. Baseline and ongoing

#### Nursing Diagnosis and Management

***Respiratory failure***

- Impaired Gas Exchange related to alveolar hypoventilation secondary to (specify), p. 475
- Impaired Gas Exchange related to ventilation-perfusion inequality secondary to (specify), p. 474
- Ineffective Breathing Pattern related to chronic airflow limitations, p. 470
- Ineffective Breathing Pattern related to respiratory muscle deconditioning secondary to mechanical ventilation, p. 471
- Ineffective Airway Clearance related to excessive secretions, p. 466
- Ineffective Airway Clearance related to impaired cough secondary to loss of glottic closure with cuffed endotracheal/tracheostomy tube, p. 468
- High Risk for Aspiration risk factors: reduced level of consciousness, depressed cough, and gag reflexes, presence of tracheostomy or endotracheal tube, p. 476
- Decreased Cardiac Output related to decreased preload secondary to mechanical ventilation with or without PEEP, p. 457
- Altered Nutrition: Less Than Body Protein-Calorie Requirements related to lack of exogenous nutrients and increased metabolic demand. (See also discussion of metabolic results from carbohydrate overfeeding, Chapter 6.)
- High Risk for Infection risk factor: invasive monitoring devices, p. 465
- Sensory-Perceptual Alterations related to sensory overload, sensory deprivation, sleep pattern disturbance, p. 489
- Sleep Pattern Disturbance related to circadian desynchronization, p. 455
- High Risk for Impaired Skin Integrity risk factors: immobility, nutritional deficit, steroid therapy, enteral tube feedings, stool incontinence, p. 499
- Body Image Disturbance related to actual change in body structure, function, and appearance, and/or functional dependence on life-sustaining technology, p. 443
- Powerlessness related to health care environment or illness-related regimen, p. 445
- Ineffective Individual Coping related to situational crisis and personal vulnerability, p. 447

respiratory assessment should include airway patency, respiratory rate and depth, pattern of respirations, presence of or changes in adventitious lung sounds, arterial blood gas analysis, and secretion production and clearance.

Establishing the baseline state of the patient's monitoring parameters is important, since it is the reference point from which progress or deterioration is judged. Next, the nurse should establish the levels of change necessary to trigger alterations in intervention. For example, if arterial blood gases are being periodically assessed, what goal is desired? Once this is established, the intervention techniques can be preplanned. In this situation, the nurse knows in advance what to do for specific blood gas results without having to recontact the physician. When clear plans are articulated in advance, unnecessary loss of time and effort is eliminated.

## ADULT RESPIRATORY DISTRESS SYNDROME (ARDS)

### Description

Adult respiratory distress syndrome (ARDS) is a well-recognized syndrome erupting as the final common pathway of various insults that cause damage to the alveolar-capillary interface (see the box below, right and Fig. 11-1). Despite the advancement in techniques available to monitor and support critically ill patients, the outcome for patients with ARDS has improved little. Mortality rates remain at 50% to 60%.[8,11,38,62] A National Institutes of Health (NIH) study reports that mortality rates increase significantly when organ failure is present: one organ (lung only), 40%; two organs, 54%; four organs, 84%; and with five organs failing, 100%.[11] No clear understanding of the pathology or the approach to treatment exists, making ARDS a challenging and frustrating phenomenon estimated to affect 150,000 patients annually.[58]

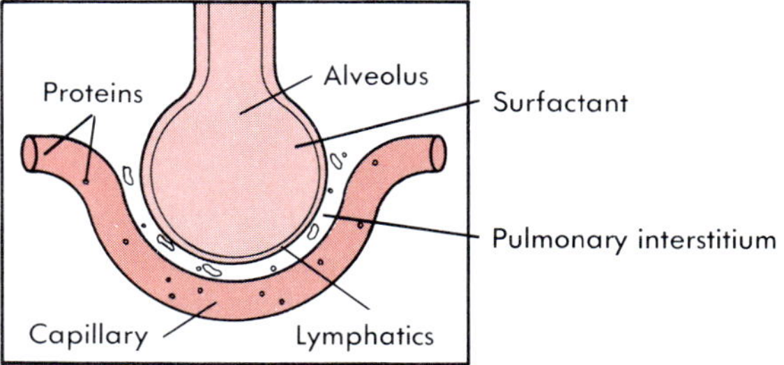


***Fig. 11-1*** Normal dynamics at the alveolar-capillary membrane. In the normal lung, small amounts of fluid may leave the capillary space and enter the pulmonary interstitium where the lymphatic system removes the fluid and returns it to the capillary space. The normal capillary membrane is relatively impermeable to protein; therefore protein does not usually enter the interstitial space. The normal alveolar membrane is rather impermeable to fluid; therefore fluid does not usually enter the alveolar space. Surfactant, produced by type II alveolar epithelial cells, lines the interior of each alveolus and acts to maintain alveolar stability and to prevent alveolar collapse (see the box on p. 259).

In 1967 Ashbaugh and others[1] described the criteria for diagnosing ARDS. They identified a syndrome preceded by a catastrophic event, such as multiple trauma, followed by increased intrapulmonary shunting, increased dead space, and loss of pulmonary compliance with resulting hypoxemia despite increasing levels of $FIO_2$. Changes revealed by chest x-ray evaluation, with the appearance of diffuse bilateral infiltrates, confirmed the diagnosis. Studies continue to be done to clarify the etiological factors related to ARDS and to find treatment modalities that will lower the mortality.

### Cause

Many factors have been implicated as causative agents of ARDS, but the mechanisms of pulmonary injury are often unclear. The box on p. 259 lists situations frequently leading to adult respiratory distress syndrome. Of those implicated, patients with direct lung injury and/or systemic sepsis are at highest risk of developing ARDS.[8,38] Fein and others[26] demonstrated in a retrospective study that 18% of all patients admitted to the hospital with sepsis developed ARDS. In a study by Hudson[38], 40% of patients with sepsis developed ARDS. When sepsis is associated with trauma, the incidence of ARDS is probably higher. Hudson[38] found that simultaneous occurrence of more than one predisposing condition more than doubled the incidence of ARDS. Patients with indirect lung injury should be carefully monitored for early signs of respiratory insufficiency, which may signal the development of ARDS.

### ALVEOLAR CAPILLARY MEMBRANE

The vessels of the alveolar-capillary membrane form a network around each alveolus that is so dense it forms an almost continuous sheet of blood covering the alveoli. The interior diameter of each capillary segment is approximately 10 μm, just large enough to allow red blood cells to squeeze by in single file so that their cell membranes touch the capillary walls, as illustrated in Fig. 11-2. In this way, oxygen and carbon dioxide need not pass through significant amounts of plasma when diffusing into and out of the alveoli, making a highly efficient vehicle for gas exchange.[35]

The alveolar-capillary membrane is composed of several layers of cells: the alveolar epithelium, the alveolar basement membrane, the interstitial space, the capillary basement membrane, and the capillary endothelium. Oxygen and carbon dioxide traverse easily across these layers, which present no barrier to diffusion because the membrane is less than 0.5 μg thick. However, there are pulmonary disorders—such as cardiogenic pulmonary edema and ARDS—which increase the thickness of the membrane enough that a barrier to diffusion results.

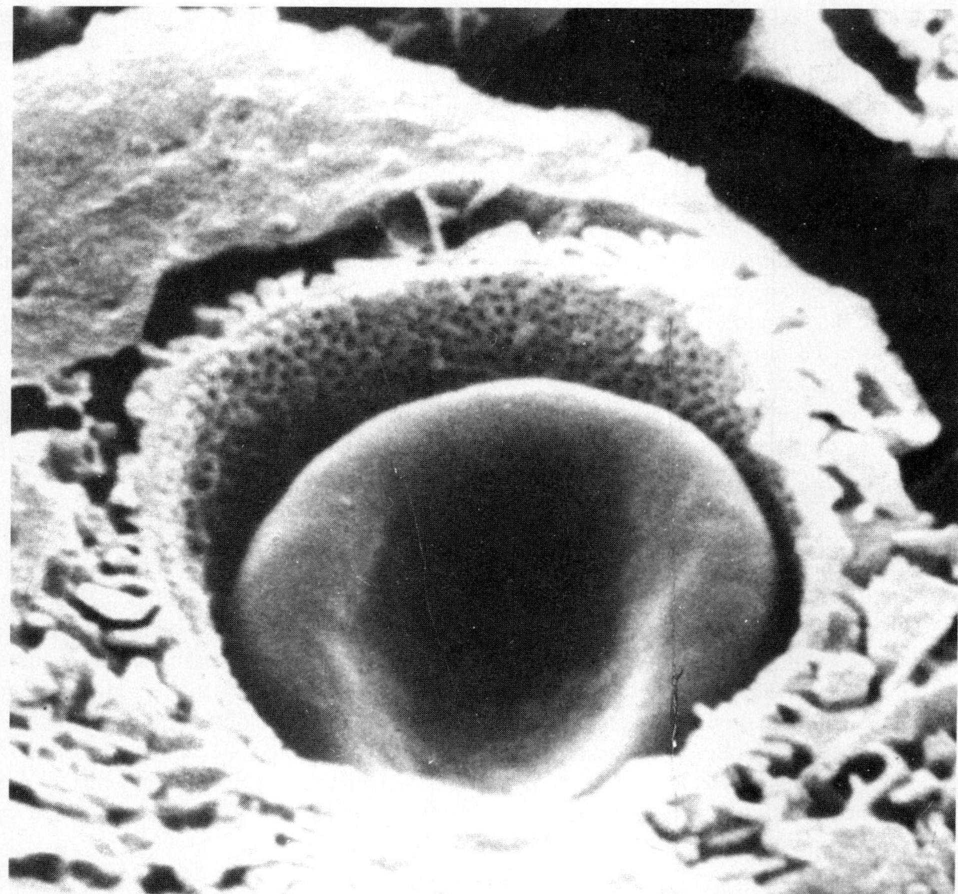

*Fig. 11-2* Scanning electron micrograph of a red blood cell in a capillary. Note that the diameters of both are similar. In many instances the red blood cells course through even smaller capillaries, often through capillaries that are one half the diameter of the red blood cell. This is possible because the cells are pliable, mainly as a result of their biconcave disk shape. (From Martin DE: Respiratory anatomy and physiology, St Louis, 1988, Mosby–Year Book, Inc.)

## Pathophysiology

Research on the biochemical processes involved in the pathological states related to ARDS has resulted in diverse theories. No single element or common mechanism has yet been identified. Some areas being studied include arachidonic acid, the complement system, free radicals, and platelet and neutrophil activity.[4,8,12,59]

After the precipitating injury, changes in the alveolar-capillary endothelium allow for larger than normal amounts of fluid and protein to leak into the pulmonary interstitium and eventually into the alveoli, causing noncardiogenic (increased permeability versus increased pressure) pulmonary edema. The process of pulmonary noncardiogenic edema is a progressive one with fluid and proteins first accumulating in the interstitium, which in itself does not interfere with gas exchange.[4,12] However, as the interstitial fluid overwhelms the local controlling factors (oncotic pressure, capillary hydrostatic pressure, lymphatic drainage), the increased hydrostatic pressure compresses the alveoli. At this point, diminished gas exchange occurs and hypoxemia is seen. Eventually, fluid and protein enter the alveoli, decrease the activity of surfactant, and promote alveolar collapse (Fig. 11-3, *A* and *B*). Pulmonary shunting increases, and the hypoxemia worsens. In severe ARDS, shunting can involve 50% of blood flow through the lungs that is reflected in arterial blood gas results showing acidosis, hypercapnia, and hypoxemia despite supplemental $FIO_2$. As fluid continues to flood the pulmonary interstitium and alveolar spaces, lung compliance and functional residual capacity decrease, while the work of breathing, oxygen consumption, and dead space area increase.[2,8] Eventually, the protein that has leaked out of the vascular space into the interstitium and alveoli forms hyaline membranes (an eosinophilic substance), further decreasing compliance and increasing the hypoxemia as seen by a widening alveolar-arteriole $O_2$ gradient and

## CONDITIONS LEADING TO ARDS

### DIRECT PULMONARY INJURY

Aspiration of gastric contents or other toxic substances
Near-drowning
Inhalation of toxic substances
Diffuse viral pneumonia
Diffuse mycoplasmal pneumonia
Diffuse rickettsial pneumonia
Pulmonary contusion secondary trauma
Drugs: heroin, panaquat, salicylates
Embolism: fat, air, amniotic fluid

### INDIRECT PULMONARY INJURY

Sepsis—especially gram-negative
Severe pancreatitis
Multiple emergency blood transfusions
Multiple trauma
Disseminated intravascular coagulation (DIC)
Shock from any cause
Neurogenic states: head trauma, increased intracranial pressure
Nonpulmonary systemic diseases
Postcardiopulmonary bypass
Anaphylaxis

Modified from Bernard G and Brigham K: Ann Rev Med 36:195, 1985.

## SURFACTANT

Surfactant is a phospholipid composed of fatty acids bound to lecithin. Like other surfactants such as detergents and soaps, pulmonary surfactant functions to lower surface tension. Whereas with detergents and soaps this decrease in surface tension cleans clothes, within the lungs it stabilizes the alveoli, increases lung compliance, and eases the work of breathing. When pulmonary disease disrupts the normal synthesis and storage of surfactant, the lungs become less compliant, and the work of breathing increases. Severe loss of surfactant results in alveolar instability, collapse (atelectasis), and impairment of diffusion. The classic example of this pathology occurs in adult respiratory distress syndrome (ARDS), in which the increased permeability of the alveolar-capillary bed allows vascular fluid to move into the alveoli, interfering with the production of surfactant. The refractory hypoxemia, tissue hypoxia, and mortality from ARDS result from altered alveolar-capillary permeability, disruption of surfactant production, alveolar instability, and atelectasis.

Sighing is thought to contribute to the spread of surfactant throughout the lungs because the large volume of air generated by the sigh opens otherwise partially closed alveoli and spreads surfactant over their walls.[59] This theory is supported by studies that have shown that continuous ventilation with the same volume of air, as in controlled mechanical ventilation, can result in decreasing lung compliance, meaning that the lungs become "stiffer" and more difficult to inflate.[14,33]

Surfactant has a half-life of only 14 hours; this short time period accounts for the high metabolic activity of the type II cells. Because of its function in lipid metabolism, thyroxine is thought to play a role in surfactant production. Studies in animals and humans have shown an increased production and storage of surfactant when thyroxine has been administered. Acetylcholine, prostaglandins, and estradiol are also known to increase surfactant synthesis.[64]

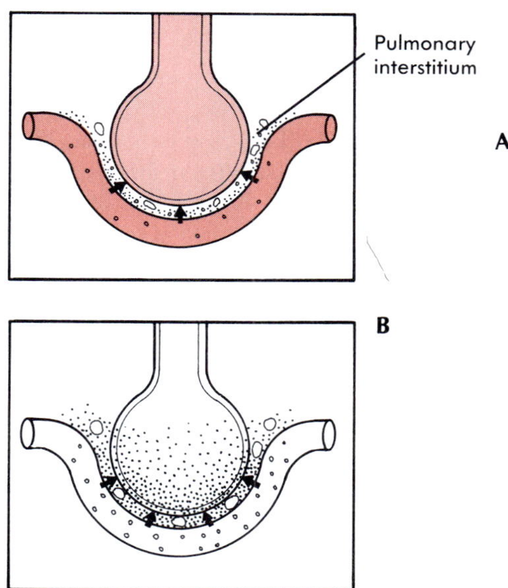


***Fig. 11-3*** Dynamics at the alveolar-capillary membrane during ARDS. **A,** Damage to the alveolar-capillary membrane can cause a change in membrane permeability so that excessive amounts of fluid and protein leak out of the capillary space into the interstitial space. If the leak persists, the lymphatic system will become overwhelmed as the fluid accumulation grows. Alveolar and respiratory bronchial compression occur due to the mounting accumulation of interstitial fluid and protein. **B,** As the pulmonary interstitium becomes overwhelmed, fluid is forced into the alveolar space. Fluid in the alveolar space disrupts the function of both the type I and the type II alveolar epithelial cells. Disruption of the type I cells, which maintain alveolar wall structure, causes breaks in the junctions between type I cells and enhances the movement of fluid into the alveoli. Disruption of the type II cells, which synthesize surfactant, causes alveolar instability and collapse. The overall clinical effects are severe atelectasis, impairment of gas exchange, and intrapulmonary shunting.

hypoxemia that is unresponsive to increasing the $FIO_2$ (refractory hypoxemia).

### Assessment and Diagnosis

The clinical picture, depending on the precipitating event, may be one of acute full-blown pulmonary edema with frothy sputum, air hunger, tachypnea, tachycardia, and hypotension or one of gradually increasing respiratory insufficiency and hypoxemia. Generally, during the early phase of ARDS, the patient will exhibit hyperventilation. Crackles may be present over the lung fields, and patchy infiltrates may be seen on chest x-ray. As the syndrome progresses, the patient will demonstrate a persistent low $PaO_2$ despite high inspired oxygen concentrations. The $PaCO_2$ will remain low at first, as a result of the hyperventilation. Eventually, however, $PaCO_2$ retention will accompany the hypoxemia. Signs and symptoms of tissue hypoxia will be evident as the condition worsens. Increasing pulmonary vascular resistance has been found to be a poor prognostic sign.[59] With significant lung involvement, the clinical picture reflects severe respiratory failure. Chest x-ray evaluation reveals a "white out" of the lung. Table 11-9 correlates the clinical features of ARDS with x-ray and pulmonary function findings.

Some patients will develop pulmonary fibrosis with permanent pulmonary disability if they survive the event.

Diagnosis of ARDS is based on clinical and laboratory criteria, as reviewed in the box at right. In all cases, though, the clinical hallmark of ARDS is *severe refractory arterial hypoxemia,* a result of intrapulmonary right-to-left shunting.[62]

#### CRITERIA FOR DIAGNOSING ARDS

- A compatible clinical history of a precipitating event
- Hypoxemia—$PaO_2$ less than 50 mm Hg on an $FIO_2$ of 0.6;[59] other authorities recommend a $PaO_2$ less than 60 mm Hg at an $FIO_2$ of 0.50 or more[82]
- Decreased pulmonary compliance of less than 50 ml/cm $H_2O$
- Radiological evidence of diffuse bilateral alveolar infiltrates
- Absence of underlying cardiogenic pulmonary edema and lung disease evidenced by a pulmonary capillary wedge pressure of no greater than 18 mm Hg[59]
- Increased shunt fraction and increased dead space ventilation (Vd/Vt)[59]

### Treatment

Currently, major therapy for ARDS involves treating the underlying cause, preventing further alveolar capillary membrane damage, and supporting tissue oxygenation through the use of positive pressure ventilation, with careful attention to perfusion.

Recognition of the patient at risk for developing ARDS should be part of any therapeutic approach. At this time, instituting prophylactic, positive pressure breathing modalities in patients has not prevented development of the syndrome, yet early recognition and aggressive treatment of hypoxemia is warranted.

Arterial blood gases should be closely monitored in at-risk patients (review the box on p. 259). Progressive deterioration in $PaO_2$ represents incipient respiratory failure requiring early ventilatory support. Criteria for establishment of ventilatory support in at-risk patients, as outlined by Norwood and Civetta,[67] include (1) respiratory rate >30 to 35 breaths per minute, and (2) $PaO_2$ <55 mm Hg with $FIO_2$ of 21%. Retention of $CO_2$ would be a further indication that ventilatory support is needed.[67]

***Table 11-9*** Clinical presentation of adult respiratory distress syndrome

| Clinical features | X-ray findings | Pulmonary function |
|---|---|---|
| Tachypnea and dyspnea | Diffuse or localized condensation images, interstitial pattern with increased vascular shadows | Reduced $PaO_2$<br>Reduced $PaCO_2$ |
| Progressive dyspnea, irritability, cyanosis, confusion, hypoxemia (partially reversible with $FIO_2$) | Alveolar edema pattern, normal vascular shadows, normal heart size | Reduced $PaO_2$<br>Reduced $PaCO_2$<br>Reduced compliance<br>Reduced functional residual capacity |
| Severe hypoxemia despite $FIO_2$ of 1.0 | Alveolar edema pattern with progression to massive fibrosis in some cases | Increased A-$aDO_2$<br>Reduced functional residual capacity<br>Reduced compliance<br>Reduced $PaO_2$<br>Increased $PaCO_2$ |

From Cadierno-Carpintero M and others: Cardiovasc Rev Rep 8(3):35, 1987.
$FIO_2$, concentration of inspired oxygen; $PaO_2$, arterial oxygen pressure; $PaCO_2$, arterial carbon dioxide pressure; A-$aO_2$, alveolar-arterial oxygen gradient.

Ventilatory support should be as physiological as possible to avoid gas exchange problems, alkalemia, and progressive respiratory muscle weakness. Norwood and Civetta[67] feel that controlled mandatory ventilation (CMV) should never be used alone, because it is not similar to normal breathing. They recommend intermittent mandatory ventilation (IMV) or synchronized IMV (SIMV). IMV/SIMV diminishes the side effects associated with CMV by permitting spontaneous ventilation in addition to intermittent mechanical support. When the IMV/SIMV modality is used, the mechanically delivered ventilations should be administered in one to two breath increments up to a level per minute that maintains a normal blood pH and $Paco_2$. The tidal volume of the ventilator inhalation is usually equal to 5 ml/pound or 10 to 15 ml/kg of body weight.[67] Since the IMV/SIMV mode allows the patient to breathe spontaneously by means of a circuit that bypasses the machine, the patient's respiratory rate indirectly reflects adequacy of ventilation. Generally, the number of ventilator-derived breaths (IMV/SIMV) should be increased when the patient's spontaneous rates become tachypneic (>30/min) or if the patient's breathing becomes labored. Subjective complaints by the patient of difficulty breathing, breathlessness, or increasing anxiety may indicate need for an IMV/SIMV rate adjustment. The

***Table 11-10*** Ventilator modes used during the treatment of ARDS

| Ventilator modes | Application |
|---|---|
| Assist control (A/C) with PEEP | Allows for adjustment for varying volumes and high minute ventilation<br>Decreases the work of breathing over IMV/SIMV<br>With PEEP and effective tidal volume, recruits alveoli<br>Generally, requires only mild sedation<br>Commonly used, available on all models and generations of ventilators<br>Patient can influence rate of ventilation, not tidal volume |
| IMV/SIMV | Control mode ventilator with a circuitry that permits uninhibited spontaneous ventilation by the patient<br>For $\dot{V}E$ to increase the patient's spontaneous breaths must increase<br>Is associated with lower mean airway pressure than A/C[59]<br>Increases the work of breathing over A/C<br>Usually requires only mild sedation<br>SIMV—synchronizing the ventilator-delivered breath with the patient's own ventilation prevents competition between the patient's respiratory rhythm and the ventilator rhythm<br>Allows for partial ventilator support; that is, the patient and ventilator provide a portion of the required ventilation |
| Pressure-controlled inverted ratio ventilation | Increases the inspiratory time of the ventilator to 50% of the respiratory cycle with an inspiratory pause of 20-30%[59]<br>Has been shown to improve $Pao_2$ and $PaCo_2$ in ARDS patients<br>Allows for more even gas distribution in lungs<br>May require significantly more sedation than for A/C or IMV/SIMV |
| High-frequency jet ventilation (HFV) | Uses small volumes (less than dead space volume) at high-frequency rates to achieve gas exchange |
| High-frequency positive pressure ventilation (HFPPV) | Creates lower peak and mean airway pressures than conventional volume ventilation |
| High-frequency oscillation (HFO) | Can be used with PEEP<br>Bronchospasm unresponsive to medications can require termination of HFV<br>Generally requires only mild sedation<br>No proven benefits seen in ARDS |
| Differential lung ventilation (DLV)—selective PEEP | Useful for patients with severe unilateral lung disease when conventional means have failed<br>Different rates, tidal volumes, and PEEP are selected for each lung<br>Requires double-lumen endotracheal tube and two ventilators for manipulation of several parameters |
| Extracorporeal membrane oxygenation (EMO) | Used with conventional ventilator support for partial hypoxemia and hypercapnia<br>Studies showed no long-term improvement in survival and therefore not recommended at this time[59] |

additional modality of PEEP with IMV/SIMV is one mode of respiratory support. Table 11-10 outlines methods of ventilator support used in ARDS.

Depending on the severity of the disease process, institution of therapy to reverse the hypoxemia may initially necessitate an $FIO_2$ >0.5 to achieve a satisfactory level of oxygenation ($PaO_2$ >70 mm Hg). When this occurs, measures should be taken to recruit alveoli by the use of PEEP. PEEP is used to reduce the loss of functional residual capacity by opening alveoli. PEEP provides an airway pressure greater than atmospheric pressure at the end of exhalation and thus holds the alveoli open. This decreases pulmonary shunting, which reduces hypoxemia and may allow for a reduction in $FIO_2$ to nontoxic levels ($FIO_2$ <50%). Institution of PEEP should begin at 2 to 3 cm $H_2O$.[67] (PEEP as a ventilator modality is explained in Chapter 12.)

Caution must be used in applying PEEP, because the intrathoracic pressure changes created can decrease cardiac output. Most authorities recommend a gradual increase in PEEP and use of the minimal PEEP pressure that will still allow for adequate oxygenation ($PaO_2$ >70 mm Hg with $FIO_2$ <0.5).[90]

Individual investigators have used different parameters to decide when PEEP is sufficient. Suter and others[90] adjusted PEEP levels to the point at which the greatest improvement in pulmonary compliance was experienced. They, as well as others,[7,67,90] do not recommend the use of PEEP >15 cm $H_2O$. Optimal PEEP has been described as the amount that reduces intrapulmonary shunt fraction (Qsp/Qt) to less than 20%.[59] Regardless of the method used, the goal of ventilatory support is adequate oxygenation by means of nontoxic levels of $FIO_2$. A reduction of $FIO_2$ below 0.50% is desired as soon as the patient's condition permits. Maintaining higher levels of $FIO_2$ fosters absorption atelectasis, disruption of surfactant production, and oxygen toxicity.

Once PEEP has been instituted, the intrapulmonary shunt should be calculated every 10 to 15 minutes after each increase in the PEEP level until significant improvement in clinical status has been achieved. Hemodynamic monitoring of the cardiac output should be implemented in most patients to adequately assess cardiac function. Reductions in cardiac output associated with PEEP may be lessened by increasing preload and by the use of inotropic agents. If a pulmonary artery catheter is not available for Qsp/Qt measurements, the PEEP can be increased until the $PaO_2/FIO_2$ ratio is 250 to 300:1. This ratio has been found to correspond to a 15% to 25% shunt fraction.

Ventilatory support should be maintained until correction of the cause has occurred and respiratory involvement has been corrected. Blood gas analyses and chest x-rays should be evaluated for attainment of normal values and resolutions of pulmonary congestion. Weaning before reaching these clinical goals will generally be unsuccessful. All parameters including $FIO_2$, IMV/SIMV rate, and PEEP should be serially reduced as opposed to sudden termination. Support is considered minimal when the $FIO_2$ is 0.4 or less, the IMV/SIMV rate is 2 per minute, and PEEP is about 5 cm.[59,67] At this point, with satisfactory arterial blood gases, weaning can begin.

If the patient does not require intubation on the basis of maintaining airway patency, extubation at the end of the weaning process can proceed. Successful weaning, according to Norwood and Civetta,[67] exists when the patient can maintain pH >7.35, $PaCO_2$ <45, respiratory rate <30/minute, a $PaO_2$ >55, and $FIO_2$ of 0.21 on a constant positive airway pressure of 5 cm $H_2O$ without any supplemental IMV/SIMV breaths.

Medical teams worldwide are beginning to re-study the effects of extracorporeal membrane oxygenation (ECMO) on ARDS patients. Encouraging results have been shown in several research settings.[62]

### Other Therapeutic Approaches

Little evidence shows that administration of glucocorticoids improves the outcome of ARDS. In animal studies, steroids have caused a reduction in free oxygen radicals, and use early in the syndrome may be efficacious but is still debatable.[15,98] Several well-conducted clinical trials have failed to demonstrate any benefit of steroids in the treatment of ARDS.[8,52,96] Large doses of steroids have been effective in treating a small number of patients with ARDS associated with fat emboli, but only if administered early in the syndrome.[28] Investigation continues in the use of imidazole and indomethacin in the treatment of ARDS. These agents have been shown to reduce production of arachidonic acid, a cellular element believed to be a mediator of lung injury. Presently, the use of these agents is considered experimental.

Because prostaglandins appear to play a role in the pathological changes associated with ARDS, experimental use of $PGE_1$ infusions is being studied.[59] Though the preliminary outcomes of using prostaglandin are encouraging, larger clinical trials need to be completed before it can be considered an appropriate part of ARDS management.

Fluid therapy is aimed at maintaining adequate intravascular volume to provide sufficient cardiac output and tissue perfusion, yet minimize contribution to lung edema. Hemodynamic monitoring is recommended as a way to accurately assess fluid needs. A pulmonary wedge pressure in the range of 10 to 12 mm Hg is desired, and the use of fluid challenges, or diuretics, depending on the direction of the pressure alteration, should be used to achieve this range.

Although disagreement exists about the use of crystalloids versus colloids, various studies fail to show that colloids are more advantageous. Supporting the cardiovascular system with crystalloid fluids is acceptable, unless severe protein depletion (50% of normal) exists.

### Summary of Nursing Care

The nursing diagnoses and management of adult respiratory distress syndrome are summarized in the box on p. 263. Throughout the course of ARDS, respiratory moni-

**Nursing Diagnosis and Management**

***Adult respiratory distress syndrome***

- Impaired Gas Exchange related to ventilation-perfusion inequality secondary to increased alveolar capillary membrane permeability, p. 474
- Ineffective Airway Clearance related to impaired cough secondary to loss of glottic closure with cuffed endotracheal/tracheostomy tube, p. 468
- High Risk for Aspiration risk factors: presence of tracheostomy or endotracheal tube, p. 476
- Decreased Cardiac Output related to decreased preload secondary to mechanical ventilation with or without PEEP, p. 457
- Altered Nutrition: Less Than Body Protein-Calorie Requirements related to lack of exogenous nutrients and increased metabolic demand. (See also discussion of metabolic results from carbohydrate overfeeding, Chapter 6.)
- High Risk for Infection risk factor: invasive monitoring devices, p. 465
- Sensory-Perceptual Alterations related to sensory overload, sensory deprivation, sleep pattern disturbance, p. 489
- Hopelessness related to failing or deteriorating physical condition, p. 446
- Anxiety related to threat to biological, psychological, and/or social integrity, p. 448

toring is an important nursing responsibility. Identification of patients at risk for developing ARDS should activate a plan of frequent purposeful respiratory assessment. Sophistication of the type of data achievable varies with the respiratory support being provided to patients, since the newer computer-operated ventilators can monitor multiple ventilatory function parameters.

Even when mechanical ventilatory support and intubation are not necessary, indirect data about gross lung compliance and hypoxemia can be obtained at the bedside. Ear or pulse oximetry measurements of $Sao_2$ and incentive spirometry measurements should be evaluated on all patients at risk for ARDS. Initial arterial blood gas values are essential. A complete physical examination of the patient's respiratory system should be performed initially and once each shift, with more frequent assessment of lung sounds and respiratory rate. An elevated respiratory rate and falling $Pao_2$ should warn the nurse of a change in the patient's condition and the need for further assessment.

In ARDS, as the lungs "stiffen" from pathophysiological changes, incentive spirometer performance as it reflects functional residual capacity (FRC) will decline. Vital capacity measurements will decrease in ARDS and a vital capacity below 1.5 L or 20 ml/kg may indicate impending respiratory failure.[59,72]

Patients receiving ventilatory therapy should have additional parameters reflecting lung mechanics routinely monitored. Some ventilators have inline pneumotachographs available that constantly measure lung volume and pressures. These measurements are used to provide a pressure-volume curve that indicates lung compliance. A gas sample port may also be available for measuring exhaled carbon dioxide, which allows determination of adequacy of ventilation.

Tidal volume and airway pressures can be monitored by observing various ventilator dials and the spirometer. When automatic measurements of compliance are not available as part of the ventilator data, manual measurements can be taken by the respiratory therapist. In the ARDS patient, decreasing compliance reflects a worsening of the syndrome.

Ongoing gas monitoring will be needed to manage the patient with ARDS. This includes arterial blood gases, oximetry, and mixed venous sampling if available. Continuous monitoring of the $Paco_2$ is not as useful as continuous $O_2$ monitoring in ARDS victims.

During mechanical ventilation, the best oxygenation at lowest airway pressures is desired. The initial maximal inspiratory pressure (Pmax), except when severe pulmonary disease is present, is usually $<50$ cm $H_2O$. If higher pressures are generated, this can indicate that excessive flow rates or excessive tidal volumes have been established on the ventilator settings. High inspiratory pressures increase the risk of barotrauma. In severe ARDS the pressure needed to adequately ventilate the patient may be significantly above normal; however, if excessive pressure is the only means of ensuring adequate gas exchange, the risk of barotrauma must be accepted. Mean airway pressure is more important than peak pressure in considering risks for barotrauma. In some cases, especially during emergencies, the trachea is intubated with too small a tube, which creates unnecessary air flow resistance. The critical care nurse should consider this factor during initial evaluation of the patient's airway.

Suctioning the patient with ARDS on a PEEP modality may necessitate special consideration to technique and equipment. When possible, suctioning should occur by means of a closed suctioning system to avoid ventilator disconnection and loss of PEEP.[79] If this cannot be achieved as a result of the equipment available, use of a PEEP valve is recommended. When a manual resuscitation bag is used, it must be able to deliver a volume 1½ times the patient's Vt to assure hyperinflation and prevent alveolar collapse.

The nurse must titrate fluid replacements accurately to ensure adequate cardiac output and avoid overhydration. All infusions should be delivered through a mechanical volume device. Hemodynamic lines require close monitoring, and, when several invasive pressures are being followed, the PA wave line should be chosen for continuous visualization.

Establishing a baseline patient weight and following the weight on a daily or alternate-day basis is an accurate and efficient way to evaluate fluid balance. Generally, weight gains of >0.5 kg (1.1 pounds)/day or >2.5 kg (5 pounds)/ week indicate fluid retention.[44]

### COMPLICATIONS ASSOCIATED WITH ADULT RESPIRATORY DISTRESS SYNDROME

**PULMONARY**

Pulmonary emboli
Pulmonary barotrauma
Pulmonary fibrosis
Pulmonary complications of ventilatory and monitoring procedures
- Mechanical ventilation
  - Right main stem intubation
  - Alveolar hypoventilation
- Pulmonary artery catheter
  - Pulmonary infarction
  - Pulmonary hemorrhage
- Tracheal intubation
  - Laryngeal injury
  - Tracheal stenosis

**GASTROINTESTINAL**

Gastrointestinal hemorrhage
Ileus
Gastric distention
Pneumoperitoneum

**RENAL**

Renal failure
Fluid retention

**CARDIAC**

Dysrhythmia
Hypotension
Low cardiac output

**INFECTION**

Sepsis
Nosocomial pneumonia

**HEMATOLOGICAL**

Anemia
Thrombocytopenia
Disseminated intravascular coagulation

**OTHER**

Hepatic
Endocrine
Neurological
Psychiatric

Complications can result from the ARDS syndrome itself or from the treatment modalities. Decreased cardiac output as a result of PEEP and pulmonary infarction from pulmonary artery catheterization are examples of the latter. Early recognition of complications allows for intervention and hopefully lessens the morbidity (see the box at left).

Development of renal failure in the ARDS patient is an ominous sign as mortality rises to the 60th percentile. Careful monitoring of urinary output, urine specific gravity, and body weights can alert the nurse to renal insufficiency and allow for prompt aggressive treatment that may prevent renal failure. Creatinine clearance should be used in place of the BUN or serum creatinine, since these may be normal in renal insufficiency. When the volume of urinary output per hour is relatively constant, a secondary urinary creatinine clearance measurement correlates well with 24-hour clearance and can be used.[59] Since it is known that inappropriate antidiuretic hormone (ADH) secretion can occur with mechanical ventilation, especially associated with PEEP >10 cm $H_2O$, this complication should be considered.[59]

Nosocomial infections can be fatal for ARDS patients. Meticulous hand washing and use of aseptic techniques when suctioning and caring for any indwelling catheters are mandatory. Minimizing the number of invasive lines is recommended. Pneumonia is a frequent development among ARDS patients; self-colonization of the lower respiratory tract by organisms located in the oropharynx is a likely cause. Use of prophylactic antibiotics is not recommended, because this practice seems to encourage the growth of more virulent organisms. A major contributing factor in the development of infections is malnutrition, which should be avoided or corrected in ARDS patients as quickly as possible. In a majority of patients, enteral alimentation will generally suffice. When enteral feedings are contraindicated, parenteral hyperalimentation should be initiated.

## THORACIC SURGERY

Surgery of the lung is performed to remove tumors, benign and malignant, for pleurodesis in repeated pneumothoraxes, and to resect abscesses or empyemas unresponsive to antibiotic therapy. Surgical resection of tumors is the most frequent reason for a thoracotomy.

### Description/Cause

Cancer of the lung represents 22% of all cancers in men and 10% of cancers in females.[6] In 1986, it was estimated that 149,000 new lung cancers were diagnosed. Because of the late stage at which many lung cancers are diagnosed, only 20% to 25% can be treated surgically.[6]

Surgical treatment may involve wedge resection, segmentectomy, lobectomy, or pneumonectomy depending on the site, extent of lung tissue involvement, and tumor cell type involved. A wedge resection indicates part of a lobe has been surgically removed, a lobectomy indicates an entire lobe has been removed, and a pneumonectomy indicates removal of an entire lung.

### Assessment and Diagnosis

Before surgery, a complete evaluation of the patient is needed to determine the appropriateness of surgery as a treatment and to determine whether removal of lung tissue can be done without jeopardizing respiratory function. This is especially important when a lobectomy or pneumonectomy is being considered.

When resection is being undertaken for tumor treatment, preoperative evaluation of the type and extent of tumor must be performed. Tumor type may be determined by cytology or tissue biopsy. The preoperative evaluation should include pulmonary function tests to determine the patient's ability to lose lung tissue.

### Treatment

A pneumonectomy is required when a tumor involves the lobar and hilar lymph nodes or when a lobectomy would not remove all of the tumor. Pneumonectomy permits a wide resection of the lymphatic drainage system, but it is also associated with higher morbidity, because the loss of such a large amount of lung tissue can result in inadequate lung capacity and pulmonary hypertension.

For a lobectomy to be performed, the tumor must be isolated to a lobe and the lymph nodes must be free from metastasis. Less lung tissue is resected with this procedure, reducing the complications and morbidity and maintaining greater functional ability for the patient.

Segmentectomy and wedge resection remove the least amount of lung tissue. To be effective, the tumor must be peripherally located without chest wall involvement or other metastasis. These procedures are associated with a low operative mortality of about 2% to 5%.[85]

Various complications are associated with pulmonary resection. The loss of parenchyma can result in respiratory insufficiency and pulmonary hypertension. Hemodynamic monitoring with balloon-tipped catheters is not routine in thoracotomy patients but should be implemented in patients with compromised cardiac function. Changes in pulmonary artery pressures can be used to evaluate cardiac function, fluid status, and intrathoracic changes.

Postoperative development of a bronchopleural fistula is a chief cause of mortality. This develops when a suture line fails to secure occlusion of the bronchial stump.[27] During surgery, careful attention is given to isolating and closing the bronchus in attempts to secure a lasting seal with subsequent stump healing.

### Summary of Nursing Care

Refer to the box above for nursing diagnoses and management of thoracic surgery. Nursing care of the post thoracotomy patient involves interventions aimed at (1) supporting ventilation and gas exchange, (2) monitoring the patient for signs and symptoms of complications, and (3) assisting the patient to return to an adequate activity level.

Postoperatively, strict attention must be given to avoidance of respiratory depression caused by narcotics used to control pain. The patient's rate may be normal, but the tidal volume can be depressed as a side effect of narcotic administration. This can be evaluated by periodic measurement of the tidal volume. Shortness of breath in the first few days following pneumonectomy or lobectomy may be related to hypoxemia, retained secretion, hypoventilation, or other causes.

Careful evaluation of the mediastinal position is required regularly in the postoperative period as an indication of intrathoracic pressure. As with a tension pneumothorax, deviation of the mediastinum can lead to cardiorespiratory insufficiency and failure. The mediastinal position can be determined by (1) palpating for tracheal deviation, (2) palpating and auscultating the position of the apex of the heart, and (3) chest x-ray examination. If a mediastinal shift occurs, correction by injecting or withdrawing air/fluid should be performed. Chest x-rays used to evaluate the mediastinal

**Nursing Diagnosis and Management**

***Thoracic surgery***

- Ineffective Breathing Pattern related to thoracic pain, p. 472
- Ineffective Airway Clearance related to thoracic pain, p. 469
- Impaired Gas Exchange related to ventilation-perfusion equality secondary to (specify), p. 474
- Acute Pain related to transmission and perception of noxious stimuli secondary to thoracic surgery, p. 485
- Activity Intolerance related to knowledge deficit of energy-saving techniques, p. 463
- Knowledge Deficit: Activity Restrictions related to lack of previous exposure to information, p. 441
- Sleep Pattern Disturbance related to fragmented sleep and/or circadian desynchronization, p. 455
- Altered Nutrition: Less Than Body Protein-Calorie Requirements related to lack of exogenous nutrients and increased metabolic demand.
- High Risk for Infection risk factors: protein-calorie malnourishment, central intravenous line, p. 465
- Body Image Disturbance related to actual change in body structure, function, and appearance, p. 443
- Altered Role Performance related to physical incapacity to resume usual or valued role, p. 444
- Ineffective Individual Coping related to situational crisis and personal vulnerability, p. 447
- Sexual Dysfunction related to activity intolerance secondary to chronic lung disease, p. 451

position must avoid any oblique proliferation of the x-ray, because this may cause erroneous interpretation.

Deep breathing exercises should be performed regularly with all post thoracotomy patients. These exercises help reexpand collapsed lung tissue, thus promoting early resolution of the pneumothorax in patients with partial lung resections. Coughing, which should only be encouraged when secretions are present, assists in mobilizing secretions for removal. Because of intraoperative positioning and preoperative and perioperative medications, atelectasis and secretion pooling are common during the postoperative period. Furthermore, as a result of postoperative pain, the patient's ventilations may be shallow, thereby encouraging the development of atelectasis and secretion stasis.[27] Respiratory infections can occur from retained secretions and incomplete lung expansion. Deep breathing and, when appropriate, coughing should be encouraged in the first few days after surgery.

Positioning the patient should take into account the surgical incision site, the surgery, and the perioperative position. Frequent turning helps to improve ventilation and perfusion in the lungs. The patient should not be turned directly onto the unaffected side during the initial period after a pneumonectomy, because the bronchial stump incision is fresh and there is an increased risk of disruption of the suture line. Tilting the patient slightly toward the unaffected side is possible, but the surgeon should indicate when free side-to-side positioning is safe.

Except following a pneumonectomy, chest tubes are placed to remove air and fluid. When auscultating lungs, air leaks should be evaluated. In the early phase, an air leak is commonly heard over the affected area, because the pleura has not yet tightly sealed. As healing occurs, this leak should disappear. An increase in an air leak or appearance of a new air leak should prompt investigation of the thoracic drainage system to discover whether air is leaking into the system from outside or whether the leak originates from the patient's incision. A significant air leak can result in a tension pneumothorax. Increased air leaks not related to the thoracic drainage system may indicate disruption of sutures.

Hemorrhage is an early life-threatening complication that can occur in thoracotomy. In all patients, except those with pneumonectomy, an increase in chest tube drainage can signal excessive bleeding. During the immediate postoperative period, chest tube drainage should be measured every 15 minutes and this frequency decreased as the patient stabilizes. When chest tube loss is >100 ml/hour, when fresh blood is noted, or when a sudden increase in drainage occurs, hemorrhage should be suspected.[27]

Resections of a large lung area or pneumonectomies may be followed by a rise in the central venous pressure. With the loss of one lung, the right ventricle must empty its stroke volume into a vascular bed that has been reduced by 50%. This means a higher pressure system is created, which may tax the limit of the right ventricle leading to right ventricular heart failure. Depending on previous heart function, acute decompensation of both ventricles can result. Measures are aimed at supporting cardiac function and avoiding intravascular volume excess.

Within a few days of surgery, range of motion to the shoulder on the operative side should be performed. The patient frequently splints the operative side and avoids shoulder movement because of pain. If immobility is allowed, stiffening of the shoulder joint can result. This is referred to as "frozen shoulder" and may require physical therapy and rehabilitation to regain satisfactory range of motion of the shoulder joint.

Usually on the day after surgery, the patient will be able to sit in a chair. Activity should be systematically increased, with attention to the patient's activity tolerance. With adequate pulmonary function present before surgery and a surgical approach designed to preserve respiratory function, full return to previous activity levels is possible. This may take as much as 6 months to 1 year, depending on tissue resected and the patient's general condition.

## REFERENCES

1. Ashbaugh DG and others: Acute respiratory distress in adults, Lancet 2:319, 1967.
2. Baehrendtz S and Hedenstierns G: Differential ventilation and selective positive end-expiratory pressure: effects on patients with acute bilateral lung disease, Anesthesiology 61:511-517, 1984.
3. Baker S and Young D: Methemoglobinemia: the hidden diagnosis, Critical Care Nurse 10(3):50, 1990.
4. Balk R and Bone R: Adult respiratory distress syndrome, Med Clinics North Am 62:551, 1983.
5. Bartlett RH: Respiratory therapy to prevent pulmonary complications of surgery, Resp Care 29(6):667, 1984.
6. Baum G and Wolinsky E: Textbook of pulmonary disease, ed 3, Boston, 1983, Little Brown & Co.
7. Bernard G and Brigham K: The adult respiratory distress syndrome, Ann Rev Med 85:195, 1985.
8. Benard GR and others: High dose cortico steroids in patients with ARDS, N Eng J Med 317:1565, 1987.
9. Bone R: Adult respiratory distress syndrome, Clin Chest Med 3(1): 42, 1982.
10. Boucher BA, Witt WO, and Foster TS: The postoperative adverse effects of inhaled anesthetics, Heart Lung 15(1):63, 1986.
11. Brandstetter R: The adult respiratory distress syndrome, Heart Lung 15(2):155, 1986.
12. Brigham K: Mechanisms of lung injury, Clin Chest Med 3:9, 1982.
13. Burns SM: Advances in ventilator therapy: high frequency, pressure support and nocturnal positive pressure ventilation, Focus Crit Care 17(3):227, 1990.
14. Burton GG and Hodgkin JE: Respiratory care: guide to clinical practice, Philadelphia, 1984, JB Lippincott Co.
15. Cadierno-Carpintero M and others: Adult respiratory distress syndrome, Cardiovasc Rev Report 8(3):35, 1987.
16. Chase RA and Gordon J: Overwhelming pneumonia, Med Clin North A 70(4):945, 1986.
17. Chokshi S, Asper R, and Khandheria B: Aspiration pneumonia: a review, Am Fam Physician 33:195, 1986.
18. Cole A, Weller S, and Sykes M: Inverse ratio ventilation compared with PEEP in adult respiratory failure, Intensive Care Med 10:227, 1984.
19. Cooper K and Wetstein L: Emergency management of acute infiltrative pulmonary disease, Emerg Decis 2:53, 1986.
20. Crocker P and Quick G: Acute respiratory failure, Emerg Med 18:26, 1986.

21. Culver BH: Pulmonary responses to sleep, Resp Care 34(6):510, 1990.
22. Dal Santo G: Acid aspiration: pathophysiological aspects, prevention and therapy, Int Anesthesiol Clin 24:49, 1986.
23. Didier EP: Some effects of anesthetics and the anesthetized state of the respiratory system, Resp Care 29(5):463, 1984.
24. East T, Pace N, and Westenskow D: Lateral position with differential lung ventilation and unilateral PEEP following unilateral acid aspiration in the dog, Acta Anesthesiol Scand 28:529, 1984.
25. Fahey P, Harris K, and Vanderwarf C: Clinical experience with continuous monitoring of mixed venous oxygen saturation in respiratory failure, Chest 85(5):748, 1984.
26. Fein A and others: The risk factors, incidence and prognosis of ARDS following septicemia, Chest 1:40, 1983.
27. Finkelmeier B: Difficult problems in postoperative management, Crit Care Q 9(3):59, 1986.
28. Flick M and Murray J: High-dose corticosteroid therapy in the adult respiratory distress syndrome, JAMA 251:1054, 1983.
29. Frame P: Acute infectious pneumonia in the adult, Basics Resp Disease 10(3):2, 1982.
30. Fulmer JD and Snider GL: American College of Chest Physicians/ National Heart, Lung and Blood Institute National Convergence on Oxygen Therapy, Heart Lung 13(5):550, 1984.
31. Gantz N: Respiratory infections in the elderly, Geriatric Med Today 6(12):13, 1987.
32. Griffin DE and Wallace RJ: Bacterial pneumonia in the adult: diagnosis and therapy, Hosp Med 24:188, 1988.
33. Grum CM and Chauncey JB: Conventional mechanical ventilation, Clin Chest Med 9(1):37, 1988.
34. Guenter C and Welch M: Pulmonary medicine, ed 2, Philadelphia, 1982, JB Lippincott Co.
35. Guyton AC: Textbook of medical physiology, Philadelphia, 1986, WB Saunders Co.
36. Hanley MV and Tyler ML: Ineffective airway clearance related to airway infection, Nurs Clin North Am 22(1):135, 1987.
37. Hodgkin JE and Petty TL: Chronic obstructive pulmonary disease: current concepts, Philadelphia, 1987, WB Saunders Co.
38. Hudson LD: The prediction and prevention of adult respiratory distress syndrome, Resp Care 35(2):161, 1990.
39. Hurst J and others: Combined use of high-frequency jet ventilation and induced hypothermia in the treatment of refractory respiratory failure, Crit Care Med 85:771, 1985.
40. Johnson MA: Bronchitis and common pneumonias: pathogenic causes and treatment, Fam Pract Recertification 8(8):49, 1986.
41. Johnson NT and Pierson DJ: The spectrum of pulmonary atelectasis: pathophysiology, diagnosis, and therapy, Resp Care 31(11):1107, 1986.
42. Johnson W: Nosocomial infection of respiratory tract with gram negative bacillus, Ann Int Med 77:701, 1972.
43. Kirilloff L and others: Does chest physical therapy work? Chest 88(3):436, 1985.
44. Lane G, Cronin K, and Peirce A: Flow charts: clinical decision making in nursing, Philadelphia, 1983, JB Lippincott Co.
45. Lane G and Peirce A: When persistence pays off, Nursing 82 12:44, January 1982.
46. Lareau S and Larson JJ: Ineffective breathing pattern related to airflow limitations, Nurs Clin North Am 22(1):170, 1987.
47. Leedom JM and Yu VL: Pneumonia in compromised patients, Patient Care, February 15, 1988.
48. Levison M and others: Clindamycin compared with penicillin for the treatment of anaerobic lung abscess, Ann Int Med 98:466, 1983.
49. Lockhart G: Thoracic trauma, Critical Care Quart 9(3):32, 1986.
50. Lough MD: Pulmonary responses to exercise, Resp Care 34(6):517, 1990.
51. Luce JM: Clinical risk factors for postoperative pulmonary complications, Resp Care 29(5):484, 1984.
52. Luce JM, Tyler ML, and Pierson DJ: Intensive respiratory care, Philadelphia, 1984, WB Saunders Co.
53. Luce JM and others: Ineffectiveness of high dose methylprednisolone in preventing parenchymal lung injury and improving mortality in patients with ARDS, Am Rev Resp Dis 138:62, 1988.
54. Mackenzie C and Shin B: Cardiorespiratory function before and chest physiotherapy in mechanically ventilated patients with post-traumatic respiratory failure, Crit Care Med 13(6):483, 1985.
55. MacNee W: Treatment of respiratory failure: a review, J Royal Society Med 78:61, 1985.
56. Marini JJ: Postoperative atelectasis: pathophysiology, clinical importance and principles of management, Resp Care 29(5):516, 1984.
57. Martin L: Pulmonary physiology in clinical practice: the essentials for patient care and practice, St Louis, 1987, Mosby–Year Book, Inc.
58. Maunder RJ and Hudson LD: Pharmacologic strategies for treating the adult respiratory distress syndrome, Resp Care 35(3):241, 1990.
59. McDonnell K, Fahey P, and Segal M: Respiratory intensive care, New York, 1987, Little Brown & Co.
60. Methany N, Spies M, and Eisenberg P: Frequency of nasoenteral tube displacement and associated risk factors, Res Nurs Health 9:241, 1986.
61. Molloy D and others: Hemodynamic management in clinical acute hypoxemic respiratory failure. Dopamine vs. dobutamine, Chest 90:636, 1986.
62. Morris AH and others: Extracorporeal $CO_2$ removal therapy for adult respiratory distress syndrome patients, Resp Care 35(3):224, 1990.
63. Moser KM and others: Shortness of breath: a guide to better living and breathing, St Louis, 1983, Mosby–Year Book, Inc.
64. Murray JF: The normal lung, Philadelphia, 1986, WB Saunders Co.
65. Neff TA and others: Indications for oxygen therapy, Heart Lung 13(5):553, 1984.
66. Norton L and Conforti C: The effect of body position on oxygenation, Heart Lung 14(1):45, 1985.
67. Norwood S and Civetta J: Ventilatory support in patients with ARDS, symposium on critical care, Surg Clinics North Am 65(4):895, 1985.
68. O'Bryne C: Post-operative care and complications in the thoracotomy patient, Crit Care Q 7:4, 1985.
69. O'Donohue WJ: National survey of the usage of lung expansion modalities for the prevention and treatment of postoperative atelectasis following abdominal and thoracic surgery, Chest 87(1):76, 1985.
70. Oakes R: Ventilatory failure, Prim Care Emerg Descis 2(6): 25, 1986.
71. Peitzman A and others: Pulmonary acid injury, effects of positive end-expiratory pressure and crystalloid vs. colloid fluid resuscitation, Arch Surg 117:662, 1982.
72. Petty T: Adult respiratory distress syndrome: definition and historical perspective, Clin Chest Med 3(1):3, 1982.
73. Roberts J and others: Diagnostic accuracy of fever as a measure of postoperative pulmonary complications, Heart Lung 17(2):166, 1988.
74. Rosenow E, Wilson V, and Cockerill F: Pulmonary disease in the immunocompromised host, Mayo Clin Proc 60:473, 1985.
75. Rossi A and others: Measurements of static compliance of the total respiratory system in patients with acute respiratory failure during mechanical ventilation, Am Rev Resp Dis 131:672, 1985.
76. Rossi A and others: Respiratory mechanics in mechanically ventilated patients with respiratory failure, New York, 1985, The American Physiological Society.
77. Scanlan CL, Spearman CB, and Sheldon RL: Egan's fundamentals of respiratory care, St Louis, 1990, Mosby–Year Book, Inc.
78. Schoene RB: The control of ventilation in clinical medicine: to breathe or not to breathe, Resp Care 34(6):500, 1990.
79. Schumann L and Parsons G: Tracheal suctioning and ventilator tubing changes in adult respiratory distress syndrome: use of a positive end-expiratory pressure valve, Heart Lung 14(4):362, 1985.
80. Scuderi J and Olsen GN: Respiratory therapy in the management of post operative complications, Resp Care 34(4):281, 1989.
81. Shackford SB: FACS: Blunt chest trauma: the intensivist's perspective, J Inten Care Med 1(3):125, 1986.
82. Shapiro BA: Respiratory critical care: state of the art—controversies—new horizons, vol 8, Chicago, 1988, Respiratory Care Seminars, Inc.

83. Shapiro BA, Harrison RA, and Walton JR: Clinical application of blood gases, St Louis, 1982, Mosby–Year Book, Inc.
84. Shapiro BA and others: Clinical application of respiratory care, St Louis, 1985, Mosby–Year Book, Inc.
85. Shields TW: Carcinoma of the lung. In Shields TW, editor: General thoracic surgery, Philadelphia, 1983, Lea & Febiger.
86. Snapper JR and Brigham KI: Pulmonary edema, Hosp Prac 2(5):87, 1986.
87. Spray SB, Zudema GD, and Cameron JL: Aspiration pneumonia, incidence of aspiration with endotracheal tubes, Am J Surg 131:70, 1976.
88. Stock CM and others: Prevention of postoperative pulmonary complications with CPAP, incentive spirometry, and conservative therapy, Chest 87(2):151, 1985.
89. Sukumarin M and others: Evaluation of corticosteroid treatment in aspiration of gastric contents: a controlled clinical trial, Mt Sinai J Med 47:335, 1980.
90. Suter PM, Fairly AB, and Isenburg MD: Optimum end-expiratory airway pressure in patients with acute pulmonary failure, N Engl J Med 292:284, 1975.
91. Timberlake GA: Trauma in the golden hour, Emerg Med 18(20):78, 1986.
92. Tobin MJ: Physiology in medicine: update on strategies in mechanical ventilation, Hosp Prac 21(6):69, 1986.
93. Traver GA: Respiratory nursing: the science and the art, New York, 1982, John Wiley & Sons.
94. Tyler ML: The respiratory effects of body position and immobilization, Resp Care 29(5):472, 1984.
95. Vasbinder-Dillon D: Understanding mechanical ventilation, Crit Care Nurse 8(7):42, 1988.
96. Weigelt JA and others: Early steroid therapy for respiratory failure, Arch Surg 120:536, 1985.
97. West JB: Respiratory physiology, Baltimore, 1985, Williams & Wilkins.
98. West JB: Pulmonary pathophysiology, Baltimore, 1987, Williams & Wilkins.
99. Wolfe J, Bone R, and Ruth W: Effects of corticosteroids in the treatment of patients with gastric aspiration, Am J Med 63:719, 1977.

CHAPTER 12

# Pulmonary Therapeutic Management

## CHAPTER OBJECTIVES

- *Summarize the important aspects of the nursing care of a patient undergoing oxygen therapy.*
- *Describe how nursing interventions may help prevent the complications associated with artificial airways.*
- *Identify suctioning guidelines that will assist in preventing hypoxemia, atelectasis, and infection.*
- *Discuss how the various modes of mechanical ventilation alter ventilatory dynamics.*
- *Describe important aspects of the nursing care of a patient receiving mechanical ventilation and of a patient being weaned from devices providing mechanical ventilation.*

## KEY TERMS

absorption atelectasis, p. 272
oxygen toxicity, p. 272
hyperbaric oxygen therapy, p. 274
tracheal necrosis, p. 277
mechanical ventilation, p. 280
modes of mechanical ventilation, p. 281
positive end-expiratory pressure (PEEP), p. 281
criteria for weaning, p. 287
intrapleural pressure, p. 288
chest physiotherapy (CPT), p. 289

## OXYGEN THERAPY

### Goals of Therapy

Normal cellular function depends on a supply of oxygen adequate to meet metabolic needs. Along with oxygen, all cells require energy to maintain their function or biochemical reactions, many of which are life sustaining. Cellular energy is derived from high-energy phosphate bonds such as those in adenosine triphosphate (ATP). Most cellular energy is used, transported, and stored in the form of these high-energy phosphate bonds, which, when broken, release their tremendous energy supply.

Energy is normally stored and released from the high-energy phosphate bonds by what is called oxidative metabolism. Oxygen must be available in the cell so that cellular processes continue to release the energy needed for biochemical processes. The level of cellular oxygen tension at which necessary cellular functions decrease is called the critical oxygen tension. Tissue hypoxia exists when cellular oxygen tensions are inadequate.

The primary indications for oxygen administration are hypoxemia and tissue hypoxia. The goal of oxygen administration, in all cases, is to provide a sufficient concentration of inspired oxygen to permit full use of the oxygen-carrying capacity of the arterial blood, thus ensuring adequate tissue oxygenation if the cardiac output is adequate and if the hemoglobin concentration and structure are normal. Restoring adequate tissue oxygen tension will eliminate the compensatory responses to hypoxia. Increased ventilatory work is a normal response to hypoxemia and/or tissue hypoxia, as is increased myocardial work. Both of these increased work loads can be decreased or prevented by the use of appropriate oxygen therapy.

### Principles of Therapy

Oxygen is an atmospheric gas that must also be considered a drug because, like most other drugs, oxygen has detrimental as well as beneficial effects. Oxygen is one of the most commonly used and misused drugs. As a drug, it must be administered for good reason and in a proper, safe manner. Oxygen is generally ordered either in liters per minute or as a concentration of oxygen expressed as a percent, such as 40%, or as a fraction of inspired oxygen ($FIO_2$), such as 0.4.

The amount of oxygen administered depends on the pathophysiological mechanisms affecting the patient's oxygenation status and should ideally provide an arterial partial pressure of oxygen ($PaO_2$) of 70 to 100 mm Hg so that a hemoglobin saturation of greater than 90% is achieved. The concentration of oxygen given to an individual patient is a clinical judgment that is based on the many factors that influence oxygen transport, such as hemoglobin concentration, cardiac output, and the arterial oxygen tension. Once oxygen therapy has begun, the patient should be continuously assessed for level of oxygenation and the factors affecting it. Arterial blood gas values should be evaluated several times daily until the desired $PaO_2$ is reached and has stabilized. If the desired response to the amount of oxygen delivered is not achieved, the oxygen supplementation should be adjusted and the patient's condition reevaluated. It is important to use this dose-response method so that the lowest possible level of oxygen is administered that will still achieve a satisfactory $PaO_2$.

More recently, alternatives to frequent arterial punctures or arterial line withdrawals have been developed, including continuous monitoring of arterial hemoglobin saturation with an oximeter (various probe sites available) or monitoring of mixed venous oxygen saturation ($S\bar{v}O_2$) through a pulmonary artery catheter.[5] The introduction of the fiberoptic pulmonary artery catheter has provided continuous monitoring of $S\bar{v}O_2$.

## Hazards of Oxygen

Oxygen is a colorless, tasteless, and odorless gas that, although seemingly innocuous, is actually quite hazardous. Oxygen does not burn but does support combustion, a matter of importance to its use in the hospital. A mere spark can become a large, hot flame in the presence of an oxygen-enriched environment, and the burning speed increases as the partial pressure of oxygen in the environment increases. Thus the higher the oxygen within the environment, the faster and hotter is the fire. The "No Smoking" signs that are posted are extremely important for this reason.

## Methods of Delivery

Oxygen therapy can be delivered by many different devices. The devices most often seen in the hospital and home are nonrebreathing systems. These systems are either high flow or low flow and are of variable degrees of complexity. With a high-flow system, the gas flows out of the device into the patient's airways in amounts sufficient to meet all inspiratory volume requirements, and the concentration of the oxygen delivered is not affected by the ventilatory pattern of the patient. A low-flow system supplies a gas flow that is insufficient to meet all inspiratory volume requirements and is dependent on the existence of a reservoir of oxygen, its dilution with room air, and the patient's ventilatory pattern. The anatomical reservoir in this case is composed of the nasopharynx and the oropharynx. As the patient's ventilatory pattern changes, the inspired oxygen concentration varies because of the different amount of air used to mix with the reservoir gas and the constant flow of oxygen. A common misconception is that a low-flow system delivers only low concentrations of oxygen and a high-flow system delivers only high concentrations of oxygen.

### Low-flow systems

***Nasal cannula and catheter.*** Low concentrations of oxygen can be successfully delivered through a nasal cannula or prongs. The nasal cannula has the advantages of being lightweight, economical, disposable, and easily applied. Cannulas are generally well tolerated by patients and are one of the most commonly used devices for oxygen administration. Nasal cannulas do have the disadvantage of instability, resulting in displacement by a restless or unobservant patient. Pathological conditions such as deviated septum, mucosal drainage and edema, and nasal polyps can interfere with the oxygen intake.

The cannula is made of soft plastic and has two prongs that insert 1 cm into each nare. Oxygen flow from 1 to 6 L per minute can be delivered comfortably with the $FIO_2$ ranging from 24% to 44%. Higher flows such as 7 and 8 L per minute should be avoided because of the irritating and drying effect on the nasal mucosa.

Controversy exists about the efficacy of oxygen administration through a nasal cannula in mouth-breathing patients. Studies have shown that the final delivery of oxygen to the blood is not significantly affected by mouth breathing,[56,58] because the inspired ambient air flow in the oral pharynx entrains oxygen from the nasopharynx. Other studies, however, have shown tracheal concentration differences with mouth breathers.[56]

Since the nasal cannula is a low-flow system in which the oxygen concentration delivered relies on a mixture of ambient air and oxygen, the overall oxygen concentration will be altered by tidal volume and ventilatory pattern. For example, when a patient has a large tidal volume, the $FIO_2$ delivered to the alveoli will be low because more air from the atmosphere mixes with the oxygen. Conversely, when the tidal volume is small, the $FIO_2$ will be high. When a patient has a regular breathing pattern with consistent rate and tidal volume, cannulas can provide controlled oxygen therapy.

The nasal catheter is another low-flow device. It is inserted through the nasal passage until its tip lies in the oropharynx. It has several holes in its terminal 1 inch. More reliable control of $FIO_2$ can be achieved by using a nasal catheter, but its successful use depends on proper insertion and maintenance. There actually is little indication for catheter use because of its tendency to irritate the nasal passage and because of the need to move the catheter every day to the alternate nare so that pharyngeal damage is minimized.

***Transtracheal oxygen catheters.*** Transtracheal oxygen therapy is a relatively new system that delivers oxygen directly into the trachea through a small hole in the neck called a tract. It is generally used for patients requiring chronic oxygen therapy who are admitted to the critical care unit with exacerbations of their lung disease.

Some of the situations in which transtracheal oxygenation would be recommended include the following:

- Need for continuous, 24-hour oxygen
- $PaO_2 \leq 55$ mm Hg
- Complications of nasal cannula use such as dry, sore, bleeding nose or ears
- Evidence of cor pulmonale
- Erythrocythemia
- Motivation and ability to care for the catheter

Benefits of transtracheal oxygen therapy include decreased oxygen flow rates (sometimes as much as one fourth to one half of the flow for nasal cannula oxygen), improved appearance and thus self-concept, decreased pulmonary hypertension, renewed sense of taste and smell, improved compliance with the oxygen therapy, greater mobility, and better general health.[1]

Patients who are admitted to the critical care unit with a transtracheal catheter should continue to receive oxygen through their transtracheal catheter unless they require intubation. If a higher $FIO_2$ than can be achieved with the transtrachael method is needed, the transtracheal catheter can be used in conjunction with another method such as an oxygen mask. It is important to maintain the catheter in its tract because the tract can close within hours if the catheter is removed. If the tract closes, the procedure must be repeated, if appropriate. The catheter can be sutured in place if the bead chain must be removed.

***Oxygen masks.*** There are several different types of oxygen masks, which vary in construction and purpose. Most masks are made of soft plastic and are disposable. Masks can be uncomfortable because of the tight fit required on the face and because of the head strap that is necessary to hold the mask in place. Masks can also become hot because of the heat generated from the face around the nose and mouth. Some patients, especially those in severe respiratory distress, complain of claustrophobic feelings when wearing a mask. Despite the oxygen flow into the mask, patients feel "air hunger" because of the close fit of the mask and the heat trapped within it.

Care and close observation should be used when masks are on patients who are likely to vomit since the flow of vomitus can be blocked, thus increasing the chance of aspiration. Masks should also be used with care on the unconscious patient. An oral airway should always be in place to prevent airway obstruction by a flaccid tongue.

**SIMPLE MASKS.** The usual simple, open-face mask is a disposable plastic unit that does not have any valves or reservoir bag. It covers the nose and mouth, has vents for exhaled air, and can deliver oxygen concentrations up to 60%. Oxygen flow rates at a minimum of 5 to 6 L per minute should be used to wash out the exhaled carbon dioxide that accumulates within the mask. Controlled oxygen therapy is difficult with an open-face mask because it does not provide precise inspired oxygen concentrations. However, this mask is a convenient and relatively comfortable device for delivering moderate oxygen concentrations over short periods and thus is widely used, especially in areas such as the recovery room. One of the main uses for simple masks is to deliver humidification or aerosol therapy. Limitations are similar to those of all masks and include discomfort and frequent removal of the mask for activities such as eating, expectorating, and coughing.

**PARTIAL REBREATHING MASK.** The partial rebreathing mask is similar to the rebreathing mask that is used for delivery of anesthesics in the operating room. The partial rebreathing mask is a tight-fitting mask with a reservoir bag that is always open to the mask. The reservoir bag allows delivery of concentrations of oxygen greater than 60% to nonintubated patients. The purpose of the mask is to conserve oxygen by having the patient rebreathe some of his or her exhaled air. The oxygen source flows into the neck of the mask, allowing oxygen to flow directly into the mask during inhalation and into the bag during exhalation. A liter flow into the bag of at least 5 to 6 L per minute is required to prevent deflation of the reservoir bag. Because of the constant filling of the reservoir bag, only the first one third of the exhaled air volume enters the bag. This exhaled air is high in oxygen and low in carbon dioxide, because it is the volume of air that ventilated the anatomical dead space. Because minimal room air enters the mask, the concentration of delivered oxygen is fairly predictable, even if the patient's ventilatory pattern exceeds the flow rate of the oxygen source (see Chapter 10, Table 10-10, for the predicted oxygen concentrations of oxygen delivery systems).

**NONREBREATHING MASKS.** The nonrebreathing mask is another mask and reservoir bag system similar to the partial rebreathing system. With this mask, however, there is a one-way valve between the bag and mask, and no air enters the bag during exhalation. The exhaled air is diverted to the atmosphere through a flap valve in the facepiece. If the oxygen source fails or the patient's needs suddenly exceed the flow of oxygen, a flap or spring-loaded valve either in the neck or in the mask itself permits the intake of room air. When the nonrebreathing mask has a tight seal over the face, it is designed to deliver 90% to 100% oxygen. However, studies have shown that the mask delivers an average of 63% oxygen.[56] Factors responsible for this decreased concentration of oxygen include entrainment of room air because of a loose-fitting mask and open exhalation ports that allow room air to dilute the oxygen from the reservoir bag.

**High-flow systems.** High-flow systems provide a flow rate and reservoir capacity that are adequate to provide the total inspired volume required by the patient. Both high and low oxygen concentrations can be delivered by these systems; the oxygen concentrations are much more controlled and can be delivered in a range of 24% to 100%. One advantage of a high-flow system is that changes in the patient's ventilatory pattern do not affect the $FIO_2$ as long as the device is properly applied and a consistent oxygen flow can be delivered. The temperature and humidity of the gas can also be controlled since the entire inspired volume is being supplied.

***Venturi mask.*** The most reliable control of $FIO_2$ can be achieved by using a Venturi mask, which controls the oxygen concentration by flowing 100% oxygen at high velocity through a narrowed orifice or "jet." This high velocity causes entrainment of air at the orifice. The higher the velocity, the more the air is entrained; this is what is referred to as the Bernoulli principle, and it is one of the most accurate means of delivering a prescribed concentration of oxygen. Venturi masks currently in use can deliver 24%, 28%, 35%, and 40% oxygen. The recommended flow rates for these percentages are, respectively, 6 L, 6L, 10L, and 10 L per minute.

Venturi masks are especially efficacious in patients who are chronically hypoxemic and hypercapnic, such as occurs with chronic obstructive pulmonary disease (COPD). An excessive concentration of oxygen could cause respiratory depression in these patients because their respiratory center is no longer responsive to hypercapnia and is dependent on a low $Pa{O_2}$ for stimulation to breathe. The Venturi mask can provide a COPD patient with a precise oxygen concentration that does not change with ventilatory pattern and hence offers more control for an oxygen-sensitive patient.

Venturi masks cause all the discomfort of other masks and are also very wasteful of oxygen. The high air flow produced by the mask can be drying to the mucous membranes. Attempts to humidify the gas have not been very successful because of the large amount of entrained air.

### Complications of Oxygen Therapy

Oxygen, like most drugs, has adverse effects and complications resulting from its use. The old adage, "if a little is good, a lot is better," does not apply to oxygen. The lung is designed to handle a concentration of 21% oxygen, with some adaptability to higher concentrations, but adverse effects and oxygen toxicity can result if a high concentration is administered too long.

**Hypoventilation.** The first adverse effect of oxygen administration is hypoventilation. The hypoxemic, hypercapnic patient who has chronic lung disease is at potential risk of hypoventilation with oxygen supplementation. In this type of patient and those patients with a depressed respiratory drive (such as a patient with drug-overdose), the administration of oxygen may actually cause abolition of the hypoxemia that is responsible for driving the ventilation, resulting in hypoventilation and an increase in the arterial partial pressure of carbon dioxide ($Pa{CO_2}$). An elevated $Pa{CO_2}$ will cause hyperventilation in most patients because carbon dioxide is the stimulus to breathe. But in patients who rely on hypoxemia as their main respiratory drive (for example, in patients who are chronically hypercapnic), the $Pa{CO_2}$ may continue to rise as hypoventilation progresses. Eventually, the patient becomes somnolent and even obtunded because of carbon dioxide narcosis. Because of this risk of hypoventilation and carbon dioxide accumulation, all chronically hypercapnic patients require careful low-flow oxygen administration.

**Absorption atelectasis.** Another adverse effect of high concentrations of oxygen is **absorption atelectasis.** Breathing high concentrations of oxygen washes out the nitrogen that normally fills the alveoli. The higher the $FI{O_2}$ delivered to the alveoli, the lower will be the amount of nitrogen. Since nitrogen does not diffuse from an alveolus into the pulmonary capillary, it is responsible for holding open the alveolus. Therefore gradual shrinking of the alveolus can occur if a patient receives a high $FI{O_2}$ and is ventilating minimally. In this situation, oxygen in the alveolus is absorbed into the bloodstream faster than it can be replaced by ventilation, and collapse of the alveolus can result.

The effect high concentrations of oxygen have on surfactant also contributes to atelectasis. It has been postulated that surfactant, although not destroyed by hyperoxia, is redistributed and removed from close contact with the alveolar walls where it functions to keep the alveoli open.

**Oxygen toxicity.** The most detrimental effect of breathing a high concentration of oxygen is the development of **oxygen toxicity,** which is dependent on the oxygen tension and the duration of exposure. No significant damage occurs to the lung exposed to an $FI{O_2}$ of 0.5 or less at sea level for extended periods,[8,10,69] and 100% oxygen can be breathed for 24 hours or less by healthy and even by cardiopulmonary-diseased patients with little evidence of pulmonary dysfunction[58] or clinical signs of oxygen toxicity.[69] However, there are wide variations to oxygen tolerance among individuals, and scientific study is lacking. The patients most likely to develop oxygen toxicity are those that require intubation, mechanical ventilation, and high oxygen concentrations for extended periods.

The pathogenesis of lung injury by oxygen toxicity is attributed to biochemical reactions of oxygen-free radicals on the lung parenchyma and microvasculature.[8] The first symptom is substernal chest pain that is exacerbated by deep breathing. A dry cough and tracheal irritation follow. Eventually, there is definite pleuritic pain on inhalation, followed by dyspnea. Upper-airway changes may include a sensation of nasal stuffiness, sore throat, and eye and ear discomfort. Chest radiographs and pulmonary function tests remain normal until symptoms are severe. Complete, rapid reversal of these symptoms will occur as soon as normal oxygen concentrations return. This stage in the development of oxygen toxicity can affect many organs other than the lungs, including the central nervous system, vascular system, hematopoietic system, and the heart (Table 12-1).

As oxygen toxicity progresses, objective pulmonary damage becomes evident. A chest radiograph reveals atelectatic streaks and patches of bronchopneumonia, and bronchoscopy reveals tracheobronchitis but no infection. There is also a definite decrease in vital capacity, decreased compliance, reduced functional residual capacity, and evidence of pulmonary shunting. These abnormalities are reversible several days after return to normal oxygen concentrations. If high oxygen concentrations are still needed, permanent damage may occur. There are individual susceptibilities to oxygen toxicity and even variances within an individual (Table 12-2).

The pathological features of oxygen toxicity can be di-

***Table 12-1*** Acute effects of high concentrations of normobaric oxygen*

| Part affected | Site of action | Result | Outcome |
|---|---|---|---|
| Ear, sinuses | Air in body cavities | Replacement of air by oxygen, which is then absorbed | Sinus and ear pain |
| Airways | Mucosa of nose, throat, trachea, and bronchi | Irritation | Decreased mucociliary clearance; mucosal swelling and inflammation |
| Lung parenchyma | Poorly ventilated areas | Nitrogen is washed out and oxygen is absorbed | Atelectasis, microatelectasis |
| Ventilation | Peripheral chemoreceptors | Depressed ventilatory drive | Increased tissue carbon dioxide and $Paco_2$, which stimulate the ventilatory drive |
| | Deoxygenated hemoglobin—decreased | Decreased carbon dioxide carriage | Same as for peripheral chemoreceptors |
| | Hypoxic drive—abolished | Carbon dioxide narcosis | Hypoventilation, apnea |
| Pulmonary function | Airways and parenchyma | Decreased compliance | Reduced vital capacity |
| Heart | Vagal receptors | Slight bradycardia | Decreased cardiac output† |
| | Cardiac muscle | Slightly depressed | Decreased cardiac output† |
| Regional circulation | Coronary and cardiac vessels | Arteriolar constriction | Uncertain† |
| | Peripheral circulation | Arteriolar constriction | Slight hypertension† |
| | Retinal circulation | Arteriolar constriction | Impaired visual fields |
| | Conjunctival vessels | Vasodilation | Conjunctivitis |
| | Pulmonary circulation | Vasodilation | Improved ventilation/perfusion (V/Q) mismatch, decrease in pulmonary hypertension |
| Blood | Erythrocyte membrane | Damage | Hemolysis |
| | Kidneys | Fluid retention‡ | Decreased serum albumin and hematocrit |

Modified from Ziment I: Respiratory pharmacology and therapeutics, Philadelphia, 1978, WB Saunders Co.
*Time for the effects to develop is variable.
†Clinical significance is rare.
‡Initial fluid retention is usually followed by diuresis.

vided into an early exudative stage and a late proliferative stage. Within 24 to 48 hours of oxygen exposure, exudative changes appear. Initially, the capillary endothelial cells become damaged, and they leak serum protein and fluid into the interstitial space of the alveolar wall. This fluid is collected by the lymphatic system, which empties it into the general circulation.

As the capillary damage progresses, the flow of fluid out of the capillaries increases and may exceed the lymphatic system's ability to drain it. There is minimal gas exchange impairment at this point; however, with continued exposure to hyperoxia, alveolar cells become damaged, allowing the escaped alveolar capillary fluid to pass directly into the alveolar spaces and causing gas exchange impairment.

Oxygen-induced damage to the cells of the alveolar wall initiates a self-sustaining process of ongoing injury. The byproducts of the injured cells attract inflammatory cells, especially the polymorphonuclear leukocytes (PMNs). While PMNs ingest the inflammatory debris, they release proteolytic enzymes and oxygen free radicals that further damage the alveolar tissue.

The lung will respond with cellular proliferation if it

***Table 12-2*** Factors affecting oxygen toxicity

| Hastened onset or increased severity | Delayed onset or decreased severity |
|---|---|
| Adrenocortical hormones | Acclimatization to hypoxia |
| Adrenocorticotropic hormone | Adrenergic blocking drugs |
| Carbon dioxide inhalation | Anesthesia |
| Convulsions | Antioxidants |
| Dexamethasone | Chlorpromazine |
| Dextroamphetamine | Gamma-aminobutyric acid |
| Disulfiram (ATA base) | Ganglionic blocking drugs |
| Epinephrine | Glutathione |
| Hyperthermia | Hypothermia |
| Insulin | Hypothyroidism |
| Norepinephrine | Immaturity |
| Paraquat | Intermittent exposure |
| Thyroid hormones | Reserpine |
| Vitamin E deficiency | Starvation |
| X-irradiation | Tris (hydroxymethyl) aminomethane |
| | Vitamin E |

From Scanlan CL, Spearman CB, and Sheldon RN, Egan's fundamentals of respiratory care, St Louis, 1990, Mosby–Year Book, Inc.

survives the aforementioned process and the disease process originally responsible for the hypoxemia. Cellular proliferation occurs as an attempt to repair the alveolar damage, and the alveolar walls become filled with fibroblasts. Alveolar type II cells, which are relatively tolerant to hyperoxia,[10] replicate and reestablish the damaged alveolar wall. Endothelial cell repair and replacement occurs, and the pulmonary edema is reabsorbed. The final result is irregular scarring. Clinically, other complications such as infection must also resolve.

**Summary.** Oxygen is an extremely beneficial drug if used correctly, but it is sometimes taken for granted. Oxygen administration requires close patient observation and continuous application of the oxygen device to ensure controlled oxygen therapy. Use of supplemental oxygen is especially important during activities that will decrease the blood oxygen level such as turning, dangling, coughing, walking, eating, and even just talking.

Other modalities of therapy may also be used along with oxygen therapy for the hypoxemic patient, including aerosol therapy, chest physiotherapy, medications, and assisted-breathing techniques (for example, intermittent positive pressure breathing). By using these other measures, the concentration of oxygen necessary to provide adequate oxygenation may be decreased to a minimum, thus reducing the chances of oxygen toxicity.

### Hyperbaric Oxygen Therapy

**Hyperbaric oxygen therapy** is a medical intervention whereby 100% oxygen is breathed at increased atmospheric pressure in an enclosed pressure chamber. Hyperbaric chambers date back 300 years when Henshaw built the first chamber, in which air was compressed using a bellows.[40] Previously, there was no sound physiological basis for hyperbaric oxygen therapy nor was there any animal or clinical research to direct its use. However, since the 1930s there have been studies establishing the appropriate indications and guidelines for the use of hyperbaric oxygen therapy.

The Undersea and Hyperbaric Medical Society (UHMS) was founded in 1967 and initially used its specialized talents for the support of persons engaged in undersea activities. UHMS is the one body of scientists and physicians with the combined expertise to guide hyperbaric medicine activities. In 1983, the Hyperbaric Medical Committee of UHMS developed a report on hyperbaric oxygen therapy.[22] The committee organized disorders for which hyperbaric oxygen therapy is effective into two categories (Table 12-3). Category 1 conditions are disorders for which hyperbaric oxygen therapy is the primary mode of treatment. Also in this category are conditions in which it is an important adjunct to other primary therapy measures. The efficacy of hyperbaric oxygen therapy in these disorders has been shown through research and clinical experience. Category 2 conditions represent disorders for which hyperbaric oxygen therapy is considered experimental. This category concerns life-threatening or limb-threatening cases in which evidence is strong that hyperbaric oxygen may be of value.

Although hyperbaric chambers are not in many medical centers, the number of chambers in the United States, as well as the number of patients being treated, is growing.

***Table 12-3*** Conditions known to be effectively treated by hyperbaric oxygen (category 1) or for which such treatment is considered experimental (category 2)

| Category 1 | Category 2 |
|---|---|
| Radiation necrosis: osteoradionecrosis, soft-tissue radiation necrosis | Head and spinal cord injury (traumatic) |
| Decompression sickness | Bone grafts |
| Carbon monoxide poisoning (acute): smoke inhalation | Carbon tetrachloride poisoning (acute) |
| Gas embolism (acute) | Cerebrovascular accident, either thrombotic or embolic (acute): stroke; frostbite |
| Gas gangrene | Fractures |
| Osteomyelitis (refractory) | Hydrogen sulfide poisoning |
| Soft-tissue infection and tissue necrosis caused by mixed aerobic and anaerobic organisms; Bacteroides infection | Abscess, either intraabdominal or intracranial |
| Crush injury with traumatic ischemia | Lepromatous leprosy |
| Compromised skin grafts or flaps; selected problem wounds | Meningitis |
| Selected mycotic infections (refractory: mucormycosis, actinomycosis, canibolus coronato) | Pseudomembranous colitis (antimicrobial agent-induced) |
| Cyanide poisoning (acute) | Radiation, myelitis, cystitis, enteritis, proctitis |
| Cerebral edema (acute) | Sickle cell crisis and/or hematuria (sickle cell anemia) |
| Thermal burns | Mutliple sclerosis |
| Anemia from exceptional blood loss | Retinal arterial insufficiency (acute) |
| | Retinopathy adjunctive to scleral buckling procedures in patients with sickle cell peripheral retinopathy and retinal detachment |
| | Pyoderma gangrenosum |
| | Selected anaerobic infections (refractory): actinomycosis |

From the Hyperbaric Medicine Committee of the Undersea Medical Society, Revised classification, 1986, Bethesda, Md, The Committee.

Two types of chambers are in use—the monoplace and the multiplace. The monoplace chamber holds only one patient and is compressed with 100% oxygen. The maximal compression depth is approximately 66 feet of sea water. The multiplace chamber can hold multiple patients, as well as staff, with the number dependent on the chamber size. The chamber is compressed with air, and the patients breathe 100% oxygen by mask or hood or by ventilator through an artificial airway. A multiplace chamber can reach a depth of 165 feet of sea water, which is the maximal depth needed to treat decompression sickness (bends) or air embolism.

Hyperbaric oxygen therapy works in many ways to provide its therapeutic effects. The hyperbaric state improves the oxygen-carrying capacity of the blood, possibly improving the oxygenation of ischemic tissue. The increased barometric pressure in the chamber greatly increases the amount of oxygen that is dissolved into plasma. At sea level (1 atmosphere) there is normally 0.3 cc of oxygen dissolved per 100 ml blood; at 3 atm 6 cc of oxygen will be dissolved per 100 ml blood. Thus a low hemoglobin count is compensated by the increased oxygen dissolved in plasma. During treatment, a patient's $Pa_{O_2}$ may be as high as 800 to 2000 mm Hg. As well as increasing oxygen delivery to the tissues, hyperbaric oxygen therapy treatments enhance leukocyte function and cause neovascularization, which is the growth of new blood vessels. All of these processes promote wound healing, especially in diabetic ulcers, osteoradionecrosis (damage and death to tissue and bone as a result of radiation therapy), nonhealing wounds, or traumatic injuries. Further, the increased pressure within the hyperbaric chamber reduces the size of gas emboli, possibly accounting for restoration of blood flow to anoxic areas.

High oxygen levels in the tissues will prevent toxin production and eventually kill bacteria such as *Clostridium perfringens* (gas gangrene). Hyperbaric oxygen therapy also shortens the half-life of carboxyhemoglobin (with carbon monoxide poisoning) and provides sufficient tissue oxygenation for normal aerobic metabolism despite a high carboxyhemoglobin level.

Each disorder treated by hyperbaric oxygen therapy has a specific protocol that uses the Navy's hyperbaric treatment tables to determine depth, time at depth, and decompression time. Most routine treatments such as for wound healing compress or "dive" to 45 to 60 feet of sea water and stay at that depth for approximately 90 to 120 minutes.

The chamber is staffed by specially trained technicians, nurses, and doctors. A well-trained staff is essential because the chamber presents some situations that are unique to the hyperbaric state. The multiplace chamber must always have a technician or a nurse inside with the patient(s). This person is responsible for monitoring the patient, as well as for monitoring those items that are affected by pressure such as air volume in the cuff of an endotracheal tube, intravenous (IV) drip chambers, and blood pressure cuffs. The physical status of the patient must be closely observed. Problems such as respiratory difficulty, ear pain, decreasing blood sugar (specifically in diabetics), bradycardia, and symptoms of oxygen toxicity may arise that result from the hyperoxic state or from the pressure changes the patient undergoes while in the chamber.

Some risks and adverse effects of hyperbaric oxygen therapy are inherent with the therapy. Barotrauma to the middle ear and paranasal sinuses is probably the most frequently seen problem that occurs when care is not taken to equalize the pressure in these areas during descent. Administering vasoconstrictor sprays or pills may help. Presence of sinus problems or an upper respiratory infection (URI) may preclude diving. Performing bilateral myringotomies may be necessary to prevent ear trauma to a patient who is unable to clear his ears or sinuses, especially when the patient is unconscious.

A major concern during hyperbaric therapy is the development of oxygen toxicity. Hyperbaric oxygen toxicity has some distinguishing features from normal barometric toxicity and is actually an acceleration in the development of various syndromes of normobaric oxygen toxicity. Clinical pulmonary oxygen toxicity is not a threat during hyperbaric oxygen therapy as long as standard Navy hyperbaric treatment tables are used. Central nervous system (CNS) oxygen toxicity is of concern at oxygen partial pressures greater than 3 atm. The effects of CNS toxicity are dose related and almost always reversible. Therefore patients must have air breaks interspersed with breathing the 100% oxygen in a multiplace chamber to prevent oxygen toxicity at depth. Generally, CNS oxygen toxicity is manifested by signs of CNS hyperexcitability, with the most dramatic symptom oxygen convulsion. The seizure may even be the first sign of oxygen toxicity. The treatment of CNS oxygen toxicity includes removal of the oxygen, use of a bite block, seizure precautions, and protection of the patient. Conditions that affect the development of oxygen toxicity at normobaric oxygen levels (see Table 12-2) also apply to the hyperbaric oxygen therapy setting.

## ARTIFICIAL AIRWAYS

### Endotracheal Intubation

An endotracheal tube is the most commonly used artificial airway for providing short-term airway management. The endotracheal airway may be placed through the orotracheal or nasotracheal route. In most situations involving emergency placement the orotracheal route is used since the approach is simpler and affords use of a larger diameter endotracheal tube.[75] Nasotracheal intubation provides greater patient comfort over time and is preferred in situations in which the patient has suffered a jaw fracture or when it is anticipated that the endotracheal tube may be needed for more than 48 hours.[60,75]

Indications for endotracheal intubation are as follows: (1) respiratory insufficiency or failure, (2) airway maintenance in patients who develop obstruction despite the presence of a pharyngeal airway, (3) prevention of massive aspiration of stomach contents in a compromised patient, (4) removal of airway secretions, and (5) need to provide a fraction of inspired oxygen ($FIO_2$) >60% (relative indication).

Successful intubation should result in (1) auscultation of breath sounds in both lungs, (2) warm, exhaled air felt at the end of the exhalation port in spontaneously breathing patients, and (3) bilateral movement of the upper chest wall when mechanical ventilation is instituted.

Tube placement should be verified by a chest x-ray examination. The tip of the endotracheal tube should be 2 cm above the carina to achieve equal bilateral ventilation.[75] After the chest x-ray exam, tube placement may need adjustment. Once final adjustment of the position is complete, the level of insertion (marked in centimeters on side of tube) should be noted and the tube securely anchored.

### Tracheal Intubation

Tracheostomy is a life-saving procedure used only when other choices are not feasible, and it is preferred in patients in whom long-term problems contraindicate the use of an endotracheal tube. The following are indications for its use: (1) to prevent or reverse upper airway obstruction,[44] (2) to prevent aspiration in a patient with anticipated long-term swallowing problems, (3) to facilitate secretion removal in a patient with long-term pulmonary problems,[44] (4) to provide a closed system for mechanical ventilation, (5) for a patient with intolerance for an endotracheal tube, and (6) for a patient in whom passage of an endotracheal tube is undesirable or impossible (laryngeal or pharyngeal obstruction).[33]

A tracheostomy provides the best route for long-term airway maintenance and avoids the oral, nasal, pharyngeal, and laryngeal complications of endotracheal intubation.[44] The tube is shorter, wider, and less curved than the endotracheal tube; thus the resistance to airflow is less, and breathing is easier. The tracheostomy has other advantages over endotracheal intubation, including (1) easier secretion removal, whether by suctioning or by patient cough, (2) increased patient acceptance and comfort, (3) the possibility of the patient's eating and talking, and (4) the facilitation of ventilator weaning since a tracheostomy tube is easier to breathe through when the patient is off the ventilator.

### Problems Associated with Artificial Airway Placement

Significant problems can be associated with tracheostomy or endotracheal tube placement. The tubes impair the respiratory defense system by bypassing the upper airway system; thus the warming and humidifying of air must be performed by external means. Cleansing or filtering the air is not feasible, but suctioning and tracheostomy care can remove some particles. There is great potential for tracheobronchial tree infection after the placement of an artificial airway.[44] Studies show that once an artificial airway is placed, contamination of the lower airways will follow within 24 hours.[33,58] This results from colonization of the lower airways with bacteria commonly found in the upper airways. The patient's general condition and the presence or absence of pulmonary trauma or disease significantly affect the likelihood that an infection will ensue.

Other consequences of artificial airway placement include an altered body image and loss of independence. Nutrition is impaired during the acute stage of airway placement because of loss of oral feeding. Supplemental enteral or parenteral nutrition is mandatory. Verbal communication is impaired until the trachea can be plugged or a talking trach is inserted. Endotracheal tubes preclude talking; further, tube movement when patients attempt to talk increases local irritation and should be discouraged. Careful attention must be given to minimize tracheal damage resulting from tube movement. Flexible mounts and swivels should be used to lessen the transmission of ventilator tube movement to the airway. The patient's tracheal tube requires adequate support

***Table 12-4*** Factors that predispose damage to the airways by artificial tubes

| General factors | Site-specific factors |
|---|---|
| Duration of intubation | **LARYNGEAL** |
| Duration of mechanical ventilation | Multiple orotracheal or nasotracheal intubations |
| Inadequate patient sedation | Inexperienced larynoscopist, an emergency intubation, or self-extubation |
| Repeated flexion and extension of the neck | Too large a translaryngeal tube |
| Decerebrate or decorticate movements | Tube material |
| Patient out of phase with controlled mechanical ventilation ("bucking" the ventilator) | **TRACHEAL** |
| Traction on the tube during turning, suctioning, and ventilator connection and disconnection | Cuff overinflation |
| Previous prolonged intubation | Combination of high positive end-expiratory pressure (PEEP) and low lung compliance |
| Chronic airway or lung disease (especially sputum-producing disease) requiring frequent suctioning procedures | Too small or large a cuff in relation to the tracheal size |
| Airway infection | Noncircular cross-sectional tracheal shape |
| Hypotension | Cuff material |

Modified from MacKenzie C: Heart Lung 12(5):485, 1983.

during turning, positioning, and suctioning. When necessary, sedation should be used to control prolonged coughing, agitation, or uncontrolled movements.[44]

### Complications Resulting from Use of Artificial Airways

Tracheal damage from cuff pressure is a frequent complication of endotracheal or tracheal intubation. Research studies have demonstrated superficial lesions occurring less than 12 hours after tube placement, with more severe erosion occurring over time. Mackenzie[44] summarized the factors that precipitate laryngotracheal damage and the complications seen in artificial airways (Table 12-4). The box below outlines nursing interventions that decrease the complications of intubation.

**Tracheal necrosis.** Cuffed artificial airway tubes that have been in place as few as 3 to 5 days have caused early necrosis in the tracheal cartilage.[62] When this necrosis occurs in the posterior tracheal mucosa, a tracheoesophageal fistula results. The fistula allows air to escape into the stomach, causing distention. It also allows gastric aspiration of stomach contents into the trachea. This complication occurs more commonly when both an artificial airway and a standard size nasogastric tube are present. Using small gastric feeding tubes decreases chances of formation of tracheoesophageal fistula.

Anterior wall tracheal necrosis may cause erosion of the tracheal tube into the innominate artery, a rare but life-threatening complication.[47] It is suspected when a pulsating tracheostomy tube is observed or if bright red blood is expelled. Immediate intervention is necessary since exsanguination can occur. Continuous bleeding through a tracheostomy tube may be an early sign of innominate artery erosion, and it should be evaluated by the physician.

**Tracheal dilation.** A prolonged intubation period may allow pressure from an artificial airway cuff to distort and dilate the tracheal wall. Suspicions should arise when increasing amounts of cuff air are needed to create a seal or when bulging of the tracheal wall is seen at the cuff site on the x-ray film.

**Tracheal stenosis.** Tracheal stenosis is a narrowing of the trachea that occurs 1 week to 2 years after endotracheal intubation or tracheostomy. It results from healing of the inflamed area in which the tube cuff was located.

Stenosis is more common with a tracheostomy than with an endotracheal intubation, with the incidence 65% and 19%, respectively.[33,62,75] Symptoms occur when 50% or more of the tracheal diameter is reduced and include dyspnea, loss of exercise tolerance, stridor, and recurrent pulmonary infections. The severity of stenosis can be reduced by tube choice, maintenance of proper cuff pressure, the use of shorter intubation periods, and prevention of respiratory infection and excessive tube movement.

**Infections.** Tracheostomy requires an open incision into the trachea, which is associated with risk of wound infection and possible sepsis. Aseptic care of the site and proper suction technique reduce the infection risks.

**Airway obstruction.** Airway obstruction is a potential complication associated with the kinking of an endotracheal tube, secretion buildup, or slippage of a soft cuff over the end of the artificial airway. If obstruction is suspected, repositioning the patient's head, neck, or tube should be attempted. Other methods to reduce the obstruction include deflating the cuff, attempting to pass a suction catheter, or removing the inner cannula. If none of the maneuvers is successful and the patient cannot breathe through the tube, it must be removed.

**Subcutaneous emphysema.** Subcutaneous emphysema, or mediastinal emphysema, occurs when air escapes from the tracheostomy incision into the tissues, dissects fascial planes under the skin, and accumulates around the face, neck, and throat. These areas may then appear puffy, and slight finger pressure reveals a crackling sensation (crepitation) under the skin where the air is present. Subcutaneous emphysema can occur immediately after the tracheostomy tube is inserted or anytime later, particularly if the tube is too short. Generally, this is not a serious complication be-

#### NURSING INTERVENTIONS TO MINIMIZE TRACHEAL DAMAGE RESULTING FROM ARTIFICIAL AIRWAY PLACEMENT

- Stabilize the tube as much as possible to prevent movement within the larynx.
- Avoid frequent retaping since this involves unnecessary manipulation of tube.
- Note the depth of the tube at placement and periodically thereafter to avoid displacement.
- Avoid overinflation of the cuff—maintain pressure <25 mm Hg.
- Do not engage in periodic deflation or inflation of cuff.
- Do not use high pressure–low volume cuffs; use only high volume–low pressure cuffs.
- When nasotracheal intubation is present, inspect nares every day for signs of septal ischemia.
- Provide frequent mouth cleansing to decrease infection.
- Take measures to avoid traumatic extubation by patient (sedate or restrain).
- Follow strict aseptic technique when giving artificial airway care and when suctioning (use proper universal blood and body secretion precautions; gloves and goggles should be worn by the nurse(s)).
- Avoid excessive negative pressure during suctioning; use only amount necessary to remove secretions (keep below 120 mm Hg).
- Support ventilator tubing to avoid traction on the patient's airway tube.
- Take measures to avoid excessive movement by patient (i.e., repeated flexion and extension of head, coughing, chewing, tonguing the tube).

cause the air will eventually be reabsorbed. Rarely, mediastinal subcutaneous emphysema is associated with pneumothorax.

Other known complications are presented in the box at right.

## AIRWAY MANAGEMENT

### Humidification

Humidification of air is normally performed by the mucosal layer of the upper respiratory tract. When this area is bypassed such as occurs in endotracheal intubation and tracheostomy or when supplemental oxygen is used, humidification by external means is necessary. Various humidification devices add water to inhaled gas to prevent drying and irritation of the respiratory tract, to prevent undue loss of body water, and to facilitate secretion removal by expectoration or by suctioning.

Bubble diffusion humidifiers are commonly used to provide moisture to inhaled gas. They may be warm or cold humidifiers. With a cold humidifier, the gas diffuses out of a stem submerged in water. The gas breaks into small bubbles and vaporizes. At room temperature, the gas provides only approximately 50% of the humidification needed by the body; hence this method of humidification can lead to drying and irritation of mucous membranes when used for a significant time period. Diffusion humidifiers are unable to adequately humidify gas at higher rates of flow, making them more suitable for low-flow oxygen delivery over short time spans. Cold humidifiers are relatively simple and reliable devices and are available as disposable units, thus decreasing maintenance time and eliminating potential infections associated with reusable equipment.

Warm humidifiers provide better humidification than do cold humidifiers since warm humidification supplies heat as well as moisture and breaks gas into smaller particles at higher flow rates. Heated cascade humidifiers are preferred for use with intubated patients since 100% humidification of inhaled gas can be ensured.

### Suctioning

Tracheal suctioning is a method of clearing secretions from the airways and is performed through an artificial airway (endotracheal or tracheal tube) either nasotracheally or orotracheally. Suctioning through the oral or nasal passages is difficult and is limited to clearance of the upper airway.

Tracheal suctioning is a frequently performed procedure for removing secretions from the trachea in patients with a compromised cough reflex. It involves the use of sterile technique and is performed in a manner that is effective yet minimizes associated complications (see the box, "Complications of Tracheal Suctioning"). Although no standard procedure exists, certain common techniques of tracheal suctioning are described in the literature and include the following: (1) preoxygenation of the patient,[4,15,18,46,60] (2) use of sterile, disposable suction trays equipped with gloves, catheter, and solution, (3) limiting the suctioning period to 15 seconds or less, (4) periodic instillation of sterile saline solution to liquify secretions, and (5) wearing masks and goggles as part of universal precaution techniques. Three of these practices require further scrutiny to apply a suctioning technique based on tested clinical rationale.

***Preoxygenation.*** Hypoxemia is a serious side effect of tracheal suctioning and, if not minimized, can lead to tissue hypoxia. Many studies have explored ways to lessen hypoxia associated with tracheal suctioning. Barnes and

#### COMPLICATIONS OF ARTIFICIAL AIRWAYS

**TUBE (OROTRACHEAL AND NASOTRACHEAL)-RELATED COMPLICATIONS**

Trauma during insertion
Sinusitis (nasotracheal)
Supraglottic and epiglottic edema
Laryngeal ulcerations or granuloma
Inability to vocalize
Vocal cord paralysis or immobility
Laryngitis, stridor, or hoarseness on extubation
Subglottic stenosis
Tracheal erosion from the tip of the tube
Tracheal granuloma
Endobronchial intubation
Airway infection
Necrosis of nasal septum (nasotracheal)
Pneumothorax
Posterior laryngeal abscess with obstruction

**TRACHEOSTOMY STOMAL COMPLICATIONS**

Incorrect position—too low, too high, or not in midline
Surgical complications during and after stomal creation
Rupture of the posterior tracheal membrane during insertion of the tracheostomy tube through the stoma
False passage of the tube into the subcutaneous tissue anterior to the tracheal stoma
Innominate artery erosion from an incorrectly positioned stoma or erosion from the tip of the tracheostomy tube
Persistent fistula or scarring on healing
Stenosis at the level of the stoma because of granuloma formation
Infection

**CUFF-RELATED COMPLICATIONS**

Trauma during insertion through larynx or during accidental extubation (orotracheal and nasotracheal)
Tracheal wall erosion
Tracheomalacia
Tracheoesophageal fistula
Tracheal stenosis
Tracheal granuloma
Tracheitis
Cuff leak with loss of airway seal, leading to inadequate ventilation
Aspiration past an improperly sized or inflated cuff

## COMPLICATIONS OF TRACHEAL SUCTIONING

### HYPOXEMIA

Suctioning removes oxygen from the airways and may lead to hypoxemia. Hypoxemia can be minimized by preoxygenation and by keeping the wall suction pressure as low as possible while still allowing effective mucus removal. Many techniques of preoxygenation exist—manual resuscitator bagging, ventilator breath sighing, and providing a ventilator breath with regular tidal volume. Currently hyperinflation (1½ times the usual tidal volume) and high $FIO_2$ (0.6-1.0) are recommended for the ventilator-dependent patient. Manual resuscitator bagging may not deliver an $FIO_2$ of 1.0.[15]

### TRAUMATIC AIRWAY ULCERATION

Traumatic airway is directly related to the amount of wall suction pressure used. The wall suction should be set at a level that allows easy removal of secretions but not so high that trauma to the airways is induced. Suction should be kept below 120 mm Hg. Excessively high suction does not mean better secretion clearance.

### CARDIAC DYSRHYTHMIAS

Cardiac dysrhythmias include premature ventricular contractions, tachycardia, bradycardia, and sudden death. The dysrhythmias result from hypoxemia and/or vagal receptor stimulation that can occur with suctioning. Preoxygenation may lessen dysrhythmia formation. The cardiac monitor should be observed during suctioning, and suctioning should be interrupted if significant dysrhythmias occur (as per unit protocol).

### BRONCHOSPASMS

Bronchospasms are associated with catheter irritation of the tracheal membranes and with coughing; use of bronchodilators may be effective.

### INFECTION

Infection is related to placement of an artificial airway and/or a break in sterile technique while suctioning.

### ATELECTASIS

Atelectasis is created by excessive wall suction pressure and/or by suctioning too long and/or by using a catheter too large. The suction catheter should be no greater than one half of the internal diameter of the tracheal tube, and wall suction should be kept at the lowest level (<120 mm Hg) that will still support effective suctioning.

Kirchhoff[4] concluded that preoxygenation should be provided to all ventilated patients and that the methodology used to provide oxygen should be tailored to the patient's clinical situation, whether by hyperinflation, hyperventilation, hyperoxygenation, or insufflation (see the box above).

## TECHNIQUES TO PREVENT HYPOXEMIA RESULTING FROM SUCTIONING

### INSUFFLATION

Insufflation refers to supplemental oxygen delivered by a double-lumen suctioning catheter or by the side arm on the endotracheal or tracheal adapter. It provides simultaneous oxygen delivery during suctioning.

### HYPEROXYGENATION

Hyperoxygenation refers to increasing the fraction of inspired oxygen ($FIO_2$), usually to 100%, before, during, and after suctioning. This may be achieved by turning the ventilator oxygen setting to 100% or by using a resuscitation bag to provide the patient with 100% oxygen. If increasing the oxygen is accomplished by changing the ventilator setting, sufficient time must elapse to achieve that oxygen concentration in the system. The time lapse varies with the type of ventilator used.

### HYPERINFLATION

Hyperinflation refers to increasing the patient's tidal volume, usually by 150%. This can be achieved by using the sigh component of the ventilator or by using some resuscitation bags. When the patient is being ventilated at high tidal volumes, regular resuscitation bags may not be able to provide the volume necessary to achieve hyperinflation. Hyperinflation does not refer to changes in $FIO_2$, although increasing the $FIO_2$ frequently accompanies hyperinflation.

### HYPERVENTILATION

Hyperventilation refers to an increase in ventilatory rate without necessarily changing the tidal volume or oxygen level delivered.

They further concluded that spontaneously breathing patients may require only a few breaths of room air or supplemental oxygen before suctioning and that no single procedure is beneficial for all patients.

Preventing hypoxemia has also led to the development of suctioning equipment and techniques that avoid removing the patient from ventilator support. This is referred to as closed system suctioning. The benefits include maintaining pressure ventilation, maintaining oxygenation, and continuation of positive end-expiratory pressure (PEEP).[67] Care must be taken to ensure that proper ventilator settings are selected to prevent negative airway pressure from occurring during closed system suctioning, leading to mucosal injury and airway collapse.[67] Carlon, Fox, and Ackerman[13] found no clinically significant improvement of oxygenation results when they compared closed and open suction methods.

Since closed suction systems are many times more expensive than regular systems, cost effectiveness should be considered when deciding about generalized use, as should the fact that closed suction systems prevent dissemination of contaminated secretions—an important factor when choosing equipment and technique.

**Duration of suctioning.** The effect of limiting the duration of suctioning is not as clear-cut as it once seemed. Medical personnel have been admonished to limit suctioning to 10-second periods, but some studies have indicated little change in the fall of the $PaO_2$ after the initial 5 seconds of suctioning, even when periods ranging from 10 to 45 seconds in duration were used.[4] Recent advances in fiberoptic pulmonary catheters allow continuous measurements of mixed venous oxygen saturations; when available, the effects of suctioning duration can be readily monitored, allowing moment-to-moment variation of suctioning time. When mixed venous oxygen saturation monitoring is unavailable, oximetry can be used, even though its response to changes in oxygenation is somewhat delayed.

**Saline solution instillation.** One practice commonly used to manage tenacious secretions is the instillation of 2 to 5 ml of sterile saline solution through an artificial airway into the tracheobronchial tree. Hanley[30] found normal saline solution instillations resulted in an unpredictable distribution of saline solution within the lungs and that blind suctioning removed little of the instilled saline solution from the airways. Because mucus and saline solution do not easily mix, instilling saline solution acts more as a lavage.[60] The concept of bronchial lavage during suctioning has further been explored by Muto.[49] He also found saline solution injected at the opening of the endotracheal or tracheostomy tube did not result in liquefying secretions and was not all retrieved by regular suctioning methods. In an attempt to improve suctioning technique, he developed Irri-Cath™, a double-lumen catheter that irrigates and suctions simultaneously.[49] Muto and his colleagues have used this technique on intubated patients at Massachusetts General Hospital and believe the Irri-Cath reduces the tracheobronchial irritation associated with suctioning, significantly decreases the incidence of bronchoscopy for retained secretions, and speeds the recovery of patients who have secretion problems.[49] This technique has not been widely adopted as of this writing, and further investigation by other practitioners is needed to determine its efficacy versus that of saline solution instillations.

**Suctioning guidelines.** The use of suctioning can be hazardous in unstable critically ill patients. Factors that signal a higher risk for side effects from suctioning are the presence of a $PaO_2 < 70$ mm Hg, a wide alveolar to arterial (A-a) gradient, shock, dysrhythmias, or acid-base imbalances.

Since, at best, no clear procedure exists to eliminate the hazards of tracheal suctioning, the procedure should be performed only when necessary. Routine suctioning should be avoided because it increases respiratory tract trauma, stimulates secretion production, increases the risk of infection, and exposes the patient to other complications previously outlined.

## MECHANICAL VENTILATION

**Mechanical ventilation** is used to treat hypoxemia and tissue hypoxia, to maintain positive pressure in the airways throughout the respiratory cycle, to lessen the work of breathing, and to provide ventilation for patients who cannot, themselves, effectively ventilate. The most common indication for mechanical ventilation is impending or actual acute ventilatory failure defined as an arterial partial pressure of carbon dioxide ($PaCO_2$) >50 mm Hg with a pH less than 7.25. Reversal of this process is desired while minimizing the complications of mechanical ventilation. Mechanical ventilators work through either negative or positive pressure applied to the chest.

### Negative Pressure Ventilators

Negative pressure ventilators were the first type developed. The iron lung, or tank ventilator, fits over the patient's entire body except for his or her head and generates a negative pressure gradient that moves air into the lung. These ventilators prohibit access to the patient and are not practical for this reason. However, negative pressure therapy can benefit patients with (1) hypoventilation caused by mechanical (chest wall or neuromuscular) abnormalities, (2) hypoventilation caused by central respiratory system abnormalities, and (3) hypoxemic respiratory failure.[7]

Some of the benefits of negative pressure ventilation include the following[7]:

- Avoidance of an artificial airway—especially advantageous when long-term ventilation is needed
- Improved arterial oxygenation in spontaneously breathing adults with progressive pulmonary disease
- Decreased need for sedation and muscle relaxants
- Decreased work of breathing when used as intermittent therapy
- Alternative to electrophrenic pacing for some patients with primary alveolar hypoventilation

### Positive Pressure Ventilators

Positive pressure ventilators achieve lung inflation by applying intermittent positive pressure ventilation (IPPV) or continuous positive pressure ventilation (CPPV) to the airway. This requires a relatively airtight seal between the patient and the ventilator, which is usually achieved by a balloon-cuffed tracheal or endotracheal tube. Positive pressure ventilators may be subdivided into volume-cycled, pressure-cycled, and time-cycled machines. Some newer generation ventilators can vary the cycling mechanism.

Volume ventilators are designed to deliver a preset volume of gas to the patient. The machine can deliver the volume of gas despite changes in pressure within the patient's lungs. To avoid barotrauma to the lungs, pressure limits can be programmed into the ventilator. When the pressure limit is exceeded, the ventilator will "spill" the remaining volume of gas out of the system, but barring this situation, the ventilator will deliver the set volume throughout considerable pressure ranges.

Pressure ventilators deliver gas until a preset pressure is reached; thus the volume delivered varies when the pressure within the patient's lungs increases or decreases for any reason. Pressure ventilators are not useful for ventilation of critically ill patients because pressure ventilators do not adapt well to changes in lung compliance and resistance. Also, many pressure-cycled ventilators cannot deliver positive end-expiratory pressure (PEEP), limiting their application.

Time-cycled ventilators deliver gas during a preset time interval. They are less popular because of the difficulty in delivering consistent tidal volumes in the presence of changing respiratory dynamics.

Newer generation ventilators are equipped with computers, internal mechanisms that allow the choice of various modes of ventilation, and built-in features that provide continuous compliance measurements and display of volume pressure curves. Most modern ventilators allow application of various modes of therapy and fine adjustment of inspired oxygen. Oxygen delivery can vary precisely from 21% (room air) to 100%.

High-frequency ventilation, a new addition to the positive pressure family, delivers small tidal volumes at a high ventilatory rate in an effort to reduce the barotrauma and the cardiac complications associated with normal-frequency mechanical ventilation. Three systems have evolved using high-frequency ventilation—high-frequency jet ventilation, high-frequency positive pressure ventilation, and high-frequency oscillation (Table 12-5).

**Modes of application.** The term ventilator mode refers to how the machine ventilates for the patient. Selection of a particular **mode of ventilation** determines how much the patient will participate in his own ventilatory pattern (see the box, "Modes of Mechanical Ventilation," p. 282). Choice depends on the patient's situation, as well as the personal biases and experiences of the clinicians.

Intermittent mandatory ventilation (IMV) has many advocates. This mode allows the spontaneously breathing patient to continue breathing while the ventilator periodically gives a selected breath. Proponents of IMV argue that it reduces the need for muscle paralysis and sedation, prevents a patient's "bucking" the ventilator, and achieves a more normal ventilation/perfusion (V/Q) matching.

IMV may relieve the detrimental reduction in cardiac output associated with positive pressure ventilation. This is more likely true if the patient is not exposed to significant increases in the work of breathing as a result of IMV. Synchronized intermittent mandatory ventilation (SIMV) was developed to prevent "stacking" of respirations, which could occur when random periodic breaths were given by the ventilator to spontaneously breathing patients. The SIMV system depends on a demand valve, which senses a fall in airway pressure as the patient begins to inhale and opens to allow spontaneous inhalation. Some demand valves require too much inspiratory effort on the part of the patient and greatly increase the work of breathing to the patient's detriment.

Various settings on the ventilator allow individualizing the parameters to a patient requiring support. The basic group of settings found on most modern ventilators is outlined in the box, "Definitions of Basic Ventilator Settings," p. 283.

**Positive end-expiratory pressure.** One of the most controversial areas of ventilator setting is the **positive end-expiratory pressure (PEEP)** adjustment.[39] When PEEP is used it maintains an airway pressure greater than atmospheric pressure at the end of exhalation. This pressure increases alveolar volume and/or recruits previously collapsed alveoli. The overall effect is to increase the FRC. In patients with diffuse infiltrative pulmonary disease, application of PEEP decreases hypoxemia and often allows reduction of $FIO_2$ to less toxic levels. Statements about PEEP's reducing or redistributing lung fluid in patients with noncardiogenic edema have not been supported by current studies.[47] In some circumstances, PEEP has been effective in improving oxygenation and reducing intrapulmonary shunts.

PEEP indicates positive airway pressure at the end of exhalation. Various forms of breathing circuits achieve this state (see the box, "Forms of Positive Expiratory Pressure,"

***Table 12-5*** Modes of high-frequency ventilation

| Mode | Respiratory rate per minute | Tidal volume | Peak inspiratory pressure | Comment |
|---|---|---|---|---|
| High-frequency positive pressure ventilation | 60 to 100 | 3 to 5 ml/kg body weight | Low | Similar to conventional IPPV |
| High-frequency jet ventilation | 100 to 200 | 3 to 5 ml/kg body weight | Low | Short bursts delivered into upper airways; requires a special "jet" ventilator |
| High-frequency oscillation | 60 to 3600 | Less than 3 ml/kg body weight | Low | Uses piston, or audio loud-speaker, or flow interrupter to oscillate column of gases in airway |

From Scanlan CL, Spearman CB, and Sheldon RL: Egan's fundamentals of respiratory care, St Louis, 1990, Mosby–Year Book, Inc.

## MODES OF MECHANICAL VENTILATION

### CONTROLLED MECHANICAL VENTILATION (CMV)

Delivery of a preset number of breaths per minute at a preset volume. Breathing cannot be triggered by the patient. *Use:* apneic patient secondary to brain damage, muscle paralysis, sedation.

### ASSISTED MECHANICAL VENTILATION (AMV)

Ventilator triggered by the patient's inspiratory effort. Patient controls the rate of breathing while the ventilator controls the tidal volume ($V_T$) and performs the work. The patient continues to perform a significant amount of the work of breathing (WOB) rather than passively inhaling; excessive inspiratory effort can occur.

### ASSIST-CONTROL VENTILATION (ACV)

Delivery of a breath triggered by the inspiratory effort of the patient after a preselected time interval has elapsed. A back-up rate is set, which will support the patient if his or her respiratory efforts fall below the set ventilator rate. *Use:* wide range of patients who are spontaneously breathing but who have ventilatory failure or gas exchange inefficiency.

### INTERMITTENT MANDATORY VENTILATION (IMV) AND SYNCHRONIZED INTERMITTENT MANDATORY VENTILATION (SIMV)

Receipt by spontaneously breathing patient of periodic positive pressure breaths at a selected rate. SIMV is a modification that synchronizes the mechanical breath and patient's spontaneous breathing. *Uses:* wide range of patients with need for ventilator support and as a method of systematic weaning.

### PRESSURE SUPPORT VENTILATION (PSV)

Also called inspiratory flow assistance. To decrease the WOB, PSV combines the features of assisted ventilation and continuous positive airway pressure (CPAP). When triggered, the ventilator applies a small amount of positive pressure to the airways. It is intended to overcome resistance and thereby decrease the WOB, improve mixed venous oxgyen saturation ($S\bar{v}O_2$), and lower minute ventilation ($\dot{V}_E$), respiratory rate, and oxygen consumption ($\dot{V}O_2$). *Uses:* spontaneously breathing patient and weaning.[47]

### PRESSURE-CONTROLLED INVERTED RATIO VENTILATION (PC-IRV) AND INVERSE INSPIRATORY TO EXPIRATORY VENTILATION (IVR)

Also called prolonged inspiratory time ventilation. *Uses:* inspiratory:expiratory (I:E) ratios as high as 3:1 or 4:1 in treating hypoxemic patients not responding to other mechanical ventilatory forms; adult respiratory distress syndrome (ARDS); limited study—still considered experimental.

### DIFFERENTIAL LUNG VENTILATION (DLV)

Also known as independent lung ventilation and selective PEEP. A modified technique of one-lung ventilation is used in surgery. DLV requires intubation with a double-lumen endotracheal tube (Carlen, Ravanian, Robertshaw, Univent, or Broncho-cath) and allows establishment of separate ventilator parameters for each lung. It can be arranged by using (1) one ventilator with adjustable circuits, (2) two asynchronous ventilators independently delivering ventilation, (3) two synchronized ventilators using separate circuits, (4) one volume ventilator and one high-frequency ventilator, (5) two CPAP circuits, or (6) one ventilator and one CPAP circuit. *Uses:* severe unilateral asymmetric lung disease such as in patients with trauma, bronchopleural fistula, pneumonia, or an aspiration lung disorder.[47]

p. 284). When PEEP is used with intermittent mandatory ventilation, the patient receives continuous positive pressure ventilation (CPPV) with ventilator breaths and continuous positive airway pressure (CPAP) with spontaneous breaths.

PEEP should be instituted and discontinued in a planned, systematic manner in which (1) PEEP is the only variable manipulated, (2) adjustments in PEEP are made at 3 to 5 cm $H_2O$ at a time, and (3) the time interval between change and evaluation is held at more than 20 minutes to judge responses adequately.[47]

The patient response to PEEP is evaluated in various ways. Some clinicians use changes in shunt fraction, some use level of $FIO_2$, whereas others use mixed venous oxygen (see box, "Bases for Selection of Best Level of PEEP," p. 284). Abrupt institution or withdrawal of high levels of PEEP can create problems associated with cardiac output and hypoxemia.

When PEEP is used, the risk of barotrauma is increased, especially in patients with unilateral lung disease or emphysema. It is not generally used in patients with chronic obstructive pulmonary disease (COPD), but improper adjustment of ventilator settings can result in "auto-PEEP." Auto-PEEP occurs with incomplete emptying of a lung area, which can occur when the respiratory rate is fast and the I:E ratio is too short. The presence of auto-PEEP can be evaluated by occluding the exhalation port at the end of exhalation and reading the pressure dial. A positive pressure reading indicates auto-PEEP is occurring.

### Summary of Nursing Care for the Patient on Mechanical Ventilation

**Routine assessments.** Refer to the box on p. 286 for nursing diagnoses and management of controlled mechanical ventilation. Routine monitoring of ventilator function

## DEFINITIONS OF BASIC VENTILATOR SETTINGS

### RESPIRATORY RATE

Number of breaths the ventilator will deliver per minute. It may be exceeded by a spontaneously breathing patient in assist-control and intermittent mandatory ventilation (IMV) modes. Total respiratory rate equals patient rate plus ventilator rate. Common starting rate is 12 to 14 per minute. Adjust rate to pH and $Paco_2$.

### TIDAL VOLUME

Volume delivered to patient during a normal ventilator breath. Usual volume is selected 5 to 15 cc/kg.

### INSPIRATORY:EXPIRATORY (I:E) RATIO

#### Peak flow rate

Maximal flow rate that machine delivers during tidal breath.

#### Inspiratory flow rate

Some machines allow separate adjustment of flow rate, whereas in other machines, flow rate is determined by tidal volume, respiratory rate, and I:E ratio. Majority of ventilators deliver a square flow wave pattern (⎍), with a rapid rise in flow that remains constant throughout inhalation. Some ventilators have tapered flow patterns (⋀_). The I:E ratio should be 1:1.5 or 1:2 to allow complete exhalation and to avoid air trapping.

#### I:E ratio

Adjusted directly on time-cycled ventilators. It is determined by tidal volume and rate of inspiratory flow on volume-regulated ventilators. Usually a 1:2 ratio is sought unless inverse ratio ventilation is in use.

### SENSITIVITY

A control that adjusts the ventilatory response to patient respiratory effort. In the control mode, sensitivity is off, so the machine does not respond to spontaneous patient effort. Otherwise, sensitivity is adjusted to allow the patient to initiate a ventilator (AC mode) breath or to breathe spontaneously (IMV mode).

### SIGHS

Allows periodic selection of a larger-than-normal tidal volume. This feature substitutes for the normal sighing reflex. It is purported to prevent microatelectasis and intrapulmonary shunting. Usually sigh volumes are 1½ to 2 times tidal volume. Frequency can be individualized. If regular tidal volume is >7 cc/kg, sighing may not be necessary.

### POSITIVE END-EXPIRATORY PRESSURE (PEEP)

Available on most ventilators. PEEP maintains greater than atmospheric pressure in airways at the completion of exhalation, serving to increase the functional residual capacity (FRC). It is adjusted up to 20 cm $H_2O$. Greater amounts are not recommended because of adverse effect on cardiac output.

### PRESSURE LIMITS

Adjustable setting to regulate the maximal pressure the machine can generate to deliver the tidal volume. Once the pressure limit is reached, ventilator will spill undelivered tidal or sigh volume to the atmosphere to protect the patient from barotrauma. Limit is usually established as 12 to 20 cm $H_2O$ above the normal ventilating pressure. Audible and visual alarms are used to signal excess pressure.

### OXYGEN CONCENTRATION ($FIo_2$)

Selects delivery of oxygen between 21% and 100%. The concentration of oxygen should be kept at the lowest possible level to prevent oxygen toxicity. Concentrations <50% are desirable.

### MONITORS/ALARMS

Devices on ventilators to track the volumes and $FIo_2$ delivered. Many ventilators have a spirometer to monitor tidal volumes. Audible and visual alarms signal improper amounts.

is important to patient safety. This task is generally performed by respiratory therapists on an hourly or as-needed basis. Even so, the nursing staff needs to verify respiratory settings, monitors, and alarms as part of patient assessment and care. Table 12-6 reviews ventilator alarms.

Monitoring should also encompass evaluation of the patient's status in relationship to desired outcomes of ventilation and to prevent or minimize complications associated with respiratory therapy. Bedside evaluation of vital capacity, minute ventilation, arterial blood gas (ABG) values, and other pulmonary function tests may be warranted, according to the patient's condition.

Static and dynamic compliance should be monitored. Some newer generation ventilators give a continuous display of volume-pressure curves and exhaled carbon dioxide, allowing moment-to-moment evaluation of respiratory function and immediate intervention as needed. Compliance and resistance can be approximated on older ventilators by excluding the exhalation port at the end of exhalation.

**Assessment for complications of mechanical ventilation.** Mechanical ventilation is often lifesaving, but like other interventions, it is not without its own complications. Some complications are preventable, whereas others can be minimized but not eradicated (see the box, "Complications

## FORMS OF POSITIVE EXPIRATORY PRESSURE

### CONTINUOUS POSITIVE AIRWAY PRESSURE (CPAP)

Used in the spontaneously breathing patient who may or may not be intubated.

***Advantages***

- Keeps airway pressure greater than ambient pressure throughout inhalation and exhalation
- Provides patient with alternative to mechanical ventilatory support; may be useful in treating cardiac pulmonary edema because CPAP improves oxygenation and decreases venous return
- Does not require intubation

***Disadvantages***

- Aerophagia and gastric distention
- Aspiration of stomach contents
- Decreased cardiac output
- Barotrauma
- Facial erosion and irritation from CPAP mask
- Patient discomfort and poor tolerance

The CPAP mask requires a light, airtight seal; its recommended time for use is 6 to 12 hours. The CPAP mask is used intermittently as a postoperative treatment and as a nighttime prevention of acute respiratory failure in the patient with neurological disease.

### Expiratory positive airway pressure (EPAP)

Used in spontaneously breathing patients. It has greater swings in airway pressure and thus increases the work of breathing significantly over that with CPAP and for that reason is not widely used.

### Continous positive pressure breathing (CPPB)

Term used when the patient is in the assist-control mode. CPPB triggers inhalation by creating ventilator sub-PEEP pressure rather than subatmospheric pressure. CPPB implies a small decrease in positive pressure before inhalation, but airway pressure remains above atmospheric pressure.

### Continuous positive pressure ventilation (CPPV)

Patient ventilated throughout controlled mechanical ventilation mode. It allows application of PEEP without a fall in airway pressure.

***Disadvantages***

- Cardiac output can fall more than with other forms of mechanical support associated with PEEP.

### POSITIVE END-EXPIRATORY PRESSURE (PEEP)

Maintains pressure in the airway above atmospheric pressure at end of exhalation, therefore adding to FRC with PEEP up to 15 cm $H_2O$. PEEP increases alveolar diameter and improves arterial oxygenation. Most popular methods of application involve the following:

1. Best PEEP (best compliance as seen by pressure-volume curve)[47]
2. Optimal PEEP (lowest shunt fraction [$Q_S/Q_T$])[39,47]
3. Least PEEP (lowest pressure in cm $H_2O$ that provides arterial partial pressure of oxygen [$Pa_{O_2}$] >60 mmHg with $F_{IO_2}$ <0.60)[39,47]

***Advantages***

- Increases FRC
- Decreases shunting
- Allows use of lower levels of $F_{IO_2}$

***Disadvantages***

- Increases risk of barotrauma
- Reduces cardiac output
- Generally contraindicated in patients with unilateral lung disease[39]

Associated With Mechanical Ventilation," p. 286, for common side effects).

Changes in cardiac output become more pronounced in hypoxemic patients. Ensuring adequate vascular volume will negate the decreased cardiac output in some patients. Continuous positive pressure ventilation (CPPV) or positive pressure ventilation with PEEP has the most dramatic effect on decreasing cardiac output. This decrease in cardiac output relates to the positive pressure that is maintained in the thoracic cavity throughout the respiratory cycle, which serves to decrease venous return and cardiac filling. PEEP also increases right-ventricular afterload, which causes dilation of the right ventricle and subsequent shifting of the intraventricular septum leftward.[47]

The displaced septum, in addition to compression of the left ventricle by distended lungs, further reduces cardiac output. Decreased cardiac output is not always associated with impaired tissue perfusion and hypoxemia. Adequacy

## BASES FOR SELECTION OF BEST LEVEL OF PEEP

1. Greatest oxygenation as determined by $Pa_{O_2}$ or $Pa_{O_2}/F_{IO_2}$ fraction
2. Best compliance as seen by pressure volume curve
3. Lowest dead space/tidal volume ratio ($V_D/V_T$); lowest $V_D/V_T$ occurs at greatest compliance
4. Lowest pulmonary vascular resistance
5. Lowest shunt fraction ($Q_S/Q_T$); a shunt of 15% or a $Pa_{O_2}$ to $F_{IO_2}$ ratio of 300 or more is frequently chosen
6. Lowest $PA_{CO_2}$-$Pe_{CO_2}$ gradient; when dead space increases, cardiac output decreases
7. Least amount of PEEP to provide $Pa_{O_2}$ >60 mm Hg, with $F_{IO_2}$ <0.6

Modified from MacDonnell K, Fahey P, and Segal M: Respiratory intensive care, Boston, 1987, Little, Brown & Co, Inc.

**Table 12-6** Ventilator alarms and nursing actions

| Tidal volume less than pre-set | Low-pressure alarm | High-pressure alarm | PEEP (low alarm) | Auto (intrinsic PEEP) | Apnea alarm |
|---|---|---|---|---|---|
| Partial or complete disconnection from ventilator<br>Leak in patient breathing circuit (tubing)<br>Malfunction in the exhaled Vt spirometer<br>Lack of seal at tracheostomy or endotracheal tube<br>Malfunction in the volume ventilator<br>1. If discrepancy between measured Vt and preset value is greater than 20%, or if there is an alteration in clinical state ( agitation, obtundation, decrease BP), disconnect patient from ventilator.<br>2. Manually "hand bag" the patient.<br>3. If leaks persist with hand-bag system, endotracheal or tracheostomy tube is malfunctioning. Air may be felt or heard escaping, the patient may talk or make sounds.<br>4. If leak is positional (i.e., seen with tracheal dilation), reposition tube and/or patient.<br>5. If not positional, recheck pilot balloon.<br>6. If leak remains, endotracheal tube should be replaced, contact physician and coordinate arrangements.<br>7. If leak resolves with "bagging," the problem is in ventilator system. Check all connections and tubing. Correct and reconnect patient to ventilator.<br>8. If malfunction cannot be easily corrected, contact respiratory therapy. Maintain patient ventilation. | Alarm indicates leak<br>1. Employ same schemas as low Vt state.<br>2. If patient is receiving CPAP, then the low-pressure alarm system is the only indication of a disconnection or major leak. | Indicates change either in "system" resistance (e.g., $H_2O$ in breathing circuit or secretions, bronchospasm, or obstruction in the endotracheal tube) or change in lung compliance<br>1. Inspect tubing, check for kinks in tubing, patient clamping down on tube, and suction patient.<br>2. Observe ease or difficulty in passing catheter through the endotracheal or tracheostomy tube.<br>3. Listen for bilateral lung sounds, check level of tube for depth or insertion; if questions remain about tube placement, check chest x-ray film.<br>4. Patient may be "bucking" the ventilator—assess need to sedate, give support and reassurance. If anxiety and agitation exist, rule out hypercapnia and hypoxemia before sedating the patient. | Indicates leaks in system or mechanical failure of PEEP mechanism<br>1. Check "system" similar to Vt leak.<br>2. Call respiratory therapy personnel. | Ventilator pressure manometer reads zero during exhalation; therefore must check during no-flow state. Occlude exhalation port at end exhalation; manometer should read zero.<br>1. If auto PEEP is present, allow more time for exhalation. "Stacking" (inhalation occurring while patient is still exhaling) can be detected if a volume displacement spirometer is in use. | Can be triggered by IMV/SIMV or CPAP modes when patient does not initiate breath within preset time unit.<br>1. Assess patient for fatigue or change in status. Frequent periods of apnea may necessitate more controlled breaths. |

*Always ensure that an adequate $FIO_2$ is used; use $FIO_2$1.0 if in doubt. When in doubt, manual resuscitation should be used and ventilator replaced.*

Modified from MacDonnell K, Fahey P, and Segal M: Respiratory intensive care, Boston, 1987, Little, Brown & Co.

**Nursing Diagnosis and Management**
***Controlled mechanical ventilation***

- Ineffective Breathing Pattern related to respiratory muscle deconditioning secondary to mechanical ventilation, p. 471
- Ineffective Airway Clearance related to impaired cough secondary to loss of glottic closure with cuffed endotracheal/tracheostomy tube, p. 468
- High Risk for Aspiration Risk Factors: Tracheostomy or endotracheal tube, impaired swallowing, facial/oral/neck surgery or trauma, wired jaws, p. 476
- Decreased Cardiac Output related to decreased preload secondary to mechanical ventilation with or without PEEP, p. 457
- Sleep Pattern Disturbance related to fragmented sleep and/or circadian desynchronization, p. 455
- Body Image Disturbance related to functional dependence on life-sustaining technology, p. 443
- Powerlessness related to health care environment or illness-related regimen, p. 445
- Ineffective Individual Coping related to situational crisis and personal vulnerability, p. 447
- Anxiety related to threat to biological, psychological, or social integrity, p. 448

of cardiac output can be monitored by evaluating the mixed venous oxygen and by assessing the patient. Retarded venous return to the heart has been implicated as a causative factor in hepatic dysfunction and in increased intracranial pressure associated with mechanical ventilation. Further studies must focus on these complications to determine if mechanical ventilation is the only cause involved.

**Weaning from mechanical ventilation.** Weaning patients from mechanical ventilation can be a painstaking, lengthy task. Some of the factors that may contribute to this difficulty are continued lung disease or dysfunction, respiratory muscle fatigue, pharmacological interventions, and alterations in ventilatory drive.[57] Weaning should begin only after the acute disease(s) requiring ventilator support for the patient have been corrected and patient stability has been achieved.[38] Once this stage of illness has been reached, spontaneous breathing mechanics should be evaluated.

Patients who can maintain an arterial oxygen saturation at 90% on an $FIO_2$ of 0.21 while breathing spontaneously with a continuous positive airway pressure (CPAP) of $<5$ cm $H_2O$ have a 94% success rate for weaning.[47] Many physiological parameters are followed during the course of mechanical ventilation to gauge the patient's readiness for weaning.

**COMPLICATIONS ASSOCIATED WITH MECHANICAL VENTILATION**

**UPPER AIRWAY TRAUMA CAUSED BY INTUBATION**

Dental damage
Nasal damage
Vocal cord hematoma
Laryngeal edema
Tracheal ulcers
Tracheal dilation
Tracheal stenosis
Tracheoesophageal fistula
Laryngeal stenosis
Tracheomalacia

**INCREASED WORK OF BREATHING**

Caused by decreased lumen size of artificial airways
Caused by breathing through synchronized intermittent mandatory ventilator circuitry or by presence of auto-PEEP

**INFECTION**

From equipment contamination
From colonization of lower tract through artificial airway tube

**BAROTRAUMA**

Pneumomediastinum
Subcutaneous emphysema
Pneumothorax
Pneumoperitoneum

**REDUCED CARDIAC OUTPUT**

Caused by decreased venous return
Caused by increased right-ventricular afterload
Caused by decreased left-ventricular distensibility
Leads to subsequent alteration in renal, hepatic, cerebral function

The box, "Criteria for Weaning," lists the parameters and describes values most authorities believe are necessary before weaning from mechanical ventilation can be attempted.

***General principles of weaning.*** The success of weaning is dependent on the underlying disease of the patient and the length of ventilator support. Patients with several underlying diseases, with severe chronic obstructive pulmonary disease (COPD), or who have been ventilated in excess of 30 days can pose special problems during weaning.[47] However, before attempting to discontinue mechanical ventilation, certain factors should be considered.

The patient should be stable without support of vasopressors for 12 to 24 hours before weaning. Some clinicians may use low-dose dopamine to augment renal blood flow or low-dose nitroglycerin to prevent cardiac decompensation resulting from a sudden increase in venous return, which

### CRITERIA FOR WEANING

**DEGREE OF SHUNT**

Less than 0.20 or P(A-a) $O_2$ gradient <350 mm Hg (or 100%)[10]

**DEAD SPACE TO TIDAL VOLUME**

Dead space less than 0.6 of tidal volume ($V_D/V_T$ ratio <0.6)[64]

**VITAL CAPACITY (VC)**

VC >10 cc/kg or 20% to 25% of predicted normal[38,64]

**MAXIMAL VOLUNTARY VENTILATION (MVV)**

Patient able to double minute ventilation on demand, generally indicating a reserve for breathing independently[64]

**INSPIRATORY FORCE**

Patient able to generate at least −20 to −25 cm $H_2O$ pressure for adequate spontaneous ventilation[42]

**FORCED EXPIRATORY VOLUME IN ONE SECOND ($FEV_1$)**

Needs to move 10 cc/kg for successful weaning[10]

**RESPIRATORY RATE (RR)/MINUTE VENTILATION ($\dot{V}_E$)**

Resting, spontaneous RR <30/minute and resting, spontaneous $\dot{V}_E$ <10 L/minute

will occur when positive pressure ventilation is discontinued.[47] The patient should be clear of any significant infection before weaning proceeds.

Special attention should be given to the patient's nutritional status. Often, ventilator patients, because of their overall condition and inability to take food orally, are receiving parenteral or enteral feedings. Studies have demonstrated excessive carbon dioxide production from carbohydrate calories can create hypercapnia during weaning.[20] Recent studies suggest critically ill hospitalized patients require approximately 2000 cal/day, which is much less than previously believed. Some sources recommend reducing caloric intake by 50% once weaning is instituted.[20]

The patient's pH, $Paco_2$, and $Pao_2$ should be comparable to baseline, preintubation levels before weaning is undertaken.

Weaning difficult patients such as those with COPD or on long-term ventilator support should be a systematic purposeful process that takes advantage of the patient's best energy level and allows rest and sleep because sleep deprivation interferes with weaning. Early daytime weaning will probably be more successful.

Weaning difficult patients requires their cooperation. Discrete, attainable goals should be set to avoid overexertion and respiratory muscle fatigue on the part of the patient. Failure at weaning attempts may result in patient depression or despondency.

While weaning is in process, the patient should be monitored for signs of fatigue, hypoxemia, and tissue hypoxia.

Once the patient has been weaned, the endotracheal or tracheal tube should be removed unless some condition is present that contraindicates this action.

### INDICATIONS FOR CHEST TUBE DRAINAGE

Pneumothorax >20%
- Traumatic
- Spontaneous
- Tension pneumothorax

Hemothorax >500 cc

Pneumohemothorax
- Surgically induced
- After chest surgery
- Traumatic

Pleural effusion

Mechanically ventilated patients with any size pneumothorax or hemothorax

## CHEST TUBES

Chest tubes are inserted into the pleural space to remove fluid or air and reinstate the negative intrapleural pressure and reexpand collapsed lungs or portions of the lungs. The box, "Indications for Chest Tube Drainage," outlines the major indications for chest tubes. A review of pleural membrane physiology is presented in the boxes on p. 288.

When chest tubes are needed for removal of air, insertion is at the second or third intercostal space of the anterior thoracic wall. This location best removes air which rises to the top of the pleural space, as opposed to the fluid, which gravitates to the lowest level of the space. Placement of chest tubes to drain fluid is low in the thoracic cavity at the sixth, seventh, or eighth intercostal space. Some patient situations call for placement of tubes at both locations to evacuate both air and fluid. Once the chest tube is placed, it is connected to a water-seal drainage system.

Water-seal drainage systems have evolved from separate glass bottles of one, two, or three containers into a self-contained disposable plastic unit that can be used in various modes.

The drainage system is aseptically prepared for use, with sterile water placed in the water seal and suction control chambers. Usually the water-seal chamber is filled at the 2-cm to 3-cm level, and the suction-control chamber is filled with 15 to 25 cm of water. When only air is being evacuated, lower levels of suction can be used. Connection points of the drainage tubing should be sealed with tape and an oc-

## WHY THE LUNGS STAY INFLATED

The lungs stay inflated because the pressure surrounding them (intrapleural) is always less than the pressure within them (intrapulmonary).

### WHY IS THE INTRAPLEURAL PRESSURE LESS THAN THE INTRAPULMONARY PRESSURE?

The intrapleural pressure is always (1) less than intrapulmonary pressure, (2) less than atmospheric pressure, and (3) considered negative because of the "pull" of the two pleural membranes in opposite directions. The parietal pleura is pulled outward by forces within the chest wall, whereas the visceral pleural is pulled inward by the force of the elastic fibers within the lungs.

### WHY DO THE TWO PLEURAL MEMBRANES "PULL" IN OPPOSITE DIRECTIONS?

The parietal pleura, attached to the chest, is pulled outward because the elastic fibers within the intercostal muscles exert outward pressure on the ribs. These fibers are in a relaxed state when the rib cage is fully expanded such as during a deep inhalation. The visceral pleural, attached to the lungs, is pulled inward because the elastic fibers within the lungs, responsible for elastic recoil, exert pressure to make the lungs smaller. Elastic fibers in the lungs are only in a relaxed position when the lung is at its smallest configuration such as occurs with a pneumothorax. Hence, because of the opposite pull of the chest wall and the lung and because the pleural membranes are attached to these structures, there is a constant pull of the two membranes in opposite directions. The subatmospheric pressure, which results within the pleural space, plus the greater than atmospheric intrapulmonary pressure within the lungs allow the lungs to remain inflated. Anything that causes the pressure within the pleural space to rise to atmospheric pressure or above will cause the lung(s) to collapse—a pneumothorax.

clusive dressing applied at the chest tube sight. Petroleum (Vaseline) gauze, once used at all chest tube insertion sites, has been eliminated from use except when the tube is inadvertently removed, and the use of only a dry sterile gauze with tape is necessary because the suction is believed to remove any air leak from around the chest tube insertion point.

Once the chest tubes are placed, efforts are directed at maintaining the patency and sterility of the system. The one-unit disposable system improves the maintenance of sterility. When drainage occurs in excess of the system's capacity, a new setup is used, or, in the case of some systems, the drainage container can be easily removed and replaced. The disposable systems also have self-sealing sampling ports that allow obtaining drainage for examination without interruption of the integrity of the unit.

## PLEURAL MEMBRANES

The pleural membranes consist of two serous membranes—the parietal and visceral pleurae. The parietal pleura is attached to the thoracic wall; the visceral pleura is attached to the lungs and covers them completely. Both surfaces have a blood and lymphatic supply through which they secrete and absorb fluid. In healthy individuals, there is a continuous filtration of fluid from the capillaries of the parietal pleura into the capillaries of the visceral pleura. However, since pleural fluid is constantly being secreted and absorbed, at any one time there are only 3 to 5 ml within the pleural space, and excess fluid is removed by the lymphatic system.[55] Pleural fluid allows the visceral and parietal pleural membranes to glide against each other during inhalation and exhalation. Patients who have experienced a loss of pleural fluid or inflammation of the pleural space (pleuritis) often report severe, painful breathing.

### PLEURAL SPACE

There are two main issues of importance regarding the pleural space. First, the pleural space has a pressure within it called *intrapleural pressure,* which differs in value from intraalveolar and atmospheric pressures. Second, the pleural space has the capacity to hold much more fluid than its normal volume of a few milliliters.

### INTRAPLEURAL PRESSURE

Normally, intrapleural pressure is less than intra-pulmonary pressure* and less than atmospheric pressure. Atmospheric pressure, in pulmonary physiology, is assigned a value of zero; any pressure less than atmospheric pressure is negative, and any pressure greater than atmospheric pressure is positive.[45] Zero is used in reference to atmospheric pressure to simplify terminology. Atmospheric pressure at sea level is approximately 760 mm Hg; intrapleural pressure and intrapulmonary pressure vary from slightly above to slightly below 760 mm Hg.

Since under normal conditions intrapleural pressure is less than atmospheric pressure, it is recorded as a negative number, with a normal range of $-4$ cm $H_2O$ to $-10$ cm $H_2O$ during exhalation and inhalation, respectively. A deep inhalation can generate intrapleural pressures of $-12$ to $-18$ cm $H_2O$.

This negative intrapleural pressure results because forces within the chest wall exert pressure to pull the parietal pleura (attached to the chest wall) outward and away from the visceral pleura (attached to the lungs) while the elastic fibers within the lungs exert pressure to pull the visceral pleura inward away from the parietal pleura. The constant "pull" of the two pleural membranes in opposite directions from each other causes the pressure within the space to be subatmospheric.

This subatmospheric pressure functions in a very important manner—it keeps the lungs inflated (see the box at left). If atmospheric pressure enters the pleural space, all or part of a lung will collapse, producing a pneumothorax (frequently, a pneumothorax affects only a portion of one lung).

*Intrapulmonary pressure is also known as intraalveolar pressure and reflects pressure inside the lungs.

Maintaining drainage involves careful attention to the suction applied and to maintenance of unobstructed drainage tubes. Kinks and large loops of tubing should be avoided because they prevent drainage and air evacuation, which may prevent timely lung reexpansion or may result in a tension pneumothorax. Retained drainage also becomes an excellent medium for multiplication of bacteria.

The water-seal chamber must be routinely observed for unexpected bubbling caused by an air leak in the system. When suspicious bubbling is present, the source must be identified. To determine if the source is within the system or within the patient, systematic brief clamping of the drainage tube should be performed. Staying as close to the occlusive dressing as possible, the nurse should place a padded clamp on the drainage tubing. If the air bubbling stops, the air leak is located between the patient and the clamp. The leak can be within the patient or at the insertion site. Therefore the clamp is removed and the chest tube site exposed. The tube is inspected as it enters the chest to make sure all the eyelets are within the patient. If an eyelet port is outside the chest, it can be a source of air leaking into the system and must be occluded, possibly requiring the attention of the physician. When the insertion site has been eliminated as a leakage source, the chest dressing is reapplied, with it completely and securely covering the site.

If the air bubbling does not stop when a clamp is placed on the chest tube, the leak is located between the clamp and the drainage collector. By releasing the clamp and moving down the tubing a few inches at a time until the bubbling stops, the leak is located. If this action is practical, the area of the leak can be taped to reestablish a seal. If this technique proves unreliable or impossible, the system or tubing should be replaced.

Padded clamps and sterile petroleum gauze should be kept at the patient's bedside at all times. If the chest tube or system is inadvertently interrupted, the clamp is applied to the chest tube as close to the insertion site as possible while the drainage system is reestablished. Sterile petroleum gauze is applied to the chest wall if the chest tube is accidentally removed. Implementing both these techniques immediately in such cases will minimize or prevent the formation of a pneumothorax and avoid greater complications.

When a hemothorax is present, drainage must be carefully assessed and measured to avoid the presence of unrecognized bleeding. When the chest tubes are placed after surgery or traumatic injury, fresh blood may be expected immediately. Both the amount and characteristics of the blood should change within a few hours if the bleeding has stopped. Drainage of more than 100 ml/hour for 2 consecutive hours or a sudden change in amount of bloody drainage requires further investigation.[17] The patient should be completely assessed and the physician consulted. In some cases surgical intervention may be necessary. Routine milking or stripping of chest tubes is not recommended because excessive negative pressure can be generated in the chest.[43] Pressures as high as −350 cm $H_2O$ have been recorded using chest strippers, a manual device. If blood clots are present in the drainage tubing or obstruction is present, careful milking of the chest tubes may be performed.

**Nursing Diagnosis and Management**
***Chest tubes***

- Ineffective Breathing Pattern related to modifiable chest wall restrictions secondary to pneumothorax and/or pleural effusion, p. 470
- Ineffective Breathing Pattern related to thoracic pain, p. 472
- Ineffective Airway Clearance related to thoracic pain, p. 469
- Impaired Gas Exchange related to ventilation-perfusion inequality secondary to (specify), p. 474
- Body Image Disturbance related to actual change in body structure, function, or appearance, p. 443

Throughout the duration of chest tube placement, the patient should be periodically assessed for reexpansion of the lung and for complications of chest tube drainage. The nurse should assess the thorax and lungs, paying particular attention to any tracheal deviation, asymmetry of chest movement, presence of subcutaneous emphysema, characteristics of breathing, quality of lung sounds, and presence of tympany or percussion sounds, which are indicative of pneumothorax. Nursing diagnoses and management related to chest tubes are summarized in the box above.

## CHEST PHYSIOTHERAPY

Historically, **chest physiotherapy (CPT)** has been used to supplement the patient's coughing effort or to substitute for it in absent cough states. CPT is directed at improving mucus and sputum clearance and airway function and includes all or various combinations of chest percussion, chest vibration, postural draining, coughing, or suctioning.

Recently, the efficacy of these techniques has been questioned. In an effort to evaluate their overall and specific usefulness in clinical situations, Kirilloff and others[41] completed an extensive review of the investigative studies involving CPT interventions. Their findings and conclusions are briefly summarized in Table 12-7. The reader is encouraged to refer to their original work for a more detailed discussion. The outcomes of their review are pertinent to the nurse clinician because they indicate CPT is not appropriate in every patient population or situation.

Proper application of CPT requires knowledge of the anatomical arrangement of lung segments so that positioning for gravity drainage will result. When positioning a patient, the area of lung to be drained should be uppermost, with the airway as vertical as possible. Because the patient's condition affects his or her ability to tolerate postural drainage, the length of percussion or vibration time will vary. In

***Table 12-7*** Effects of chest physiotherapy on patients with respiratory complications

| Acutely ill patients | Intervention | Outcomes |
|---|---|---|
| With chest radiograph changes and increased secretions | Postural drainage<br>Percussion, deep breathing, coughing, or suctioning | Increased $PaO_2$ 30 minutes after chest physiotherapy (CPT) and at 1 hour<br>Increased sputum expectoration |
| With scant secretions | Same | No improvement in arterial blood gas (ABG) values or volume of sputum<br>No improvement in VC, FEV, FRC<br>Decrease in $PaO_2$ after chest percussion and greater decrease 30 minutes after CPT<br>No improvement in chest radiograph or length of hospital stay |
| **CONCLUSIONS** | | |
| Beneficial to acutely ill patients with increased volume of secretions<br>Beneficial to patients with lobar atelectasis<br>No benefit to patients with status asthmaticus<br>May cause bronchospasm and hypoxemia in acutely ill patients | | |
| With a large volume of secretions (e.g., with cystic fibrosis or bronchiectasis) | CPT versus coughing alone or with forced expiration technique | Coughing and CPT produced approximately equal results in sputum amount and radioaerosol clearance<br>Sputum and radioaerosol clearance increased with forced exhalation techniques over that with cough alone or in combination with postural drainage |
| | CPT | Increased FRC |
| With small volume of secretions | CPT | No improvement in FVC, FEV, or sputum production |
| **GENERAL CONCLUSIONS** | | |
| CPT improves mucous clearance in chronic patients with copious sputum production; directed, coached coughing may be as beneficial as postural drainage in these patients.<br>Forced exhalation techniques may increase sputum clearance with or without postural drainage in patients with chronic copious sputum production.<br>Patients with chronic lung disease who are producing small amounts of sputum show no beneficial changes with CPT. | | |

*VC, Vital capacity; FEV, forced expiratory volume; FRC, functional residual capacity; FVC, forced vital capacity.

critically ill patients, CPT may be required every 2 to 4 hours, but often a routine of performing early morning and late evening CPT is established.[68] CPT should not be performed within 1 hour of eating because of patient discomfort and the possibility of regurgitation and aspiration.[68]

Percussion and vibration, along with postural drainage, constitute CPT. Percussion and vibration help dislodge mucus from airway walls, making its removal by postural drainage and coughing more effective. Percussion uses the nurse's hands in a cupped configuration to clap rhythmically on the patient's chest wall. Percussion (or clapping, as it is also called) is performed for approximately 2 minutes over the thorax of the lung segment requiring drainage.[74] The chest should be covered with a towel during percussion.

Vibration can be performed manually or with the aid of a mechanical vibrator or percussor. When manual vibration is performed, the nurse's flat hands are placed firmly against the chest wall. As the patient exhales, the nurse shakes her arms while pressing on the patient's chest, creating a gentle vibratory sensation in the patient's chest. This technique is repeated two to three times in an area. Vibration or percussion can be used alone or with postural drainage. Vibration is as effective as percussion and may be better tolerated in some critically ill patients.

CPT may be contraindicated in patients with recent hemoptysis or severe hypertension and in patients with unstable hemodynamics. Central nervous system problems such as cerebral aneurysm and edema contradict the use of CPT.[27]

## REFERENCES

1. Adamo JP and others: The Cleveland Clinic's initial experience with transtracheal oxygen therapy, Resp Care 35(2):153, 1990.

2. Albert R: Least PEEP: Primum non nocere (Editorial), Chest 87(1):2, 1987.
3. Aubier M and others: Effect of hypophosphatemia on diaphragmatic contractility in patients with acute respiratory failure, N Engl J Med 313(7):420, 1985.
4. Barnes CA and Kirchhoff KT: Minimizing hypoxemia due to endotracheal suctioning: a review of the literature, Heart Lung 15(2):164-176, 1986.
5. Bernard G and Bradley R: Adult respiratory distress syndrome: diagnosis and management, Heart Lung 15(3):250, 1986.
6. Bernhard W and others: Intracuff pressures in endotracheal and tracheostomy tubes: related cuff physical characteristics, Chest 87(6):720-725, 1985.
7. Blaufuss J and Wallace C: Two negative pressure ventilators: current clinical application and nursing care, Crit Care Nurs Q 9(4):14, 1987.
8. Brown LH: Pulmonary oxygen toxicity, Focus Crit Care 17(1):68, 1990.
9. Burns SM: Advances in ventilator therapy: high frequency, pressure support, and nocturnal nasal positive pressure ventilation, Focus Crit Care 17(3):227, 1990.
10. Burton G and Hodgkin J: Respiratory care: a guide to clinical practice, ed 2, Philadelphia, 1984, JB Lippincott Co.
11. Cane RD and Shapiro BA: Mechanical ventilatory support: concepts in emergency and critical care, JAMA 254(1):87, 1985.
12. Capps J and Schade K: Work of breathing: clinical monitoring and considerations in the critical care setting, Crit Care Nurs Q 11(3):1, 1988.
13. Carlon G, Fox S, and Ackerman N: Evaluation of a closed-tracheal suction system, Crit Care Med 15(5):522, 1987.
14. Christopher K and others: Transtracheal oxygen therapy for refractory hypoxemia, JAMA 256(4):494, 1986.
15. Chulay M and Graeber G: Efficacy of a hyperinflation and hyperoxygenation suctioning intervention, Heart Lung 17(1):15, 1988.
16. Cosenza JJ and Norton LC: Secretion clearance: state of the art from nursing perspective, Crit Care Nurse 6(4):23, 1986.
17. Cowley RA and Dunham CM: Shock trauma/critical care manual: initial assessment and management, Baltimore, 1982, University Park Press.
18. Crabtree GS: Reducing tracheal injury and aspiration, DCCN 7(6):324, 1988.
19. Crabtree-Goodnough SK: The effects of oxygen and hyperinflation on arterial oxygen tension after endotracheal suctioning, Heart Lung 14(1):11, 1985.
20. Dark D, Pingleton M, and Kerby G: Hypercapnia during weaning: a complication of nutritional support, Chest 88(1):141, 1985.
21. Davidson L and Brown S: Continuous $Svo_2$ monitoring: a tool for analyzing hemodynamic status, Heart Lung 15(3):287, 1986.
22. Davis J: Hyperbaric oxygen therapy: a committee report, Bethesda, Md, 1983, Undersea Medical Society, Inc.
23. Demers B: The impact of technology on the risks associated with endotracheal suctioning and airway management: the changes the decade has wrought, Resp Care 34(5):339, 1989.
24. Earl J: Full ventilatory support: a point of view, Resp Care 34(8):741, 1989.
25. East TD: The ventilator of the 1990's, Resp Care 35(3):233, 1990.
26. Fuchs P: Before and after chest surgery: stay right on respiratory care, Nursing 83, 13(5):46, 1983.
27. Gaskell DV and Webber BA: The Brompton hospital guide to chest physiotherapy, ed 4, Oxford, 1980, Blackwell Scientific Publications.
28. Gregg BL: What's new in respiratory care: more choices on the ventilator menu, Crit Care Choices 11:30, 1990.
29. Gruden MA: High-frequency ventilation: an overview, Crit Care Nurse 5(1):36, 1985.
30. Hanley MV: Normal saline intratracheal instillation in intubated patients and dogs, master's thesis, 1977, University of Washington.
31. Harper R: A guide to respiratory care, Philadelphia, 1981, JB Lippincott Co.
32. Heffner JE, Miller KS, and Sahn S: Tracheostomy in the intensive care unit. Part I, Chest 90(2):269-274, 1987.
33. Heffner JE, Miller KS, and Sahn S: Tracheostomy in the intensive care unit. Part II, Complications, Chest 90(3):430, 1987.
34. Heimlich H: Respiratory rehabilitation with transtracheal oxygen system, Ann Otol Rhinol Laryngol 91(6):643, 1982.
35. Heimlich H and Carr G: Transtracheal catheter technique for pulmonary rehabilitation, Ann Otol Rhinol Laryngol 94(5):502, 1985.
36. Henneman EA: Effect of nursing contact on the stress response of patients being weaned from mechanical ventilation, Heart Lung 18(5):483, 1989.
37. Herve P and others: Hypercapnic acidosis induced by nutrition in mechanically ventilated patients: glucose versus fat, Crit Care Med 13(7):537-540, 1986.
38. Hess D: Perspectives on weaning from mechanical ventilation: with a note on extubation, Resp Care 32(3):167, 1987.
39. Hess D: Controversies in respiratory critical care, Crit Care Nurs Q 11(3):62, 1988.
40. Jacobson J, Morsch J, and Rendell-Baker L: The historical perspective of hyperbaric therapy, Ann NY Acad Sci 117:651-670, 1965.
41. Kirilloff LH and others: Does chest physical therapy work? Chest 88(3):436, 1985.
42. Kline JL and others: The use of calculated relative inspiratory effort as a predictor of outcome in mechanical ventilation weaning trials, Resp Care 32(1):870, 1987.
43. Lane G, Cronin K, and Pierce A: Flow charts: clinical decision-making in nursing, Philadelphia, 1983, JB Lippincott Co.
44. MacKenzie C: Compromises in the choice of orotracheal or nasotracheal intubation and tracheostomy, Heart Lung 12(5):485, 1983.
45. Martin L: Pulmonary physiology in clinical practice, St Louis, 1987, Mosby–Year Book, Inc.
46. Massaro D: Oxygen: toxicity and tolerance, Hosp Pract 21(7):95, 1986.
47. McDonnell K, Fahey P, and Segal M: Respiratory intensive care, Boston, 1987, Little, Brown & Co.
48. Meijer K, van Saene HK, and Hill JC: Infection control in patients undergoing mechanical ventilation: traditional approach versus a new development—selective decontamination of the digestive tract, Heart Lung, 19(1):11, 1990.
49. Muto R: Personal communication, November 1988.
50. Pepe P and Marini J: Occult positive end-expiratory pressure in mechanically ventilated patients with airflow obstruction, Am Rev Resp Dis 126(1):166, 1982.
51. Peruzzi WT: Full and partial ventilatory support: the significance of ventilator mode, Resp Care 35(2):174, 1990.
52. Petty TL: The use, abuse and mistique of positive end expiratory pressure, Am Rev Resp Dis 138(2):475, 1988.
53. Preusser B and others: Effects of two methods of preoxygenation on mean arterial pressure, cardiac output, peak airway pressure and post-suctioning hypoxemia, Heart Lung 17(3):290, 1988.
54. Rashkin M and Davis T: Acute complications of endotracheal intubation, Chest 89(2):165, 1986.
55. Sahn S: The pleura, Am Rev Resp Dis 138(1):184, 1988.
56. Scanlan CL, Spearman CB, and Sheldon R: Egan's fundamentals of respiratory therapy, ed 5, St Louis, 1990, Mosby Year–Book, Inc.
57. Schoene RB: The control of ventilation in clinical medicine: to breathe or not to breathe, Resp Care 34(6):500, 1989.
58. Shapiro B and others: Clinical application of respiratory care, ed 3, Chicago, 1985, Mosby–Year Book, Inc.
59. Siskind MM: A standard care for the nursing diagnosis of ineffective airway clearance, Heart Lung, 18(5):477, 1989.
60. Skelton M and Nield M: Ineffective airway clearance related to artificial airway, Nurs Clin North Am 22(1):167, 1987.
61. Smith RA, Novak RA, and Venus B: End-tital $CO_2$ monitoring utility during weaning from mechanical ventilations, Resp Care 34(11):972, 1989.

62. Snowberger P: Prevention of complications: decreasing tracheal damage due to excessive cuff pressures, Dimens Crit Care Nurs 5(3):136, 1986.
63. Spofford B and others: Transtracheal oxygen therapy: a guide for the respiratory therapist, Resp Care 32(5):345, 1987.
64. Sporn P and Marganroth M: Discontinuation of mechanical ventilation, Clin Chest Med 9(1):113, 1988.
65. Stone KS and others: Effects of lung hyperventilation on mean arterial pressure and postsuctioning hypoxemia, Heart Lung 18(4):377, 1989.
66. Suter PM, Fairly AB, and Isenburg MD: Optimum end-expiratory airway pressure in patients with acute pulmonary failure, N Engl J Med 292(6):284, 1975.
67. Taggart J, Dorinsky N, and Sheahan J: Airway pressures during closed system suctioning, Heart Lung 17(5):536, 1988.
68. Tecklin JS: Positioning, percussing and vibrating patients for effective bronchial drainage, Nursing 79 9(3):64, 1979.
69. Tisi G: Pulmonary physiology in clinical medicine, ed 2, Baltimore, 1983, Williams & Wilkins.
70. Toben B and Lewandowski V: Nontraditional and new ventilatory techniques, Crit Care Nurs Q 11(3):12, 1988.
71. Tobin MJ: Physiology in medicine: update on strategies in mechanical ventilation, Hosp Prac 21(6):69, 1986.
72. Traver GA: Ineffective airway clearance: physiology and clinical application . . . cough effectiveness, Dimens Crit Care Nurs 4(4):198, 1985.
73. Trout C: Artificial airways: tubes and tracks, Resp Care 21(6):513, 1976.
74. Waterson M: Teaching your patients postural drainage, Nursing 78 8(3):51, 1978.
75. Wu W and Huang S: Tracheal intubation, Consultant 26(5):34, 1986.

UNIT V

# NEUROLOGICAL ALTERATIONS

CHAPTER 13

# Neurological Assessment and Diagnostic Procedures

## CHAPTER OBJECTIVES

- *List the five components of the neurological assessment.*
- *Describe the pathway of pupillary response.*
- *Define the respiratory patterns associated with neurological deterioration.*
- *State the changes in vital sign changes associated with neurological deterioration.*
- *Define brain death and persistent vegetative state.*
- *Describe the differences in cerebral angiography and digital subtraction angiography.*
- *State the differences in the two types of dye used in myelography.*
- *Explain the differences in electroencephalography and evoked potentials.*
- *Discuss the patient positioning required for lumbar puncture.*

## KEY TERMS

Glasgow Coma Scale, p. 296
decorticate posturing, p. 296
decerebrate posturing, p. 296
lateralizing signs, p. 297
oculocephalic reflex (doll's eyes), p. 298
cold caloric test, p. 299
brain death, p. 300
persistent vegetative state, p. 301
cerebral angiogram, p. 302

## COMPONENTS OF NEUROLOGICAL ASSESSMENT

There are five major components of neurological assessment in the critically ill patient. They are evaluation of (1) level of consciousness, (2) motor movements, (3) pupils and eye signs, (4) respiratory patterns, and (5) vital signs. Until all five of these parameters have been assessed, a complete neurological examination has not been performed.

### Level of Consciousness

Assessment of the level of consciousness is the most important aspect of the neurological assessment. In most situations a patient's level of consciousness will deteriorate before any other changes in neurological assessment are noted. These deteriorations are often subtle and must be monitored carefully.

**Components of consciousness.** There are two major components of consciousness: *arousal or alertness* and *content of consciousness or awareness.*[10]

***Arousal.*** Assessment of the arousal component of consciousness is an evaluation of the reticular activating system and its connection with the thalamus and the cerebral cortex. Arousal is the lowest level of consciousness, and observation is centered around the patient's ability to respond to verbal or noxious stimuli in an appropriate manner.

***Awareness.*** Content of consciousness is a higher level function and is concerned with assessment of the patient's orientation to person, place, and time. Assessment of content of consciousness requires the patient to give appropriate answers to a variety of questions. Changes in the patient's answers indicating increasing degrees of confusion and disorientation may be the first sign of neurological deterioration.

**Categories of consciousness.** The following categories, though vague, are often used to describe the patient's level of consciousness[10]:

*Alert*—Patient responds immediately to minimal external stimuli.

*Lethargic*—State of drowsiness or inaction in which the patient needs an increased stimulus to be awakened.

*Obtunded*—A duller indifference to external stimuli exists and response is minimally maintained.

*Stuporous*—The patient can be aroused only by vigorous and continuous external stimuli.

*Comatose*—Vigorous stimulation fails to produce any voluntary neural response.

Patients are frequently difficult to categorize under these descriptions. Also, the levels of consciousness are not defined in enough detail, and communication of patient condition is often misinterpreted. For example, one clinician might describe a patient's response as obtunded, whereas the next clinician might describe the same response as stuporous. Because of this difficulty in communicating level of consciousness, a variety of assessment tools have been devised to assist in this evaluation.

***Table 13-1*** Glasgow coma scale

| Category | Score | Response |
|---|---|---|
| Eye opening | 4 | Spontaneous—eyes open spontaneously without stimulation |
| | 3 | To speech—eyes open with verbal stimulation but not necessarily to command |
| | 2 | To pain—eyes open with noxious stimuli |
| | 1 | None—no eye opening regardless of stimulation |
| Verbal response | 5 | Oriented—accurate information about person, place, time, reason for hospitalization, and personal data |
| | 4 | Confused—answers not appropriate to question, but correct use of language |
| | 3 | Inappropriate words—disorganized, random speech; no sustained conversation |
| | 2 | Incomprehensible sounds—moans, groans, and mumbles incomprehensibly |
| | 1 | None—no verbalization despite stimulation |
| Best motor response | 6 | Obeys commands—performs simple tasks on command; able to repeat performance |
| | 5 | Localizes to pain—organized attempt to localize and remove painful stimuli |
| | 4 | Withdraws from pain—withdraws extremity from source of painful stimuli |
| | 3 | Abnormal flexion—decorticate posturing spontaneously or in response to noxious stimuli |
| | 2 | Extension—decerebrate posturing spontaneously or in response to noxious stimuli |
| | 1 | None—no response to noxious stimuli; flaccid |

**Assessment of consciousness.** The general rule for evaluation of an altered level of consciousness is to systematically determine the type and degree of noxious stimuli required to produce a response. This concept is incorporated into a variety of clinical assessment tools.

The most widely recognized level of consciousness assessment tool is the **Glasgow Coma Scale** (GCS).[15] This scored scale is based on evaluation of three categories: eye opening, verbal response, and best motor response (Table 13-1).

The best possible score on the GCS is 15, and the lowest score is 3. Generally a score of 7 or less on the GCS indicates coma. The GCS is a level of consciousness assessment tool only and should never be considered a complete neurological examination. It is not a sensitive tool for evaluation of an altered sensorium. The GCS does not account for possible aphasia. The GCS is not a good indicator of lateralization of neurological deterioration. Lateralization involves decreasing motor response on one side or changes in pupillary reaction.

### Motor Movements

**Levels of motor movements.** A simple way of organizing the assessment of motor movements is to use the categories defined in the Glasgow Coma Scale[15] as a guide. The difference in this part of the assessment is that now each extremity is evaluated and recorded individually.

*Obeys commands*—Performs simple tasks on command. Able to repeat performance.

*Localizes to pain*—Organized attempt to localize and remove painful stimuli.

*Withdraws from pain*—Withdraws extremity from source of painful stimuli.

*Abnormal flexion*—**Decorticate posturing** spontaneously or in response to noxious stimuli (Fig. 13-1).

*Extension*—**Decerebrate posturing** spontaneously or in response to noxious stimuli (see Fig. 13-1).

*Flaccid*—No response to noxious stimuli; flaccid.

In addition, a comparison of function is made with that of the opposite extremity. If a patient with spinal cord injury or dysfunction is being evaluated, a separate scale should be used with more detail about motor strength of particular muscle groups.

**Motor assessment techniques**

***Obeys commands.*** Next to the assessment of orientation and awareness, the assessment of the patient's ability to follow commands is one of the highest levels of functioning evaluated. In assessing the ability to follow commands, there are several points that must be recognized. Commands given to a patient with an altered level of consciousness must be simple and direct statements such as, "Show me your thumb." A common error made by clinicians in assessing the patient's ability to respond to commands is to include the simple command along with other verbal communication. To prevent sensory overload and therefore the patient's inability to respond to command, the command should not

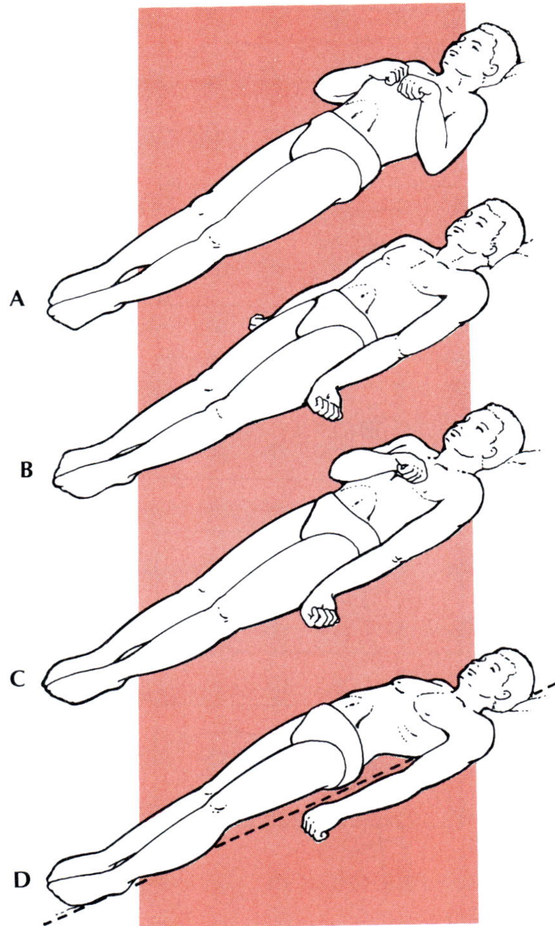


***Fig. 13-1*** Abnormal motor responses. **A,** Decorticate posturing. **B,** Decerebrate posturing. **C,** Decorticate posturing on right side and decerebrate posturing on left side of body. **D,** Opisthotonic posturing.

be included as part of any other verbal conversation. As a patient is emerging from an unconscious state, the brain is less capable of processing and sorting multiple stimuli simultaneously. The key to assessment of the patient's ability to follow commands is to reduce surrounding stimuli or distractors and to keep the command simple and direct.

Another error commonly made in the assessment of the patient's ability to follow commands involves the type of command given. Appropriate commands are those not calling for random or reflex responses. "Squeeze my hand" is a common command used by caregivers and family alike. In the low levels of consciousness, the reflex of hand grasp may be present and is initiated when the assessor's hand is placed within the patient's hand. If this is the case, it is often difficult to accurately assess whether the patient is responding to command or exhibiting a reflex response.

Acceptable commands include "Show me your thumb" or "Stick out your tongue." When using these commands, care must be taken that the command is not followed by visual or tactile stimuli. It is not uncommon to observe an assessment in which the nurse asks the patient "show me your thumb" while the nurse is tapping the thumb. With this scenario it is impossible to determine whether the patient is following a verbal command or withdrawing from tactile stimuli.

***Noxious stimuli.*** Once it has been determined that the patient is incapable of comprehending and following a simple command, the use of noxious stimuli is required to determine the motor responses of the body.

**ACCEPTABLE NOXIOUS STIMULI**

1. *Nail bed pressure* is an acceptable form of noxious stimuli. It requires use of an object such as a pen to apply firm pressure to the nail bed. Pressure applied to each extremity allows for evaluation of individual extremity function. The patient's movement must not be interrupted while the nurse is applying the nail bed pressure. Although this pressure is classified as noxious stimuli, if no response is elicited from nail bed pressure other noxious stimuli measures should be employed.

2. *Trapezius pinch* is another acceptable method of delivering noxious stimuli. Performed by squeezing the trapezius muscle, this method allows for observation of total body response to stimuli. Trapezius pinch is often difficult to perform on large or obese adults.

3. *Pinching of the inner aspect of the arm or leg* is the final acceptable form of administering noxious stimuli. A small portion of the patient's tissue on the sensitive inner aspect of the arm or leg is pinched firmly and each extremity is evaluated independently. Although this form of noxious stimuli is the most apt to cause bruising, it is also the most sensitive for eliciting a movement response.

**UNACCEPTABLE NOXIOUS STIMULI**

1. *Sternal rub* is often used as a form of noxious stimuli. Firm pressure is applied to the sternum in a rubbing motion usually with the assessor's knuckles. When used repeatedly the sternum could become excoriated, open, and infected. Open-handed firm patting of the sternal area to arouse the patient is acceptable.

2. *Supraorbital pressure* is another form of noxious stimuli that should be avoided. Patients with head injuries, frontal craniotomies, or facial surgeries should not be evaluated with this method because of the possibility of underlying fractured or unstable cranium. Therefore it is better not to develop the habit of applying supraorbital pressure to deliver noxious stimuli.

3. *Nipple pinching* and *testicle pinching* has been used for many years. Although never described in texts as an acceptable method for delivering noxious stimuli, it can often be observed in the clinical setting. For obvious reasons this type of noxious stimuli is inappropriate and unnecessary.

**Assessment of lateralizing signs. Lateralizing signs** are a difference in neurological assessment findings on one side of the body and include unilateral deterioration in motor movements or changes in pupillary response. Lateralizing signs help to localize the lesion to one side of the brain. The occurrence of lateralizing signs indicates an emergency situation. Unilateral deterioration of motor movements and pupillary response may herald herniation. Notification of the physician and immediate intervention is imperative.

### Pupil and Eye Assessment

The assessment of pupillary function and eye movement is an important component of the neurological assessment.[18] Especially in the unconscious patient or the patient receiving neuromuscular blocking agents and sedation, pupillary response is one of the few neurological signs that can be assessed. Serial evaluation, appropriate technique, recognition of abnormalities, and good documentation are all important.

**Anatomy of pupil response.** Pupil reaction is a function of the autonomic nervous system. Parasympathetic control of pupil reaction occurs through innervation of the oculomotor nerve (CN III), which exits from the brainstem in the midbrain area. When the parasympathetic fibers are stimulated, the pupil constricts. Sympathetic control of the pupil originates in the hypothalamus and travels down the entire length of the brainstem. When the sympathetic fibers are stimulated, the pupil dilates.

Pupil changes provide a valuable tool to assessment because of pathway location. The oculomotor nerve lies at the junction of the midbrain and the tentorial notch. Any increase of pressure that exerts force down through the tentorial notch compresses the oculomotor nerve. Oculomotor nerve compression results in a dilated, nonreactive pupil. Sympathetic pathway disruption occurs with involvement in the brainstem. Loss of sympathetic control leads to pinpoint, nonreactive pupils. Pupillary reactivity is also affected by medications, particularly sympathetic and parasympathetic agents, direct trauma, and eye surgery. Pupil reactivity is relatively resistant to metabolic dysfunction and can be used to differentiate between metabolic and structural causes of decreased levels of consciousness.

**Anatomy of eye movement.** Control of eye movements occurs with interaction of three cranial nerves: oculomotor (CN III), trochlear (CN IV), and abducens (CN VI). The pathways for these cranial nerves provide integrated function through the internuclear pathway of the medial longitudinal fasciculus (MLF) located in the brainstem. The MLF provides coordination of eye movements with the vestibular and reticular formation.

**Assessment of pupillary response.** Evaluation of pupillary response includes assessment of size, shape (round, irregular, or oval), and degree of reactivity to light. Comparison should be made between the two pupils for equality. Any of these components of the pupil assessment could change in response to increasing pressure on the oculomotor nerve at the tentorium.

The technique for evaluation of direct pupillary response involves use of a narrow-beamed bright light shone into the

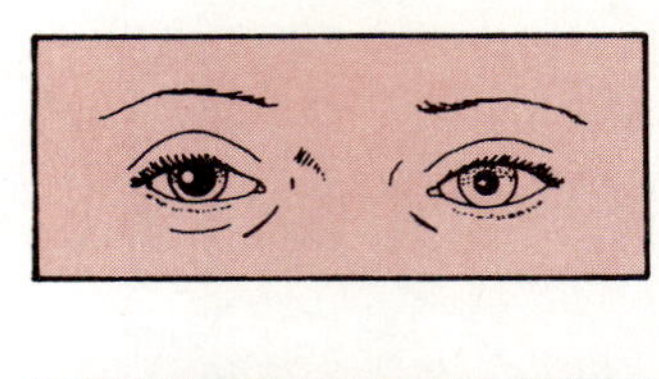

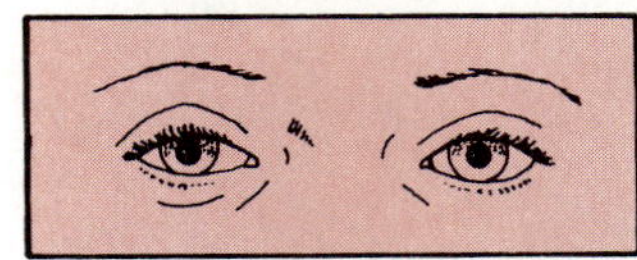

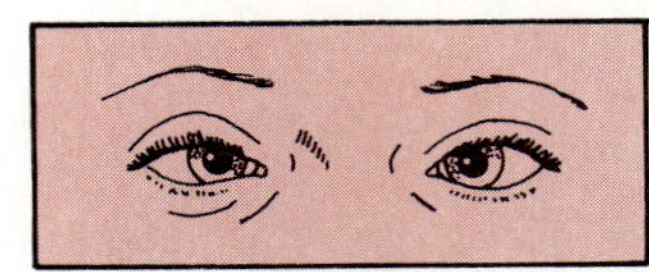

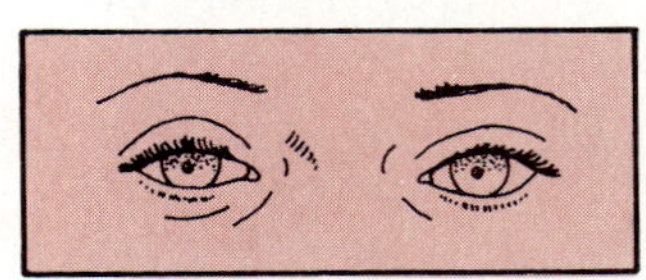

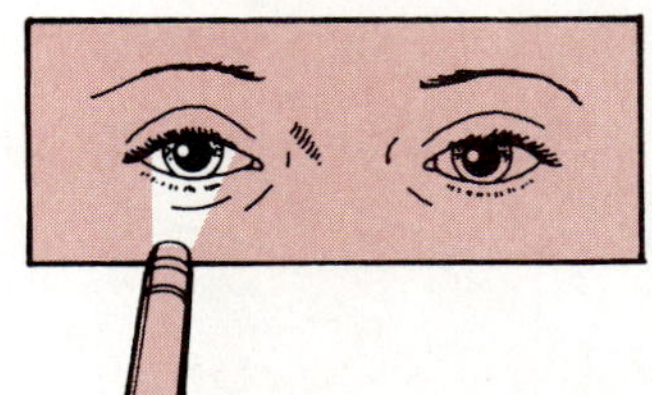

***Fig. 13-2*** Abnormal pupillary responses.

pupil from the outer canthus of the eye (Fig. 13-2). If the light is shone directly onto the pupil, glare or reflection of the light may prevent the assessor proper visualization. Consensual pupillary response is the constriction of the pupil in response to a light shone into the opposite eye.

**Assessment of eye movements**

***Extraocular movements.*** In the conscious patient, the function of the three cranial nerves of the eye and their innervation with the MLF can be assessed by the nurse's asking the patient to follow a finger through the full range of eye motions. If the eyes move together into all six fields, extraolcular movements (EOM) are intact.[2]

***Oculocephalic reflex (doll's eyes).*** In the unconscious patient, assessment of ocular function and the innervation of the MLF is done by eliciting the doll's eyes procedure. If the patient is unconscious as a result of trauma, the nurse should ascertain that there is no cervical injury before performing this examination.

To assess the **oculocephalic reflex,** the nurse should hold the eyelids open and briskly turn the patient's head to one side while observing the eye movements, then briskly turn the patient's head to the other side and observe. If the oculocephalic reflex is intact, doll's eyes are present. The eyes deviate to the opposite direction than that to which the head is turned. If the oculocephalic reflex is not intact, doll's eyes are absent. This lack of response in which the eyes remain midline and move with the head indicates significant brainstem injury. If the oculocephalic reflex is abnormal, doll's eyes are abnormal. In this situation the eyes rove or move in opposite directions. Abnormal oculocephalic reflex indicates some degree of brainstem injury.

***Oculovestibular reflex (cold caloric test).*** The oculovestibular reflex is usually performed by a physician as one of the final clinical assessments of brainstem function. Twenty to 50 ml of ice water is injected into the external auditory canal. The normal eye movement response is a rapid nystagmus/like deviation toward the irrigated ear. This response indicates brainstem integrity. The **cold caloric test** is an extremely noxious stimulation and may produce a decorticate or decerebrate posturing response in the comatose patient. It is not recommended to perform this procedure on a conscious patient. An abnormal response would be dysconjugate eye movement, which indicates a brainstem lesion, or no response, which indicates little to no brainstem function.

### Respiratory Patterns

**Control of respirations.** The activity of respirations is a highly integrated function receiving input from the cerebrum, brainstem, and metabolic mechanisms. There is a close correlation in clinical assessment between altered levels of consciousness, the level of brain or brainstem injury, and the respiratory pattern noted (Fig. 13-3).

Under the influence of the cerebral cortex and the diencephalon, three brainstem centers control respirations. The lowest center, the medullary respiratory center, sends impulses through the vagus nerve to innervate muscles of inspiration and expiration. The apneustic and pneumotaxic centers of the pons are responsible for the length of inspiration and expiration and the underlying respiratory rate.

**Respiratory patterns.** Changes in respiratory patterns assist in identifying the level of brainstem dysfunction or injury. The respiratory patterns are defined in Table 13-2.

Evaluation of respiratory pattern must also include evaluation of the effectiveness of gas exchange in maintaining adequate oxygen and carbon dioxide levels. Hypoventilation is not uncommon in the patient with an altered level of consciousness. Alterations in oxygenation or carbon dioxide levels can result in further neurological dysfunction. Intracranial pressure (ICP) will increase with hypoxemia or hypercapnia.

Finally, assessment of the respiratory function in a patient with neurological deficit must also include assessment of airway maintenance and secretion control. Cough, gag, and swallow reflexes responsible for protection of the airway may be absent or diminished.

### Vital Signs

**Cardiac.** The brain's tremendous metabolic demand requires an adequate supply of blood to continually perfuse the brain. Evaluation of the cardiovascular system identifies inappropriate supply for the known cerebral demand.

***Decreased cardiac output.*** For whatever the reason (vasodilation, bradycardia, tachycardia, hypovolemia, or inadequate pump), decreased cardiac output will lead to decreased perfusion of cerebral tissue, hypoxia, and neurological injury. In the presence of increased ICP, decreased

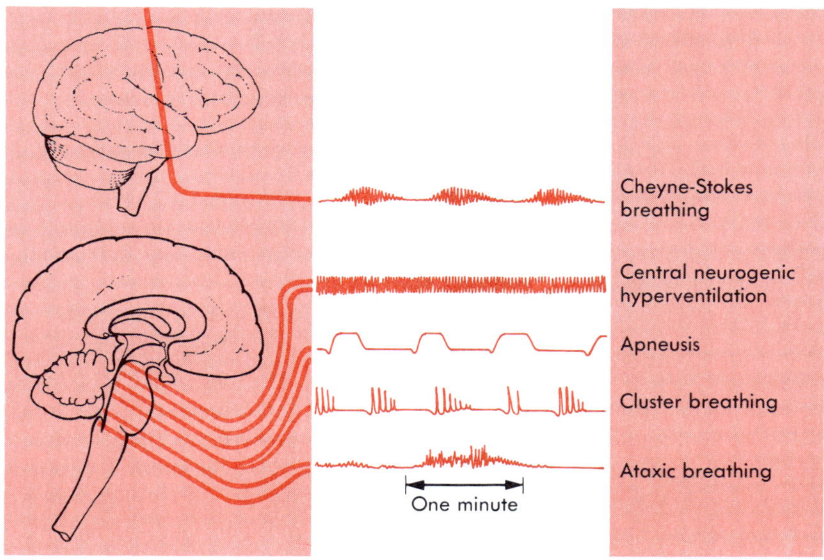


***Fig. 13-3*** Abnormal respiratory patterns with corresponding level of central nervous system activity.

**Table 13-2** Respiratory patterns

| Pattern of respiration | Description of pattern | Significance |
|---|---|---|
| Cheyne-Stokes | Rhythmic crescendo and decrescendo of rate and depth of respiration; includes brief periods of apnea | Usually seen with bilateral deep cerebral lesions or some cerebellar lesions |
| Central neurogenic hyperventilation | Very deep, very rapid respirations with no apneic periods | Usually seen with lesions of the midbrain and upper pons |
| Apneustic | Prolonged inspiratory and/or expiratory pause of 2-3 seconds | Usually seen in lesions of the mid to lower pons |
| Cluster breathing | Clusters of irregular, gasping respirations separated by long periods of apnea | Usually seen in lesions of the lower pons or upper medulla |
| Ataxic respirations | Irregular, random pattern of deep and shallow respirations with irregular apneic periods | Usually seen in lesions of the medulla |

cardiac output is even more detrimental because low blood pressure must overcome the additional resistance of intracranial pressure to provide blood to the brain.

***Hypertension.*** A common manifestation of the intracranial injury is systemic hypertension. Cerebral autoregulation, responsible for the control of cerebral blood flow, is frequently lost with any type of intracranial injury. After cerebral injury, the body is often in a hyperdynamic state (increased heart rate, blood pressure, and cardiac output) as part of a compensatory response. With the loss of autoregulation and as blood pressure increases, cerebral blood flow and volume increase, and therefore intracranial pressure increases. Control of systemic hypertension is necessary to stop this cycle.

***Bradycardia.*** The medulla and the vagus nerve provide parasympathetic control to the heart. When stimulated, this lower brainstem system produces bradycardia. Increasing intracranial pressure frequently causes bradycardia. Abrupt intracranial pressure changes can also produce dysrhythmias, such as premature ventricular contractions (PVC), atrioventricular (A-V) block, or ventricular fibrillation.

*Cushing's triad* is a set of three signs/symptoms (bradycardia, systolic hypertension, and bradypnea) that are related to pressure on the medullary area of the brainstem. These signs often occur in response to intracranial hypertension or a herniation syndrome.

The appearance of Cushing's triad is a *late* finding that may be absent in neurological deterioration. Attention should be paid to alteration in each component of the triad and intervention initiated accordingly.

### Neurological Changes Associated with Intracranial Hypertension

Assessment of the patient for signs of increasing intracranial pressure is an important function of the critical care nurse. Increasing ICP can be identified by changes in level of consciousness, pupillary reaction, motor response, vital signs, and respiratory patterns.

**Level of consciousness.** As ICP increases, the level of consciousness deteriorates. Increased restlessness and confusion, agitation, or decreased responsiveness could all be indicators of deterioration in neurological status. For the most part, level of consciousness is the first sign of deterioration in a conscious patient. Subtle changes that are identified and acted on may prevent the serious consequences associated with neurological decline.

**Pupillary reaction.** Any changes in pupillary size, shape, or reactivity are ominous signs. In the unconscious patient, pupils are the most sensitive indication that deterioration is in progress.

**Motor response.** Deterioration in motor strength or the appearance of lateralizing signs may indicate increasing ICP. Even subtle changes in motor response can be highly predictive of neurological deterioration.

**Vital signs.** As described, vital signs play a variable role in the evaluation of deteriorating neurological status. Increasing systolic blood pressure and/or development of bradycardia should signal the evaluator to further assess for potential deterioration in function.

**Respiratory patterns.** Change in respiratory patterns can be a sensitive indicator of decreasing levels of function. The assessment of this parameter is usually lost, because most patients with critical neurological injury are intubated and ventilated to prevent the serious neurological damage caused by hypoxia and hypercapnia.

### Brain Death and Persistent Vegetative State

The assessment of patients for brain death and persistent vegetative state (coma) remain controversial. Brief review of some of the issues surrounding both of these topics will be discussed.

**Brain death.** As the result of technological advances, death—as defined by cessation of heart beat and respirations—may not occur despite the presence of irreversible loss of brain function. Life can be supported almost indefinitely provided the proper mechanical support is accompanied by physical care. **Brain death** is defined as an irreversible loss of all brain function. In 1968, the Harvard Medical School defined the first set of clinical criteria to aid in the diagnosis of brain death.[1] These criteria included unresponsive coma, apnea, absent brainstem reflexes, absent spinal reflexes, two isoelectric electroencephalograms 24 hours apart, absence of drug intoxication, and absence of hypothermia. In the years following 1968, the Harvard Criteria as well as other proposed groups of criteria were developed and researched in the clinical setting. Although no one set of criteria exists for all patients, an array of acceptable methods for establishing brain death have been described.

The legal issue involves the recognition of cessation of brain function as an equal definition with the cessation of cardiopulmonary function in the determination of death. California and Alaska were two states that first adapted the definition of death to include brain death. Since then, virtually all states developed some statutory change in law to recognize the existence of brain death.

The American Medical Association House of Delegates defines brain death in the following way:

> An individual who has sustained either (a) irreversible cessation of circulatory and respiratory functions, or (b) irrreversible cessation of all functions of the entire brain, should be considered dead. A determination of death shall be made in accordance with accepted medical standards.[16]

In 1980, the Uniform Determination of Death Act—identical to the AMA bill—was passed by the National Conference of Commissioners of Uniform State Laws. Even those states that have not changed statutes to recognize the existence of brain death accept the existence of the phenomena.

The actual criteria used in any health care setting is usually developed by an agency-based ethics committee. Review of the criteria at the institution in which the critical care nurse is employed allows a better understanding of the process and procedures of the institution.[7]

**Persistent vegetative state.** From the advancing technology of modern medicine came another entity described as **persistent vegetative state.** This comatose condition does not result in death if mechanical support is withdrawn but also does not include any recovery of consciousness. In brain death, all functions of the brain including the brainstem have ceased. In persistent vegetative state the higher cortical functions of the cerebral hemisphere have been irreversibly damaged, but the lower functions of the brainstem remain intact.[6] With brainstem function comes spontaneous respirations, as well as cardiovascular control. Also seen are some of the brainstem signs such as involuntary chewing, lip-smacking, and roving eye movements.

The emotional and financial strain to both family and society for a patient in a persistent vegetative state is enormous. Although the laws are now generally supportive of brain death, the issue of withdrawing support from a patient in a persistent vegetative state or even withholding additional support, is still controversial. Several courts have ruled that it is lawful to reduce care for patients in persistent vegetative state but have described differing standards and procedures for implementing such decisions.[3]

## RADIOLOGIC PROCEDURES

### Skull and Spine Films

The purpose of radiographs of the skull or spine are to identify fractures, anomalies, or possibly tumors. The role of skull radiographs in trauma has diminished with the advent of computerized axial tomography (CT scan). If the patient is to be sent for CT scan during the initial assessment process, a skull radiograph may not be necessary.

Nursing care involves positioning of the patient to obtain adequate films. Any situation in which traumatic injury, especially head injury, is the cause of the patient's admission to the critical care unit, the cervical spine should be treated as unstable until proved otherwise.

### Computerized Axial Tomography

Computerized axial tomography (CT scan) provides the clinician with a mathematically reconstructed view of multiple sections of the head and body. This is accomplished by passage of intersecting x-ray beams through the examined area and measurement of the density of substances through which the x-ray beam passes. The more dense the substance the x-ray beam passes through, the whiter it will appear on the finished film. The less dense a substance, the blacker it will appear. Therefore in a normal CT scan of the head, bone appears white, blood appears off-white, brain tissue appears shaded gray, CSF appears off-black, and air appears black (Fig. 13-4).

The purpose of the CT scan is to obtain rapid, noninvasive visualization of structures. CT scan is indicated in the diagnostic work-up of severe headache, head trauma with associated loss of consciousness, seizures, hydrocephalus, suspicion of space-occupying lesions, hemorrhage, or vascular lesions and edema. There are two types of CT scans—contrast and noncontrast scans. The noncontrast scan is

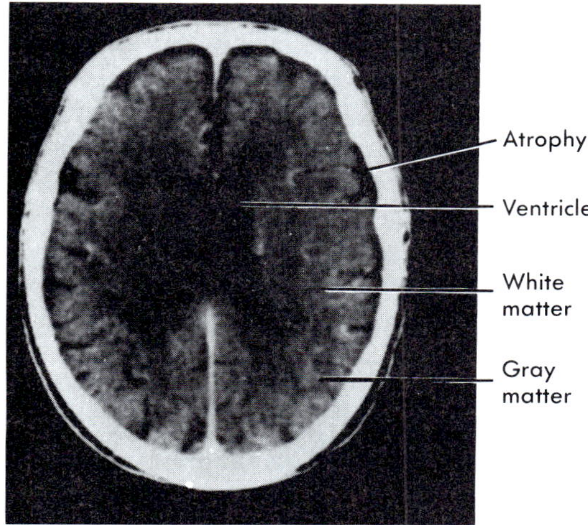


***Fig. 13-4*** CT scan image. (From Ballinger PW: Merrill's atlas of radiographic positions and radiologic procedures, ed 7, St. Louis, 1990, Mosby–Year Book, Inc.)

noninvasive, requires no premedication of the patient, and is good for analysis and location of normal brain structures. Noncontrast CT scans of the head are appropriate in trauma patients in whom the goal is to view the intracranial area for evidence of intracranial hemorrhage, cerebral edema, or shift of structures. Noncontrast CT scan is also appropriate in the diagnosis of hydrocephalus.[8,11]

Contrast CT scan involves the use of an intravenously injected contrast medium. The use of contrast enhances the vascular areas and allows for detection of vascular lesions or the further definition of lesions noted on a noncontrast scan.

Nursing care of the patient receiving a CT scan can be divided into two areas of focus: observation of patient tolerance of procedure and observation of patient reaction to the dye in contrast scanning. Because of the associated activity and positioning, transporting and scanning of a critically ill patient with known or suspected intracranial hypertension can cause a deterioration in the patient's condition. The nurse must always remain with the patient during CT scan and closely observe the neurological status, vital signs, and intracranial pressure, if monitored.

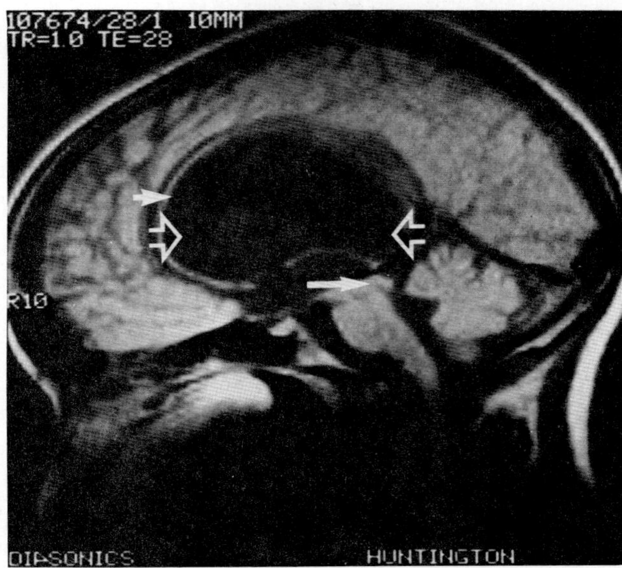


*Fig. 13-5* Magnetic resonance image of the brain. Sagittal section demonstrating marked enlargement of the lateral ventricle *(open arrow)* with stretching of the corpus callosum *(arrowhead)* as a result of aqueductal stenosis *(arrow)* (SE 1000/28). (From Stark D and Bradley WG: Magnetic resonance imaging, ed 2, St Louis, 1991, Mosby–Year Book, Inc.)

## Magnetic Resonance Imaging

Magnetic resonance imaging (MRI) is a relatively new procedure. The patient is placed in a large magnetic field. The nuclei of the atoms of the body are stimulated and momentarily absorb some of the energy generated by the magnetic field. Different tissue densities absorb and subsequently release differing amounts of energy. The release of the energy (resonance frequency) is then measured and plotted (Fig. 13-5).[4]

In MRI small tumors that have tissue densities different from those of the surrounding cells can be identified before they would be visible by any other radiographic test. MRI can also identity small hemorrhages deep in the brain that are invisible on CT scan. Finally, MRI is able to identify areas of cerebral infarct within a few hours of the incident, as well as small areas of plaque in patients with multiple sclerosis.

Nursing care of these patients involves patient teaching and preparation. The procedure is lengthy and requires the patient to lie motionless. Removal of all metal from the patient's body and clothing is essential, as the basis of MRI is a magnetic field. Any questions about specific devices or metals should be directed to the neuroradiologist before testing. The test is considered relatively safe and noninvasive, but the procedure is still too new to have all risks identified.

## Cerebral Angiogram

**Cerebral angiogram**[11] involves the injection of radiopaque contrast medium into the intracranial or extracranial vasculature. With the use of serial radiologic filming, angiography traces the flow of blood from the arterial circulation through the capillary bed to the venous circulation. Cerebral angiography allows visualization of the lumen of vessels to provide information about patency, size (narrowing or dilation), any irregularities, or occlusion. Angiography is necessary in the diagnosis of cerebral aneurysm, arteriovenous malformation, carotid artery disease, and some vascular tumors.

The procedure involves placement of a catheter in the femoral artery and threading it up the aorta and into the origin of the cerebral circulation. Other injection sites include a direct carotid or vertebral artery puncture or placement of a catheter in the brachial, axillary, or subclavian artery. Several views of vessels can be studied on angiogram. A four-vessel angiogram involves injections into the right and left internal carotid arteries and the right and left vertebral arteries. If the area of suspected disease has already been identified, a single vessel study may be all that is required. This is particularly true when angiography is used as a follow-up in the evaluation of intracranial vascular surgery. Also, if carotid artery disease is a working diagnosis, angiogram may include views of the arch of the aorta, plus the external and internal carotid arteries.

Once the catheter is appropriately placed, the contrast medium is injected. Following this, a rapid succession of radiographs are taken as the contrast medium progresses through the cerebral circulation. Separate contrast medium injections occur for each vessel being studied.

In preparation of the patient, patient instruction and education are essential. A hot, burning sensation is often experienced when the contrast medium is injected. This is especially true if the contrast is injected into the external carotid system. Preparation of patients for this burning sensation assures them that it is not an abnormal occurrence. Before and after the procedure the patient must be well hydrated to assist the kidneys in clearing the heavy dye load. If the patient is unable to tolerate oral fluids, an intravenous line should be placed before the procedure is begun.

Complications associated with a cerebral angiogram include (1) cerebral embolus caused by the catheter dislodging a segment of atherosclerotic plaque in the vessel, (2) hemorrhage or clot formation at the insertion site, (3) vasospasm of a vessel caused by the irritation of catheter placement, (4) thrombosis of the extremity distal to the injection site, or (5) allergic reaction to the contrast medium.

Post procedure assessment involves vital sign measurement every 15 minutes, neurological evaluation, observation of the injection site, and assessment of neurovascular integrity distal to the injection site. Any abnormalities noted must be immediately reported.

### Digital Subtraction Angiography

Digital subtraction angiography[11] is a method of visualizing the arteriovenous circulation of the intracranial space. Radiographic dye is injected either into the venous or the arterial circulation, but significantly less dye is necessary for this procedure than for arterial angiography. Films taken before and after dye injection are superimposed on each other and all matching images are subtracted. This leaves only the dye enhanced cerebral vessels present for study and evaluation. Digital subtraction angiography eliminates the shadows and distortions of bone or other material that sometimes block the viewing of the cerebral vessels. With venous injection of dye for the digital subtraction angiography, intracranial and extracranial vessels are enhanced. With arterial injection of dye, the same complications are possible as with cerebral angiography.

### Myelography

Myelography[8] is the radiography of the spinal cord and vertebral column following injection of a contrast material into the subarachnoid space by lumbar or cisternal puncture. Myelography allows visualization of the spinal canal, the subarachnoid space around the spinal cord, and the spinal nerve roots through the use of radiograph. Indications for myelography include identification of spinal canal blockage caused by herniated intervertebral discs, spinal cord tumors, bony fragments or growths, or congenital anomalies.

The procedure involves a lumbar or cisternal puncture followed by an injection of contrast medium. Done under fluoroscopy, the infusion of the dye is observed and radiographic films are taken. Two basic types of contrast medium are used—an oil-based preparation (Pantopaque) or a water-based preparation (metrizamide). Use of an oil-based preparation, which is heavier than the cerebrospinal fluid (CSF), allows the radiologist to place the patient in a variety of positions while observing the flow of dye through the spinal subarachnoid space. Pantopaque must be removed at the end of the procedure. Use of an oil-based preparation is associated with a higher incidence of severe postprocedure headache as a result of loss of cerebrospinal fluid. For this reason, the patient must remain flat in bed for 4 to 6 hours to prevent headache and CSF leak from the puncture site.

Use of the water-based preparation allows for better visualization of nerve roots and projections off the spinal cord. Because of the potential toxicity of water-based preparations to the cerebral tissue, care must be taken to ensure that a large dye load does not reach the surface of the brain. This is accomplished by keeping the patient's head elevated 30 to 45 degrees after the procedure. Toxicity is evidenced by grand mal seizures. Patients receiving a metrizamide myelogram should be kept well hydrated to assist in clearing of the dye through the urine. Use of phenothiazines is to be avoided after metrizamide myelography because of the increase in symptoms of toxicity.

Possible risks involved with myelography include injection of the dye outside of the subarachnoid space, arachnoiditis as a result of irritation of the arachnoid membranes from a foreign material, allergic reactions to the dye that may cause confusion, disorientation or an anaphylactic reaction, headache, or grand mal seizure.[9]

## CEREBRAL BLOOD FLOW STUDIES

The goal of cerebral blood flow studies[11] is to measure the amount of blood flow overall or in regions of the brain to detect areas of increased or decreased cerebral circulation. Normal cerebral blood flow values average 50 to 55 ml of flow per 100 g of cerebral tissue per minute.

Methods of determining cerebral blood flow range from intracarotid injection of radioisotopes to intravenous injection to inhalation of isotopes or nitrous oxide. The most clinically acceptable method of cerebral blood flow analysis involves inhalation of xenon-133 for 3 to 5 minutes. Clearance of this isotope from brain tissue is then monitored from 16 to 32 probes that are placed externally around the head. Information from the probes is passed to a computer that calculates regional cerebral blood flow. This is the least invasive of all techniques. The difficulty with this method is that all body tissues take up xenon and then clear it, including the skin and muscles of the scalp under detectors. Although mathematical calculations are factored in, cerebral blood flow results are an estimated value at best. Further research and development are necessary to make this valuable diagnostic tool clinically acceptable and accurate.

## ELECTROENCEPHALOGRAPHY

Electroencephalography (EEG)[4,12] is the recording of electrical impulses, commonly called brain waves, generated by the brain. The purpose of the EEG is to detect and localize abnormal electrical activity. This abnormal activity can be defined as slowing, which occurs in areas of injury or infarct, or spikes and waves seen in irritated tissue. Indications for the use of an EEG include seizure focus identification, infarct, metabolic disorders, confirmation of brain death (electrocerebral silence), and some head injuries.

Electrodes are placed noninvasively on the head and the electrical impulses detected are transferred to a central recording device that records the information in wave form. There are five types of waves or rhythms that may be present: alpha, theta, beta, sleep spindles, and spike and wave rhythms. For further discussion on EEG, see Chapter 5.

Continuous EEG monitoring has become common in the critical care environment. The goal of continuous EEG monitoring is to identify changes in electrical activity that could indicate inadequate vascular supply to an area or provide evidence of subclinical seizures. Subclinical seizures are evidenced by sharp spike and wave electrical activity that is not in evidence by visual observation of the patient. Detection and treatment of subclinical seizures may prevent secondary brain injury.

## EVOKED POTENTIALS

Evoked potentials[4,8] involve the recording of electrical impulses generated by a sensory stimulus as it travels through the brainstem and into the cerebral cortex. Evoked potentials are used to assess the status of sensory pathways. Another use of evoked potentials is in the determination of the existence of brainstem or spinal cord injury in the traumatically injured patient.

There are three types of evoked potential tests: (1) visual evoked responses (VER), (2) brainstem auditory evoked responses (BAER), and (3) somatosensory evoked responses (SSER). VER involves monitoring of the visual pathways through the brainstem and cortex in response to viewing a shifting geometric pattern on a screen or placing a mask over the eye that sends a flashing light stimulus. BAER involves monitoring the auditory pathway through the brainstem and cortex in response to a rhythmic clicking sound sent through earphones placed over the patient's ears. SSER involves monitoring of sensory pathways from the extremities ascending the spinal cord through the brainstem and into the cortex. This is done by administering a small electrical shock to a nerve root in the periphery such as the ulnar or radial nerve.

## LUMBAR PUNCTURE

The main purpose of lumbar puncture (LP) is to enter the subarachnoid space to obtain diagnostic information or provide therapeutic intervention. Diagnostic information comes from samples of cerebrospinal fluid evaluated for the presence of subarachnoid blood, infection, or laboratory analysis. Pressure readings are also obtained for use diagnostically. Therapeutic modalities of an LP include removal of bloody or purulent CSF, injection of medications into the subarachnoid space to bypass the blood-brain barrier (antibiotics or analgesics), or the introduction of spinal anesthesics.

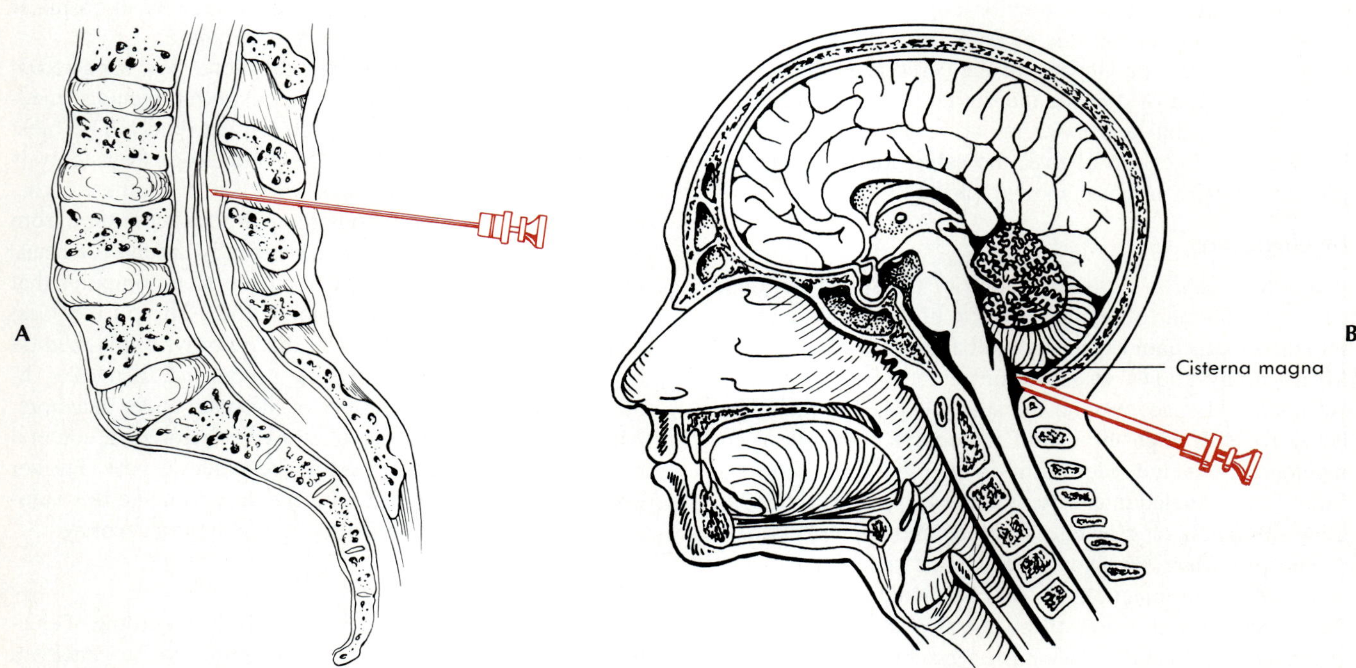


***Fig. 13-6*** **A,** Lumbar puncture. **B,** Cisternal puncture. (From Long BC and Phipps WJ: Medical-surgical nursing: a nursing process approach, ed 2, St Louis, 1989, Mosby–Year Book, Inc.)

An LP involves the introduction of an 18 to 22 gauge hollow needle into the subarachnoid space at L4 to L5 below the end of the spinal cord that is usually at L1 to L2. The patient can be placed either in the lateral recumbent position with the knees and head tightly tucked or in the sitting position leaning over a bedside table or some other support (Fig. 13-6).

Risks associated with a lumbar puncture include possible brainstem herniation if intracranial pressure is elevated or respiratory arrest associated with neurological deterioration.

Cisternal puncture which is the introduction of a needle into the cisterna magna at the C1 to C2 level is another method for obtaining access to the subarachnoid space. Risks of cisternal puncture are slightly higher than those associated with an LP, but it is a necessary procedure if there is inability to enter the lumbar space because of scar tissue or some other physical barrier or if there is a total blockage of the CSF pathway somewhere along the spinal column.

**REFERENCES**

1. Ad Hoc Committee of the Harvard Medical School to Examine the Definition of Brain Death: A definiton of irreversible coma, JAMA 205:337, 1968.
2. Bates B: A guide to physical exam, ed 4, Philadelphia, 1991, JB Lippincott Co.
3. Beresford HR: Severe neurologic impairment: legal aspects of decision to reduce care, Ann Neurol 15(5):409, 1984.
4. Borel C and Hanley D: Neurologic intensive care unit monitoring. In Rogers MC and Traystman RJ, editors: Critical care clinics: symposium on neurologic intensive care, vol 1, no 2, Philadelphia, 1985, WB Saunders Co.
5. Brophy vs. New England Sinai Hospital, Inc., J Am Geriatr Soc 35(7):669, 1987.
6. Cranford R: The persistent vegetative state: the medical reality (getting the facts straight), Hastings Cent Rep 18:27, 1988.
7. Davis KM and others: Brain death: nursing roles and responsibilities, J Neurosci Nurs 19(1):36, 1987.
8. Hickey JV: The clinical practice of neurologic and neurosurgical nursing, ed 2, Philadelphia, 1986, JB Lippincott Co.
9. Jones AG: Side effects following metrizamide myelography and lumbar laminectomy, Neurosci Nurs 19(2):90, 1987.
10. Plum F and Posner J: The diagnosis of stupor and coma, ed 3, Philadelphia, 1980, FA Davis Co.
11. Ricci MM: Core curriculum for neuroscience nursing, Chicago, 1984, American Association of Neuroscience Nurses.
12. Rudy EB: Advance neurological and neurosurgical nursing, St Louis, 1984, Mosby–Year Book, Inc.
13. Samuels MA: A systematic approach to the comatose patient, Emerg Med 22(8):16, 1990.
14. Steinbrook R: Artificial feeding—solid ground not a slippery slope, N Engl J Med 318(5):286, 1988.
15. Teasdale G and Jennett W: Assessment of coma and impaired consciousness: a practical scale, Lancet 2:81, 1974.
16. Ventura MG and Masser PG: Defining death: developments in recent law. In Rogers MC and Traystman RJ, editors: Critical care clinics: symposium on neurologic intensive care, vol 1, no 2, Philadelphia, 1985, WB Saunders Co.
17. Wilberger JE: Emergency burr holes: current role in neurosurgical acute care, Top Emerg Med 11(4):16, 1990.
18. Wilson SF and others: Determining interater reliability of nurses' assessment of pupillary size and reaction, J Neurosci Nurs 20(3):189, 1988.

CHAPTER 14

# Neurological Disorders

## CHAPTER OBJECTIVES

- *Define the concept of "malignant tumors" in the intracranial space.*
- *Define the treatment dilemmas of aneurysm rupture associated with vasospasm and rebleeding.*
- *Discuss the pathophysiology of Guillain-Barré syndrome.*

## KEY TERMS

astrocytoma, p. 306
meningioma, p. 307
cerebrovascular accident, p. 308
ischemic stroke, p. 308
hemorrhagic stroke, p. 308
berry aneurysm, p. 309
rebleeding, p. 309
arteriovenous malformation (AVM), p. 311
intracerebral hemorrhage, p. 312
Guillain-Barré syndrome, p. 312

## CENTRAL NERVOUS SYSTEM (CNS) TUMORS

### Description

Primary CNS tumors are classified as benign or malignant, but the definition of these terms varies from the tumor classification system of the rest of the body. Benign CNS tumors are those growths lying in accessible areas of the CNS with slow growth and lack of invasiveness. These can be completely removed without significant neurological deficit. Malignant tumors are neoplasms such as glioblastoma multiforme, which have multiple fingerlike projections into normal tissue. Attempts to completely remove all of the tumor would cause unacceptable neurological damage. Another type of CNS malignancy is the presence of a usually benign growth that lies deep in vital structures of the CNS where attempt at removal would cause severe neurological deficit. Tumors are malignant by location not by histological classification. Generally, CNS tumors do not metastasize outside of the CNS. Metastatic cells from the body do reproduce in the CNS. Primary lesions of the lung, breast, and prostate contribute most significantly to metastatic lesions in the brain.

### Cause

In the adult population, the most common tumor is glioblastoma multiforme, followed by meningioma and astrocytoma. Glioblastomas represent more than one half of all primary intracranial lesions.[39]

### Pathophysiology

A variety of classification systems have been developed over the years to categorize CNS tumor cells. For discussion here, tumors will be grouped in order of frequency.[48] Tumors of the CNS are competing with normal tissue for space inside the enclosed environment of the cranium or spinal column.

#### Classification

***Gliomas.*** Gliomas arise from the four neuroglial cells: astrocytes, oligodendroglia, ependymal cells, and microglia. Gliomas compose more than 50% of all primary tumors of the CNS.

ASTROCYTOMAS. A range of tumors from benign to highly malignant arise from the astrocyte cell. These tumors are graded from I to IV. **Astrocytoma** grade I is a slow-growing tumor with a life expectancy for the patient of up to 15 years. Astrocytoma grade II is a less well-differentiated cell that grows more rapidly, and the patient has a life expectancy of 8 to 10 years. Astrocytoma grade III has increasing malignant cytological features. Life expectancy of the patient with this tumor group is 2 to 5 years. The final most severe astrocytoma, grade IV, is also known as glioblastoma multiforme. It is characterized by grossly undifferentiated cells, significant necrosis, and a high incidence of hemorrhage into the lesion. Life expectancy of the patient with glioblastoma multiforme is 6 to 18 months.[26]

**OLIGODENDROGLIOMAS.** Oligodendrogliomas are usually benign but are occasionally malignant. They are slow growing, fairly solid, and discrete from surrounding brain tissue. Oligodendrogliomas are likely to have calcification as part of the mass. Frequently oligodendroglioma cells are found mixed with astrocytoma cells. The presence of a significant number of oligodendroglioma cells in an astrocytoma is a good prognostic sign.

***Meningiomas.*** The majority of **meningiomas** are noninvasive and considered benign. They are encapsulated and well demarcated from surrounding tissue. Meningiomas are most often found around the venous sinuses, over the convexities of the brain, or on the sphenoid ridge. These extremely slow-growing tumors can become quite large before symptoms appear. Meningiomas are the most common extramedullary CNS tumor.

***Acoustic neuromas or Schwannomas.*** These tumors are frequently small and considered benign, but they grow in the brainstem area that is difficult to access. Morbidity and mortality of these tumors is usually associated with pressure and damage to surrounding brainstem structures.

***Pituitary tumors.*** Pituitary tumors are made up of three types that arise from the adenohypophysis or anterior lobe of the pituitary. These three tumor types are chromophobic, eosinophilic, and basophilic adenomas.

The chromophobe adenoma responsible for 90% of pituitary tumors is a nonsecretory space-occupying tumor. These tumors produce their effect by putting pressure on surrounding secretory cells, which causes decreased production of stimulating hormones. This produces symptoms of hypopituitarism: irregular menses, amenorrhea, decreased libido, impotence, decreased body hair, and decreased production of other stimulating hormones.

There are two recognized hormone-secreting pituitary tumors. Eosinophilic adenomas secrete growth hormone (GH) that results in *giantism* before puberty and *acromegaly* after puberty. Basophilic adenomas secrete adrenocorticotropic hormone (ACTH), which results in Cushing's syndrome. Further alteration of this classification system is required because it has become clear that other pituitary hormone–producing tumors, such as prolactin-secreting adenoma, also occur.

***Vascular tumors.*** Vascular tumors of the CNS include hemangioma, hemangioblastoma, and, in some classifications, the arteriovenous malformation (AVM). A hemangioma is a closely packed group of abnormally dilated blood vessels. The hemangioblastoma contains a mixture of capillaries and large stromal cells. Both tumors are usually small and considered benign unless hemorrhage occurs. These lesions are found in both the brain and spinal cord.

The arteriovenous malformation is a tangled mass of arterial and venous vessels that may present as a mass lesion or CNS hemorrhage. AVMs will be discussed in the section on cerebral vascular disease in this chapter.

***Metastatic lesions.*** Lesions that most commonly give rise to metastases in the CNS are lung and breast lesions. Tumor cells are spread by blood or the lymphatic system. Metastatic lesions are generally well circumscribed with a defined margin. However, lesions are usually multiple. The incidence of metastatic tumors of the CNS is on the increase as therapy for limiting growth at other tumor sites improves.[26] Generally the blood-brain barrier remains intact with metastatic lesions so treatment with chemotherapeutic agents is difficult.

### Assessment and Diagnosis

Assessment of a patient with suspected CNS tumor is focused around the specific neurological abnormalities presented by the patient. Patients may initially have focal neurological deficit, history of increasing headaches that are worse in the morning than in the evening, seizure activity, hormonal changes, or personality changes.

Physical examination serves to further define the focal neurological deficit. If the tumor is large enough to create a mass effect, papilledema may be found. Papilledema is present in 70% to 75% of all brain tumors.

Depending on the suspected pathology, diagnostic workup may include a CT scan, MRI, EEG, neuroendocrine tests, cerebral angiogram, chest x-ray examination, or bone scan. After a specific lesion has been identified a biopsy is frequently performed for a histologic diagnosis. Once the type of tumor has been diagnosed, medical management can be planned.

### Treatment

Treatment of CNS tumor is centered around surgery, radiation, and chemotherapy. Depending on the type and location of the tumor, any or all of these treatment modalities may be employed.

If there is a major component of cerebral edema associated with the identified tumor, steroids are often the beginning point of medical management. The use of steroids, particularly dexamethasone (Decadron), can result in a significant reversal of neurological symptoms temporarily. Steroids, believed to reduce cerebral edema by strengthening the cell membrane, reduce neurological deficit by reducing intracranial pressure.

**Surgery.** Surgical removal of the entire lesion is the goal but not always the outcome. In benign, well-defined lesions, surgical removal may be the only treatment necessary. In invasive, poorly defined lesions, surgery is the beginning point of treatment. Even though it is well recognized that a craniotomy will not remove 100% of an invasive tumor, "debulking" of the tumor mass reduces pressure on surrounding structures and may slow the growth process.

**Radiation.** With incompletely excised tumors, radiation is often the next step of medical management. Some tumors that occur in functionally critical areas, such as the brainstem, hypothalamus, or thalamus, are not surgically accessible without resulting in significant neurological deficit. Radiation may be the primary medical management of these tumors.

**Chemotherapy.** Until recently, chemotherapy was unavailable to patients with malignant brain tumors because it was believed that chemotherapeutic agents did not cross the blood-brain barrier. Although that is still of primary concern, other factors also limit the effects of chemotherapy on brain tumors. Tumors of the CNS are small by nature. Although mitosis of abnormal cells in the tumor bed is occurring, it may not occur at a fast enough rate for a course of chemotherapy to be effective.[41] Also, with further study it appears that the microenvironment of the tumor area is not heterogeneous and therefore not 100% sensitive to any one chemotherapeutic agent.[41] In all considerations of chemotherapy, attention must be focused on protection of the normal delicate cerebral tissue.

### Nursing Diagnosis and Management
#### *Cerebral tumors*

- Altered Cerebral Tissue Perfusion related to increased intracranial pressure secondary to brain tumor, edema, p. 480
- Unilateral Neglect related to stroke involving the right cerebral hemisphere, p. 482
- Impaired Verbal Communication: Aphasia related to cerebral speech center injury, p. 488
- High Risk for Aspiration risk factors: depressed cough and gag reflexes, decreased gastrointestinal motility secondary to anesthesia, impaired swallowing, p. 476
- High Risk for Infection risk factor: invasive monitoring devices, p. 465
- High Risk for Impaired Skin Integrity risk factors: steroid therapy, reduced mobility, p. 499
- Sleep Pattern Disturbance related to fragmented sleep, p. 455
- Sensory-Perceptual Alterations related to sensory overload, sensory deprivation, sleep pattern disturbance, p. 489
- Anxiety related to threat to biological, psychological, and/or social integrity, p. 448
- Ineffective Individual Coping related to situational crisis and personal vulnerability, p. 447
- Body Image Disturbance related to actual change in body structure, function, and appearance, p. 443
- Altered Role Performance related to physical incapacity to resume usual or valued role, p. 444
- Knowledge Deficit: Prognosis, Medications, Activity Restrictions, Reportable Symptoms related to lack of previous exposure to information, p. 441
- Hopelessness related to perceptions of failing or deteriorating physical condition, p. 446

### Summary of Nursing Care

Most nursing management of the patient with a CNS tumor does not occur in the critical care environment. Generally, patients are in the critical care unit during the postoperative stage of craniotomy. With the advent of steroids, the cerebral edema associated with brain tumors and craniotomy has virtually been eliminated. Patients with an uncomplicated craniotomy for removal of a brain tumor often remain in the critical care unit only overnight, if at all. Patients who have had excision of a cervical or high thoracic spinal cord tumor will be in the unit postoperatively for close observation of respiratory status and motor/sensory function of the extremities. Refer to the box titled "Nursing Diagnosis and Management, Cerebral Tumors."

## CEREBROVASCULAR DISEASE

### Cerebrovascular Accident

**Description. Cerebrovascular accident,** commonly known as stroke, is a descriptive term for the onset of neurological symptoms caused by the interruption of blood flow to the brain. There are two basic types of stroke: ischemic and hemorrhagic. **Ischemic stroke** is a stroke that produces symptoms resulting from an occlusion of a blood vessel. This can be either thrombotic or embolic in nature. The majority of thrombotic strokes are the result of the accumulation of atherosclerotic plaque in the vessel lumen, especially at bifurcations or curves of the vessel. An embolic stroke occurs when a small embolus from the left side of the heart or lower cerebral circulation travels distally and lodges in a small vessel resulting in loss of blood supply. **Hemorrhagic strokes** are divided into intracerebral hemorrhage and subarachnoid hemorrhage. Intracerebral hemorrhage is most often caused by hypertensive rupture of a cerebral vessel. Subarachnoid hemorrhage can be caused by aneurysm rupture or arteriovenous malformation (AVM) rupture.

**Cause.** The risk of having a stroke before reaching age 70 is one in 20.[21] The major risk factors related to stroke are associated with factors that lead to the development of atherosclerosis. The major risk factors include hypertension, cardiac impairments, or diabetes mellitus.

### Cerebral Aneurysm

**Description.** An aneurysm is an outpouching of the wall of a blood vessel that results from weakening of the wall of the vessel. Most cerebral aneurysms are saccular or berrylike with a stem and neck. Aneurysms are usually small, 2 to 6 mm in diameter, but may be as large as 6 cm. Clinical concern arises if an aneurysm ruptures or becomes large enough to exert pressure on surrounding structures.

**Cause.** Ninety percent of aneurysms are congenital. The other 10% can be a result of traumatic injury (that stretches and tears the muscular middle layer of the arterial vessel),

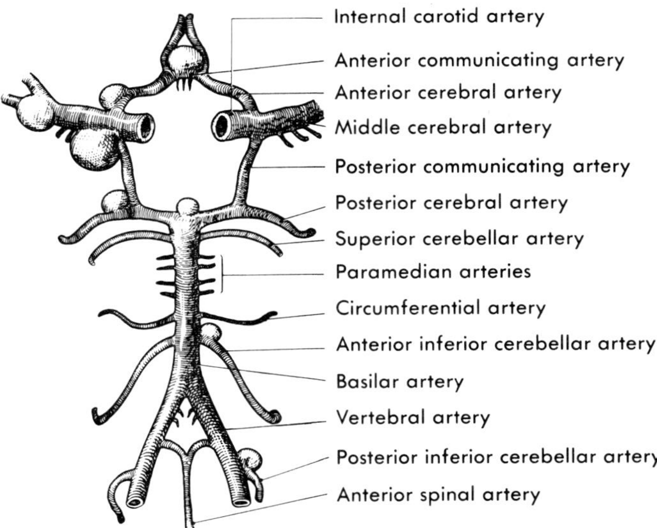


***Fig. 14-1*** The common sites of **berry aneurysms**. The size of the aneurysm in the drawing is proportional to the frequency of occurrence at the various sites. (From Wyngaarden JB and Smith LH, editors: Cecil textbook of medicine, ed 18, Philadelphia, 1987, WB Saunders.)

infectious material (most often from infectious vegetation on valves of the left side of the heart after subbacterial endocarditis) that lodges against a vessel wall and erodes the muscular layer, or of undetermined cause. Multiple aneurysms occur in 20% to 25% of the cases and are often bilateral, occurring in the same location on both sides of the head. Common sites of aneurysms are illustrated in Fig. 14-1.

**Pathophysiology.** The cause of the vessel development defect that occurs in the congenital aneurysm is unknown. A small portion of the inner muscular or elastic layer of the vessel is poorly developed, leaving a thin vessel wall. As the individual matures, blood pressure rises and more stress is placed on this thin vessel wall. Ballooning out of the vessel occurs, which gives the aneurysm its berrylike appearance.

The aneurysm becomes clinically significant when the vessel wall becomes so thin that it ruptures, sending arterial blood at a high pressure into the subarachnoid space. For a brief moment of aneurysm rupture, intracranial pressure is believed to approach mean arterial pressure and cerebral perfusion falls.[32] In other situations, the aneurysm expands and places pressure on surrounding structures. This is particularly true with the posterior communicating artery aneurysm that puts pressure on the oculomotor nerve (CN III) causing ipsilateral pupil dilation and ptosis.

**Assessment and diagnosis.** The initial presentation of a patient with an aneurysm is usually following subarachnoid hemorrhage (SAH). SAH becomes the working diagnosis until the cause of the hemorrhage is determined. Signs and symptoms of SAH range from sudden onset of "worst headache of my life" to coma or death.

Forty-five percent of the patients who survive SAH report sudden brief loss of consciousness followed by severe headache, 45% report severe headache associated with exertion but no loss of consciousness, and in 10% the bleeding was severe enough to cause loss of consciousness for up to several days.[13] Vomiting, nuchal rigidity (stiff neck), photophobia, seizure, hemiplegia, or other focal neurological deficits are also common.

A review of histories shows that the patient often reports one or more incidents of sudden onset of headache with vomiting in the weeks preceding major SAH. These are "warning leaks" of the aneurysm in which small amounts of blood ooze from the aneurysm into the subarachnoid space. This irritation causes headache, stiff neck, and photophobia. These small "warning leaks" are seldom detected because the condition is not severe enough for the patient to seek medical attention. If a neurological deficit, such as third cranial nerve palsy, develops before aneurysm rupture, medical intervention is sought and the aneurysm may be surgically secured before the devastation of rupture can occur.

Diagnosis of SAH is based on clinical presentation, as well as CT scan and lumbar puncture. If CT scan is unequivocal, a lumbar puncture is performed to obtain CSF for analysis. Cerebrospinal fluid after SAH is bloody in appearance with a red cell count >1,000. If lumbar puncture is performed more than 5 days after the SAH, CSF fluid is xanthochromic (dark amber) as blood products are broken down. Cloudy CSF usually indicates some type of infectious process such as bacterial meningitis, not subarachnoid hemorrhage.

Once the SAH has been documented, a cerebral angiogram is necessary to identify the exact cause of the SAH. If a cerebral aneurysm rupture is the cause, angiogram is also essential to define the exact location of the aneurysm in preparation for surgery (Fig. 14-2).

**Treatment.** Treatment of patients with SAH is complex. Decisions about surgical intervention and the timing of that intervention are based on the patient's clinical presentation. The two major complications following a subarachnoid hemorrhage from aneurysm rupture are rebleeding and vasospasm.

**Rebleeding** is another major subarachnoid hemorrhage that may occur at any time in an unsecured aneurysm. The incidence of rebleeding is as great as 50% in the first few months, with the highest incidence being in the first few days after hemorrhage.[19] Definitive treatment for prevention of rebleeding is surgical clipping of the aneurysm. Because of the patient's clinical condition and the technical difficulty of the surgery, early surgical repair of the aneurysm is not always possible.

Antifibrinolytic agents (aminocaproic acid) have been suggested in situations in which early surgery is not an option. Antifibrinolytic agents act by preventing the pro-

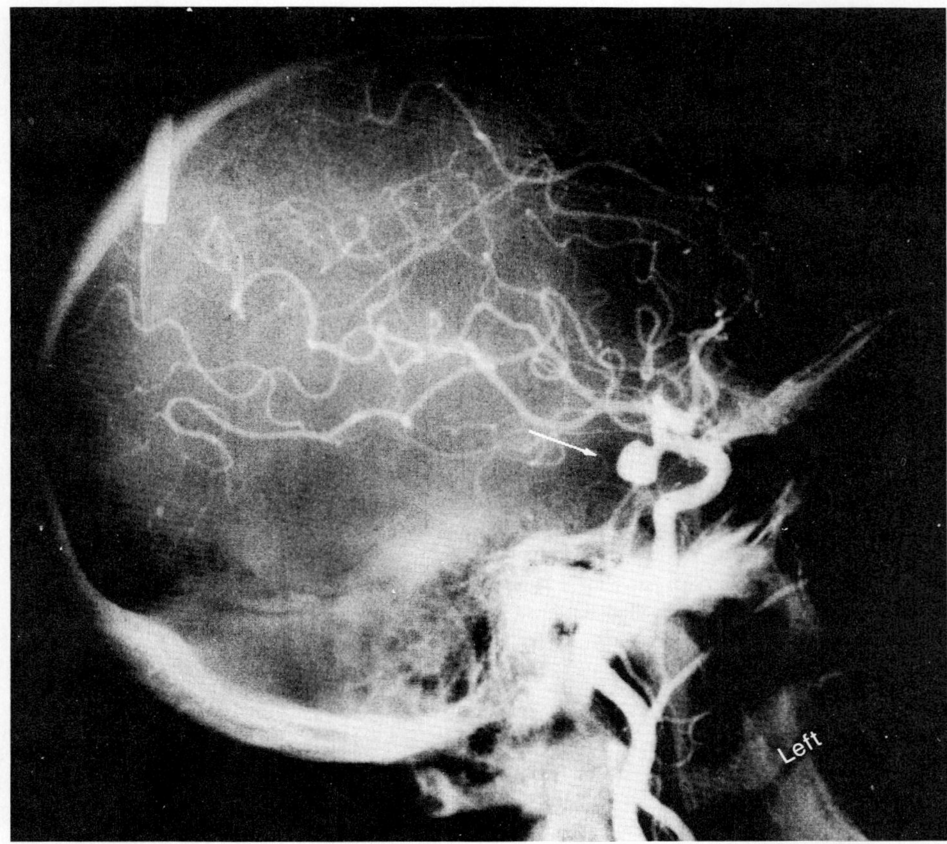


***Fig. 14-2*** Cerebral angiography showing location of aneurysm at posterior communicating artery. (From Tortorici M: Fundamentals of angiography, St Louis, 1982, Mosby–Year Book, Inc.)

duction of fibrin responsible for resolving the clot at the tip of the aneurysm. There is a tendency for these drugs to increase the incidence and severity of the other common SAH complication—vasospasm. Clinical trials continue to evaluate the efficacy of this treatment.[7,23]

The presence or absence of cerebral vasospasm has a significant effect on the outcome of a patient after SAH. Vasospasm is the narrowing of the lumen of the vessel either from actual spastic constriction of the vessel or an inflammatory swelling of the vessel wall that narrows the lumen. Vasospasm is a critical issue because of its location in the cerebral vasculature. Because aneurysms occur at the circle of Willis, the major vessels responsible for feeding cerebral circulation are affected by vasospasm. Decreased arterial flow occurs in large areas of the cerebral hemispheres depending on the arterial vessels involved in the vasospasm reaction. Ischemic stroke is the outcome of this decreased flow. The peak period for vasospasm is 7 to 14 days after rupture.

*Hypervolemic hypertension* involves increasing the patient's blood pressure and cardiac output through the use of fluid and volume expanders such as plasma. Systolic blood pressure is maintained between 150 and 160 mm Hg. This increase in volume and pressure forces blood at higher pressures through the vasospastic area. The obvious deterrent to use of induced hypertension is the risk of rebleed in an unsecured aneurysm. This therapy can be used safely only after surgery for aneurysm clipping. The second complication associated with hypervolemic hypertension therapy is the risk of pulmonary edema associated with fluid overload.

The second therapy for the treatment of vasospasm is the use of calcium channel blockers. Although the exact role of calcium channel blockers in the prevention of vasospasm is not known, evidence is mounting in clinical research trials of its effectiveness if begun immediately after the initial hemorrhage.[1,7,33]

Timing of surgery is a key medical management issue. Since the introduction of microsurgery and improved surgical techniques, patients are frequently taken to the operating room within the first 48 hours after rupture. This early surgical intervention to secure the aneurysm eliminates the risk of rebleeding and allows hypertensive therapy to be used in the postoperative period for the treatment of vasospasm. Early surgery also allows the neurosurgeon to flush out the excess blood and clots from the basal cisterns (reservoir of CSF around the base of the brain and circle of Willis) to reduce the risk of vasospasm.

*Aneurysm clipping* is the surgical procedure that is performed for repair of the aneurysm. This procedure involves a craniotomy to expose the area of aneurysm. The aneurysm itself is isolated and a clip is placed over the neck of the aneurysm to eliminate the area of weakness.

Development of hydrocephalus is a late complication that frequently occurs after SAH. Blood that has circulated in the subarachnoid space and has been absorbed by the arachnoid villi may obstruct these villi and reduce the rate of CSF absorption. Over time, increasing volumes of CSF in the intracranial space produce communicating hydrocephalus. Treatment for this is placement of a drain to remove CSF. This can be temporary with a catheter placed into the lateral ventricle and attached to an external drainage bag or permanent with the placement of a ventriculoperitoneal shunt. Nursing care is summarized after discussion of intracerebral hemorrhage, p. 312.

### Arteriovenous Malformation

**Description. Arteriovenous malformation (AVM)** is a tangled mass of arterial and venous blood vessels that shunt blood directly from the arterial side into the venous side, bypassing the capillary system. AVMs may be small, focal lesions or large lesions that occupy almost an entire hemisphere.

**Cause.** The cause of an AVM is always congenital. The exact embryonic reason for the development of this malformation is unknown. AVMs are not confined to the cerebral circulation. AVMs can be found in the spinal cord and in the renal, gastrointestinal, or integumentary system; Port wine stains of the skin may be caused by small superficial AVMs.

**Pathophysiology.** Once the embryonic dysfunction that resulted in the AVM has occurred, the pathophysiology is related to the size and location of the malformation. The AVM can be fed by one or more cerebral arteries. Called feeders, these arteries tend to enlarge over time and increase the volume of blood shunted through the malformation as well as increase the overall mass effect. Large, dilated tortuous draining veins also develop as a result of the increasing flow of blood. Blood flowing into the venous side of the AVM does so at a higher than normal pressure. Because there is no muscular layer in the vein as there is in the artery, veins become extremely engorged.

As a result of the shunting of blood through the AVM and away from normal cerebral circulation, poor perfusion occurs in the underlying cerebral tissues. This decreased perfusion produces a chronic ischemic state that results in cerebral atrophy.

**Assessment and diagnosis.** Initial assessment of the patient depends on the presenting symptoms. Although SAH is one of the most common and severe presenting symptoms, there are other signs and symptoms that also may occur before subarachnoid hemorrhage.

The onset of seizures is frequently a reason for the patient with an AVM to seek medical attention. As the mass of the AVM enlarges and the flow of blood increases, the pulsation of the blood vessel against the cerebral tissue surface causes a disturbance of the electrical activity of the area. Seizures can be focal or generalized.

Headaches are another common symptom of patients with an AVM. Headache may occur as a result of the increasing mass effect of the lesion or be associated with vascular changes in response to the shunted blood.

A very small percentage of the patients demonstrate a bruit and will report a constant swishing sound in the head with each heart beat. In other patients, the bruit can be auscultated with a stethoscope placed over the skull.

Other symptoms of AVM may include motor/sensory defects, aphasia, dizziness, or fainting. Since a majority of patients are under the age of 30, symptoms such as these would not likely be attributed to atherosclerotic vascular disease.

Diagnostic evaluation includes CT scan, EEG, and angiogram. CT scan is performed initially as a noninvasive study to begin the diagnostic process. If an AVM is suspected from the results of the noncontrast scan, a contrast scan is performed. EEG is done to attempt to localize any seizure focus or to define areas of cortical injury caused by cerebral ischemia or atrophy.

Finally, for confirmation and definition of the AVM, an angiogram is performed. If surgical intervention is planned, an angiogram is required to identify the feeding arteries and draining veins of the AVM.

**Treatment**

***Surgical excision.*** Treatment of the patient has traditionally involved surgical excision of the AVM or conservative management of the symptoms such as seizures and headache. The decision for surgical excision depends on the location and size of the AVM. Some malformations are located so deep in cerebral structures (the thalamus or midbrain) that attempts to remove the AVM would cause severe neurological deficits. The history of previous hemorrhage, the age, and general condition of the patient are also taken into account in the decision about surgical intervention.

Surgical excision of large AVMs include the risk of reperfusion bleeding. As feeding arteries of the AVM are clamped off, the arterial blood that usually flowed into the AVM is now diverted into the surrounding circulation. In many cases the surrounding tissue has been in a state of chronic ischemia and the arterial vessels feeding these areas are maximally dilated. As arterial blood begins to flow at a higher volume and pressure into these dilated arteries, seeping of blood from the vessels may occur. In the postoperative phase, low blood pressure is maintained to prevent further reperfusion bleeding. In large AVMs, two to four stages of surgery might be required over a 6- to 12-month period.

***Embolization.*** Embolization is another method of reducing the size of an AVM. It may also be used on surgically inaccessible AVMs. Embolization is an interventional radiology technique in which a catheter is placed in the groin or other site, similar to that done in an angiogram. Under fluoroscopy, the catheter is threaded up to the internal carotid artery. Small silastic beads or a variety of other materials such as glue are then slowly introduced through the catheter. The increased flow to the AVM should carry the blocking material into the AVM. The purpose of this procedure is to block the feeding arterial portion of the AVM and therefore eliminate the AVM. Frequently, embolization and surgery are combined. The patient receives one to three sessions of embolization to reduce the size of the lesion and then has a craniotomy for total excision.

Risks to the procedure include lodging of the substance in a vessel feeding normal tissue. This creates an embolic stroke. Onset of neurological symptoms occurs immediately. Another risk involves passage of the embolic substance right through the lesion out the venous system and into the lung. If that should occur the patient experiences a pulmonary embolus. Nursing care is summarized after discussion of intracerebral hemorrhage, next column.

### Intracerebral Hemorrhage

**Description. Intracerebral hemorrhage** is the escape of blood into cerebral tissue. Causes of intracerebral hemorrhage are aneurysm or AVM rupture, trauma, or hypertensive hemorrhage. This section will concentrate on hypertensive hemorrhage. Hemorrhage destroys cerebral tissue, causes cerebral edema, and increases intracranial pressure.

**Cause.** The cause of hypertensive stroke is largely a longstanding history of hypertension. Blood dyscrasia (leukemia, hemophilia, sickle cell disease), anticoagulation therapy, and hemorrhage into brain tumors are other possible causes of intracerebral hemorrhage. Frequently on questioning, the patient with a hypertensive hemorrhage will admit to having discontinued antihypertensive medication 2 to 3 weeks before the hemorrhage.

**Pathophysiology.** The pathophysiology of intracerebral hemorrhage is caused by continued elevated blood pressure exerting force against smaller arterial vessels that have become damaged from arteriosclerotic changes. Eventually this artery breaks, and blood bursts from the vessel into the cerebral tissue, creating a hematoma. Intracranial pressure rises precipitously in response to the increased overall intracranial volume.

**Assessment and diagnosis.** Initial assessment usually reveals a critically ill patient. The patient is often unconscious and requires ventilatory support. History from a relative or significant other describes a sudden onset of severe headache with rapid neurological deterioration.

Vital signs usually reveal a severely elevated blood pressure (200/100 to 250/150), slow pulse, and deep, labored respirations. The patient arrives in the emergency room with many of the signs of increased intracranial pressure.

**Treatment.** Administration of an antihypertensive medication is usually begun immediately to reduce the blood pressure to relatively normal pressure. If the hemorrhage is significant enough to cause increased ICP, the blood pressure should not be allowed to drop rapidly or too low. If blood pressure drops below 140 systolic and ICP remains high, cerebral perfusion may be compromised.

Surgical removal of the clot is dependent on the size and location of the clot, the patient's ICP, and other neurological symptoms. If the hematoma is large and causes a shift in structures or ICP is elevated despite routine methods to lower it, a craniotomy for removal of the hematoma is performed. Nonsurgical management includes measures to maintain the ICP within normal limits and support of all other vital functions until the patient regains consciousness.

**Summary of nursing care.** Nursing management of the patient with cerebrovascular disease is summarized in the box on p. 313.

If the patient is comatose after the cerebrovascular insult, all interventions for caring for the immobile patient should be initated. Immobility is implicated in many patient complications so intervention to reduce the effects of immobility should occur as soon as possible.

Emotional support to the patient and family is, as always, important. Especially if the patient is dealing with a neurological deficit such as hemiplegia, aphasia, or any significant neurological deficit, fear of dependency and of becoming a burden are issues that must be faced. Both the patient and family should be involved in all aspects of planning of care.[8]

## GUILLAIN-BARRÉ SYNDROME

### Description

**Guillain-Barré syndrome (GBS)**, also known as Landry-Guillain-Barré syndrome, is a postinfectious peripheral polyneuritis characterized by a rapidly progressive ascending peripheral nerve dysfunction leading to paralysis. It is 90% to 100% reversible and is one of the most common peripheral nervous system diseases. Because of the ventilatory support required for these patients, GBS is one of the few peripheral neurological diseases requiring a critical care environment.

### Cause

The cause of GBS is unknown, but more than 50% of patients reported a mild febrile illness, either respiratory or gastrointestinal, 1 to 3 weeks before the onset of signs and symptoms. The result is a possible autoimmune response of the peripheral nervous system.

### Pathophysiology

This disease affects the motor and sensory pathways of the peripheral nervous system as well as the autonomic nervous system functions of the cranial nerves. The major finding in GBS is a segmental demyelination process of the peripheral nerves. Inflammation around this demyelinate area causes further dysfunction.

**Nursing Diagnosis and Management**

***Cerebrovascular disease***

- Altered Cerebral Tissue Perfusion related to increased intracranial pressure secondary to brain hemorrhage, edema, stroke, hydrocephalus, p. 480
- Altered Cerebral Tissue Perfusion related to vasospasm secondary to subarachnoid hemorrhage after ruptured intracranial aneurysm or arteriovenous malformation, p. 478
- Unilateral Neglect related to right cerebral hemisphere stroke, p. 482
- Impaired Verbal Communication: Aphasia related to cerebral speech center injury, p. 488
- High Risk for Aspiration risk factors: reduced level of consciousness, presence of endotracheal tube, gastrointestinal tube, tube feedings, situation hindering elevation of upper body (vasospasm after subarachnoid hemorrhage), decreased gastrointestinal motility secondary to anesthesia, impaired swallowing, p. 476
- High Risk for Altered Peripheral Tissue Perfusion risk factor: vasopressor therapy (vasospasm after cerebral artery aneurysm rupture), p. 462
- Impaired Gas Exchange related to alveolar hypoventilation secondary to decreased level of consciousness, p. 475
- Ineffective Breathing Pattern related to respiratory muscle deconditioning secondary to mechanical ventilation, p. 471
- Ineffective Airway Clearance related to impaired cough secondary to loss of glottic closure with cuffed endotracheal tube, p. 468
- Activity Intolerance related to postural hypotension secondary to prolonged immobility, p. 463
- Altered Nutrition: Less Than Body Protein-Calorie Requirements related to lack of exogenous nutrients and increased metabolic demand. (See also discussion of metabolic results from carbohydrate overfeeding, Chapter 6.)
- High Risk for Infection risk factors: invasive monitoring devices, p. 465
- High Risk for Impaired Skin Integrity risk factors: reduced mobility protein-calorie malnourishment, steroid therapy, altered cutaneous sensation, p. 499
- Anxiety related to threat to biological, psychological, and /or social integrity, p. 448
- Ineffective Individual Coping related to situational crisis and personal vulnerability, p. 447
- Sensory-Perceptual Alterations related to sensory deprivation, sensory overload, sleep pattern disturbance, p. 489
- Sleep Pattern Disturbance related to fragmented sleep, p. 455
- Body Image Disturbance related to actual change in body structure, function, and appearance, p. 443
- Powerlessness related to health care environment and illness-related regimen, p. 445
- Altered Role Performance related to physical incapacity to resume usual or valued role, p. 444
- Self-Esteem Disturbance related to feelings of guilt over physical deterioration, p. 442
- Knowledge Deficit: Physical Rehabilitation, Medications, Reportable Symptoms related to lack of previous exposure to information, p. 441

GBS is believed to be an autoimmune response to antibodies formed against the recent febrile illness. Immune reactions from the T cells and B cells of the lymphatic system set up a local inflammatory reaction that triggers further inflammation.

Once the temporary inflammatory reaction stops, myelin-producing cells begin the process of reinsulating the demyelinated portions of the peripheral nervous system. When remyelination occurs, normal neurological function should return. In some instances the axon may be damaged during the inflammatory process. The degree of axonal damage is responsible for the extent of neurological dysfunction that persists after recovery.

### Assessment and Diagnosis

The usual course of GBS begins with an abrupt onset of lower extremity weakness that progresses to flaccidity and ascends over a period of hours to days. Motor loss is usually symmetrical. In the most severe cases, complete flaccidity of all peripheral nerves, including spinal and cranial nerves, occurs. The ascending paralysis plateaus for 1 to 4 weeks. This is followed by descending paralysis and return to normal or near-normal function.

Admission to the hospital occurs when lower extremity weakness prevents mobility. Admission to the critical care unit occurs when progression of the weakness threatens respiratory muscles. As the patient's weakness progresses, close observation is essential. Frequent assessment of the respiratory system, including ventilatory parameters such as inspiratory force and tidal volume, are necessary. The most common cause of death in GBS patients is from respiratory arrest.

As the disease progresses and respiratory effort weakens, intubation and mechanical ventilation are necessary. Con-

## Nursing Diagnosis and Management
### *Guillain-Barré syndrome*


- Ineffective Airway Clearance related to respiratory muscle dysfunction and impaired cough secondary to Guillain-Barré syndrome, p. 469
- Sensory-Perceptual Alterations related to sensory overload, sensory deprivation, sleep pattern disturbance, p. 489
- Acute Pain related to transmission and perception of noxious stimuli secondary to reestablishment of myoneural activity, p. 485
- Ineffective Airway Clearance related to impaired cough secondary to loss of glottic closure with tracheostomy or endotracheal tube, p. 468
- Impaired Gas Exchange related to alveolar hypoventilation secondary to respiratory muscle paralysis, p. 475
- High Risk for Aspiration risk factors: depressed cough and gag reflexes, presence of tracheostomy or endotracheal tube, gastrointestinal tube, tube feedings, decreased gastrointestinal motility secondary to immobility, impaired swallowing, p. 476
- Ineffective Breathing Pattern related to respiratory muscle deconditioning secondary to mechanical ventilation, p. 471
- Altered Nutrition: Less Than Body Protein-Calorie Requirements related to lack of exogenous nutrients, (See also discussion of metabolic results from carbohydrate overfeeding, Chapter 6.)
- High Risk for Infection risk factors: protein-calorie malnourishment, invasive monitoring devices, p. 465
- High Risk for Impaired Skin Integrity risk factors: protein-calorie malnourishment, immobility, steroid therapy, stool and urine incontinence, p. 499
- Activity Intolerance related to postural hypotension secondary to prolonged immobility, p. 463
- Body Image Disturbance related to functional dependence on life-sustaining technology, p. 443
- Powerlessness related to health care environment and illness-related regimen, p. 445
- Anxiety related to threat to biological, psychological, and/or social integrity, p. 448
- Ineffective Individual Coping related to situational crisis and personal vulnerability, p. 447
- Knowledge Deficit: Course of Treatment, Prognosis related to lack of previous exposure to information, p. 441


tinued, frequent assessment of neurological deterioration occurs until the patient reaches the peak of the disease and plateaus.

The diagnosis of GBS is based on clinical findings plus CSF analysis and nerve conduction studies. CSF analysis demonstrates a normal protein initially that elevates in the fourth to sixth week. No other changes in CSF occur. Nerve conduction studies that test the velocity at which nerve impulses are conducted are significantly reduced as would be expected with the demyelinating process of the disease.

### Treatment

The treatment of GBS is limited. No curative treatment exists for this disease. It simply must run its course. The main focus of medical management is the support of bodily functions and the prevention of complications. Some physicians support the use of steroids for their antiinflammatory effect. The effectiveness of steroids are difficult to assess. If steroids are prescribed, all usual precautions associated with steroid use should be followed. Plasmapheresis has also been used, which involves plasma exchanges or washes that remove the antibodies causing the GBS.

### Summary of Nursing Care

The nursing management of the patient with GBS is extensive. The goal of nursing management is to support all normal body functions until such time as the patient can do so on his or her own. Nursing management focuses on immobility, pulmonary care, nutritional support, pain management, and, very importantly, emotional support. See the box at left for nursing management of patients with Guillain-Barré syndrome.

Total ventilatory support and pulmonary toilet are required at the peak level of the illness. As the patient's symptoms recede, weaning from the ventilator and initiation of deep breathing exercises will be important in prevention of pulmonary complications.

Implementing nutritional support should occur early in the course of the disease. Since it is known that GBS recovery is a long process, adequate nutritional support will be a problem for an extended period of time. Nutritional support is usually accomplished through the use of enteral feeding.

Pain control is an important component in the care of patients with GBS. Although the patient has minimal to no motor function, most sensory functions are maintained. The patient feels considerable muscle ache and pain.

The emotional support required by these patients is extensive. Although the illness is almost 100% reversible, the total helplessness of the patient, the constant pain or discomfort, plus the length of the course of the disease makes this a difficult experience with which to deal. It is important to remember that GBS does not affect the level of consciousness or cerebral function. Interaction and communication are necessary elements of the nursing plan of care.

**REFERENCES**


1. Adams HP: Early management of the patient with recent aneurysmal subarachnoid hemorrhage, Stroke 17(6):1068, 1986.
2. Adornato BT and Glasberg MR: Disease of the spinal cord. In Rosenberg RN, editor: Neurology, New York, 1988, Grune & Stratton.
3. Albin MS: Acute cervical spinal injury. In Rogers MC and Traystman RJ, editors: Critical care clinics: neurologic intensive care, Philadelphia, 1985, WB Saunders Co.
4. Albright AL, Price RA, and Guthkelch AN: Brainstem gliomas of children: a clinicopathological study, Cancer 52:2313, 1983.
5. Ammons AM: Cerebral injuries and intracranial hemorrhages as a result of trauma, Nurs Clin North Am 25(1):23, 1990.
6. Baker SP, O'Neill B, and Karpf RS: The injury fact book, Lexington, Mass, 1984, DC Heath & Co.
7. Beck DW and others: Combination of aminocaproic acid and nicardipine in treatment of aneurysmal subarachnoid hemorrhage, Stroke 19(1):63, 1988.
8. Bernstein LP: Family-centered care of the critically ill neurologic patient, Crit Care Clin North Am 2(1):41, 1990.
9. Browner CM: Halo immobilization brace care: an innovative approach, J Neurosci Nurs 19(1):24, 1987.
10. Cooper JD, Tabaddor K, and Hauser WA: The epidemiology of head injury in the Bronx, Neuroepidemiology 2:70, 1983.
11. Dacey RG and Dikmen SS: Mild head injury. In Cooper PR, editor: Head injury, Baltimore, 1987, Williams & Wilkins.
12. Farwell JR, Dohrmann GJ, and Flannery JT: Medulloblastoma in childhood: an epidemiological study, J Neurosurg 61:657, 1984.
13. Fisher CM: Clinical syndromes in cerebral thrombosis, hypertensive hemorrhage and ruptured aneurysm, Clin Neurosurg 22:117, 1975.
14. Flynn EP: Cerebral vasospasm following intracranial aneurysm rupture: a protocol for detection, J Neurosci Nurs 21(6):348, 1990.
15. Fretag E: Autopsy findings in head injuries from blunt forces: statistical evaluation of 1367 cases, Arch Path 75:402, 1963.
16. Graham DI, Adams JH, and Gennarelli TA: Pathology of brain damage in head injury. In Cooper PR, editor: Head injury, Baltimore, 1987, Williams & Wilkins.
17. Gresham GE and others: Epidemiologic profile of long-term stroke disability: the Framingham study, Arch Phys Med Rehab 60:487, 1979.
18. Hunt WE and Hess RM: Surgical risks as related to time of intervention in the repair of intracranial aneurysms, J Neurosurg 28:14, 1968.
19. Jane JA, Winn HR, and Richardson AE: The natural history of intracranial aneurysms; rebleeding rates during acute and long-term period and implication for surgical management, Clin Neurosurg 24:176, 1977.
20. Jankovic J: Differential diagnosis of stroke. In Meyer JS and Shaw T, editors: Diagnosis and management of stroke and TIAs, Menlo Park, Calif, 1982, Addison-Wesley Publishing Co.
21. Kannel WB and others: Components of blood pressure and risk of atherothrombotic brain infarction: the Farmingham study, Stroke 7:327, 1976.
22. Kassell NF, Haley EC, and Torner JC: Antifibrinolytic therapy in the treatment of aneurysmal subarachnoid hemorrhage, Clin Neurosurg 33:137, 1986.
23. Kassell NF and others: Treatment of ischemic deficits from vasospasm with intravascular volume expansion and induced arterial hypertension, Neurosurgery 11(3):337, 1982.
24. Keenlyside R and Brezman D: Fatal Guillian-Barré syndrome after the national influenza immunization program, Neurology 30:929, 1980.
25. Klauber MR, Marshall LF, and Barrett-Conner E: Prospective study of patients hospitalized with head injury in San Diego County, 1978, Neurosurgery 9:26, 1981.
26. Kornblith PL, Walker MD, and Cassady JR: Neurologic oncology, Philadelphia, 1987, JB Lippincott Co.
27. Kraus JF: Epidemiology of head injury. In Cooper PR, editor: Head injury, Baltimore, 1987, Williams & Wilkins.
28. Kraus JF and others: The incidence of acute brain injury and serious impairment in a defined population, Am J Epidemiol 119:186, 1984.
29. Locksley HB: Natural history of subarachnoid hemorrhage, intracranial aneurysm and AVM. In Sachs AL and others: Intracranial aneurysms and subarachnoid hemorrhage: a cooperative study, Philadelphia, 1969, JB Lippincott Co.
30. Marshall LF, Toole BM, and Bowers SA: The national traumatic coma data bank. Part 2. Patients who talk and deteriorate: implications for treatment, J Neurosurg 59:285, 1983.
31. National Center for Health Statistics: Monthly Vital Statistics Report. Advanced Report of Final Mortality Statistics, 1982, Hyattsville, Md, Public Health Service. Dec. 20, 1984. 33(9):Supp DHHS Pub. No. (PHS) 85-112.
32. Normes H and Magnaes B: Intracranial pressure in patients with ruptured saccular aneurysm, J Neurosurg 36:536, 1972.
33. Petruk KC and others: Nimodipine treatment in poor-grade aneurysm patients: results of a multicenter double blind placebo-controlled trial, J Neurosurg 68(4):505, 1988.
34. Phonprasert C and others: Extradural hematoma: analysis of 138 cases, J Trauma 20:679, 1980.
35. Piepmeier JM: Cervical fracture. In Long DM, editor: Current therapy in neurological surgery, ed 2, St Louis, 1989, Mosby–Year Book, Inc.
36. Plyar PA: Management of the agitated and aggressive head injury patient in an acute hospital setting, J Neurosci Nurs 21(6):358, 1990.
37. Rimel RW and others: Disability caused by minor head injury, Neurosurgery 9:221, 1981.
38. Sances A and others: The biomechanics of spinal injuries, CRC Crit Rev Biomech Eng 11:1, 1984.
39. Schoenberg BS: Epidemiology of primary nervous system neoplasms. In Schoenberg BS, editor: Advances in neurology, vol 19, New York, 1978, Raven Press.
40. Seelig JM and others: Traumatic acute epidural hematoma: unrecognized high lethality in comatose patients, Neurosurgery 15:617, 1984.
41. Shapiro WR and others: Heterogeneous response to chemotherapy of human gliomas grown in mice, Cancer Treat Rep 65(suppl 2):55, 1981.
42. Spinal Cord Injury, No. 81-160. Bethesda, 1981, US Dept of Health and Human Services, National Institutes of Health.
43. Susi EA and others: Traumatic cerebral vasospasm and secondary head injury, Crit Care Clin North Am 21(1):15, 1990.
44. Tindall RSA: Cerebrovascular disease. In Rosenberg RN, editor: Neurology, New York, 1980, Grune & Stratton.
45. Welsh DM: Volumetric insterstitial hyperthermai: nursing implications for brain tumor treatment, J Neurosci Nurs 20(4):229, 1988.
46. Wolf P and Kannel W: Controllable risk factors for stroke: preventive implications of trends in stroke mortality. In Meyer JS and Shaw T, editors: Diagnosis and management of stroke and TIAs, Menlo Park, Calif, 1982, Addison-Wesley Publishing Co.
47. Wrobel CJ and Marshall LF: Closed head injury management dilemmas. In Long DM, editor: Current therapy in neurological surgery, ed 2, St Louis, 1989, Mosby–Year Book, Inc.
48. Zulch DJ: Principles of the New World Health Organization (WHO) Classification of Brain Tumors, Neuroradiology 19:59, 1980.

CHAPTER 15

# Neurological Therapeutic Management

## CHAPTER OBJECTIVES

- *Discuss the concept of cerebral autoregulation.*
- *Calculate cerebral perfusion pressure.*
- *Describe the therapies commonly used to treat intracranial hypertension.*
- *Discuss the complications associated with high-dose barbiturate therapy.*
- *List the four supratentorial herniation syndromes.*

## KEY TERMS

volume-pressure curve, p. 316
autoregulation, p. 317
cerebral profusion pressure, p. 317
ventriculostomy, p. 317
barbiturate therapy, p. 320
uncal herniation, p. 321
central herniation, p. 322

Despite the diversity of neurological pathologies, one aspect of the critical care management of the neurosurgical patient is common to a wide variety of these pathological conditions. This chapter focuses on the concepts of intracranial pressure (ICP) and the types of ICP monitoring. Also discussed are the therapies for management of intracranial hypertension.

## ASSESSMENT OF INTRACRANIAL PRESSURE

### Monro-Kellie Hypothesis

The intracranial space comprises three components: brain substance (80%), cerebrospinal fluid (CSF) (10%), and blood (10%). Under normal physiological conditions, the ICP is maintained below 15 mm Hg mean pressure. Basic to understanding the pathophysiology of ICP is the Monro-Kellie hypothesis.[11] This hypothesis proposes that an increase in volume of one intracranial component must be compensated by a decrease in one or more of the other components so that total volume remains fixed. This compensation, although limited, includes displacing CSF from the intracranial vault to the lumbar cistern, increasing CSF absorption, and compressing the low-pressure venous system.

### Volume-Pressure Curve

When the brain is capable of compliance, significant increases in intracranial volume can be tolerated without much increase in ICP. However, the amount of intracranial compliance is limited. Once this limit has been reached, a state of decompensation with increased ICP results. As the ICP rises, the relationship between volume and pressure changes, and small increases in volume may cause major elevations in ICP. The exact configuration of the **volume-pressure curve** and the point at which the steep rise in pressure occurs vary with individual patients.[16] The configuration of this curve is also influenced by the cause and the rate of volume increases within the intracranial vault; for example, a patient with an acute epidural hematoma will neurologically deteriorate more rapidly than the patient with a meningioma of the same size. Monitoring these changes in intracranial dynamics and continuous clinical assessment of the patient's neurological status have proven beneficial in diagnosing and treating sustained rises in ICP. Such elevations of ICP often precede evidence of neurological deterioration obtained through the clinical assessment.

### Cerebral Blood Flow and Autoregulation

Cerebral blood flow is proportional to meet the metabolic demands of the brain. Although the brain is only 2% of body weight, it requires 15% to 20% of the resting cardiac output and 15% of the body's oxygen demands.[17] The normal brain has a complex capacity to maintain a constant

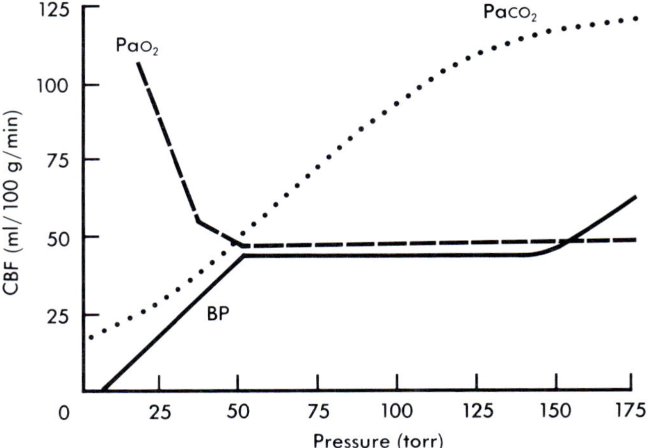


***Fig. 15-1*** Effects of arterial blood pressure, oxygen, and carbon dioxide on cerebral blood flow.

blood flow despite wide ranges in arterial pressure—an effect known as **autoregulation** (Fig. 15-1). Mean arterial pressure (MAP) of 50 to 150 mm Hg does not alter cerebral blood flow when autoregulation is present.[17] Outside the limits of this autoregulation, cerebral blood flow becomes passively dependent on the perfusion pressure. Other factors besides arterial blood pressure that affect cerebral blood flow are conditions that result in acidosis, alkalosis, and changes in metabolic rate.[9] Conditions that cause acidosis (hypoxia, hypercapnia, and ischemia) result in cerebral vascular dilation. Conditions causing alkalosis (hypocapnia) result in cerebrovascular constriction. Normally, a reduction in metabolic rate (for example, from hypothermia or barbiturates) decreases cerebral blood flow, and increases in metabolic rate (for example, from hyperthermia) result in an increase in cerebral blood flow.

### Cerebral Perfusion Pressure

**Cerebral perfusion pressure** (CPP), an estimated pressure, is the blood pressure gradient across the brain and is calculated as the difference between the incoming MAP and the opposing ICP on the arteries[6,17]:

$$\text{CPP} = \text{MAP} - \text{ICP}$$

The CPP in the average adult is approximately 80 to 100 mm Hg, with a range of 60 to 150 mm Hg. The CPP should be maintained near 60 mm Hg to provide adequate blood supply to the brain. If the CPP drops below this point, ischemia may develop. A sustained CPP of 30 mm Hg or less usually will result in neuronal hypoxia and cell death. When the mean systemic arterial pressure equals the ICP, cerebral blood flow may cease.

### Monitoring Techniques

The type of monitor placed in the ventricular system is usually a small catheter known as a **ventriculostomy** catheter. It is inserted through a burr hole with the patient under local anesthesia and is usually placed in the anterior horn of the lateral ventricle. If at all possible, the side chosen for placement of the ventriculostomy is the nondominant hemisphere (Fig. 15-2, *A*).

The second type of monitor frequently used is the *subarachnoid bolt or screw*. This small, hollow device is placed in a patient under local anesthesia through a burr hole, with the distal end lying in the subarachnoid or subdural space. The insertion of this device is easier than insertion of the ventriculostomy (Fig. 15-2, *B*).

Another type of device commonly used is the *epidural monitor*. It too is placed through a burr hole while the patient is under local anesthesia. It is essential for the physician to strip the dura away from the inner table of the skull before inserting the epidural monitor. The most common type of epidural monitor is the fiberoptic or pneumatic sensor, although there are other implantable epidural transducers that are often used for long-term monitoring (Fig. 15-2, *C*).

A new type of ICP monitoring system is the *fiberoptic transducer-tipped catheter* (Fig. 15-2, *D*). This small (4 Fr) catheter can be placed intraventricularly, intraparenchymally, in the subarachnoid space, or in the subdural space.

There are advantages and disadvantages to each of these systems.[7] The type of monitor chosen depends on both the suspected pathology and physician's preference. Table 15-1 lists the specific advantages and disadvantages of these methods for monitoring ICP.

## MANAGEMENT OF INTRACRANIAL HYPERTENSION

Once intracranial hypertension is documented, therapy must be prompt to prevent secondary insults. All therapies are directed toward reducing one or more of the components (blood, brain, CSF) that lie within the intracranial vault. A

**MANAGEMENT OF INTRACRANIAL HYPERTENSION**

1. Keep patient's head elevated 30-45 degrees and in neutral plane.
2. Maintain controlled ventilation to an arterial partial pressure of carbon dioxide ($Paco_2$) of 25-30 torr with adequate sedation and muscle relaxants.
3. Maintain arterial partial pressure of oxygen ($Pao_2$) >70 torr.
4. Maintain systemic arterial pressure between 140 and 160 mm Hg systolic.
5. Maintain normothermia.
6. Use prophylactic anticonvulsants.
7. Perform ventricular drainage if possible.
8. Administer lidocaine intravenous (IV) bolus as pretreatment for suctioning.
9. Administer mannitol (0.25-1 mg/kg) as needed.
10. Administer high-dose barbiturate therapy as needed.

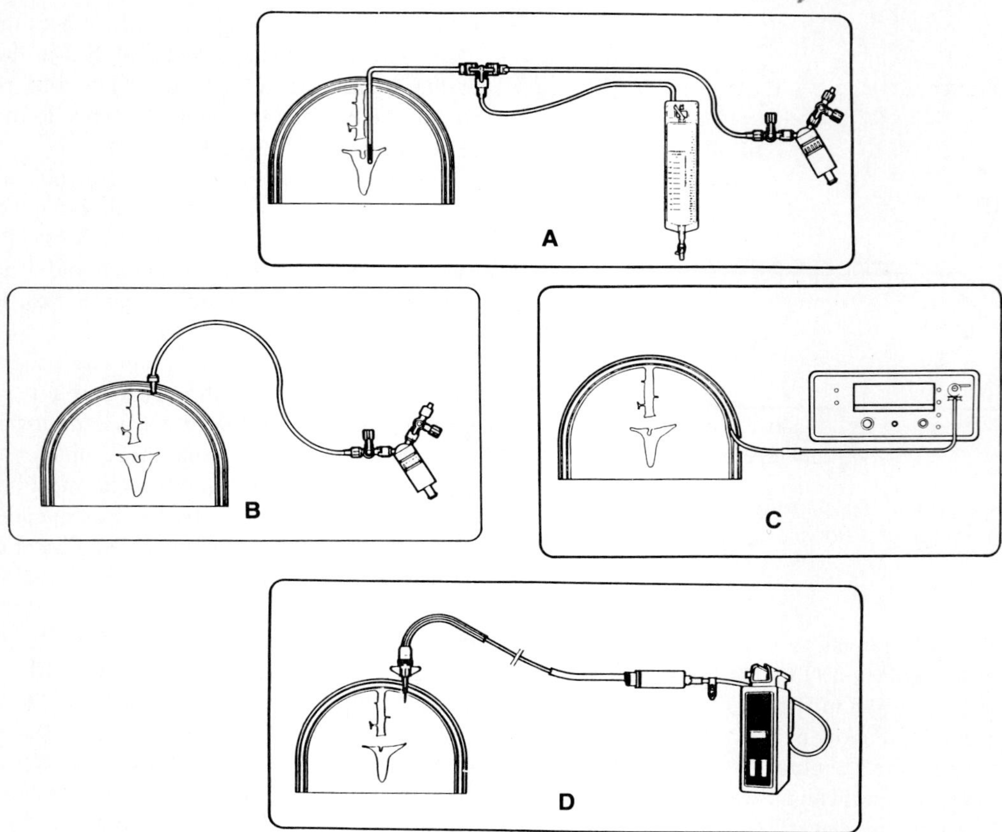


*Fig. 15-2* **A,** Ventricular pressure monitoring system. **B,** Subarachnoid pressure monitoring system. **C,** Epidural pressure monitoring system. **D,** Intraparenchymal pressure monitoring system. (Courtesy Camino Laboratories, San Diego, Calif.)

major goal of therapy is to determine the cause of the elevated pressure and, if possible, remove the cause.[27] Computed tomography becomes invaluable in identifying mass lesions that can be surgically evacuated.[3] In the absence of a surgically treatable mass lesion, intracranial hypertension is treated medically. Nurses play an important role in rapid assessment and implementation of appropriate therapies for reducing ICP (see the box on p. 317).

## Patient Positioning

Positioning of the patient is a significant factor in both the prevention and treatment of elevated ICP. Positions that allow proper venous return are ones that maintain the head and neck elevated 30 to 45 degrees and in a neutral position at all times. In these positions, gravity enhances venous drainage from the brain and head.[15,24]

## Controlled Ventilation

Controlled hyperventilation is an important adjunct of therapy for the patient with increased ICP. If the carbon dioxide pressure ($P_{CO_2}$) can be reduced from its normal level of 35 to 40 mm Hg to a range of 25 to 30 mm Hg in the patient with intracranial hypertension, vasoconstriction of cerebral arteries, reduction of cerebral blood flow, and increased venous return will result. Reducing the intracranial blood volume results in a general reduction in ICP.[27]

The brain requires a constant supply of oxygen adequate to meet the demands of cerebral metabolism. Therefore maintaining uninterrupted oxygenation is of utmost importance in the management of the brain injured. In addition, hypoxia is a profound stimulus to increase cerebral blood flow and cerebral blood volume; therefore inadequate oxygenation in the presence of poor intracranial compliance will increase ICP.[18]

## Sedation and Muscle Relaxants

Any treatment modality that increases the incidence of noxious stimulation to the patient carries with it the potential for increasing ICP. Such noxious stimuli include pain secondary to injuries sustained with the initial trauma, the presence of an endotracheal tube, coughing, suctioning, repositioning, bathing, and many routine nursing care procedures. Even patients who do not seem to move may respond to paralysis with decreased ICP, presumably because of improved chest wall compliance.[21]

The use of muscle relaxants without sedation is not recommended. Agents such as pancuronium bromide, for example, have no analgesic effect and do not adequately pro-

***Table 15-1*** Comparison of ICP monitoring systems

| System | Advantages | Disadvantages |
|---|---|---|
| Ventricular catheter | Reliable measurement within CSF<br>Access for CSF drainage and sampling<br>Access for determination of volume-pressure curve | Difficulty locating lateral ventricle<br>Risk of intracerebral bleeding or edema at cannula track<br>Risk of infection<br>Need for transducer repositioning with head movement |
| Subarachnoid bolt/screw | Useful if ventricles are small<br>No penetration of brain<br>Decreased risk of infection | Unable to drain CSF<br>Unreliable pressure when high ICP herniates brain into bolt<br>Requires intact skull<br>Need for transducer repositioning with head movement |
| Epidural sensor | Ease of insertion<br>No dural penetration<br>Lower risk of infection<br>No adjustment of transducer needed with head movement | Unable to drain CSF<br>Unable to recalibrate or rezero after placement<br>Questionable accuracy of sensing ICP through dura<br>Separate large monitoring system required |
| Fiberoptic transducer-tipped catheter | Versatile system<br>Able to be placed in three different areas of cerebrum<br>Able to monitor intraparenchymal pressure<br>Access for CSF drainage with ventricular system<br>No adjustment of transducer needed with head movement | Catheter relatively fragile<br>Unable to recalibrate or rezero after placement<br>Separate monitoring system required |

tect patients from pain and the physiological responses that can occur from pain-producing procedures and, most importantly, from stimulation originating in the larynx. The need to have an endotracheal tube in place for long periods of time makes it necessary to sedate most and paralyze many of these patients.[12]

### Temperature Control

Cerebral metabolic rate is directly proportional to body temperature, and it increases 5% to 7% per degree centigrade of increase in body temperature.[13] This fact is significant because as the cerebral metabolic rate increases, blood flow to the brain must increase to meet the tissue demands. To avoid the increase in blood volume that is associated with an increased cerebral metabolic rate, hyperthermia must be prevented in the brain-injured patient. Antipyretics and cooling devices should be used when appropriate while the source of the fever is sought. Conversely, hypothermia reduces cerebral metabolic rate. Maintenance of body temperature between 30° and 37° C may be beneficial if full cardiopulmonary support is given and if shivering, which greatly increases the body's metabolic requirements, is prevented. Sedation and neuromuscular blocking agents or phenothiazines are used to control shivering when hypothermia is used.

Persistent fluctuation and/or hypothermia or hyperthermia in conjunction with head injury is a grave prognostic sign and has usually been associated with death or a persistent vegetative state. These patients may represent a group with severe hypothalamic injury.[13]

### Blood Pressure Control

Sustained systolic arterial hypertension (>160 mm Hg) in conjunction with elevated ICP should be vigorously treated. Control of systemic arterial hypertension may require nothing more than the administration of a sedative agent. In cases in which sedation has proven inadequate in controlling systemic arterial hypertension, primary antihypertensive agents are used. Care must be taken in choosing antihypertensive agents because many of the peripheral vasodilators are also cerebral vasodilators (for example, nitroprusside and nitroglycerin). It is believed, however, that all antihypertensives cause some degree of cerebral vasodilation. To reduce this vasodilating effect, it has been suggested that cotreatment with beta blockers (for example, propranolol and labetalol) may be beneficial.[18]

### Seizure Control

Seizures cause metabolic requirements to increase, resulting in elevated cerebral blood flow, cerebral blood volume, and ICP even in paralyzed patients. If blood flow cannot match demand, ischemia will develop, cerebral energy stores will be depleted, and irreversible neuronal destruction will occur.[18]

The usual anticonvulsant regimen for seizure control includes phenytoin and/or phenobarbital in therapeutic doses. The loading dose for phenytoin is 15 to 18 mg/kg, and the loading dose for phenobarbital is 4 to 8 mg/kg. Maintenance doses of phenytoin are administered to achieve a therapeutic blood level of 10 to 20 μg/ml. Maintenance doses of phenobarbital are administered to keep the blood level at 2 to 3 mg%.[2]

### Lidocaine

Various forms of sensory stimulation (including tracheal intubation, laryngoscopy, and endotracheal suctioning) may provoke marked increases in ICP and MAP. One therapy used to prevent cerebral ischemia and acute intracranial hypertension has been the administration of lidocaine through an endotracheal tube or intravenously before nasotracheal suctioning.[27]

Administering lidocaine prophylactically before endotracheal suctioning has been widely practiced. In most cases, 50 to 100 mg is administered intravenously approximately 2 minutes before suctioning the patient. If the endotracheal route is chosen, 2 cc of 4% lidocaine is the preferred dose, and suctioning must be completed within 5 minutes of administering the drug. It is believed that adherence to this procedure protects the patient from the associated increases in ICP that occur with suctioning.

### Cerebrospinal Fluid Drainage

CSF drainage for intracranial hypertension may be used along with other treatment modalities. CSF drainage is accomplished by the insertion of a pliable catheter into the anterior horn of the lateral ventricle, preferably on the nondominant side. Such drainage can help support the patient through periods of cerebral edema by controlling spikes in ICP. One of the major advantages of the ventriculostomy is its dual role as both a monitoring device and a treatment modality. Because CSF provides a favorable medium for the development of infection, it is essential that flawless aseptic technique be followed during insertion and maintenance of the system. The ventricular system is connected to a drainage bag and is then maintained as a closed system for the period of time the ventriculostomy remains in place—usually 3 to 5 days.

When using this system for treatment, there are two ways to accomplish removal of CSF: it can be removed intermittently when ICP becomes elevated, or it can be removed continuously, with the ventriculostomy bag at a predetermined level above the lateral ventricle. Intermittent drainage involves draining CSF for brief periods (30 to 120 seconds) when ICP exceeds the upper limits of normal. Frequent periods of drainage (more than four times per hour) should be reported to the physician. Continuous drainage is most often ordered when the patient has significant amounts of blood in the subarachnoid space (for example, with a subarachnoid hemorrhage). The ventricular drainage bag is placed 10 to 15 cm above the level of the third ventricle so that if ICP exceeds 10 to 12 mm Hg, CSF will be shunted into the drainage bag. One very important concept to keep in mind is that when intracranial hypertension or a mass lesion is suspected, a lumbar puncture is contraindicated because of the risk of downward herniation.

### Diuretics

**Osmotic agents.** The three best-known osmotic diuretics are urea, mannitol, and glycerol. Although urea is still used in some clinical settings, mannitol has gained wide acceptance as the osmotic diuretic of choice. Mannitol, a larger molecule than urea, is retained almost entirely in the extracellular compartment and has little to none of the rebound effect noted with urea. It has also been suggested that mannitol in particular improves perfusion to ischemic areas of the brain, producing cerebral vasoconstriction and resulting in a reduction of ICP.[12] Glycerol, the effect of which is similar on the brain to that of mannitol, has the advantage of oral administration. It is also apparently a safe drug for long-term use. The fact that glycerol can be administered orally has no real benefit in the medical treatment of the severely brain-injured patient.

The usual dose of mannitol is 0.5 to 1.5 g/kg. Recent data suggest that small doses (0.25 g/kg) decrease ICP as rapidly and profounding as higher doses (1 g/kg), but the effect is somewhat less prolonged (4 to 6 hours).[18] Smaller doses of mannitol simplify fluid and electrolyte management, and their use is encouraged whenever possible.[12,27]

**Nonosmotic agents.** Nonosmotic diuretics have also been used to decrease ICP. Furosemide, one such nonosmotic diuretic, may act differently from osmotic agents by pulling sodium and water from edematous areas and, perhaps, by decreasing CSF production. One advantage of furosemide administration over the use of osmotic diuretics is that its effect is not generally associated with increases in serum osmolality. Therefore electrolyte imbalances may not be as severe with the use of nonosmotic diuretics.

Another diuretic in this category is acetazolamide. The action of this drug is to reduce the rate at which CSF is produced in the choroid plexus. Generally, the use of acetazolamide in head-injured patients is contraindicated because of its cerebral vasodilative effect.

### High-Dose Barbiturate Therapy

**Barbiturate therapy** is a treatment protocol developed for the management of uncontrolled intracranial hypertension that has not responded to the conventional treatments previously described. Uncontrolled ICP is described in the literature as follows[13,14,20]:

1. ICP >20 mm Hg for 30 minutes or more, with unresponsiveness to aggressive use of conventional therapies
2. ICP >40 mm Hg for 15 minutes or more, CPP <50 mm Hg, or both

Although the specific action of barbiturates in the reduction of ICP is unclear, several theories exist to explain their effect on the central nervous system and the subsequent cerebral protection they provide. Barbiturates increase the cerebrovascular resistance and therefore decrease cerebral blood flow, resulting in a reduction in intracranial volume. Systemic blood pressure is also lowered, reducing hydrostatic pressure in the damaged cerebral tissue and helping arrest edema formation.[25] Barbiturates also slow cerebral metabolism by reducing the functional electrical generation of the neurons. This decreased cerebral metabolism thus lessens the glucose and oxygen demands of the brain.[1,23] Barbiturates are also effective anticonvulsants and may suppress subclinical seizure activities. Finally, it has been postulated that barbiturates are scavengers of free radicals and thereby prevent cell membrane damage and destruction.[23,25]

The two most commonly used drugs in high-dose barbiturate therapy are pentobarbital and thiopental. Pentobarbital, a longer-acting barbiturate, is administered in a loading dose of 3 to 5 mg/kg of body weight over a 15-minute period, with a maintenance dose of 1 to 2 mg/kg/hour. Thiopental, a shorter-acting barbiturate, is administered in a loading dose of 1 to 5 mg/kg of body weight and a maintenance dose of 1 to 3 mg/kg/hour. The goal with either of these drugs is a reduction of ICP to 15 to 20 mm Hg while maintaining a MAP of 70 to 80 torr. A therapeutic serum blood level for high-dose barbiturate therapy is 3 to 5 mg%. Patients are maintained on high-dose barbiturate therapy until ICP has been controlled within the normal range for 24 hours. Barbiturates should never be stopped abruptly but should be tapered slowly over approximately 4 days.[12] The complications most frequently encountered are hypotension, hypothermia, and decreased cardiac output.

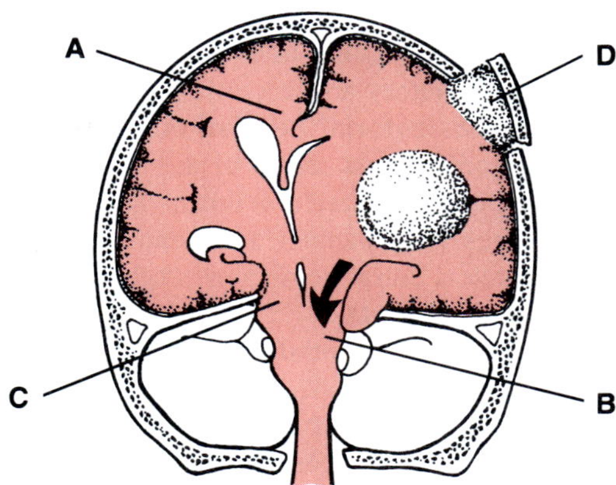


***Fig. 15-3*** Supratentorial herniation. *A,* Cingulate. *B,* Uncal. *C,* Central. *D,* Transcalvarial.

The major unresolved issue in the use of high-dose barbiturates is their effect on outcome after head injury. The small subset of patients who fail to achieve ICP control with standard therapy does benefit from the judicious and carefully monitored and administered high-dose barbiturate therapy.[4] Nursing management of increased intracranial pressure is summarized in the box below.

### Nursing Diagnosis and Management

***Increased intracranial pressure***

- Altered Cerebral Tissue Perfusion related to increased intracranial pressure secondary to brain trauma, hemorrhage, edema, infection, tumor, stroke, or hydrocephalus, p. 480
- Altered Cerebral Tissue Perfusion related to vasospasm secondary to subarachnoid hemorrhage after ruptured intracranial aneurysm or arteriovenous malformation, p. 478
- High Risk for Infection risk factors: invasive monitoring devices, p. 465
- High Risk for Aspiration risk factors: reduced level of consciousness, depressed cough and gag reflexes, presence of tracheostomy or endotracheal tube, gastrointestinal tube, tube feedings, delayed gastric emptying, and decreased gastrointestinal motility secondary to immobility, p. 476
- Ineffective Airway Clearance related to impaired cough secondary to loss of glottic closure with cuffed tracheostomy or endotracheal tube, p. 468
- Ineffective Breathing Pattern related to respiratory muscle deconditioning secondary to mechanical ventilation, p. 471

## HERNIATION SYNDROMES

The goal of neurological evaluation, ICP monitoring, and treatment of increased ICP is to prevent herniation. Herniation of intracerebral contents results in the shifting of tissue from one compartment of the brain to another and places pressure on cerebral vessels and vital function centers of the brain. If unchecked, herniation rapidly causes death as a result of the cessation of cerebral blood flow and respirations.

### Supratentorial Herniation

There are four types of supratentorial herniation syndromes: central or transtentorial, uncal, cingulate, or transcalvarial (Fig. 15-3).

**Uncal herniation. Uncal herniation** is the herniation syndrome most often noted. In uncal herniation, a unilateral, expanding mass lesion, usually of the temporal lobe, increases ICP, causing the tip of the temporal lobe (uncus) to displace laterally. Lateral displacement pushes the uncus over the edge of the tentorium, puts pressure on the oculomotor nerve (cranial nerve III) and posterior cerebral artery ipsilateral to the lesion, and flattens the midbrain against the opposite side.

Signs and symptoms of uncal herniation include ipsilateral pupil dilation, respiratory pattern changes leading to respiratory arrest, and contralateral hemiplegia leading to decorticate or decerebrate posturing. If no intervention occurs, uncal herniation results in fixed and dilated pupils, flaccidity, and respiratory arrest.

**Central or transtentorial herniation.** In **central herniation** an expanding mass lesion of the midline, frontal, parietal, or occipital lobes results in downward displacement of the hemispheres, basal ganglia, and diencephalon through the tentorial notch. Central herniation is often preceded by uncal and cingulate herniation.

Signs and symptoms of central or transtentorial herniation include loss of consciousness; small, reactive pupils progressing to fixed, dilated pupils; respiratory changes leading to respiratory arrest; and decorticate posturing progressing to flaccidity. In the late stages, uncal and central herniation syndromes are similar in their effects on the brainstem.

**Cingulate herniation.** Cingulate herniation occurs when an expanding lesion of one hemisphere shifts laterally and forces the cingulate gyrus under the falx cerebri. Cingulate herniation occurs frequently. Whenever a lateral shift is noted on a computed tomographic (CT) scan, cingulate herniation has occurred. Little is known about the effects of cingulate herniation, and there are no signs and symptoms that assist in its diagnosis. Cingulate herniation is not life-threatening on its own, but if the expanding mass lesion that caused cingulate herniation is not controlled, uncal or central herniation will follow.

**Transcalvarial herniation.** Transcalvarial herniation is the extrusion of cerebral tissue through the cranium. In the presence of severe cerebral edema, transcalvarial herniation occurs through an opening from a skull fracture or craniotomy site.

### Infratentorial Herniation

There are two infratentorial herniation syndromes: upward transtentorial herniation and downward cerebellar herniation.

**Upward transtentorial herniation.** Upward transtentorial herniation occurs when an expanding mass lesion of the cerebellum causes protrusion of the vermis (central area) of the cerebellum and the midbrain upward through the tentorial notch. Compression of the third cranial nerve and diencephalon occurs. Obstruction of CSF flow occurs with blockage of the central aqueduct and distortion of the third ventricle. Deterioration occurs rapidly.

**Downward cerebellar herniation.** Downward cerebellar herniation occurs when an expanding lesion of the cerebellum exerts pressure downward, sending the cerebellar tonsils through the foramen magnum. Compression and displacement of the medulla oblongata occurs, rapidly resulting in respiratory and cardiac arrest.

#### REFERENCES

1. Anderson BJ: The metabolic needs of head trauma victims, J Neurosci Nurs 19(4):211, 1987.
2. Commission for the Control of Epilepsy and Its Consequences: Plan for nationwide action on epilepsy, vol 4, DHEW Pub No (NIH) 78-279, Bethesda, Md, 1978, National Institutes of Health.
3. Eisenberg HM, Weiner RN, and Tabaddor K: Emergency care: initial evaluation. In Cooper PR, editor: Head injury, ed 2, Baltimore, 1987, The Williams & Wilkins Co.
4. Eisenberg HM and others: High-dose barbiturate control of elevated intracranial pressure in patients with severe head injury, J Neurosurg 69:15, 1988.
5. Guillaume J and Janny P: Monometrie intracranienne continue; interet physio-pathologique et clinique de la methode, Presse Med 59:953, 1951.
6. Hickey JV: The clinical practice of neurological and neurosurgical nursing, ed 2, Philadelphia, 1986, JB Lippincott Co.
7. Hopkins CC: Infection: pathogenesis, prevention, and treatment. In Ropper AH, Kennedy SK, and Zervas NT, editors: Neurological and neurosurgical intensive care, Baltimore, 1983, University Park Press.
8. Javid M: Urea in intracranial surgery: a new method, J Neurosurg 18:51, 1961.
9. Jennett B and Teasdale G: Management of head injuries, Philadelphia, 1981, FA Davis Co.
10. Lundberg N: Continuous recording and control of ventricular fluid pressure in neurosurgical practice, Acta Psychiatr Neurol Scand Suppl 149:1, 1960.
11. Marmarou A and Tabaddor K: Intracranial pressure: physiology and pathophysiology. In Cooper PR, editor: Head injury, ed 2, Baltimore, 1987, The Williams & Wilkins Co.
12. Marshall LF and Marshall SB: Medical management of intracranial pressure. In Cooper PR, editor: Head injury, ed 2, Baltimore, 1987, The Williams & Wilkins Co.
13. Marshall LF, Smith RW, and Shapiro HM: The outcome with aggressive treatment in severe head injuries, J Neurosurg 50:20, 1979.
14. Miller JD: Barbiturates and raised intracranial pressure, Ann Neurol 6(3):189, 1979.
15. Mitchell PH: Intracranial hypertension: influence of nursing care activities, Nurs Clin North Am 21(4):563, 1986.
16. Mitchell PH, Amos D, and Astley C: Nursing and ICP: studies of two clinical problems. In Miller JD, editor: Intracranial pressure VI, New York, 1986, Springer-Verlag.
17. Rockoff MA and Kennedy SK: Physiology and clinical aspects of raised intracranial pressure. In Ropper AH, Kennedy SK, and Zerfas NT, editors: Neurologic and neurosurgical intensive care, Baltimore, 1983, University Park Press.
18. Rockoff MA and Ropper AH: Treatment of intracranial hypertension. In Ropper AH, Kennedy SK, and Zervas NT, editors: Neurologic and neurosurgical intensive care, Baltimore, 1983, University Park Press.
19. Rockoff MA, Marshall LF, and Shapiro HM: High dose barbiturate therapy in humans: a clinical review of 60 patients, Ann Neurol 3:83, 1979.
20. Rudy EB: Advanced neurological and neurosurgical nursing, St Louis, 1984, Mosby–Year Book, Inc.
21. Shapiro HM: Intracranial hypertension: therapeutic and anesthetic considerations, Anesthesia 43:445, 1975.
22. Shapiro HM, Wyte SR, and Loeser J: Barbiturate-augmented hypothermia for reduction of persistent intracranial hypertension, J Neurosurg 40:90, 1974.
23. Siesjo BK and others: Brain metabolism in the critically ill, Crit Care Med 4:283, 1976.
24. Snyder M: Relation of nursing activities to increases in intracranial pressure, J Adv Nurs 8:273, 1983.
25. Swann KW: Management of severe head injury. In Ropper AH, Kennedy SK, and Zervas NT, editors: Neurologic and neurosurgical intensive care, Baltimore, 1983, University Park Press.
26. Wilberger JE: Emergency burr holes: current role in neurosurgical acute care, Top Emerg Med 11(4):69, 1990.
27. Wrobel CJ and Marshall LF: Closed head injury management dilemmas. In Long DM, editor: Current therapy in neurological surgery, ed 2, vol 2, St Louis, 1989, Mosby–Year Book, Inc.

UNIT VI

# RENAL ALTERATIONS

CHAPTER 16

# Renal Assessment and Diagnosis

## CHAPTER OBJECTIVES

- *Discuss the rationale involved in developing a consistent, sequential format for performing renal nursing assessment.*
- *Perform a thorough nursing assessment of the renal system on a critically ill patient and interpret the results.*
- *Identify methods for assessing normal skin turgor.*
- *Describe the pathophysiological mechanism responsible for the development of edema and ascites and identify the proper method for assessing each one.*
- *Describe the pathophysiological mechanism responsible for orthostatic hypotension.*
- *Describe the effect of decreased serum albumin levels on fluid dynamics within the body.*
- *Identify how alterations of both the hemoglobin and the hematocrit levels can signal fluid volume deficit or excess.*
- *Explain why elevations of blood urea nitrogen and creatinine can signal renal dysfunction.*
- *Describe the relationship between serum osmolality and antidiuretic hormone.*

## KEY TERMS

volume deficit, p. 326
volume excess, p. 326
fluid wave, p. 327
normal serum electrolyte values, p. 328
blood urea nitrogen, p. 329
creatinine, p. 329
anion gap, p. 330
proteinuria, p. 331
renal computed tomographic (CT) scan, p. 331
renal ultrasonography, p. 331
renal biopsy, p. 331

## RENAL ASSESSMENT

The body presents a variety of signs and symptoms that demonstrate fluid and electrolyte disorders. A methodical way of examination presents data that help pinpoint the actual problem. The following section explains the process of taking a fluid and electrolyte history and performing the physical assessment of fluid and electrolyte balance. An outline of this information is presented in the box, "Important Aspects of the Fluid and Electrolyte Assessment."

### History

A renal history should begin with a description of the chief complaint, written in the patient's own words. Included in the description of the chief complaint should be its onset, location, and duration and factors that lessen or aggravate the problem.[2] Descriptions of any treatment sought by the individual, medications taken to alleviate symptoms, or procedures performed to ameliorate the problem are often helpful in delineating the extent of the current complaint.

Of particular concern in gaining a complete renal and fluid history is the patient's past medical history. Similar symptoms, problems, or treatment for complaints in the past may give important clues to current treatment or may aid in establishing the cause of the problem. The family history may also provide important information to aid in identifying and treating the patient's disorder. A history is investigative and usually progressive in nature, with one question often leading to another.

### Clinical Assessment

**Inspection.** Physical assessment begins with looking at neck veins and hand veins. For inspection of the patient's neck veins, he or she should be in the supine position, in which normal venous distention is usually noted. If neck veins do not distend with the patient in the supine position, hypovolemia is suspected. After supine inspection, the head of the bed should be elevated to 45 to 90 degrees. If with the bed at 45 degrees the veins remain distended more than 2 cm above the sternal notch, fluid overload may be suspected.[9]

Hand vein inspection is performed simply by observing for venous distention, the expected response, when the hand

### IMPORTANT ASPECTS OF THE FLUID AND ELECTROLYTE ASSESSMENT

**NURSING HISTORY**

1. Chief complaint
2. History of present problem
   a. Onset
   b. Duration
   c. Signs/symptoms
   d. Treatments
3. Past history of fluid or renal problems or familial history of fluid or renal problems
4. Dietary likes/dislikes/intake each day
5. Fluid likes/dislikes/intake each day
6. Dentures: if used, oral condition/hygiene
7. Cultural background
8. Educational background

**NURSING ASSESSMENT**
**Fluid status (Deficit/Excess)**

1. Skin turgor
2. Mucous membranes
3. Intake and output
4. Presence of edema/ascites
5. Neck and hand vein engorgement
6. Lung sounds—crackles
7. Blood pressure (hypertension or hypotension)
8. Vertigo on rising
9. Blurred vision
10. Diaphoresis
11. Behavioral changes
12. Low grade fever
13. Tachycardia

is held in the dependent position. Venous filling that takes longer than 5 seconds suggests hypovolemia. When the hand is elevated, the distention should disappear within 5 seconds. If distention does not disappear within 5 seconds after the hand is elevated, fluid overload is suspected.

The skin and mucous membranes, when inspected, present readily visible signs of fluid alterations. When a fluid **volume deficit** exists, skin loses elasticity and mucous membranes become sticky. If a fluid **volume excess** exists, edema is sometimes present, particularly in dependent areas of the body. However, without further assessment the imbalance cannot be positively identified. Other disorders and contributing factors might lead to an inaccurate assumption of a fluid volume disorder. For instance, mouth breathing can dry the oral mucous membranes temporarily. A more accurate way to assess the fluid status of the oral cavity is to inspect the mouth, using a tongue blade. Stickiness of this area is more indicative of fluid volume deficit than complaints of a dry mouth.[9]

Assessment of skin turgor provides additional data for identifying fluid-related problems. As the skin over the forearm is picked up and released, the rapidity of its return to its normal position should be observed. Normal elasticity and fluid status allow almost immediate return to shape once the skin is released. However, in fluid volume deficit the skin remains raised and does not return to its normal position for several seconds. Because of the usual loss of skin elasticity in the elderly, this test is not accurate for fluid assessment of this age-group. The elderly individual's skin turgor can be assessed in the shoulder area, which retains elasticity.[9]

Changes in skin texture and overall appearance reveal much about fluid status. For example, the patient with renal failure has rough, dry skin and deposits of urate crystals on the skin, called *uremic frost*. These patients frequently have scratch marks because of the pruritis associated with renal failure.

Edema is defined as the presence of excess fluid in the interstitial space. However, the presence of edema does not always indicate true fluid overload; a loss of albumin from the vascular space can cause peripheral edema, yet the patient may be hypovolemic.

Edema is usually assessed by applying fingertip pressure on the skin over a bony prominence such as the ankles, pretibial areas (shins), and the sacrum. If the indentation made by the fingertip does not disappear within 30 seconds, "pitting" edema is present. Pitting edema is indicative of increased interstitial volume and is not in evidence until approximately a 10% weight gain has occurred.[5] It is gauged by a subjective scale of 1 to 4, with +1 indicating only minimal pitting and +4 indicating severe pitting. Edema may also appear in hands and feet, around the eyes, and in the cheeks. Dependent areas such as the sacrum are the most likely to demonstrate edema in patients chronically confined to a wheelchair or bed. Skeletal muscles do not usually reflect changes in fluid status but do reflect changes in electrolyte levels. A skeletal muscle change to weakness or paralysis usually signals a deficit of an electrolyte, particularly of a major cation (potassium and sodium). However, a calcium deficit leads to the opposite extreme—severe cramping and muscle spasm.

**Palpation.** Although palpation of the kidneys is not directly linked to fluid and electrolyte assessments, any subtle changes in kidney function can result in problems with fluids and electrolytes. Palpation of the kidneys is achieved through the bimanual capturing approach. *Capturing* is accomplished by placing one hand posteriorly under the flank of the supine patient with fingers pointing to the midline, while placing the opposite hand just below the rib cage anteriorly. The patient is asked to inhale deeply, while pressure is exerted to bring the hands together. As the patient exhales, the kidney should be felt between the hands. After each kidney is palpated in this manner, they should be compared for size and shape. Each should be firm, smooth, and of equal size.[5]

**Percussion.** Percussion is performed to detect pain in the area of an organ or to determine excess accumulation of air, fluid, or solids in a body cavity. Although percussion of the kidneys per se does not give direct evidence of fluid and electrolyte level abnormalities, it can provide information about kidney location, size, and possible problems that could lead to future fluid and electrolyte level abnormalities.

Percussion of the kidney is performed with the patient in a sidelying or sitting position, with the examiner's hand placed over the costovertebral angle (lower border of the rib cage on the flank). Striking the back of the hand with the opposite fist will produce a dull thud, which is normal. Pain may be indicative of infection.

Observation and percussion of the abdomen is of value in assessing fluid status also. Percussing the abdomen (using the same procedure as for the kidneys but placing the patient supine) can result in a dull sound (solid bowel contents or fluid) or a hollow sound (gaseous bowel).[2]

Ascites, defined simply as severe fluid distention of the abdominal cavity, is an important observation in determining fluid imbalances. Differentiating ascites from distortion caused by solid bowel contents is done by producing what is called the **fluid wave.** The fluid wave is elicited by exerting pressure to the abdominal midline while one hand is placed on the right or left flank. Tapping the opposite flank produces a wave in the accumulated fluid that can be felt under the hands. Other signs of ascites are a protuberant, rounded abdomen and abdominal striae.

Ascites may or may not represent fluid volume excess. Individuals with a compromised hepatic system may have severe ascites but actually by hypovolemic. On the other hand, individuals suffering from renal failure may be plagued with ascites caused by true volume overload, which forces fluid into the abdomen because of increased capillary hydrostatic pressures.

**Auscultation.** Although auscultation is perhaps the most difficult area of assessment to master, it provides more accurate information about extracellular fluid (ECF) changes than the areas of assessment previously discussed. Listening for specific sounds in the heart and lungs provides information about the presence or absence of increased fluid in the interstitium or vascular space. Increased heart rate alone does not offer much data about fluid volume, but combined with a low blood pressure, it may indicate hypovolemia. Often hypertension is accompanied by a third or fourth heart sound, which may indicate the presence of fluid overload.

Hypertension may be indicative of fluid overload but may also be caused by atherosclerotic or arteriosclerotic vessel changes. Blood pressure readings should be taken at rest with the patient lying, sitting, and standing. A drastic drop in pressure from lying to sitting or from sitting to standing represents an "orthostatic" drop known as orthostatic hypotension. A 20 mm Hg drop in pressure may represent a fluid volume deficit and occurs when the venous circulation is so volume depleted that a sufficient preload is not immediately available after the position change. Vascular sounds heard by auscultating major vessels are called *bruits* (Fig. 16-1). A bruit is a blowing or swishing sound, much like cardiac murmurs.[2] Fluid volume excess, coupled with stenosis or any impediment to vascular flow, will produce a loud bruit.

Lung assessment is extremely important in gauging fluid status. Dyspnea with any mild exertion or dyspnea at night that prevents sleeping in a supine position may indicate fluid overload. Shallow, gasping breaths punctuated by periods of apnea may indicate severe acid-base imbalances. Since the lungs are one of the primary controllers of acid-base balance, it is important to identify the types of respiratory changes associated with each condition.

**Weight.** The single most important assessment of fluid status is the patient's weight. Significant fluctuations in body weight over a 1- to 2-day period are indicative of fluid gains and losses. However, this important sign is often forgotten or ignored when assessing the individual's renal and fluid status.

When possible, the patient should be weighed during admission to the critical care unit. It is important to note whether the current weight differs significantly from the weight 1 to 2 weeks before admission. Thereafter, the patient should be weighed daily for comparison with the previous day. The weight should be obtained at the same time each day, with the patient wearing the same amount of clothing. One liter of fluid equals 1 kg, or approximately 2.2 pounds.

**Intake and output.** Intake and output can be compared with the patient's weight to evaluate accurately the gain or loss of fluid. Urinary output plus insensible fluid losses (perspiration and water vapor from the lungs) can range widely from 750 to 2400 ml daily. When intake exceeds output, a positive fluid state exists. If disorders such as renal failure perpetuate the positive fluid gain, fluid overload results. Conversely, if output exceeds intake (fever, increased respiration, profuse sweating, vomiting, diarrhea, gastric suction), a negative fluid state exists.

Abnormal output of body fluids not only creates fluid imbalances, but also creates electrolyte and acid-base disturbances. For example, gastrointestinal suction or loss by diarrhea can result in fluid deficit, sodium and potassium deficits, and metabolic acidosis (from excessive loss of bicarbonate). During a 24-hour period, fever can increase skin and respiratory losses by as much as 75 ml per degree Fahrenheit rise.[9]

**Clinical observations.** Disturbances in fluid and electrolyte levels are often accompanied by signs and symptoms less measurable than those previously mentioned but that are, nonetheless, indicative of serious change.

Changes in mental status such as disorientation are often a result of acidosis. Lethargy, coma, and confusion may result from sodium, calcium, or magnesium excess or deficit. Apprehension may be secondary to sodium deficit or to a shift of fluid from the plasma to the interstitium.[12] Also, individuals with respiratory changes secondary to fluid volume overload are frequently apprehensive.

Apathy and withdrawal often accompany hypovolemic states.[12] Renal failure patients with systemic increases in

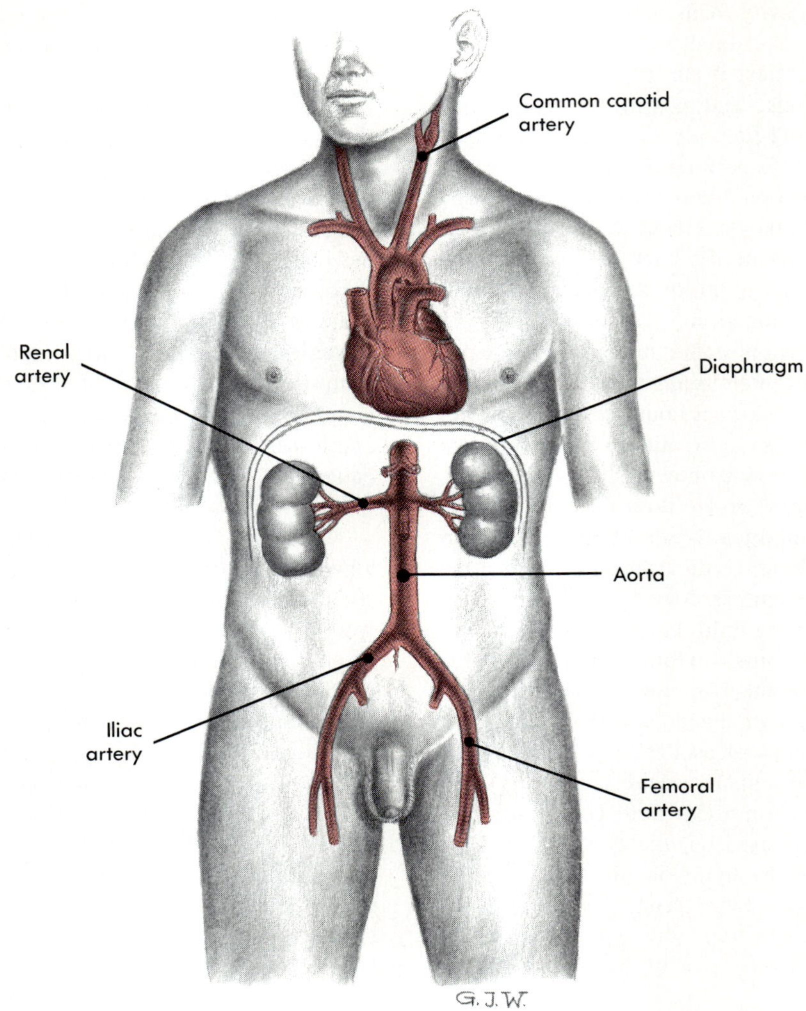


***Fig. 16-1*** Sites for auscultation of bruits.

electrolytes, fluids, and nitrogenous waste products can also exhibit apathy, restlessness, confusion, and withdrawal. It is often difficult to separate the emotional component from the actual physiological mechanism. Nonetheless, the importance of considering a fluid or electrolyte disorder as the cause of a mental or emotional change must be emphasized.

Thirst is one of the first subjective cues to fluid volume changes in the patient. Thirst results from actual fluid loss and increased serum osmolality or is driven by usual habits of the patient. It is important for the critical care nurse to recognize the presence of thirst and to design the appropriate interventions aimed at the cause. Of particular concern are patients who are comatose, immobile, confused, or elderly, all of whom may have difficulty recognizing and/or satisfying thirst.[16]

## Laboratory Assessment

A number of laboratory tests and diagnostic procedures are used to assess renal and fluid status.[4,6] The most definitive tests are explained in the following narrative and are summarized in Table 16-1.

**Assessment of blood**

***Serum electrolytes.*** **Normal serum electrolyte values** and functions are summarized in Table 16-2.[4,6,7,15]

***Serum albumin.*** Serum albumin is manufactured in the liver and composes slightly more than 50% of the total plasma protein. Albumin is primarily implicated in the maintenance of colloid osmotic pressure, which functions to hold fluid in the vascular space. The blood vessel walls, because of their impermeability to plasma proteins, prevent albumin from leaving the vascular space.

Decreased albumin levels result in plasma-to-interstitial fluid shift, which creates peripheral edema. A decreased albumin level can occur as a result of protein-calorie malnutrition in which available stores of albumin are depleted, oncotic pressure is decreased, and fluid is shifted from the vascular space to the interstitial space. Liver disease can also cause a fall in albumin levels as the diseased liver fails

***Table 16-1*** Serum tests for diagnosing renal and fluid disorders

| Substance | Normal values |
|---|---|
| Albumin | 3.5-5.5 g/dl |
| Hemoglobin (Hgb) | Males: 13.5-17.5 g/dl<br>Females: 12-16 g/dl |
| Hematocrit (Hct) | Males: 40-54%<br>Females: 37-47% |
| Blood urea nitrogen (BUN) | 9-20 mg/dl |
| Creatinine | 0.7-1.5 mg/dl |
| Osmolality | 275-295 mOsm/L[2] |

to synthesize sufficient albumin. Further, severe portal hypertension can force albumin and other plasma proteins into the abdominal cavity, creating ascites.

***Hemoglobin and hematocrit.*** The hemoglobin (Hgb) and hematocrit (Hct) levels can be indicative of increases or decreases in intravascular fluid volume. An increase in the hematocrit often indicates a severe fluid volume deficit, which results in hemoconcentration—hence, the elevated Hct level. Conversely, a decreased Hct level can indicate fluid volume excess because of the dilutional effect of the extra fluid load. The history and bedside assessment will aid in determining whether fluid imbalances and/or disease states are responsible.

***Blood urea nitrogen and creatinine.*** **Blood urea nitrogen** (BUN) and **creatinine** are both by-products of protein metabolism. The importance of these two serum tests is not with normal levels but with increases or decreases. Both BUN and creatinine levels become elevated when renal function deteriorates.

Creatinine is a by-product of normal cell metabolism and appears in serum in amounts proportional to the body muscle mass. Creatinine is easily excreted by the renal tubules. Tracing the amount of creatinine in the excreted urine and the amount of creatinine in the blood over 24 hours provides accurate information about kidney function. Creatinine excess occurs most often in individuals with renal failure in

***Table 16-2*** Normal electrolyte values and functions

| Electrolyte | Normal serum value | Functions |
|---|---|---|
| Sodium | 135-145 mEq/L | Maintains extracellular osmolality<br>Maintains the active transport mechanism in conjunction with potassium<br>Controls body fluids (largely responsible for water movement and retention)<br>Aids in maintaining neuromuscular activity<br>Aids in some enzyme activities (helping to create energy)<br>Influences acid-base balance |
| Potassium | 3.5-5.0 mEq/L | Promotes transmission of nerve impulses<br>Maintains intracellular osmolality<br>Activates several enzymatic reactions<br>Aids in regulation of acid-base balance<br>Promotes myocardial, skeletal, and smooth muscle contractility |
| Chloride | 98-108 mEq/L | Maintains body osmolality (in conjunction with sodium)<br>Aids in body water balance (in conjunction with sodium)<br>Competes with bicarbonate for recombination with sodium to maintain acid-base balance<br>Maintains acidity of body fluids (gastric juice) |
| Calcium | 8.5-10.5 mg/dl or 4.5-5.8 mEq/L | Maintains hardness of bone and teeth (crystalline in nature)<br>Contracts skeletal muscle<br>Coagulates blood<br>Maintains cellular permeability<br>Contracts heart muscle |
| Phosphorus | 2.7-4.5 mg/dl | Aids in structure of cellular membrane<br>Helps deliver oxygen to the tissues<br>Is integral part of intracelluiar energy production (ATP)<br>Helps maintain bone hardness<br>Aids in enzyme regulation (ATPase) |
| Magnesium | 1.5-2.5 mEq/L | Aids in neuromuscular transmission<br>Aids in contraction of heart muscle<br>Activates enzymes for cellular metabolism of carbohydrates and proteins<br>Aids in maintaining the active transport mechanism at the cellular level<br>Aids in transmission of hereditary information to offspring |
| Bicarbonate | 24-28 mEq/L | Buffers the acidity of body fluids (controls the hydrogen ion concentration and combines with other body salts to maintain acid-base balance) |

whom the diminished renal function impairs creatinine excretion.

BUN levels are not as accurate an indicator of renal failure as creatinine because BUN levels fluctuate greatly with protein intake, whereas creatinine levels are relatively unaffected by protein intake. Elevations in the BUN level can be correlated with the signs and symptoms of uremia; as the BUN value rises, symptoms of uremia become more pronounced as a result of the irritation this metabolite produces on bodily membranes. Increased levels of BUN (often called *urea*) also occur with fluid volume deficit (hemoconcentration), infection, excessive protein intake, and renal failure.

***Serum osmolality.*** The serum osmolality level reflects the concentration or dilution of vascular fluid. Antidiuretic hormone (ADH) plays an important role in maintaining the serum osmolality level. When the serum osmolality level increases (for example, with insufficient fluid intake), ADH is released from the pituitary gland and stimulates increased water reabsorption, which expands the vascular space and brings the serum osmolality level back to normal. A more concentrated urine also results. The opposite occurs with a decreased serum osmolality level, which inhibits the production of ADH and results in increased excretion of water through the kidneys, producing a dilute urine and bringing the serum osmolality level back to normal.

***Anion gap.*** The **anion gap** is a calculation of the difference between the measurable cations (sodium and potassium) and the measurable anions (chloride and bicarbonate). The value represents the remaining unmeasurable anions present in the extracellular fluid (for example, phosphates, sulfates, ketones, pyruvate, lactate). The normal value is 10 to 12 mEq/L and should not exceed 14 mEq/L. An increased anion gap level reflects an overproduction and/or poor excretion of acid products.[10]

Renal failure can increase the anion gap value because of retention of acids and altered bicarbonate reabsorption. Diabetic ketoacidosis results in ketone production, which also elevates the level of the anion gap. The measurement of the anion gap is a rapid, effective method for identifying acid-base imbalance, but it cannot be used to pinpoint the actual acid-base disturbance specifically.

**Assessment of urine.** Urinary volume, contents, color, clarity, acidity, alkalinity, and odor provide excellent information about the patient's condition relative to fluids and electrolytes. Specific tests are presented in Table 16-3; several are discussed in greater detail to clarify certain disorders.

***Urine pH.*** Urine pH indicates the acidity or alkalinity of the urine. An increase in urinary acidity (decreased level of pH) indicates retention of sodium and acids by the body. Conversely, a decrease in urinary acidity (increased pH or more alkaline level) means the body is retaining bicarbonate. However, urinary pH levels are greatly affected by diet and medications.

***Specific gravity.*** Specific gravity measures the density or weight of urine compared with distilled water. Decreases in specific gravity values reflect inability of the kidneys to excrete the usual solute load into the urine (less dense with fewer solutes). Increases in specific gravity values (a more concentrated urine) occur with a body fluid volume deficit as the result of fever, vomiting, or diarrhea. An increased specific gravity value can also occur with diabetes or glomerular membrane permeability changes, which allow glucose and protein in the urine, thereby increasing the urine concentrations.[4]

**Table 16-3** Urinalysis tests for diagnosing renal disorders

| Substance | Normal values |
|---|---|
| Specific gravity | 1.003-1.030 |
| Urinary osmolality | 300-1200 mOsm/L |
| Urinary pH | 4.5-8.0 |
| Urinary electrolytes | |
| Sodium | 80-180 mEq/24 hr |
| Potassium | 40-80 mEq/24 hr |
| Chloride | 110-200 mEq/24 hr |
| Calcium | 50-300 mEq/24 hr |

***Osmolality.*** The urinary osmolality value more accurately pinpoints fluid balance than does the serum osmolality value, because the serum osmolality value is actually a reflection of serum sodium concentration and is therefore subject to far more influences than the urinary osmolality value. However, the simultaneous measurement of both the serum and urinary osmolality levels provides a more accurate assessment of fluid status. The urinary osmolality level increases during fluid volume deficit because of the retention of fluid by the body. Conversely, the urinary osmolality level decreases during volume excess because fluid is excreted by the kidneys. In late renal failure, the urinary osmolality value is usually quite low because solutes and fluids are being abnormally retained.[14]

***Glucose.*** Glucose is normally reabsorbed by the renal tubules; therefore urine should be free of glucose. However, the appearance of glucose in the urine may be transient in nature, brought on by ingestion of a heavy carbohydrate load or caused by stress, or resulting from the renal changes accompanying pregnancy.

Consistent appearance of glycosuria occurs during hyperglycemic episodes of diabetes when the renal threshold for glucose is exceeded and the excess glucose is spilled into the urine. However, when renal failure accompanies hyperglycemia, glycosuria cannot be considered indicative of the level of hyperglycemia because of the erratic excretion of glucose by the damaged nephrons.

***Protein.*** Protein, like glucose, is normally absent from the urine because the large protein molecule cannot pass across the normal glomerular capillary membrane. Thus consistent appearance of protein in the urine suggests compromise of the glomerular membrane and possible renal disease.

Transient appearance of protein in the urine can occur as the result of efferent arteriole constriction caused by stress, extreme exercise, or extreme cold. Also, **proteinuria** can occur after ingestion of a high protein meal or can accompany the renal changes associated with pregnancy.

Levels of proteinuria of 0.5 to 4.0 g/day indicate renal compromise, and the amount excreted directly correlates with the severity of the damage.[4]

***Electrolytes.*** Levels of urinary electrolytes are not as frequently measured as are serum electrolytes because of the lesser significance of urinary findings. To measure urinary electrolyte levels, a 24-hour urine sample is required. The electrolyte levels are highly variable, and the electrolytes depend on the kidneys for adequate excretion. Consequently, decreases in urinary electrolyte levels are highly suggestive of renal failure. The urinary sodium level, on the other hand, may increase because of the inability of aldosterone to effect sodium reabsorption in the damaged nephrons.[4]

***Urinary sediment.*** The presence of epithelial cells and *casts* aids in identifying problems related to the kidneys. The consistent appearance of epithelial cells shed by the nephron may indicate *nephritis*. Casts differ in composition and size, and both characteristics correlate to the severity and type of renal damage. White blood cell casts indicate pyelonephritis and also occur during the exudative stage of acute glomerulonephritis. Red blood cell casts indicate glomerulonephritis, whereas hyaline casts are associated with renal parenchymal disease and glomerular capillary membrane inflammation.

***Table 16-4*** Renal imaging tests

| Test | Comments |
|---|---|
| Intravenous pyelography (IVP) | Intravenous injection of contrast, followed by visualization of the internal renal structures<br>Determines kidney size and shape and presence of tumors or obstructions<br>Hypersensitivity to contrast media in some patients |
| Renal CT scanning | Injections of radioisotope, followed by scintillation photography<br>Determines presence of tumors, cysts, hemorrhages, necrosis, or calcification<br>May be employed instead of renal biopsy |
| Renal ultrasonography | High-frequency sound waves are transmitted to the kidneys<br>Determines fluid accumulation, obstruction, or structural changes due to disease process |

## DIAGNOSTIC PROCEDURES

### Radiologic Assessment

Radiologic assessment serves to supplement laboratory assessment in the confirmation or clarification of renal and urological disorders. Although many procedures are available, Table 16-4 describes the most frequently employed diagnostic measures, including **renal computed tomographic (CT) scan** and **renal ultrasonography.**

### Renal Biopsy

**Renal biopsy** is the definitive diagnostic measure for confirming renal disease. Percutaneous needle biopsy includes obtaining a specimen of kidney tissue via the introduction of a cannula through the skin over the flank. Biopsy, although rarely employed, is used to determine the presence of diseases such as glomerulonephritis, amyloidosis, and lupus erythematosus.

#### REFERENCES

1. Ames SW and Kneisl CR: Essentials of adult health nursing, Menlo Park, Calif, 1988, Addison-Wesley Publishing Co.
2. Bates B: A guide to physical examination, ed 5, Philadelphia, 1991, JB Lippincott Co.
3. Eisenberg M: Electrolyte measurements during inhospital cardiopulmonary resuscitation, Critic Care Med 18:25, 1990.
4. Fischbach F: A manual of laboratory diagnostic tests, ed 3, Philadelphia, 1988, JB Lippincott Co.
5. Grimes J and Burns E: Health assessment in nursing practice, ed 2, Boston, 1987, Jones & Bartlett Publishers, Inc.
6. Innerarity S: Electrolyte emergencies in the critically ill renal patient, Crit Care Nurs Clin North Am 2:89, 1990.
7. Insel J and Elwyn DH: Body composition. In Askanazi J, Starker PM, and Weissman C, editors: Fluid and electrolyte management in critical care, Boston, 1986, Butterworth and Co (Publishers), Ltd.
8. Malasanos L and others: Health assessment, ed 4, St Louis, 1989, Mosby–Year Book, Inc.
9. Metheny NM: Fluid and electrolyte balance—nursing considerations, Philadelphia, 1987, JB Lippincott Co.
10. Narins RG Jr and others: Metabolic acid-base disorders: pathophysiology, classification and treatment. In Arieff AI and DeFronzo RA, editors: Fluid, electrolyte and acid-base disorders, vol 1, New York, 1985, Churchill Livingstone, Inc.
11. Poyss AS: Assessment and nursing diagnosis in fluid and electrolyte disorders, Nurs Clin North Am 22(4):773, 1987.
12. Rice V: Problems of water regulation: diabetes insipidus and syndromes of inappropriate anti-diuretic hormone, Crit Care Nurse 32:64, 1983.
13. Richard C: Assessment of renal structure and function. In Lancaster L: Core curriculum for nephrology nursing, Englewood Cliffs, NJ, 1987, AJ Janetti, Inc.
14. Shorecki KL and Brenner BM: Edema forming states: congestive heart failure, liver disease, and nephrotic syndrome. In Arieff AI and DeFronzo RA, editors: Fluid, electrolyte and acid-base disorders, vol 1, New York, 1985, Churchill Livingstone, Inc.
15. Tilkian SM, Conover MB, and Tilkian AG: Clinical implications of laboratory tests, ed 4, St Louis, 1987, Mosby–Year Book, Inc.
16. Woodtli AO: Thirst: a critical care nursing challenge, DCCN 9:6, 1990.

CHAPTER 17

# Renal Disorders and Therapeutic Management

## CHAPTER OBJECTIVES

- *List signs and symptoms of each of the serum electrolyte disturbances discussed in this chapter.*
- *Identify clinical manifestations of acute and chronic renal failure.*
- *Describe important aspects of the nursing care of a patient with acute renal failure.*
- *Describe important aspects of the nursing care of a patient with chronic renal failure.*
- *Identify and describe the various types of vascular access for hemodialysis.*
- *Explain the differences—including advantages, disadvantages, and nursing care—between peritoneal dialysis, continuous ambulatory peritoneal dialysis, and continous cycling peritoneal dialysis.*
- *Describe essential aspects of the nursing care for a patient with a renal transplant.*

## KEY TERMS

hypokalemia, p. 332
hyperkalemia, p. 332
hyponatremia, p. 335
water intoxication, p. 335
hypocalcemia, p. 336
hypoproteinemia, p. 338
metabolic acidosis, p. 338
metabolic alkalosis, p. 338
acute tubular necrosis, p. 338
acute renal failure, p. 340
chronic renal failure, p. 342
uremic syndrome, p. 343
arteriovenous (A-V) fistula, p. 346
continuous arteriovenous hemofiltration (CAVH), p. 349

## RENAL DISORDERS

### Electrolyte Disturbances

The specific contributions of the electrolytes to the successful maintenance of overall body functioning are important. Very often, changes in the electrolytes can initiate serious organ dysfunction. Their replacement or reduction is required to restore the necessary equilibrium. Table 17-1 summarizes electrolyte disturbances.

**Hypokalemia. Hypokalemia** is a potassium deficit of the extracellular fluid (ECF) and occurs as a result of the body's tendency to excrete potassium. It is complicated by secondary conditions such as vomiting, gastric suction, and excess aldosterone production and by use of potent diuretics, which further enhance potassium losses.[19,59]

Clinical assessment of hypokalemia necessitates looking at the serum potassium level, since it is impossible to look at actual total body stores of potassium. The most significant clinical sign related to potassium changes occurs in the electrocardiogram (ECG). Hypokalemia slows depolarization of the cells and thereby slows conduction velocity of the heart.[14] Hypokalemia has also been implicated in cases of sudden cardiac death in individuals who have cardiac compromise.

Treatment of hypokalemia is through oral or parenteral replacement. Parenteral potassium replacement should not exceed 20 mEq/hr or 150 mEq/L/day in adults or 3 mEq/kg in children. Additionally, potassium is *always* diluted for parenteral use. Potassium levels should be monitored carefully during potassium supplementation. Observation of renal function is also necessary to prevent hyperkalemia as a result of potassium retention.[59] Observation of intravenous (IV) sites for extrusion into the tissues is essential, since potassium is very caustic to the tissues.

**Hyperkalemia. Hyperkalemia** is an excess of potassium in the ECF that often occurs secondary to kidney failure. Additionally, cell damage resulting from surgery, burns, or myocardial infarction releases potassium into the ECF.[19,55,67]

ECG findings in hyperkalemia are also of value in confirming a diagnosis of hyperkalemia. The appearance of tall, peaked T waves, a lengthening PR interval, widening QRS

***Table 17-1*** Electrolyte disturbances

| Disturbance | Serum value | Causes | Findings |
|---|---|---|---|
| Hypokalemia | Less than 3.5 mEq/L | Metabolic alkalosis<br>Decreased potassium intake<br>Use of diuretics without potassium supplementation<br>Loss of gastrointestinal (GI) fluids (suction, nausea and vomiting, diarrhea)<br>Hyperaldosteronism (primary and secondary Cushing's syndrome) | Muscular weakness<br>Cardiac irregularities<br>Abdominal distention and flatulence<br>Paresthesia<br>Decreased reflexes<br>Anorexia<br>Dizziness<br>Confusion<br>Increased sensitivity to digitalis<br>ECG changes |
| Hyperkalemia | Greater than 5.0 mEq/L | Acute or chronic renal failure<br>Excess intake of potassium<br>Excess intake through infusions<br>Burns<br>Crushing injuries<br>Potassium-sparing diuretics<br>Metabolic acidosis<br>Transfusions of old blood | Irritability and restlessness<br>Anxiety<br>Nausea and vomiting<br>Abdominal cramps<br>Weakness<br>Numbness and tingling (fingertips and circumoral)<br>Cardiac irregularities (first tachycardia, then bradycardia)<br>ECG changes |
| Hyponatremia | | | |
| Water intoxication | May be less than 125 mEq/L (very mild to severe); serum sodium value of 110-115 mEq/L known to occur | Excess $D_5W$ solution intravenously<br>Excess plain water intake<br>Renal failure | Disorientation<br>Muscle twitching<br>Nausea and vomiting<br>Abdominal cramps<br>Headaches<br>Seizures |
| True hyponatremia | Less than 135 mEq/L | Gastric suction<br>Vomiting<br>Burns<br>Use of potent diuretics<br>Heat exhaustion (excessive sweating)<br>Loss from wounds and drainage<br>Use of tap-water enemas<br>Diarrhea<br>Adrenal insufficiency | Apprehension<br>Dizziness<br>Postural hypotension<br>Cold, clammy skin<br>Decreased skin turgor<br>Tachycardia<br>Oliguria |
| Syndrome of inappropriate release of ADH (SIADH) | Less than 120 mEq/L | Central nervous system (CNS) disorders<br>Major trauma (stress)<br>Malignancies (lung, pancreas, thymus)<br>Certain drugs (oral hypoglycemics, antineoplastics, diuretics, analgesics, bronchodilators) | Anorexia<br>Nausea and vomiting<br>Abdominal cramps<br>Lethargy and withdrawal<br>Convulsions<br>Coma<br>Urinary osmolality greater than plasma |
| Hypernatremia | Greater than 145 mEq/L | Inability to respond to thirst (decreased fluid intake)<br>Heatstroke<br>Diarrhea (excess fluid loss)<br>Severe insensible loss (ventilation, sweating)<br>Diabetes insipidus | Extreme thirst<br>Fever<br>Dry, sticky mucous membranes<br>Altered mentation<br>Seizures (later stages) |

*Continued.*

***Table 17-1*** Electrolyte disturbances—cont'd

| Disturbance | Serum value | Causes | Findings |
|---|---|---|---|
| | | Excessive administration of sodium solutions (e.g., hypertonic saline, sodium bicarbonate)<br>Hypertonic tube feedings without water supplement<br>NOTE: Hypermatremia is usually the result of dehydration of the ECF and subsequent hyperconcentration of the sodium. | |
| Hypocalcemia | Less than 8.5 mg/dl or 4.5 mEq/L | Protein malnutrition (decreased albumin causes decreased calcium)<br>Decreased calcium intake<br>Burns or infection<br>Decreased parathyroid function (PTH controls serum calcium availability)<br>Decreased GI absorption of calcium (diarrhea)<br>Excessive antacid use (prevents absorption)<br>Renal failure (decreased vitamin D available to stimulate absorption) | Irritability<br>Muscular tetany<br>Muscle cramps<br>Decreased cardiac output (decreased contractions)<br>Bleeding (decreased ability to coagulate)<br>ECG changes |
| Hypercalcemia | Greater than 10.5 mg/dl or 5.8 mEq/L | Increased parathyroid activity (increases bone resorption of calcium)<br>Multiple fractures<br>Prolonged immobilization<br>Bone tumors<br>Other malignancies<br>Decreased phosphorus (inverse relationship between calcium and phosphate) | Deep bone pain<br>Excessive thirst<br>Anorexia<br>Lethargy<br>Weakened muscles |
| Hypomagnesemia | Less than 1.4 mEq/L | Malnutrition<br>Chronic alcoholism (malnutrition)<br>Diuretics (prolonged use)<br>Severe diarrhea<br>Severe dehydration | Choroid and athetoid muscle activity<br>Facial tics<br>Spasticity<br>Cardiac dysrhythmias |
| Hypermagnesemia | Greater than 2.5 mEq/L | Excessive intake of magnesium products (antacids and laxatives)<br>Renal failure<br>Severe dehydration if oliguria is present | CNS depression (especially respiratory)<br>Lethargy<br>Coma<br>Bradycardia<br>ECG changes |
| Hypophosphatemia | Less than 3.0 mg/dl | Diabetic ketoacidosis (renal wasting)<br>Malabsorption disorders<br>Renal wasting of phosphorus<br>Prolonged use of IV dextrose infusions<br>Low-phosphate diets in patients with renal failure<br>Phosphate-poor total parenteral nutrition solutions | Hemolytic anemias<br>Depressed white cell function<br>Bleeding (decreased platelet aggregation)<br>Nausea, vomiting, and anorexia |

***Table 17-1*** Electrolyte disturbances—cont'd

| Disturbance | Serum value | Causes | Findings |
|---|---|---|---|
| Hyperphosphatemia | Greater than 4.5 mg/dl | Renal failure<br>Lactic acidosis<br>Catabolic stress<br>Chemotherapy for certain malignancies | Tachycardia<br>Nausea<br>Diarrhea<br>Abdominal cramps<br>Muscle weakness<br>Flaccid paralysis<br>Increased reflexes |
| Hypochloremia | Less than 98 mEq/L | Loss of gastric contents (vomiting, suction)<br>Diarrhea (prolonged)<br>Excessive diuretic use<br>Excessive sweating<br>Prolonged use of IV dextrose<br>Metabolic alkalosis | Hyperirritability<br>Tetany or muscular excitability<br>Slow respirations<br>Decreased blood pressure (with fluid loss) |
| Hyperchloremia | Greater than 108 mEq/L | Severe diarrhea<br>Urinary diversions<br>Renal failure<br>Metabolic acidosis<br>Excessive parenteral administration of isotonic saline solution | Weakness<br>Lethargy<br>Deep, rapid breathing<br>Possible unconsciousness (later stages) |
| Hypoalbuminemia | Less than 3.8 g/dl | Protein-deficient diet<br>Burns<br>Starvation<br>Surgeries (major, with prolonged recovery phase)<br>Digestive diseases | Muscle wasting<br>Peripheral edema (fluid shift)<br>Decreased resistance to infection<br>Poorly healing wounds |
| Metabolic acidosis | Bicarbonate level less than 22 mEq/L<br>Partial pressure of carbon dioxide ($PCO_2$) normal or less than 35 mm Hg to compensate for the low bicarbonate level<br>pH below 7.35 | Diabetic ketoacidosis<br>Lactic acidosis<br>Uremia<br>Ingestion of acids (e.g., salicylates, alcohol, boric acid)<br>Starvation<br>Diarrhea<br>Some diuretics | Weakness<br>Dizziness<br>Rapid respirations<br>Coma (later stages) |
| Metabolic alkalosis | Bicarbonate level greater than 26 mEq/L<br>$PCO_2$ level normal or greater than 45 mm Hg to compensate for the elevated bicarbonate level<br>pH level greater than 7.45 | Vomiting (with loss of chloride)<br>Excessive intake of alkalies<br>Primary aldosteronism (because of loss of potassium)<br>Diuretic use in patient with congestive heart failure (CHF)(on occasion) | Hyperexcitability of muscles<br>Bradycardia<br>Bradypnea<br>Numbness and tingling |

complexes, and flattening P waves indicate elevations of potassium.[28]

Potassium supplementation should be discontinued. Administration of calcium parenterally will temporarily block the effects of hyperkalemia in the heart muscle, but further measures are required to actually decrease serum levels, including sodium bicarbonate injection and the use of a mixture of hypertonic dextrose and insulin. However, eventual excretion of potassium is necessary, particularly in the presence of renal failure. Consequently, cation-exchange resins (for example, sodium polystyrene sulfonate [Kayexalate]) are administered, and hemodialysis should be initiated.[55]

**Hyponatremia. Hyponatremia** is a deficiency of sodium in the ECF when compared with water. Hyponatremia can be deceptive because in several disorders there is not an actual deficit of sodium but an excess of water in relationship to the sodium. At least three scenarios offer further explanation of the possible alterations in sodium and ECF balance.

The first scenario is hyponatremia associated with an increase in the ECF volume and is commonly known as **water**

**intoxication** or dilutional hyponatremia. A concomitant inability to excrete the excess volume leads to dilution of the existing sodium.

For example, in an individual with renal compromise, ingestion of water or infusion of IV solutions beyond the excretion capacity of the kidney results in dilutional hyponatremia. The decrease in glomerular filtration rate (GFR) is implicated as the primary mechanism for this occurrence.

A second picture of hyponatremia is a loss of both sodium and ECF. Implicated in the development of this disturbance are the loss of sodium-rich gastrointestinal (GI) fluids, overuse of potent diuretics, and aldosterone insufficiency. In the case of GI losses, not only sodium and water are depleted, but potassium is also. With less potassium available for excretion by the distal tubule, the stimulus to release aldosterone is partially lost and sodium is not sufficiently reabsorbed.[2]

Treatment for both cases of hyponatremia involves treating the underlying conditions, administering IV sodium chloride solutions, and discontinuing diuretic therapy. Correction of the hyponatremic states with IV saline solutions may prevent the problem of fluid shifts from the ECF to the intracellular fluid (ICF) when sodium is lost.[21]

Finally, hyponatremia can result from the syndrome of inappropriate secretion of ADH (SIADH).The condition results from oversecretion of ADH (vasopressin), which permits the continuous reabsorption of water from the renal tubular system. Sodium excretion is high in the urine, whereas large amounts of water are retained under the influence of ADH secretion. Fluid restriction, sodium replacement, mild diuretics, and drugs to control ADH secretion (demeclocycline) represent current treatment for the disorder.[25,31]

**Hypernatremia.** Sodium excess of the ECF is extremely dangerous and can arise from an actual increase in sodium or from losses of water. Hypernatremia can occur with a loss of both ECF sodium and water, but the water loss far exceeds the amount of sodium loss. Watery diarrhea or profuse sweating can cause severe hypotonic fluid loss.

True hypernatremia can be caused by administration of high sodium content tube feedings without sufficient water intake and by administration of hypertonic saline solutions for correction of sodium imbalance or administration of sodium bicarbonate during cardiac arrest.[43,54]

Finally, hypernatremia can result from only water loss such as occurs with diabetes insipidus. This disorder is classified as either central diabetes insipidus (arising from central nervous system causes) or nephrogenic diabetes insipidus, which results in a loss of the renal response to ADH, causing no reabsorption of water in the collecting ducts. As water is lost, sodium in the ECF rises.[72]

Regardless of the causes of hypernatremia, one particular characteristic remains common—thirst. Thirst is the main defense against hyperconcentration of the fluid compartments. The same osmoreceptors that trigger ADH release are responsible for stimulation of thirst and are stimulated when the serum osmolality rises to 294 mOsm/kg.[25,64] An enormous intake of fluid, however, helps maintain the serum osmolality near normal.

**Hypocalcemia.** Calcium deficit can be misleading because of the three different ways calcium is held within the body. Ninety-eight to ninety-nine percent of the calcium within the body is bound in bone and is not readily available. The remainder is either protein bound or ionized in the bloodstream.[16] Since serum calcium is primarily protein bound, changes in serum protein values will lead to changes in serum calcium values.

The serum calcium level is affected by the inverse relationship that exists between calcium and phosphorus. When phosphorus levels are high, calcium absorption is inhibited; the reverse is also true.[70] Further, serum calcium levels are influenced by the pH of the arterial blood. In acidosis, the lower pH results in the release of more calcium from protein binding, which elevates the ionized calcium. Conversely, an elevated pH results in calcium becoming more highly bound to protein, reducing the ionized calcium.[16] Thus when correcting acidosis, care must be taken to monitor calcium and replace it as needed.

The person experiencing **hypocalcemia** may display facial muscle twitching (Chvostek's sign) or carpophalangeal spasm (Trousseau's sign). Cardiac changes are also present with hypocalcemia and are reflected as prolonged QT segments on the ECG and decreased left-ventricular contractility.[16] Both problems result from the decreased availability of calcium to perform its role in cell depolarization and consequent neurotransmission. Treatment for hypocalcemia depends on whether the disorder is acute or chronic. Acute hypocalcemia is treated with IV administration of calcium. An initial bolus of 200 mg is given over 10 minutes, followed by 1 to 2 mg/kg/hour until levels are normal (6 to 12 hours).[70] However, the success of treatment of hypocalcemia often depends on normalizing the levels of other electrolytes. For example, the administration of calcium in the presence of hyperphosphatemia usually results in little success in correcting the original calcium imbalance. If magnesium levels are low, infusion of calcium only results in its excretion from the kidney in favor of magnesium retention. Drugs that predispose to or prolong hypocalcemia should also be discontinued.[70]

**Hypercalcemia.** An excess of calcium in the ECF is known as hypercalcemia. Hypercalcemia is mediated almost exclusively from abnormalities in bone activity rather than absorption and release of calcium into the ECF.[15]

Treatment of acute hypercalcemia involves dilution of the calcium using IV fluids and concomitant use of "loop" diuretics (furosemide) to enhance calcium excretion.[15] Thiazide diuretics inhibit excretion of calcium and should not be used in cases of hypercalcemia.[40] Oral phosphorus preparations may be given to increase bone deposition of calcium.[15] However, phosphorus preparations should not be given to those patients with renal failure. Additionally, the diarrhea and/or constipation caused by phosphorus may be undesirable in some individuals. IV phosphate administration is used as a last resort because of the potential for developing soft-tissue calcification from calcium-phosphate precipitates.[40]

**Hypomagnesemia.** Magnesium is involved in enzymatic reaction, cellular permeability, and the maintenance of neuromuscular excitability. However, the causes of magnesium deficit are lead by those involving loss from the GI tract.[17] Nutritional deficits such as result from administering parenteral nutrition or tube feedings that are magnesium poor can lead to hypomagnesemia. The administration of loop diuretics such as furosemide also can enhance magnesium losses.

The signs and symptoms of hypomagnesemia involve the role magnesium plays in neuromuscular excitability. Severe respiratory muscle depression may occur, rendering the individual in need of mechanical ventilation. Mental apathy and confusion may also be present. Finally, life-threatening dysrhythmias can result from magnesium depletion.[20]

Treatment for hypomagnesemia usually involves IV replacement with magnesium sulfate. However, before treatment is initiated, determination of adequate renal function should be undertaken. Individuals with severe hypomagnesemia may be given 2 g as a 10% solution over 2 minutes, followed by 12 g in 1 L of fluid over 12 hours.[20] Moderate decreases may be treated with 24 to 40 mEq of magnesium sulfate administered parenterally for several days. Oral or nasogastric (NG) supplementation should approach 16 mEq/day.[16]

**Hypermagnesemia.** The development of excess levels of magnesium in the ECF, although rare, goes hand in hand with chronic renal disease. The renal tubules can no longer excrete magnesium, and dialysis is quite ineffective in removing magnesium.[38]

The signs and symptoms associated with hypermagnesemia demonstrate profound central nervous system (CNS) involvement. The individual may exhibit muscle weakness, inability to swallow, hyporeflexia, hypotension, and cardiac dysrhythmias.[38] The ECG will demonstrate a prolonged PR interval, wide QRS, tall T waves, atrioventricular (A-V) block, and premature ventricular contractions (PVCs).

Treatment for magnesium excess should be vigorous and immediate, with discontinuance of all magnesium-containing drugs, replacement of ECF volume (if secondary to dehydration), and administration of calcium gluconate to counteract the effects of the magnesium.[43] Individuals with severe hypermagnesemia may suffer from respiratory depression secondary to the effect of magnesium on the respiratory centers of the brain. Mechanical ventilation may become necessary to sustain ventilation until the excess is corrected.

**Hypophosphatemia.** Hypophosphatemia is a deficit of phosphorus in the ECF. Phosphorus shares an inverse relationship with calcium, and losses or gains in either electrolyte cause the kidneys to retain or excrete the other.

The individual with hypophosphatemia develops bleeding disorders from defective platelets and fragile red blood cell (RBC) membranes. Muscular weakness, paresthesia, and GI distress result from reduced energy and oxygen transport to cells, which phosphorus helps accomplish.[5]

Replacement of phosphorous stores is generally done very slowly because the actual serum level may not reflect a deficit in the intracellular compartment. Oral supplementation is usually achieved through ingestion of skim milk. Fleet's Phospho-Soda can be mixed in water and administered either orally or by NG or feeding tube. Parenteral phosphorus is usually not given unless the serum phosphorus reaches 1.0 mg/dl.[5] Parenteral preparations of phosphorus must be diluted, and care must be taken to monitor levels of phosphorus to prevent precipitation with calcium. Phosphate solutions should be administered in quantities no greater than 1 g over 24 hours.[31]

**Hyperphosphatemia.** Phosphorus excess of the ECF usually occurs in cases of chronic renal failure. The renal tubules no longer excrete phosphorus as before, but uptake continues in the GI tract.

The signs and symptoms of hyperphosphatemia closely parallel those of hypocalcemia, since these disorders are likely to occur simultaneously. However, muscle tetany and soft-tissue calcifications are usually the more prominent signs of this disorder.[34]

Treatment for hyperphosphatemia may range from simple dietary restriction of phosphorus to ingestion of aluminum antacids, which bind phosphate in the intestine. Adequate hydration and correction of any existing hypocalcemia can enhance the renal excretion of the excess phosphate.[70]

**Hypochloremia.** Hypochloremia is a deficit of chloride in the ECF. Hypochloremia develops as a result of loss of fluids rich in chloride. These fluids can also be rich in sodium, since chloride combines with sodium. Hypochloremia can be associated with acid-base disorders, particularly metabolic alkalosis, since the retention of bicarbonate, which occurs with metabolic alkalosis, leads to the excretion of chloride ions. The signs and symptoms of hypochloremia primarily result, not from the loss of chloride, but from the loss of potassium and ionized calcium.[50]

Treatment for hypochloremia usually involves chloride replacement with a variety of medications such as ammonium chloride tablets or a parenteral solution containing chloride.[50] Treatment of the causative disorder should proceed immediately.

**Hyperchloremia.** Hyperchloremia is an excess of chloride ions in the ECF. Just as a deficit of chloride is related to acid-base imbalance, so is hyperchloremia. In patients with metabolic acidosis in whom bicarbonate ions are lost excessively, chloride ions are retained. Treatment for hyperchloremia is based on first treating the underlying cause and correcting the acidosis. Additionally, parenteral administration of sodium bicarbonate can restore bicarbonate stores.[50]

**Hypoproteinemia.** A reduction in protein of the ECF may be rapid or insidious and is a difficult-to-treat malady.

Loss of protein can be sudden, such as with burns or surgery, or very slow and steady, such as with renal insufficiency (undetected), malnutrition, bleeding, or liver disease.[50]

The edema associated with **hypoproteinemia** results from a plasma-to-interstitial fluid shift from a lack of oncotic pressure in the vascular space. For example, in patients with liver disease, insufficient amounts of albumin are produced, thereby lowering oncotic pressure within the vascular system.

Treatment is difficult because the individual may no longer be able to ingest orally the high amounts of protein needed to replace stores. NG feedings or total parenteral nutrition (TPN) can be used to replace stores, but the course of protein replacement is often lengthy. Human serum albumin can be used to treat hypoalbuminemia. However, albumin must be administered slowly (2 to 3 ml/min) to avoid fluid overload as a result of normalizing oncotic pressure.[50]

**Bicarbonate deficit.** A primary base bicarbonate deficit is referred to as **metabolic acidosis.** The arterial pH is decreased as a result of loss of bicarbonate.

Bicarbonate deficit occurs in patients with renal failure because the GFR decreases and the available buffers are insufficient to allow acid secretion into the renal tubules. Therefore hydrogen ions are retained in place of bicarbonate, which is lost in the urine.[4] As bicarbonate levels in the ECF drop, potassium exits the cells and floods the ECF, leading to a hyperkalemic state.

Treatment of bicarbonate deficit is achieved by treating the cause and administering oral or parenteral bicarbonate.[50] Replacement of bicarbonate is calculated on the basis of body weight and the desired increment of increase in bicarbonate.[43]

**Bicarbonate excess.** An excess of bicarbonate or excess loss of acid in the ECF is referred to as **metabolic alkalosis.** Metabolic alkalosis can develop from severe fluid and acid losses, causing the retention of bicarbonate, or it can develop from excessive addition of bicarbonate to the body.

Potassium levels should also be carefully monitored; metabolic alkalosis causes hydrogen ion release from the cells and a subsequent exchange for potassium, leading to potassium deficit of the ECF.[59]

Treatment of bicarbonate excess primarily involves increasing excretion through the kidney. However, if the patient is taking excessive medications containing bicarbonate, withdrawal of these medications will be necessary. Also, if the cause is a loss in chloride, replacement of the chloride will produce bicarbonate excretion.

### Acid-Base Abnormalities

**Carbonic acid deficit in ECF.** Carbonic acid deficit in the ECF is usually referred to as *respiratory alkalosis*. The deficit results from any situation causing hyperventilation such as pain, CNS lesions, fever, or assisted ventilation.[51]

The individual who is hyperventilating loses carbon dioxide, which is required to formulate carbonic acid, but retains bicarbonate. The body attempts to compensate for the lost carbon dioxide by allowing excretion of bicarbonate through the kidneys, possibly inducing a deficit of bicarbonate.[37] Also, chloride may be exchanged for bicarbonate at the cellular level, thereby decreasing the available bicarbonate in the ECF.[37]

Besides rapid breathing, the individual may experience tetany (because of the pH and calcium relationship), paresthesia, tingling and numbness (especially around the mouth), blurred vision, diaphoresis, dry mouth, and coma (later stages).[37] Laboratory findings reveal a serum pH level greater than 7.45 and $P_{CO_2}$ level below 35 mm Hg.

Treatment is aimed at reducing the hyperventilation if the cause is known. For instance, sedating the patient may be helpful. Parenteral administration of chloride solutions are helpful in reducing the bicarbonate while the respiratory problem is treated.[4]

**Carbonic acid excess in ECF.** Carbonic acid excess is known commonly as respiratory acidosis. This disorder develops when the lungs fail to rid the body of the appropriate amount of carbon dioxide, resulting in formation of excess carbonic acid from the excess carbon dioxide. Hypoventilatory effort or obstruction to ventilations results in respiratory acidosis. Drugs, anesthetics, CNS damage, neurological disease, or musculoskeletal diseases may be implicated in the development of this disorder. The kidneys compensate for the problem by excreting hydrogen, reabsorbing bicarbonate, and regenerating bicarbonate from the excess carbon dioxide. This process is slow, however (5 days for maximal effect), and other support measures are usually required.[37]

Treatment is aimed at correcting the cause of the hypoventilation or ventilatory distress. Oxygen or mechanical ventilation may be helpful.

### Renal Disturbances

#### Acute tubular necrosis

***Description.*** **Acute tubular necrosis** refers to damage occurring within the epithelium of the tubular portions of the nephron. Acute tubular necrosis is sometimes used synonymously with acute renal failure but is, in fact, a cause of acute renal failure. Damage to the cellular structures in this area prevents normal concentration of urine, filtration of wastes, and regulation of acid-base, electrolyte, and water balance.[56] A number of disorders can result in ATN, and several contributing factors may work together to bring about tubular damage.[56]

***Causes.*** Common causes of acute tubular necrosis, listed in Table 17-2, are broken into two categories—ischemic and toxic.

***Pathophysiology.*** There are several theories, often discussed and researched, to explain the pathophysiology behind acute tubular necrosis. The *back-leak* theory suggests that tubular injury, whether ischemic or toxic, leads to return

***Table 17-2*** Causes of acute tubular necrosis

| Ischemic | Toxic |
|---|---|
| Hemorrhage | Rhabdomyolysis |
| Excessive diuretic use | Gout |
| Burns | Hypercalcemia |
| Peritonitis | Gram-negative sepsis |
| Sepsis | Radiocontrast media |
| Congestive heart failure | Methanol |
| Myocardial ischemia | Carbon tetrachloride |
| Pulmonary emboli | Heavy metals |
| | Insecticides |
| | Drugs ("street type" phencyclidine [PCP]) |
| | Aminoglycoside antibiotics |
| | Analgesics containing phenacetin |

of metabolites (for example, creatinine) to the peritubular circulation. This causes decreased urinary production with retention of wastes, water, and electrolytes.[46,54]

Another theory refers to *tubular obstruction* from interstitial edema or from an accumulation of casts and sloughing tissue creating an obstruction. Filtration ceases when tubular hydrostatic pressure reaches that of glomerular filtration pressure. This decreases the formation of urine because of the nonavailability of filtrate to process.[46,54]

The *vascular* theories suggest that damage to the tubules is primarily mediated by obstruction in the renal capillary beds. Prolonged ischemia results in afferent arteriolar constriction and a reduction of GFR, which decreases the available filtrate. The exchange between tubules and capillaries is obliterated, and tubular cells fail to receive the necessary blood flow and oxygen to sustain them.[54] *Decreased glomerular membrane permeability* is suggested as a fourth explanation. It restricts filtration but occurs at the cellular level and is independent of blood flow.[46]

Finally, the last theory suggests that *vasoconstriction* reduces renal perfusion and reduces capillary flow in the cortical region of the kidney (site of most of the glomeruli), resulting in acute tubular necrosis.

***Assessment and diagnosis.*** Assessment of acute tubular necrosis involves tracking disturbances in fluid volume, electrolyte and acid-base disturbances, and problems with elimination of metabolic wastes. Accurate documentation of intake and output, as well as daily weights, serve to track not only fluid losses contributing to ischemic tubular damage, but also the eventual fluid gains resulting from oliguria. Such additional signs and symptoms as increased serum BUN, creatinine, and potassium levels; cardiac dysrrhythmias; thirst; and apathy reflect the disturbances in body fluid balance.[46]

***Treatment.*** Treatment for acute tubular necrosis depends, for the most part, on the phase of the disease. If the patient is oliguric, treatment may include dialysis to remove fluids and toxins, drugs to combat infections and prevent complications, and fluid and dietary regulation with increased nutrients and fluid restrictions to decrease the metabolite load. In the early diuresis phase, output may be stimulated by use of loop diuretics such as furosemide to enhance water excretion.[4]

**TOXINS ASSOCIATED WITH ACUTE TUBULAR NECROSIS**

**DRUGS**

**Antibiotics**

Cephalosporins
Aminoglycosides
Tetracyclines

**Antineoplastics**

Methotrexate
Cisplatin

**Nonsteroidal antiinflammatory drugs (NSAID)**

**CHEMICALS**

Ethylene glycol

**PIGMENTS**

Myoglobin (rhabdomyolysis)

**CONTRAST MEDIA**

***Summary of nursing care.*** Because many experts consider acute tubular necrosis as part of acute renal failure, the nursing care would be the same. However, the nurse may actually provide additional preventive care for acute tubular necrosis alone. The nurse is in a unique position to identify individuals at high risk for renal insult, and patients who have been exposed to toxins associated with acute tubular necrosis should be identified. (See the box above, "Toxins Associated with Acute Tubular Necrosis.")

The critical care nurse must be vigilant of hemodynamic parameters that provide early information about fluid balance and perfusion of the kidneys. Not only must the nurse be alert for dehydration, but for fluid overload as well. Postoperative or trauma patients receiving fluid replacement require as strict attention to output as to intake. Subtle decreases in urinary output may not be observed unless comparisons of intake to output are made on a consistent basis.

Monitoring blood pressures and hemodynamics is helpful in assessing the fluid changes associated with the progressive course of acute tubular necrosis. Measurement of the abdominal girth for ascites and testing for pitting edema over body prominences and in dependent body areas should be frequent. Finally, cardiac outputs and pulmonary artery

**Nursing Diagnosis and Management**

***Acute tubular necrosis and acute renal failure***

- High Risk for Fluid Volume Excess risk factor: renal failure, p. 496
- Anxiety related to threatened biological, psychological, and/or social integrity, p. 448
- High Risk for Infection risk factors: protein-calorie malnourishment, invasive monitoring devices, p. 465
- Body Image Disturbance related to functional dependence on life-sustaining technology, p. 443
- Knowledge Deficit: Fluid Restriction, Reportable Symptoms, and Medications related to lack of previous exposure to information, p. 441
- Sensory-Perceptual Alterations related to sensory overload, sensory deprivation, and sleep pattern disturbance, p. 489
- Ineffective Individual Coping related to situational crisis and personal vulnerability, p. 447

**CAUSES OF ACUTE RENAL FAILURE**

**PRERENAL**

Hemorrhage
Severe GI losses
Burns
Renal trauma
Volume depletion (actual loss or "third-spacing")
Congestive heart failure, causing decreased renal perfusion
Hypoxia

**INTRARENAL**

Thrombus
Stenosis
Hypertensive sclerosis
Glomerulonephritis
Pyelonephritis
Acute tubular necrosis
Diabetic sclerosis
Toxic damage

**POSTRENAL**

Obstructions (stenosis, calculi)
Prostatic disease
Tumors

pressure (PAP) measurements can indicate a fall in intravascular volume. Cardiac output can decrease with a severe enough initial insult (for example, hemorrhage). Nursing diagnoses and management of acute tubular necrosis and acute renal failure are summarized in the box above.

**Acute renal failure**

***Description.*** **Acute renal failure** can be defined as any rapid decline in GFR with subsequent development of retention of metabolic waste products (azotemia). Acute renal failure is caused by a variety of insults. Mortality rates for it are still very high at approximately 50%, even with advanced critical care and dialysis techniques.[30,46,68] GI bleeding, sepsis, and CNS changes are often implicated in deaths related to ARF.[4]

***Causes.*** Causes for acute renal failure are broken into three categories, which are also the categories used to describe causes of chronic renal failure (see the box above). *Prerenal* causes are usually associated with any insult that reduces vascular perfusion to the kidney. *Intrarenal* causes are insults to the kidney tissue. *Postrenal* causes are usually obstructive disorders occurring beyond the kidney in the remainder of the urinary tract.

***Pathophysiology.*** Little is known about the exact pathophysiology of acute renal failure. It is suspected that decreased renal perfusion results in renin-angiotensin release, aldosterone release, and vasoconstriction of the blood supply to the nephron. Increased water and sodium uptake further reduces the available filtrate, whereupon renal tubular cells necrose and slough.[54]

***Assessment and diagnosis.*** Assessment for acute renal failure and chronic renal failure are essentially the same. Indeed, acute renal failure may eventually become chronic renal failure, depending on the extent of damage to the renal tubules.[56] The assessment can be divided into laboratory (blood and urine), radiological, and fluid areas (Table 17-3).

Finally, general assessment of the individual can reveal the effects that renal failure has on other body systems. For instance, hemodynamic monitoring during treatment for prerenal causes is valuable in tracking fluid balance and the need for fluid removal (dialysis) or replacement (IV fluids).[68] The remaining areas of assessment should include a general review of the body systems.

***Treatment.*** Medical interventions for acute renal failure are directed toward three basic goals: (1) correcting the causative mechanism, (2) promoting regeneration of the remaining functional renal capacity, and (3) preventing complications. Medical management is based on the three categories of causes of acute failure. Prerenal failure, involved with perfusion problems and often with fluid losses and shifts, requires two specific methods of management: fluid replacement and stimulation of output with diuretics. Also, the defect causing the initial perfusion problem must be corrected.

Intrarenal failure involves the introduction of increased amounts of water, solutes, and potential toxins into the

***Table 17-3*** Assessment in acute renal failure

| Assessment area | Findings |
|---|---|
| **LABORATORY** | |
| **Blood** | |
| Hgb and Hct | Decreased |
| Electrolytes | Increased potassium, decreased calcium, decreased sodium |
| Plasma osmolality | Variable, usually increased |
| BUN and creatinine | Increased |
| **Urine** | |
| Specific gravity | Decreased (fixed in chronic renal failure) |
| Urinary sediments | Normal to increased |
| Osmolality | Decreased |
| Creatinine clearance | Decreased |
| Sodium concentration | Decreased |
| **RADIOLOGICAL** | |
| Renal scan | All radiological findings depend on the specific pathology involved |
| IVP | |
| Angiographies | |
| **FLUID** | |
| Urinary output | Decreased |
| Skin turgor | Variable |
| Edema | Usually present |

circulation, so prompt measures are needed to decrease their levels. Hemodialysis is the usual treatment of choice, particularly if volume overload creates pulmonary and cardiac compromise. Severe hyperkalemia almost always necessitates hemodialysis because of the life-threatening cardiac dysrhythmias resulting from hyperkalemia. Dialysis may also be initiated for cases of uremic pericarditis or severe azotemia in which other treatments are contraindicated.[4]

Other forms of dialysis such as continous ambulatory peritoneal dialysis (CAPD) and continuous cycling peritoneal dialysis (CCPD) may be used to attempt correction of the renal failure. Continuous arteriovenous hemofiltration (CAVH) is sometimes used—mainly to remove fluid accumulation but also to reduce the solute load. It is used for patients who cannot tolerate the cardiovascular strain that hemodialysis often produces.[67]

Drugs, fluid restriction, and dietary control constitute a large part of the medical treatment for renal failure. Fluid restriction is used to prevent circulatory overload and interstitial edema associated with ARF and is calculated on the basis of daily urinary volumes and insensible losses. Patients are usually restricted to 1 L of fluid if urinary output is 500 ml or less and insensible losses range from 500 to 750 ml per day. However, if the patient is nonoliguric, fluid intake may be liberalized on an individual basis, determined by matching the daily fluid outputs.[54]

Electrolyte levels require frequent observation, especially in the initial critical phases of failure. Potassium may quickly reach levels of 6.0 mEq/L and above. Other than through hemodialysis, hyperkalemia can be treated temporarily by IV infusion of insulin and glucose. An infusion of 100 ml of 50% dextrose accompanied by 20 units of regular insulin will force potassium back into the cells.[14] Sodium bicarbonate (40 to 160 mEq) may be infused to promote higher excretion of potassium in the urine.[14] Finally, sodium polystyrene sulfonate (Kayexalate), a cation-exchange resin, is mixed in water and sorbitol and given orally, rectally, or through an NG tube.[11] The resin captures potassium in the bowel, which eliminates it in the feces.

Dilutional hyponatremia, associated with renal failure, can be corrected with fluid restriction. However, if sodium stores are actually depleted, 3% normal saline solution is usually administered intravenously as a replacement.[50] In addition, sodium levels may be raised during dialysis by changing the amount of sodium in the dialysate bath.

Calcium levels are reduced in renal failure, and, as previously described, the reduction is related to multiple factors, among which is hyperphosphatemia. Aluminum hydroxide preparations are administered to bind phosphorus in the bowel and thereby lower its level. Calcium may also be increased by use of calcium supplements, vitamin D preparations, and synthetic calcitriol (Rocaltrol).[70]

The nutritional aspect of renal failure may involve replacement as well as restriction. With the availability of refined products, it has become quite easy to provide total parenteral nutrition (TPN) while the patient is undergoing dialysis. If the patient is anorexic and malnourished, TPN can be provided, and renal formulas are even available.

The renal diet prescription is quite restrictive. Protein, potassium, sodium, and phosphorus are usually limited. For instance, protein restriction may vary from 0.5 to 1.0 g/kg/day to limit azotemia.[56] Carbohydrates are encouraged, primarily to provide needed energy for healing (35 to 45 kcal/kg/day).[29,46]

***Summary of nursing care.*** The actual nursing care for the individual with acute renal failure focuses on prevention or control of complications secondary to the disease process. In preventing infection, the nurse must not only frequently monitor for signs of infection but must maintain the patient's pulmonary hygiene, skin integrity, and nutrition. Consideration must be given to limiting invasive procedures and providing strict asepsis when performing dressing changes, catheterizations, or any such invasive procedures.[46] Should the individual be immobile, frequent turning and observation of potential sites for skin breakdown enhance the chances of avoiding infection. If the individual has developed significant anasarca, the use of a circulating air or air-fluid mattress may help prevent skin breakdown.

Frequent assessment of intake and output, particularly the output in response to any administered diuretics, is a necessary part of the nursing care for the patient in renal failure. Daily patient weights correlate with the intake and output to confirm fluid overloads. The nurse should take great care to note the return of urinary output and to seek replacement for the fluids and electrolytes that can be rapidly lost during this phase.

Hyperkalemia, hypocalcemia, hyponatremia, and hyperphosphatemia may all occur during acute renal failure. The nurse must be aware of the signs and symptoms of these electrolyte imbalances and prevent or control their associated side effects. The imbalances with the most potential hazard are hyperkalemia and hypocalcemia, which can result in life-threatening cardiac dysrhythmias.[46] The nurse is involved not only in monitoring signs and symptoms of these imbalances, but in teaching the patient and family ways to avoid imbalances and consequences of the imbalances.

Although the nurse can do little to prevent hyponatremia, nursing care must include frequent assessment for its signs and symptoms. The astute nurse also must remember that as fluid overload worsens in the oliguric patient, dilutional hyponatremia may also develop. Finally, hyperphosphatemia results most often in severe pruritus. Nursing care is subsequently directed at soothing the itching by performing frequent skin care with emollients, discouraging scratching, and administering phosphate-binding medications.

Care in preventing blood loss in the individual with renal failure centers on observation. Irritation of the GI tract from metabolic waste accumulation should be expected, and stools, NG drainage, and emesis should be tested for occult blood.

The nurse must give accurate, uncomplicated information to the patient and family about acute renal failure, including its prognosis, treatment, and possible complications. The nurse should be aware that sleep-rest disorders and emotional upset can occur as complications of acute renal failure and should encourage the patient and family to voice concerns, frustrations, and fears. Searching for ways to allow the patient to control some aspects of the acute care environment or treatment is also essential. However, at times the patient may be disoriented, severely fatigued, or incapable of participating in care.

### Chronic renal failure

***Description.*** Current health care literature suggests a steady rise in the number of individuals who will face renal failure, either requiring acute or chronic care. Therefore caregivers must be aware of the necessary components of care for these individuals.

**Chronic renal failure** is defined as *insidious* and *irreversible* damage to the kidneys. Often signs and symptoms develop over a period of years, and the patient will have been treated for a variety of suspected disorders before renal failure is diagnosed. Treatment is usually based on the degree of residual kidney function.

***Causes.*** The causes of chronic renal failure are basically the same as those for acute renal failure. The Public Health Department revealed at least three main causes of chronic

## MANIFESTATIONS OF CHRONIC RENAL FAILURE

**CARDIOVASCULAR**

Hypervolemia
Hypertension
Dysrhythmias
Congestive heart failure
Pericarditis
Cardiomegaly

**PULMONARY**

Adventitious lung sounds (crackles)
Dyspnea
Pulmonary edema
Uremic pleuritis

**NEUROLOGICAL**

Insomnia
Apathy
Confusion
Short-term memory loss
Lethargy
Behavior changes
Peripheral neuropathy
Paraesthesia—asterixis

**GASTROINTESTINAL**

Nausea and vomiting
Ulcerations
GI bleeding
Uremic fetor
Diarrhea
Constipation

**INTEGUMENTARY**

Pallor
Pruritus
Color changes (uremic bronzing)
Decreased turgor
Skin fragility

**SKELETAL**

Joint pain
Joint swelling
Gait changes
Reduced range of motion

**HEMATOLOGICAL**

Anemia
Platelet defects
Decreased white blood count

renal failure: (1) glomerulonephritis, (2) diabetes mellitus, and (3) primary hypertensive disease.[52]

***Pathophysiology.*** Glomerulonephritis is initiated in various ways but is characterized as an *immune complex disorder*. Little is known about the initiation of the immune response in glomerulonephritis. However, it is known that certain antigens specific to glomerular tissue are circulated to the glomeruli and, in turn, initiate an inflammatory response in the glomerular basement membrane. The antigens may work to decrease antiglomerular basement antibodies, rendering the glomerulus vulnerable to invasion by infectious agents.[54]

As the glomeruli are damaged and the GFR decreases as a result of sclerosis of the glomerular membrane, protein passes into the tubular filtrate and is eventually excreted in the urine. Sodium and water retention occur, in part because of the body's response in an attempt to alleviate the hypovolemia that results from the protein loss. Interstitial edema develops as a result of decreased protein in the vascular space.[54]

Hypertensive kidney damage can be the sole cause of renal failure or can occur secondary to another disease such as diabetes mellitus. In the hypertensive state, the increased vascular resistance of diseased vessels predisposes to high pressure entering the glomerulus and results in damage to the membrane. Hypertension causes glomerular and tubular problems through malfunction of the renin-angiotensin system. Ischemia and decreased blood volume stimulate the renin-angiotensin system to reabsorb water and sodium from the tubules in an effort to increase volume and thereby the GFR. This creates volume overload, which scleroses the glomeruli by producing a higher vascular pressure. The resulting sclerosis destroys the ability of the glomerular membrane to filter selectively and often reduces available filtrate, leading to eventual necrosis of the tubular structures.[51]

Diabetes mellitus does not directly attack the nephron itself but mediates the damage through thickening arterial walls and eventual thickening of the glomerular basement membrane from the resultant high pressure.[51] Diabetic damage often results not only in renal failure, but in blindness (retinal damage) and cardiac failure because of major blood vessel involvement.

***Assessment and diagnosis.*** The patient assessment for chronic renal failure involves evaluation for many of the same signs and symptoms that occur in patients with acute renal failure (see the box, "Manifestations of Chronic Renal Failure"). However, the progression of chronic renal failure differs from acute renal failure and is characterized by three phases.

The first phase, *diminished renal reserve,* involves the appearance of protein in the urine and elevations of the blood pressure. Mild elevations in BUN and creatinine levels may also be observed. However, for the most part, with fluid and sodium restrictions, the remaining regulatory functions continue within normal limits.[51]

### SIGNS AND SYMPTOMS OF END-STAGE RENAL DISEASE (UREMIC SYNDROME)

- "Restless legs" and burning sensation of soles of feet
- Apathy
- Confusion
- Stupor
- Flapping tremor of hands (asterixis)
- Insomnia
- Anorexia
- Nausea and vomiting
- Uremic fetor (breath odor)
- Melena
- Dyspnea
- Crackles on auscultation of lungs
- Cardiac dysrhythmias
- Pericardial rub on auscultation
- Additional heart sounds (fluid overload)
- Cardiomegaly
- Edema (dependent areas)
- Poor skin turgor (generalized)
- Pruritis
- Brittle nails and hair
- Anemia (normocytic, normochromic)
- Easy bruising
- Bleeding (gums, nose, GI tract)
- Oliguria or anuria

*Renal insufficiency,* the second phase, is a worsening of kidney function characterized by increases in serum BUN and creatinine levels, mild elevation of the potassium level, impaired concentrating ability, and anemia.

The third phase, *end-stage renal disease,* is often characterized by a set of signs and symptoms known as **uremic syndrome.** At the point end-stage renal disease is reached, the GFR is usually less than 6 ml/min.[12] The signs and symptoms of end-stage renal disease result from the severely elevated BUN, creatinine, potassium, and phosphate levels, as well as the decreased sodium, calcium, Hb, and Hct levels, and fluid retention.[11] (See the box, "Signs and Symptoms of End-Stage Renal Disease.")

***Treatment.*** Medical and nursing treatment of end-stage renal disease are aimed at preserving as much kidney function as possible, correcting fluid and electrolyte imbalances, correcting problems with the body's organ systems, postponing or eliminating the need for dialysis or transplantation, and providing the patient with the knowledge and support that will enhance the quality of life while coping with the disease.

Correcting fluid and electrolyte problems is of prime concern in treating patients with renal failure. Fluid overload is frequently present, and fluid excess can be removed through hemodialysis or peritoneal dialysis. Fluid and sodium restrictions help control fluid overload. The patient is usually restricted to 1000 to 1500 ml/24 hours of fluid intake, depending on current urinary output.[26] On occasion, patients will experience *nocturnal dehydration,* which can be eliminated by spreading the allotted fluid over the 24-hour period.

Hypertension and congestive heart failure are controlled by providing medications that increase cardiac output and lower blood pressure, allowing less cardiac strain and reducing the risk of hypertensive damage to the remaining nephrons.

Normalizing serum electrolytes is often difficult in patients with renal failure. Elevations in potassium may require emergent dialysis or simple alteration in dietary restriction of potassium. Calcium and phosphorous regulation becomes "tricky," depending on the role PTH is playing in maintaining the calcium levels. Phosphorous binders, calcium supplements, and calcium absorption stimulators (calcitriol) are used to normalize calcium and phosphorus. Sodium is usually controlled with a 2-gm sodium (no added salt) dietary restriction.[29]

In the past, androgens were used to stimulate RBC production in the patient with CRF. Recently, recombinant DNA technology has made it possible to synthesize erythropoietin (epoietin alfa). Similar to erythropoietin, epoietin alfa stimulates RBC production, but with fewer side effects. Hematocrit levels usually rise within 2 weeks, with levels of 30% to 33% as a goal.[41]

Care of the patient receiving epoietin alfa involves monitoring the levels of serum iron, ferritin, total iron-binding capacity (TIBC), hemoglobin, hematocrit, and reticulocytes. The patient must typically ingest iron, B vitamins, and folic acid to support RBC maturation. Blood pressures may rise due to increased vascular volume, and vascular access clotting may result from increased blood viscosity.[7]

Transfusions are used as a last resort to provide additional RBCs. Multiple transfusions can further depress bone marrow function and are associated with risks such as hepatitis B and acquired immunodeficiency syndrome. Packed RBCs are given to limit the fluid load of whole blood. "Washed" cells, which limit cytotoxic antibody formation, may be given to those patients seeking transplant.[6]

***Summary of nursing care.*** The nursing care for the patient with chronic renal failure is multifaceted. The key to understanding much of the care for this patient is in understanding the following treatments: hemodialysis, peritoneal dialysis, and kidney transplantation. The treatments and their possible associated complications require intense observation and careful management by the nurse.

First, the nurse must be aware of the fluid and electrolyte balances associated with chronic renal failure. Assessment for fluid overload and the signs and symptoms of hyperkalemia remain foremost on the list of nursing care. Daily weights, intake and output measurements, auscultation of the lungs, and assessment of the skin for edema provide a general picture of the fluid status of the patient. In addition, an important part of the nurse's care centers on patient teaching about adherence to fluid and dietary restrictions and the consequences of nonadherence. Nursing diagnoses and management of chronic renal failure are summarized in the box below.

The nurse frequently collaborates with the physician and dietician in maintaining the nutritional intake of the patient with chronic renal failure. The nurse can aid the patient in

**Nursing Diagnosis and Management**

***Chronic renal failure***

- High Risk for Fluid Volume Excess risk factor: renal failure, p. 496
- High Risk for Infection risk factors: protein-calorie malnourishment, invasive monitoring devices, p. 465
- High Risk for Impaired Skin Integrity risk factors: reduced mobility, poor subcutaneous tissue support (peripheral and sacral edema), uremic pruritis, steroid therapy, p. 499
- Activity Intolerance related to postural hypotension secondary to prolonged immobility, p. 463
- Ineffective Individual Coping related to situational crisis and personal vulnerability, p. 447
- Anxiety related to threatened biological, psychological, and/or social integrity, p. 448
- Body Image Disturbance related to functional dependence on life-sustaining technology and/or actual change in body structure, function, and appearance, p. 443
- Knowledge Deficit: Dialysis Routine, Fluid Restrictions, Medications, Fluid and Dietary Restrictions, Vascular Access Assessment and Care, Reportable Symptoms related to lack of previous exposure to information, p. 441
- Sensory/Perceptual Alterations related to sensory overload, sensory deprivation, and sleep pattern disturbance, p. 489
- Self-Esteem Disturbance related to feelings of guilt over physical deterioration, p. 443
- Altered Role Performance related to physical incapacity to resume usual or valued role, p. 444
- Powerlessness related to health care environment or illness-related regimen and/or physical deterioration despite compliance, p. 445
- Hopelessness related to perceptions of failing or deteriorating physical condition, p. 446
- Altered Health Maintenance related to lack of perceived threat to health, p. 439
- Noncompliance: Self-Care Routine related to lack of resources, p. 440

complying with dietary restrictions and in gaining the needed nutrition by obtaining dietary histories from the patient, determining the patient's desires for ethnic choices in the diet, and assessing areas of patient difficulty in compliance with restrictions. In addition, the nurse can reinforce the teaching of the dietician with explanations about the need for adequate nutrition and the consequences of insufficient intake.

The patient with chronic renal failure often copes with pruritis, brittle hair, and skin color changes (pallor, uremic bronzing). The nurse should not only provide skin care, but should teach the individual to provide self-care on a consistent basis. Teaching the patient the reasons behind development of skin-care problems may provide the impetus for the patient to adhere to the medication and dietary regimen that helps eliminate the problems.

Fatigue and activity intolerance are often voiced as among the most frustrating of complications for the individual with chronic renal failure. Although the usual cause of the fatigue is anemia, fluid overload or secondary cardiac complications can also contribute to the problem. The nurse should monitor Hb and Hct levels for any sudden changes. Patient teaching should include explanations about renal anemia, fluid overload, and cardiac disease and their relationship to fatigue. A discussion with the patient and family about an activity and exercise schedule that allows frequent rest may help alleviate the patient's frustration.

Teaching the patient about the various medications prescribed to control chronic renal failure's complications can be a challenging aspect of nursing care. Of particular importance is the nurse's care in instructing the patient in the avoidance of overmedication and the use of over-the-counter preparations that might create further complications (for example, kaolin and pectin [Kaopectate], magnesium antacids, and phosphate laxatives).

Finally, as with acute renal failure, focusing attention on the emotional needs of the patient and family coping with chronic renal failure is important. The nurse must be aware that the patient often responds to chronic disease by passing through stages of coping much like those of the grief process. The nursing care involved in providing emotional support should include the following: (1) emphasizing listening to the patient's frustrations, needs, and fears, (2) emphasizing to the patient and family the normalcy of the emotional response to chronic renal failure, (3) providing an avenue for the patient and family to seek professional counseling, (4) suggesting support groups that consider problems of those coping with renal failure, and (5) encouraging the patient and family to take active roles in the treatment process.

## THERAPEUTIC MANAGEMENT

### Hemodialysis

Although other methods of dialysis treatment for chronic renal failure have become more sophisticated, hemodialysis remains the treatment most widely used. The wide availability of hemodialysis equipment and the ability to use it rapidly during emergencies predisposes physicians to the selection of hemodialysis as the primary mode of treatment.

Hemodialysis roughly translates as "separating from the blood."[23] As a treatment, hemodialysis literally separates and removes from the blood the excess electrolytes, fluids, and toxins. Although efficient in regulating chemicals, it does not remove all metabolites. Furthermore, electrolytes, toxins, and fluids increase between treatments, requiring performance of dialysis on a regular basis.

The treatment works by circulating blood outside the body through synthetic tubing to a *dialyzer*, which consists of several membrane pockets (flat-plate type) or tubes (hollow-fiber type). While the blood flows through the membranes, which are semipermeable, a fluid known as the dialysate bath bathes the membranes and, through osmosis and diffusion, performs exchanges of fluid, electrolytes, and toxins from the blood to the bath. The blood and bath are shunted in opposite directions (countercurrent flow) through the dialyzer to maintain the osmotic and chemical gradients at their highest.

To remove fluid, a positive hydrostatic pressure is applied to the blood, and a negative hydrostatic pressure is applied to the dialysate bath. Heparin is added to the system just before the blood enters the dialyzer. Without the heparin, the blood would clot since its presence outside the body and its passage through foreign substances initiate the clotting mechanism. Heparin can be administered by bolus injection or intermittent infusion.[61]

After leaving the dialyzer, the blood continues through synthetic tubing and is returned to the body. Since the systemic blood pressure is not sufficient to propel the blood through this *extracorporeal* (outside the vessels) circuit, a pump is used to provide a consistent flow of blood (200 to 400 ml/minute) through the system. Various monitoring devices prevent blood loss, air embolus, access collapse, or high pressure destruction of the dialyzer or access.

The dialysate bath is composed of electrolytes, blood buffers, and water in quantities that create a diffusion gradient across the membranes. For instance, the potassium content may be 2.0 mEq/L in the dialysate to enhance diffusion from the hyperkalemic blood of the renal patient to the dialysate. Calcium absorption is also enhanced by this process. Higher amounts of ionized calcium are placed in the dialysate than are present in the patient's serum. The calcium travels from the dialysate to the patient's vascular space, thereby enhancing calcium stores.

Tap water is not safe for use in dialysis; the prevalence of calcium, magnesium, organic and inorganic matter, bacteria, and chloramines in tap water can jeopardize effective dialysis. Therefore purification methods must be undertaken to remove these materials, as well as salts contained in the tap water. Distillation, reverse osmosis purification, and carbon filtering are currently used as methods for obtaining safe water for use in the dialysis treatment.[18]

**Vascular access for hemodialysis.** Hemodialysis can

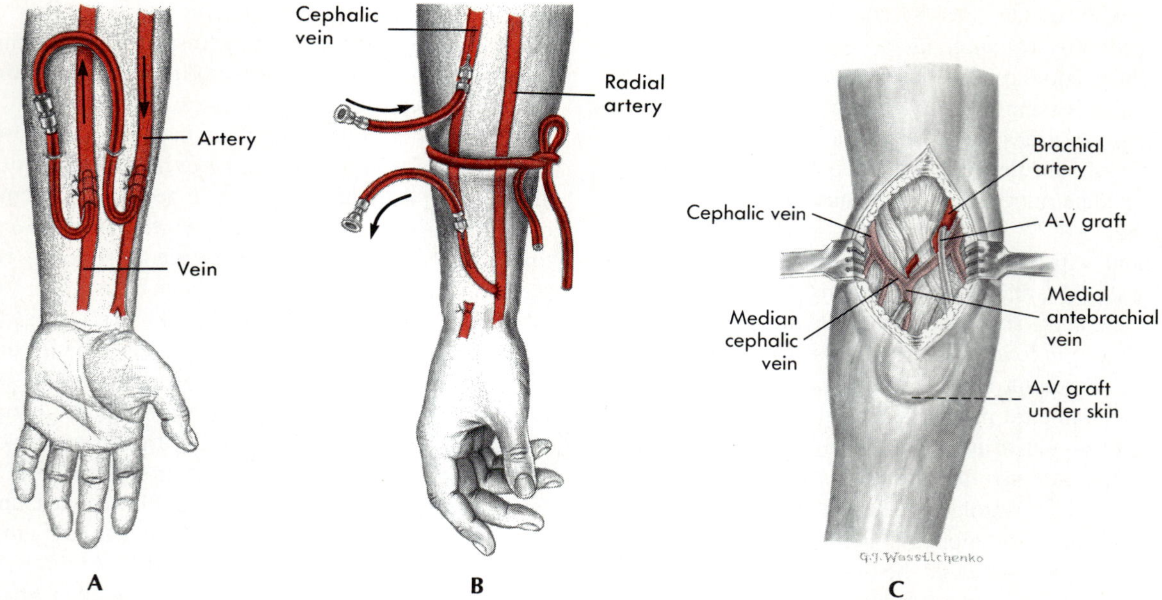


***Fig. 17-1*** Circulatory access for hemodialysis. **A,** External (temporary) arteriovenous cannula (shunt). **B,** Internal (permanent) arteriovenous fistula. **C,** Internal (permanent) arteriovenous graft. (**A** and **B** from Thompson JM and others: Mosby's manual of clinical nursing, ed 2, St Louis, 1989, Mosby–Year Book, Inc.)

only be performed by obtaining access to the bloodstream. Over many years, various types of accesses such as arteriovenous (A-V) fistulas, A-V shunts, A-V grafts, and femoral and subclavian catheters have been created. The common denominator in most accesses is access to the arterial circulation and return to the venous circulation; femoral and subclavian catheters access the venous circulation only.

It is essential for the nurse to become familiar with each type of access, the potential problems that each can develop, and the nursing interventions each requires. The dialysis patient is often taught that the access is a "lifeline," so care on the part of patient and nurse can prevent complications.

***A-V shunt.*** An A-V shunt is seldom used today as a result of the advent of subclavian and femoral catheters. However, if the temporary catheters cannot be used, access can rapidly be obtained through an A-V shunt. The shunt consists of Teflon vessel tips, Silastic tubing, and a connection joint for creating the circuit between the arterial and venous tubing[33] (Fig. 17-1, *A*). The shunt requires a peripheral artery, usually radial or ulnar, and a peripheral vein such as the cephalic or basilic. A cutdown is performed on each vessel, with the vessel tips inserted and sutured in place. Tubing extends from each vessel tip (outside the body) and is connected, when not being used for dialysis, by a straight connector or a heparin-T device. Blood flows in a U-shaped fashion from artery to vein. Shunts may also be inserted in the thigh or ankle areas. Complications common to A-V shunts are thrombosis, infection, and skin erosion. Nursing care considerations for A-V shunts are listed in Table 17-4.

***A-V fistula.*** The **A-V fistula** is created by surgically visualizing a peripheral artery and vein, creating an opening in the artery and the vein, and anastomosing the two open areas. Anastomoses may be side-to-side, end-to-side, or end-to-end. The high arterial flow creates swelling of the vein, or a *pseudoaneurysm,* at which point (when healed) a large-bore needle can be inserted to obtain outflow. Inflow is accomplished through a second large-bore needle inserted into a peripheral vein distal to the fistula (Fig. 17-1, *B*).

Fistulas are the preferred mode of access if the vessels are of quality because of the durability of the individual's own vessels and the relatively few complications in comparison with the other accesses. However, development of sufficient flow to the fistula may require weeks to months. Attempting to obtain flow from the underdeveloped fistulas often causes painful vascular spasm and reduced flow. In addition, internal accesses have the potential for creating arterial insufficiency because of the high arterial blood flow diverted for dialysis purposes. The arterial insufficiency produces a set of symptoms known as *vascular steal syndrome* (pale, cold distal extremity with severe spasmodic pain). Additional complications such as thrombosis, infection (low rate), or venous hypertension can occur with A-V fistulas.[10] The care of the fistula and nursing considerations are listed in Table 17-5.

***A-V grafts.*** Currently, A-V grafts are, by far, the most frequently used access for treating chronic renal failure. Synthetic materials such as Goretex or biological materials such as human umbilical veins provide a wide range of lumen sizes and graft lengths. The graft is a tube formed

***Table 17-4*** Care of the A-V shunt

| Complications | Nursing Care |
|---|---|
| Clotting<br>Dislodgment<br>Skin erosion<br>Infection<br>Bleeding | 1. Monitor for signs and symptoms of infection.<br>2. Monitor for signs and symptoms of thrombosis (darkening of blood, separation of serum or cellular compartment blood in tubing, decreased temperature of tubing).<br>3. Assess insertion site daily for erosion around insertion sites.<br>4. Use strict aseptic technique during dressing changes at insertion sites.<br>5. Teach patient to avoid sleeping on or prolonged bending of accessed limb.<br>6. Keep two shunt clamps attached to patient's clothing or access dressing at all times. |

***Table 17-5*** Care of the A-V fistula

| Complications | Nursing care |
|---|---|
| Thrombosis<br>Infection<br>Pseudoaneurysm<br>Vascular steal syndrome<br>Venous hypertension<br>Carpal tunnel syndrome<br>Inadequate blood flow | 1. Teach patient to avoid wearing constrictive clothing on limb containing access.<br>2. Teach patient to avoid sleeping on or prolonged bending of accessed limb.<br>3. Use aseptic technique when cannulating access.<br>4. Avoid repetitious cannulation of one segment of access.<br>5. Offer comfort measures such as warm compresses or ordered analgesics to lessen pain of vascular steal.<br>6. Teach patient to develop the blood flow in the fistulas through exercises (squeezing a rubber ball) while applying mild impedance to flow just distal to the access (at least once per day for 10 to 15 minutes). |

of the desired material (usually Goretex), which is surgically implanted in the limb. The area is surgically opened, and an artery and vein are located. A tunnel is created (either straight or U-shaped) in the tissue in which the graft is placed. Anastamoses are made with the graft ends connected to the artery and vein. The blood is allowed to flow through the graft, and the surgical area is closed. The graft creates a raised area (looking like a vein) just under the skin and peripheral tissue layers (Figure 17-1, *C*). Two large-bore needles are used for outflow and inflow to the graft. For both grafts and fistulas after needle removal at the end of the hemodialysis treatment, pressure must be applied to stem bleeding. Nursing care for and complications of the A-V graft are listed in Table 17-6.

***Subclavian and femoral vein catheters.*** Sublcavian and femoral vein catheters are used most often in cases of acute renal failure when short-term access is required or when vascular access is nonfunctional in a patient requiring immediate hemodialysis.[61] Both subclavian and femoral catheters can be inserted at the bedside.

Femoral catheters may be single lumen, requiring insertion of two catheters into the same vessel, with the outflow catheter placed distal to the inflow catheter.[33] The subclavian catheter, however, usually has two lumens with a central partition running the length of the catheter. The outflow catheter pulls the blood flow through openings that are proximal to the inflow openings on the opposite side. This design avoids dialyzing the same blood just returned to the area (recirculation), which can severely reduce dialysis' efficiency.

### Peritoneal Dialysis

Peritoneal dialysis has existed as a treatment for renal failure approximately 20 years longer than hemodialysis. Because of problems with equipment, technique, and practical, long-term application, peritoneal dialysis was used for cases of acute renal failure only when hemodialysis was not possible. However, in 1978 peritoneal dialysis for chronic renal failure was successfully established.

Peritoneal dialysis involves the introduction of sterile dialyzing fluid through an implanted catheter into the abdominal cavity. The dialysate bathes the peritoneal membrane,

***Table 17-6*** Care of the A-V graft

| Complications | Nursing care |
|---|---|
| Bleeding<br>Thrombosis<br>False aneurysm formation<br>Infection<br>Arterial or venous stenosis<br>Vascular steal syndrome | 1. Avoid too early cannulation of new access.<br>2. Teach patient to avoid wearing constrictive clothing on accessed limb.<br>3. Avoid repeated cannulation of one segment of access.<br>4. Use aseptic technique when cannulating access.<br>5. Monitor for changes in arterial or venous pressure while patient is on dialysis.<br>6. Provide comfort measures to reduce pain of vascular steal (e.g., warm compresses, analgesics as ordered). |

**Table 17-7** Peritoneal dialysate solutions and fluid removal characteristics

| Standard solution* | | Solution type | Fluid removal characteristics: Acute PD (1-hr dwell time) | CAPD (4-hr dwell time) |
|---|---|---|---|---|
| Sodium | 132 mEq/L | 1.5% | 50-100 ml | −40-600 ml |
| Calcium | 3.5 mEq/L | 2.5% | 100-200 ml | 200-300 ml |
| Magnesium | 1.5 mEq/L | 4.25% | 300-400 ml | 150-1100 ml |
| Chloride | 102 mEq/L | | | |
| Lactate | 35 mEq/L | | | |

Modified from Schoenfeld P: Care of the patient on peritoneal dialysis. In Cogan M and Garavoy M, editors: Introduction to dialysis, New York, 1985, Churchill Livingstone, Inc.

*Available in 1.5, 2.5, 4.25% dextrose concentrations. For continuous ambulatory peritoneal dialysis (CAPD), bags are sterile, prepackaged, and premixed (250 ml to 3L sizes). For acute peritoneal dialysis (PD), sterile bottles of solution are premixed.

which covers the abdominal organs and overlies the capillary beds supporting the organs. By the processes of osmosis, diffusion, and active transport, excess fluid and solutes travel from the peritoneal capillary fluid through the capillary walls, through the peritoneal membrane, and into the dialyzing fluid. After a selected time period, the fluid is drained out of the abdomen by gravity. The process is then repeated.

The volume of dialysate instilled into the abdomen affects the clearance. Research has shown that during acute peritoneal dialysis, 3.5 L/hour will provide a urea clearance of 26 ml/minute.[53] During chronic continuous peritoneal dialysis, 2-L exchanges every 4 hours provide a clearance of 7 ml/minute.[53] The dialysate should be instilled at body temperature for comfort and to provide some vasodilation and increased solute transport in the peritoneum.

The length of time the solution remains in the peritoneal cavity (dwell time) and the solution composition affect the outcome. The dwell time affects the amount of fluid removed from the peritoneal capillaries, although a longer dwell time will not remove proportionately more fluid because of osmotic equilibration across the membranes.[42] The various glucose concentrations of the dialysate provide for different rates of fluid removal. Dialysate solution and fluid removal characteristics are listed in Table 17-7.

**Catheters.** Peritoneal access has changed dramatically over a period of years from the straight, rigid catheters used in acute peritoneal dialysis to the highly sophisticated permanent peritoneal catheters used at present for chronic peritoneal dialysis. All the catheters require surgical implantation; their purpose is delivery to and drainage from the peritoneal cavity. Most catheters have an external segment, a tunnel segment passing through subcutaneous tissue and muscle, a cuff for stabilization at the peritoneal membrane, and an internal segment with numerous holes to quickly deliver and drain dialysate (Fig. 17-2).

**Complications.** Complications of peritoneal dialysis can be numerous. However, with the exception of peritonitis, the complications from peritoneal dialysis are less severe than those associated with hemodialysis. The complications and nursing care related to peritoneal dialysis are listed in Table 17-8.

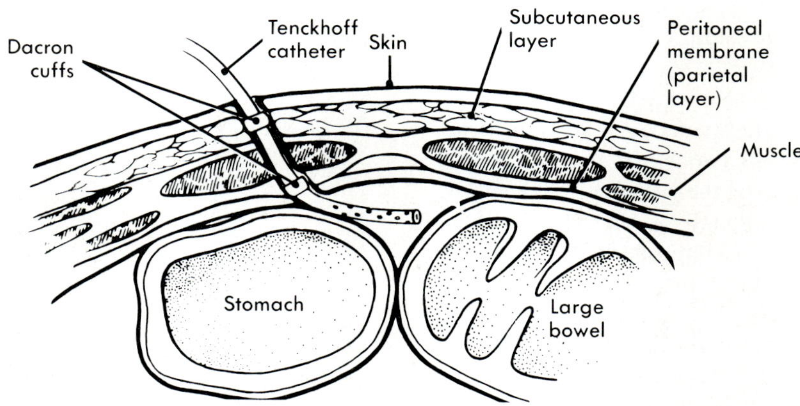


*Fig. 17-2* Peritoneal catheter. (From Lewis S and Collier I: Medical-surgical nursing, ed 3, St Louis, 1992, Mosby–Year Book, Inc.)

***Table 17-8*** Complications of peritoneal dialysis

| Complications | Nursing care |
|---|---|
| Peritonitis | Assess for signs and symptoms: cloudy effluent, abdominal pain, rebound tenderness, nausea and vomiting, and fever.<br>Obtain effluent sample for culture.<br>Administer antibiotics as ordered.<br>Teach patient and family signs and symptoms and their prevention. |
| Exit site infection | Monitor site daily for signs and symptoms of infection: enduration, erythema, purulence, and hyperthermia.<br>Increase daily cleaning of site.<br>Apply topical antibiotics as ordered (this is a controversial practice).<br>Teach patient and family to avoid items such as creams and lotions around exit site. |
| Catheter tunnel infection | Assess for signs and symptoms of infection: pain along tunnel, enduration for several centimeters away from catheter, erythema leading away from the exit site, and drainage at exit site or as tunnel is "milked" toward exit site.<br>Teach patient and family signs and symptoms of infection.<br>Teach patient and family to avoid pulls or tugs on the catheter or trauma to the exit site.<br>Emphasize the need to maintain cleansing regimen at exit site. |
| Fluid obstruction | Change position of the patient (i.e., standing, lying, side-lying, knee-chest).<br>Relieve patient's constipation.<br>Irrigate the catheter.<br>Ensure sufficient fluid is in abdomen (sometimes requires a residual reservoir of approximately 50 ml). |
| Rectal pain | Ensure a sufficient reservoir of fluid.<br>Use slow infusion rate. |
| Shoulder pain | Ensure that all air is primed from infusion tubing.<br>Attempt draining the effluent with the patient in knee-chest position.<br>Administer mild analgesics as ordered. |
| Hernias | Monitor for increase in size of or pain in area of hernia.<br>Decrease volume of exchanges as ordered.<br>Dialyze with the patient in the supine position.<br>Use abdominal binder or support for the patient (as long as not binding on catheter exit site).<br>Avoid initiation of peritoneal dialysis until exit site healing has taken place (approximately 1 to 2 weeks if possible). |
| Fluid overload | Increase use of hypertonic solutions.<br>Decrease by mouth (PO) fluid intake.<br>Shorten dwell times.<br>Weigh patient frequently.<br>Monitor lung sounds and peripheral edema. |
| Dehydration | Assess patient for decreased skin turgor, muscle cramps, hypotension, tachycardia, and dizziness.<br>Discontinue hypertonic solutions.<br>Increase PO fluid intake.<br>Lengthen dwell times. |
| Blood-tinged effluent | Monitor for change in effluent color (clear yellow to pink or rusty).<br>Administer heparin, as ordered, to avoid fibrin formation.<br>Obtain patient history about catheter trauma and patient activity before appearance of complication. |

### Continuous Arteriovenous Hemofiltration

**Continuous arteriovenous hemofiltration (CAVH)** was developed in the late 1970s as an alternative to hemodialysis for treatment of certain cases of acute renal failure. It accomplishes the water and solute removal needed in the acutely ill patient while providing the advantage of decreased stress on the cardiovascular system. Additionally, continuous arteriovenous hemofiltration does not require dialysate or the technical equipment necessary for dialysis. It works by using simple convection, and it provides continuous dialysis.[69] Continuous arteriovenous hemofiltration is usually used on patients with acute renal failure and hy-

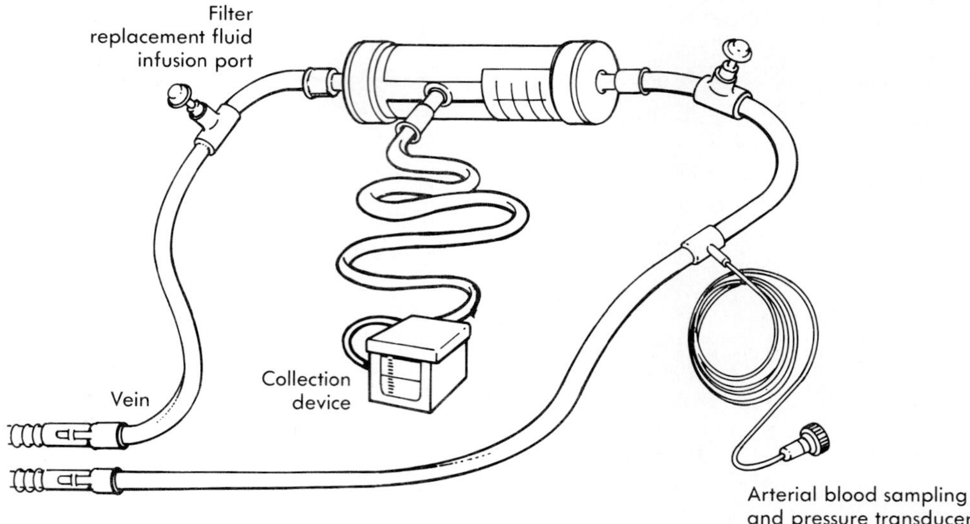


*Fig. 17-3* Continuous arteriovenous hemofiltration circuit.

pervolemia who cannot tolerate the cardiovascular instability associated with hemodialysis.[13,32,47]

In the early 1980s, continuous arteriovenous hemodialysis (CAVHD) was introduced as a modification of CAVH. The CAVHD process includes the delivery of low-flow dialysate in a countercurrent direction to the blood flow. The system components of CAVH and CAVHD are similiar, with the addition of a pump to deliver dialysate in CAVHD. Nursing care in both procedures focuses on maintaining hemodynamic stability, electrolyte balance, and system patency.[39]

At the vascular access (frequently a temporary femoral catheter), tubing is attached, allowing blood flow to the hemofilter (Fig. 17-3). An arterial sampling port and a heparin infusion line are present before the hemofilter is reached. The hemofilter is constructed like the hollow-fiber dialyzer used for hemodialysis except for having a single outflow port for filtrate and no dialysate ports. The blood enters and exits the hemofilter, with the filtrate flowing from the outflow port into the collection device. After exiting the hemofilter, the blood passes through tubing containing the intravenous replacement port and travels back to the vein. The blood is propelled by the systemic blood pressure.[48] A mean arterial pressure of 60 mm Hg is required for continuous arteriovenous hemofiltration to function.[69]

Hemofilters are designed to clear solutes and unbound molecules of 500 to 10,000 daltons. Typical hemodialysis can only clear particles of up to 5000 daltons.[23] Therefore the hemofilter clears many drugs that dialysis cannot remove, along with large amounts of fluids that cannot be removed in as great a quantity through hemodialysis. It has been reported that as much as 14 L of fluid can be removed through the hemofilter in a 24-hour period.[10] Significant fluid removal alone can be accomplished by simply allowing the blood pressure to push the blood continuously through the circuit.[48] A screw clamp applied to the ultrafiltrate port controls the fluid removal.[47]

Anticoagulation is important, since blood is traveling through an extracorporeal circuit. Commonly, a 20-units/kg dose of heparin is given before initiation of the continuous arteriovenous hemofiltration. Thereafter, 500 units per hour are infused throughout the treatment.[47] Clotting times are frequently determined to monitor anticoagulation.

Nursing care is multifaceted for the patient receiving continuous arteriovenous hemofiltration treatment and is summarized in Table 17-9.

### Renal Transplantation

Renal transplantation is another form of treatment for chronic renal failure. Recent developments in the area of immunosuppression have made this treatment a less risky option.[24] However, the posttransplant lifestyle requires ongoing medication and dietary regimens that may burden the individual with lifestyle limitations. Therefore careful pretransplant evaluation and teaching are necessary to provide a greater chance of long-term success. The nurse is instrumental in educating the patient and family, meeting care needs, and monitoring progress of the individual with a renal transplant.

The presurgical preparation involves a thorough medical examination and a psychological and socioeconomic evaluation. The risks of transplantation and the potential complications must be thoroughly discussed with the patient and family. Before the actual surgery, a hemodialysis treatment may be performed to achieve acceptable fluid and electrolyte levels and to keep uremic toxins at low levels.

**Immunosuppression.** A series of *tissue-matching* tests must be performed to prevent, as much as possible, rejection of the foreign kidney. Even though tissue-matching tests are

***Table 17-9*** Nursing care during continuous arteriovenous hemofiltration

| Complications | Nursing care |
|---|---|
| Fluid and electrolyte changes | Observe for changes in central venous pressure or pulmonary capillary wedge pressure.<br>Observe for changes in vital signs.<br>Observe electrocardiogram for changes as result of electrolyte abnormalities.<br>Monitor output values every hour.<br>Control ultrafiltration. |
| Clotting of hemofilter and circuit | Observe filter and lines once every hour for signs of clotting (dark spots).<br>Monitor blood pressure for decreased flow through filter. |
| Bleeding | Monitor accelerated clotting time (ACT) no less than once every hour.<br>Adjust heparin dose within specifications to maintain ACT.<br>Observe dressing on vascular access for blood loss.<br>Observe for blood in filtrate (filter leak). |
| Access dislodgment or infection | Observe access site at least once every 2 to 4 hours.<br>Ensure that clamps are available within easy reach at all times.<br>Observe strict sterile technique when dressing vascular access. |

performed, immunosuppression is still required after surgery. Other tests performed before renal transplant are listed in Table 17-10.

Immunosuppressive therapy includes a number of medications such as corticosteroids (prednisone), purine analogues (azathioprine), antilymphocyte globulin, and cyclosporine, which can be used in combination or supplemented with radiation to effect immunosuppression.

***Cyclosporine.*** Introduced in 1983 and a product of soil fungus, cyclosporine has become the leading immunosuppressant for use in all forms of organ transplantation. Despite its powerful immunosuppression capability, cyclosporine can induce nephrotoxicity, hepatotoxicity, hyperkalemia, and other life-threatening side effects, as well as several less threatening but annoying side effects. The acute side effects of cyclosporine are usually managed by switching the therapy to azathioprine.[3]

***Orthoclone.*** Orthoclone (OKT3) is a new immunosuppressant that acts to reverse cell-mediated rejection in renal transplant. Clinical trials have demonstrated a promising 94% to 95% success rate in reversal of rejection. However, several adverse reactions such as fever, nausea, vomiting, diarrhea, and pulmonary edema have been observed as early as 1 hour past administration of the first dose of OKT3.[44]

***Table 17-10*** Renal tissue-matching tests

| Test | Explanation |
|---|---|
| ABO compatibility | 1. Donor and recipient must have same blood type.<br>2. Compatibility is same as for blood transfusion crossmatching: O, universal donor; AB, universal recipient. |
| Histocompatibility (antigen matching) | 1. Genes determine antigen production and structure.<br>2. Antigens on the WBCs human leukocyte antigens (HLAs) are of concern in renal transplantation (matches may be achieved between donors and recipients).<br>3. Identification of the antigens, which occur in pairs (one inherited from each parent), determines the shared antigens between parents, siblings, and children and therefore determines success of crossmatching.<br>4. Test is performed on venous blood. |
| Tissue typing, lymphocytotoxicity | 1. Lymphocytes are separated and exposed to antisera with known antibodies.<br>2. Lysis of the lymphocytes indicates that the tissue *will not* match; thus a transplantation will not be successful. |
| Mixed lymphocyte culture (MLC) | 1. Test is performed only in cases of living, related donor transplants (because of lengthy processing time).<br>2. Lymphocytes of donors and recipients are combined and cultured in a medium.<br>3. Growth of cells indicates a successful crossmatch.<br>4. Lysis areas in culture indicate cell death and unsuccessful crossmatch. |
| WBC crossmatch | 1. Identifies antigens between WBCs (process similar to ABO crossmatch). |

**Rejection.** Rejection of the transplanted kidney can occur during the actual surgical implantation or months to years later. Rejection has been classified into three types: hyperacute, acute, and late. The types of rejection and characteristics of each are summarized in Table 17-11.

**Implantation.** The actual surgical implantation of the kidney occurs at the iliac fossa of the recipient (Fig. 17-4). This placement allows ease of attachment to the renal vessels and implantation of the ureter into the bladder. Before the transplant, care is taken to minimize all abnormalities and preexisting disturbances. For example, hypertension is carefully controlled through the use of medications. Gastroin-

**Table 17-11** Types of renal transplant rejection

| Type | Characteristics |
|---|---|
| Hyperacute | 1. It occurs promptly after transplant.<br>2. Condition is untreatable.<br>3. Occurrence is rare if careful pretransplant crossmatching is undertaken. |
| Acute | 1. It occurs 1 to 6 months after transplant.<br>2. Signs and symptoms are fever, graft tenderness, hypertension, increased creatinine levels, and decreased urinary output.<br>3. Condition may result from surgical complications (e.g., obstruction, thrombus, urological stenosis) or medical complications (e.g., acute tubular necrosis [ATN], hypovolemia, urinary tract infection).<br>4. Treatment is undertaken with steroids, antilymphocyte sera, graft irradiation, monoclonal antibodies. |
| Late | 1. Condition occurs 6 months to years after transplant.<br>2. It is a slow process, with signs and symptoms of fluid retention, hypertension, and steady rise in blood urea nitrogen and creatinine levels.<br>3. It may result from urinary tract infections, vascular complications of the graft, urinary tract obstruction, or a recurrence of the original renal disease.<br>4. Treatment usually is aimed at continuing immunosuppressive therapy and measures to support remaining renal function until patient requires dialysis. |

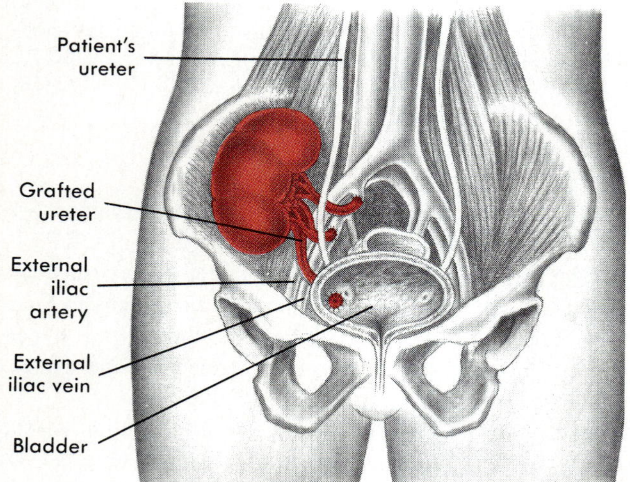


***Fig. 17-4*** Renal transplant. (From Thompson JM and others: Mosby's manual of clinical nursing, ed 2, St Louis, 1989, Mosby–Year Book, Inc.)

**Nursing Diagnosis and Management**

***Renal transplantation***

- High Risk for Infection risk factors: immunodeficiencies, invasive lines, p. 465
- High Risk for Fluid Volume Excess risk factor: renal failure, p. 496
- Sensory-Perceptual Alterations related to sensory overload, sensory deprivation, sleep pattern disturbance, p. 489
- Body Image Disturbance related to actual change in body structure, function, and/or appearance, p. 443
- Altered Health Maintenance related to lack of resources and/or lack of perceived threat to health, p. 439

testinal lesions may be treated by drugs or surgical intervention. Prophylactic antibiotic therapy may be initiated. Finally, dialysis is usually performed to remove excess fluid, electrolytes, and waste products to optimize the internal environment.[3]

**Donor preparation.** Careful preparation and care of the kidney donor must also be performed.[8,9] The living, related donor must undergo psychological, social, and physical evaluations, and these may prove to be extensive. However, the donor will be placed at no greater surgical risk than the recipient.

**Summary of nursing care.** Equally careful consideration must be given the cadaver donor and any of his or her family or significant others.[49] Foremost in the mind of the nurse must be the provision of compassionate care to the family. Ensuring that all criteria for donation have been met and obtaining informed consent are other important aspects of nursing care.

Nursing care for the individual considering or actually undergoing renal transplantation ranges from initial explanation of the pros and cons of the surgery to clinical follow-up of compliance to the posttransplant regimen and management of problems. Nursing care of the transplant recipient is directed toward the nursing diagnoses listed in the box above.

## SUMMARY

An overview of the available treatments for chronic renal failure provides the nurse with information with which to guide practice. The challenge to the nurse comes from the rapidity with which technology is altering the treatments described herein. However, the nurse is uniquely able to provide the teaching, intervention, and support that are often omitted in the technological realm.

**REFERENCES**


1. Adler S and Fraley DS: Acid-base regulations cellular and whole body. In Arieff AI and DeFronzo RA: Fluid, electrolyte and acid-base disorders, vol 1, New York, 1985, Churchill Livingstone, Inc.
2. Aluis R, Geheb M, and Cox M: Hypo- and hyperosmolar states: diagnostic approaches. In Arieff AI and DeFronzo RA: Fluid, electrolyte and acid-base disorders, vol 1, New York, 1985, Churchill Livingstone, Inc.
3. Amend JC and others: Immunosuppression following renal transplantation. In Garovoy MR and Guttmann RD: Renal transplantation, New York, 1986, Churchill Livingstone, Inc.
4. Appel GB and Stern L: Acute and chronic renal failure. In Askanazi J, Starker PM, and Weissman C: Fluid and electrolyte management in critical care, Boston, 1986, Butterworth & Co (Publishers), Ltd.
5. Baker W: Hypophosphatemia, Am J Nurs 22(4):999, 1985.
6. Bass: Common complications of immunosuppression in the renal transplant patient, ANNA J 13(4):196, 1986.
7. Binkley L and others: Epoetin alfa: a keystone in the treatment of the anemia of end stage renal disease, ANNA 16(5):341, 1989.
8. Bodenham A and Park GR: Care of the multiple organ donor, Intensive Care Med 15:340, 1989.
9. Brown M: Clinical management of the organ donor, Dimens Crit Care Nurs 8:134, 1989.
10. Butt MH: Vascular access for chronic hemodialysis. In Nissensen AR and Fine RN: Dialysis therapy, St Louis, 1986, Mosby–Year Book, Inc.
11. Carbone V and Bonato J: Nursing implications in the care of the chronic hemodialysis patient in the critical care setting, Heart Lung 14(6): 570, 1985.
12. Chambers JK: Fluid and electrolyte problems in renal and urologic disorders, Nurs Clin North Am 22(4):815, 1987.
13. Coloski D, Mastrianni J, and Brown L: Continuous arteriovenous hemofiltration patient: nursing care plan, Dimens Crit Care Nurs 9:130, 1990.
14. Commerford PJ and Lloyd EA: Arrhythmias in patients with drug toxicity, electrolyte, and endocrine disturbances, Med Clin North Am 68(5):1051, 1984.
15. Coward DD: Cancer-induced hypercalcemia, Cancer Nurs 9(3):125, 1986.
16. Desai TK, Carlson RW, and Geheb MA: Hypocalcemia and hypophosphatemia in acutely ill patients, Crit Care Clin 5(4):927, 1987.
17. Dickerson RN and Brown RO: Hypomagnesemia in hospitalized patients receiving nutritional support, Heart Lung 14(6):561, 1985.
18. Easterling RE: Water treatment for in-center hemodialysis, including verification of water quality and disinfection. In Nissenson AR and Fine RN: Dialysis therapy, St Louis, 1986, Mosby–Year Book, Inc.
19. Feluer L and Pendarius J: Electrolyte imbalances: intraoperative risk factors, AORN J 49(4):992, 1989.
20. Flink EB: Magnesium deficiency, Hosp Pract 15:116I, 1987.
21. Forse RA: Sodium regulation. In Askanazi J, Starker PM, and Weissman C: Fluid and electrolyte management in critical care, Boston, 1986, Butterworth & Co (Publishers), Ltd.
22. Gotch FL and Keen M: Dialysis and delivery systems. In Cogan M and Garovoy M, editors: Introduction to dialysis, New York, 1985, Churchill Livingstone, Inc.
23. Gutch CF and Stoner MH: Review of hemodialysis for nurses and dialysis personnel, ed 4, St Louis, 1983, Mosby–Year Book, Inc.
24. Harasyko C: Kidney transplantation, Nurs Clin North Am 24:851, 1989.
25. Heitkemper M and Bond E: Fluid and electrolytes: assessment and interventions, J Enterostom Ther 15:18, 1988.
26. Hoffart N: Nutrition in renal failure, dialysis, and transplantation. In Core curriculum for nephrology nursing, Pitman, New Jersey, 1987, AJ Janetti, Inc.
27. Horwood CH and Cook CV: Cyclosporine in transplantation, Heart Lung 14(6):529, 1985.
28. Huerta BJ and Lemberg L: Potassium imbalance in the coronary care unit, Heart Lung 14(2):193, 1985.
29. Hui YH: Essentials of nutrition and diet therapy, Monterey, Calif, 1987, Wadsworth, Inc.
30. Jochimsen F and others: Impairment of renal function in medical intensive care: predictability of acute renal failure, Crit Care Med 18:480, 1990.
31. Johndrow PD and Thornton S: Syndrome of inappropriate antidiuretic hormone—a growing concern, Focus Crit Care 12(5):29, 1985.
32. Kaplow R and Bendo K: QA in continuous arteriovenous hemofiltration, Dimens Crit Care Nurs 8:170, 1989.
33. Krupski and others: Access for dialysis. In Cogan M and Garovoy M, editors: Introduction to dialysis, New York, 1985, Churchill Livingstone, Inc.
34. Kurokawa K and others: Physiology of phosphorus metabolism and pathophysiology of hypophosphatemia and hyperphosphatemia. In Arieff AI and DeFronzo RA: Fluid, electrolyte and acid-base disorders, vol 1, New York, 1985, Churchill Livingstone, Inc.
35. Lancaster LE: Anatomy and physiology for the renal system. In Core curriculum for nephrology nursing, Pitman, NJ, 1987, AJ Janetti, Inc.
36. Lancaster LE: Nursing process and care planning in nephrology nursing. In Core curriculum for nephrology nursing, NJ, 1987, AJ Janetti, Inc.
37. Laski ME and Kurtzman NA: Acid-base disturbances in pulmonary medicine. In Arieff AI and DeFronzo RA: Fluid, electrolyte and acid-base disorders, vol 1, New York, 1985, Churchill Livingstone, Inc.
38. Lau K: Magnesium metabolism: normal and abnormal. In Arieff AI and DeFronzo RA: Fluid, electrolyte and acid-base disorders, vol 1, New York, 1985, Churchill Livingstone, Inc.
39. Lawyer LA and Velasco A: Continuous arteriovenous hemodialysis in the ICU, Crit Care Nurs 9(1):19, 1989.
40. Levine MM and Kleeman CR: Hypercalcemia: pathophysiology and treatment, Hosp Pract 22(7):93, 1987.
41. Lundin AP: Epogen®: Combats the anemia of renal disease, Nephrol Nurs Update 1(6):1, 1989.
42. Manji N and others: Peritoneal dialysis for acute renal failure: overfeeding resulting from dextrose absorbed during dialysis, Crit Care Med 18:29, 1990.
43. Metheny NM: Fluid and electrolyte balance: nursing considerations, Philadelphia, 1987, JB Lippincott Co.
44. Moir EJ: Nursing care of patients receiving orthoclone OKT3, ANNA J 16(5):327, 1989.
45. Narins RG and others: Metabolic acid-base disorders: pathophysiology, classification, and treatment. In Arieff AI and DeFronzo RA: Fluid, electrolyte and acid-base disorders, vol 1, New York, 1985, Churchill Livingstone, Inc.
46. Norris MK: Acute tubular necrosis: preventing complications, Dimens Crit Care Nurs 8:16, 1989.
47. Palmer JC and others: Nursing management of CAVH for acute renal failure, Focus Crit Care 13(5):21, 1986.
48. Paradiso C: Hemofiltration: an alternative to dialysis, Heart Lung 18(3):11, 1989.
49. Peele A: The nurse's role in promoting rights of donor families, Nurs Clin North Am 24:939, 1989.
50. Plumer AL and Cosentino F: Principles and practice of intravenous therapy, Boston, 1987, Little, Brown & Co, Inc.
51. Richard CJ: Causes of renal failure, Core curriculum for nephrology nursing, Pitman, New Jersey, 1987, AJ Janetti, Inc.
52. Rubin RJ: Epidemiology of end stage renal disease and implications for public policy, Public Health Rep 99(5):492, 1984.
53. Schoenfeld P: Care of the patient on peritoneal dialysis. In Cogan M and Garovoy M, editors: Introduction to dialysis, New York, 1985, Churchill Livingstone, Inc.
54. Schrier R: Renal and electrolyte disorders, ed 3, Boston, 1986, Little, Brown & Co, Inc.
55. Schwartz MW: Potassium imbalances, Am J Nurs 87(10):1292, 1987.

56. Sillix DH and McDonald FD: Acute renal failure, Crit Care Clin 5(4):909, 1987.
57. Sondheimmer JH and Migdal SD: Toxic nephropathies, Crit Care Clin 5(4):883, 1987.
58. Spencer H and others: Calcium requirements in humans, Clin Orthop 184:270, 1984.
59. Stanaszek WF and Romankiewicz JA: Current approaches to management of potassium deficiency, Drug Intell Clin Pharm 19:176, 1985.
60. Starker PM and Gump FE: Gastrointestinal disorders. In Askanazi J, Starker PM, and Weissman C: Fluid and electrolyte management in critical care, Boston, 1986, Butterworth & Co (Publishers), Inc.
61. Taylor T: Preventing complications from hemodialysis, DCCN 9(4): 172, 1990.
62. Thompson JM and others: Mosby's manual of clinical nursing, ed 2, St Louis, 1989, Mosby–Year Book, Inc.
63. Tilney NL and Strom TB: Surgical aspects of kidney transplantation. In Garovoy MR and Guttmann RD: Renal transplantation, New York, 1986, Churchill Livingstone, Inc.
64. Tonnensen AS: Water balance and control of osmolality. In Askanazi J, Starker PM, and Weissman C: Fluid and electrolyte management in critical care, Boston, 1986, Butterworth & Co, Publishers, Inc.
65. Ulrick BT and Irwin BC: Renal transplantation. In Core curriculum for nephrology nursing, Pitman, NJ, 1987, AJ Janetti, Inc.
66. Valladares BK and Lemberg L: Catecholamines, potassium, and beta-blockade, Heart Lung 15(1):105, 1986.
67. Weisberg LS, Szerlip HM, and Cox M: Disorders of potassium homeostasis in critically ill patients, Crit Care Clin 5(4):835, 1987.
68. Whittaker AA: Acute renal dysfunction, Focus Crit Care 12(3):12, 1985.
69. Winkelman C: Hemofiltration: a new technique in critical care nursing, Heart Lung 14(3):265, 1985.
70. Zaloga GP and Chernow B: Hypocalcemia in critical illness, JAMA 256(4):1924, 1986.
71. Zappacosta AR and Perras ST: Continuous ambulatory peritoneal dialysis, Philadelphia, 1984, JB Lippincott Co.
72. Zucker AR and Chernow B: Diabetes insipidus and SIADH, Crit Care Q 6(3):63, 1983.

UNIT VII

# GASTROINTESTINAL ALTERATIONS

CHAPTER 18

# Gastrointestinal Assessment and Diagnostic Procedures

## CHAPTER OBJECTIVES

- *Perform a thorough nursing assessment of the gastrointestinal system on a critically ill patient and interpret the results.*
- *Outline the impact surgery has on a critically ill patient's nutritional status.*
- *Detail the relevant nursing care before, during, and after liver biopsy.*
- *List important diagnostic procedures for detection of large bowel disorders.*

## KEY TERMS

liver biopsy, p. 359
liver-spleen scan, p. 360
endoscopy, p. 360
fistulogram, p. 361

## CLINICAL ASSESSMENT

### History

There are two specific considerations in obtaining and using the history and results of the physical examination of the patient with an alteration in the gastrointestinal (GI) system. First, because alterations in nutritional status can be either causative or resultant, an accurate nutritional assessment should be incorporated into the assessment process to provide better patient care. Second, as the population grows increasingly older, the percent of elderly patients admitted to critical care units is increasing, having implications for this area of nursing practice.

Patients with suspected or confirmed GI disorders should have their health history reviewed for the following:

1. Past health history, including any previous surgery (Table 18-1), diseases (Table 18-2), or hospitalizations

***Table 18-1*** Surgical impact on nutritional status

| Organ(s) resected | Nutritional implications |
|---|---|
| Oropharynx | Tube dependency (loss of gastrointestinal access) |
| Esophagus | Malabsorption of fat, loss of normal swallowing function, decreased motility, obstruction |
| Stomach | Dumping syndrome, anemia, delayed emptying, malabsorption |
| Pancreas | Exocrine and/or endocrine insufficiency |
| Small bowel | Steatorrhea, bile acid depletion, fat malabsorption, anemia ($B_{12}$ malabsorption), short gut syndrome |

Modified from Knox LS: Nurs Clin North Am 18(1):103, 1983.

***Table 18-2*** Gastrointestinal disorders associated with micronutrient disorders

| Disease state or historical feature | Associated deficiency |
|---|---|
| Pancreatic insufficiency | Vitamins A, D, E, K |
| Gastrectomy | Vitamins A, D, E, $B_{12}$; folic acid, iron, calcium |
| Liver disease, alcoholism | Vitamins A, C, D; riboflavin, niacin, thiamine, folic acid, magnesium, zinc |
| Short bowel syndrome, ileal resection | Vitamin $B_{12}$, folic acid, calcium, magnesium |
| Blind loop syndrome | Vitamin $B_{12}$ |
| Bile salt depletion, cholestyramine ingestion | Vitamins A, K |
| Obstructive jaundice | Vitamins A, K |
| Prolonged antacid therapy, peptic ulcer disease | Thiamine, vitamin C |
| Miscellaneous disorders: | |
| Prolonged antibiotic therapy | Vitamin K |
| Fever | Vitamins A, C; thiamine, riboflavin, folic acid |

## CLINICAL ASSESSMENT OF THE ADULT GASTROINTESTINAL SYSTEM

### INSPECTION

Lips: symmetry, color, edema, surface abnormalities.
Tongue: swelling, variation in size or color, coating, ulceration, ability to move.
Gums: inflammation, bleeding.
Gag reflex: intact.
Mouth odors or exudate.
Abdomen: Perform inspection in warm, well-lighted environment with patient in comfortable position with abdomen exposed; view from slightly above and to one side of patient's abdomen. Observe skin (pigmentation, lesions, striae, scars, dehydration venous pattern), contour, movement (respiratory, symmetry, peristalsis).

#### Normal findings

Skin: pigmentation varies considerably within normal range because of race, ethnic background, occupation exposure; however, abdomen is generally lighter in color than other exposed areas.
Contour: slightly concave or slightly round appearance.
Movement: symmetrical; no visible pulsations or peristaltic waves.

#### Abnormal findings

Skin: jaundice, skin lesions, tenseness, glistening, stretch marks, scars (keloids), masses.
Contour: distended (asymmetrical/generalized).

#### Related information

Chart findings, using one of two anatomical maps (four quadrants or nine sections).

#### *Geriatric*

Connective tissue changes and lower total body water make determining dehydration through skin assessment difficult.
Difficulty in chewing and dysphagia: salivary production slows and thickens; problems can be related to temporomandibular joint degeneration or loose, lost, or worn teeth.
Dry mouth, halitosis: salivary production drops and becomes more alkaline.
Pale gums: capillary blood supply diminishes.
Vermillion border of mouth missing: skin loses elasticity.
Yellow papules on oral mucosa: sebaceous glands enlarge (Fordyce's granules).

### AUSCULTATION

Listen below and to the right of umbilicus for bowel sounds; proceed methodically through all quadrants, lifting and placing diaphragm of stethoscope lightly.

#### Normal findings

Sounds in small intestine are high pitched and gurgling; colonic sounds are low pitched and have a rumbling quality.
Bowel sounds occur at a rate of 5 to 35/minute.

#### Abnormal findings

Lack of bowel sounds throughout 5-minute period, extremely soft and widely separated sounds, and increased sounds with characteristically high-pitched, loud rushing sound (peristaltic rush).
Bruits, peritoneal friction rubs, venous hums.

2. Potential nonspecific problems that may affect the GI system—changes in weight, appetite, or activity level
3. Location and description of symptoms, including the site, pain characteristics, and temporal relationship to events (for example, food intake, time of day)
4. Intake and output (food elimination)—diet (food patterns), nutritional status, bowel characteristics (stool descriptions), use of medication and alcohol

To help ascertain the nutritional status of a patient, the nurse should review the history, focusing on weight loss, edema, anorexia, vomiting, diarrhea, decreased or unusual food intake, and chronic illness.

A compounding problem is the nonspecificity of symptoms as they relate to the GI system; that is, there are systemic manifestations of GI disorders as well as other disorders that have a GI manifestation. The patient's history should be examined for information about multiple drug intake, GI alterations potentially caused by normal aging, and changes in psychosocial parameters that could result in physical problems (for example, lack of money for dentures—dysphagia).

### Physical Examination

The physical examination of the critically-ill GI patient is summarized in the box above.

## LABORATORY ASSESSMENT

The value of various laboratory procedures used to diagnose and treat diseases of the GI system has often been emphasized. However, no single test provides an overall picture of the various organs' functional state. Also, no single value is predictive by itself. More than 100 laboratory tests have been proposed for the study of the liver and biliary tract alone. For example, in a patient with cirrhosis, the values for prothrombin time, bilirubin, alkaline phosphatase, alanine aminotransferase (ALT), and aspartate ami-

**Related information**

Normal venous hum is audible at times but is abnormal when heard in periumbilical region and accompanied by a palpable thrill.

Decreased bowel sounds are not significant without added data (for example, nausea, vomiting, digestion).

***Geriatric***

Pediatric chest piece on stethoscope is useful with emaciated patient.

Aging leads to lessened peristalsis (listen for full 5 minutes) and diminished mucus secretion in esophagus ("popping" sound as food is pushed down dry esophagus).

Laxative intake can cause loud gurgling sounds.

Bell of stethoscope is used to listen to vascular sounds; not uncommon to hear cardiac murmurs over abdominal area.

Because of decreased secretion of digestive enzymes, normal bowel sounds may sound "less combustible."

**PERCUSSION**

Proceed systematically to percuss lightly the entire abdomen, including the liver and spleen.

**Normal findings**

Stomach: tympanic when empty.

Intestine: tympanic or hyperresonant.

Liver and spleen: dull.

**Abnormal findings**

Flatness over stomach.

Solid masses and distended bladder: dull sound.

Liver and spleen: dull sounds beyond anatomical borders.

**Related information**

**Geriatric**

Upper liver border usually is found in fourth or fifth intercostal space (adults) but in elderly drops to fifth to seventh intercostal space; liver span shrinks to 6 to 12 cm.

Changes in tonal quality in elderly is caused by changes in connective tissue and diminished muscle mass.

**PALPATION**

Perform both light (tender) and deep palpation of each organ and each quadrant of abdomen.

Light: assesses depth of skin and fascia (depth approximately 1 cm).

Deep: assesses beneath rectus abdominis muscle; perform bimanually (4 to 5 cm deep).

Examine any areas in which patient complains of tenderness last.

**Normal findings**

No areas of tenderness or pain.

No bulges, masses, or hardening.

**Abnormal findings**

Rebound tenderness, rigidity.

If enlarged, gallbladder (right upper quadrant) palpable as small mass attached to liver.

Spleen palpable only if enlarged.

**Related information**

Liver sometimes cannot be palpated in healthy adult; however, in extremely thin but healthy adult, it may be felt at the coastal margin.

***Geriatric***

Palpation of abdominal organs is easier because of relaxed abdominal musculature.

Loss of muscle tone is apparent, especially in diaphragm and costal margin.

Abdomen is preferred site for palpating skin to assess hydration because of wrinkling and loss of turgor elsewhere.

notransferase (AST) all elevate, but hemoglobin and hematocrit values drop (secondary to red blood cell destruction and/or GI bleed). In a patient with hepatitis, serum transaminase values rise early then fall as bilirubin rises. Jaundice occurs as the total bilirubin value goes above 2.5 mg/dl. Mild prolongation of prothrombin time and elevation of alkaline phosphatase may occur. With hepatic coma, in addition to those values reflecting the underlying liver disease, a plasma aminogram shows altered amino acid patterns, and serum ammonia levels rise but do not correlate well with level of encephalopathy.

## DIAGNOSTIC PROCEDURES

### Liver Biopsy

**Liver biopsy** is a bedside procedure, usually performed for diagnosis of primary liver disease. Morphological, biochemical, bacteriological, and immunological studies can be performed on the tissue sample. It can also yield information about the progression of the patient's disease and response to therapy. It is performed less frequently for diagnosis of metabolic disease or malignancy or in patients with multisystem organ failure. The procedure requires patient compliance if performed without significant sedation. Generally it involves the following:

1. Anesthetizing the pericapsular tissue
2. Insertion of either a coring or suction needle between the eighth and ninth intercostal space while the patient either breathes lightly or holds his or her breath
3. Withdrawal of the needle with the sample
4. Positioning the patient on his or her right side for several hours (he or she must remain flat for 24 hours after the procedure)

The procedure is brief; however, it is not uncommon for the patient to experience some pain as a result of irritation to the liver tissue. Abdominal or radiating pain from the epigastric area should be reported immediately. Hemorrhage is a rare but serious complication, thus requiring monitoring of vital signs every 30 minutes for 4 hours and every hour for the next 8 hours. Other complications include damage to neighboring organs, bile peritonitis, infection at the needle site, and shock. This procedure is generally not undertaken if the patient is severely debilitated, is unable to cooperate, has bleeding tendencies or sepsis, or if liver dullness cannot be detected. Because of its invasive nature, possible complications, limited total organ assessment ability, and requirement of patient involvement, other techniques (liver scans, endoscopy) have evolved to partially replace the biopsy.

### Liver Scans

Liver scans are currently used in assessing a patient's hepatic status. A **liver-spleen scan** involves intravenous (IV) injection of radioisotopes, the uptake of which is primarily in the liver and spleen with little or no uptake occurring in patients with cirrhosis or splenomegaly secondary to portal hypertension. A liver scan yields information about the size, vascularity, and blood flow of the organs. The scan requires IV injection of radionuclides. These short-lived isotopes concentrate in the bile, allowing visualization of the biliary system and gallbladder, along with emptying into the duodenum; nonvisualization indicates obstruction. The patient is not sedated but must be able to lie flat for 30 to 90 minutes during the scanning. Uptake results can indicate cirrhosis, hepatitis, tumors, abscesses, and cyst.

### Endoscopy

Several forms of **endoscopy** are available for the direct visualization and evaluation of the lower GI tract. The main difference between them is the length of the colon that can be examined.

The proctoscope allows evaluation of only the few centimeters at and above the rectum. The flexible fiberoptic sigmoidoscope can view the anal canal, rectum, and sigmoid colon (up to 60 cm). With this instrument, approximately 60% of the polyps and colorectal cancers are detectable. Lastly, the colonoscope permits direct visualization of the entire colon and often the lower part of the small intestine.

The main value of the various lower GI scopes is their diagnostic potential. However, they also have a therapeutic benefit in that they allow removal of some suspicious lesions (for example, polyps), thus averting surgery.

Invasive tests have risks for the patient. Potential complications include bowel perforation (abdominal pain and distention, rectal bleeding, fever, mucopurulent drainage), hemorrhage, vasovagal stimulation, and oversedation. Fortunately, these complications are rare in the hands of an experienced physician.[12]

### Plain and Abdominal X-Ray Studies

Numerous radiologic studies are available to investigate large bowel disease further. The most noninvasive are the plain films such as the chest and the abdominal x-ray. Air in the bowel serves as a contrast media to aid in the visualization of the bowel as shown in Fig. 18-1. Gas patterns (the presence of gas inside or outside the bowel lumen and the distribution of gas in dilated and nondilated bowel) are best revealed by plain films. These studies detect bowel obstruction, perforation, foreign bodies, and calcifications. An erect chest x-ray film or an erect abdominal flat-plate film can demonstrate free gas, suggesting a pneumoperitoneum such as that shown in Fig. 18-2. The supine abdominal x-ray film (abdominal flat plate) also demonstrates the caliber of the bowel, which is an important determination in monitoring megacolon. When a patient is unable to sit or stand for erect films, a left-lateral decubitus radiograph is a good substitute. No special preparation is required for plain films.

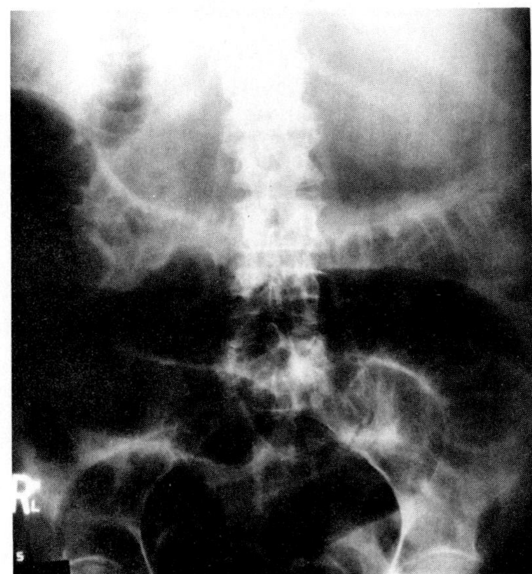

***Fig. 18-1*** Abdominal flat-plate film demonstrates a grossly dilated large bowel *(darker shadows)* and small bowel *(lighter contrast above colon)*. The air in the colon serves as the contrast agent.

### Barium Enema

When clearer visualization of the colon is needed, a radiopaque liquid barium suspension is introduced into the colon through the rectum or through a colostomy. A barium enema in indicated when investigating colon cancer, colonic obstruction, diverticular disease, polyps, and inflammatory bowel disease.

### Air-Contrast Barium Enema

To enhance the detail of the mucosal surface, air can also be introduced into the colon with the barium. This is called a double-contrast study.

When bowel perforation is suspected, a water-soluble contrast agent such as diatrizoate meglumine (Gastrografin) is the contrast medium used in place of barium. Its use is

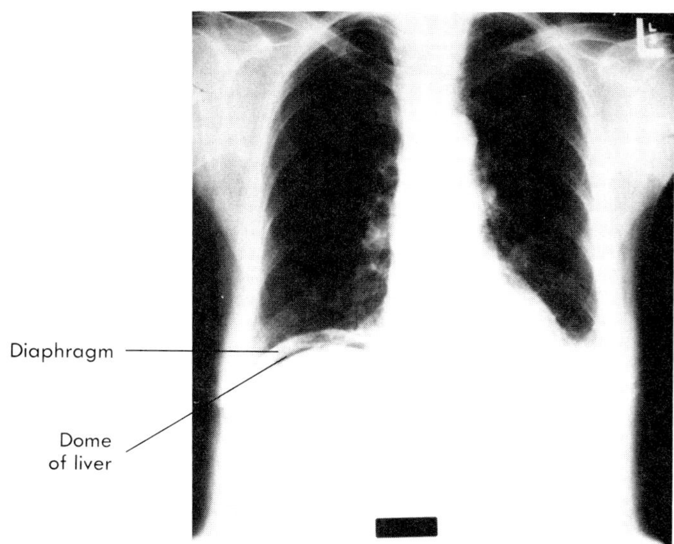


***Fig. 18-2*** Upright chest radiograph reveals free air in the chest as the result of a perforation. Intraperitoneal air is located beneath the right diaphragm *(arrow)* and the dome of the liver *(arrow)*.

necessary because barium leakage into the abdominal cavity can cause peritonitis. No preparation is required for this test.

### Fistulogram

A **fistulogram** is performed to visualize a fistulous tract and to identify communicating organs. A water-soluble contrast medium is instilled into the fistula. No special preparation is required for this test.

### Ultrasound

Ultrasound is not often used to investigate bowel disorders. When used, the patient usually must have a full bladder.

### Computed Tomography

Computed tomography (CT scan) is a radiographic examination that provides cross-sectional images of internal anatomy. It detects mass lesions more than 2 cm in diameter. However, it does not distinguish between benign and malignant tumors, cysts, or abscesses; therefore this type of scan has limited application for colonic disease. It has proven particularly effective in assessing lymph node enlargement and recurrence of colorectal carcinoma.

### Magnetic Resonance Imaging

Magnetic resonance imaging (MRI) is a radiologic examination that provides multiplanar images of the internal anatomy. This is a relatively new technique based on the emission or absorption of electromagnetic radiation by nuclei when exposed to particular magnetic fields. Since MRI involves use of a powerful magnet, patients with metal implants or cardiac pacemakers cannot undergo this examination.

#### REFERENCES


1. Al JAS: Upper abdominal pain: identifying gastrointestinal causes, Consultant 24(12):67, 1984.
2. Bates B: A guide to physical examination, ed 4, Philadelphia, 1991, JB Lippincott Co.
3. Block GJ and Noland JW: The abdomen. In Health assessment for professional nursing: a developmental approach, Norwalk, Conn, 1986, Appleton-Century-Crofts.
4. Carpenito LJ: Nursing diagnosis: application to clinical practice, Philadelphia, 1989, JB Lippincott Co.
5. Englert DA: Gastrointestinal system. In Kennedy-Caldwell C and Guenter P, editors: Nutrition support nursing-core curriculum, ed 2, Silver Spring, Md, 1985, American Society for Parenteral and Enteral Nutrition.
6. Field S: Plain films: the acute abdomen, Clin Gastroenterol 13(1):3, 1984.
7. Fischbach F: A manual of laboratory diagnostic tests, ed 3, Philadelphia, 1988, JB Lippincott Co.
8. Greenberger NJ: Gastrointestinal disorders: a pathophysiological approach, ed 2, Chicago, 1981, Mosby–Year Book, Inc.
9. Kastrup EK: Drug facts and comparisons, Philadelphia, 1987, JB Lippincott Co.
10. Lang CE and Shulte CV: Nutritional assessment in critical care—the adult patient. In Lang CE, editor: Nutritional support in critical care, Rockville, Md, 1987, Aspen Publishers.
11. Mansell E and others: Patient assessment: examination of the abdomen, Am J Nurs 74(9):1679, 1974.
12. McAloose B and others: Society of gastroenterology nurses and associates: standards for practice, Gastroenterol Nurs 12(4):229, 1990.
13. Meir HB: Ultrasound in gastroenterology, Clin Gastroenterol 13(1):183, 1984.
14. Patras AZ and Brozenec SA: Gastrointestinal assessment: identifying significant problems, AORN J 40(5):726, 1984.
15. Price SA and Wilson LM: Pathophysiology: clinical concepts of disease processes, ed 3, New York, 1986, McGraw-Hill Book Co.
16. Stafford R: Gastrointestinal diagnostic tests, J Enterostom Ther 13(6):242, 1986.
17. Swedberg J, Driggers DA, and Deiss F: Screening for colorectal cancer: the role of the primary care physician, Postgrad Med 79:67, 1986.
18. Thompson JM and others, editors: Mosby's manual of clinical nursing, ed 2, St Louis, 1989, Mosby–Year Book, Inc.
19. Varella LD and Kennedy-Caldwell C: Nursing care and specialized nutritional support—the adult patient. In Lang CE, editor: Nutritional support in critical care, Rockville, Md, 1987, Aspen Publishers.
20. Wallach J: Interpretation of diagnostic tests, ed 2, Boston, 1974, Little, Brown & Co.
21. Widmann FK: Clinical interpretation of laboratory tests, ed 9, Philadelphia, 1983, FA Davis Co.

CHAPTER 19

# Gastrointestinal Disorders and Therapeutic Management

## CHAPTER OBJECTIVES

- *Discuss causes, medical treatment, and nursing care for stress ulcer.*
- *Discuss the high-risk causes, medical treatment, and nursing care of acute gastrointestinal bleeding.*
- *Describe the pathophysiology of acute pancreatitis.*
- *Describe important aspects of the nursing care of patients with acute intestinal obstruction, perforated viscus, and fistula.*

## KEY TERMS

dysphagia, p. 362
odynophygia, p. 362
stress ulcer, p. 362
pancreatitis, p. 364
intestinal ischemia, p. 365
functional obstruction, p. 365
mechanical obstruction, p. 365
perforated viscus, p. 367
therapeutic effect tubes, p. 369

## GASTROINTESTINAL DISORDERS

### Dysphagia

**Description, cause, and pathophysiology.** When a patient experiences difficulty during swallowing or within a few seconds after swallowing, he or she is diagnosed as having **dysphagia.** When the sensation is described as painful, it is called **odynophagia.** Dysphagia can be caused by a number of physiologic and psychologic alterations and frequently results from central nervous system damage from a cerebrovascular accident, trauma, or a progressive degenerative disease. In patients with head injury, stroke, motor neuron diseases, and myasthenic disorders, the impairment is usually part of a more widespread disorder. Dysphagia may, however, occur as a fairly isolated problem.

**Assessment and diagnosis.** Immediate difficulty swallowing is associated with the thoracic section of the esophagus. Dysphagia can be experienced after intake of either liquids or solids. Assessment and medical diagnosis are based on site of occurrence, type and temperature of food that initiates the symptoms (liquids, semisolids, hot or cold), length of time the symptom has existed, and results from endoscopy, manometry, or a barium x-ray study.

**Treatment.** Some patients with dysphagia are managed by a diet change to semisolid foods. However, critically ill patients with dysphagia who are at risk for aspiration should receive parenteral or enteral nutrition. Enteral nutrition should be initiated after cardiovascular and respiratory stabilization and after the risk of generalized ileus (for example, from spinal injury and trauma) has receded. Tube insertion in the patient with a head injury (especially anterior basal skull fractures) should proceed with great caution because penetration of the intracranial cavity by GI tubes and feeding tubes has been reported.[2] In the patient with cervical spinal injury, nasoenteric tubes must be inserted without moving the neck. Refer to the box below for specific nursing diagnosis and management of dysphasia.

### Stress Ulcer

**Description, cause, and pathophysiology.** The term **stress ulcer** (erosive gastritis) covers a spectrum of diseases ranging from superficial mucosal erosions to discrete, mature ulcers. Stress ulcers, which are usually multiple, are located mainly in the fundus of the stomach, although they

**Nursing Diagnosis and Management**
***Dysphagia***

- High Risk for Aspiration risk factor: impaired swallowing, p. 476

may involve the entire GI tract. It is the most common cause of upper GI bleeding and the most frequent pathological process within the stomach. Patients at risk include those in high physiologic stress situations such as occur with thermal injury, head trauma, extensive surgery, shock, or acute neurological disease.

Several pathophysiologic mechanisms have been suggested as operative in stress ulcer formation, including gram-negative septicemia, steroid and catecholamine intake, and mucosal ischemia. The onset can be very rapid (2 to 10 days), and hemorrhage can begin without pain. If hemorrhage goes untreated, mortality can exceed 50%. Patients at risk for development of stress ulcers should be assessed for the presence of hematemesis (red blood or coffee-ground emesis), bloody nasogastric aspirate, and melena (black or dark red stools).

**Treatment.** Pharmacological gastric acid neutralization is the accepted treatment for stress ulcers and may even be used prophylactically in high-risk settings. A common regimen includes administering liquid antacids (30 ml every 4 hours) in an attempt to establish and maintain an alkaline gastric environment. At a pH of 5.0, 99.9% of the gastric acid is neutralized, and pepsin activity is essentially nonexistent. Antacids frequently will plug small feeding tubes; therefore a patient may require a 14-French or larger nasogastric tube when antacid administration becomes necessary. Some patients will receive alternating courses of antacids and gastric suctioning. An attempt should be made to keep the pH in the 4.0 to 4.5 range, with additional dosages of antacids given when the pH falls below 4.0. In addition, courses of cimetidine (Tagamet) or other new hydrochloric acid ($H_2$) blockers may be used. Although they would seem useful, continuous enteral feedings apparently do not prevent stress ulceration in critically ill patients.[1]

### Acute Gastrointestinal Bleeding

**Description, cause, and pathophysiology.** Hemorrhage can be a serious symptom or complication of several medical problems (see the box, "Causes of Upper Gastrointestinal Bleeding"). If unrecognized or treated too late, GI hemorrhage can lead to acute GI perforation, peritonitis, sepsis, hypovolemic shock, and ultimately death. In more than one third of patients with GI disease, bleeding will be the initial symptom, and in more than 70% of them, none will have a history of previous bleeding. Generally, gastric surgery patients are not at high risk for postoperative hemorrhage, which, when it does occur, is usually the result of splenic injury or slippage of a suture. Mortality is highest for those patients with bleeding esophageal varices, whereas mortality decreases in those patients with gastric ulcers.

**Assessment and diagnosis.** Hematemesis and melena are hallmark manifestations of GI bleeding. Because it is difficult to estimate the amount of blood in emesis or stool, a description of the sample and the patient's clinical picture are the initial sources for a differential medical diagnosis. Laboratory tests help determine the extent of the bleeding by showing a decrease in the hemoglobin, hematocrit, or blood urea nitrogen (BUN) levels or a change in clotting factors. Diagnostic procedures (endoscope) and radiological studies (radionuclide imaging) aid in establishing the site of the bleeding.[15]

Gastric perforation constitutes a surgical emergency. When it occurs, the patient will suddenly complain of severe generalized abdominal pain with significant rebound tenderness and rigidity. Other symptoms include fever, tachycardia, dehydration, and ileus. Gastric perforation most often occurs when hemorrhaging results from duodenal ulcer. Mortality is approximately 10% to 20%, with death caused by peritonitis and septicemia.

**Treatment.** In addition to gastric acid neutralization, other treatments include gastric lavage cooling, administration of vasopressin, and surgical repairs such as those procedures used to treat GI hemorrhage (gastroenterostomy,

#### CAUSES OF UPPER GASTROINTESTINAL BLEEDING*

Peptic ulceration (gastric and duodenal ulcers)—50%-75%
Acute mucosal lesions (gastritis and erosions [stress ulcers])—1%-33%
Unknown—approximately 16%
Esophagogastric varices—approximately 10%
Reflux esophagitis—approximately 2%
Miscellaneous <8%; examples: gastric neoplasms, hepatic trauma, esophagogastric trauma

*Reported occurrence ranges.

#### Nursing Diagnosis and Management
***Acute gastrointestinal bleeding***

- Fluid Volume Deficit related to active blood loss, p. 495
- High Risk for Infection risk factor: invasive monitoring devices, p. 465
- High Risk for Aspiration risk factors: gastrointestinal tube, increased intragastric pressure, p. 476
- Anxiety related to threatened biological, psychological, and/or social integrity, p. 448
- Sensory-Perceptual Alterations related to sensory overload, sensory deprivation, and sleep pattern disturbance, p. 489
- Ineffectual Individual Coping related to situational crisis and personal vulnerability, p. 447

gastroduodenostomy [Billroth I], gastrojejunostomy [Billroth II or subtotal gastrectomy], partial gastric resection, vagotomy, antrectomy, and pyloroplasty).

**Summary of nursing care.** Nursing care for GI hemorrhage is similar despite the specific cause (refer to box on p. 363). Priorities include the control of bleeding, maintenance of fluid and electrolyte balance, and pharmacological gastric acid neutralization (see "Stress Ulcer"). All patients should be monitored for impending complications of shock, vasovagal responses (especially the elderly), and gastric perforation.

### Acute Pancreatitis

**Description. Pancreatitis,** which may be acute or chronic, is an autodigestive process that results from premature activation of the pancreatic digestive enzymes. These digestive enzymes are normally inactive while housed in the pancreas and become active only in the small intestine. During acute pancreatitis they become active within the pancreas and, in effect, begin the process of digestion before reaching the small intestine. Hence the term *autodigestion* of the pancreas.

**Cause and pathophysiology.** Acute pancreatitis is caused chiefly by biliary disease (most commonly gallstones) and by alcoholism. Other causes include reflux of duodenal contents, penetrating duodenal ulcer, surgical trauma (especially of the organs surrounding the pancreas), hyperparathyroidism, vascular disease, and the use of certain drugs (opiates, steroids, thiazide diuretics, sulfonamides, and oral diuretics). Pancreatitis occurs more frequently in women than in men.

Although the common pathogenic mechanism in acute pancreatitis is autodigestion, it is unclear how or why the pancreatic enzymes are activated before reaching the small intestine.

During acute pancreatitis, trypsin, normally inactive in the pancreas, becomes active and triggers the secretion of the proteolytic enzymes, phospholipase A, elastase, and killikrein. Phospholipase A, in the presence of bile, digests the phospholipids of cell membranes, causing severe pancreatic parenchymal and adipose tissue necrosis. Elastase activation causes dissolution of the elastic fibers of blood vessels and ducts, leading to hemorrhage. Kallikrein activation causes the release of bradykinin and kallidin, resulting in vasodilation and increased vascular permeability. The effects are fluid shifts, hypotension, and pain.

**Assessment and diagnosis.** The most prominent symptom of acute pancreatitis is sudden epigastric to midabdominal pain. The pain may vary from mild and tolerable to severe and incapacitating. It is often reported as a "boring" sensation that radiates to the back. Nausea and/or vomiting may accompany the pain. The patient may obtain some comfort by leaning forward or by lying down with knees drawn up. Pancreatic pain is usually steady and lasts 1 to several days. The pathogenesis of this pancreatic pain relates to extravasation of plasma and red blood cells in the area surrounding the pancreas, release of digested protein and lipids of the pancreas, and ductal swelling.

Physical examination may show tachypnea, leukocytosis, hypocalcemia, tachycardia, and/or some degree of shock. The hypocalcemia is thought to result from marked fat necrosis, which results in the release of free fatty acids. They combine with calcium to form calcium soaps. Neuromuscular irritability and tetany may develop. Palpation of the abdomen will reveal tenderness, guarding, and, if peritonitis is present, rigidity. Bowel sounds may or may not be present.

The diagnosis is confirmed by an acute, severely elevated serum amylase level frequently exceeding 250 Somogyi units/dl, and sometimes reaching 400 to 500 Somogyi units (normal is 60 to 180 Somogyi units/dl). Serum lipase levels will also be elevated. Other findings may include hyperglycemia and elevated bilirubin and decreased serum albumin levels.

**Treatment.** Treatment includes relief of pain, reduction of pancreatic secretions, and prevention or treatment of complications.

Pain relief is achieved with meperidine rather than opiates since meperidine causes less spasm of the sphincter of Oddi. The patient is placed on nothing-by-mouth (NPO) status, and gastric suction is begun to place the pancreas "at rest" and to eliminate any undue secretion of the digestive enzymes. Total parenteral nutrition will be required for prolonged, severe cases of pancreatitis. Antibiotics are administered to treat secondary infection and/or to prevent pancreatic abcess. Plasma and electrolytes infusion are ordered to treat the fluid shifts.

**Nursing Diagnosis and Management**

***Acute pancreatitis***

- Acute Pain related to transmission and perception of noxious stimuli secondary to acute pancreatitis, p. 485
- Ineffective Breathing Pattern related to abdominal pain, p. 472
- Fluid Volume Deficit related to wound drainage, p. 495
- Altered Nutrition: Less than Body Protein-Calorie Requirements related to lack of exogenous nutrients and increased metabolic demand.
- Anxiety related to threatened biological, psychological, and/or social integrity, p. 448
- Sensory-Perceptual Alterations related to sensory overload, sensory deprivation, and sleep pattern disturbance, p. 489
- Ineffectual Individual Coping related to situational crisis and personal vulnerability, p. 447

**Summary of nursing care.** Nursing diagnoses of the patient with acute pancreatitis are summarized in the box on p. 364. Nursing care concerns treating the pain related to acute pancreatitis. Analgesics should be liberally provided, because pancreatic pain can be immobilizing. Because of the pain and the need for high doses of analgesic, the patient's ventilatory pattern should be assessed for depth and rate. Abdominal pain often results in shallow rapid breathing, which can precipitate atelectasis and pneumonia, and high doses of analgesic may further impair the ventilatory pattern. The nursing objective regarding pain control should be achieving pain relief while maintaining ventilations at normal depth and rate. Measures used to rest the pancreas, the NPO status, and gastric suctioning also assist in pain control. Relaxation techniques may augment analgesia. Potential or actual fluid volume deficit is another nursing care concern. Parenteral nutrition may be required for prolonged cases of pancreatitis in which NPO status must be maintained (usually longer than 5 days). The nurse should be alert for development of complications of pancreatitis. Leukocytosis may signal infection or pancreatic abscess. Pulmonary crackles, previously not found, may mean development of atelectasis, pneumonia, or ARDS.

### Intestinal Ischemia

**Description and cause. Intestinal ischemia** can result from either transient or prolonged insufficient mesenteric vascular supply of the splanchnic vessels (the celiac axis, the superior mesenteric artery, and the inferior mesenteric artery). Sometimes the progressive increase in collateral circulation compensates for ischemia. See the box below for a list of pathological conditions commonly associated with intestinal ischemia.

Intestinal ischemia occurs in patients older than 50 years of age who also have a history of arteriosclerosis, cardiac failure, or hemodynamic disorders (for example, multiple myeloma). Ischemic damage can also occur after angioplastic surgery for a ruptured aortic aneurysm or vascular ligations associated with colonic resections.

**Assessment and diagnosis.** A confusing array of manifestations accompany intestinal ischemia. There are no specific features and no satisfactory clinical test to confirm the diagnosis. Initially, the patient complains of diffuse or medial abdominal pain. Later, bloody diarrhea, tenesmus, fever, and hyperleukocytosis can develop. Symptoms are insidious; therefore intestinal ischemia should be suspected in any patient more than 50 years of age who has vague abdominal complaints and a history of heart disease or hemodynamic disorders.

When the sensitive intestinal mucosa becomes hypoxic, mucosal lesions, ulcerations, edema, and hemorrhage develop. The mucosal lesions can heal quickly if the ischemia is brief. However, most of the time the lesions become infected with pathogenic colonic flora. The resulting inflammatory response may conceal the vascular origin and confuse the clinical picture with Crohn's disease or ulcerative colitis. Elevated serum alkaline phosphatase and amylase levels and metabolic acidosis indicate intestinal infarction and evolving gangrenous necrosis.

Radiographic examination of the ischemic colon may reveal "thumbprints" characteristic of mucosal ischemia. Mesenteric arteriography can pinpoint the location of the vascular compromise.

**Treatment.** Rapid recognition of the disease and rapid treatment are essential. Prognosis is poor because these patients are generally not good surgical candidates due to age and concurrent pathological conditions such as arteriosclerosis and heart disease. When ischemia is transient, revascularization can be accomplished. Suspected ischemia and necrosis warrant an emergency resection of the involved bowel.

**Summary of nursing care.** The nurse should evaluate signs that would indicate intestinal perforation. They might include a change in the pain pattern, increased abdominal girth and rigidity, and a marked deterioration in vital signs. An elevated temperature may indicate an infection secondary to pathogenic colonic flora or perforation.

When diarrhea occurs along with intestinal ischemia, accurate intake and output measurements are necessary. Perianal skin should be evaluated and protection provided to prevent a break in skin integrity. A nasogastric tube and bowel rest are needed to avoid stress on an already compromised bowel.

**PATHOLOGIC CONDITIONS ASSOCIATED WITH INTESTINAL ISCHEMIA**

Thrombosis or embolus in splanchnic bed
Cardiopathy or impaired cardiac output
Polyarteritis nodosa
Buerger's disease
Vasculitis secondary to collagen diseases
Strangulation obstruction (e.g., sigmoid volvulus)

### Acute Intestinal Obstruction

**Description and cause.** Acute intestinal obstruction occurs when bowel contents fail to move forward. **Functional obstruction,** also known as paralytic ileus, results from the absence of peristalsis and frequently occurs with hypokalemia. **Mechanical obstruction** results from occlusion of the bowel lumen and is most often the result of neoplasms. The box, "Causes of Colonic Obstruction," on the following page lists examples of both types of obstruction.

Bowel necrosis and perforation are potential complications of colonic obstruction, and both can progress to sepsis. Bowel necrosis occurs as a result of impaired circulation associated with volvulus and closed-loop obstruction and with sustained excessive intraluminal pressure. Bowel perforation often results from overdistention of the bowel lumen and is also a sequelae to bowel necrosis. These complica-

### CAUSES OF COLONIC OBSTRUCTIONS

**FUNCTIONAL OBSTRUCTION**

Prolonged intestinal distention
Hypokalemia
Peritonitis
Narcotic use
Intestinal ischemia
Sepsis

**MECHANICAL OBSTRUCTION**

**Contained within lumen**

Intussusception
Large gallstones
Meconium
Bezoars
Neoplasms

**Extending into bowel wall**

Congenital atresia
Congenital stenosis
Inflammatory bowel disease
Diverticulitis
Radiation
Neoplasms

**Outside the bowel**

Adhesions
Hernias
Neoplasms
Abscesses
Volvulus
Stomal stenosis

tions carry a high mortality rate and can be avoided by astute observations and prompt surgical intervention.

**Assessment and diagnosis.** Colonic obstructions have minimal forewarning. Typically, patients are initially seen in acute distress, with abdominal distention, obstipation, constipation, cramping abdominal pain, and high-pitched bowel sounds. Emesis is seen only if the ileocecal valve is incompetent or the obstruction prolonged. Hypokalemia may occur when the obstruction is prolonged. Initially, dehydration is unusual and is the result of insufficient intake. When the obstruction is prolonged, dehydration may develop secondary to the movement of fluid and electrolytes into the bowel lumen above the obstruction.

The obstructed bowel lumen accumulates fluid and gas proximal to the point of obstruction. Trapped fluids cause bowel distention, which triggers the secretion of fluid and electrolytes into the lumen and perpetuates the distention. As the distention progresses, the bowel wall edema can ultimately impede venous and arterial supply and cause bowel necrosis and perforation.

A chest x-ray film and serial abdominal flat-plate films taken with the patient standing or sitting and supine will reveal dilated loops of gas-filled bowel. Barium or diatrizoate meglumine (gastrografin) enemas are used to locate the exact site and the degree of obstruction.

**Treatment.** Medical interventions include replacement of fluids and immediate decompression of the obstruction with nasogastric suction. Use of long GI tubes is contraindicated for colonic obstruction. A sigmoid volvulus can be nonsurgically reduced by inserting a rectal tube during sigmoidoscopy or barium enema, thus relieving the obstruction. Because the volvulus can recur, elective resection at a later date is desirable.

Surgical intervention is required when the obstruction fails to resolve within 24 hours. When the patient is not acutely ill, surgical resection can be a one-stage procedure with reanastomosis of the bowel, therefore eliminating the need for a temporary colostomy. More often a two- or three-stage procedure is used and a temporary colostomy created.

**Summary of nursing care.** Nursing diagnoses of the patient with acute intestinal obstruction are summarized in the box below. The patient should be observed for signs of bowel obstruction such as abdominal distention, nausea, vomiting, and elevated blood phosphorous or amylase levels. Bowel sounds may be absent or faint and tinkling, depending on the extent of the obstruction. A nasogastric tube should be inserted for decompression. Placement and patency should be checked as needed (prn) to ensure adequate decompression. Outputs greater than 1000 ml/8 hours

### Nursing Diagnosis and Management
***Acute intestinal obstruction***

- Acute Pain related to transmission and perception of noxious stimuli secondary to acute intestinal obstruction, p. 485
- Ineffective Breathing Pattern related to abdominal pain, p. 472
- Decreased Cardiac Output related to decreased preload secondary to fluid volume deficit, p. 459
- Decreased Cardiac Output related to decreased preload secondary to septicemia, p. 460
- High Risk for Aspiration risk factors: gastrointestinal tube, increased intragastric pressure, decreased GI motility, increased gastric residual, delayed gastric emptying, p. 476
- High Risk for Impaired Skin Integrity risk factor: prolonged immobility, p. 499
- Anxiety related to threatened biological, psychological, and/or social integrity, p. 448
- Ineffective Individual Coping related to situational crisis and personal vulnerability, p. 447

can occur. Administration of antipyretics will be necessary for treatment of fever. The patient should be monitored for electrolyte imbalance (hyponatremia and hypokalemia) and fluid deficit. Accurate intake and output must be maintained. IV fluids should be administered to prevent dehydration.

### Perforated Viscus

**Description and cause.** A **perforated viscus** is a hole in the bowel that results in the spillage of contents into the peritoneal cavity. It is an abdominal crisis that requires an expeditious evaluation, an organized approach, and mature surgical judgment for a successful outcome. A bowel perforation can be spontaneous, can result from a diagnostic or therapeutic procedure or can be related to trauma (see the box, "Causes of Colorectal Perforations").

The contamination of the peritoneal cavity results in peritonitis, which is an inflammation of the peritoneum caused by bacterial or chemical irritation. The most common bacteria involved are *Escherichia coli, Streptococcus, Staphylococcus, Pneumococcus, Pseudomonas aeruginosa,* and *Clostridium perfringens*. Of them, *E. coli* is the most frequent cause, and *Streptococcus* is the most virulent type. Chemical irritation is caused by the enzymes or the pH of the spilled contents.

**Assessment and diagnosis.** The hallmarks of a perforated viscus include abdominal pain and "boardlike" rigidity, hypoactive bowel sounds, leukocytosis, and free air in the abdominal cavity. Other symptoms vary with the extent of the peritonitis, its severity, and the type of organism responsible. If left unchecked, the peritonitis will result in sepsis with high fever, dehydration, shock, oliguria, and eventually death.

In addition to a history and abdominal assessment, numerous laboratory tests and flat and upright abdominal x-ray films will be ordered. The films will confirm the presence of free air in the abdomen.

**Treatment.** Medical interventions are initiated to minimize additional complications. GI decompression is necessary to reduce further contamination of the peritoneum and to decrease the risk of vomiting and aspiration. Nothing is given by mouth to provide bowel rest and eliminate further spillage of GI contents. IV fluids are initiated to correct hypovolemia and electrolyte imbalance, and antibiotics are administered. Oxygen may be useful to decrease intestinal hypoxia and, along with proper patient positioning (head up), to assist oxygenation, which may be impaired because of abdominal distention and pain. Pain control must also be provided.

Surgery is almost always indicated in the treatment of a perforated viscus, and the surgical procedure undertaken is dictated by the primary cause and the patient's overall condition. The aim of surgical intervention is to close the perforation, prevent septicemia, and prevent or drain abscesses. A temporary colostomy may be required to divert intestinal contents away from the perforation and/or infection or to protect a questionable bowel anastomosis.

**Summary of nursing care.** Nursing diagnoses related to perforated viscus are summarized in the box above. Vital signs require assessment every hour. The patient should be checked for signs of peritonitis such as abdominal pain, rigidity, fever, elevated white blood cell (WBC) count, hypotension, tachycardia, and tachypnea. The patient with documented peritonitis should be observed for signs of acute bleeding, including hypotension, tachycardia, tachypnea, decreased urinary output, sudden drop in hemoglobin and hematocrit, warm, dry flushed skin, increased lethargy or drowsiness, restlessness, and changes in sensorium.

#### Nursing Diagnosis and Management
***Perforated viscus***

- Acute Pain related to transmission and perception of noxious stimuli secondary to perforated viscus, p. 485
- Ineffective Breathing Pattern related to abdominal pain, p. 472
- Decreased Cardiac Output related to decreased preload secondary to fluid volume deficit, p. 459
- Decreased Cardiac Output related to decreased preload secondary to septicemia, p. 460
- Anxiety related to threatened biological, psychological, and/or social integrity, p. 448
- High Risk for Aspiration risk factors: GI tube, decreased GI motility, delayed gastric emptying, increased gastric residual, p. 476
- High Risk for Infection risk factors: invasive monitoring devices, protein-calorie malnourishment, p. 465
- Ineffectual Individual Coping related to situational crisis and personal vulnerability, p. 447

#### CAUSES OF COLORECTAL PERFORATIONS

Ruptures (e.g., diverticulum, appendix, pericolic abscess)
Surgical procedures involving the bowel or contiguous organs
Diagnostic tests (e.g., endoscopy, barium enema)
Therapeutic procedures (e.g., polypectomy with endoscopy, insertion of an enema tip, explosions with use of cautery during proctosigmoidoscopy)
Ingested foreign bodies (e.g., pits, bones)
Chronic constipation
Trauma (e.g., gunshot, knife wound)

### Fistula

**Description and cause.** A fistula is an abnormal communication between two or more structures or spaces. Fistulas are more specifically categorized according to location, involved structures, and volume of output as demonstrated in Table 19-1.

Complications such as fluid and electrolyte imbalance, malnutrition, and sepsis are responsible for the mortality associated with fistulas. High-output fistulas (more than 500 ml per 24 hours) have a poor prognosis because of fluid and electrolyte imbalance. Advances in nutritional support, however, have improved the prognosis.[18]

Several conditions predispose to fistula formation, including Crohn's disease, trauma, diverticulitis, small bowel obstruction, cancer, ulcerative colitis, and irradiation. Failure of the suture line after an abdominal surgical procedure is the most common cause for fistula formation. Fistulas can develop in irradiated tissue immediately after the therapy or many years later.

**Assessment and diagnosis.** An external fistula is usually quite obvious because of the drainage of fluid, feces, or urine through an aperture in the skin. Internal fistulas communicating with the bladder or vagina result in passage of gas, feces, or urine from the urethra or vagina. The patient may also have a fever of unknown origin.

Collection of the effluent and accurate measurements are essential in fistula management. Volume of output and laboratory analysis of the output can aid in identifying the location of the fistula. To identify accurately the fistulous tract, the involved organs, and the associated pathological conditions, radiographic studies using a water-soluble dye should be conducted (for example, fistulogram or diatrizoate meglumine [gastrografin] enema).

**Treatment.** Medical management requires strict attention to fluid and electrolyte balance, infection control, and nutritional support. Laboratory analysis of the output makes accurate replacement of electrolytes possible. When fever is persistent, an abscess should be suspected, and external drainage of the abscess must be established.

Nutritional support is provided either enterally or parenterally. Because oral intake stimulates bowel activity, the patient should be placed on bowel rest when the fistula involves the GI tract. Bowel rest can be achieved with parenteral and specific types of enteral nutrition. In the early treatment phase, parenteral nutrition is preferred. Once the location of the fistula is identified and the patient is stabilized, enteral nutrition may be initiated for colonic fistulas. With intense nutritional support, approximately 50% of the high-volume fistulas will close spontaneously, although doing so may take at least 2 months.

Specific situations can delay or prevent spontaneous fistula closure, thus requiring surgical intervention (see the box below). It is best to delay any surgical procedures until the patient is infection free and well nourished. Bowel necrosis or abscess, however, requires immediate surgical attention. Several techniques are used to treat fistulas: diversion, resection, or "patching." The procedure used depends on the location, size, and cause of the fistula and the patient's surgical risks. Irradiation- or neoplastic-induced fistulas rarely heal spontaneously because of the local tissue fibrosis and hypoxia typical of radiation and surgery.[18,20,22]

**Summary of nursing care.** A patient with a high-output intestinal fistula must be monitored carefully for fluid and electrolyte disturbances. Clinical assessment, including accurate measurement of intake and output, is essential for prompt identification of malabsorption. Dehydration can result in decreased temperature, increased heart rate, oliguria, and postural hypotension. Hypokalemia can result in a drop in blood pressure; a weak, irregular pulse; electrocardiographic (ECG) changes; and paresthesia; and hyponatremia can result in confusion, apprehension, hypotension, and shock.

Sepsis is a major cause of death in patients with enterocutaneous fistulas. Abscess formation should be suspected in

***Table 19-1*** Nomenclature for fistulas

| Category | Terminology | Meaning |
|---|---|---|
| Location | Internal | Tract contained within body |
| | External | Tract exits through skin |
| Involved structures | Colo- | Colon |
| | Entero- | Small bowel |
| | Vesico- | Bladder |
| | Vaginal | Vagina |
| | Cutaneous | Skin |
| | Recto- | Rectum |
| Volume | High output | More than 500 ml/24 hours |
| | Low output | Less than 500 ml/24 hours |

Modified from Boarini JH, Bryant RA, and Irrgang SJ: Semin Oncol Nurs 2:287, 1986.

**FACTORS THAT DELAY OR PREVENT SPONTANEOUS CLOSURE OF FISTULAS**

- Complete disruption of bowel continuity
- Distal obstruction
- Foreign bodies in the fistulous tract
- Epithelial-lined tract contiguous with the skin
- Cancer in the site
- Previous irradiation
- Crohn's disease
- Presence of large abscess

Modified from Irrgang SJ and Bryant RA: J Enterostomal Ther 6(2):211, 1984.

the presence of an elevated temperature and clinical deterioration. Vital signs should be monitored every 2 hours or more frequently. Antipyretics should be administered as ordered.

### Pseudomembranous Enterocolitis

**Description and cause.** Pseudomembranous enterocolitis is an antibiotic-associated diarrhea in which the bowel mucosa and submucosa become inflamed and necrosis ensues. Because normal bowel flora is altered by antibiotic therapy commonly used in critical care, the environment is conducive for the proliferation of opportunistic microorganisms such as *Clostridium difficile*. As *C. difficile* multiplies, it produces a cytopathic toxin that damages the epithelial cells in the mucosa. A number of antimicrobial agents have been implicated as inciting pseudomembranous enterocolitis, including clindamycin, lincomycin, some cephalosporins, penicillin G, chloramphenicol, tetracycline, and ampicillin.

**Assessment and diagnosis.** Patients with pseudomembranous enterocolitis exhibit severe diarrhea, abdominal tenderness, leukocytosis, and fever. Stools are profuse but do not contain blood. The onset of symptoms may begin during antibiotic therapy or may be delayed until after discontinuation of it. As bowel wall necrosis progresses, the patient loses fluid, electrolytes, and albumin. Toxic megacolon, perforation, and peritonitis are potential complications.

Plain abdominal films and colonoscopy will reveal an edematous distended colon, distorted haustra, an erythematous, friable mucosa, yellow-white plaques, and ulcerations. Stool analysis may reveal *C. difficile*, although a negative culture does not absolutely rule out the disease.

**Treatment.** To prevent the disease from fulminating, antibiotics sensitive to *C. difficile* should be initiated. Colectomy or constructing a diverting ileostomy may be necessary when the symptoms are intractable to medical management or if toxic megacolon develops.

**Summary of nursing care.** Profuse diarrhea is a significant problem in the management of these patients. Refer to the box below. Vital signs should be monitored frequently to evaluate fluid and electrolyte imbalances secondary to losses. An elevated temperature is common, and administration of antipyretics may be indicated.

Because of the risk of toxic megacolon and perforation, regular abdominal assessments are important. Any increases in abdominal girth or abdominal rigidity should be reported immediately to the physician.

**Nursing Diagnosis and Management**
***Pseudomembranous enterocolitis***

Fluid Volume Deficit related to diarrhea, p. 495

## THERAPEUTIC MANAGEMENT

### Gastrointestinal Intubation

Because GI intubation is so common in intensive care patients, it is important for nurses to know the clinical indications and responsibilities inherent in their use. There are four categories of GI tubes based on function: nasogastric suction tubes, long intestinal tubes, therapeutic effect tubes, and feeding tubes (discussed in Chapter 6).

**Nasogastric suction tubes.** Nasogastric suction tubes (Levin, Salem-Sump) remove fluid regurgitated into the stomach, prevent accumulation of swallowed air, may partially decompress the bowel, and reduce the patient's risk for aspiration. The tube is passed through the nose into the nasopharynx and then down through the pharynx into the esophagus and stomach. The length of time the nasogastric tube remains in place depends on its use. Nursing care should prevent the complications common to this therapy, which include the following: ulceration and necrosis of the nares, esophageal reflux, esophagitis, esophageal erosion and stricture, gastric erosion, and dry mouth and parotitis from mouth breathing; interference with ventilation and coughing; and loss of fluid and electrolytes.

**Long intestinal tubes.** *Miller-Abbott, Cantor, Johnston, and Baker* tubes are all examples of long intestinal tubes that are placed either preoperatively or intraoperatively. The long length allows removal of contents from the intestine that cannot be accomplished by a nasogastric tube. These tubes can also decompress the small bowel. In addition, they can splint the small bowel intraoperatively or postoperatively. Because progression of the tubes is dependent on bowel peristalsis, their use is contraindicated in patients with paralytic ileus and severe mechanical obstruction. In addition to monitoring for the complications associated with nasogastric tubes, nurses should monitor the patient for gaseous distention of the balloon section, making removal difficult; rupture of the balloon or spillage of mercury into the intestine; overinflation of balloon, leading to intestinal rupture; and reverse intussusception if the tube is removed rapidly.

**Therapeutic effect tubes. Therapeutic effect tubes** most commonly refer to those designed to compress bleeding esophageal and gastric varices. They include the *Sengstaken-Blakemore tube*, and *Linton-Nachlus tube*, the *Edlich tube*, and the *Boyce* modification of the Sengstaken-Blakemore tube. This treatment modality stops acute variceal hemorrhage 85% to 90% of the time. Because the esophagus is totally occluded and rupture of the gastric balloon may result in complete airway obstruction (because of the tube's rising into the nasopharynx), rupture of the esophagus and pulmonary aspiration are major complications that can be fatal.

Because accumulation of secretions in the esophagus is a problem with the Sengstaken-Blakemore tube, a Linton-Nachlus tube may be used instead because it is designed with one gastric balloon and one lumen for aspiration that ends in the stomach and another lumen that ends in the

***Table 19-2*** Gastrointestinal surgical procedures

| Surgical procedure | Synonymous terms | Description | Fecal diversion | Indications | Nursing concerns |
|---|---|---|---|---|---|
| Abdominoperinal resection | APR<br>Miles' procedure | Wide resection of the rectum, surrounding tissues, and lymph nodes is accomplished by an abdominal and perineal approach. | Permanent sigmoid or descending colostomy | Rectal cancer | Patient has both an abdominal and perineal wound.<br>Impotency results in almost every case.<br>Stoma care. |
| Total proctocolectomy | Panproctocolectomy | Colon and rectum are removed. | Permanent ileostomy | Chronic ulcerative colitis<br>Familial polyposis<br>Crohn's disease | Patient has both an abdominal and perineal wound.<br>Stoma care. |
| Hartmann's pouch | | Distal bowel is closed, and end stoma is created. | Temporary or permanent colostomy, depending on disease | Trauma<br>Incontinence<br>Diverticulitis<br>Rectal cancer (palliative)<br>Obstruction<br>Hirschsprung's disease | Patient may experience long-term mucus discharge from rectal stump.<br>Stoma care. |
| Subtotal colectomy | Segmental resection | Diseased portion of the colon is removed—may be a one-, two-, or three-staged procedure.<br>One-stage procedure: diseased colon is removed, and bowel is reanastomosed; no stoma is created.<br>Two-stage procedure: diseased colon is removed, and temporary stoma is created; later (usually 6-8 weeks), stoma is taken down.<br>Three-stage procedure: stoma is created to resolve immediate problem (e.g., obstruction); next, diseased colon is removed; finally, stoma is taken down. | Possibly a temporary colostomy | Diverticulitis<br>Colon cancer<br>Perforation<br>Trauma<br>Crohn's disease<br>Intestinal ischemia<br>Obstruction<br>Intestinal fistulas<br>Chronic ulcerative colitis (not curative)<br>Familial polyposis (not curative) | |

| | | | | | |
|---|---|---|---|---|---|
| Ileorectal anastomosis | | Colon is removed, and ileum is anastomosed to rectum. | Temporary ileostomy if performed in two stages | Crohn's disease<br>Chronic ulcerative colitis (not curative)<br>Familial polyposis (not curative) | Patient experiences frequent, liquid stools.<br>Numbers of stools decreases over time as bowel adapts.<br>Perianal skin care is important. |
| Ileoanal anastomosis | | Colon and rectum are removed, and ileum is sutured to the anal canal. | Temporary ileostomy if performed in two stages | Chronic ulcerative colitis<br>Familial polyposis<br>Atonic colon | Patient experiences frequent, liquid stools.<br>Number of stools decreases over time as bowel adapts.<br>Perianal skin care is important. |
| Continent ileostomy | Kock's pouch | Colon and rectum are removed; approximately 45 cm of the distal ileum is used to construct internal reservoir and nipple valve. | Permanent continent ileostomy, usually flush with the skin | Chronic ulcerative colitis<br>Familial polyposis | Stoma care (temporary).<br>Postoperatively, stoma is catheterized continuously to avoid overdistention of pouch and tension on the many suture lines.<br>Approximately 14-21 days after surgery, catheter is removed, and patient must intubate stoma to empty the reservoir. |
| Ileoanal reservoir | Restorative proctocolectomy<br>IAR<br>J pouch<br>S pouch<br>Park's pouch<br>Endorectal ileal pouch–anal anastomosis | Procedure is usually performed in two stages.<br>Stage 1: abdominal excision of colon and part of rectum; mucosectomy of rectal stump to dentate line; construction of terminal ileal reservoir; ileostomy.<br>Stage 2: ileostomy takedown. | Temporary ileostomy (usually 6-8 weeks) | Chronic ulcerative colitis<br>Familial polyposis | Reoperation rate is relatively high.<br>Stoma care.<br>High ileostomy results in large volume output and potential fluid and electrolyte depletion.<br>After Stage 2, patient experiences frequent, liquid stools, transient incontinence, and perianal skin irritation. Conditions improve with pouch adaptation. |
| Low anterior resection | | Wide resection of upper portion of rectum includes at least a 2-cm distal margin from tumor to anal verge.<br>Procedure includes a hypogastric lymph node dissection in addition to the mesenteric dissection.<br>Splenic flexure may be mobilized. | Possibly a temporary colostomy with a questionable anastomosis | Rectal cancer (upper one third of rectum) | Long-term results are not known.<br>Stoma care (temporary). |

**Nursing Diagnosis and Management**
***Intestinal Tubes***

High Risk for Aspiration risk factor: gastrointestinal tube, p. 476

esophagus. In addition, its gastric balloon applies pressure to the intragastric veins because of its larger size; thus esophageal compression is not necessary. Nursing diagnosis and management related to intestinal tubes is listed in the box above.

## Surgical Procedures

Numerous surgical procedures are used in the treatment of lower GI diseases or conditions. Some of the more common surgical procedures are described in Table 19-2. Surgery may be the primary therapy or may be reserved for the management of complications of a particluar disorder.

### REFERENCES


1. Anderson C and Cerda JJ: Nutrition in GI disease: diets for patients with esophageal and gastric disorders, part 1, Consultant 26(5):25, 1986.
2. Boarini JH, Bryant RB, and Irrgang SJ: Fistula management, Semin Oncol Nurs 2(4):287, 1986.
3. Buschiazzo L and Possanzo C: A 57-year-old man with bleeding esophageal varices, JPEN 12(3):131, 1986.
4. Corman MC: Colon and rectal surgery, Philadelphia, 1984, JB Lippincott Co.
5. Decker SI: The life-threatening consequences of a GI bleed, RN 48(10):18, 1985.
6. Dusek JL: Iced gastric lavage slows bleeding in gastric hemorrhage, Crit Care Nurse 4(4):8, 1984.
7. Eastwood GL: Upper GI bleeding. II. Differential diagnosis and management, Hosp Med 23(3):44, 1987.
8. Falconer MW: Falconer's the drug, the nurse, the patient, ed 7, Philadelphia, 1982, WB Saunders Co.
9. Fischer JE: The pathophysiology of enterocutaneous fistulas, World J Surg 7:446, 1983.
10. Fleischer D: The therapeutic use of lasers in GI disease, SGA-J 7(2):8, 1984.
11. Fleischer D: Gastrointestinal endoscopy: a look into the future, SGA-J 9(4):171, 1987.
12. Fuller E: Managing a lower GI bleed, Patient Care 18(6):118, 1984.
13. Gaber A: Endoscopic control of upper gastrointestinal bleeding with bipolar coagulation, SGA-J 7(2):20, 1984.
14. Goldberg SM, Gordon PH, and Nivatvongs S: Injuries to the anus and rectum. In Essentials of anorectal surgery, ed 2, Philadelphia, 1989, JB Lippincott Co.
15. Grove KL and others: Acute gastrointestinal hemorrhage, Topic Emerg Med 12(2):9, 1990.
16. Guenter P and Slowm B: Hepatic disease: nutritional implications, Nurs Clin North Am 18(1):71, 1983.
17. Hoppe MC, Descalso J, and Kapp SR: Gastrointestinal disease: nutritional implications, Nurs Clin North Am 18(1):47, 1983.
18. Irrgang SJ and Bryant RA: Management of the enterocutaneous fistula, J Enterostom Ther 6(2):211, 1984.
19. Kagan BM: Antimicrobial therapy, ed 3, Philadelphia, 1980, WB Saunders Co.
20. Kurtz RS, Heimann TM, and Aufses AH: The management of intestinal fistulas, Am J Gastroenterol 76:377, 1981.
21. Larson G and others: Upper gastrointestinal bleeding: predictors of outcome, Surgery 100(4):765, 1985.
22. MacFadyen BV, Jr, Dudrick SJ, and Ruberg RL: Management of gastrointestinal fistulas with parenteral hyperalimentation, Surgery 74:100, 1973.
23. Maloney JP: Surgical intervention in the alcoholic patient with portal hypertension, Cleve Clin Q 8(4):63, 1986.
24. Meeroff JC: Algorithm for managing patients with severe GI hemorrhage, Hosp Pract 19(3):186, 1984.
25. Meeroff JC: Management of massive gastrointestinal bleeding, part 2, Hosp Pract 21(5):93, 1986.
26. Padilla GV and others: Subjective distresses of nasogastric tube feeding, JPEN 3:53, 1979.
27. Peppercorn MA: Acute gastrointestinal hemorrhage: pinpointing the source of defining its treatment, Consultant 27(6):61, 1987.
28. Price SA and Wilson LM: Pathophysiology: clinical concepts of disease processes, ed 3, New York, 1986, McGraw-Hill Book Co.
29. Quinless FW: Severe liver dysfunction: client problems and nursing actions, Focus Crit Care 12(1):24, 1985.
30. Rottenberg R: GI bleeding, emergency handbook, Patient Care 20(14):72, 1986.
31. Sabiston DC, editor: Davis-Christopher textbook of surgery: the biological basis of modern surgical practice, ed 13, Philadephia, 1986, WB Saunders Co.
32. Saegesser F: II: Acute abdomen from vascular disorders in the elderly, Clin Gastroenterol 13(1):145, 1984.
33. Smith JL and Graham DY: Variceal hemorrhage: problems of selecting therapy that reduces risk of death, Consultant 23(10):85, 1983.
34. Solomon J, Harrington D , and Gogel HK: When the patient suffers from esophageal bleeding, endoscopic sclerotherapy, RN 50(2):24, 1987.
35. Thomas RJ: The response of patients with fistulas of the gastrointestinal tract to parenteral nutrition, Surg Gynecol Obstet 153:77, 1981.
36. Webb WA: Management of foreign bodies of the upper gastrointestinal tract, SGA-J 9(1):9, 1986.
37. Wetzel DA: Gastrointestinal complications following renal transplantation: nursing implications, J Enterostom Ther 14(1):16, 1987.
38. Winters G: Coping with the massive GI bleeder: one method—esophga-gastric tamponade, SGA-J 8(2):24, 1985.
39. Yussen PS and LaManna MM: Anatomic localization of acute GI hemorrhage by radionuclide angiography, SGA-J 10(1):12, 1987.

# UNIT VIII

# ENDOCRINE ALTERATIONS

CHAPTER 20

# Endocrine Assessment and Diagnosis

## CHAPTER OBJECTIVES

- *Perform a thorough nursing assessment of the endocrine system on a critically ill patient, interpret the results, and plan nursing interventions that will treat any abnormal findings.*
- *List the criteria for a health history that would be specific in assessing for diabetic ketoacidosis and hyperglycemic hyperosmolar nonketotic coma.*
- *Compare and contrast at least three clinical and laboratory manifestations of diabetes insipidus and syndrome of inappropriate antidiuretic hormone.*
- *List the laboratory tests that will differentiate central diabetes insipidus from nephrogenic diabetes insipidus.*

## KEY TERMS

gluconeogenesis, p. 377
glycosylated hemoglobin, p. 378
ketonemia, p. 378
ketonuria, p. 378
antidiuretic hormone (ADH), p. 378
computerized axial tomography (CAT), p. 379
magnetic resonance imaging (MRI), p. 379

The endocrine system controls and communicates through the distribution of potent hormones throughout the body (see Fig. 20-1 for a listing of the endocrine glands, hormones, target tissue, and action). When stimulated, the endocrine organ secretes hormones into surrounding body fluids. Once in circulation, these hormones travel to a specific target tissue where they exert a pronounced effect on specialized cells. Receptors found on the cell surfaces or within the cells are equipped with molecules that recognize and bind the hormone to the cell and produce a specific response.[3]

Diabetic ketoacidosis (DKA) is an endocrine emergency. It is perhaps the most common endocrine disorder for which the patient is admitted to the critical care unit. Hyperglycemic hyperosmolar nonketotic coma (HHNC) is another endocrine dysfunction involving carbohydrate metabolism. This potentially lethal disorder has a mortality rate greater than 40%[13] and is often seen in the critical care unit as a complication of other serious health problems.

Diabetes insipidus (DI) and syndrome of inappropriate antidiuretic hormone (SIADH) are two pituitary disorders that disrupt the body's regulation of plasma osmotic pressure and circulating blood volume. Each disease is rarely seen alone but rather develops secondary to a precipitating illness.

This chapter will focus on the assessment and diagnosis of these four metabolic disorders.[6]

## ENDOCRINE ASSESSMENT

The majority of the endocrine glands are located deep within the protective encasement of the human body. Although the placement of the glands provides security for the glandular functions, their inaccessibility prevents the glands from being physically appraised. Most endocrine glands cannot be assessed by palpation, percussion, or auscultation. The endocrine glands that are not assessed by physical inspection can nevertheless be assessed by the clinician who understands the metabolic actions of the hormones involved.[1] Therefore, since percussion or palpation cannot be used, the nurse monitors the functioning of the target tissue.

Frequently the initial focus of the hormonal disturbance is not on the gland itself but rather on the specific cell receptor or target for the hormonal action. For example, posterior pituitary dysfunction is suspected when the patient has decreased urine output, clinical signs of hypervolemia. Similarly, pancreatic disorders are often recognized by first noting imbalances in the beta cell hormone, insulin, and its systemic effects. A dysfunctioning pancreas is suspected when the patient is lethargic and has hot dry skin, oliguria, and a sweet-smelling odor to the breath.[36,41]

Collecting clues that may signal a dysfunctioning gland poses a challenge to the nurse clinician because target tissues of insulin (adipose and muscle cells) and antidiuretic hor-

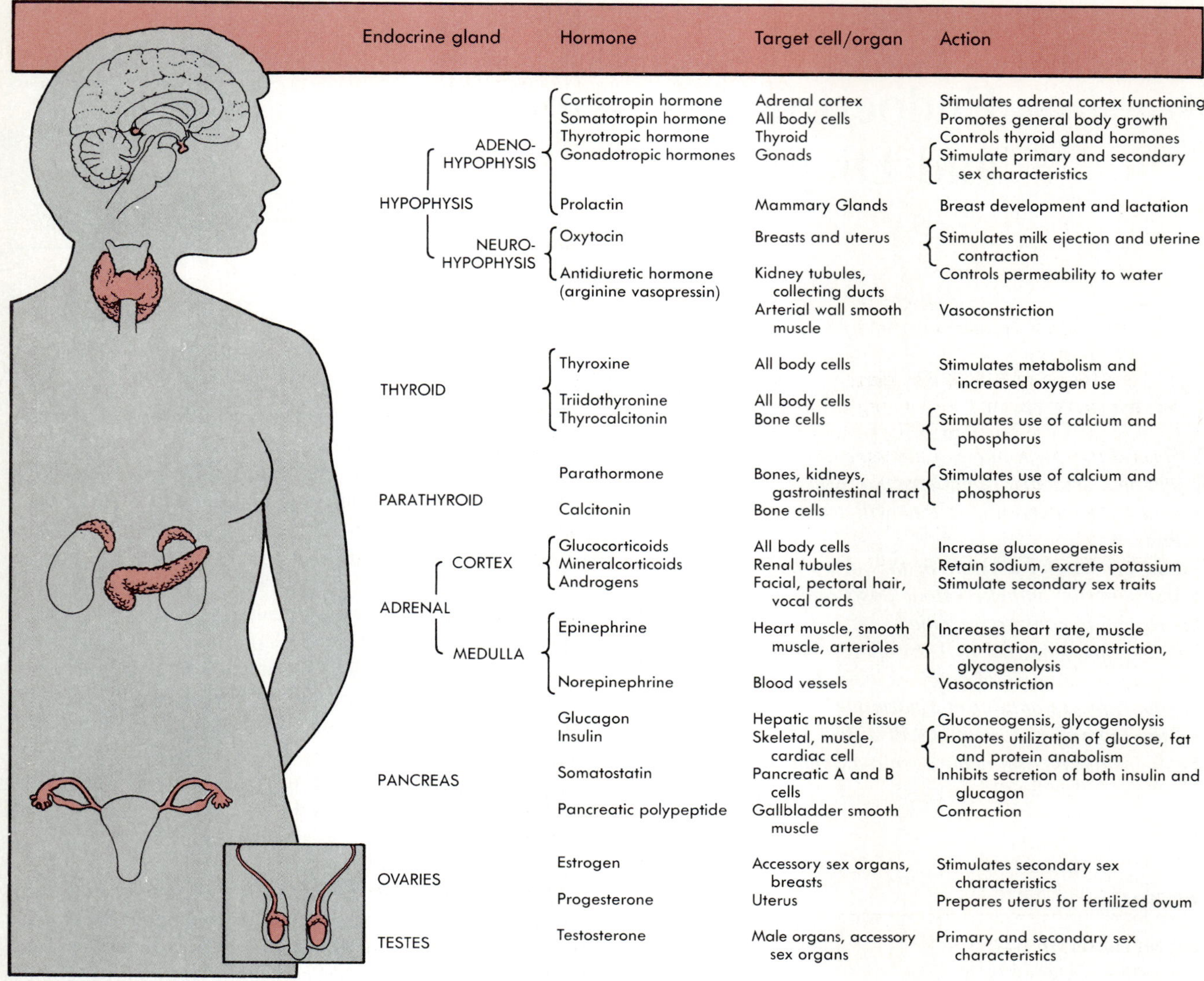

| Endocrine gland | | Hormone | Target cell/organ | Action |
|---|---|---|---|---|
| HYPOPHYSIS | ADENO-HYPOPHYSIS | Corticotropin hormone | Adrenal cortex | Stimulates adrenal cortex functioning |
| | | Somatotropin hormone | All body cells | Promotes general body growth |
| | | Thyrotropic hormone | Thyroid | Controls thyroid gland hormones |
| | | Gonadotropic hormones | Gonads | Stimulate primary and secondary sex characteristics |
| | | Prolactin | Mammary Glands | Breast development and lactation |
| | NEURO-HYPOPHYSIS | Oxytocin | Breasts and uterus | Stimulates milk ejection and uterine contraction |
| | | Antidiuretic hormone (arginine vasopressin) | Kidney tubules, collecting ducts | Controls permeability to water |
| | | | Arterial wall smooth muscle | Vasoconstriction |
| THYROID | | Thyroxine | All body cells | Stimulates metabolism and increased oxygen use |
| | | Triidothyronine | All body cells | |
| | | Thyrocalcitonin | Bone cells | Stimulates use of calcium and phosphorus |
| PARATHYROID | | Parathormone | Bones, kidneys, gastrointestinal tract | Stimulates use of calcium and phosphorus |
| | | Calcitonin | Bone cells | |
| ADRENAL | CORTEX | Glucocorticoids | All body cells | Increase gluconeogenesis |
| | | Mineralcorticoids | Renal tubules | Retain sodium, excrete potassium |
| | | Androgens | Facial, pectoral hair, vocal cords | Stimulate secondary sex traits |
| | MEDULLA | Epinephrine | Heart muscle, smooth muscle, arterioles | Increases heart rate, muscle contraction, vasoconstriction, glycogenolysis |
| | | Norepinephrine | Blood vessels | Vasoconstriction |
| PANCREAS | | Glucagon | Hepatic muscle tissue | Gluconeogensis, glycogenolysis |
| | | Insulin | Skeletal, muscle, cardiac cell | Promotes utilization of glucose, fat and protein anabolism |
| | | Somatostatin | Pancreatic A and B cells | Inhibits secretion of both insulin and glucagon |
| | | Pancreatic polypeptide | Gallbladder smooth muscle | Contraction |
| OVARIES | | Estrogen | Accessory sex organs, breasts | Stimulates secondary sex characteristics |
| | | Progesterone | Uterus | Prepares uterus for fertilized ovum |
| TESTES | | Testosterone | Male organs, accessory sex organs | Primary and secondary sex characteristics |

***Fig. 20-1*** Location of endocrine glands with hormones, target cell/organ, and hormone action.

mone (kidney tubule) are influenced by numerous other factors. Therefore, the nurse starts with a pertinent data base including history (when available) and precipitating factors. The patient in the critical care unit may not be able to provide an adequate history for the nurse's assessment data base. Changes in level of consciousness and urgent medical/nursing procedures may delay the patient from providing a personal perspective of the current problem. This initial phase of the nursing process should not be ignored, however, and sources other than the patient (family, friends, previous medical records) should be used to supply vital information.

### History

A complete health history would include the patient's chief complaint and current health history. Chronic as well as episodic diseases are discussed (acute stress could increase endogenous glucose). Also included in the medical history are questions about the past history and any pertinent family history. An outline of this information is presented in the box, "Important Aspects of Endocrine Assessment."

### Physical Assessment

Antidiuretic hormone controls the amount of fluid lost and retained within the body. The nurse uses a hydration assessment to determine the effectiveness of ADH function. A hydration assessment includes skin integrity, skin turgor, and buccal membrane moisture. Intake and output, when performed accurately and conscientiously on *all* routes of fluid intake and loss, provides information about the body's fluid balance. A balanced intake and output, absence of

### IMPORTANT ASPECTS OF ENDOCRINE ASSESSMENT

#### NURSING HISTORY

1. Chief complaint
2. History of present problem
   a. Onset
   b. Duration
   c. Signs/symptoms
   d. Treatments
3. History of pancreatic problems, surgery, diabetes, carbohydrate imbalances, thyroid disease, or kidney problems
4. Head or neurological disorders
5. Recent severe infection or surgical trauma
6. Past or current treatments using hyperalimentation, peritoneal dialysis, or hemodialysis
7. Recent, unexplained changes in weight, thirst, hunger, or urination patterns
8. Changes in mental abilities, i.e., memory loss, momentary disorientation, difficulty concentrating, lethargy
9. Recent changes in daily levels of activities, e.g., decreased endurance level, fatigue, weakness
10. Usage of prescription or over-the-counter drugs
11. Presence of acute stress
12. Family history of present illness, e.g., carbohydrate imbalance

#### NURSING ASSESSMENT

1. Skin turgor
2. Mucous membranes
3. Intake and output
4. Presence of edema
5. Blood pressure, i.e., hypertension, hypotension, orthostatic hypotension
6. Behavioral changes
7. Decreased muscle strength or muscle coordination
8. Mental confusion
9. Weight changes
10. Presence of thirst

thirst, absence of edema, and stable weight all provide the nurse with information indicating the patient's hydration status is adequate for the patient's metabolic demands.

Blood pressure and pulse are frequently monitored. Decreased blood pressure with an increased pulse is characteristic of hypovolemia, whereas elevated blood pressure and rapid, bounding pulse may indicate hypervolemia. Orthostatic hypotension occurs when there is a decrease in extracellular fluid volume.

The patient's neurological system is frequently evaluated when assessing the pituitary gland. Alterations in serum sodium levels have an adverse effect on brain tissue and disrupt the patient's behavioral patterns. Muscle coordination, deep tendon reflexes, and muscle strength are included in this neurological assessment. A summary of important assessment aspects is provided in the box at left.

***Table 20-1*** Laboratory assessment of endocrine disorders

| Substance | Normal value |
|---|---|
| **SERUM** | |
| Insulin | 5-20 μU/ml |
| Glucose | 70-110 mg/dl (fasting)<br>85-125 mg/dl (nonfasting) |
| Glycosylated hemoglobin | 4.0%-7.0% of total hemoglobin |
| Ketones | 2-4 ml/100 ml (ketones)<br>0.3-2 mg/100 ml (acetone) |
| Osmolality | 285-300 mOsm/L |
| Antidiuretic hormone (ADH) | 1.5 picograms/ml or <1.5 mg/L |
| **URINE** | |
| Ketones | Negative |
| Glucose | Negative |
| Osmolality | 300-1600 mOsm/L |
| Specific gravity | 1.005-1.030 |

### Laboratory Assessment

Diagnosis of pancreatic and pituitary dysfunction is made through a combination of laboratory tests, in conjunction with the clinical picture. A summary of serum and urine diagnostic tests is provided in Table 20-1.

**Insulin.** The release of insulin is dependent on the concentration of blood glucose; when glucose levels rise, insulin levels also rise. Conversely, when serum glucose levels are low, insulin secretion is inhibited. A fasting blood sample is preferred for evaluation of serum insulin levels, because it portrays the body's ability to balance glucose levels with the body's glucose needs.

**Glucose.** Circulating blood glucose is derived from three sources: exogenous intake of glucose, release of glycogen stores, and breakdown of non-carbohydrate sources, known as **gluconeogenesis.** A fasting blood sample identifies glucose as a simple, numerical value, but it actually measures many complex, interrelated processes. The glucose reading measures the ability of the pancreatic A cells to balance the release of glucagon with the B cell release of insulin. Circulating glucose is also dependent on the peripheral uptake of glucose and the functioning of the liver and its role in gluconeogenesis. Consistently elevated glucose levels signal an increase in glucagon production and an insufficient amount of effective insulin.[7]

**Glycosylated hemoglobin.** During the 120-day lifespan of erythrocytes the hemoglobin within each cell binds to the available blood glucose through a process known as glycosylation. Increased levels of circulating glucose cause an increase in glycosylation.

**Glycosylated hemoglobin** provides information about the degree of hyperglycemia, including the actual increased values over a specific period of time. This test eliminates many variables that could normally affect the accurate interpretation of a glucose test. Fasting state, exercise, stress, and medications do not interfere with this test result.[15]

**Ketones.** Ketones are byproducts of fat metabolism. Normally, when the body utilizes carbohydrate as its main source of energy, fat metabolism is complete and only a trace of ketones is found in the blood. In the absence of glucose, fats are burned for energy. Lipolysis (fat breakdown) occurs so rapidly that fat metabolism is incomplete, and ketone bodies collect in the blood **(ketonemia)** and are excreted in the urine **(ketonuria)**. Ketonemia is observed by a fruity, sweet-smelling odor on the exhaled breath. Ketonemia is the result of the body's attempt to maintain the pH level within normal range.[36] Both blood and urine specimens can be tested in the laboratory or with reagent strips. Urine samples can also be tested with specially prepared tablets.

**Osmolality**

***Serum osmolality.*** Serum osmolality refers to the number of dissolved particles in a solution. An accumulation of ketone bodies and ketoacids in the hyperglycemic blood sample results from the rapid, incomplete breakdown of fat and protein. The ketone bodies and ketoacids collect in the plasma as metabolic "debris" and, along with the increasing levels of glucose that cannot enter the cell, drastically increase the number of particles that normally circulate in the plasma. This increase in circulating particles coupled with the fluid loss from osmotic diuresis significantly raises the plasma osmolality.

***Urine.*** Osmolality of urine refers to the number of dissolved particles in a urine sample. This reading depends on the ability of the kidney tubules to absorb or block reabsorption of fluids. This dilution or concentration of urine depends on the presence of ADH, the permeability of the kidney nephron, and the relative osmolality of the circulating serum.

Increased serum osmolality will stimulate the release of ADH, which in turn will reduce the amount of water lost at the tubules. Body fluid is thereby retained to dilute the particle concentration in the blood stream. Decreased serum osmolality inhibits the release of ADH, the kidney tubules increase their permeability, and fluid is eliminated from the body in an attempt to regain normal concentration of particles in the bloodstream.[15,36]

The most accurate results of the body's ability to maintain a fluid balance are obtained when urine and blood samples are collected simultaneously.

**Antidiuretic hormone.** The presence of **antidiuretic hormone (ADH)** in the blood stream is measured by radioimmunoassay. This diagnostic procedure provides accurate results and, when available, is used in preference to water load and water deprivation tests (discussed later).

To prepare a patient for this test, all drugs that may alter the release of antidiuretic hormone are withheld for a minimum of 8 hours. Medications that affect ADH levels are morphine sulfate, lithium carbonate, chlorothiazide, carbamazeprine, oxytocin, and certain neoplastic and anesthetic agents. Nicotine, alcohol, both positive and negative pressure ventilation, and emotional stress can also influence the ADH levels and must be considered when interpreting the values.

The test is read by comparing serum antidiuretic hormone levels with the blood and urine osmolality. The presence of increased ADH in the bloodstream compared with a low serum osmolality and elevated urine osmolality confirms the diagnosis of syndrome of inappropriate antidiuretic hormone (SIADH). Reduced levels of serum ADH in a patient with high serum osmolality, hypernatremia, and reduced urine concentration signal central diabetes insipidus.[7]

**Water deprivation test.** The water deprivation test is based on the premise that the antidiuretic hormone is released to conserve urinary water when a patient is at risk of becoming dehydrated. This procedure purposely withholds all fluid while laboratory tests determine the body's response to the pending dehydration.

Usually, all fluids are withheld for 24 hours or until a patient has lost up to 5% of his or her body weight.[19] Normally, such a deprivation of fluids would stimulate the release of ADH to conserve urine to maintain serum osmolality. In a balanced state, the serum osmolality would remain constant while the urine osmolality increased.

Patients with reduced levels of ADH are unable to curtail fluid losses through the urine despite increases in blood osmolality. Elevated serum osmolality with a urine osmolality that is either equal to or less than the serum concentration would indicate continued loss of urinary fluid despite hemoconcentration.[7,15]

The nurse must carefully evaluate the patient's response to this dehydration test to prevent serious fluid imbalances. The patient must be weighed frequently to detect the amount of fluid lost. Blood pressure is taken every 1 to 2 hours to identify decreased blood volume that could indicate pending vascular collapse. Serum sodium levels are also monitored for a disproportionate rise in sodium compared with the reduced blood volume. Diabetes insipidus is suspected when reduced levels of ADH occur with increased serum osmolality and reduced urine concentration.

Water deprivation test results are usually followed up with a subcutaneous injection of aqueous Pitressin (synthetic antidiuretic hormone). This phase of testing will provide information to differentiate the type of diabetes insipidus. Serial urine samples are collected for 2 hours, and the urine volume and osmolality is measured.

The patient with normal hypophyseal functioning would respond to the exogenous ADH by reabsorbing water at the tubule and raising the urine osmolality slightly less than 5%.[15] Test results in which urine osmolality remains unchanged are suspicious for nephrogenic diabetes insipidus indicating that the target tissue or cell receptor sites are no longer receptive to the ADH.

**Water load test.** The water load test is based on the premise that changes in the concentration of particles in the blood stream will affect the release of ADH as the body strives to maintain a homeostatic balance. This test overhydrates the patient and then provides a series of blood and urine tests to monitor the sequence of physiological events leading to a fluid balance.

The patient is given nothing by mouth overnight. He or she is instructed not to smoke (nicotine can stimulate ADH release) and not to take medications that alter ADH levels. The patient is asked to drink 20 ml of water per kilogram of body weight within 15 to 30 minutes. Intravenous 5% dextrose in water is given over 8 to 10 minutes if oral fluid cannot be taken.

Serial urine samples are collected for 4 to 5 hours and tested for volume, osmolality, and specific gravity. A serum osmolality is also done at the end of the test and its result is compared with the entire volume of urine collected during the test.[15,36]

This hypotonic fluid load test would decrease the urine osmolality in a healthy subject. Patients with excessive antidiuretic hormone would have decreased serum osmolality while maintaining either a constant or elevated urine concentration.

This test subjects patients with cardiac or renal dysfunctions to circulatory overload and requires frequent assessment for the signs of cardiac decompensation, such as dyspnea, chest pain, moist breath sounds, jugular vein distension, and elevated central venous pulmonary artery pressures. Because of the inherent risks associated with the water load test, the test is performed on select patients.

Decreasing the patient's serum osmolality with overhydration has a dilutional effect on the serum sodium level, resulting in a mild dilutional hyponatremia. Because of this, the patient should be carefully monitored for sodium changes, including gastrointestinal stimulation, cramps, diarrhea, apprehension, and changes in personality.

## DIAGNOSTIC PROCEDURES

In addition to the laboratory tests, radiographic examination, computerized tomography, and magnetic resonance imaging are useful in diagnosing hypothalamic-hypophyseal disease. Although these tests may not definitively diagnose diabetes insipidus or syndrome of inappropriate antidiuretic hormone, they are useful in diagnosing the primary causes of these diseases.

**Radiologic examination.** A basic x-ray examination of the inferior skull views the sella turcica and surrounding bone formation. Bone fractures, or tissue swelling at the base of the brain, apparent on a radiograph, suggests interference with the vascular supply and nerve impulses to the hypothalamo-pituitary system. Dysfunction may occur if the hypophysis, infundibular stalk, or the neurohypophysis is impaired.

**Computerized axial tomography. Computerized axial tomography** of the base of the skull (sella turcica) identifies pituitary tumors, blood clots, cysts, nodules, or other tissue masses. A skull CT scan provides more definitive results than a radiograph and whenever possible is done in preference to a skull radiograph.

**Magnetic resonance imaging. Magnetic resonance imaging (MRI)** is a noninvasive diagnostic scanning device that uses a magnetic field rather than ionizing radiation used by x-ray examinations or CAT scans. The MRI enables the radiologist to visualize internal organs as well as examine the cellular characteristics of specific tissue.[33] The soft fluid tissue in and immediately surrounding the brain makes the brain especially responsive to MRI scanning. Although the MRI is not a definitive diagnostic test for posterior pituitary hormonal imbalance, its use identifies anatomical disruption of the gland and the surrounding area suggestive or primary causes of DI and SIADH.

### REFERENCES

1. Braundwald E and others, editors: Harrison's principles of internal medicine, ed 11, New York, 1987, McGraw-Hill Book Co.
2. Bullock B and Rosendahl P: Pathophysiology, adaptations and alterations in function, ed 2, Glenview, Illinois, 1988, Scott Foresman & Company/Little, Brown College Division.
3. Burch W: Endocrinology, ed 2, Baltimore, 1988, Williams & Wilkins.
4. Butts D: Fluid and electrolyte disorders associated with diabetic ketoacidosis and hyperglycemic hyperosmolar nonketotic coma, Nurs Clin North Am 22(4):827, 1987.
5. Chanson P and others: Ultra-low doses of vasopressin in the management of diabetes insipidus, Crit Care Med 15(1):44, 1987.
6. DeGroot L: Endocrinology, ed 2, Philadelphia, 1989, WB Saunders Co.
7. Fischbach F: A manual of laboratory diagnostic tests, ed 3, Philadelphia, 1988, JB Lippincott Co.
8. Germon K: Fluid and electrolyte problems associated with diabetes insipidus and syndrome of inappropriate antidiuretic hormone, Nurs Clin North Am 22(4):785, 1987.
9. Grindlinger G and Boylan M: Amelioration by indomethacin of lithium-induced polyuria, Crit Care Med 15(5):538, 1987.
10. Guyton A: Textbook of medical physiology, ed 7, Philadelphia, 1986, WB Saunders Co.
11. Hadley M: Endocrinology, ed 2, Englewood Cliffs, NJ, 1988, Prentice-Hall.
12. Hall R and Evered D: Color atlas of endocrinology, ed 2, St Louis, 1990, Mosby–Year Book, Inc.
13. Harris M and Hamman R, editors: Diabetes in America, Bethesda, Md, 1985, US Department of Health and Human Services, Public Health Service, National Institutes of Health, National Institute of Arthritis, Diabetes and Digestive and Kidney Diseases.
14. Hemmer M and others: Urinary ADH excretion during mechanical ventilation and weaning in man, Anesthesiology 52(5):395, 1980.
15. Henry J, editor: Todd, Sanford, Davidsohn, clinical diagnosis and management by laboratory methods, ed 17, Philadelphia, 1984, WB Saunders Co.
16. Hollinshead W and Rosse C: Textbook of anatomy, ed 4, Philadelphia, 1985, Harper & Row Publishers.

17. Hudak C: Critical care nursing: a holistic approach, Philadelphia, 1990, JB Lippincott Co.
18. Kirby R: Pocket companion of critical care: immediate concerns, Philadelphia, 1990, JB Lippincott Co.
19. Kohler P, editor: Clinical endocrinology, New York, 1986, John Wiley & Sons.
20. Krall L and others: Joslin's diabetes mellitus, ed 12, Philadelphia, 1988, Lea & Febiger.
21. Lubin M and others, editors: Medical management of the surgical patient, Boston, 1988, Butterworths.
22. Martin C: Endocrine physiology, New York, 1985, Oxford University Press.
23. McEvoy G, McQuarrie G, and DiPietro J, editors: Drug information '87, Bethesda, Md, 1987, American Society of Hospital Pharmacists.
24. Mercer M: Myths & facts . . . about diabetes insipidus, Nursing '90, 20(5):20, 1990.
25. Methany N and Snively WD: Nurse's handbook of fluid balance, ed 4, Philadelphia, 1983, JB Lippincott Co.
26. Nerozzi D, Goodwin F, and Costa E, editors: Neuropsychiatric disorders, New York, 1987, Raven Press.
27. Newman R: Bedside blood sugar determinations in the critically ill, Heart Lung 17(6):667, 1988.
28. Nikas, D: Critical aspects of head trauma, Crit Care Nurs Q 10(1):19, 1987.
29. Patterson L and Noroian E: Diabetes insipidus versus syndrome of inappropriate antidiuretic hormone, Dimens Crit Care Nurs 8(4):226, 1989.
30. Polak J and Bloom S: Endocrine tumours, the pathobiology of regulatory peptide-producing tumours, London, 1985, Churchill Livingstone.
31. Potgieter P: Inappropriate ADH secretion in tetanus, Crit Care Med 11(6):417, 1983.
32. Powers M: Handbook of diabetes nutritional management, Rockville, Md, 1987, Aspen Publishers.
33. Rudy E: Magnetic resonance imaging, new horizon in diagnostic technique, J Neurosurg Nurs 17(6):331, 1985.
34. Sabo C and others: Diabetic ketoacidosis: pathophysiology, nursing diagnoses and interventions, Focus Crit Care 16(1):21, 1989.
35. Schroeder S: Current medical diagnoses and treatment, Norwalk, Conn, 1989, Appleton & Lange.
36. Schroeder S, Krupp M, and Tierney L: Current medical diagnosis and treatment, Norwalk, Conn, 1988, Appleton & Lange.
37. Slaunwhite R: Fundamentals of endocrinology, New York, 1988, Marcel Dekker, Inc.
38. Staller A: Systemic effects of severe head trauma, Crit Care Nurs Q 10(1):58, 1987.
39. Swearingen P, Sommers M, and Miller K: Manual of critical care: applying nursing diagnosis to adult critical illness, ed 2, St Louis, 1991, Mosby–Year Book, Inc.
40. Tepperman J and Tepperman H: Metabolic and endocrine physiology, ed 5, Chicago, 1987, Mosby–Year Book, Inc.
41. Tobin M: Essentials of critical care medicine, New York, 1989, Churchill Livingstone.
42. Vokes T and Robertson G: Disorders of antidiuretic hormone, Endocrinol Metab Clin North Am 17(2):281, 1988.
43. Williams C: Lung cancer, Oxford, New York, 1984, Oxford University Press.
44. Yeates S and Blaufuss J: Managing the patient in diabetic ketoacidosis, Focus Crit Care 17(6):240, 1990.

CHAPTER 21

# Endocrine Disorders and Therapeutic Management

## CHAPTER OBJECTIVES

- *Discuss why and how osmotic diuresis occurs with plasma hyperosmolality.*
- *Explain the pathophysiology of diabetes ketoacidosis and list at least four signs or symptoms that identify both early and late stages of this disorder.*
- *List the priorities of nursing care for a patient with early signs or symptoms of diabetic ketoacidosis.*
- *Identify at least three factors that compose a high-risk profile for the patient with hyperglycemic hyperosmolar nonketotic coma.*
- *List the priorities of nursing care a patient with diabetes insipidus and syndrome of inappropriate antidiuretic hormone.*

## KEY TERMS

diabetic ketoacidosis, p. 381
glycogenolysis, p. 381
"fruity" breath odor, p. 382
hyperglycemic hyperosmolar nonketotic coma, p. 385
diabetes insipidus, p. 388
Pitressin, p. 391
desmopressin acetate, p. 391
syndrome of inappropriate antidiuretic hormone, p. 392
Kussmaul's breathing, p.382

## DIABETIC KETOACIDOSIS

### Description

**Diabetic ketoacidosis** (DKA) is a serious complication of diabetes mellitus. It poses a life-threatening situation to the type I, insulin-dependent diabetic patient, although it rarely affects the type II insulin-independent diabetic patient. Ketoacidosis may develop over several hours in a person who has had diabetes for a period of time. In an undiagnosed diabetic patient, it may take days to develop and be an abrupt signal of the onset of the disease. Ten percent of all deaths attributed to diabetes result from DKA.[13] It is estimated, however, that these deaths occur not from the ketoacidotic state alone, but rather from late complications (pneumonia, myocardial infarction, infection) resulting from DKA.[1]

### Cause

Ketoacidosis results from an alteration in the insulin-glucagon levels in the body. Potential causes of diabetic ketoacidosis are listed in the box on p. 382.

Recently, diabetic ketoacidosis has been seen in patients who use insulin pump devices that aim to provide tighter glucose control. Improper functioning resulting in insulin leakage or pump failure[36] initially causes subtle changes in glucose levels. The patient, believing his or her glucose was aptly controlled by the pump, attributes the physical symptoms to extraneous health problems. Tending to trust the functioning of the pump, the patient delays testing serum glucose and urine ketones while DKA is progressively developing.

### Pathophysiology

Insulin is the metabolic key to the transfer of glucose from the bloodstream into the cell where it can be immediately used for energy or stored to be used at a later time. Without the necessary insulin, glucose remains in the bloodstream and cells are deprived of their energy source. A complex pathophysiological chain of events follows (Fig. 21-1). The release of glucagon is stimulated when insulin is ineffective in providing the cells with glucose for energy. Glucagon increases the amount of glucose in the bloodstream by breaking down stored glucose **(glycogenolysis)** and converting noncarbohydrate molecules into glucose (gluconeogenesis). Blood glucose levels for the patient in diabetic ketoacidosis typically range from 300 to 800 mg/dl blood. The hyperglycemia increases the plasma osmolality, and blood becomes hyperosmolar.

Excessive urination and glycosuria occur as a result of the osmotic diuresis. The excess glucose filtered at the glo-

**POTENTIAL CAUSES OF DIABETIC KETOACIDOSIS**

**DECREASED EXOGENOUS INSULIN INTAKE**

Lack of knowledge, poor compliance
- Omitting dose
- Insufficient dose to meet glucose requirement

Malfunctioning insulin pump
Pharmacological drugs
- Phenytoin
- Thiazide/sulfonamide diuretics

**INCREASED ENDOGENOUS GLUCOSE**

Diabetes management changes
- Decreased exercise without decreasing food or increasing insulin
- Increased dietary intake

Sympathetic nervous system responses
- Stressful events
  - Injury
  - Surgery
  - Infections
    - Respiratory tract
    - Urinary tract
    - Pancreatitis
  - Emotional trauma

Increased glucagon
Increased growth hormone
Pharmacological drugs
- Steroid therapy
- Epinephrine/norepinephrine

merulus cannot be reabsorbed at the renal tubule and "spills" into the urine. Large amounts of water, along with sodium, potassium, and phosphorus, are excreted in the urine.[34]

Polydipsia occurs as the decrease in the circulating blood volume stimulates the osmoreceptors in the hypothalamus and promotes the release of angiotensin II. This initiates a strong thirst sensation intended to curtail the loss of fluids and replenish the circulating blood volume. The fluid volume deficit also stimulates vasoconstriction as a means to preserve blood pressure.

Both the vasoconstriction and the extremely elevated levels of glucose impair the delivery of oxygen to the peripheral cells and impede the removal of metabolic wastes.

As DKA progresses, gluconeogenesis continues to convert noncarbohydrate molecules into glucose. Ketoacidosis occurs as ketoacid end products accumulate in the blood and rapid, incomplete fatty acid metabolism releases highly acidic substances into the bloodstream (ketonemia) and the urine (ketonuria).

The acid ketones dissociate and yield hydrogen ions ($H^+$) that accumulate and cause a drop in serum pH. The patient with gluconeogenesis has ketones accumulating in the bloodstream faster than can be metabolized. The bicarbonate and sodium loss through osmotic diuresis prevents the formation of sodium bicarbonate needed to buffer the increasing carbonic acid. The respiratory rate is altered in an attempt to compensate for the carbonic acid build-up. Breathing becomes deep and rapid (**Kussmaul's breathing**) to blow off carbonic acid in the form of $CO_2$. Acetone is exhaled, giving the breath its characteristic **"fruity" breath odor**.

Gluconeogenesis stimulates mobilization of protein and protein catabolism increases. Protein is broken down and converted to glucose in the liver.

Nitrogen accumulates as protein is metabolized. Urea, added to the bloodstream, increases the osmotic diuresis and accentuates the dehydration. Loss of muscle mass and reduced resistance to infection occur with impaired protein utilization. The combined states of acidosis and osmotic diuresis lead to a loss of phosphorus, further compromising peripheral tissue perfusion. Hypophosphatemia impairs the oxygen function of the hemoglobin by increasing hemoglobin's affinity for oxygen and thereby reducing delivery of oxygen to the cells.[40,19]

### Assessment and Diagnosis

Considering the complexity and potential seriousness of DKA, the diagnosis is straightforward. With a known diabetic patient, a diagnosis of DKA is determined by heavy ketonuria and glycosuria in the presence of hyperglycemia and ketonemia. If the patient is not known to have diabetes, other causes of metabolic acidosis must be differentiated before a course of therapy is begun. Starvation, alcoholism, certain toxic chemicals, lactic acid, and uremia may result in a ketoacidotic state.[1] The treatment plan would vary depending on the cause. DKA diagnostic considerations are presented in the box on p. 384.

### Treatment

Once diagnosed, diabetic ketoacidosis requires aggressive medical and nursing management to prevent progressive decompensation.[44] Treatment is needed to:

1. Reverse dehydration
2. Restore the insulin-glucagon ratio to promote cellular use of glucose; reduce the counterregulatory hormone, glucagon; and break the ketotic cycle
3. Treat and prevent circulatory collapse
4. Replenish electrolytes

The diabetic ketoacidotic patient is significantly dehydrated, may have lost 5% to 10% of body weight in fluids, and may have a fluid deficit of 3 to 5 L.[36] Initially, normal physiological saline may be given to reverse the vascular deficit, hypotension, and extracellular fluid losses. The rate is varied depending on urinary output, secondary illnesses, and precipitating factors. To dilute the serum osmolality, infusions of half-strength sodium chloride may follow the initial saline replacement.

Once serum glucose is decreased to 250 to 300 mg/dl blood, a 5% dextrose solution is infused.[36] Intravenous glu-

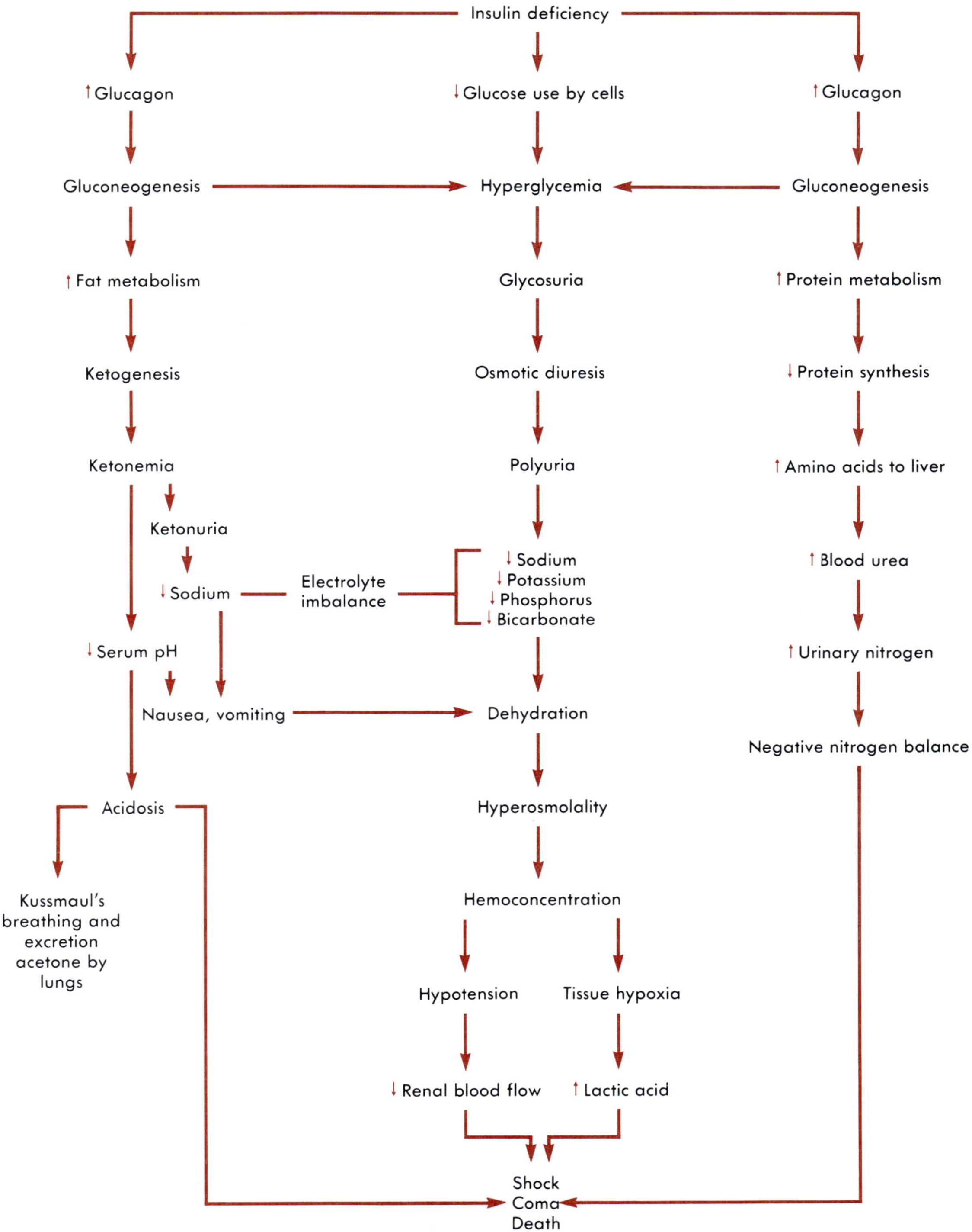


***Fig. 21-1*** Pathosphysiology of diabetic ketoacidosis (DKA). A carbohydrate derangement affects the metabolism of both protein and fat.

### DIAGNOSTIC CONSIDERATIONS OF DIABETIC KETOACIDOSIS

**ONSET**

Malaise
Headache
Polyuria
Polydipsia
Polyphagia
Nausea and vomiting
Extreme fatigue
Dehydration
Weight loss
Changes in level of consciousness (leading to coma)

**PHYSICAL EXAMINATION**

Dehydration, i.e., flushed dry skin, dry buccal membranes, decreased skin turgor
Tachycardia
Hypotension
Kussmaul's breathing
Subnormal temperature
"Fruity breath"
Stupor or unconsciousness

**LABORATORY FINDINGS**

| | |
|---|---|
| Serum glucose | 300-800 mg/dl |
| Serum ketones | Strongly positive |
| Serum pH | <7.3 |
| Serum osmolality | <350 mOsm/L |
| Serum sodium | Normal or low |
| Serum potassium | Low, normal, or elevated (total body K is depleted) |
| Serum bicarbonate | <15 mEq/L |
| Serum phosphorus | Low, normal, or elevated |
| Urine glucose* | 3% to 4% |
| Urine acetone | Strong |

*Clinitest, two-drop method

cose is necessary to replenish glucose stores, and to prevent hypoglycemia and cerebral edema. Intravenous glucose is maintained until the patient no longer requires intravenous fluids and is taking liquids by mouth.

Insulin is given simultaneously with intravenous fluids. A reversal of the ketoacidotic metabolic abnormalities gradually occurs as the patient is hydrated and given insulin. The serum glucose level falls as large quantities of glucose are perfused through the kidneys and removed in the urine. Insulin inhibits the release of glucagon and glucose is no longer poured into circulation. The ketoacidotic cycle is gradually broken, since ketoacids are no longer produced as a byproduct of incomplete fat metabolism. The serum osmolality is reduced with vigorous fluid replacement coupled with the reduction of glucose, urea, and ketones circulating in the bloodstream. Osmotic diuresis is reversed as the continuous fluids replace fluid losses, and serum glucose levels return to normal.

The traditional use of large doses of insulin has slowly given way to lower, continuous intravenous doses of insulin. A bolus of 0.3 U/kg may be given to saturate the insulin cell receptor sites and compete with any insulin resistance at the cell receptor site. Replacement of low-dose insulin, 0.1 U/kg/hr (approximately 6 to 10 U/Hour), is given intravenously or intramuscularly depending on circulatory perfusion until acidosis is reversed.

Hypokalemia may occur as insulin promotes $K^+$ return to the cell, and acidosis is reduced. Unless the initial hypokalemia is severe, potassium may not be given for 3 to 4 hours after treatment begins or until the potassium shift stabilizes. Insulin treatment also precipitates hypophosphatemia as serum phosphate returns to the cell. Although the need to administer phosphate is currently debated, its use does seem to improve tissue oxygenation and promote the renal excretion of hydrogen ions.[1]

The replacement of lost bicarbonate is also controversial. While intravenous bicarbonate promotes the rapid acidotic reversal leading to alkalinization, the sudden shift in electrolytes may cause deprivation of oxygen. It is generally agreed that bicarbonate is started for critically severe acidotic states (pH <7 and bicarbonate <5 mE/L) and stopped when the pH level reaches 7.2.[36] An indwelling arterial line provides access to hourly sampling of blood gases.

Some comatose patients may require gastric intubation to decompress stomach contents and prevent vomiting and subsequent aspiration. The use of a nasogastric tube also reduces impaired ventilation resulting from abdominal distention.

In addition to vigorous medical treatment the practitioner investigates the precipitating causes of ketoacidosis. Unless the precipitating factors are known and resolved, DKA will probably recur. After 10 to 12 hours of effective treatment, the patient's hydration and neurological and metabolic status should drastically improve.

#### Summary of Nursing Care

Nursing diagnoses and management related to diabetic ketoacidosis are listed in the box on p. 385.

Rapid intravenous fluid replacement requires the use of a volumetric pump when possible. Accurate intake and output must be maintained to record the body's use of fluid. Skin assessment for moisture content provides information about the body's distribution and use of fluid within body tissues. Although the patient complains of intense thirst, it may be unwise for the conscious patient to drink large quantities of water if there is a concurrent problem with abdominal distention. Ice chips may be used as an alternative to quench the patient's thirst, along with reassurance that the intravenous fluids will soon satisfy the need for fluids. Oral care including lip balm will help keep lips supple and prevent them from cracking. Prepared sponge sticks or moist gauze pads can be used to moisten oral membranes of the unconscious patient.

**Nursing Diagnosis and Management**

***Diabetic ketoacidosis***

- Decreased Cardiac Output related to decreased preload secondary to fluid volume deficit, p. 459
- Anxiety related to threat to biological, psychological, and/or social integrity, p. 448
- Knowledge Deficit: Self-Care of Diabetes Mellitus related to lack of previous exposure to information, and/or cognitive/perceptual learning limitations, p. 441
- Potential Impaired Skin Integrity risk factor: Alterations in tissue perfusion.
- Body Image Disturbance related to functional dependence on life-sustaining technology, p. 443
- Ineffective Individual Coping related to situational crisis and personal vulnerability, p. 447
- Altered Health Maintenance related to lack of perceived threat to health, p. 439
- Self-Esteem Disturbance related to feelings of guilt over physical deterioration, p. 442
- Powerlessness related to physical deterioration despite compliance, p. 445
- Hopelessness related to perceptions of failing or deteriorating physical condition, p. 446

Vital signs, especially heart rate, hemodynamic findings, and blood pressure, are constantly monitored to assess cardiac response to the fluid replacement. Reduction in the rate and volume of infusion, elevation of head, and oxygen and oronasalpharyngeal suctioning as needed may be required to assist the patient to manage the increased intravascular volume.

Urine tests for glucose, ketones, specific gravity, and blood glucose are done every 30 to 60 minutes at the bedside. Serum osmolality is monitored and blood urea nitrogen and creatinine levels are assessed for possible renal impairment related to decreased renal perfusion.

Insulin is given intravenously to the severely dehydrated patient to ensure absorption when inadequate circulation is present. It is suggested that 25 U regular human insulin be added to 250 ml of 0.9% saline; 50 ml of this solution is then used to prime the tubing. The prepared solution provides maximum absorption for the container and tubing before starting the infusion.[23] As dehydration and hypotension diminish, insulin is given intramuscularly or subcutaneously. Throughout the insulin therapy, both patient response and laboratory data are assessed for changes relating to glucose levels. Respirations are frequently assessed for changes in rate, depth, and fruity "acetone" odor. When the blood glucose level falls to 250 to 300 mg/100 ml blood a 5% dextrose solution is infused to prevent hypoglycemia. Regular insulin may be decreased as the glucose level reaches a range of 250 to 300 mg. Should hypoglycemia occur, insulin is stopped and the physician notified.

Electrolytes fluctuate throughout the rehydration phase. Standard protocols to administer electrolytes based on laboratory criteria routinely used in the critical care unit may or may not be followed. The nurse must be aware of the obvious and obscure signs indicative of changing electrolyte levels.

Skin care takes on new dimensions for the patient with diabetic ketoacidosis. Dehydration, hypovolemia, and hypophosphatemia interfere with oxygen delivery at the cell site and contribute to inadequate perfusion and tissue breakdown. Patients must be repositioned every hour to relieve capillary pressure and promote adequate perfusion to body tissues.

Lung sounds are assessed every 8 hours or as needed. Encouraging the conscious patient to cough and deep breathe every hour promotes full ventilation of the lungs and helps prevent pulmonary complications. Strict sterile technique is used to maintain all intravenous systems. All venipuncture sites are checked every 4 hours for signs of inflammation, phlebitis, or infiltration. Strict surgical asepsis is used for all invasive procedures.

Neurological assessments performed every 4 hours or as needed coupled with serum osmolality values serve as an index of the patient's response to the rehydration therapy.

Throughout the treatment, the precipitating causes of the patient's DKA are examined and treated. If the patient is newly diagnosed as having diabetes, teaching about the disease process and self-care is provided. Comprehensive instruction for patients and families involve various health care personnel including the nurse, dietician, and physician.

For previously diagnosed diabetics, the knowledge level and compliance history are important in formulating a teaching plan. Learning objectives include definition of hyperglycemia and its causes, harmful effects, and symptoms. Additional objectives include a definition of ketoacidosis and its causes, symptoms, and harmful consequences. The patient and family are expected to learn the principles of diabetes management during illness. They are also expected to know the warning signs that must be brought to the attention of a health care practitioner.

## HYPERGLYCEMIC HYPEROSMOLAR NONKETOTIC COMA

### Description

The condition known as **hyperglycemic hyperosmolar nonketotic coma** (HHNC) is a frequently lethal complication of diabetes mellitus. The hallmarks of HHNC are extremely high levels of plasma glucose with resulting elevations in hyperosmolality and osmotic diuresis. Inability to replace fluids lost through diuresis or severe diarrhea leads to profound dehydration and changes in level of conscious-

## POTENTIAL CAUSES OF HHNC

**Insufficient insulin**

Diabetes mellitus
Pancreatic disease
Pancreatectomy
Pharmacological
  Phenytoin
  Thiazide/sulfonamide diuretics

**Increased endogenous glucose**

Acute stress
  Extensive burns
  Myocardial infarction
  Infection
High-calorie enteral feedings
Pharmacological
  Glucocorticoids
  Steroids
  Sympathomimetics
  Thyroid preparations

**Increased exogenous glucose**

Hyperalimentation (total parenteral nutrition)
Hemodialysis
Peritoneal dialysis
High-calorie enteral feedings

ness. Hyperglycemic hyperosmolar nonketotic coma has a 40% to 50% mortality rate.[13]

## Cause

HHNC occurs when the pancreas produces a relatively insufficient amount of insulin for the high levels of glucose that floods the bloodstream (see the box above, "Potential Causes of HHNC"). The disorder occurs mainly, although not exclusively, in elderly, obese individuals who have underlying conditions requiring medical treatment. The individual may be a patient with type II insulin-dependent diabetes who is treated with diet and hypoglycemic agents. HHNC can also occur in previously undiagnosed and therefore untreated diabetic persons.[4]

## Pathophysiology

The syndrome of hyperglycemic hyperosmolar nonketotic coma represents a deficit of insulin and an excess of glucagon. Fig. 21-2 schematically presents the pathophysiology. Reduced insulin levels prevent the movement of glucose into the cells, thus allowing glucose to accumulate in the plasma. Excessive glucose, along with the end products of incomplete fat and protein metabolism, collect as debris in the bloodstream. As the number of particles increase in the blood, hyperosmolality increases.[4]

Hemoconcentration persists despite removal of large amounts of glucose in the urine (glycosuria) by the kidneys.

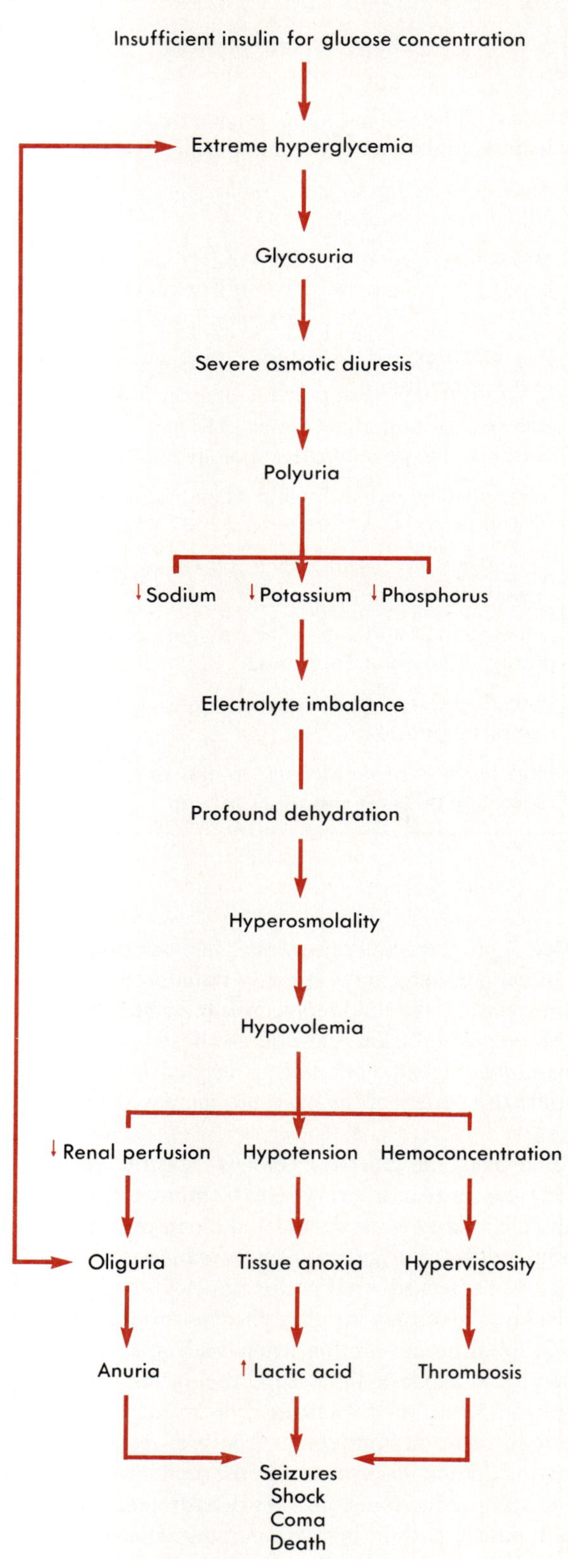


***Fig. 21-2*** Pathophysiology of hyperglycemic hyperosmolar nonketotic coma (HHNC).

The hyperosmolality and reduced blood volume stimulates the release of antidiuretic hormone to increase tubular reabsorption of water. ADH, however, is powerless in overcoming the osmotic pull exerted by the glucose load. Excessive fluid volume is lost at the kidney tubule with simultaneous loss of potassium, sodium, and phosphate in the urine.

Hypovolemia reduces renal circulation, and oliguria develops. Although this conserves water and preserves the blood volume, it prevents further glucose loss and hyperosmolality increases.

Ketoacidosis is absent or very mild in HHNC despite the level of free fatty acids resulting from gluconeogenesis. The reasons for lack of ketoacidosis are unclear.[36] It is surmised that the patient may have either a glucagon resistance or sufficient insulin present to prevent the liver from converting fatty acids into ketones.[32]

In an effort to restore homeostasis, the sympathetic nervous system reacts to the body's stress response. Epinephrine, a potent stimulus for gluconeogenesis, is released and additional glucose is added to the bloodstream. Unless the glycemic diuresis cycle is broken with aggressive fluid replacement, the intracellular dehydration affects fluid and oxygen transport to the brain cells. Central nervous system dysfunctioning may result and lead to coma. Hemoconcentration increases the blood viscosity, which may result in clot formation, thromboemboli, and cerebral, cardiac, and pleural infarcts.[1]

### Assessment and Diagnosis

HHNC has a slow, subtle onset. Initially, the symptoms may be nonspecific and may be ignored or attributed to concurrent disease processes in the patient. Medical attention may not be obtained for these nonspecific, nonacute symptoms until the patient is unable to take sufficient fluids to offset the fluid losses. HHNC diagnostic considerations are listed in the box at right.

**DIAGNOSTIC CONSIDERATIONS OF HYPERGLYCEMIC HYPEROSMOLAR NONKETOTIC COMA**

**HISTORY**

Polyuria
Polydipsia
Advancing weakness
Progressive dehydration
Mental confusion
Convulsions
Coma

**PHYSICAL EXAMINATION**

Obtunded patient
Profound fluid deficit
Severe dehydration, i.e., longitudinal wrinkles in the tongue, decreased salivation, decreased CVP, increased pulse and respirations

**LABORATORY FINDINGS**

| | |
|---|---|
| Serum glucose | 600-2000 mg/dl |
| Serum ketones | Normal or mildly elevated |
| Serum pH | Normal |
| Serum osmolality | >350 mOsm/L |
| Serum sodium | Normal or elevated |
| Serum potassium | Low, normal, or elevated |
| Serum bicarbonate | Normal |
| Serum phosphorus | Low, normal, or elevated |
| Urine glucose* | 4% or highest concentration |
| Urine acetone | Absent or mild |

*Clinitest, two-drop method

### Treatment

Treatment is necessary to interrupt the glycemic diuresis and to prevent vascular collapse. The underlying cause of HHNC must then be sought. The same basic principles used to treat diabetic ketoacidosis are used for the patient with hyperglycemic hyperosmolar coma: rehydration, electrolyte replacement, restoration of insulin/glucagon ratio, and prevention/treatment of circulatory collapse.

Rapid rehydration is the primary intervention. The fluid deficit may be as much as 25% of the patient's total body water. Current debate exists regarding whether isotonic or hypotonic solutions are more appropriate for treating the severe fluid deficit. The general consensus is to use physiological normal saline (0.9%) for the first 3 L during the first 2 hours of treatment, especially for the patient in circulatory collapse.[1] Half-strength hypotonic saline (0.45%) can subsequently be used to reduce the serum osmolality. The patient may need replacement of 6 to 10 L of fluid in the first 10 hours.[3] Sodium input should not exceed that required to replace the losses. Careful monitoring for sodium and water balance is required to prevent hemolysis as hemoconcentration is reduced.[36] To prevent relative hypoglycemia, the hydrating solution is changed to 5% dextrose in water, in 0.9% saline or in 0.45% saline when the serum glucose levels fall to 250 to 300 mg/dl.

Vigorous fluid therapy alone can reverse hyperosmolar coma. However, intravenous insulin is usually given to facilitate the cellular use of glucose and decrease the serum osmolality more rapidly.[1] Muscle, liver, and adipose cells are usually quite receptive to exogenous insulin levels in the patient with HHNC, and the insulin needs are minimal. Ten to fifteen units of regular insulin is given intravenously as a bolus. Maintenance doses of insulin to control hyperglycemia may range from 0.1 U/kg/hr intravenously until glucose falls to 250 mg to a one time administration of 15 U subcutaneously.[36] Once glucose levels are at 250 mg/dl, insulin treatment is usually discontinued. Aggressive treatment of the underlying causes of HHNC (severe infection, therapeutic procedures, medications) are included in the medical treatment to prevent HHNC recurrence.

**Nursing Diagnosis and Management**
***Hyperglycemic hyperosmotic nonketotic coma***

- Decreased Cardiac Output related to decreased preload secondary to fluid volume deficit, p. 459
- Anxiety related to threat to biological, psychological, and/or social integrity, p. 448

### Summary of Nursing Care

Nursing diagnoses and management related to HHNC are listed in the box above. Since hyperglycemic hyperosmolar coma occurs most frequently in the patient with a precipitating stressor or illness, it is not unlikely that the nurse would be the first person to recognize its development. Nursing management of the patient at risk for HHNC involves prompt recognition of changes in the patient's osmolar state. The nurse assesses hydration status and monitors blood values that might indicate HHNC (refer to the box on p. 387). Changes in the patient's personality provide neurological clues to the impact of fluid imbalance on the central nervous system. When unexplained behavior changes are coupled with changing laboratory values and other signs of dehydration, hyperosmolality is to be suspected.

Once HHNC is identified, the nurse plans care to manage the alterations brought about by the fluid deficit, the increase in glucose, and the electrolyte imbalances. Because HHNC occurs most often in the elderly, special care of the elderly is emphasized. Throughout the critical care period, the nurse collects information necessary to identify the precipitating cause of HHNC and educates the patient and family in prevention of its recurrence. Hemodynamic monitoring, including central venous pressure, pulmonary arterial wedge pressure, and pulmonary artery pressure, reveals the degree of dehydration and the effectiveness of the hydration therapy. Because a preexisting cardiopulmonary or renal problem may exist in the elderly patient, the hemodynamic parameters must be based on the values normal for that patient's age and current medical condition. The nurse is alerted to symptoms of fluid overload while vigorously rehydrating the older patient. Cardiac monitoring for sinus rhythm, central venous pressure, and pulmonary arterial readings continue to provide an evaluation of the patient's fluid tolerance.

Rigorous fluid replacement and low-dose insulin administration are best controlled with electronic volumetric pump devices. Electrolyte replacement orders are based on the patient response to the treatment plan. Bedside serum glucose monitoring and urine tests for ketones are done every 30 to 60 minutes to determine effectiveness of treatment.

Neurological assessments, including level of consciousness, pupillary response, motor function, and reflexes, are done frequently to monitor the patient's response to treatment. Seizure precautions include nursing actions to protect the patient from injury and provide an open airway. Oxygen is administered via nasal cannula. Anticonvulsants, with the exception of phenytoin (interferes with endogenous insulin), may be ordered. Documentation of seizures includes onset, duration, and description of seizure activity.

Fluid replacement, range of motion exercises, frequent positioning, and assessing skin turgor, color, temperature, and peripheral pulses are used to maintain and monitor skin integrity. Elastic support hose, elastic wraps or antiembolotic stockings may be used in an effort to prevent lower extremity venous stasis.

Combined alertness to the signs and symptoms identifying the underlying cause of the disease is needed to prevent its recurrence. Diabetic teaching plans are necessary if the hyperglycemic coma is the result of untreated diabetes.

## DIABETES INSIPIDUS

### Description

**Diabetes insipidus** (DI) occurs when there is an insufficiency or a hypofunctioning of antidiuretic hormone

**CAUSES OF DIABETES INSIPIDUS**

**CENTRAL DIABETES INSIPIDUS**
**Primary**

ADH deficiency from hypothalamic-hypophyseal malformation
- Congenital defect
- Idiopathic

**Secondary**

ADH deficiency from destruction to the hypothalamic-hypophyseal system
- Trauma
- Infection
- Surgery
- Primary neoplasms
- Metastatic malignancies
- Autoimmune response

**NEPHROGENIC DIABETES INSIPIDUS**

Inability of kidney tubules to respond to circulating antidiuretic hormone
- Decrease or absence of ADH receptors
- Cellular damage to nephron, especially loop of Henle
- Kidney damage, i.e., hydronephrosis, pyelonephritis, polycystic kidney
- Untoward response to drug therapy, i.e., lithium carbonate, demeclocycline

**PSYCHOGENIC DIABETES INSIPIDUS**

Rare form of water intoxication
- Compulsive water drinking

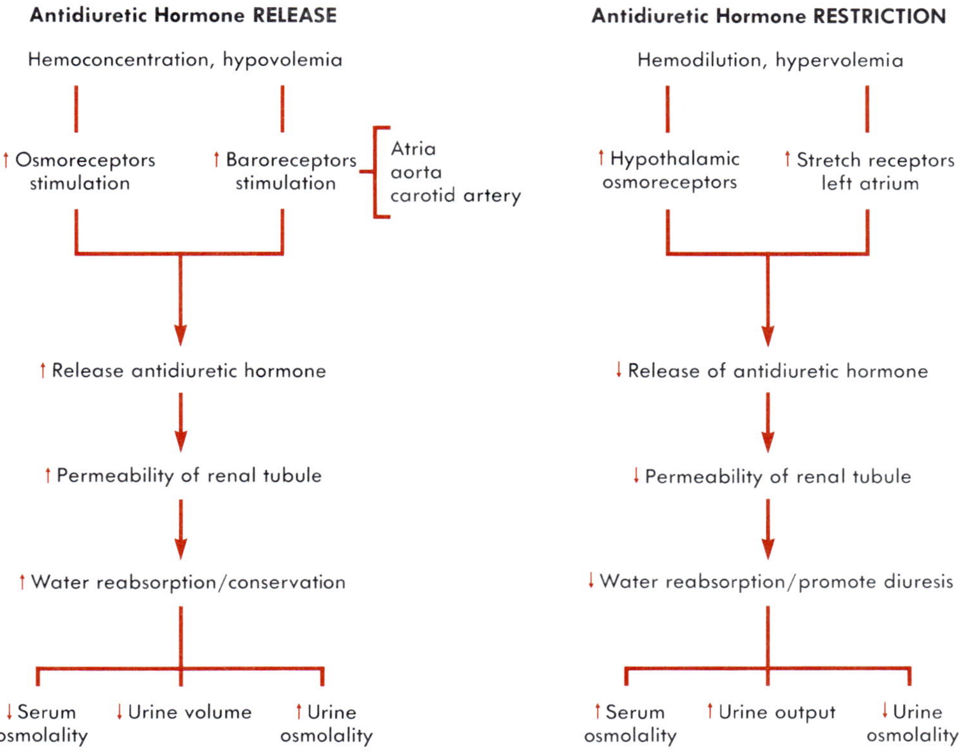


***Fig. 21-3*** Physiology of the release and restriction of antidiuretic hormone (ADH).

(ADH). Antidiuretic hormone normally stimulates the kidney tubules to reabsorb filtered water when the body needs to increase fluid stores. ADH stimulates the tubules to increase permeability to water when particles in the bloodstream increase in number (rising osmolality) or when blood pressure falls.[8] Figure 21-3 schematically presents the physiology of the release and restriction of antidiuretic hormone. Persons without adequately functioning antidiuretic hormone develop unrestricted serum hyperosmolality. An intense thirst and the passage of excessively large quantities of very dilute urine adds to the characteristics of the disease.

## Cause

Diabetes insipidus is categorized into three types according to cause: central diabetes insipidus, nephrogenic diabetes insipidus, and psychogenic diabetes insipidus (see the box on p. 388).[8,24,29] Central diabetes occurs when there is an interruption in the synthesis and release of antidiuretic hormone. It is further divided into primary and secondary categories. Primary DI occurs when structural abnormalities within the hypothalamus, infundibular stalk, and neurohypophysis prevent the release of ADH according to the body's inherent signals. Primary DI may result from an inherited familial disorder or from a neurohypophyseal system that fails to develop at birth. Primary DI may also be "idiopathic" or sporadic and occur without apparent cause.[2] Secondary diabetes insipidus occurs as a result of trauma to the neurohypophyseal functioning unit. Nephrogenic diabetes insipidus (NDI) results from the inability of the kidney nephrons to respond to circulating ADH. Psychogenic diabetes insipidus is a rare form of the disease that occurs with compulsive water drinking.

## Pathophysiology

ADH is the controlling force in the maintenance of fluid balance. Damage to the hypothalamus, infundibular stalk, or posterior pituitary can lead to a disruption in the normal neuroendocrine communication system, and resulting secretion of ADH.[8] (Fig. 21-4 is a diagram of the events postulated to occur with primary diabetes insipidus.)

A decreased amount of circulating ADH decreases the kidney tubules' reabsorption of water and leads to excessive water excretion in the urine. As free water is lost from the bloodstream, the serum osmolality rises and elevations in serum sodium stimulate the thirst receptors. Patients who are responsive and able will drink excessive amounts of water to relieve their thirst. This reduces the serum osmolality to a more normal level and prevents dehydration. The disease is debilitating. It interrupts all activities, including sleep, since the patient experiences extreme thirst and constant need to empty the urinary bladder.[22] If the patient is unable to replace lost fluids, severe extracellular dehydration will result.

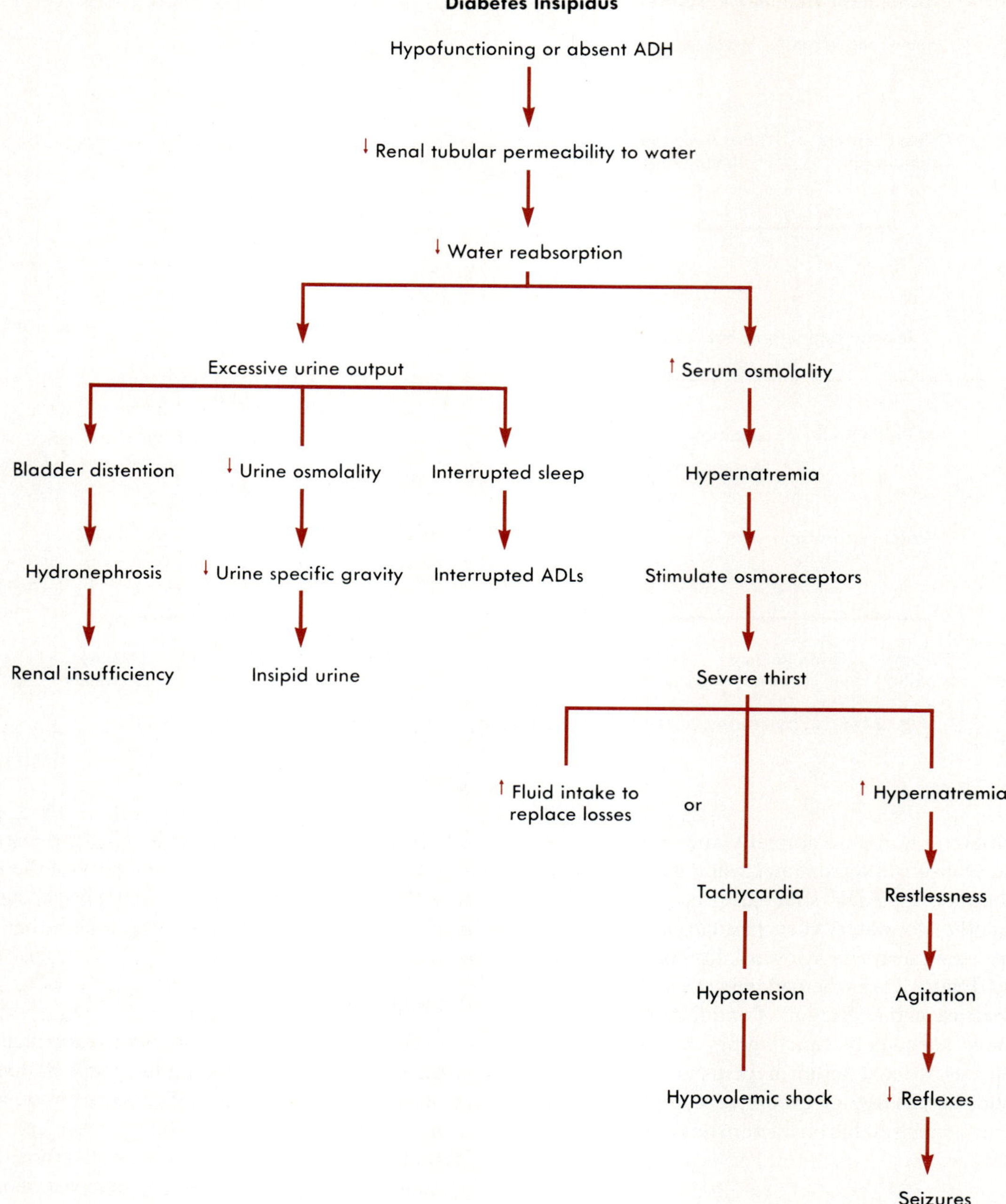


***Fig. 21-4*** Pathophysiology of diabetes insipidus (DI).

## Assessment and Diagnosis

Clinical manifestations of DI may develop gradually or may occur suddenly after head injury or other precipitating disease. Initially, urine production may exceed 300 ml/hour accompanied by an abnormally low urine osmolality.[21]

Diagnostic tests used to establish the presence of DI evaluate the body's innate ability to balance fluid and electrolytes. Although these tests are early markers for the disease, most are routinely performed and not specific to the endocrine system (see the box on p. 391). The tests done most frequently include a comparison of serum osmolality, urine osmolality, and serum sodium levels.[29]

Further tests are useful in differentiating DI according to cause. Using a water deprivation or dehydration test, the patient is deprived of fluids for a 24-hour period. During this time, urine and plasma osmolality measurements are taken. Adequate ADH functioning would maintain the plasma osmolality level within normal limits, while the urine osmolality level would increase to as high as 800 mOsm/L. Patients with ADH deficiency minimally concentrate the

### DIAGNOSTIC VALUES OF DIABETES INSIPIDUS

| | |
|---|---|
| Serum ADH | Decreased in primary DI, but may be normal if neurogenic or psychogenic |
| Serum osmolality | >300 mOsm/L |
| Serum sodium | >145 mEq/L |
| Urine osmolality | <300 mOsm/L |
| Urine specific gravity | <1.005 SI units |
| Urine output | 30-40 L/24 hours |
| Fluid intake | ≥50 L/24 hours |

urine following dehydration, while plasma osmolality level rises above 300 mOsm/kg and serum sodium >145 mEq/L.

Alternate tests may include quantitative analysis of serum antidiuretic hormone level. Absent or decreased levels of serum ADH in the presence of hyperosmolar serum and hypoosmolar urine would indicate primary and secondary ADH deficiency. Normal serum ADH levels (1 to 5 pg/ml or <1.5 mg/L)[7] accompanying clinical manifestations of diabetes insipidus may indicate nephrogenic diabetes insipidus (NDI) in which the kidney tubule is insensitive to ADH. Normal ADH levels with elevated blood osmolality and increased urine output may also suggest pharmacologically induced DI or excessive or compulsive water drinking. The ADH concentration level may be measured to differentiate the type of diabetes insipidus present. Exogenous ADH is given parenterally, after which urine and blood osmolality tests are recorded. Water retention and overhydration are risks with this test and it is contraindicated in patients with cardiac dysfunction.[24,29]

#### Treatment

Medical intervention is based on the underlying pathological conditions. When possible, treatment involves management of the primary diseased condition that is creating the interference in ADH circulation. Fluid replacement is provided in the initial phase of the treatment to prevent circulatory collapse. Patients who are able are given voluminous amounts of fluid orally to balance output. For those unable to take sufficient fluids orally, hypotonic intravenous solutions are rapidly infused and carefully monitored to restore the hemodynamic balance.

Medications have been used successfully to treat diabetes insipidus. Patients with primary and secondary DI who are unable to synthesize antidiuretic hormone require exogenous ADH replacement therapy.

One form of the hormone available for short-term substitution is aqueous, synthetic **Pitressin**. It is administered intramuscularly, subcutaneously, or applied topically to the nasal mucosa. Onset of antidiuresis is rapid and lasts up to 8 hours. Chronic DI may be treated with a more potent substitute. Pitressin Tannate is a pituitary extract in oil. The drug is given intramuscularly and never intravenously. The onset of antidiuresis is slow, with the peak activity occurring after 48 hours. The effects of this drug last for several days. Both drugs will constrict smooth muscle and can elevate systemic blood pressure. Water intoxication can also occur if the dose is higher than the therapeutic level.

Another drug for patients with mild forms of DI is a synthetic analogue of ADH, **desmopressin acetate** (DDAVP). It is administered parenterally or via the nasal mucosa (not inhaled). The drug has fewer side effects than other ADH preparations. It has minimal effects on the smooth muscle tissue and does not cause hypertension.[5]

Minute dosages of pituitary extract provide greater control of patient's fluid balance with minimal side effects. Recent trial studies have found that ultra-low doses of pituitrin (bovine posterior pituitary extract of combined oxytocin and vasopressin) have satisfactorily regulated urine output and promoted cardiovascular stability. The dosage is critically measured with a syringe pump to ensure the exact amount of the hormone for the patient's hydration status.[5]

Various drugs have been found that stimulate the production and release of endogenous antidiuretic hormone for patients who have ADH present, although in insufficient quantities. These drugs include carbamazepine, an anticonvulsive; clofibrate, a hypolipidemic; and chlorpropamide, an oral hypoglycemic agent.

Nephrogenic diabetes insipidus does not respond to hormonal replacement treatment or to administration of an anticonvulsive or hypolipidemic drug. However, chlorpropamide and tolbutamide have been found to be effective in increasing the responsiveness of the nephron site to circulating antidiuretic hormone. Trial studies have shown indomethacin, a nonsteroidal antiinflammatory, is therapeutic in the treatment of lithium-induced polyuria and polydipsia.[9] Certain thiazide diuretics are also used in the treatment of nephrogenic DI. It is not known why diabetes insipidus responds paradoxically to a thiazide diuretic.[22]

#### Summary of Nursing Care

While the basic nursing management of the patient with diabetes insipidus involves a continual, conscientious assessment of the patient's hydration status, diabetes insipidus may be complicated by the primary reason for which the patient was admitted to the critical care unit. Nursing care may then include management of several dysfunctioning systems. Nursing diagnoses and management related to DI are summarized in the box on p. 392.

Critical assessment and management of the patient's fluid status is the most important concern for the patient with DI. Intake and output measurement, condition of buccal membranes, skin turgor, daily weights, presence of thirst, and temperature form a basic assessment list that becomes paramount for the patient unable to regulate fluid needs and fluid lost. A hypotonic intravenous solution (to reduce the

**Nursing Diagnosis and Management**
***Diabetes insipidus***

- Fluid Volume Deficit related to decreased antidiuretic hormone secretion secondary to diabetes insipidus, p. 502
- Potential Impaired Skin Integrity risk factor: poor subcutaneous tissue perfusion, p. 499
- Potential Alteration in Peripheral Tissue Perfusion risk factor: vasopressor therapy (vasopressin), p. 462
- Anxiety related to threat to biological, psychological, and/or social integrity, p. 448
- Sensory-Perceptual Alterations related to sensory overload, sensory deprivation, and sleep pattern disturbance, p. 489

serum hyperosmolality) may be ordered to replace loss[39] plus 50 ml/hr to replace insensible losses.[38] Urine and blood should be simultaneously collected for osmolality studies. Bedside specific gravity analysis gives immediate information regarding variations in kidney tubules' reabsorption of water. If the patient has an indwelling Foley catheter, scrupulous asepsis is required to prevent a nosocomial infection as the closed system is repeatedly entered. Serum sodium and potassium levels are monitored and relayed to the physician as necessary.

Meticulous skin care is necessary to preserve skin integrity and prevent breakdown caused by dehydration. Alterations in elimination are frequently experienced by the patient with DI. Constipation results from fluid loss and, depending on the patient's status, is treated with dietary fiber and/or stool softeners. Diarrhea may accompany the abdominal cramping and intestinal hyperactivity associated with ADH drug therapy. Untoward effects are brought to the attention of the physician for dosage modification. Antidiuretic hormone replacement is accomplished with extreme caution in the patient with a history of cardiac disease, since vasopressin tannate may cause hypertension and overhydration. At the first signs of cardiovascular impairment, the drug is discontinued and fluid intake is restricted until urine-specific gravity is less than 1.015 and polyuria resumes.

The patient who is unable to satisfy sensations of thirst and who is unable to complete any task or self-care activity without the need to urinate is confused and frightened. For patients who are able to verbalize their fears, having someone who is interested and nonjudgmental may help reduce the emotional turmoil. The nurse must recognize the patient's reluctance to engage in any activity because of the polyuria. Having a bedpan or commode constantly in attendance will reduce anxiety for the alert patient.

Educating the patient and the family about the disease process and how it affects thirst, urination, and fluid balance will encourage patients to participate in their care and reduce the feelings of hopelessness. Patients who are discharged with the disease are taught, along with their families, the signs and symptoms of dehydration and overhydration. They are taught to correctly weigh themselves daily and to take urine-specific gravity measurements. Printed information pertaining to drug actions, side effects, dosages, and time table is given to the patient, as well as an outline of parameters that need to be reported to the physician.

## SYNDROME OF INAPPROPRIATE ANTIDIURETIC HORMONE

### Description

Opposite of diabetes insipidus is the **syndrome of inappropriate antidiuretic hormone** (SIADH). SIADH occurs when there is an increase in the release of the antidiuretic hormone. The excess antidiuretic hormone secreted in the bloodstream exceeds the amount needed to maintain blood volume and serum osmolality.

### Cause

There are many causes of SIADH, many of which are seen in patients who are critically ill.[6,12] Causes of SIADH are outlined in the box on p. 393.

### Pathophysiology

In SIADH, antidiuretic hormone continues to be released into the blood stream despite the feedback mechanism signaling a normal serum osmolality and blood volume (Fig. 21-5). Hypersecretion of ADH results in hyponatremia and hemodilution.

ADH release increases the kidney tubule reabsorption of water that in turn increases the circulating blood volume. Dilutional hyponatremia occurs as the expanded plasma volume dilutes the previously normal serum levels. The hyponatremia is further aggravated as aldosterone release (normally released to retain sodium at the tubules) is suppressed.[19] Serum hypoosmolality leads to a shift of fluid into the intracellular fluid compartment in an attempt to equalize osmotic pressure. Because there is minimal sodium present in this fluid, edema does not usually result. Without ADH and aldosterone, water is retained, urine output is diminished, and further sodium is excreted in the urine. Patients with the syndrome of inappropriate antidiuretic hormone usually excrete a urine that is more concentrated than would be expected for the corresponding concentration of blood.[8,29]

### Assessment and Diagnosis

The patient with SIADH becomes water intoxicated. The clinical manifestations of this condition are related to the

## POTENTIAL CAUSES OF SYNDROME OF INAPPROPRIATE ANTIDIURETIC HORMONE

**Malignant disease associated with autonomous production of ADH**

Bronchogenic oat cell carcinoma
Pancreatic adenocarcinoma
Duodenal, bladder, ureter, prostatic carcinomas
Lymphosarcoma, Ewing's sarcoma
Acute leukemia, Hodgkin's disease
Cerebral neoplasm, thymoma

**Central nervous system diseases that interfere with the hypothalamic-hypophyseal system and increase the production and/or release of ADH**

Head injury
Brain abscess
Hydrocephalus
Pituitary adenoma
Subdural hematoma
Subarachnoid hemorrhage
Cerebral atrophy
Guillain-Barré syndrome
Tuberculous meningitis
Purulent meningitis
Herpes simplex encephalitis
Acute intermittent porphyria

**Neurogenic stimuli capable of increasing ADH**

- Decreased glomerular filtration rate
- Physical and/or emotional stressors
  - Pain
  - Fear
  - Trauma
  - Surgery
  - MI
  - Acute infection
  - Hypotension
  - Hemorrhage
  - Hypovolemia

**Pulmonary diseases believed to stimulate the baroreceptors and increase ADH**

Pulmonary tuberculosis
Viral and bacterial pneumonia
Empyema
Lung abscess
Chronic obstructive lung disease
Status asthmaticus
Cystic fibrosis

**Endocrine disturbances that hormonally influence ADH**

Myxedema
Hypothyroidism
Hypopituitarism
Adrenal insufficiency—Addison's disease

**Medications that mimic, increase the release of, or potentiate ADH**

- Hypoglycemics
  - Insulin
  - Tolbutamide
  - Chlorpropamide
- Potassium-depleting thiazide diuretics
- Tricyclic antidepressants
  - Imipramine
  - Amitriptyline
- Phenothiazine
  - Fluphenazine
  - Thioridazine
- Thioxanthenes
  - Thiothixene
  - Chlorprothixene
- Chemotherapeutic agents
  - Vincristine
  - Cyclophosphamide
- Narcotics
- Carbamazepine
- Clofibrate
- Acetaminophen
- Nicotine
- Oxytocin
- Vasopressin
- Anesthetics

excess fluid in the extracellular compartment and the proportionate dilution of the circulating sodium. Although edema is not usually present, there may be slight weight gain from the expanded extracellular fluid volume.

Hyponatremia may initially be asymptomatic. Early signs and symptoms of dilutional hyponatremia include lethargy, anorexia, nausea, and vomiting. As the water and sodium imbalance progresses, neurological signs of hyponatremia predominate. Inability to concentrate, mental confusion, apprehension, and seizures may progress to loss of consciousness and death.

The medical diagnosis is based on various factors.[36,41] Primary disorders (oat cell carcinoma, CNS disturbance), clinical manifestations, and laboratory tests provide data to substantiate SIADH. Laboratory values are listed in the box on p. 394.

To confirm the diagnosis, a water load test is done. After a period of fasting, a dehydrated patient is overhydrated

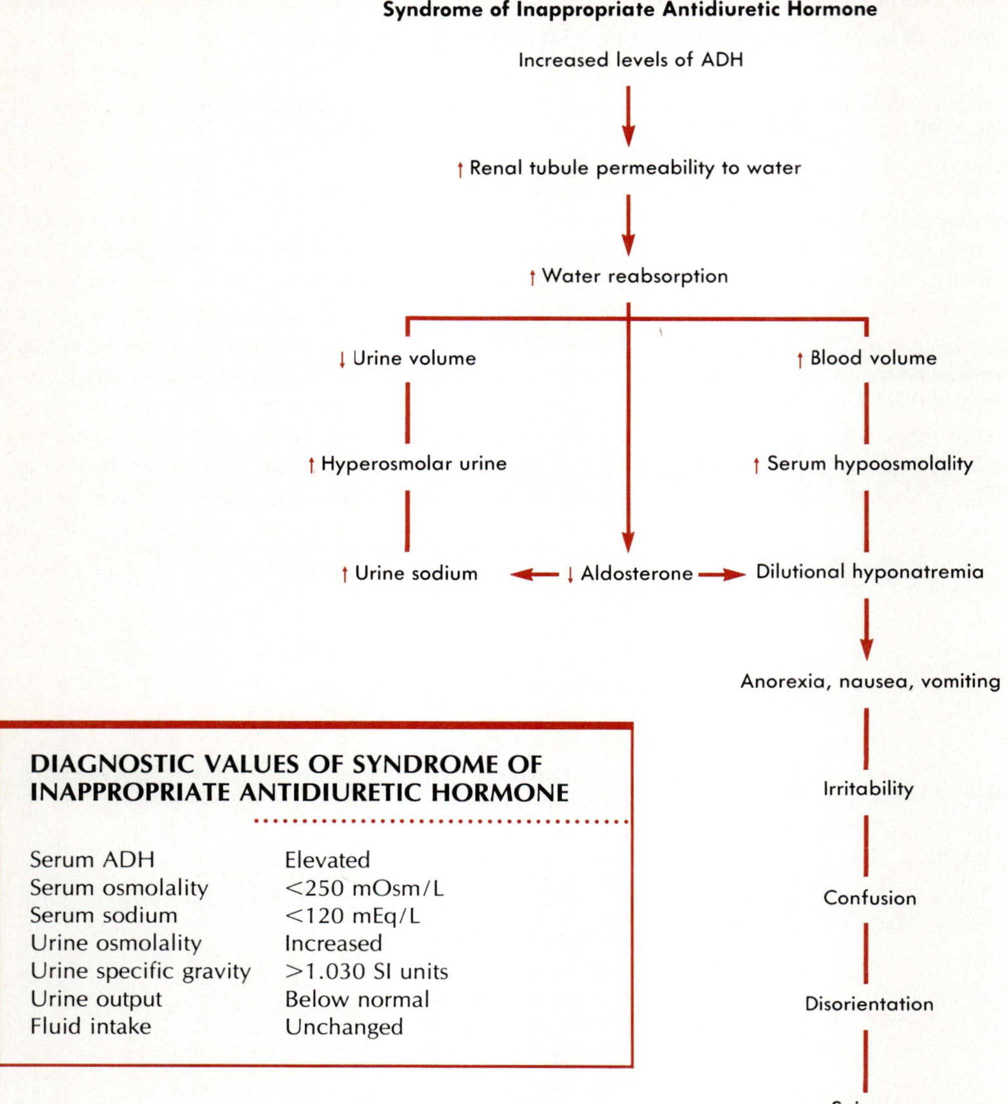


**DIAGNOSTIC VALUES OF SYNDROME OF INAPPROPRIATE ANTIDIURETIC HORMONE**

| | |
|---|---|
| Serum ADH | Elevated |
| Serum osmolality | <250 mOsm/L |
| Serum sodium | <120 mEq/L |
| Urine osmolality | Increased |
| Urine specific gravity | >1.030 SI units |
| Urine output | Below normal |
| Fluid intake | Unchanged |

***Fig. 21-5*** Pathophysiology of syndrome of inappropriate antidiuretic hormone (SIADH).

with water. The urine output and serum osmolality level are carefully monitored to discover a decline in serum osmolality level resulting from peak moments of overhydration. Patients with SIADH show a decrease in serum osmolality level regardless of the fasting state and an inability to secrete dilute urine despite the hydration resulting from the water load.[7]

### Treatment

In the critical care unit, SIADH often occurs as a secondary disease. Ideally, recognition and treatment of the primary disease will reduce the production of ADH. If the patient is receiving any of the chemical agents suspected of causing the disease, discontinuing the drug, if possible, may return ADH levels to normal. The medical therapy that is the most successful (along with treatment of the primary disease) is simple reduction of fluid intake[36] to less than 1000 ml/day.[43] Patients with severe hyponatremia <115 mEq/L or those with seizures are infused with 3% to 5% hypertonic saline[42] for rapid but temporary correction of the hemodilution caused by the retention of fluid at the tubules and severe sodium loss. Furosemide is added to further increase the diuresis and prevent risk of pulmonary edema related to the hypertonic saline solution. Hypertonic saline solution is administered very slowly and with extreme caution (0.1 mg/kg/min) until the patient's serum sodium level is increased to 125 mEq/L.[42] Treatment with a hypertonic solution is temporary, as the sodium is continuously removed from the body through the urine.

Narcotic agonists such as oxilorphan and butorphanol

reduce the secretion of ADH in many patients with SIADH. However, the drugs do not seem to be effective in patients with SIADH caused by lung malignancies. Patients with lung malignancies are treated with demeclocycline hydrochloride, an antibacterial tetracycline, and lithium carbonate, an alkali metal salt primarily used to alter psychogenic behavior. These drugs inhibit the tubule response to ADH and decrease the water reabsorption at the tubules.[3]

### Summary of Nursing Care

Thorough, astute nursing assessments are required for care of the patient with SIADH while attempting to correct the fluid and sodium imbalance: the systemic effects of hyponatremia occur rapidly and can be lethal. Evaluation of the patient's neurological status, especially level of consciousness, is done every 1 to 2 hours. Seizure precautions for the patient with SIADH are provided regardless of the degree of hyponatremia. Assessment of the patient's hydration status is frequently monitored with serial assessment of urine output, blood and urine sodium, urine-specific gravity, and urine and blood osmolality levels. Elimination patterns are assessed since constipation may occur when fluids are restricted.

Accurate measurement of intake and output is required to calculate fluid replacement for the patient with excessive antidiuretic hormone. All fluids are restricted as ordered, providing only a sufficient intake to equal urine output. Frequent mouth care may provide comfort during the period of fluid restriction through moistening the buccal membrane. Weights may be taken every 12 hours to gauge fluid retention or loss. Hemodynamic monitoring, including blood pressure, central venous pressure, and pulmonary arterial wedge pressures, are performed frequently to assess for fluid overload (refer to the box below).

Hypertonic saline is infused very cautiously. A volumetric pump is used to deliver 0.1 mg/kg/min[42] or set to deliver a flow rate determined by the serum sodium levels. The saline infusion is usually discontinued when the patient's serum sodium levels reach 125 mEq/L. The hypertonic solution is discontinued if signs or symptoms of bounding pulse, increased thirst (to replace depleted cellular fluid), hand vein emptying longer than 5 seconds when the hand is elevated, coupled with increased serum sodium levels, occur.

Signs and symptoms of congestive heart failure and pulmonary edema such as elevated blood pressure, PAWP, or CVP are also causes to discontinue the hypertonic saline infusion. Apprehension, abrupt position changes to an upright position to breathe, dyspnea, moist cough, and increased respiratory and heart rates also indicate the inability of the cardiopulmonary system to accommodate the increased fluid load.

An alteration in bowel elimination resulting in constipation may occur from decreased fluid intake and inactivity. Cathartics or low volume hypertonic enemas may be given to stimulate peristalsis. Tap water or hypotonic enemas should *not* be given, because the water in the enema solution may be absorbed through the bowel and potentiate water intoxication.

Rapidly occurring changes in the patient's neurological status may frighten visiting family members. Sensitivity to the family's unspoken fears can be shown by words of empathy and providing time for the patient and family to express their feelings. The nurse should discuss the course of the disease and its affect on water balance with the patient and family. The nurse should also explain the fluid restrictions and the family's role in treating SIADH. Teaching the patient and the family to measure the intake and output will encourage independence and instill a sense of usefulness.

**Nursing Diagnosis and Management**

***Syndrome of inappropriate antidiuretic hormone (SIADH)***

- Fluid Volume Excess related to increased antidiuretic hormone secretion secondary to SIADH, p. 501

#### REFERENCES


1. Braundwald E and others, editors: Harrison's principles of internal medicine, ed 11, New York, 1987, McGraw-Hill Book Co.
2. Bullock B and Rosendahl P: Pathophysiology, adaptations and alterations in function, ed 2, Glenview, Illinois, 1988, Scott Foresman & Company/Little, Brown College Division.
3. Burch W: Endocrinology, ed 2, Baltimore, 1988, Williams & Wilkins.
4. Butts D: Fluid and electrolyte disorders associated with diabetic ketoacidosis and hyperglycemic hyperosmolar nonketotic coma, Nurs Clin North Am 22(4):827, 1987.
5. Chanson P and others: Ultra-low doses of vasopressin in the management of diabetes insipidus, Crit Care Med 15(1):44, 1987.
6. DeGroot L: Endocrinology, ed 2, Philadelphia, 1989, WB Saunders Co.
7. Fischbach F: A manual of laboratory diagnostic tests, ed 3, Philadelphia, 1988, JB Lippincott Co.
8. Germon K: Fluid and electrolyte problems associated with diabetes insipidus and syndrome of inappropriate antidiuretic hormone, Nurs Clin North Am 22(4):785, 1987.
9. Grindlinger G and Boylan M: Amelioration by indomethacin of lithium-induced polyuria, Crit Care Med 15(5):538, 1987.
10. Guyton A: Textbook of medical physiology, ed 7, Philadelphia, 1986, WB Saunders Co.
11. Hadley M: Endocrinology, ed 2, Englewood Cliffs, NJ, 1988, Prentice-Hall.
12. Hall R and Evered D: Color atlas of endocrinology, ed 2, St Louis, 1990, Mosby–Year Book, Inc.
13. Harris M and Hamman R, editors: Diabetes in America, Bethesda, Md, 1985, US Department of Health and Human Services, Public Health Service, National Institutes of Health, National Institute of Arthritis, Diabetes and Digestive and Kidney Diseases.
14. Hemmer M and others: Urinary ADH excretion during mechanical ventilation and weaning in man, Anesthesiology 52(5):395, 1980.
15. Henry J, editor: Todd, Sanford, Davidsohn, clinical diagnosis and management by laboratory methods, ed 17, Philadelphia, 1984, WB Saunders Co.
16. Hollinshead W and Rosse C: Textbook of anatomy, ed 4, Philadelphia, 1985, Harper & Row, Publishers.

17. Hudak C: Critical care nursing: a holistic approach, Philadelphia, 1990, JB Lippincott Co.
18. Kirby R: Pocket companion of critical care: immediate concerns, Philadelphia, 1990, JB Lippincott Co.
19. Kohler P, editor: Clinical endocrinology, New York, 1986, John Wiley & Sons.
20. Krall L and others: Joslin's diabetes mellitus, ed 12, Philadelphia, 1988, Lea & Febiger.
21. Lubin M and others, editors: Medical management of the surgical patient, Boston, 1988, Butterworths.
22. Martin C: Endocrine physiology, New York, 1985, Oxford University Press.
23. McEvoy G, McQuarrie G, and DiPietro J, editors: Drug information '87, Bethesda, Md, 1987, American Society of Hospital Pharmacists.
24. Mercer M: Myths & facts . . . about diabetes insipidus, Nursing 90, 20(5):20, 1990.
25. Methany N and Snively WD: Nurse's handbook of fluid balance, ed 4, Philadelphia, 1983, JB Lippincott Co.
26. Nerozzi D, Goodwin F, and Costa E, editors: Neuropsychiatric disorders, New York, 1987, Raven Press.
27. Newman R: Bedside blood sugar determinations in the critically ill, Heart Lung 17(6):667, 1988.
28. Nikas D: Critical aspects of head trauma, Crit Care Nurs Q 10(1):19, 1987.
29. Patterson L and Noroian E: Diabetes insipidus versus syndrome of inappropriate antidiuretic hormone, Dimens Crit Care Nurs 8(4):226, 1989.
30. Polak J and Bloom S: Endocrine tumours, the pathobiology of regulatory peptide-producing tumours, London, 1985, Churchill Livingstone.
31. Potgieter P: Inappropriate ADH secretion in tetanus, Crit Care Med 11(6):417, 1983.
32. Powers M: Handbook of diabetes nutritional management, Rockville, Md, 1987, Aspen Publishers.
33. Rudy E: Magnetic resonance imaging, new horizon in diagnostic technique, J Neurosurg Nurs 17(6):331, 1985.
34. Sabo C and others: Diabetic ketoacidosis: pathophysiology, nursing diagnoses and interventions, Focus Crit Care 16(1):21, 1989.
35. Schroeder S: Current medical dianoses and treatment, Norwalk, Conn, 1989, Appleton & Lange.
36. Schroeder S, Krupp M, and Tierney L: Current medical diagnosis and treatment, 1988, Norwalk, Conn, 1988, Appleton & Lange.
37. Slaunwhite R: Fundamentals of endocrinology, New York, 1988, Marcel Dekker, Inc.
38. Staller A: Systemic effects of severe head trauma, Crit Care Nurs Q 10(1):58, 1987.
39. Swearingen P and Keen JH: Manual of critical care: applying nursing diagnosis to adult critical illness, ed 2, St Louis, 1991, Mosby–Year Book, Inc.
40. Tepperman J and Tepperman H: Metabolic and endocrine physiology, ed 5, Chicago, 1987, Mosby–Year Book, Inc.
41. Tobin M: Essentials of critical care medicine, New York, 1989, Churchill.
42. Vokes T and Robertson G: Disorders of antidiuretic hormone, Endocrinol Metab Clin North Am 17(2):281, 1988.
43. Williams C: Lung cancer, Oxford, New York, 1984, Oxford University Press.
44. Yeates S and Blaufuss J: Managing the patient in diabetic ketoacidosis, Focus Crit Care 17(6):240, 1990.

UNIT IX

# MULTISYSTEM ALTERATIONS

CHAPTER 22

# Trauma

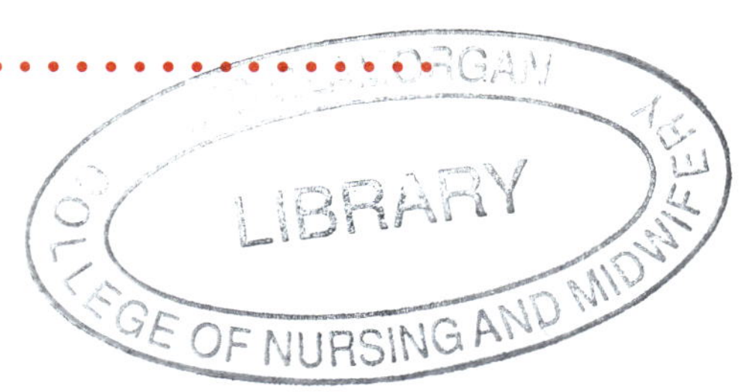


## CHAPTER OBJECTIVES

- *Compare and contrast the current methodologies of trauma patient classification systems.*
- *Plan a systematic approach to the physical assessment of and intervention for trauma patients, using primary and secondary surveys.*
- *Discuss the mechanisms of injury for head trauma and spinal cord trauma.*
- *Describe the pathophysiology of epidural, subdural, and intracerebral hematomas.*
- *State the difference between complete and incomplete injury in spinal cord trauma.*
- *Discuss common abdominal injuries.*
- *Differentiate between immediately life-threatening thoracic injuries and potential life-threatening thoracic injuries.*

## KEY TERMS

Anatomical Injury Scale (AIS), p. 401
Trauma Score, p. 401
concussion, p. 402
contusion, p. 403
epidural hematoma, p. 403
subdural hematoma, p. 404
missile injuries, p. 404
open pneumothorax, p. 407
flail chest, p. 407
pulmonary contusion, p. 407
peritoneal lavage, p. 408
complete injury of the spinal cord, p. 410
Brown-Sequard syndrome, p. 410
spinal shock, p. 411
neurogenic shock, p. 411

Trauma care in the twentieth century advanced through the work of George Crile,[15] who was involved in the study of hemorrhagic shock. During World War I the time lapse between injury and surgery averaged 12 to 18 hours, with a mortality rate of 8.5%. This time lapse was decreased by 33% in World War II, and the decrease was reflected by a 5.8% mortality rate. Over the 10-year period of the United States involvement in Vietnam, the time from injury to definitive care was reduced to a mere 65 minutes, reducing mortality to 1.7%. This "golden hour of trauma" remains a standard for acute resuscitation. The 60-minute time frame incorporates activation of the emergency medical system, stabilization and transportation in the prehospital setting, and rapid resuscitation on arrival in the emergency department. Thus getting the *right patient* to the *right facility* at the *right time* is essential in combating impairments in circulation and respiration.[6,35]

## RESUSCITATION PRIORITIES

The patient suffering multiple injuries requires an aggressive, predetermined approach to treatment. The American College of Surgeons (ACS) has developed programs such as the Advanced Trauma Life Support Course (ATLS) to address the need for rapid assessment. A similar nursing model, the Trauma Nurse Core Course (TNCC), has been introduced by the Emergency Nurses Association (ENA). Other programs include the Basic Trauma Life Support Course (BTLS) and the Prehospital Trauma Life Support Course (PHTLS). All of these programs emphasize the need for a systematized approach to the assessment and resuscitation of the multiple trauma patient.

Fortunately, only 10% to 20% of all injuries are classified as immediately or potentially life-threatening injuries.[12] Using the assessment techniques taught in the trauma programs, the practitioner can rapidly assess for the presence of these injuries, using the primary survey, secondary survey, and resuscitation and management.

### Primary Survey

The primary survey includes the following hallmarks of assessment: the *ABCs*—A, Airway; B, Breathing; C, Circulation *and* Cervical spine immobilization; plus *D* and *E*—D, Disability (minineurological examination); E, Exposure (removal of clothes).

**Airway.** During this preliminary survey, airway patency and mode of oxygen delivery are evaluated. The most common form of obstruction is caused by the tongue, followed in descending order by blood, teeth, vomitus, and foreign objects. If there is loss of consciousness, intubation should strongly be considered for airway maintenance. Patients who have suffered massive facial injuries or fractures of the facial bones and who require airway protection should undergo cricothyroidotomy. Likewise, the conscious patient or the patient with suspected or proven midface or basilar skull fracture should *not* have nasotracheal intubation attempted. Because of possible disruption of the cribriform plate, *any* nasally placed tube can penetrate the intracranial contents.[1]

**Breathing.** Respiratory rate and quality should be recorded and continually assessed. Supplemental oxygenation should be used in all trauma patients, since aerobic metabolism is dependent on saturation of hemoglobin with oxygen. "Supersaturation" with supplemental oxygen may be necessary for the patient with hemorrhage.

**Circulation.** During the primary survey the systemic blood pressure can be rapidly evaluated by using the *80-70-60* method. If a radial pulse is palpable, the minimal systolic pressure is 80 mm Hg. A systolic pressure of 70 mm Hg should be present with a carotid pulse and a systolic pressure of 60 mm Hg with a femoral pulse.[28,29] Capillary refill should be determined, as should skin temperature and pulse quality.[28,29] Capillary refill time greater than 3 seconds indicates that the capillary beds are not receiving adequate circulation.

Cardiac monitoring should also be initiated to detect rhythm disturbances. Placement of large-bore catheters (14 to 16 gauge) should be used for IV access. Primary peripheral access should be at a level above the diaphragm (upper extremities). Central venous access should be used as a secondary site in most instances. Restoration of volume can be accomplished through administration of crystalloid (lactated Ringer's solution or 0.9% saline solution), colloid (plasma or albumin), and/or blood products. Using the pneumatic antishock garment should be considered.

**Disability.** After the ABCs have been assessed, a brief neurological assessment should be performed. It is designed as a brief assessment of level of consciousness (LOC) only. During the secondary survey a more detailed assessment is emphasized; during the primary survey, time is essential. By using the AVPU mnemonic, which was devised by the American College of Surgeons,[1] confusing terminology can be avoided:

A, Alert
V, Verbal
P, Pain
U, Unresponsive

Once venous access and laboratory specimens are obtained, 50% dextrose, thiamine, and naloxone can be administered to reverse metabolic causes of depressed mental status. When preparing the site for venous access, isopropyl alcohol preparations interfere with the serum ethanol results. A povidone-iodine solution is recommended to prevent this occurrence.

**Exposure.** All clothing should be removed from the trauma patient as quickly as possible, and all body surfaces should be inspected for the presence of injury. Once the clothes have been cut down the center of both legs and arms, the patient can be logrolled (while cervical spine immobilization is maintained through in-line cervical traction), and his or her undersurface can be inspected and the clothing and all jewelry removed.

### Secondary Survey

A more detailed head-to-toe assessment is performed after the primary survey. During the secondary survey, adjuncts such as 12-lead electrocardiography (ECG); cervical spine, thoracic, and pelvic radiographs; arterial blood gas determination; contrast-enhanced radiography; and diagnostic peritoneal lavage can be used. The history is one of the most important aspects of the secondary survey. The prehospital providers (paramedics, emergency medical technicians [EMTs], first responders) can usually provide most of the vital information pertaining to the accident. It is suggested that a member of the trauma team (nurse, physician, or both) should meet the transporting vessel and help "unload" the patient. While this is being performed, a thorough description of the accident scene can be obtained. The first question that should be answered relates to the mechanism of injury—is it *blunt* or *penetrating?* If a penetrating mechanism is responsible for the injury, the following issues should be addressed:

- Weapon used (handgun, shotgun, rifle, knife)
- Caliber of weapon (if known and applicable)
- Number of shots fired (if applicable)
- Gender of assailant (if known)
- Position of victim and assailant when injury occurred

If the injury mechanism is blunt, the following should be addressed:

- Length of fall (greater than or equal to 15 feet)
- Temperature extremes (hot or cold)
- Motor vehicle accident (MVA) extrication time
- Passenger compartment intrusion (in MVA)
- Ejection
- Location in automobile (passenger, driver; frontseat, backseat)
- Restraint status (lapbelt, shoulder harness, lapbelt–shoulder harness combination, unrestrained)
- Speed of involved automobile(s)
- Occupants (number of and morbidity status)
- Amount of external damage
- Amount of internal damage
- Speed of automobile if pedestrian accident

The AMPLE mnemonic, developed by Freeark and Baker of the Cook County Hospital in Chicago, is a quick, dependable method of obtaining the patient's history[11]:

A, Allergies
M, Medications (current)
P, Past illness and surgeries
L, Last meal/Loss of Consciousness
E, Events preceding the accident

## DIAGNOSTIC STUDIES

Treatment should not be delayed for the sole purpose of obtaining specimens for laboratory analysis. For medicolegal purposes, serum ethanol and toxicology screening cannot not be randomly performed without patient consent. In some institutions, serum ethanol screening is performed on all trauma admissions; to prevent "selection bias" and its possible legal implications, ethanol levels must be determined on *all* admissions. In settings in which determination of serum ethanol levels cannot be rapidly obtained, the formula described by Unkle, Clements, and Ross[36] ($-1.055 + 0.00365 \times$ Serum *osmolality* = *Ethanol*) can used to predict accurate ethanol levels.

The multiple trauma patient should have the following laboratory studies performed:

1. Complete blood count (CBC) with differential
2. Serum electrolyte profile to include sodium, potassium, chloride, carbon dioxide, glucose, urea nitrogen, and creatinine levels
3. Platelet count
4. Coagulation parameters (prothrombin time, partial thromboplastin time)
5. Type and screen (ABO compatibility)
6. Urinalysis with microscopic examination
7. Serum amylase level
8. Serum osmolality level
9. Serum ethanol level
10. Liver function study (serum glutamic-pyruvic transaminase [SGPT] level)

### Radiographic Studies

Radiological examination of the trauma patient is a tertiary concern, following the subjective response and objective physical assessment. Only after these two phases have been completed can other diagnostic tools be used. In all patients with traumatic injury, one should automatically assume that the cervical spine is injured until proven otherwise. For the cervical spine to be considered "cleared," or without anatomical injury, it should be evaluated from the following three radiological views: (1) cross-table lateral, (2) opened-mouth odontoid, and (3) anterior-posterior (A-P).

The next series of films that should be obtained are either the supine pelvis or the upright chest view. Points can be made for choosing either first, since they both detect life-threatening injury. If pelvic fracture is suspected and the patient is hemodynamically stable, it has been suggested that the pelvis view be chosen first. Unstable bony fragments can worsen or initiate arterial and venous hemorrhage. The upright chest film should be the first view taken of the chest. Mediastinal widening greater than 8 cm indicates great vessel injury and can be appropriately demonstrated in this view. Should a supine chest view be chosen, a false-positive mediastinal widening will be seen in the majority of cases.

After the above-mentioned views have been obtained, the following studies may be performed: contrast enhanced CT, arteriography or angiography, IV pyelography, retrograde cystogram, or plain film examination of extremities or other injury sites.

## PATIENT CLASSIFICATION

Numerous clinical methods for patient classification are in existence today. For purposes of this chapter, the tools that are pertinent to the trauma population are discussed. The described methodology has many implications in the acute setting: triage of patients, standardization of injury, and prediction of morbidity and mortality. The reader is encouraged to refer to the references for a more extensive review of these tools.

### Anatomical Injury Scale (AIS)

Both the **Anatomical Injury Scale (AIS)**[26] and its spinoff, the Injury Severity Score (ISS),[27] have been recognized as indicators of the magnitude of traumatic injury and as predictors of mortality. The AIS divides the body into six anatomical regions: head/neck, face, thorax, abdomen, extremities, and external (integumentary). Injuries are classified on a sliding scale, with 1 a minor injury and 5 a critical injury with survival uncertain. The anatomical regions with the three highest scores are then squared. The sum is considered the ISS. An injury that is classified as *non-survivable* is assigned an AIS = 6, with an automatic score of 75.

### Trauma Score

The **Trauma Score** devised by Champion and associates[6] (Table 22-1) is a physiological method of categorizing the multiple trauma patient. It incorporates the Glasgow Coma Scale (GCS), as well as the variables of respiration and circulation. The ranges of the Trauma Score are from a high of 16 and to low of 1. The probability of survival can be estimated using the Trauma Score. Other tools such as the Trauma Index[21] have proven less accurate as predictors of injury severity and are used infrequently.

## CEREBRAL TRAUMA

Injuries of the brain are described by the functional changes or losses that occur. Some of the major functional abnormalities seen in head injury will be described in the following section.

***Table 22-1*** Trauma score

| Category | Value | Points |
|---|---|---|
| A. Respiratory rate | 10-24 | 4 |
| | 25-35 | 3 |
| | >35 | 2 |
| | <10 | 1 |
| | 0 | 0 |
| B. Respiratory effort | Normal | 1 |
| | Shallow or absent | 0 |
| C. Systolic blood pressure | 90 | 4 |
| | 70-90 | 3 |
| | 50-69 | 2 |
| | <50 | 1 |
| | 0 | 0 |
| D. Capillary refill | Normal | 2 |
| | Delayed | 1 |
| | None | 0 |
| E. Glasgow Coma Scale (GCS) | | |
| 1. Eye opening | Spontaneous | 4 |
| | To voice | 3 |
| | To pain | 2 |
| | None | 1 |
| 2. Verbal response | Oriented | 5 |
| | Confused | 4 |
| | Inappropriate words | 3 |
| | Incomprehensible words | 2 |
| | None | 1 |
| 3. Motor response | Obeys commands | 6 |
| | Purposeful movement (pain) | 5 |
| | Withdrawal (pain) | 4 |
| | Flexion (pain) | 3 |
| | Extension (pain) | 2 |
| | None | 1 |
| **Total GCS points** | **Score** | |
| 14-15 | 5 | |
| 11-13 | 4 | |
| 8-10 | 3 | |
| 5-7 | 2 | |
| 3-4 | 1 | |
| TOTAL GCS POINTS ______ (1 + 2 + 3) | TRAUMA SCORE ______ (TOTAL POINTS = A + B + C + D + E) | |

Modified from Champion HR and others: Crit Care Med 9:672, 1981.

## Concussion

A **concussion** is a mild form of diffuse brain injury, occurring as the consequence of the acceleration-deceleration and rotational motion of the head. They are associated with a global disruption but have no macroscopically visible lesion.

A concussion syndrome involves a temporary reversible disturbance of neurological function with or without loss of consciousness. If loss of consciousness occurs, it may last for seconds to an hour. The neurological dysfunctions present as confusion, disorientation, and sometimes a period of posttraumatic amnesia.

Other symptoms seen after concussion are headache, dizziness, irritability, inability to concentrate, impaired memory, and fatigue.[14] A few patients develop postconcussion syndrome and continue to complain of the headaches, dizziness, inability to concentrate, and memory difficulties for

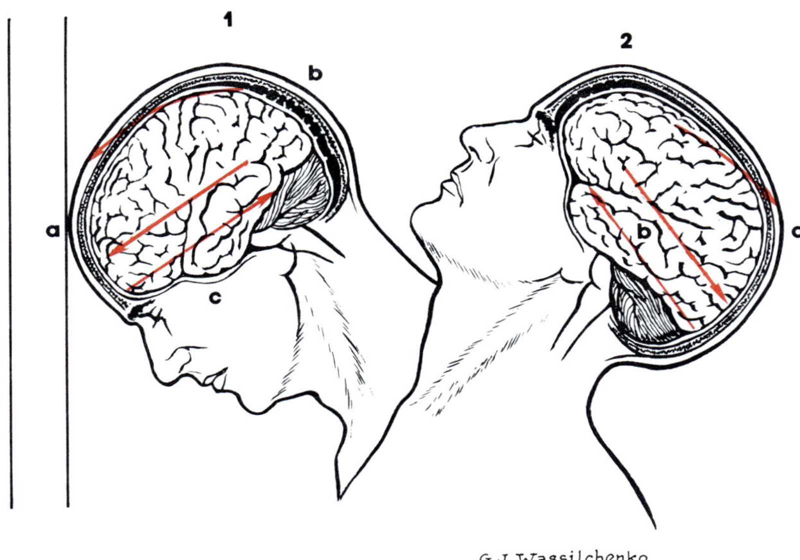


***Fig. 22-1*** Coup and contrecoup head injury following blunt trauma. *1,* Coup injury: impact against object. *a,* Site of impact and direct trauma to brain; *b,* Shearing of subdural veins; *c,* Trauma to base of brain. *2,* Contrecoup injury: impact within skull. *a,* Site of impact from brain hitting opposite side of skull; *b,* Shearing forces throughout brain. These injuries occur in one continuous motion—the head strikes the wall (coup), then rebounds (contrecoup).

more than a year. This indicates that a concussion may not be as benign an injury as previously believed.

### Contusion

Cerebral **contusion** is the most frequently encountered lesion of all head injuries.[16] Cerebral contusion is described as bruising of the brain without puncture or tearing of the *pia membrane*. The "bruised" area is made up of edematous cells of the gray matter with petechiae or hemorrhage as well as necrosis. Underlying white matter is affected to a varying degree depending on the severity of the contusion. Contusion occurs from the absorption of energy into the cerebral tissue upon impact. Two forms of lesions are noted (Fig. 22-1). *Coup injury* is injury to the cerebral tissue directly under the point of impact. *Contrecoup injury* is distant from the site of impace and occurs because of the motion of the cerebral contents inside the skull.

The signs and symptoms of contusion are related to the location and degree of the contusion and the presence of other associated lesions. Contusions can be small, localized areas of dysfunction resulting in a focal neurological deficit, or they can be larger, in which case over 2 to 3 days following the impact injury the area increases in size as a result of edema and further hemorrhages. This large contusion produces a mass effect that causes significant increases in ICP.

Diagnosis of contusion is made by CT scan. If the CT scan indicates contusion, especially in the temporal area, the nurse must pay particular attention to neurological assessment and look for subtle changes in pupillary signs or vital signs irrespective of a stable ICP.

Treatment of cerebral contusion is controversial. Since contusion continues to progress over 3 to 5 days after the primary injury, contusions—particularly large ones—can be a significant factor in secondary injury. If contusions are small, focal, or multiple, they are treated medically with serial assessments and ICP monitoring. Larger contusions that produce considerable mass effect are surgically removed early to prevent the increased edema and intracranial pressure found as contusion matures.[38]

### Hematomas

Hematomas resulting from head injury form a mass lesion and lead to increased intracranial pressure. Three types of hematomas will be discussed here (Fig. 22-2).

**Epidural hematoma. Epidural hematoma** (EDH) is a collection of blood between the inner table of the skull and the outermost layer of the dura. Epidural hematoma is frequently associated with injury to the middle meningeal artery. A blow to the head that causes a linear skull fracture on the lateral surface of the head may tear the middle meningeal artery. As the artery bleeds, it pulls the dura away from the skull, creating a pouch that expands into the intracranial space.

EDH may occur as a result of low-impact injuries such as falls or high-impact injuries such as motor vehicle accidents. EDH occurs from trauma to the skull and meninges, not the acceleration-deceleration forces seen in other head

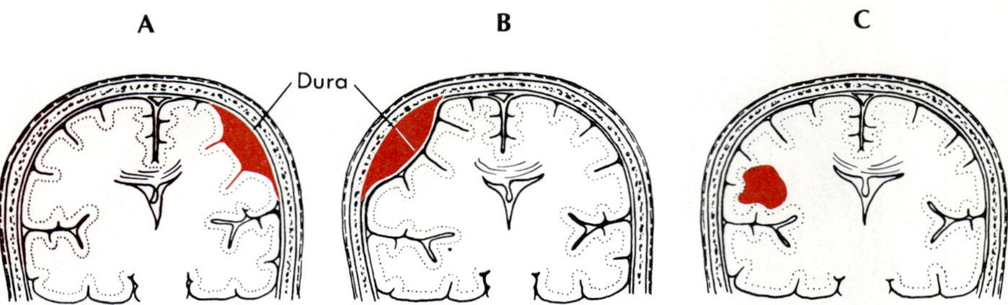


*Fig. 22-2* Different types of hematomas. **A,** Subdural hematoma. **B,** Epidural hematoma. **C,** Intracerebral hematoma.

trauma. Patients with EDH make up a significant percentage of the "talk and die" or "talk and deteriorate" population. These groups are composed of patients whose primary injury was not severe enough to disrupt cerebral functioning but with time and the development of secondary injury may deteriorate or die.[23]

The "classic" signs and symptoms of a patient with EDH include brief loss of consciousness at time of impact followed by a period of lucidity that may last up to 12 hours. This lucid period is followed by rapid deterioration in neurological status from confusion to coma, with changes in pupillary reaction and onset of decerebrate or decorticate posturing. These are all signs of herniation. Rapid neurological intervention is required to save the patient's life.

Diagnosis of EDH is based on clinical symptoms and evidence of a collection of epidural blood identified on CT scan. Treatment of EDH involves surgical intervention to remove the blood and cauterize the bleeding vessels.

**Subdural hematoma. Subdural hematoma** (SDH) is the accumulation of blood between the dura and arachnoid membrane in the subdural space. Most subdural hematomas occur over the surface of the brain and result from the tearing of the bridging veins between the brain and the dura. The acceleration-deceleration and rotational forces associated with trauma are the major causes for SDH development. Subdural hematoma is often associated with underlying cerebral contusion as a result of the nature of the impact injury. Outcome or recovery after SDH is lower than that after EDH because of the increased forces and motion of the brain involved in all types of SDH except those that are chronic.

There are three types of SDH based on the timeframe during which symptoms are first identified. The three categories are acute, subacute, and chronic. Acute subdural hematomas are those hematomas which are clinically symptomatic in the first 24 to 48 hours after impact injury. Often the degree of underlying cerebral contusion or damage is so significant that unconsciousness occurs at the moment of impact and is never regained. In other situations, the patient has a lucid period before deterioration.

Subacute subdural hematomas are hematomas that develop symptomatically 3 to 20 days after trauma. In subacute hematomas the expansion of the hematoma occurs at a rate slower than that in acute SDH; therefore it takes longer for symptoms to become obvious. Clinical deterioration with subacute SDH is usually slower than that with acute SDH, but treatment by surgical intervention, when appropriate, is the same.

Chronic subdural hematoma is the term used when symptomatology occurs 20 or more days after injury. The majority of patients with chronic SDH are elderly or in late middle age. Many have a history of alcoholism, and some are on anticoagulation therapy. In up to 50% of the patients, no history of head injury exists. If a history of head injury does exist, it is often mild.[17]

**Intracerebral hematoma.** Intracerebral hematoma (ICH) is a homogenous collection of blood within the parenchyma. This is contrasted by the appearance of blood as well as contused and edematous cerebral cells in hemorrhagic contusion.

Traumatic causes of ICH include depressed skull fractures, penetrating injuries (bullet, knife, pointed objects), or sudden acceleration-deceleration motion. In sudden acceleration-deceleration, ICH occurs as the brain is lacerated across the under surfaces of the frontal bone and the sharp edges of the sphenoid wing.

Treatment of ICH is controversial in terms of surgical or nonsurgical management. It is generally believed that hemorrhages that are not causing significant ICP problems should be treated nonsurgically. Over time the hemorrhage will be reabsorbed. If significant problems with ICP occur as a result of the ICH producing a mass effect, surgical removal is necessary.

### Missile Injuries

**Missile injuries** are caused by objects that produce significant focal damage but little acceleration-deceleration or rotational injury. The injury may be depressed, penetrating, or perforating. Depressed injuries are caused by fractures of the skull with penetration of the bone into cerebral tissue. Penetrating injury is caused by a missile that enters the cranial cavity but does not exit. A low-velocity penetrating injury may involve only focal damage and no loss of consciousness. A high-velocity injury, such as a bullet, may

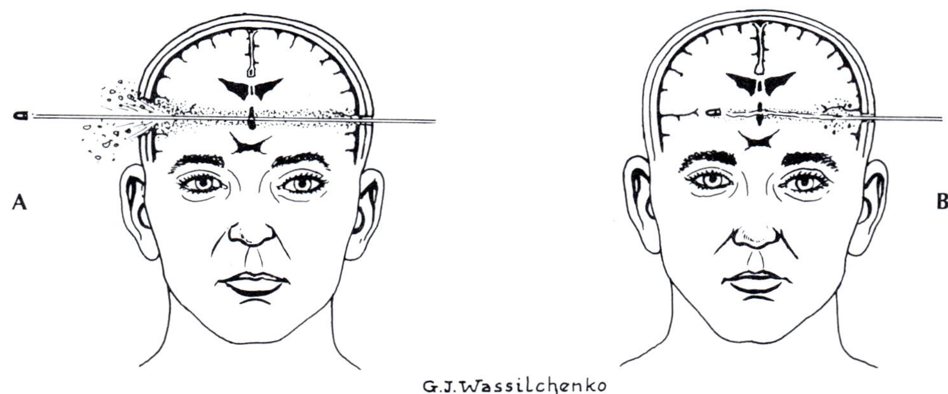


*Fig. 22-3* Bullet wounds of the head. Bullet wound or other penetrating missle will cause an open (compound) skull fracture and damage to brain tissue. Shock wave effects are transmitted throughout the brain. **A,** Perforating injury. **B,** Penetrating injury.

involve severe injury as a result of the ricocheting of the bullet through the brain. The shock waves from the high-velocity missile also cause significant cerebral disruption. Perforating injuries have much less ricochet effect but are still responsible for significant injury (Fig. 22-3).

Risk of infection and cerebral abcess is a concern in missile injuries. If fragments of the missile are embedded within the brain, careful consideration of the location and risk of increasing neurological deficit is weighed against the risk of abscess or infection. Outcome from missile injury is based on the degree of penetration and the location of the injury, as well as the velocity of the missile.

### Degree of Injury

**Mild injury.** Mild head injury is described as a GCS of 13 to 15 with loss of consciousness for 0 to 15 minutes. Patients with mild injury are often seen in the emergency room and discharged home with a family member who is instructed to routinely evaluate the patient and return the patient to the hosptial if any further symptoms appear. A small number of this group makes up the "talk and die" population. A CT scan is seldom performed unless deterioration occurs.[23,30]

**Moderate injury.** Moderate head injury is described as GCS of 9 to 12 with loss of consciousness up to 6 hours. Patients with this type of head injury are usually hospitalized. They are at high risk for deterioration from increasing cerebral edema and increasing ICP and require close observation. Hemodynamic and ICP monitoring along with ventilatory support is often not required in this group unless other systemic injuries make it necessary. Therefore constant clinical assessment is an important function of the nurse. A CT scan is usually performed initially, but otherwise only if deterioration occurs.

**Severe injury.** Severe head injury is described as GCS of 3 to 8 with loss of consciousness for longer than 6 hours. Patients with severe head injury often receive ventilatory support along with ICP and hemodynamic monitoring. A CT scan is performed to rule out any mass lesions that should be surgically removed. Patients are placed in a critical care setting for continual assessment, monitoring, and management.

### Summary of Nursing Care

Care of the patient with head injury involves continual, systematic assessments of neurological function as well as rapid intervention when deterioration is noted. Most of the care of these patients centers around maintenance of normal hemodynamic parameters and intervention for increases in ICP. These critically ill patients who have such a complex disorder require careful planning of care and continued evaluation of ICP response. Refer to the box "Nursing Diagnosis and Management: Cerebral Trauma."

## FACIAL TRAUMA

### LeFort I Fracture

LeFort I, or Guérin's, fractures are horizontal fractures of the maxilla and are the most common of LeFort's classifications.

### LeFort II Fracture

A LeFort II fracture is an extension of a LeFort I fracture into the orbit, ethmoid, and nasal bones. The cribriform plate is commonly involved, and a cerebrospinal fluid (CSF) leak can be observed.

### LeFort III Fracture

In LeFort III fracture, there is independent movement of the cranial and facial bones (craniofacial separation). CSF leaks frequently occur with these fractures, as does airway obstruction.

Soft-tissue injuries of the face caused by either blunt or penetrating mechanisms always present a challenge to the practitioner. Aggressive airway management should be in-

## NURSING DIAGNOSIS AND MANAGEMENT

### *Cerebral trauma*

- Altered Cerebral Tissue Perfusion related to increased intracranial pressure secondary to brain trauma, hemorrhage, edema, p. 480
- High Risk for Aspiration risk factors: reduced level of consciousness of tracheostomy or endotracheal tube, gastrointestinal tube, tube feedings, delayed gastric emptying, p. 476
- Ineffective Airway Clearance related to impaired cough secondary to loss of glottic closure with cuffed tracheostomy or endotracheal tube, p. 468
- Ineffective Breathing Pattern related to respiratory muscle deconditioning secondary to mechanical ventilation, p. 471
- Impaired Gas Exchange related to ventilation-perfusion inequality secondary to stasis of secretions, p. 474
- Altered Nutrition: Less Than Body Protein-Calorie Requirements related to lack of exogenous nutrients and increased metabolic demand. (See also discussion of metabolic results from carbohydrate overfeeding, Chapter 6.)
- High Risk for Infection risk factors: protein-calorie malnourishment, invasive monitoring devices, p. 465
- High Risk for Impaired Skin Integrity risk factors: reduced mobility, nutritional deficit, enteral tube feedings, stool incontinence, p. 499
- Sensory-Perceptual Alterations related to sensory overload, sensory deprivation, sleep pattern disturbance, p. 489
- Body Image Disturbance related to actual change in body structure, function, and appearance, p. 443
- Altered Role Performance related to physical incapacity to resume usual or valued role, p. 444

stituted. Cervical spine injury should also be suspected in the patient with facial trauma. Placement of tubes (nasogastric, nasotracheal) into the nasal orifice should be discouraged, since violation of the cribriform plate could result in its cranial placement. Likewise, orotracheal intubation should not be considered in the patient with massive facial injuries, since successful attempts are a rarity. Airway management should be instituted through placement of the surgical airway or cricothyroidostomy. Surgical intervention is required for all of these facial fractures.

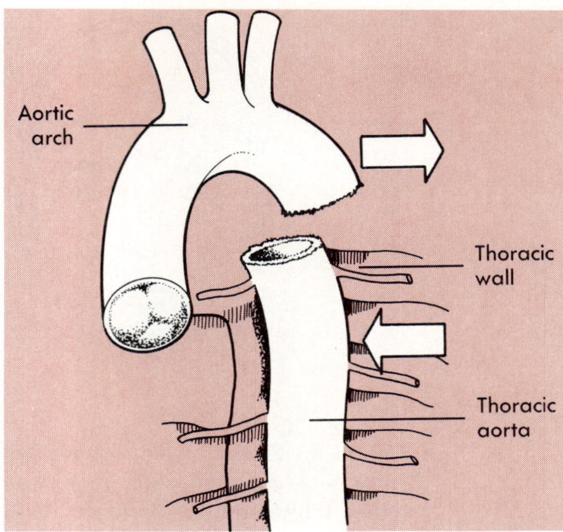


***Fig. 22-4*** Laceration of the aortic arch can result when the upper portion of the arch is thrust forward during acute deceleration because it is free to move while the lower portion of the arch remains stationary because it is fixed to the posterior thoracic wall.

## THORACIC TRAUMA

Thoracic injuries can be classified using the system established by the American College of Surgeons (ACS).[1] *Immediately life-threatening* thoracic injuries include pericardial tamponade, massive hemothorax, tension pneumothorax, open pneumothorax (sucking chest wound), and flail chest. *Potentially life-threatening* thoracic injuries include pulmonary contusion, aortic disruption, diaphragmatic hernia, tracheobronchial disruption, and myocardial contusion.

Injury to the thorax occurs as a result of either blunt, penetrating, or blast mechanisms. Blunt injury accounts for the majority of thoracic injuries and predominantly occurs secondary to motor vehicle accidents. Sudden deceleration of the human body commonly results in parenchymal injury to the lung. In addition, shearing of vessels from fixed structures such as with the aorta's tearing from the ligamentum arteriosum (Fig. 22-4), and/or compression of intrathoracic structures can occur (Fig. 22-5). Secondary intrathoracic or intraabdominal injury can occur from rib or sternal fractures.

Penetrating injury can result from use of a variety of weapons, including handguns, shotguns, rifles, and knives. Weapons are commonly classified by velocity—either low, medium, or high.

Finally, indirect forces such as the blast mechanism can result in thoracic injury that frequently involves the pulmonary parenchyma, resulting, for example, in pulmonary contusion and adult respiratory distress syndrome (ARDS).

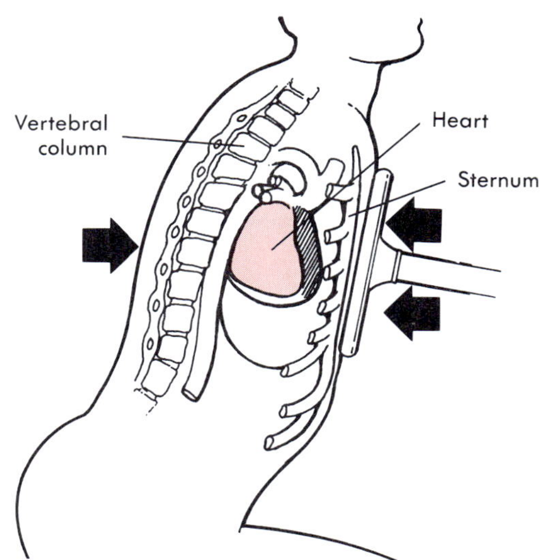


*Fig. 22-5* Myocardial contusions and rupture can result when, during sudden impact, the heart is compressed between the sternum and the vertebral column.

### Pericardial Tamponade

When myocardial trauma and injury occur, bleeding into the pericardial sac may result. The treatment of pericardial tamponade consists of relieving the congestion through either pericardiocentesis or creation of a pericardial window.

### Massive Hemothorax

Massive hemothorax indicates intrapleural blood volumes exceeding 1500 ml and is usually a result of penetrating injury. Insertion of large-bore IV lines and placement of large-bore chest tubes should be initiated in the emergency department before surgical intervention.

### Open Pneumothorax

**Open pneumothorax** ("sucking chest wound") is created when there is a communication between the atmosphere and the intrapleural space. The open pneumothorax allows free air passage during both inhalation and exhalation. Unless this situation is rapidly corrected, the patient will succumb to tissue hypoxia. Treatment consists of placing a nonocclusive dressing that is taped on three sides of the wound. Should the patient develop respiratory distress, the dressing should be "burped" to express any accumulation of air. A large-bore chest tube should also be placed distal to the site to allow for lung reexpansion.

### Flail Chest

**Flail chest** is usually the result of blunt trauma and commonly occurs in the unrestrained occupant of a motor vehicle whose chest becomes crushed under extreme force. Rib and/or sternal fractures usually occur. When two or more ribs are injured in two or more places, a flail—or "free-floating"—segment occurs, and underlying great vessel, myocardial, or pulmonary injury can result. This free-floating segment moves inward during inhalation and outward during exhalation (paradoxical breathing), leading to hypoxemia, tissue hypoxia, and respiratory failure. Negative and positive intrathoracic pressures are altered, and the resulting pain causes a decrease in tidal volume. A mediastinal shift toward the uninjured side results in a decrease in preload, thus decreasing cardiac output.

Treatment is centered on stabilizing the flail segment (usually with ventilatory support), allowing adequate exchange of oxygen and carbon dioxide and pain relief. External support of the flail segment with sterile towel clips around the flail segment are currently seldom used. If the patient develops respiratory distress or has either preexisting cardiac or pulmonary disease or acute head or orthopedic injuries, controlled ventilation should be instituted. It would also allow internal splinting through the use of positive end-expiratory pressure (PEEP) and intermittent mandatory ventilation (IMV) modalities. Pain control can be achieved through various routes such as IV, epidural, or intercostal analgesia and/or transcutaneous electrical nerve stimulation (TENS). Since an underlying injury such as pulmonary contusion may be present, fluid administration should be conservative. Diagnostic studies to detect either myocardial or great vessel trauma should be implemented.

### Pulmonary Contusion

**Pulmonary contusion,** a bruising of pulmonary parenchyma, is the most common sequela of thoracic trauma. It can be seen with or without a flail chest. Treatment of pulmonary contusion is based on the same goal as that of flail chest—ensuring adequate oxygenation. Although pulmonary contusion differs from ARDS in that contusion occurs within minutes of the injury, the latter is a commonly associated sequela.

### Aortic Disruption

Injuries to the aorta can occur through either a blunt or a penetrating mechanism and predominantly result from motor vehicle accidents. Acute deceleration leads to the shearing effects encountered in motor vehicle accidents (see Fig. 22-4).

Aortic disruption can manifest the following signs:

- Anterior or posterior thoracic pain
- Hoarseness or stridor
- Dysphagia
- Upper-extremity hypertension
- Lower-extremity hypotension
- Paraplegia
- Hypovolemic shock

Aortic injury should be highly suspected if the following are present:

- Thoracic spine fracture
- Multiple left rib fractures

- Scapular fractures
- Sternal fractures
- Fracture of rib 1, 2, or 3

The diagnosis of aortic injury is confirmed by aortography; once it is confirmed, surgical intervention is mandated.

### Diaphragmatic Injury

Blunt or penetrating injury can result in herniation of the diaphragm. If the injury results from blunt trauma, the patient will relate a history of rapid deceleration, most commonly occurring when an unrestrained driver of an automobile crashes against a steering wheel or when a backseat passenger, restrained by a lapbelt apparatus (without shoulder harness), decelerates against the belt. Direct injury to the abdomen (crush injuries, falls) can also result in herniation.

Diaphragmatic injuries from penetrating trauma are usually the result of gunshot or stab wounds. The majority of diaphragmatic injuries occur on the left side (85%) because the liver protects the diaphragm on the right. Penetrating mechanisms usually produce small rents in the diaphragm, whereas blunt injury causes larger, linear tears.

The diagnosis of diaphragmatic injury is rarely obvious. This injury should be highly suspected in patients with penetrating injuries to the anterior thoracoabdominal regions and with deceleration injuries. It should also be suspected in patients with lower rib fracture and hemothorax or lower lobe pulmonary contusion. Radiographic evaluation may reveal gastric contents in the thorax, or the hemidiaphragm may be elevated. The patient may complain of sharp shoulder pain and increasing respiratory distress. Laparotomy is indicated for all patients, regardless of the mechanism. If the herniation is discovered during thoracotomy for penetrating thoracic injury, intraabdominal involvement should be expected and a laparotomy anticipated. Use of the pneumatic antishock garment is not recommended for hypotensive patients with diaphragmatic injury because it may enlarge the tear, forcing abdominal contents into the thoracic cavity and further impeding respiration and circulation.

### Tracheobronchial Injury

Sudden increases in intrathoracic pressure against a closed glottis, massive blows to the chest (for example, in rapid deceleration), and direct injury are common causes of tracheobronchial injury.

Pain is usually present and is accompanied by severe respiratory distress and upper airway obstruction. Subcutaneous emphysema, pneumothorax, associated rib fractures, hoarseness, dysphagia, stridor, and hemorrhage may occur. Radiographic signs include pneumomediastinum, pneumothorax, free intraperitoneal air, retroesophageal air, and peribronchial air. Contrast radiography and flexible endoscopy are most commonly used for confirmation of the diagnosis. Decompression of the thorax through a chest tube and direct repair through thoracotomy are indicated.

### Summary of Nursing Care

Nursing care of the patient with intrathoracic injuries centers on maintenance of the process of ventilation (ensuring, when possible, adequate exchange of carbon dioxide and oxygen) and circulation. Providing adequate analgesia is essential for the patient with flail chest. Constant reassessment for "missed injuries" is essential regardless of the body system involved.

## ABDOMINAL TRAUMA

Intraabdominal injury can occur with either blunt or penetrating mechanisms. The majority of blunt abdominal injuries results from motor vehicle accidents. Numerous landmarks have been proposed for separating the intraabdominal and intrathoracic regions. Since thoracic and abdominal injuries frequently coincide, examination should focus on the entire thoracoabdominal region.

When determining the mechanisms of blunt injury, especially in victims of motor vehicle accidents, occupant location and restraint status are two of the most important areas to be probed. In the front-seat passenger, hepatic injury should be suspected when the point of impact is on the same side as the passenger. Likewise, a driver should be assessed for injury to the spleen in an impact on the driver's side. Use of the lapbelt, without shoulder harness, is associated with distal thoracic and proximal lumbar spine fractures (T12 to L2). In penetrating mechanisms, determining the size, shape, and configuration of the object, as well as the position of the assailant and victim, adds valuable information to the assessment.

Diagnostic **peritoneal lavage** is performed through an incision through the skin to the peritoneum. A small catheter is placed through a small opening into the peritoneum. Use of bladder decompression through urethral catheterization and gastric decompression through a nasogastric or orogastric tube is imperative to prevent secondary trauma. If gross blood is visualized on entering the peritoneal cavity, the procedure is aborted, and the patient is immediately transported to the surgical suite. If gross blood is not initially encountered, rapid infusion of either 1 L of lactated Ringer's solution or physiological solution of sodium (0.9% normal saline solution) is indicated. The IV bag is then placed in a dependent position and allowed to drain. The inability to read newspaper print through the bag is considered a positive result. This crude but accurate method detects the subtle cloudiness of blood or other contaminant in the diagnostic peritoneal fluid. Likewise, a WBC >500 high power frequency (hpf), red blood count (RBC) >100,000/hpf, or the presence of bile, bacteria, or gastric contents is criteria for further exploration.

### Spleen

The spleen remains the organ most commonly injured by blunt trauma and is second only to the liver as a source of life-threatening hemorrhage. Traditionally, splenic injury resulted in splenectomy, although currently the emphasis is shifting to splenorraphy when possible. As long as the spleen is not pulverized, attempts at repair should be made. Contraindications for repair include the presence in a patient of prolonged, severe hypotension or of a major associated injury, either intraabdominal or extraabdominal. Such a patient should not have prolonged attempts at splenic repair. Pneumococcal vaccination (Pneumovax) should be instituted after splenectomy.

### Liver

The liver is the second most commonly injured organ in blunt trauma and the primary organ injured with penetrating mechanisms. Hemoperitoneum and severe hypotension commonly occur in the presence of hepatic injury. Once the diagnosis of hepatic injury has been established, surgical therapy can usually correct the defect in the majority of cases. In massive injuries, resection of devitalized tissue is mandated. Occasionally, ligation of one of the hepatic arteries or veins is necessary to control the hemorrhage.

### Duodenum, Small Bowel, and Colon

Injuries to the duodenum, small bowel, and colon are usually the result of penetrating mechanisms. The patient who sustains hollow viscus injury from blunt trauma presents a diagnostic dilemma and requires careful abdominal assessment. Resection and direct repair are routine surgical interventions.

## SPINAL CORD TRAUMA

In decreasing order of incidence, the causes of injury are vehicular accidents, falls on or off the job, sports injuries, and penetrating or missile injuries.[2] The type of injury sustained is dependent on the mechanism of injury. Review of the mechanism of injury includes the velocity, momentum, angle of impact, and degree of abnormal motion involved in sustaining the injury. The most common mechanisms of injury are hyperflexion, hyperextension, rotation, axial loading (vertical compression), and missile or penetrating injuries.

### Mechanism of Injury

**Hyperflexion.** Hyperflexion injury is most often seen in the cervical area especially at the level of C5 to C6, the most mobile portion of the cervical spine. This type of injury is most often caused by sudden deceleration motion as in head-on collisions. Injury occurs from compression of the cord as a result of fracture fragments or dislocation of the vertebral bodies. Instability of the spinal column occurs because of rupture or tearing of the posterior muscles and ligaments.

**Hyperextension.** Hyperextension injuries involve backward and downward motion of the head often seen in rearend collisions or diving incidents. In this type of injury the spinal cord itself is stretched and distorted. Disruption of intervertebral discs occur as well as compression or fracture of the posterior elements of the vertebral column. Neurological deficits associated with this injury are often caused by contusion and ischemia of the cord without significant bony involvement. A mild form of hyperextension injury is the "whiplash" injury.

**Rotation.** Rotation injuries often occur in conjunction with a flexion or extension injury. Severe rotation of the neck or body results in tearing of the posterior ligaments and displacement (rotation) of the spinal column. The condition termed *locked facets* is a result of rotation and involves displacement of the facet junction of one or more vertebral elements, thereby producing cord compression. Cervical traction or surgery is required to return these facets to normal positions and reduce cord compression.

**Axial loading.** Axial loading or compression injuries occur from vertical force along the spinal cord. This is most commonly seen in a fall from a height in which the person lands on feet or buttocks. Compression injuries cause burst fractures of the vertebral body that often send bony fragments into the spinal canal or directly into the spinal cord (Fig. 22-6).

**Missile or penetrating injuries.** Missile or penetrating injury to the spinal cord is caused by bullet, knife, or any other object that penetrates the cord. These types of injury cause permanent damage by anatomically transecting the spinal cord.

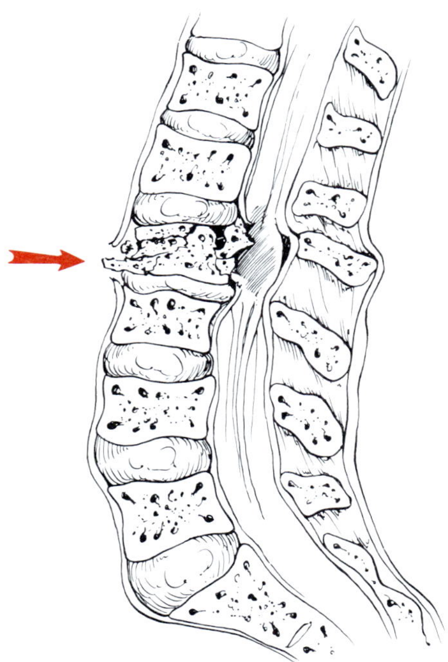

***Fig. 22-6*** Burst fracture of vertebral body causing damage to spinal cord. (From Long BC and Phipps WJ: Medical-surgical nursing: a nursing process approach, ed 2, St Louis, 1989, Mosby–Year Book, Inc.)

### Functional Injury of the Spinal Cord

Whatever the mechanism of injury or the type of vertebral column injury, the main focus of attention and intervention is toward the functional injury of the spinal cord. Functional injury refers to the degree of disruption of normal spinal cord function. Functional injuries are divided into two injury categories: complete and incomplete.

**Complete injury.** A **complete injury of the spinal cord** results in total sensory, motor, and autonomic nervous system dysfunction below the level of injury. This injury could be a result of anatomical dissection of the spinal cord or physiological dissection as a result of disruption of neurochemical pathways. More than 50% of all patients diagnosed initially as having complete injury obtain some return of function with the resolution of spinal shock (see the section entitled "Spinal Shock").

A complete injury in the cervical region results in quadriplegia. The degree of arm dysfunction is dependent on the level of injury. A complete injury in the thoracolumbar region results in paraplegia. Both quadriplegia and paraplegia involve loss of normal bowel and bladder function.

**Incomplete injury.** Incomplete injury to the spinal cord involves damage or dysfunction of one portion of the cord with normal pathways and function intact in the other portions of the cord.

***Central cord syndrome.*** Resulting from contusion, compression, or hemorrhage of the central gray matter of the cord, central cord syndrome is generally a cervical region injury. Because of the damage to gray matter, cell bodies, and nuclei at the level of injury, motor loss of the upper extremities is significant. Flaccidity, as characterized by a lower motor neuron injury (LMN), is seen. The lower extremities may exhibit upper motor neuron (UMN) injury with spasticity. Accompanying this motor injury is a varying degree of sensory loss, as well as a varying degree of bowel and bladder dysfunction (Fig. 22-7).

Hyperextension injuries, particularly if the patient has bony spurs from a preexisting degenerative disease, are the most common cause of central cord syndrome.

***Anterior cord syndrome.*** Anterior cord syndrome is caused by injury to the anterior gray horn cells (motor), the spinothalamic tracts (pain perception), and the corticospinal tracts (temperature perception). This injury results in loss of motor function below the level of the lesion. Also lost are the sensations of pain and temperature. Sensations of touch, position sense, pressure, and vibration are maintained.

Anterior cord syndromes are most often caused by flexion injuries or acute herniation of the intervertebral disc.

***Brown-Sequard syndrome.*** **Brown-Sequard syndrome** is caused by a transverse hemisection of the cord. Because of the anatomy of motor and sensory pathways of the spinal cord, Brown-Sequard syndrome results in (1) ipsilateral loss of motor function, either paralysis or paresis, (2) ipsilateral loss of touch, vibration, pressure, and position sensation, and (3) contralateral loss of pain and temperature sensation.

Brown-Sequard syndrome is caused by open, penetrating injuries such as knife or gunshot wounds or an acute ruptured intervertebral disc.

***Posterior cord syndrome.*** Posterior cord syndrome is rare. This injury results in loss of light touch and proprioception below the level of injury. Motor function and the sensation of pain and temperature remain intact. Posterior cord syndrome is usually associated with cervical hyperextension.

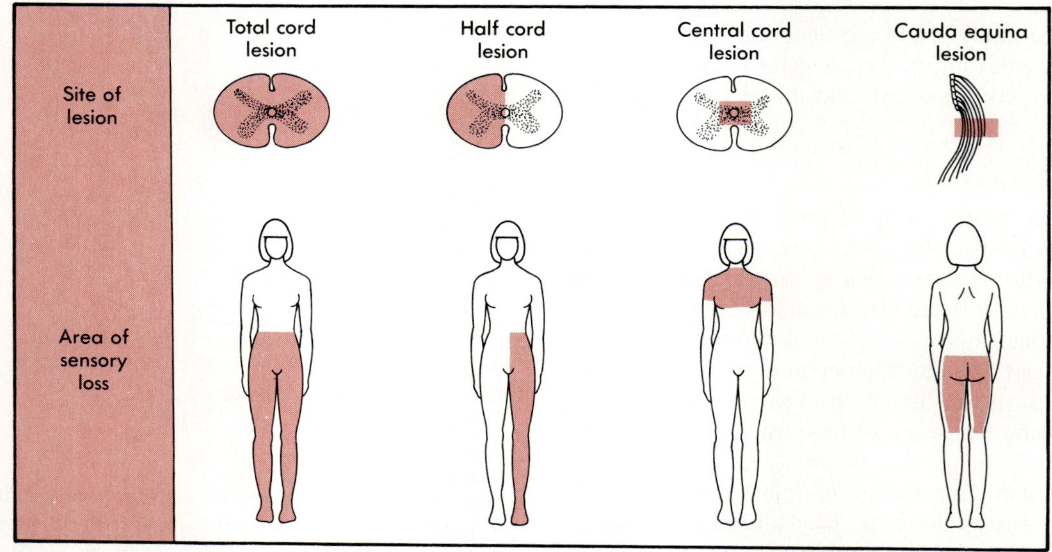


***Fig. 22-7*** Common patterns of sensory abnormality. *Upper diagrams,* site of lesion; *lower diagrams,* distribution of corresponding sensory loss.

***Cauda equina lesion.*** Injury at the levels below the end of the spinal cord at L1 are referred to as cauda equina lesions. Deficits from injury to the cauda equina vary according to the particular nerve roots involved. Damage can be bilateral or unilateral and involve both motor and sensory function. LMN lesions of the S1 to S4 area lead to flaccid bowel and bladder functions. All other lesions of the spinal cord that affect bowel and bladder function lead to UMN injury that allows for spastic control of bowel and bladder function.

### Spinal Shock

**Spinal shock** is a term applied to a condition that occurs immediately after an acute spinal cord injury. Spinal shock is the complete loss of all reflex activity below the level of injury. This includes not only loss of deep tendon reflexes, but also loss of vasomotor tone, temperature control, and bowel and bladder tone. Loss of these reflexes results clinically in bradycardia, hypotension, hypothermia, urinary retention, and paralytic ileus. Over a period of hours to months, reflex activity returns to normal.

Because of the immediate onset of spinal shock, the actual degree or permanence of any spinal cord injury is difficult to predict in the early hours after the injury. Up to 50% of all patients who appear to have complete spinal cord injury on initial evaluation regain some degree of spinal cord function after spinal shock ends.[2]

### Neurogenic Shock

**Neurogenic shock** is another symptom seen in patients with cervical injury. A portion of the sympathetic nervous system lies in the thoracolumbar region of the spinal cord and receives continuous information from the brainstem down through the cervical cord. Injury in the cervical region disrupts the pathway and leads to loss of sympathetic control. This loss results in vasodilatation of the vascular beds, bradycardia resulting from the lack of sympathetic balance to parasympathetic stimuli from the vagus nerve (CN X), and loss of the ability to sweat below the level of injury.

In assessment of a patient who presents with manifestations of shock, it is important to remember that in hypovolemic shock the patient is hypotensive and *tachycardic*. In neurogenic shock the patient is hypotensive but *bradycardic*.

### Medical Treatment

Surgical intervention is performed to provide spinal column stability in the event of an unstable injury. Unstable injuries are defined as disrupted ligaments and tendons, particularly the posterior ligamentous complex, or the inability to maintain normal alignment of the vertebral column. Identification and immobilization of unstable injuries is particularly important in the patient with incomplete neurological deficit. Without adequate stabilization, movement and dislocation of the vertebral column could cause a complete neurological deficit.

A variety of surgical procedures may be performed to achieve decompression and stabilization: laminectomy, spinal fusion, and rodding. If the injury to the spinal column is believed to be stable, nonsurgical management of the injury is the treatment of choice.

Management of the cervical injury involves immobilization of the fracture site and realignment of any dislocation. This is accomplished through skeletal traction that involves the use of tongs inserted into the skull and connected to traction weights. There are several types of cervical tongs used. Gardner-Wells and Crutchfield tongs are the most common. These tongs can be applied at the bedside with the use of local anesthetic. After the insertion of the tongs, the patient is immobilized on a kinetic treatment table, a Stryker frame, a Circ-o-lectric bed, or a regular hospital bed.

After adequate realignment of the spinal column has occurred through skeletal traction, a halo traction brace is often applied. The halo traction brace allows for the maintenance of cervical spine immobility as well as increasing mobility of the patient. With the increased mobility provided by the halo brace, the patient can also become involved in the rehabilitation process more quickly.[9]

Nonsurgical management of the patient with a thoracolumbar injury also involves immobilization. Skeletal traction may also be used in high thoracic injury. For the most part, stable injuries of the thoracolumbar spine are injuries causing no misalignment of the spinal canal. Immobilization to allow for healing of fractures is accomplished by flat bed rest with the use of a plastic or fiberglass jacket, a body cast, or a brace. Rotorest beds and Stryker frames may also be used to increase the mobility of these patients.

### Summary of Nursing Care

Nursing management of the patient with spinal cord injury centers around both the physical and psychosocial aspects of the injury. Refer to the box "Nursing Diagnosis and Management: Spinal Cord Injury" on p. 412.

## PELVIC TRAUMA

Like the thoracic cage, the pelvis is considered a ring structure. Thus, since a ring will typically break not only on the side of injury but also on its contralateral side, the patient with pelvic injury should be examined for opposing breaks. Areas with injuries associated with pelvic fractures include the abdominal viscera, perineum, retroperitoneum, and the lower extremity. The mortality rate from pelvic fractures ranges from less than 10% in patients with a simple, isolated, closed fracture to approximately 50% in patients with an open pelvic fracture. Classic signs of pelvic fracture include perineal ecchymosis (testicular or labial), pain on palpation or "rocking" of the iliac crests, and obvious deformity. Diagnostic tests include plain film examination of the pelvis, CT angiography (for diagnosis of iliac vessel injury and to control hemorrhage), and cystourethrography (to detect for genitourinary injury). Major pelvic

## NURSING DIAGNOSIS AND MANAGEMENT

***Spinal cord injury***

- Dysreflexia related to excessive automomic response to noxious stimuli secondary to spinal cord injury (T-6 or above), p. 484
- Hypothermia related to spinal cord injury, p. 481
- Decreased Cardiac Output related to vasodilation and bradycardia secondary to sympathetic blockade of neurogenic (spinal) shock following spinal cord injury (T-6 or above), p. 461
- Impaired Gas Exchange related to alveolar hypoventilation secondary to loss of accessory muscle function, p. 475
- Impaired Gas Exchange related to ventilation-perfusion inequality secondary to stasis of secretions, p. 474
- Ineffective Breathing Pattern related to respiratory muscle deconditioning secondary to mechanical ventilation, p. 471
- Ineffective Airway Clearance related to impaired cough secondary to loss of glottic closure with tracheostomy or endotracheal tube, p. 468
- Ineffective Airway Clearance related to respiratory muscle dysfunction and impaired cough secondary to quadriplegia, p. 469
- High Risk for Aspiration risk factors: depressed cough reflex (T-6 and above), presence of tracheostomy tube, gastrointestinal tube, tube feedings, situation hindering elevation of upper body, increased intragastric pressure, increased gastric residual, decreased gastrointestinal motility, delayed gastric emptying, p. 476
- Activity Intolerance related to prolonged immobility and loss of vasomotor tone, p. 463
- High Risk for Impaired Skin Integrity risk factors: immobility, loss of sensation, enteral tube feedings, stool and urine incontinence, p. 499
- Body Image Disturbance related to actual change in body structure, function, and appearance, p. 443
- Altered Role Performance related to physical incapacity to resume usual or valued role, p. 444
- Self-Esteem Disturbance related to feelings of guilt over physical deterioration, p. 442
- Powerlessness related to health care environment and illness-related regimen, p. 445
- Ineffective Individual Coping related to situational crisis and personal vulnerability, p. 447
- Hopelessness related to perceptions of failing or deteriorating physical condition, p. 446
- Knowledge Deficit: Dysreflexia, Urinary Tract Infections, Upper Respiratory Infections, Skin Care, Mobility Strategies related to lack of previous exposure to information, p. 441
- Altered Health Maintenance related to lack of perceived threat to health, p. 439

fractures should be ruled out before obtaining an upright chest film in the hemodynamically stable patient, since worsening of the stability of the fracture and increasing vascular injury can occur.

A major complication of pelvic fractures is hemorrhage. Treatment usually involves a combination of the use of a pneumatic antishock garment, fluid and blood component replacement, vessel embolization, and surgical reduction of the fracture(s). Although surgical intervention is usually necessary, some minor fractures are treated with bed rest. Application of an external fixation device allows early mobilization of the patient and assists in the prevention of deep vein thrombophlebitis and pulmonary complications.

## FEMORAL FRACTURES

The patient with a femoral fracture will initially have pain in the extremity although he or she may not necesarily have an obvious deformity. Obtaining a careful history about the mechanism of injury should alert the clinician to this possibility. Depending on the severity of injury, surgical intervention may be required. Like pelvic fractures, fractures of the femur are associated with major hemorrhagic complications. Other complications of femoral fracture include avascular necrosis of the femoral head, malunion, rejection of fixation devices, and refracture.

### REFERENCES

1. Advanced Trauma Life Support Text, Chicago, 1984, American College of Surgeons.
2. Albin MS: Acute cervical spinal injury. In Rogers MC and Traystman RJ, editors: Critical care clinics: neurologic intensive care, Philadelphia, 1985, WB Saunders Co.
3. American Association for Automotive Medicine: The abbreviated injury scale (AIS), Morton Grove, Ill, 1985, The Association.
4. Baker SP and O'Neill B: The injury severity score: an update, J Trauma 16:882, 1976.
5. Baker SP, O'Neill B, and Karpf RS: The injury fact book, Lexington, Mass, 1984, DC Heath & Co.
6. Beaver BM: Care of the multiple trauma victim: the first hour, Nurs Clin North Am 25(1):11, 1990.
7. Beskin CA: Rupture separation of the cervical trachea following a closed chest injury, J Thorac Surg 34:392, 1957.

8. Britt LD: The impact of trauma center designation: the Virginia system, Emerg Care Q 6(2):8, 1990.
9. Browner CM: Halo immobilization brace care: an innovative approach, J Neurosci Nurs 19(1):24, 1987.
10. Champion HR and others: Trauma score, Crit Care Med 9:672, 1981.
11. Collicott PE: Initial assessment of the trauma patient. In Mattox KL, Moore EE, and Feliciano DV, editors: Trauma, Norwalk, Conn, 1988, Appleton & Lange.
12. Committee on Trauma of the American College of Surgeons: Hospital and prehospital care of the injured patient, Am Coll Surg Bull 68:10, 1983.
13. Committee on Trauma Research, Commission of Life Sciences, National Research Council, and the Institute of Medicine: Injury in America: a continuing public health problem, Washington, DC, 1985, National Academy Press.
14. Dacey RG and Dikmen SS: Mild head injury. In Cooper PR, editor: Head injury, Baltimore, 1987, Williams & Wilkins.
15. Davis JH: History of trauma. In Matox KL, Moore EE, and Feliciano, DV, editors: Trauma, Norwalk, Conn, 1988, Appleton & Lange.
16. Fretag E: Autopsy findings in head injuries from blunt forces: statistical evaluation of 1367 cases, Arch Path 75:402, 1963.
17. Graham DI, Adams JH, and Gennarelli TA: Pathology of brain damage in head injury. In Cooper PR, editor: Head injury, Baltimore, 1987, Williams & Wilkins.
18. Hau T: The surgical practice of Dominique Jean Larrey, Surg Gynecol Obstet 154:89, 1982.
19. Hunter J: A treatise on the blood, inflammation, and gunshot wounds, Birmingham, England, 1982, LB Adams.
20. Jones KW: Thoracic trauma, Surg Clin North Am 60:957, 1980.
21. Kirkpatrick JR and Youmans RL: Trauma index: an aid in the evaluation of injury victims, J Trauma 11:711, 1971.
22. Madding GF, Lawrence KD, and Kennedy DA: Forward surgery of the severely injured, Second Aux Surg Group 1:307, 1942.
23. Marshall LF, Toole BM, and Bowers SA: The national traumatic coma data bank. Part 2. Patients who talk and deteriorate: implications for treatment, J Neurosurg 59:285, 1983.
24. McSwain NE: Abdominal trauma. In McSwain NE and Kerstein MD, editors: Evaluation and management of trauma, Norwalk, Conn, 1987, Appleton-Century-Crofts.
25. McSwain NE: Patient assessment and initial management. In McSwain NE and Kerstein MD, editors: Evaluation and management of trauma, Norwalk, Conn, 1987, Appleton-Century-Crofts.
26. National Safety Council: Accident facts, Chicago, 1985, The Council.
27. O'Neill B: Biomechanics of trauma, Norwalk, Conn, 1984, Appleton & Lange.
28. Prehospital Trauma Life Support Text, Educational Training, Akron, Ohio, 1986, Emergency Training.
29. Rich NM: Missile injuries, Am J Surgery 139:414, 1980.
30. Rimel RW and others: Disability caused by minor head injury, Neurosurgery 9:221, 1981.
31. Sanger PW: Evacuation hospital experience with war wounds and injuries of the chest, Ann Surg 122:147, 1945.
32. Seuvre M: Crushing injury from wheel of omnibus: rupture of the right bronchus, Bull Soc Anat (Paris) 48:680, 1873.
33. Trunkey DD: Trauma, Sci Am 249:28, 1983.
34. Trunkey DD: Torso trauma: an overview. In Trunkey DD and Lewis FR, editors: Current therapy of trauma, Philadelphia, 1986, Brian C Decker, Publisher.
35. Trunkey DD: Reflections of our origins. In Najarian JS and Delaney JP, editors: Trauma and critical care surgery, Chicago, 1987, Mosby–Year Book, Inc.
36. Unkle DW, Clements CP, and Ross SE: Osmolality as a predictor of intoxication in the trauma patient: usefulness in clinical practice, unpublished manuscript. Proceedings from the Second Annual Nursing Symposium: Management of Multiple Trauma and Burns, Cleveland, Ohio, May 19-20, 1988.
37. Walt AJ: Trauma. In Mattox KL, Moore EE, and Feliciano DV, editors: Trauma, Norwalk, Conn, 1988, Appleton & Lange.
38. Wrobel CJ and Marshall LF: Closed head injury management dilemmas. In Long DM, editor: Current therapy in neurological surgery, ed 2, St Louis, 1989, Mosby–Year Book, Inc.
39. Young W: Mechanisms underlying the acute response of central nervous system tissues to trauma, Topic Emerg Med 11(4):43, 1990.

CHAPTER 23

# Disseminated Intravascular Coagulation

## CHAPTER OBJECTIVES

- *List at least four disorders from both coagulation pathways (intrinsic and extrinsic) that can precipitate acute disseminated intravascular coagulation (DIC).*
- *Describe the most common clinical presentation of acute DIC and its cause.*
- *List important laboratory findings that are highly suggestive of DIC.*
- *Outline the medical management of DIC, including the purpose and actions of heparin, antithrombin III, epsilon-aminocaproic acid (EACA), whole blood, platelets, fresh frozen plasma, and cryoprecipitate.*
- *Discuss three nursing diagnoses and their interventions that are related to the treatment of DIC.*

## KEY TERMS

disseminated intravascular coagulation, p. 414
thrombotic process, p. 414
fibrinolytic process, p. 414
consumption coagulopathy, p. 417
aminocaproic acid (AMICAR), p. 418
fresh frozen plasma, p. 418
cryoprecipitate, p. 418
antithrombin III, p. 418
bleeding precautions, p. 419

## DESCRIPTION

**Disseminated intravascular coagulation** (DIC) is a hemorrhagic disorder produced by the effects of both **thrombotic** (clot formation) and **fibrinolytic** (clot digestion) **processes.** As the name implies, DIC causes microvascular clotting in organ systems throughout the body, but, paradoxically, its lethality stems from the profound bleeding resulting from the depletion (consumption) of clotting substances. Since both clot formation and clot digestion consume clotting factors, the most dramatic manifestation of DIC is the *acute generalized hemorrhage* secondary to the inability of blood to coagulate. The thrombotic processes of DIC can also result in infarction of major organs. The severity of DIC depends on the magnitude of the underlying disease that precipitates this syndrome of intravascular coagulation. Mortality increases with the patient's age, the extent of his or her clinical manifestations, and the severity of abnormal laboratory results.[15]

DIC can be either *acute* or *chronic*. In addition, both acute and chronic clinical forms can be designated *subclinical*. Subclinical DIC implies lack of significant clinical symptomatology; the presumptive diagnosis is based on abnormal laboratory findings.

Acute DIC, which can develop rapidly in critically ill patients, is the most serious of the acquired coagulation disorders. Mortality in acute DIC is high—estimated at 50% to 70%. Acute DIC occurs in approximately 1 in every 1000 hospital admissions, although this estimate is probably low.[16,17]

Chronic DIC is characterized by episodic changes in coagulation in the chronically ill patient. Malignancy is the most common cause, especially mucin-producing adenocarcinomas of the prostate and pancreas; solid tumors of the lung, colon, and stomach; and metastatic disease.[4,17] Chronic DIC is also associated with connective tissue diseases, renal disease, liver disease, metabolic disease, collagen vascular disease, lymphoma, and myeloma.[4,17] Unlike those with acute DIC, patients with chronic DIC manifest thrombotic complications such as thrombophlebitis, nonbacterial thrombotic endocarditis, and pulmonary embolism. Exacerbation of hemorrhage may also occur. Long-

## CAUSES OF DIC

### INFECTIONS

Bacterial
- Gram-negative sepsis (*Neisseria, Klebsiella, Pseudomonas aeruginosa, Escherichia coli)*
- Gram-positive septicemia (Staphylococcus, Streptococcus)
- Fungal (aspergillosis)

Mycobacterial (tuberculosis)
Protozoal (malaria)
Rickettsial (Rocky Mountain spotted fever)
Viral (chicken pox, measles, herpes simplex, influenza)

### MALIGNANCIES

Carcinoma (breast, colon, lung, stomach, pancreas, prostate, ovary)
Leukemia (acute promyelocytic, acute and chronic myelocytic)
Other (pheochromocytoma, polycythemia vera)

### TRAUMA

Burns
Multiple injury
Head injury
Snake bite
Fat embolism

### SURGERY

Extracorporeal circulation
Transurethral prostatectomy

### OBSTETRICAL DISORDERS

Abruptio placentae
Missed abortion
Amniotic fluid embolism
Septic abortion
Dead fetus syndrome
Toxemia of pregnancy/pregnancy-induced hypertension
Eclampsia
Hydatidiform mole
Chorioamnionitis

### IMMUNOLOGICAL DISORDERS

Incompatible transfusion reactions
Anaphylaxis
Systemic lupus erythematosis

### HEMATOLOGICAL DISORDERS

Sickle cell crisis
Use of prothrombin concentrate in patient with liver disease

### OTHERS

Pulmonary embolism
Intravenous pyelogram
Diabetic ketoacidosis
Post–cardiac arrest
Aortic aneurysm
Hyperthermia or hypothermia

Modified from Carr M: J Emerg Med 5(4):312, 1987.

term therapy is usually required, with careful monitoring of clotting studies.

## ETIOLOGY

All forms of DIC occur secondary to some underlying disease or disorder. Scores of clinical disorders cause DIC, with infection (sepsis) the most common (see the box above). Every type of infection has been implicated in the pathogenesis of DIC. The mortality rate for patients with DIC associated with severe infections is 80%.[4]

## PATHOPHYSIOLOGY

In the healthy person there is a balance between (1) clot formation (thrombosis), which is needed to minimize blood loss and to repair blood vessels, and (2) clot lysis (fibrinolysis), which maintains the patency of blood vessels. In a patient with DIC this balance is upset; *DIC is an exaggeration of the normal coagulation process*. The normal processes of thrombosis and fibrinolysis are magnified to life-threatening proportions corresponding to the severity of the precipitating disorder (Fig. 23-1).

Since DIC results from increased thrombin activity, the disorders precipitating DIC produce a systemic hypercoagulation state—thrombosis is no longer localized but is generalized *(disseminated)*. Thrombosis does not act as a protective mechanism but causes microvascular changes in major organ systems, with the possibility of organ ischemia and infarction. Thus the *initial component* of DIC is thrombosis of major vessels. The severity of the thrombosis is dependent on the intensity of the precipitating disorder.[4] Although no organ system is spared, organs with larger blood flow are more likely affected.[4] The skin, lungs, and kidneys are the organs most commonly involved and damaged during DIC.

The *second component* of DIC is hemorrhage. Lysis of clots (fibrinolysis) is naturally activated by coagulation (specifically by thrombin). In a patient with DIC the intensity of the thrombosis activates a similar intensity of lysis. Unlike what occurs in normal situations, the thrombosis in DIC is so generalized and of so great a magnitude that lysis cannot keep pace to maintain the patency of vessels.

Although the lysis is not sufficient to meet the great de-

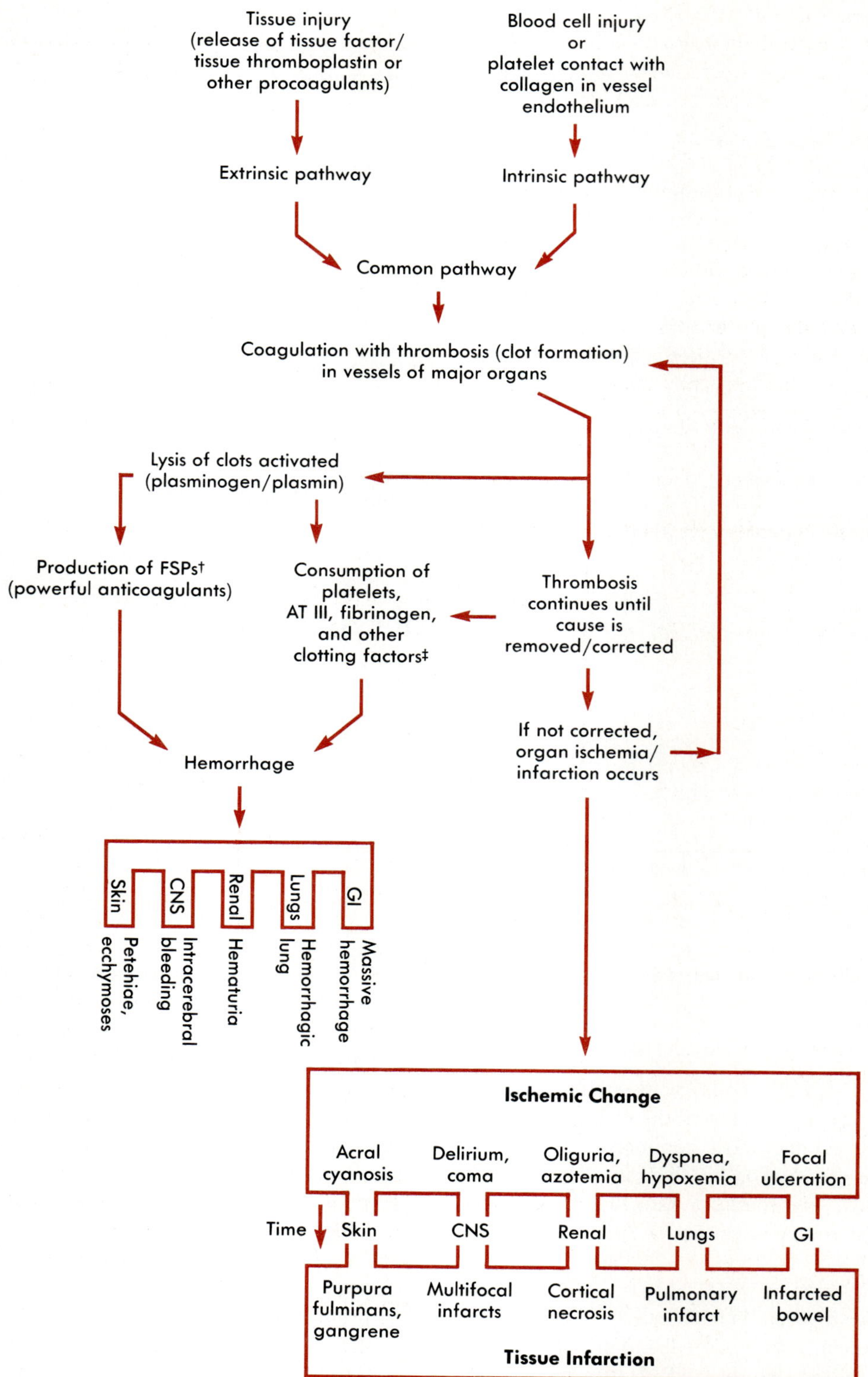


***Fig. 23-1*** Pathophysiology of DIC. Lysis of clots (fibrinolysis) is a natural consequence of and is activated by coagulation. It is intensified in patients with DIC. DIC is termed a consumption coagulopathy. During thrombosis, clotting factors are used to form clots. During fibrinolysis, clotting factors are destroyed inside the clot. The end result is a depletion of coagulation substances. *FSP,* Fibrin-split or fibrin-degradation products. (Modified from Carr M: J Emerg Med 5(4):316, 1987.)

mand, the consequences of lysis produce the classic, life-threatening hemorrhage of DIC. As fibrin and fibrinogen are digested by plasminogen during lysis, fibrin-split products are formed and exert a powerful anticoagulant effect. Their presence is a *very* characteristic feature of DIC, although fibrin-split products can appear in other disorders.

In addition, DIC is termed a **consumption coagulopathy.** The enzymes of fibrinolysis break down the clotting factors within the thrombus and platelets, fibrinogen, and thrombin are consumed in large quantities. In addition, the ongoing coagulation also consumes these same substances. The end result is a depletion of coagulation substances. The lack of clotting substances and the presence of powerful anticoagulants (fibrin-split products) produce a generalized hemorrhagic state. Ironically, this frequently fatal bleeding phenomenon is triggered by an underlying thrombotic process, and a vicious cycle of thrombosis and hemorrhage is established. The pathological consequences of fibrinolysis with

### SIGNS AND SYMPTOMS OF DIC

#### THROMBOTIC SIGNS AND SYMPTOMS

- Skin involvement
  - Red, indurated areas along vessel wall
  - Purpura fulminans (diffuse skin infarction)
  - Acral cyanosis
  - Necrosis of fingers, toes, nose, and genitalia
  - Cool, pale extremities with mottling, cyanosis, or edema
- Renal involvement
  - Renal failure
- Cerebral infarcts or hemorrhage
  - Focal neurological deficits, i.e., hemiplegia or loss of vision
  - Nonspecific changes, i.e., altered LOC, confusion, headache, or seizures
- Bowel infarction
  - Melena, hematemesis, abdominal distention, or absent or hyperactive bowel sounds
- Thrombophlebitis
- Pulmonary embolism

#### HEMORRHAGIC SIGNS AND SYMPTOMS

- Spontaneous hemorrhage into body cavities and skin surfaces
- Classic presentation of DIC is oozing or bleeding from invasive-line insertion sites or from body orifices
- Bleeding from body orifices such as the rectum, vagina, urethra, nose, and ears, as well as from the lung and GI tract
- Petechiae, purpura, or ecchymosis
- Gingival, nasal, or scleral hemorrhage on physical exam
- Hemorrhage may occur into all body cavities, including the abdomen, retroperitoneal space, cranium, and thorax

***Table 23-1*** Clotting studies in patients with DIC

| Laboratory test | Abnormality | Reason |
|---|---|---|
| Prothrombin time | >15 seconds | Elevated fibrin-split products and decreased plasma clotting factor levels |
| Platelet count | <150,00 | Platelet consumption |
| Fibrinogen | <160 mg/dl | Consumption by clotting cascade and destruction by plasmin |
| Fibrin-split Products | >One-eighth dilution | Fibrinogen destruction by plasmin |
| Antithrombin III | Decreased | Massive complex formation with active coagulation substances |

hemorrhage will continue until the precipitating cause is removed or corrected and the thrombotic process is terminated.[4,9,17]

## ASSESSMENT AND DIAGNOSIS

Since the pathologic sequelae of DIC are generalized and no organ is spared, assessment of each organ system must be accomplished. Particular attention should be paid to pathologic manifestations in the skin, since the vasculature of the skin is frequently involved in DIC and pathologic signs and symptoms are readily apparent. Although hemorrhagic signs and symptoms are the most dramatic, the critical care nurse should also note evidence of thrombotic-ischemic changes. See the box at left.

Laboratory findings also play an important role in the diagnosis and treatment of DIC. There are no generally accepted diagnostic criteria for DIC, nor is there a laboratory test that is pathognomonic for DIC. Strong indicators of DIC include thrombocytopenia (low platelet count), prolonged prothrombin time (PT), hypofibrinogenemia, and elevated levels of fibrin-split products (in the patient *without* underlying liver disease) (Table 23-1). A low platelet count occurs in nearly all DIC patients. The PT is prolonged in more than 90% of patients with DIC. The hallmark of DIC, an elevated fibrin-split/fibrin-degradation product level, strongly suggests DIC and is also found in more than 90% of DIC patients.[3,4,14] Normal or suspicious laboratory results must be viewed in the context of the clinical presentation.

## TREATMENT

Medical treatment of DIC is summarized in the box on p. 418. First and foremost, the clinician must treat the underlying illness (Fig. 23-2). In patients with septicemia and malignancies, use of antibiotics and chemotherapeutic agents is required.[14] The control of hemorrhage is accomplished in three ways: (1) through reconstitution of the patient's blood with RBCs and clotting factors, (2) through interruption of coagulation by blocking the action of throm-

**TREATMENT OF DIC**

Treat underlying illness
Reconstitute the patient's blood
  Transfuse RBCs, platelets, fresh frozen plasma, and cryoprecipitate
Interrupt coagulation by blocking the action of thrombin
  Administer heparin and antithrombin III
Terminate fibronolysis
  Administer aminiocaproic acid (AMICAR)
Treat complications

bin through antithrombotic therapy, and (3) through termination of fibrinolysis with epsilon **aminocaproic acid (AMICAR)** in extreme cases. The use of heparin and antithrombin III prevents further thrombosis and breaks the thrombosis-fibrinolysis cycle.[15] The life-threatening complications of DIC must be addressed, including hypotension, acidosis, and hypoxemia. Since acute renal failure may often develop during DIC, hemodialysis may be necessary.

### Blood Component Therapy

*RBC transfusions* and replacement of blood clotting factors may be performed. If the platelet count falls below $30{,}000/mm^3$ (or if hemorrhage is ongoing), administration of *platelets* is indicated. **Fresh frozen plasma** contains all clotting factors (V, VIII, XIII, and antithrombin III) and is also used for volume expansion.[15] Each unit of fresh frozen plasma will raise each clotting factor by approximately 5%. Appropriate laboratory tests should be monitored to determine further requirements for RBCs, platelets, and other clotting substances.[17]

Treatment of severe hypofibrinogenemia (<50 mg/dl) is the administration of **cryoprecipitate,** a concentrated source of fibrinogen and factor VIII from fresh frozen plasma. Each unit contains approximately 200 mg of fibrinogen, increasing the levels of fibrinogen and factor VIII by 2%.[15,17]

### Antithrombotic Therapy

Anticoagulants can be given to terminate the coagulation (thrombotic) process. *Heparin* produces an anticoagulant effect by potentiating the action of **antithrombin III,** which is a naturally occurring inhibitor of clotting proteins. With the formation of a heparin-antithrombin III complex, the speed of inactivation of clotting enzymes significantly increases. This complex has been shown to produce a 2000-time increase in the degradation of thrombin.[21]

**Heparin.** In the presence of intense bleeding, use of heparin therapy for DIC remains controversial. There have been no prospective randomized controlled studies to demonstrate the efficacy of using heparin in patients with DIC. Heparin is indicated, however, when there are clinical signs of thrombosis and when heparin therapy is administered concurrently with blood component therapy. General clinical indications for its use include deteriorating renal or neurological function and, under certain conditions, life-threatening bleeding unresponsive to blood product support.[12] Heparin apparently is an accepted treatment when DIC has been precipitated by amniotic fluid embolism, severe incompatible blood transfusion reactions, retained nonsurviving fetus, venous thrombosis, septic abortion, septicemia, acute promyelocytic leukemia, or heat stroke.[4,17]

Heparin is the treatment of choice in patients with chronic DIC; it is initially administered by intravenous (IV) infusion, then by subcutaneous injections for long-term maintenance. Heparin is most commonly used in these patients to treat venous thrombosis or overt skin infarction. Low-dose heparin may be given prophylactically to prevent thrombosis. Long-term heparin therapy may be necessary since use of coumarin derivatives (for example, warfarin [Coumadin] or Dicumarol) shows little effectiveness. As in patients with acute DIC, hemorrhage in patients with chronic DIC is first treated with blood products, and heparin is added if bleeding continues.[23]

**Antithrombin III.** Antithrombin III is a naturally occurring inhibitor of the active clotting process that binds with thrombin and other clotting factors to form an inactive complex. It helps produce the natural balance in the body between thrombosis and fibrinolysis. It can be administered alone or in conjunction with heparin. Administration of antithrombin III shortens the course of the disorder and decreases the complications of DIC.[21] Antithrombin III is most commonly given as a component of fresh frozen plasma (FFP). Where available, antithrombin IV can be administered as an intravenous medication. An average dose of 1 unit per kilogram will raise antithrombin III activity by 1%. In severe cases in which the level is below 50%, the antithrombin III level should be monitored every 4 hours, and antithrombin III should be administered to obtain a level of 100%. No undesirable side effects, including incompatibility reactions, have been reported with use of antithrombin III, and there have been no reported cases of hepatitis acquired from its use.[21]

### Antifibrinolytic Therapy

**Aminocaproic acid.** In approximately 5% of DIC cases, bleeding cannot be controlled with heparin. In this life-threatening situation, aminocaproic acid can be given to interrupt the fibrinolytic process through inhibition of plasmin. Aminocaproic acid is a potent inhibitor of plasminogen activators and, to a lesser degree, it inhibits fibrinolysin. It must be given only in the presence of DIC and not for other causes of fibrinolysis. There must also be reasonable certainty that the thrombotic process has already been controlled by heparin or other measures. The greatest complication—and the greatest barrier—to using aminocaproic acid is the potential for large-vessel thrombosis. Aminocaproic acid has also produced endocardial hemorrhage in laboratory animals, and it should be used with caution in

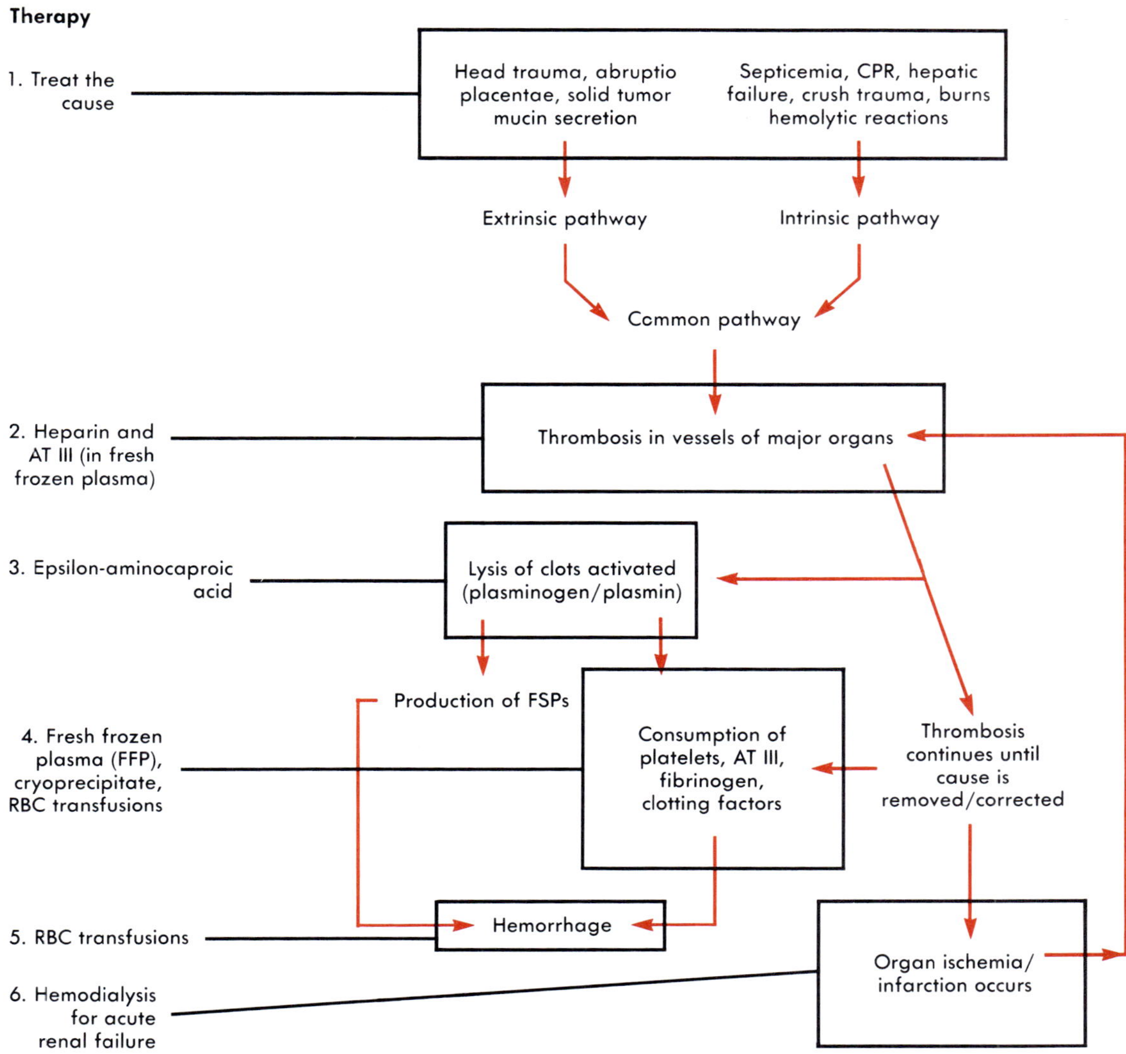


***Fig. 23-2*** Intended sites of action for therapies in DIC.

patients with cardiac dysrhythmias. Cardiac, renal, and electrolyte studies should be followed closely during its use.[1,15]

## SUMMARY OF NURSING CARE

The nursing management of a patient with DIC is directed at the prevention and/or recognition of hemorrhagic or thrombotic complications. It ranges from continuous assessment of the course of the disorder to intensive treatment maneuvers during acute hemorrhagic episodes (see the box on p. 420). Prompt attention to any sign of hemorrhage or thrombosis may spell the difference in patient morbidity and mortality.

For the patient with DIC, the nurse should institute **bleeding precautions,** which are intended to prevent blood loss. These precautions act to minimize tissue and vascular trauma, which, even in mild form, can precipitate bleeding.[8] Gentle technique is used during personal care and during turning, because exerting even normal force during these activities can produce subcutaneous bleeding. Obtaining blood pressure measurements by auscultation should be done as infrequently as possible since pressure on subcutaneous tissue can cause bleeding, with bruising or hematoma formation. An arterial line is preferable for both hemodynamic monitoring and blood sampling. Unfortunately, complications of line placement can result in significant hemorrhage. The use of intramuscular (IM) injections is avoided since the bolus of medication can rupture capillary walls from a pressure effect.[15]

Other bleeding precautions include avoiding the use of rectal temperatures, vaginal or rectal suppositories, enemas, and digital examinations of the rectum and vagina. Only paper tape should be used to secure tubes, invasive lines, and indwelling catheters since silk, plastic, and adhesive tape can cause tissue trauma and bleeding when removed.[22] Montgomery straps are a practical alternative to tape when frequent dressing changes are required. Shaving a patient

**Nursing Diagnosis and Management**
***Disseminated intravascular clotting (DIC)***

- Fluid Volume Deficit related to Hemorrhage, p. 495
- High Risk for Altered Tissue Perfusion risk factors: Cerebral, Cardiopulmonary, Renal, Gastrointestinal, Peripheral, p. 462
- Anxiety related to threat to biological, psychological, and/or social integrity, p. 448

must be performed gently with an electric razor. Use of aspirin, all aspirin-containing products, and many nonsteroidal antiinflammatory drugs (NSAIDs) is strictly contraindicated since they decrease platelet aggregation and promote bleeding. Cold compresses can be applied for pain control from bleeding into joints and tissues.

Every effort must be taken to avoid trauma to mucous membranes and to the skin. Performing frequent mouth care is necessary, since ischemia is common in the mouth. Gentle use of foam swabs for oral care, using a mild solution of saline, peroxide, or baking soda is preferable to the use of toothbrushes. Mouthwash solutions containing alcohol act as irritants and should be avoided.[15] If suctioning is required, the suction pressure should be lowered to prevent damage to the tracheal mucosa.[2]

Dry or cracking skin can become a site for bleeding or oozing. The nurse must keep the skin moist and intact through frequent application of lubricants to skin and lips, maintenance of adequate humidity in patient care areas, and prevention of patient injury.[8,17]

The potential for arterial thrombotic embolization to any major organ system is ever present in patients with DIC. The critical care nurse's contribution to the management of this problem consists of surveillance as detailed in the section, "Assessment and Diagnosis." Surveillance is meant to detect changes in organ function at the earliest possible moment; the problem is then referred to the physician for appropriate medical intervention.

## REFERENCES


1. American Medical Association Department of Drugs, Division of Drugs and Technology: Drug evaluations, ed 6, Chicago, 1986, The Association.
2. Bell TN: Disseminated intravascular coagulation and shock: multisystem crisis in the critically ill, Crit Care Nurs Clin North Am 2(2):255, 1990.
3. Carr JM, McKinney M, and McDonagh J: Diagnosis of disseminated intravascular coagulation. Role of D-dimer, Am J Clin Path 91(3):280, 1989.
4. Carr M: Disseminated intravascular coagulation: pathogenesis, diagnosis, and therapy, J Emerg Med 5(4):311, 1987.
5. Carr ME and Wolfert AI: Rewarming by hemodialysis for hypothermia: failure of heparin to prevent DIC, J Emerg Med 6(4):277, 1988.
6. Dangel R: Injury: potential for, related to disseminated intravascular coagulation (DIC). In McNally J, Stair J, and Somerville E, editors: Guidelines for cancer nursing practice, Orlando, Fla, 1985, Grune & Stratton, Inc.
7. Feinstein DI: Treatment of disseminated intravascular coagulation, Semin Thromb Hemost 14(4):351, 1988.
8. Griffin J: Hematology and immunology, concepts for nursing, Norwalk, Conn, 1986, Appleton-Century-Crofts.
9. Guyton A: Textbook of medical physiology, ed 8, Philadelphia, 1990, WB Saunders Co.
10. Johanson BC and others: Standards for critical care, ed 3, St Louis, 1988, Mosby–Year Book, Inc.
11. Miyata T and others: Disseminated intravascular coagulation caused by abdominal aortic aneurysm, J Cardiovasc Surg 29(4):494, 1988.
12. Ockelford P: Heparin 1986: indications and effective use, Drugs 31:81, 1986.
13. Pesola G and Carlon G: Pulmonary embolus-induced disseminated intravascular coagulation, Crit Care Med 15(10):983, 1987.
14. Price S and Wilson L: Pathophysiology: clinical concepts of disease processes, ed 4, St Louis, 1991, Mosby–Year Book, Inc.
15. Rooney A and Haviley C: Nursing management of disseminated intravascular coagulation, Oncol Nurs Forum 12:15, 1985.
16. Sheehy S and Barber J: Emergency nursing: principles and practices, ed 2, St Louis, 1985, Mosby–Year Book, Inc.
17. Siegrist C and Jones J: Disseminated intravascular coagulopathy and nursing implications, Semin Oncol Nurs 1(4):237, 1985.
18. Solinas S and others: Consumption coagulopathy and low-dose heparin in the surgical repair of abdominal aortic aneurysm: a study of fifteen cases, Ital J Surg Sciences 18(2):171, 1988.
19. Soloman SA and others: Severe disseminated intravascular coagulation associated with massive ventricular mural thrombosis following acute myocardial infarction, Postgrad Med J 64(756):791, 1988.
20. Suchak BA and Barbon CB: Disseminated intravascular clotting: a nursing challenge, Orthopaedic Nurs 8(6):61, 1989.
21. Vinazzer H: Clinical use of antithrombin III concentrate, Vox Sang 53(4):193, 1987.
22. Weber B, Speer M, and Swartz D: Irritation and stripping effects of adhesive tapes on skin layers of coronary artery bypass graft patients, Heart Lung 16(5):567, 1987.
23. Weitz J: Disseminated intravascular coagulation. In Brain MC and Carbone PP, editors: Current therapy in hematology-oncology, Toronto, 1988, Brian C Decker, Publisher.
24. Wilde JT and others: Association between necropsy evidence of disseminated intravascular coagulation and coagulation variables before death in patients in intensive care units, J Clin Path 41(2):138, 1988.
25. Wisecarver JL and Haire WD: Disseminated intravascular coagulation with multiple arterial thromboses responding to antithrombin III concentrate infusion, Thromb Res 54(6):709, 1989.
26. Zbilut J: Incidence of disseminated intravascular coagulation in patients admitted through the emergency department: a 5 year retrospective study, Heart Lung 9(5):833, 1980.
27. Zbilut J: Disseminated intravascular coagulation, J Emerg Nurs 7(5):213, 1981.

CHAPTER 24

# Septic Shock

## CHAPTER OBJECTIVES

- *State the theoretical and clinical definition of septic shock.*
- *List the causes and precipitating factors of septic shock.*
- *Explain the pathophysiology of septic shock.*
- *Identify the clinical manifestations of the hyperdynamic and hypodynamic phases of septic shock.*
- *Outline the important aspects of the medical management of the patient in septic shock.*
- *Summarize the nursing management of the patient in septic shock.*

## KEY TERMS

septic syndrome, p. 421
immune mediators, p. 422
multisystem organ failure, p. 424
hyperdynamic phase, p. 425
hypodynamic phase, p. 425

Septic shock is a complex pathophysiologic process that often results in multisystem organ failure and death. The multitude of causative microorganisms makes septic shock difficult to treat, and the myriad precipitating factors render it a difficult process to prevent. Often medical interventions designed to help the patient with an initial problem lead to the development of septic shock as a secondary problem. The incidence of sepsis is estimated at 70,000 to 300,000 cases annually in the United States, with 40% of these cases progressing into septic shock.[3] The mortality rate for septic shock is estimated between 40% and 95%, depending on the timeliness of identification and treatment.[11]

## DESCRIPTION

Shock is an acute, widespread process of impaired tissue perfusion resulting in cellular, metabolic, and hemodynamic derangements. Shock can be classified as hypovolemic, cardiogenic, distributive, obstructive, or combined, depending on the pathophysiologic cause. Septic shock is a form of distributive shock and is the result of microorganisms invading the body. The primary mechanism of this type of shock is the maldistribution of blood flow to the tissues, with some areas being overperfused and others being underperfused.[8,26] The result is eventual cellular damage and death.

Sepsis is the systemic state generated by the presence of invading microorganisms and their toxins in the blood or tissues. Septic *shock* is the result of the body's response to the invaders and is activated by the neurological and endocrine systems, tissue damage, and a wide variety of immune mediators. Subsequently, the patient develops cellular and metabolic derangements that produce impairment of organ and tissue perfusion. Multisystem organ failure and death ensue if this process is allowed to progress.[17,18]

The clinical description of sepsis is called the **septic syndrome.** Septic syndrome describes a clustering of clinical manifestations that, when present, are indicative of sepsis. The characteristics of septic syndrome are hypothermia or hyperthermia, tachycardia, tachypnea, clinical evidence of an infection site, and dysfunction of at least one organ system as evidenced by altered cerebral function, hypoxemia, elevated plasma lactate levels, or oliguria. The clinical description of septic shock incorporates the characteristics of the septic syndrome plus evidence of hypotension.[1,3]

## CAUSE

Sepsis and septic shock are caused by a wide variety of microorganisms (see the box, "Causative Microorganisms in Septic Shock"). These microorganisms may come from exogenous or endogenous sources. Exogenous sources include the hospital environment and members of the health care team. Endogenous sources include the patient's skin and gastrointestinal, respiratory, and genitourinary tracts. Gram-negative bacteria are responsible for approximately two thirds of the cases of septic shock. Another quarter of the cases are the result of a combination of microorganisms.[9,10,17,18,19,22]

**CAUSATIVE MICROORGANISMS IN SEPTIC SHOCK**

Gram-negative bacteria
- *Escherichia coli*
- *Klebsiella peumoniae*
- *Enterobacter*
- *Pseudomonas aeruginosa*
- *Enterococcus*
- *Serratia marcescens*
- *Bacteroides*
- *Proteus*
- *Haemophilus influenzae*

Gram-positive bacteria
- *Staphylococcus aureus*
- *Staphylococcus epidermidis*
- *Streptococcus pneumoniae*
- *Pneumococcus*
- *Clostridia*

Viruses
Fungi
Rickettsiae
Spirochetes
Protozoa
Parasites

Sepsis and septic shock are associated with a wide variety of intrinsic and extrinsic precipitating factors (see the box above, right). All of these factors interfere directly or indirectly with the body's anatomic and physiologic defense mechanisms. Several of the intrinsic factors are not modifiable or are very difficult to control. A number of the extrinsic factors are required for the diagnosis of sepsis or septic shock and the subsequent management of the patient. Therefore it becomes apparent that all critically ill patients are at risk for the development of sepsis and septic shock.[9,16,18,19,22]

## PATHOPHYSIOLOGY

Septic shock is a complex systemic response that is initiated during the entry of a microorganism into the body and the release of endotoxins or exotoxins. Endotoxins are liberated from the cell walls of the gram-negative bacteria when they are destroyed by the body's immune system. On the other hand, gram-positive bacteria and other microorganisms that are alive in the body release exotoxins.[16,17] Once a microorganism invades the body and releases the toxin a variety of mechanisms occur, including activation of the immune mediators, damage to the endothelium, and activation of the central nervous system (CNS) and the endocrine system. Consequently, a variety of physiologic and pathophysiologic events occur that affect capillary membrane permeability, clotting, the distribution of blood flow to the tissues and organs, and the metabolic state of the body. Subsequently, a systemic imbalance between cellular oxygen supply and demand develops that results in cellular hypoxia, damage, and death (Fig. 24-1).[10,11,17,18]

### Initiation of the Septic Cascade

**Immune mediators.** The septic process is initiated by the activation of **immune mediators** that are part of the inflammatory process and are released in response to invading microorganisms. These humoral, cellular, and biochemical mediators initiate a chain of complex interactions that are controlled by numerous feedback mechanisms. Eventually the immune system is overwhelmed, the feedback mechanisms fail, and a process that was designed to protect the body actually ends up harming it.[10]

The *humoral mediators* involved in septic shock are the complement system, the coagulation-fibrinolytic system, and the kallikrein-kinin system. Stimulation of these systems results in activation of cellular mediators, the formation of biochemical mediators, endothelial cell damage, peripheral vasodilation, increased capillary membrane permeability, initiation of coagulation and fibrinolysis, myocardial depression, and activation of Hageman factor (factox XII), which potentiates the effects of the humoral mediators. The *cellular mediators* involved in septic shock include polymorphonuclear granulocytes (PMNs), macrophages, lymphocytes, and platelets. Stimulation of these cells leads to the formation of biochemical mediators, stimulation of the complement and the coagulation systems, destruction of the invading microorganisms, activation of T and B cells, and the formation of microemboli. The *biochemical mediators* involved in septic shock include oxygen-free radicals, leukotrienes, prostaglandins, interleukins 1 and 2, serotonin, tumor necrosis factor, histamine, proteinases, and platelet activating factor. Stimulation of these substances results in enhancement of the cellular and humoral mediators; peripheral vasodilation; the formation of microemboli; vasoconstriction of the renal, pulmonary, and splanchnic beds;

**PRECIPITATING FACTORS ASSOCIATED WITH SEPTIC SHOCK**

| Intrinsic factors | Extrinsic factors |
|---|---|
| Extremes of age | Invasive devices |
| Coexisting diseases | Drug therapy |
| Malignancies | Fluid therapy |
| Burns | Surgical and traumatic wounds |
| AIDS | Surgical and invasive diagnostic procedures |
| Diabetes | Immunosuppressive therapy |
| Substance abuse | |
| Dysfunction of one or more of the major body systems | |
| Malnutrition | |

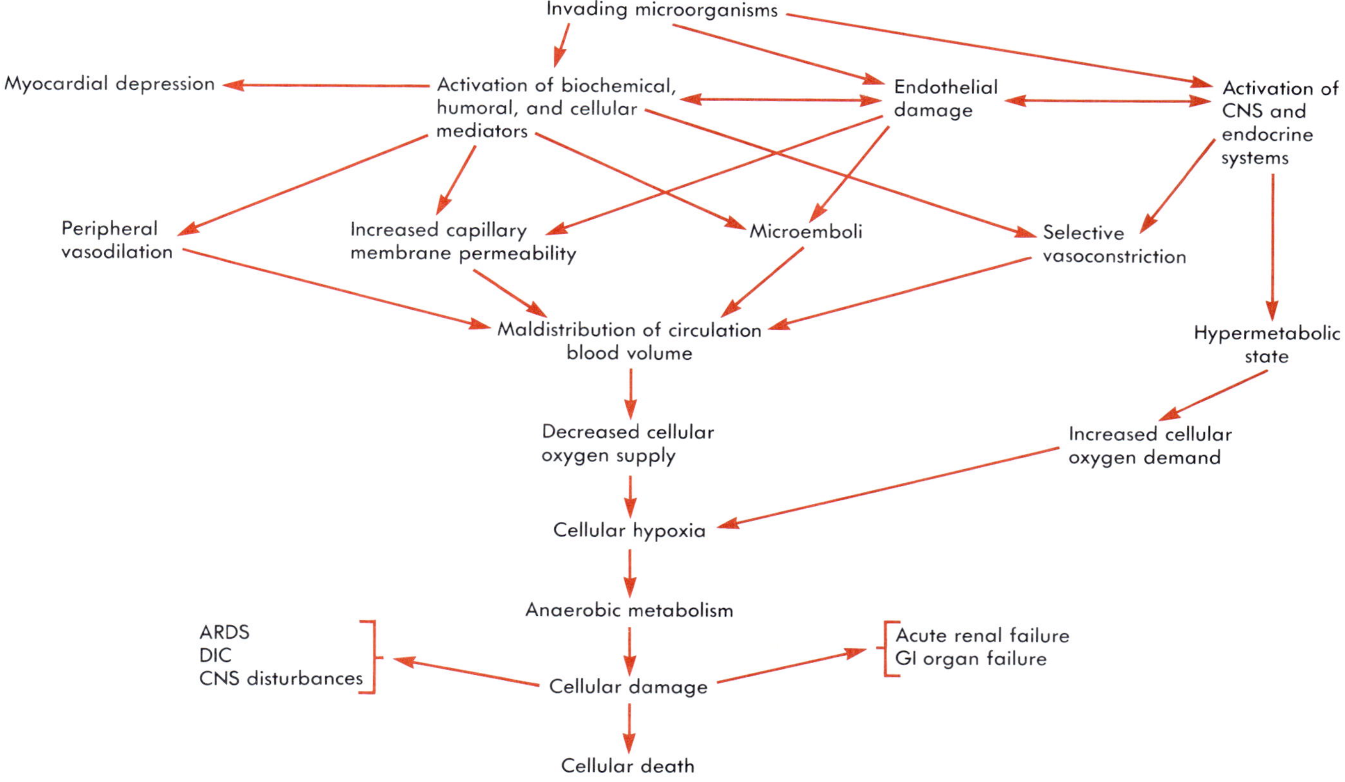


***Fig. 24-1*** The pathophysiology of septic shock.

myocardial depression; endothelial cell damage; increased capillary membrane permeability; fever; and increased metabolism.[10,15,17,23]

**Endothelial cell damage.** The septic cascade is also initiated by damage to the endothelial cells caused by the toxins released from invading microorganisms. Endothelial cell damage results in activation of the immune mediators, increased capillary membrane permeability, and the formation of microemboli. This in turn leads to disruption of blood flow to the tissues, more endothelial cell damage, and further propagation of the septic process.[10,17]

**CNS and endocrine system.** Activation of the CNS and the endocrine system also occurs as part of the primary response to invading microorganisms. This leads to stimulation of the sympathetic nervous system (SNS) and the release of adrenocorticotropic hormone (ACTH). These events trigger the release of epinephrine, norepinephrine, glucocorticoids, aldosterone, glucagon, and renin. This results in the development of a hypermetabolic state and further contributes to the vasoconstriction of the renal, pulmonary, and splanchnic beds. Activation of the CNS also causes the release of endogenous opiates, which are thought to cause vasodilation and decrease myocardial contractility.[10,16]

### Pathophysiologic Responses

Once the initial sequence of events is triggered, a series of pathophysiologic responses occur that eventually culminate in the maldistribution of circulation blood volume. These responses include massive peripheral vasodilation, formation of microemboli, selective vasoconstriction, and increased capillary membrane permeability.[10,17] The maldistribution of circulating blood volume eventually results in decreased cellular oxygen supply.[26]

**Peripheral vasodilation.** One of the major pathophysiologic responses that occurs in septic shock is massive peripheral vasodilation. Vasodilation occurs in response to the release of certain biochemical mediators, activation of the kallikrein-kinin system, and the release of endogenous opiates. Massive peripheral vasodilation leads to the development of relative hypovolemia and decreased tissue perfusion.[10,15,17]

**Microemboli.** Another major pathophysiologic response that occurs in septic shock is the formation of microemboli. Microemboli are the result of activation of the coagulation system, platelet and polymorphonuclear (PMN) granulocyte aggregation, the release of certain biochemical mediators, and damage to the endothelial cells. The formation of microemboli results in decreased tissue perfusion and further endothelial cell damage.[10,17]

**Selective vasoconstriction.** Selective vasoconstriction of the renal, pulmonary, and splanchnic beds is another pathophysiologic response to septic shock. Selective vasoconstriction occurs as the result of stimulation of the SNS and the release of renin and certain biochemical mediators. This response results in decreased tissue perfusion of the kidneys, lungs, and gastrointestinal (GI) organs, with eventual system dysfunction.[10,17]

**Increased capillary membrane permeability.** One other contributing factor to the maldistribution of circulating blood volume is increased capillary membrane permeability. This pathophysiologic derangement occurs in response to activation of the complement system and the release of certain biochemical mediators. Increased capillary membrane permeability promotes fluid loss from the intravascular space (third-spacing) and potentiates the relative hypovolemic effect induced by the massive peripheral vasodilation. The formation of microemboli is also enhanced because of the increased viscosity of the blood left in the intravascular space.[10,17]

### Pathophysiologic Result

The maldistribution of circulating blood volume decreases the amount of oxygen delivered to the cells. This situation leads to a number of cellular derangements that ultimately result in cellular death. The hypermetabolic state created by activation of the CNS and the endocrine system further enhances the situation by increasing the oxygen demands of the cells.

**Cellular derangements.** As the blood supply to the cells decreases, the cells switch from aerobic to anaerobic metabolism as a source of energy. Anaerobic metabolism produces small amounts of energy but large amounts of lactic acid. Lactic acidemia quickly develops and causes more cellular damage. The small amount of energy created by anaerobic metabolism is not enough to keep the cells functional, and irreversible damage starts to occur. The ionic pump in the cell membrane fails, causing the cell and its organelles to swell. Cellular energy production comes to a complete halt as the mitochondria swell and rupture. At this point the problem becomes one of oxygen use, instead of oxygen delivery. Even if the cell were to receive more oxygen, it would be unable to use it because of damage to the mitochondria. The cell's digestive organelles swell, resulting in leakage of destructive enzymes into the cell. Autodigestion occurs with ensuing cell death.[10,11,17]

**Metabolic derangements.** A number of metabolic derangements occur as a result of activation of the CNS and the endocrine system. A hypermetabolic state develops, which increases cellular oxygen demand and contributes to cellular hypoxia. Lactic acid production is increased as a result. Glucocorticoids, ACTH, epinephrine, and glucagon are all catabolic hormones that are released as part of this response. These hormones favor the use of fats and proteins over glucose for energy production.

The hypermetabolic state also increases the cellular metabolic needs. Increased glucose requirements, in conjunction with the high level of catabolic hormones, results in the limited ability of the cells to use glucose as a substrate for energy production. This causes glucose intolerance, hyperglycemia, relative insulin resistance, and the use of fat for energy (lipolysis). The relative insulin resistance causes the body to produce more insulin, which inhibits the use of fat as an energy substrate. This promotes the use of protein as an energy substrate and catabolism of protein stores in the visceral organs and skeletal muscles.[10,15,17]

### Organ System Dysfunction

As septic shock continues to progress and more and more cells die, the individual organ systems will malfunction and eventually fail. Every system in the body is affected by this process. **Multisystem organ failure** is defined as failure of two or more organ systems.[1]

Cardiac dysfunction is thought to develop as a result of immune mediator activation and the release of myocardial depressant factor (MDF). MDF is a substance that is released from the pancreas as it becomes ischemic. Myocardial depression is further exacerbated by myocardial hypoperfusion and lactic acidosis. Cardiogenic shock and ventricular failure eventually occur.[10,15,20] Pulmonary dysfunction occurs as a result of increased pulmonary capillary membrane permeability, pulmonary microemboli, and pulmonary vasoconstriction. Ventilatory failure and adult respiratory distress syndrome (ARDS) eventually develop.[10,25] CNS dysfunction develops as a result of immune mediator activation and cerebral hypoperfusion. Failure of the CNS leads to cardiac and respiratory depression and thermoregulatory failure.[10] Renal dysfunction develops as a result of renal vasoconstriction and renal hypoperfusion, leading to acute tubular necrosis.[10,13] Hematologic dysfunction occurs as a result of activation of immune mediators and the overstimulation of the coagulation-fibrinolytic system. Disseminated intravascular coagulation (DIC) eventually develops.[2,10] GI dysfunction occurs as a result of splanchnic vasoconstriction and splanchnic hypoperfusion, leading to failure of the gut organs. In addition, failure of the gut organs results in the release of gram-negative bacteria into the system and more immune mediators, further perpetuating the entire septic process.[6,10]

## ASSESSMENT AND DIAGNOSIS

The clinical presentation and laboratory assessment of the patient in septic shock varies, depending on whether the patient is in the early or late stages of the process. The early stage of septic shock is known as the **hyperdynamic phase,** or warm phase. The late stage is known as the **hypodynamic phase,** or cold phase, of septic shock. The hyperdynamic phase is characterized by compensatory responses, whereas the hypodynamic phase is typified by decompensatory responses (Table 24-1). Transition from one phase to another can take hours or days.[10,15,17,24]

### Hyperdynamic Phase

**Signs and symptoms.** During the hyperdynamic phase of septic shock, massive vasodilation occurs in both the venous and arterial beds. Dilation of the venous system leads to a decrease in venous return to the heart, which results in a decrease in the preload of the right and left ventricles. This is evidenced by a decline in the right atrial pressure (RAP) and pulmonary capillary wedge pressure (PCWP). Dilation of the arterial system results in a decrease in the afterload of the heart, as evidenced by a decrease in the systemic vascular resistance (SVR). The patient's blood pressure (BP) falls in response to the reduction in preload and afterload. The patient also develops pink, warm, flushed skin as a result of the massive vasodilation.[10,15,17,24]

The heart rate (HR) rises to compensate for the hypotension and in response to increased metabolic, SNS, and adrenal gland stimulation. This results in a normal-to-high cardiac output (CO) and cardiac index (CI). The diastolic BP decreases due to the vasodilation, causing the pulse pressure (PP) to widen, and the systolic BP increases due to the elevated CO. The patient develops a full, bounding pulse. As evidenced by a decline in the left ventricular stroke work index (LVSWI), myocardial contractility is decreased due to myocardial depression.[10,15,17,24] In the lungs a ventilation-perfusion mismatch develops as a result of pulmonary vasoconstriction and the formation of pulmonary microemboli. Hypoxemia occurs, and the respiratory rate (RR) increases to compensate for the lack of oxygen. The patient develops rales as increased pulmonary capillary membrane permeability leads to the development of pulmonary interstitial edema.[10,15,17,24]

Level of consciousness (LOC) starts to change as a result

***Table 24-1*** Clinical manifestations and laboratory values of septic shock

| | Hyperdynamic phase | Hypodynamic phase |
|---|---|---|
| Signs and symptoms | Increased HR | Increased HR |
| | Decreased BP | Decreased BP |
| | Wide PP | Narrow PP |
| | Full, bounding pulse | Weak, thready pulse |
| | Pink, warm, flushed skin | Pale, cool, clammy skin |
| | Increased RR | Decreased RR |
| | Rales | Rales, rhonchi, and wheezes |
| | Change in LOC | Coma |
| | Decreased UO | Anuria |
| | Increased temperature | Increased/decreased temperature |
| Hemodynamic parameters | Increased CO and CI | Decreased CO and CI |
| | Decreased SVR | Increased SVR |
| | Decreased RAP | Increased RAP |
| | Decreased PCWP | Increased PCWP |
| | Decreased LVSWI | Decreased LVSWI |
| Laboratory values | Decreased $PaO_2$ | Decreased $PaO_2$ |
| | Decreased $PaCO_2$ | Increased $PaCO_2$ |
| | Decreased $HCO_3$ | Decreased $HCO_3$ |
| | Increased $SvO_2$ | Decreased $SvO_2$ |
| | Increased PT and PTT | Increased lactate level |
| | Decreased platelet count | Increased anion gap |
| | Decreased fibrinogen level | Increased BUN and creatinine levels |
| | Decreased clotting factors | Electrolyte imbalances |
| | Increased serum glucose | Increased SGOT, SGPT, and LDH |
| | | Increased serum amylase and lipase |
| | | Decreased serum glucose |

*HR,* heart rate; *BP,* blood pressure; *PP,* pulse pressure; *LOC,* level of consciousness; *UO,* urinary output; *CO,* cardiac output; *CI,* cardiac index; *SVR,* systemic vascular resistance; *RAP,* right atrial pressure; *PCWP,* pulmonary capillary wedge pressure; *LVSWI,* left ventricular stroke work index; *PT,* prothrombin time; *PTT,* partial thromboplastin time; *BUN,* blood urea nitrogen; *SGOT,* serum glutamic oxaloacetic transaminase; *SGPT,* serum glutamic pyruvic transaminase; *LDH,* lactic dehydrogenase.

of decreased cerebral perfusion, immune mediator activation, hyperthermia, and lactic acidosis. The patient may appear disoriented, confused, combative, or lethargic. Urine output (UO) declines because of decreased perfusion of the kidneys. The patient's temperature is elevated in response to pyrogens released from the invading microorganisms, immune mediator activation, and increased metabolic activity.[10,15,17,24]

**Laboratory values.** Arterial blood gases (ABGs) drawn during this phase reveal respiratory alkalosis, hypoxemia, and metabolic acidosis. This is demonstrated by low levels of $PaO_2$, $PaCO_2$, and bicarbonate ($HCO_3$). The respiratory alkalosis is due to the patient's increased RR. The metabolic acidosis is the result of lack of oxygen to the cells and the development of lactic acidemia. The patient's lactate level may also be elevated as a result of increased lactic acid production. The mixed venous oxygen saturation ($SvO_2$) is increased. This is indicative of less oxygen being extracted from the capillary blood due to maldistribution of the circulating blood volume and impaired cellular metabolism.[10,17]

The white blood cell (WBC) count is elevated as part of the immune response to the invading microorganisms. In addition, the WBC differential reveals an increase in immature neutrophils (shift to the left). This occurs because the body has to mobilize increasing amounts of WBCs to fight the infection.[10,17] Hematologic alterations that may occur during this phase include prolongation of the prothrombin time (PT) and partial thromboplastin time (PTT), decreased platelet count, decreased fibrinogen level, decreased clotting factors, and increased fibrin split products (FSPs). These results are reflective of coagulation abnormalities that result from accelerated clotting and accelerated fibrinolysis and are indicative of the onset of DIC. An increased serum glucose level also occurs as part of the hypermetabolic response and the development of insulin resistance.[10,15,17]

### Hypodynamic Phase

**Signs and symptoms.** As the septic process progresses into the hypodynamic phase, the CO and CI decrease and profound hypotension occurs. This is the result of ventricular failure due to myocardial ischemia, lactic acidosis, myocardial depressant factor, and a rising afterload. The RAP and PCWP increase due to right and left ventricular dysfunction. Vasoconstriction occurs, as evidenced by an elevated SVR, to compensate for the falling BP. The patient develops pale, cold, clammy skin.[10,15,17,24]

The HR rises further in an attempt to compensate for the declining CO and hypotension. A variety of dysrhyth mias may occur as a result of myocardial ischemia, lactic acidosis, and circulating catecholamines. The dysrhyth mias exacerbate the reduction in CO. The PP narrows as the CO declines. The patient develops a weak, thready pulse.[10,15,17,24]

As the pulmonary system continues to deteriorate and ARDS develops, the patient exhibits rapid, shallow respirations and experiences severe shortness of breath. The RR remains high until fatigue occurs and ventilatory failure develops, which causes the RR to decline. In addition, the patient develops more adventitious breath sounds as evidenced by an increase in rales, rhonchi, and wheezes.[10,15,17,24]

The patient's LOC continues to deteriorate as the BP and cerebral perfusion fall. The patient usually becomes extremely difficult to arouse. Anuria occurs as kidney function fails due to poor renal perfusion. The patient's temperature may remain elevated or it may decline due to decreased metabolic activity and thermoregulatory failure.[10,17,24]

**Laboratory values.** ABGs drawn during this phase of septic shock reveal severe hypoxemia with a metabolic and respiratory acidosis. This is demonstrated by low $PaO_2$, high $PaCO_2$, and low $HCO_3$ levels. The respiratory acidosis is due to the decline in the patient's RR. The lactate level is elevated at this point as a result of increased anaerobic metabolism and liver failure. The patient's anion gap increases, reflecting overproduction and accumulation of lactate. The $SvO_2$ level is decreased in response to the decreased CO and severe hypoxemia.[10,17]

As multisystem organ failure develops, the patient experiences a variety of laboratory data abnormalities. As the immune system fails, the WBC count declines. The blood urea nitrogen (BUN) and serum creatinine (Cr) levels are elevated, and an assortment of electrolyte imbalances occur as the kidneys fail. Hepatic dysfunction results in elevated levels of serum glutamic oxaloacetic transaminase (SGOT), serum glutamic pyruvic transaminase (SGPT), and lactic dehydrogenase (LDH). Failure of the pancreas leads to elevated serum amylase and serum lipase levels.[10,17] As the body's supplies of glucose, fats, and proteins are exhausted the serum glucose falls.[10,15,17]

## TREATMENT

Treatment of the patient in septic shock requires a multifaceted approach. The goals of treatment are to control the infection, reverse the pathophysiologic responses, and promote metabolic support. This approach includes identifying and treating the infection, supporting the cardiovascular system and enhancing tissue perfusion, and initiating nutrition therapy. In addition, dysfunction of the individual organ systems must be treated or prevented.

### Control of the Infection

One of the first measures that must be taken in the treatment of septic shock is finding and eradicating the cause of the infection. Blood, urine, sputum, and wound cultures should be obtained to find the location of the infection. Antibiotic therapy should be initiated as soon as possible. If the microorganism is unknown, a broad-spectrum antibiotic should be administered. Once the microorganism is identified, an antibiotic more specific to the microorganism should be started. Administration of antibiotics can be particularly hazardous in gram-negative shock, because more endotoxin is released from the cell walls when the microorganisms die.[16,19] This further aggravates the entire septic process. Surgical intervention to debride infected or necrotic tissue or to drain abscesses may also be necessary to facilitate removal of the septic source.[16]

### Reverse the Pathophysiologic Responses

Another important measure that must be taken in the treatment of septic shock is supporting the cardiovascular system and enhancing tissue perfusion. Specific interventions are aimed at increasing cellular oxygen supply and decreasing cellular oxygen demand. These treatments include administering fluids, vasoactive agents, and positive inotropic agents; providing ventilatory support, controlling the patient's temperature; and reversing the acidosis.

Aggressive fluid administration is very important during the hyperdynamic phase of septic shock to augment intravascular volume and increase preload. Colloids, crystalloids, or blood products may be used, depending on the patient's condition. No one fluid has been proved better than the others. The amount of fluid that is administered may vary, but generally the goal is to restore the patient's filling pressures to the low-to-normal range. During the hypodynamic phase, fluid administration is very limited because of the potential for fluid overload and congestive heart failure.[7,10,16,17]

The administration of vasoconstrictor agents is indicated during the hyperdynamic phase of septic shock to reverse the massive peripheral vasodilation. These agents help increase the systemic vascular resistance (SVR) and augment the patient's blood pressure. Examples of these medications include epinephrine (Adrenalin), norepinephrine (Levophed), alpha-range dopamine (Intropin), metaraminol (Aramine), phenylephrine (Neo-Synephrine), and methoxamine (Vasoxyl).[4,5,7] During the hypodynamic phase, peripheral vasoconstriction is the problem and the administration of vasodilator agents is indicated. These agents help decrease the SVR and optimize the patient's CO. Examples of these medications include sodium nitroprusside (Nipride), nitroglycerin (Tridil), and phentolamine (Regitine).[4,5,7] All of these medications are titrated to the patient's response.

Myocardial depression occurs during both phases of septic shock and necessitates the administration of positive inotropic agents to increase contractility. Examples of these medications include beta-range dopamine (Intropin), dobutamine (Dobutrex), amrinone (Inocor), epinephrine (Adrenalin), norepinephrine (Levophed), isoproterenol (Isuprel), and digitalis (Digoxin).[4,5,7,20] These agents are administered in addition to the vasoactive agents, and all, except digitalis, are titrated to the patient's response.

To optimize oxygenation and ventilation, the patient should be intubated and mechanically ventilated. Ventilator settings should be adjusted to provide the patient with a $PaO_2$ level greater than 70 mm Hg and a pH level within the normal range.[16] Temperature control is also necessary to decrease the metabolic demands created by hyperthermia. Antipyretic agents and hypothermia therapy are often used. Reversal of lactic acidosis may be obligatory if the patient starts to develop associated complications. The administration of sodium bicarbonate is the most common treatment of acidosis, but it carries some risks. These risks include rebound increase in lactic acid production, development of hyperosmolar state and fluid overload due to excessive sodium, shifting of the oxyhemoglobin curve to the left, and rapid cellular electrolyte shifts.[10]

### Promotion of Metabolic Support

One more measure that must be taken in the treatment of septic shock is the initiation of nutrition therapy. The goal of nutritional support is to improve the patient's overall nutrition status, enhance the immune system, and promote wound healing. Nutrition therapy should be tailored to the individual patient's need as indicated by the underlying condition and laboratory data. The enteral route is preferred over the parental.

The nutrition supplement for the patient in septic shock should be high in protein to help offset the metabolic derangements that develop in the hypermetabolic state. The number of protein calories given depends on the patient's nitrogen balance. In early sepsis, the mix of nonprotein calories may be divided evenly between carbohydrates and fats. In the later stages of septic shock, significant alterations in fat metabolism occur and the lipid content should be limited to 10% to 15% of the total nonprotein calories. The lipid emulsion should contain medium-chain triglycerides, because these are easier to metabolize than long-chain triglycerides.[10,12]

### Experimental Therapies

There are a number of experimental therapies now being used in the treatment of septic shock. Two therapies that have been tested in humans are high-dose corticosteroids and naloxone (Narcan). High-dose corticosteroids are thought to antagonize the effects of several of the immune mediators. Extensive testing has failed to prove that this is true; therefore the use of corticosteroids is questionable for the treatment of septic shock.[16,23] Naloxone is another therapy that has been tested a number of times, with mixed results. Naloxone, an endorphin anatagonist, is thought to reverse the hypotension caused by endogenous opiates.[16,21]

More promising studies are now being done with drugs that are thought to block or alter the effects of the immune mediators. These include pulmonary vasodilating prostaglandins, free radical scavengers, cyclooxygenase inhibitors, and anticomplement antibodies. Although these therapies have demonstrated positive results in animals, their efficacy in humans needs to be more extensively tested.[16,23] One other emerging therapy is the use of monoclonal antibodies. These antibodies work directly against gram-negative microorganisms by binding with the endotoxin and blocking activation of the immune mediators. This therapy also needs more extensive testing in humans before any conclusions about its effectiveness can be made.[16]

## SUMMARY OF NURSING CARE

Prevention of septic shock is one of the primary responsibilities of any nurse in the critical care area. This includes the identification of patients at risk and reduction of their exposure to invading microorganisms. Hand washing, the use of aseptic technique, and an understanding of how microorganisms can invade the body are essential components of preventive nursing care.[9,17] Continual assessment of the patient at risk is critical in the early identification of septic shock. Early identification allows for early treatment and decreased mortality.[9]

The nursing management of a patient with septic shock is a complex and challenging responsibility. It requires an in-depth understanding of the pathophysiology of the disease and the anticipated effects of each intervention, as well as a solid understanding of the nursing process.[14,18] Assessment of a patient with septic shock includes monitoring for changes in signs and symptoms, hemodynamic parameters, and laboratory values described earlier. Frequent assessment to detect subtle changes that indicate the progression of the septic process is also very important, because the treatment varies depending on which phase the patient is in.[15,17]

### Nursing Diagnosis and Management
#### *Septic Shock*

- Decreased Cardiac Output related to decreased preload secondary to septicemia, p. 460
- Impaired Gas Exchange related to ventilation-perfusion inequality secondary to pulmonary microemboli, increased pulmonary capillary permeability, and/or pulmonary vasoconstriction, p. 474
- High Risk for Altered Tissue Perfusion risk factor: vasopresser therapy, p. 462
- Altered Nutrition: Less Than Body Requirements related to increased metabolic demands and/or lack of exogenous nutrients
- High Risk for Infection risk factor: invasive monitoring devices, p. 465
- High Risk for Impaired Skin Integrity risk factor: immobility, p. 499
- Anxiety related to threat to biological integrity, p. 448
- Sensory-Perceptual Alterations related to sensory overload, sensory deprivation, and sleep disturbance, p. 489

The patient with septic shock may have any number of disorders, depending on the progression of the process (see the box, "Nursing Diagnoses"). Nursing interventions include administering prescribed medications, monitoring the patient's response to the medications, implementing measures to prevent the development of concomitant infections and skin breakdown, and monitoring for effects and complications of nutrition therapy. Activities to decrease patient and family anxiety include explaining all procedures and treatments and allowing them to ask questions and voice concerns.[15,17]

## SUMMARY

Septic shock is a life-threatening disorder that can affect every organ system. A positive patient outcome is dependent on an early and aggressive multidisciplinary approach. The critical care nurse plays an important part in preventing, detecting, and treating this complex and challenging process.

### REFERENCES


1. Balk RA and Bone RC: The septic syndrome, Crit Care Clin 5:1, 1989.
2. Bell TN: Disseminated intravascular coagulation and shock: multisystem crisis in the critically ill, Crit Care Nurs Clin North Am 2:225, 1990.
3. Bone RC and others: Sepsis syndrome: a valid clinical entity, Crit Care Med 17:389, 1989.
4. Boyd JL, Stanford GC, and Chernow B: The pharmacotherapy of septic shock, Crit Care Clin 5:133, 1989.
5. Burns KM: Vasoactive drug therapy in shock, Crit Care Nurs Clin North Am 2:167, 1990.
6. Collins AS: Gastrointestinal complications in shock, Crit Care Nurs Clin North Am 2:269, 1990.
7. Hancock BG and Eberhard NK: The pharmacologic management of shock, Crit Care Nurs Q 11(1):19, 1988.
8. Houston MC: Pathophysiology of shock, Crit Care Nurs Clin North Am 2:143, 1990.
9. Hoyt NJ: Preventing septic shock: infection control in the intensive care unit, Crit Care Nurs Clin North Am 2:287, 1990.
10. Huddleston VB: Multisystem organ failure: a pathophysiologic approach, Lewisville, Tx, 1989, Barbara Clark Mims Associates.
11. Iverson RL: Septic shock: a clinical perspective, Crit Care Clin 4:215, 1988.
12. Kuhn MM: Nutritional support for the shock patient, Crit Care Nurs Clin North Am 2:201, 1990.
13. Lancaster LE: Renal response to shock, Crit Care Nurs Clin North Am 2:221, 1990.
14. Lancaster LE and Rice V: Nursing care planning: overview and application to the patient in shock, Crit Care Nurs Clin North Am 2:279, 1990.
15. Littletone MT: Pathophysiology and assessment of sepsis and septic shock, Crit Care Nurs Q 11(1):30, 1988.
16. Luce JM: Pathogenesis and management of septic shock, Chest 91:883, 1987.
17. Rice V: The clinical continuum of septic shock, Crit Care Nurs 4(5):86, 1984.
18. Rice V: Septic shock: nursing implications of current medical research, NITA 10:326, 1987.
19. Roach AC: Antibiotic therapy in septic shock, Crit Care Nurs Clin North Am 2:179, 1990.
20. Schremmer B and Dhainaut JF: Heart failure in septic shock: effects of inotropic support, Crit Care Med 18:S49, 1990.

21. Schumann LL and Remington MA: The use of naloxone in treating endotoxic shock, Crit Care Nurs 10(2):63, 1990.
22. Segreti J: Nosocomial infections and secondary infections in sepsis, Crit Care Clin 5:177, 1989.
23. Stroud M, Swindell B, and Bernard GR: Cellular and humoral mediators of sepsis syndrome, Crit Care Nurs Clin North Am 2:151, 1990.
24. Summers G: The clinical and hemodynamic presentation of the shock patient, Crit Care Nurs Clin North Am 2:161, 1990.
25. Vaughan P and Brooks C: Adult respiratory distress syndrome: a complication of shock, Crit Care Nurs Clin North Am 2:235, 1990.
26. Vincent JL and Van Der Linden P: Septic shock: particular type of acute circulatory failure, Crit Care Med 18:S70, 1990.

CHAPTER 25

# Anaphylaxis

## CHAPTER OBJECTIVES

- *Describe the basic mechanism for initiation of the immune response for both anaphylactic and anaphylactoid reactions.*
- *List and explain the triad of physiological effects that occur in patients with anaphylaxis.*
- *List at least two causative agents of anaphylaxis from each of the following categories: medications, food, chemicals, and animal stings or bites.*
- *Describe the medical and nursing management of patients with anaphylaxis.*

## KEY TERMS

anaphylaxis, p. 430
antigen, p. 430
true anaphylactic reactions, p. 430
anaphylactoid reactions, p. 430
mast cells, p. 432
basophils, p. 432
histamine, p. 432
leukotrienes, p. 432
prostaglandins, p. 432
bradykinin, p. 432
eosinophils, p. 432
anaphylactic shock, p. 432
distributive (low-resistance) shock, p. 432

Millions of Americans have a history of systemic or localized reactions to a variety of substances such as penicillin or bee stings. Each year an estimated 50 deaths result from bee-sting anaphylaxis. Allergic reactions to insect stings occur in approximately 0.4% of the population each year.[18,26] The realization that most anaphylaxis-related deaths occur within the *first 30 minutes* after exposure to the foreign antigen stresses the need for prompt intervention.

## DESCRIPTION

**Anaphylaxis** is a potentially life-threatening allergic reaction. It is described as a hypersensitivity reaction to an invading substance **(antigen)** that causes release of powerful vasoactive substances such as histamine and bradykinin into the bloodstream. The somatic responses to the vasoactive substance release include bronchospasm, generalized edema, hypotension, urticaria, and hives (Fig. 25-1).

Allergic reactions are categorized into four types, because their pathogenesis cannot be attributed to one mechanism (Table 25-1). Of greatest importance for this discussion is type I, also known as an anaphylactic reaction. As defined by Gell, Coombs, and Lachman,[12] **true anaphylactic reactions** (type I) occur only when immunoglobulin E (IgE) reacts with an antigen in a *previously sensitized person*. IgE is a type of antibody that is produced in response to a specific antigen; it remains inactive until rechallenged by that same antigen.

In contrast, **anaphylactoid reactions** (types II to IV), when triggered, produce allergic reactions through nonimmunologically (nonIgE) mediated mechanisms. Anaphylactoid reactions are produced in persons *not previously sensitized* and can occur with the *first exposure* to an antigen such as radiopaque dye or medication.

Vasoactive substances will, however, be liberated (with similar clinical results) in both cases. Patients with either anaphylactic or anaphylactoid reactions can manifest all of the life-threatening signs of anaphylactic shock.[23] The terms "anaphylaxis" and "hypersensitivity reaction" are used interchangeably in this chapter.

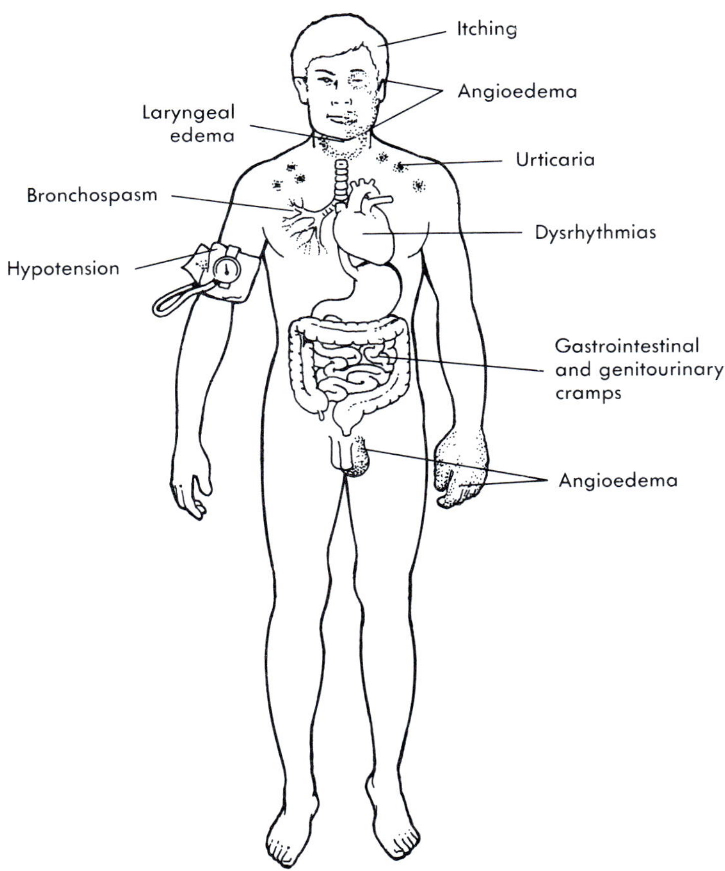


***Fig. 25-1*** Clinical manifestations of anaphylaxis. Laryngeal edema, bronchospasm, and hypotension are the major contributors to patient morbidity and mortality. (From Pr:ce S and Wilson L: Pathophysiology: clinical concepts of disease processes, ed 4, St Louis, 1991, Mosby–Year Book, Inc.)

***Table 25-1*** Classification of allergic reactions

| Type | Synonyms | Antibody | Examples |
|---|---|---|---|
| I | Anaphylactic<br>Immediate hypersensitivity | IgE | Anaphylaxis<br>Cutaneous wheal and flare<br>Extrinisic asthma |
| II | Cytotoxic | IgG<br>IgM | Transfusion reactions<br>Hemolytic anemia<br>Rh disease |
| III | Immune complex | IgG<br>IgM | Serum sickness<br>Glomerulonephritis<br>Arthus reactions |
| IV | Delayed hypersensitivity<br>Cell-mediated immunity | Not involved | Contact dermatitis<br>Tuberculin immunity |

Modifed from Levy JH and others: Spine 11(3):283, 1986.

### CAUSES OF ANAPHYLAXIS

**ANIMAL STINGS AND BITES**

Order Hymenoptera: honeybees, yellow jackets, New and Old World hornets, wasps
Jellyfish
Stingrays
Ants

**MEDICATIONS**

Antibiotics, particularly penicillin
Aspirin
Local anesthetics, e.g., lidocaine (Xylocaine)
Opiates, e.g., morphine, codeine
Tetanus antitoxin and other serums
Blood and blood products
Insulin (obtained from animals)
Radiological iodinated contrast media
Chymopapain

**FOODS**

Peanuts
Chocolate
Eggs
Seafood and shellfish
Strawberries
Milk

**CHEMICALS**

Hand lotion
Soaps
Perfume

**OTHER**

Exercise
Hemodialysis filtration membrane

## ETIOLOGY

Almost any substance can cause a hypersensitivity reaction. Such a substance, also known as antigen, is usually introduced by injection or by ingestion and is less commonly introduced through the skin or the respiratory tract. The most common offenders are listed in the box above.

## PATHOPHYSIOLOGY

The mast cell and the basophil are the primary effector cells for anaphylaxis. **Mast cells** are found in the connective tissue of all organs, particularly in small blood vessels. **Basophils** (a form of white blood cell) circulate in the bloodstream. Both type I (IgE) anaphylactic reactions and types II to IV anaphylactoid reactions act on mast cells and basophils to produce an allergic reaction.

Powerful vasoactive substances—including histamine, leukotrienes, kinins, eosinophil chemotactic factor (ECF-A), and prostaglandins—are produced inside mast cells and basophils. All of these substances are released when the mast cells or basophils swell and rupture *(degranulate)* during the anaphylactic and anaphylactoid reaction.

When released into the bloodstream, **histamine** causes vasodilation, increased capillary permeability, bronchoconstriction, coronary vasoconstriction, and cutaneous reactions (wheals, flares). Increased capillary permeability and vasodilation are largely responsible for the hypotension occurring during anaphylaxis. Fluid movement out of capillaries accounts for the characteristic edema of the face, body, and airway, as well as the pulmonary edema found in anaphylaxis. Upper-airway edema with obstruction and bronchoconstriction contributes significantly to the mortality in patients with hypersensitivity reactions. Histamine also constricts the smooth muscle in the intestinal wall, bladder, and uterus, resulting in cramping, vomiting, abdominal pain, diarrhea, incontinence, and vaginal bleeding.

The **leukotrienes** (including slow-reacting substance of anaphylaxis [SRS-A]) are more than 1000 times as potent as histamine in constricting the small airways of the bronchial tree and are potent coronary vasoconstrictors. Coronary vasoconstriction causes severe depression of myocardial contractility. **Prostaglandins** act on bronchial smooth muscle and affect mucus gland activity and the viscosity of mucus secretions. In patients with allergic reactions, prostaglandins produce inflammation, excessive mucus secretion, bronchoconstriction, peripheral vasodilation, and increased capillary permeability. Leukotrienes, prostaglandins, and chemical mediators join to stimulate nerve endings, causing itching and pain. **Bradykinin** and the other *kinins* also increase capillary permeability, cause vasodilation, and contract smooth muscles.

*(ECF-A)* promotes chemotaxis of eosinophils, thus facilitating the movement of eosinophils into the area. During allergic reactions, **eosinophils** phagocytize the antigen-antibody complex and other inflammatory debris and release enzymes that inhibit vasoactive mediators such as histamine and SRS-A.[16-18,23]

Although all of the aforementioned antigenic responses are meant to protect the body, frequently they result in serious organ dysfunction, which occurs because both the antigenic agent and the normal tissue surrounding the agent become involved in the allergic process. Further, many of the most serious responses to anaphylactic and anaphylactoid reactions are systemic in nature (increased capillary permeability, vasodilation, bronchoconstriction) and produce life-threatening consequences if not controlled. One of the most serious consequences of an anaphylactic reaction is anaphylactic shock.

## ANAPHYLACTIC SHOCK

**Anaphylactic shock** is a form of **distributive (low-resistance) shock.** With distributive shock, vascular tone is lost because of the presence of vasodilators (anaphylactic or septic shock) or the loss of autonomic nervous innervation (spinal or neurogenic shock). The end result of distributive shock is profound vasodilation of the circulatory system and a decrease in systemic vascular resistance. Profound vasodilation increases the size of the vascular bed, producing decreased venous return to the right side of the heart, decreased stroke volume and cardiac output, and decreased blood pressure.[19]

During anaphylactic shock, the three principal elements responsible for adequate perfusion (size of vascular bed, blood volume, and the pump mechanism) are all impaired. As in all forms of distributive shock, anaphylaxis results in maldistribution of the blood volume in the peripheral circulation. Vasoactive substances such as histamine and kinins produce vasodilation and poor vascular tone, particularly in the terminal arterioles. Histamine and other substances also increase capillary permeability, causing fluid shifts from the intravascular to the interstitial space. Although the total blood volume does not change, the large amount of fluid pooled in the interstitial space is not available to maintain cardiac output, creating a *relative hypovolemia*. Decreased cardiac output and hypotension follow. Lastly, the cardiovascular system is compromised by depressed myocardial contractility and coronary artery vasoconstriction produced by release of leukotrienes from degranulated mast cells and basophils.[9]

## ASSESSMENT AND DIAGNOSIS

Localized allergic reactions, anaphylaxis, and anaphylactic shock are products of the same mechanisms. The severity of each clinical situation is appraised on a continuum from localized signs, to systemic allergic reactions, to life-threatening conditions of anaphylactic shock. Each patient may manifest signs of each phase on this continuum or may progress or deteriorate during the course of the episode. It is the challenge of the clinician to monitor the patient closely for changes in status and to adjust treatment accordingly.[9,10]

The patient in *less severe anaphylaxis* will exhibit slight hypotension from vasodilation and increased capillary permeability. Smooth-muscle contraction in the bronchial tree produces wheezing, hoarseness, dyspnea, and chest tightness. The patient may feel that his or her "throat is closing" because of the laryngeal edema. In addition, the patient may have the classic symptoms of an allergic reaction: generalized pruritus (itching), urticaria (hives, wheals), angioedema (nontraumatic swelling, particularly perioral, periorbital, and in the areas of contact to the antigen), gastrointestinal (GI) upset, anxiety, and restlessness.

Patients with signs of allergic reactions or less severe anaphylaxis can deteriorate in a matter of minutes. Signs of *severe anaphylaxis* include profound hypotension, decreased level of consciousness (LOC), and respiratory distress with severe stridor and cyanosis. As vital organs become hypoxic, cardiac dysrhythmias and seizures may occur. Death may result from airway obstruction and/or cardiovascular collapse.[18,23]

### TREATMENT OF ANAPHYLAXIS

Epinepherine
Airway management
Medical antishock trousers (MAST)
Fluid resuscitation
- Lactated Ringer's or saline solution

Other medications
- Aminophylline and other bronchodilators
- Corticosteriods, e.g., hydrocortisone, dexamethasone
- Diphenhydramine (Benadryl)
- Vasopressors, e.g., dopamine
- $H_2$ antagonists, e.g., cimetidine (Tagamet)

## TREATMENT

Treatment is directed toward preservation of tissue oxygenation and normalization of blood pressure. For systemic allergic reactions and anaphylaxis, *epinephrine* (adrenaline) is the cornerstone of treatment and should be administered as quickly as possible. Its actions on peripheral vasculature and on histamine-releasing mast cells and basophils make epinephrine's role essential. Every effort must be made to administer the medication by intravenous (IV), endotracheal, or subcutaneous routes. Performing *airway management* with positive pressure and endotracheal intubation is also essential to maintain airway patency and adequate alveolar ventilation. Other modalities include the use of medical antishock trousers (MAST), diphenhydramine (Benadryl), corticosteroids, fluid resuscitation, bronchodilators, $H_2$ antagonists (cimetidine), and vasopressor drugs (dopamine). The offending substance also must be removed or discontinued as soon as possible.[28,29] Treatment for anaphylaxis is summarized in the box above.

## SUMMARY OF NURSING CARE

Nursing care of the patient with an acute hypersensitivity reaction is aimed at assessment of the respiratory and cardiovascular status, support of respiratory and cardiovascular functions, identification and removal of the offending antigen or allergen, and education and referral of the patient to prevent further life-threatening events. See the box on p. 434.

The nurse assesses the patient for signs and symptoms of a hypersensitivity reaction to establish a baseline and to monitor the patient's status on the continuum between localized, systemic, or severe anaphylactic reactions. Priority should be given to the respiratory and cardiovascular status (Table 25-2).

Upper airway or laryngeal edema may be seen as stridor, cyanosis, perioral edema, swollen tongue, facial swelling, or a subjective feeling of air hunger or panic. Bronchial or lower airway narrowing is manifested by wheezing (audible

## Nursing Diagnosis and Management
### *Anaphylaxis*

- Ineffective Airway Clearance related to laryngeal edema, subjective feeling of air hunger or panic, p. 470
- Decreased Cardiac Output related to widespread vasodilation and third spacing, p. 461
- Knowledge Deficit: Anaphylaxis related to lack of previous exposure to information, p. 441

***Table 25-2*** Signs and symptoms of anaphylaxis

| Sign/symptom | Cause |
|---|---|
| Hypotension | Vasodilation and increased capillary permeability |
| Stridor | Laryngeal edema |
| Bronchospasm | Bronchoconstriction |
| Angioedema | Increased capillary permeability |
| Itching | Leukotrienes, prostaglandins |
| Dysrhythmias | Hypoxemia, coronary vasoconstriction |

with or without a stethoscope), tachypnea, intercostal or supraclavicular retractions, and/or diminished lung sounds (indicating severe bronchoconstriction). If the patient's breathing is being assisted with positive pressure (for example, Ambu bag or mechanical ventilation), bronchoconstriction may be manifested by an increased resistance to airflow during inhalation when compressing the positive-pressure device.

The airway must be kept patent, either through proper positioning and/or insertion of an endotracheal tube or oral or nasal airway. When ventilatory failure is present, an endotracheal tube is the airway of choice since it will maintain airway patency despite upper airway edema. However, it cannot ensure ventilation past severely bronchoconstricted airways. Placement of any airway may be difficult or impossible because of upper airway edema and may actually make the swelling worse. Early and careful placement of airways is strongly advised when progression of symptoms seems likely. Suctioning of the airway may be necessary because of increased mucus production associated with allergic reactions.[19]

Although blood pressure is the most commonly practiced assessment of cardiovascular status, significant angioedema implies profound third-spacing, with extravasation of volume and relative hypovolemia. Monitoring of extremity edema (often full body), abdominal girth, and angioedema is helpful in determining the availability of body fluid.[19]

Additional swelling, despite treatment, implies unresponsiveness to treatment modalities, overaggressiveness with fluid resuscitation, or organ dysfunction (heart, kidney). Pulmonary artery catheter monitoring can be helpful in identifying, assessing, and treating these problems. Assessment then requires scrupulous attention to all organ systems and frequent monitoring of vital signs (blood pressure, pulse, and respirations), LOC, lung sounds, respiratory effort, heart sounds ($S_3$), intake and output, and arterial blood gas values. Signs and symptoms of hypersensitivity should be monitored and documented. Dysrhythmias on the electrocardiogram (ECG) may indicate hypoxemia (from a number of causes) or adverse responses to therapy (epinephrine, aminophylline).

A large-bore IV catheter must be inserted to provide a delivery route for medication and fluid resuscitation. In the patient with full-body swelling, hypovolemia, and hypotension in whom peripheral vessels are not visualized, application of the MAST suit will increase peripheral vascular resistance and blood pressure, promoting engorgement of peripheral vessels to facilitate cannulation. Fluid resuscitation is titrated to achieve a desired blood pressure (systolic = 100). Lung sounds must be monitored frequently for indications of fluid overload, often heralded by auscultation of "crackles" (rales), particularly in the posterior bases and dependent areas of the lung fields. The patient should be continuously monitored with an ECG for dysrhythmias.

The critical care nurse can play an important role in identifying knowledge deficits that may account for recurrence of severe allergic reactions. Education of the patient and family while he or she is in the critical care unit may be the first important step in safeguarding the allergic patient from further morbidity or mortality.

Avoidance of insects and known allergens, possession of emergency medication, and desensitization or venom immunotherapy are the cornerstones of prophylaxis.[26] Individuals with histories of anaphylaxis should be instructed about and should carry an *anaphylactic kit,* which contains injectable epinephrine, oral antihistamines, and a constrictive band. At the least, injectable epinephrine should be on hand at all times. These emergency self-care kits are meant for use as prompt treatment before the patient is transported to a medical facility; they are not to substitute for definitive medical care.

#### REFERENCES

1. American Heart Association: Textbook of advanced cardiac life support, Dallas, 1987, The Association.
2. Anderson J and Adkinson F: Allergic reactions to drugs and biologic agents, JAMA 258(20):2891, 1987.
3. Assem ES: Anaphylactic reactions affecting the human heart, Agents Actions 27(1):142, 1989.
4. Bickell WH and Dice WH: Military anti-shock trousers in a patient with adrenergic-resistant anaphylaxis, Ann Emerg Med 13:189, 1984.
5. Bourg P, Sherer C, and Rosen P: Standardized nursing care plans for emergency patients, St Louis, 1986, Mosby–Year Book, Inc.

6. Cahill SB and Balskus M: Intervention in emergency nursing: the first 60 minutes, Rockville, Md, 1986, Aspen Publishers, Inc.
7. Cohan R, Dunnick N, and Bashore T: Treatment of reactions to radiographic contrast material, AJR 151(2):263, 1988.
8. Corren J and Schocket AL: Anaphylaxis. A preventable emergency, Postgrad Med 87(5):167, 1990.
9. Costa AJ: Anaphylactic shock. Guidelines for immediate diagnosis and treatment, Postgrad Med 83(4):368, 1988.
10. Dickerson M: Anaphylaxis and anaphylactic shock, Crit Care Nurs Q 11:68, 1988.
11. Fincke M and Lanros N: Emergency nursing: a comprehensive review, Rockville, Md, 1986, Aspen Publishers, Inc.
12. Gell PG, Coombs RR, and Lachman PJ, editors: Clinical aspects of immunology, ed 3, Oxford, 1975, Blackwell Scientific Publications, Ltd.
13. Goldsmith SR: Comparative hemodynamic effects of antishock suit and volume expansion in normal human beings, Ann Emerg Med 12:348, 1983.
14. Granata AV, Halickman J, and Borak J: Utility of the antishock trousers (MAST) in anaphylactic schock—a case study, J Emerg Med 2(5):349, 1985.
15. Greenberger PA: Contrast media reactions, J Allergy Clin Immunol 74:600, 1984.
16. Griffin J: Hematology and immunology: concepts for nursing, Norwalk, Conn, 1986, Appleton-Century-Crofts.
17. Guyton A: Textbook of medical physiology, ed 7, Philadelphia, 1986, WB Saunders Co.
18. Keahey TM, Yancey K, and Lawley T: Immediate hypersensitivity, J Am Acad Dermatol 17:826, 1987.
19. Kuhn MA: Anaphylaxis versus anaphylactoid reactions: nursing interventions, Crit Care Nurse 10 (5):121, 1990.
20. Lantner R and Reisman RE: Clinical and immunologic features and subsequent course of patients with severe insect-sting anaphylaxis, J Allergy Clin Immunol 84(6):900, 1989.
21. Lasser EC and others: Protective effects of corticosteroids in contrast material anaphylaxis, Investigative Radiol 23(1):S193, 1988.
22. Levy JH: Anaphylactic/anaphylactoid reactions during cardiac surgery, J Clinical Anesthesia 1(6):426, 1989.
23. Levy JH, Roizen M, and Morris J: Anaphylactic and anaphylactoid reactions. A review, Spine 11(3):282, 1986.
24. Lockey RF and others: Fatalities from immunotherapy (IT) and skin testing (ST), J Allergy Clin Immunol 79(4):660, 1987.
25. Manley L, Haley K, and Dick M: Intraosseous infusion: rapid vascular access for critically ill or injured infants and children, J Emerg Nurs 14:63, 1988.
26. McLean DC: Insect sting allergy, Primary Care 14(3):513, 1987.
27. Molkhow P and Dupont C: Ketotifen in prevention and therapy of food allergy, Ann Allergy 59:187, 1987.
28. Netzel MC: Anaphylaxis: clinical presentation, immunologic mechanisms, and treatment, J Emerg Med 4(3):227, 1986.
29. Oertel T and Loehr MM: Bee-sting anaphylaxis: the use of the medical anti-shock trousers, Ann Emerg Med 13(6):459, 1984.
30. O'Leary MR and Smith MS: Penicillin anaphylaxis, Am J Emerg Med 4(3):241, 1986.
31. Orlowski JP: An animal model for anaphylactic shock (letter), Ann Emerg Med 15(8):979, 1986.
32. Price SA and Wilson LM: Pathophysiology: clinical concepts of disease processes, New York, 1987, McGraw-Hill Book Co.
33. Raper RF: Profound reversible myocardial depression after anaphylaxis, Lancet 1(8582):386, 1988.
34. Reisman R and Osur S: Allergic reactions following first insect sting exposure, Ann Allergy 59(6):429, 1987.
35. Rodman M and Others: Pharmacology and drug therapy in nursing, ed 3, Philadelphia, 1985, JB Lippincott Co.
36. Sheehy SB and Barber J: Emergency nursing: principles and practice, ed 2, St Louis, 1985, Mosby–Year Book, Inc.
37. Sheffer AL: Anaphylaxis, J Allergy Clin Immunol 81:1048, 1988.
38. Stephens GW, Bernard D, and Idelson B: Anaphylaxis: an unusual complication of hemodialysis, Clin Nephrol 24(2):99, 1985.
39. Stoelting R: Pharmacology and physiology in anesthetic practice, Philadelphia, 1987, JB Lippincott Co.
40. Szczeklik A: Adverse reactions to aspirin and nonsteroidal anti-inflammatory drugs, Ann Allergy 59:113, 1987.
41. Toogood JH: Risk of anaphylaxis in patients receiving beta-blocker drugs, J Allergy Clin Immunol 81:1, 1988.
42. Trevino RJ: Food allergies and hypersensitivities, Ear Nose Throat J 67:42, 1988.
43. Valentine MD and Lichtenstein LM: Anaphylaxis and stinging insect hypersensitivity, JAMA 258(20):2881, 1987.
44. Wayne MA: Clinical evaluation of the antishock trouser: retrospective analysis of 5 years of experience, Ann Emerg Med 12:342, 1983.
45. Weiss ME and others: Association of protamine IgE and IgG antibodies with life-threatening reactions to intravenous protamine, New Engl J Med 320(14):886, 1989.

UNIT X

# NURSING MANAGEMENT

# Nursing Management of Health Promotion

## Altered Health Maintenance

**Definition:** *The inability to identify, manage, or seek out help to maintain health.*

### *Altered Health Maintenance Related to Lack of Perceived Threat to Health and/or Lack of Resources (Financial, Interpersonal Support Systems, Health Care Access)*

#### DEFINING CHARACTERISTICS

- Denial of susceptibility to a particular disease or problem
- Denial of the seriousness of a health problem or its consequences
- Failure to assume appropriate sick role behaviors
- Lack of participation in primary and/or secondary preventive activities such as obtaining appropriate screenings, proper nutrition, routine medical and dental care
- Frequent or chronic health problems such as chronic cough, loss of teeth at an early age, frequent infections, chronic fatigue or anemia
- Physical signs of poor hygiene

#### OUTCOME CRITERIA

- Patient is able to state the health consequences of specific behaviors (for example, "Smoking is directly related to the onset of heart and lung disease").
- Patient assumes appropriate sick role behaviors.
- Patient states plans for appropriate primary and secondary preventive activities after discharge.
- Patient gains access to necessary health care.
- Patient can state self-care and health maintenance behaviors appropriate to his or her age and developmental level.

#### NURSING INTERVENTIONS *AND RATIONALE*

1. Continue to monitor the assessment parameters listed under "Defining Characteristics."
2. Assist patient to see the connection between specific behaviors and the short-term onset of symptoms or long-term progression of disease.
3. Assist patient to set short-term and long-term health management goals related to self-care and life-style.
4. Assist patient to prioritize goals and to make plans to pursue them in a manageable and realistic fashion.
5. Initiate health education *to give the patient skills necessary to meet the immediate goals.* (See nursing management of Knowledge Deficit.)
6. Initiate referrals for long-term follow-up after discharge (for example, health educators, counselors, home health personnel, primary care practitioners, or rehabilitation programs) *so that appropriate resources and assistance can be obtained.*
7. Assist patient and family in identifying social, financial, and environmental factors that limit ability to practice appropriate health maintenance measures.
8. Work with patient and family in identifying appropriate self-care and health maintenance behaviors; for example, professional dental examination and cleaning every 6 to 12 months, monthly breast self-exam for women, complete physical examinations every 2 years for adults aged 60 years or older.

## Noncompliance

**Definition:** *Personal behavior that deviates from health-related advice given by health care professionals*

### *Noncompliance: (Specify) Related to Knowledge Deficit*

#### DEFINING CHARACTERISTICS

- Lack of participation in necessary therapeutic measures
- Lack of prior experience with the recommended treatment or action
- Verbalization of inadequate knowledge or skills
- Questioning the need for the treatment or action

#### OUTCOME CRITERIA

- Patient verbalizes adequate knowledge or demonstrates adequate skills necessary for participation in treatment.
- Patient demonstrates compliance with treatment.

#### NURSING INTERVENTIONS *AND RATIONALE*

1. Continue to monitor the assessment parameters listed under "Defining Characteristics."
2. Determine specific knowledge or skills necessary *for adherence to therapeutic plan.*

For other interventions, refer to the nursing management of Knowledge Deficit on p. 441.

## Knowledge Deficit

**Definition:** *The state in which the individual experiences a decrease in cognitive knowledge or psychomotor skills that alters or may alter health maintenance.*

### *Knowledge Deficit: (Specify) Related to Lack of Previous Exposure to Information*

#### DEFINING CHARACTERISTICS

- Verbalized statement of inadequate knowledge or skills
- New diagnosis or health problem requiring self-management or care
- Lack of prior formal or informal education about the specific health problem
- Demonstration of inappropriate behaviors related to management of health problem

#### OUTCOME CRITERIA

- Patient verbalizes adequate knowledge about or performs skills related to disease process, its causes, factors related to onset of symptoms, and self-management of disease or health problem.
- Patient actively participates in health behaviors required for performance of a procedure or in those behaviors enhancing recovery from illness and preventing recurrence or complications.

#### NURSING INTERVENTIONS *AND RATIONALE*

1. Continue to monitor the assessment parameters listed under "Defining Characteristics."
2. Determine existing level of knowledge or skill.
3. Assess factors affecting the knowledge deficit:
   Learning needs, including patient's priorities and the necessary knowledge and skills for safety
   Learning ability of client, including language skills, level of education, ability to read, preferred learning style
   Physical ability to perform prescribed skills or procedures; consider effect of limitations imposed by treatment such as bedrest, restriction of movement by intravenous or other equipment, or effect of sedatives or analgesics
   Psychological effect of stage of adaptation to disease
   Activity tolerance and ability to concentrate
   Motivation to learn new skills or gain new knowledge
4. Reduce or limit barriers to learning:
   Provide consistent nurse-patient contract *to encourage development of trusting and therapeutic relationship.*
   Structure environment *to enhance learning;* control unnecessary noise, interruptions.
   Individualize teaching plan *to fit patient's current physical and psychological status.*
   Delay teaching until patient is ready to learn.
   Conduct teaching sessions during period of day when patient is most alert and receptive.
   Meet patient's immediate learning needs as they arise; for example, give brief explanation of procedures when they are performed.
5. Promote active participation in the teaching plan by the patient and family:
   Solicit input during development of plan.
   Develop mutually acceptable goals and outcomes.
   Solicit expression of feelings and emotions related to new responsibilities.
   Encourage questions.
6. Conduct teaching sessions, using the most appropriate teaching methods:
   Discussion
   Lecture
   Demonstration/return demonstration
   Use of audiovisual or printed educational materials
7. Repeat key principles and provide them in printed form *for reference at a later time.*
8. Give frequent feedback to patient when practicing new skills.
9. Use several teaching sessions when appropriate. *New information and skills should be reinforced several times after initial learning.*
10. Initiate referrals for follow-up *if necessary:*
    Health educators
    Home health care
    Rehabilitation programs
    Social services
11. Evaluate effectiveness of teaching plan, based on patient's ability to meet preset goals and objectives:
    Determine need for further teaching.

# Nursing Management of Psychosocial Alterations

## Self-Esteem Disturbance

**Definition:** *Problem that arises when a person experiences a decrease in self-worth, self-respect, self-approval, or self-confidence.*

### *Self-Esteem Disturbance Related to Feelings of Guilt About Physical Deterioration*

#### DEFINING CHARACTERISTICS

- Inability to accept positive reinforcement
- Lack of follow-through
- Nonparticipation in therapy
- Not taking responsibility for self-care (self-neglect)
- Self-destructive behavior
- Lack of eye contact

#### OUTCOME CRITERIA

- Patient verbalizes feelings of self-worth.
- Patient maintains positive relationships with significant others.
- Patient manifests active interest in appearance by completing personal grooming daily.

#### NURSING INTERVENTIONS *AND RATIONALE*

1. Continue to monitor the assessment parameters listed under "Defining Characteristics." In addition, assess the meaning of health-related situation. How does the patient feel about himself or herself, the diagnosis, and the treatment? How does the present fit into the larger context of his or her life?
2. Assess the patient's emotional level, interpersonal relationships, and feelings about himself or herself. Recognize the patient's uniqueness (how the hair is worn, preference for name used).
3. Help the patient discover and verbalize feelings and understand the crisis by listening and providing information.
4. Assist the patient to identify strengths and positive qualities that increase the sense of self-worth. Focus on past experiences of accomplishment and competency. Help patient with positive self-reinforcement. Reinforce the obvious love and affection of family and significant others.
5. Assess coping techniques that have been helpful in the past. Help the patient decide how to handle negative or incongruent feedback about the situation.
6. Encourage visits from family and significant others. Facilitate interactions and ensure privacy. Help family members entering critical care unit by explaining what they will see. Increase visitors' comfort with equipment; offer chairs and other courtesies.
7. Encourage the patient to pursue interest in individual or social activities, even though difficult in the critical care unit.
8. Reflect caring, concern, empathy, respect, and unconditional acceptance in nurse-patient relationships.
9. Remember that for the patient the nurse is a significant other who provides important appraisals of the patient and who can facilitate the change process.
10. Help the family support the patient's self-esteem.
11. Provide for continuity of nurse assignment to ensure consistent contacts that can *facilitate support of the patient's self-esteem.*

## Body Image Disturbance

**Definition:** *Problem that arises when a person fails to perceive or adapt to a change in the body's appearance, structure, or function.*

### *Body Image Disturbance Related to Actual Change in Body Structure, Function, or Appearance and/or Functional Dependence on Life-Sustaining Technology (Ventilator, Dialysis, IABP, Halo Traction)*

#### DEFINING CHARACTERISTICS

- Actual change in appearance, structure, or function
- Avoidance of looking at body part
- Avoidance of touching body part
- Hiding or overexposing body part (intentional or unintentional)
- Trauma to nonfunctioning part
- Change in ability to estimate spatial relationship of body to environment
- Verbalization of the following:
  Fear of rejection or reaction by others
  Negative feelings about body
  Preoccupation with change or loss
  Refusal to participate in or accept responsibility for self-care of altered body part
- Personalization of part or loss with a name
  Depersonalization of part or loss by use of impersonal pronouns
  Refusal to verify actual change

#### OUTCOME CRITERIA

- Patient verbalizes the meaning of the change to him or her.
- Patient requests appropriate information about self-care.
- Patient completes personal hygiene and grooming daily with or without help.
- Patient interacts freely with family or other visitors.
- Patient participates in the discussions and conferences related to planning his or her medical and nursing care in the critical care unit and transfer from the unit.
- Patient talks with trained visitors (support group representatives) about his or her loss at least twice.
- Patient verifies actual change in function.
- Patient does not refuse or fight technological intervention.
- Patient verbalizes acceptance of expected change in lifestyle.

#### NURSING INTERVENTIONS *AND RATIONALE*

1. Continue to monitor the assessment parameters listed under "Defining Characteristics." In addition, assess patient's mental, physical, and emotional state; recognize assets, strengths, response to illness, coping mechanisms, past experience with stress, support systems, and coping mechanisms.
2. Appraise the response of family and significant others. *Body image is derived from the "reflected appraisals" of family and significant others.*
3. Determine the patient's goals and readiness for learning.
4. Provide the necessary information to help the patient and family adapt to the change. Clarify misconceptions about future limitations.
5. Permit and encourage the patient to express the significance of the loss or change; note nonverbal behavioral responses.
6. Allow and encourage the patient's expression of anxiety. *Anxiety is the most predominant emotional response to a body image disturbance.*
7. Recognize and accept the use of denial as an adaptive defense mechanism when used early and temporarily.
8. Recognize maladaptive denial as that which interferes with the patient's progress and/or alienates support systems. Use confrontation.
9. Provide an opportunity for the patient to discuss sexual concerns (refer to the nursing management of Altered Sexuality Patterns on p. 453).
10. Touch the affected body part *to provide patient with sensory information about altered body structure and/or function.*
11. Encourage and provide movement of altered body part *to establish kinesthetic feedback. This enables the person to know his or her body as it now exists.*
12. Prepare the patient to look at the body part. Call the body part by its anatomic name (for example, stump, stoma, limb) as opposed to "it" or "she." *The use of impersonal pronouns increases a sense of fantasy and depersonalization of the body part.*
13. Allow the patient to experience excellence in some aspect of physical functioning—walking, turning, deep breathing, healing, self-care—and point out progress and accomplishment. *This helps to balance the patient's sense of dysfunction with function.*
14. Avoid false reassurance. Acknowledge the difficulty of incorporating the altered body part or function into one's body image. *This evidences the nurse's sensitivity and promotes trust.*
15. Talk with the patient about his or her life, generativity, and accomplishments. *Patients with disturbances in body image frequently see themselves in a distortedly "narrow" sense. Encouraging a wider focus of themselves and their life reduces this distortion.*
16. Help the patient explore realistic alternatives.
17. Recognize that incorporating a body change into body image takes time. Don't set unrealistic expectations and *thereby inadvertently reinforce low self-esteem.*
18. Suggest the use of additional resources such as trained visitors who have mastered situations similar to those of the patient. Refer patient to a psychiatric liaison nurse or psychiatrist if needed.
19. Assist patient to recognize his or her own functioning and performance in the face of technology. For example, assist the patient to distinguish spontaneous breaths from mechanically delivered breaths. *This activity will assist in weaning the patient from the ventilator when feasible. To establish realistic, accurate body boundaries, a patient needs help to separate himself or herself from the technology that is supporting his or her functioning. Any participation or function on the part of the patient during periods of dependency is helpful in preventing and/or resolving an alteration in body image.*
20. Plan for discontinuation of the treatment, for example, weaning from ventilator. Explain procedure that will be followed, and be present during its initiation.
21. Plan for transfer from the critical care environment.

## Altered Role Performance

**Definition:** *Problem that arises when a person experiences difficulty making life transitions.*

### *Altered Role Performance Related to Physical Incapacity to Resume Usual or Valued Role*

#### DEFINING CHARACTERISTICS

- Lack of acknowledgement of role change
- Change in usual patterns of responsibility
- Change in self-perception of role
- Denial of role
- Change in others' perception of role
- Conflict in roles

#### OUTCOME CRITERIA

- Patient verbalizes a beginning plan to alter life-style to meet restrictions imposed by physical incapacity.
- Patient verbalizes plans to adjust personal and family goals rather than to abandon them.
- Patient expresses willingness to interact with significant others.

#### NURSING INTERVENTIONS *AND RATIONALE*

1. Continue to monitor the assessment parameters listed under "Defining Characteristics." In addition, identify the primary, secondary, and tertiary roles of the patient. Assess the patient's developmental stage and whether there are maturational and situational crises in addition to the health-related event. *Illness disrupts role performance and makes life transitions difficult.*
2. Assess past experiences with role change, the degree of attachment to the role, and the ability or capacity to modify the role.
3. Assess the patient's perception of the role change or role loss, the responses of others, and the likelihood of a new role performance consistent with role expectations.
4. Explore with the patient the expected role change; permit patient to express his or her fears and concerns. Recognize role(s) that will continue.
5. Help the patient establish realistic goals and expectations.
6. Reinforce and support positive behaviors with verbal praise. Help the patient face any conflicts.
7. Teach the new skill(s) needed. Convey information and experience necessary to patient and family. Provide environmental supports that permit mastery of new skills (equipment and time for practice). Be sure expectations are clear. Reward mastery behavior.
8. Use role supplementation strategies (role clarifying, role-taking, role-modeling, role-rehearsal, and reference group interaction).

## Powerlessness

**Definition:** *The perception of an individual that his or her own action will not sufficiently affect an outcome. Powerlessness is a perceived lack of control over a current situation or immediate happening.*

### *Powerlessness Related to Health Care Environment or Illness-Related Regimen*

#### DEFINING CHARACTERISTICS

**Severe**

- Verbal expressions of having no control or influence over situation
- Verbal expressions of having no control or influence over outcome
- Verbal expressions of having no control over self-care
- Depression over physical deterioration that occurs despite patient's compliance with regimens
- Apathy

**Moderate**

- Nonparticipation in care or decision making when opportunities are provided
- Expressions of dissatisfaction and frustration about inability to perform previous tasks and/or activities
- Lack of progress monitoring
- Expressions of doubt about role performance
- Reluctance to express true feelings, fearing alienation from caregivers
- Passivity
- Inability to seek information about care
- Dependence on others that may result in irritability, resentment, anger, and guilt
- No defense or self-care practices when challenged

**Low**

- Passivity

#### OUTCOME CRITERIA

- Patient verbalizes increased control over situation by wanting to do things his or her way.
- Patient actively participates in planning care.
- Patient requests needed information.
- Patient chooses to participate in self-care activities.
- Patient monitors progress.
- Patient verbalizes an increased ability to cope with the stress of illness.
- Patient demonstrates commitment to option(s) selected.
- Patient recognizes that efforts to delay the progression of the disease are worth his or her effort.

#### NURSING INTERVENTIONS *AND RATIONALE*

1. Continue to monitor the assessment parameters listed under "Defining Characteristics." In addition, assess the patient's feelings and perception of the reasons for lack of power and sense of helplessness.
2. Determine as far as possible the patient's usual response to limited control situations. Determine through ongoing assessment the patient's usual locus of control, that is, whether he or she believes influence over his or her life is exerted by luck, fate, powerful persons (external locus of control) or influence is exerted through personal choices, self-effort, self-determination (internal locus of control).
3. Support patient's physical control of the environment by involving him or her in care activities; knock before entering room if appropriate; ask permission before moving personal belongings. Inform the patient that, although an activity may not be to his or her liking, it is necessary. *This gives the patient permission to express dissatisfaction with the environment and regimen.*
4. Personalize the patient's care using his or her preferred name. *This supports the patient's psychological control.*
5. Provide the therapeutic rationale for all the patient is asked to do for himself or herself and for all that is being done for and with him or her. Reinforce the physician's explanations; clarify misconceptions about the illness situation and treatment plans. *This supports the patient's cognitive control.*
6. Include patient in care planning by encouraging participation and allowing choices wherever possible, for example, timing of personal care activities and deciding when pain medicines are needed. Point out situations in which no choices exist.
7. Provide opportunities for the patient to exert influence over himself or herself and his or her body, thereby affecting an outcome. For example, share with the patient the nurse's assessment of his or her breath sounds and explain that they can be improved by self-initiated deep breathing exercises. *Feedback that the patient has been successful in helping clear his or her lungs reinforces the influence he or she does retain.*
8. Encourage family to permit patient to do as much independently as possible *to foster perceptions of personal power.*
9. Assist the patient to establish realistic short-term and long-term goals. *Setting unrealistic or unattainable goals inadvertently reinforces the patient's perception of powerlessness.*
10. Document care to provide for continuity *so the patient can maintain appropriate control over the environment.*
11. Assist the patient to regain strength and activity tolerance as appropriate, *thus increasing a sense of control and self-reliance.*
12. Increase the sensitivity of the health team members and significant others to the patient's sense of powerlessness. Use power over the patient carefully. Use the words "must," "should," and "have to" with caution *because they communicate coercive power and imply that the objects of "musts" and "shoulds" are of benefit to the nurse vs. the patient.*
13. Assist the patient to exercise physical control when possible. Provide information that patient's efforts have had desired effects. For example, suggest that the patient can reduce his or her heart rate and even dysrhythmias by performing relaxation techniques. Then provide feedback that heart rate and ectopy have decreased when true.
14. Plan with the patient for transfer from the critical care unit to the intermediate unit and eventually to home.

## Hopelessness

**Definition:** *A subjective state in which an individual sees limited or no alternatives or personal choices available and is unable to mobilize energy on own behalf.*

### *Hopelessness Related to Failing or Deteriorating Physical Condition*

#### DEFINING CHARACTERISTICS

**Major**
- Passivity
- Decreased verbalization
- Decreased affect
- Verbal cues (despondent content, "I can't," sighing)

**Minor**
- Lack of initiative
- Decreased response to stimuli
- Decreased affect
- Verbal cues (hopeless content, "I can't," sighing)
- Turning away from speaker
- Closing eyes
- Shrugging in response to speaker
- Decreased appetite
- Increased sleep
- Lack of involvement in care or passive allowance of care

#### OUTCOME CRITERIA

- Patient looks at speaker.
- Patient verbalizes, "I will try" (hopeful content).
- Patient initiates conversation with staff, family.
- Patient requests involvement in self-care activities.
- Patient's conversation reflects affect (hope, anger, disagreement, anticipation).

#### NURSING INTERVENTIONS *AND RATIONALE*

1. Continue to monitor the assessment parameters listed under "Defining Characteristics." In addition, assess the patient's total health situation realistically. Do not offer false reassurance. What is the patient's perception of treatment and the environment?
2. Assist the patient to look for alternatives. Help patient establish realistic short-term and long-term goals.
3. Offer help and assist the patient as needed, *thus conserving the patient's energy for things the patient wants to do.*
4. Encourage and help the patient to have something for which to plan. Help him or her imagine a future, even a short-term one. Support the possibilities.
5. Offer information before events occur. Facilitate control and predictability of events when possible.
6. Be careful not to create a hopeless environment. Convey hopefulness despite being helpless to alter the outcome.
7. Support the patient's sense of security and inner strengths. Enhance his or her feelings of being understood. Support what the patient finds in the situation as grounds for hope. Do not renounce hope prematurely.
8. Facilitate close personal contacts between patient and nurse, as well as between patient and family and significant others. Help them to feel involved.
9. Inspire hope. Consider the patient's religious and cultural background. *Faith and hope in God are strengthening for some patients and families.*
10. Recognize the influences of others such as family, clergy, and friends.
11. Communicate an attitude of quiet confidence, genuine interest, and mutual trust. *This does much to support the patient's hope.*
12. Help the family members not to "give up." *Their struggle, as well as that of the nurse, is important. The family can regain and sustain hope from the nurse's example.*

## Ineffective Individual Coping

**Definition:** *The impairment of a person's adaptive behaviors and problem-solving abilities for meeting life's demands and roles.*

### *Ineffective Individual Coping Related to Situational Crisis and Personal Vulnerability*

#### DEFINING CHARACTERISTICS

- Verbalization of inability to cope. EXAMPLE STATEMENTS: "I can't take this anymore." "I don't know how to deal with this."
- Ineffective problem solving (problem lumping). EXAMPLE STATEMENTS: "I have to eliminate salt from my diet; They tell me I can no longer mow the lawn; This hospitalization is costing a mint; What about my kids' future? Who's going to change the oil in the car? This is an incredible amount of time away from work."
- Ineffective use of coping mechanisms:
  *Projection:* blames others for illness or pain
  *Displacement:* directs anger and/or aggression toward family. EXAMPLE STATEMENTS: "Get out of here; leave me alone." Curses, shouts, or demands attention; strikes out or throws objects
  *Denial* of severity of illness and need for treatment
- Noncompliance. EXAMPLES: activity restriction; refusal to allow treatment or to take medications (see the nursing management of Altered Sexuality Patterns on p. 453 for interventions with patients using adaptive denial vs. patients using maladaptive denial or no denial).
- Suicidal thoughts (verbalizes desire to end life)
- Self-directed aggression. EXAMPLES: disconnects or attempts to disconnect life-sustaining equipment; deliberately tries to harm self
- Failure to progress from dependent to more independent state (refusal or resistance to care for self)

#### OUTCOME CRITERIA

- Patient verbalizes beginning ability to cope with illness, pain, and hospitalization. EXAMPLE STATEMENTS: "I'm trying to do the best I can." "I want to help myself get better."
- Patient demonstrates effective problem solving (lists and prioritizes problems from most to least urgent).
- Patient uses effective behavioral strategies to manage the stress of illness and care.
- Patient demonstrates interest or involvement in illness or environment. EXAMPLES—patient does the following:
  Requests medications when anticipating pain
  Questions course of treatment, progress, and prognosis
  Asks for clarification of environmental stimuli and events
  Seeks out supportive individuals in his environment
  Uses coping mechanisms and strategies more effectively to manage situational crisis
  Demonstrates significant reduction in impulsive, angry, or aggressive outbursts (projection, shouting, cursing) directed toward family
  Verbalizes futuristic plans, with cessation of self-directed aggressive acts and suicidal thoughts
  Willingly complies with treatment regimen
  Begins to participate in self-care

#### NURSING INTERVENTIONS *AND RATIONALE*

1. Continue to monitor the assessment parameters listed under "Defining Characteristics."
2. Actively listen and respond to patient's verbal and behavioral expressions. *Active listening signifies unconditional respect and acceptance for the patient as a worthwhile individual. It builds trust and rapport, guides the nurse toward problem areas, encourages the patient to express concerns, and promotes compliance.*
3. Offer effective coping strategies to help the patient better tolerate the stressors related to his illness and care. Give him or her permission to vent feelings in a safe setting. EXAMPLE STATEMENTS: "I don't blame you for feeling angry and frustrated." "Others who are ill like you have expressed similar feelings." "I will listen to anything you want to share with me." "We don't have to talk; I'd like to sit here with you." "It's perfectly OK to cry." *Individuals who are provided with opportunities to express their feelings will be better able to release pent-up emotions and derive a greater sense of relief and comfort. Thus they are less likely to resort to overly impulsive, aggressive acts, which may harm self or others.*
4. Inform the family of the patient's need to displace anger occasionally but that you will be working with the patient to help him or her release his or her feelings in a more constructive, effective way. *Family members who are well-informed are better equipped to cope with their loved one's emotional anguish and outbursts. They are less likely to waste energy on feelings of guilt, fear, anger, or despair and can use their strength to help the patient in more constructive ways. The knowledge that their loved one is being cared for emotionally, as well as physically, will offer family members a greater sense of comfort and understanding. They will feel nurtured and respected by the nurse's attempt to include them in the process.*

*Continued.*

## Ineffective Individual Coping—cont'd

5. With the patient, list and number problems from most to least urgent. Assist him or her in finding immediate solutions for most urgent problems, postpone those which can wait, delegate some to family members, and help him or her acknowledge problems that are beyond his control. *Listing and numbering problems in an organized fashion help break them down into more manageable "pieces" so that the patient is better able to identify solutions for those which are solvable and to suppress those which are less relevant or not amenable to interventions.*
6. Identify individuals in the patient's environment who best help him or her to cope, as well as those who do not. Validate your observations with the patient. EXAMPLE STATEMENTS: "I notice you seemed more relaxed during your daughter's visit." "After the clergy left, you were able to sleep a bit longer than usual; would you like to see him more often?" "Your grandson was a bit upset today; I'll be glad to talk to him if you like." *Supportive persons can invoke a calming effect on the patient's physiological and psychological states. Conversely, well-meaning but nonsupportive individuals can have a deleterious effect on the patient's ability to cope and must be carefully screened and counseled by the nurse.*
7. Teach the patient effective cognitive strategies to help him or her better manage the stress of critical illness and care. Help him or her construct pleasant thoughts, situations, or images that can simultaneously inhibit unpleasant realities. EXAMPLES: a day at the beach, a walk in the park, drinking a glass of wine, or being with a loved one. *Pleasant thoughts or images constructed during critical illness and care tend to inhibit or reduce the intensity of the unpleasant, stressful effects of the experience.*
8. Assist the patient in using coping mechanisms more effectively so he or she can better manage his or her situational crisis:
   - *Suppression* of problems beyond his or her control
   - *Compensation* for illness and its effects; focusing on his or her strengths, interests, family, and spiritual beliefs
   - *Adaptive displacement* of anger, fear, or frustration through healthy, verbal expressions to staff

   *Effective use of coping mechanisms helps to assuage the patient's painful feelings in a safe setting. Thus the patient is strengthened and need not resort to the use of more ineffective defenses to rid himself or herself of anxiety.*
9. Initiate a suicidal assessment if the patient verbalizes the desire to die, states that life is not worth living, or exhibits self-directed aggression. EXAMPLE STATEMENT: "We know this is a bad time for you. You're saying repeatedly that you want to die. Are you planning to harm yourself?" If the response is yes, remain with the patient, alert staff members, and provide for psychiatric consultation as soon as possible. Continue to express concern to the patient and protect him or her from harm. *Suicidal thoughts as a result of ineffective coping or exhaustion of coping devices are not an uncommon occurrence in critically ill patients. If the mood state is distressing enough, a patient may seek relief by attempting a self-destructive act. Although the patient may not imminently have the energy to succeed in his or her attempt, voicing specific plans signifies a depressed mood state and a depletion of coping strategies. Thus immediate intervention is needed since the attempt may be successful when the patient's energy is restored.*
10. Encourage the patient to participate in self-care activities and treatment regimen in accordance with his or her level of progress. Offer praise for his or her efforts toward self-care. *Patients who take an active role in their own treatment and progress are less apt to feel like helpless or powerless victims. This greater sense of control over their illness and environment will guide them more swiftly toward becoming as independent as possible.*

## Anxiety

**Definition:** *A vague, uneasy feeling, the source of which is often nonspecific or unknown to the individual.*

### *Anxiety Related to Threat to Biological, Psychological, and/or Social Integrity*

#### DEFINING CHARACTERISTICS

**Subjective**
- Verbalizations of increased muscle tension
- Expressions of frequent sensation of tingling in hands and feet
- Verbalizations of continuous feeling of apprehension
- Preoccupation with a sense of impending doom
- Verbalizations of difficulty falling asleep
- Repeated expressions of concerns about changes in health status and outcome of illness

## Anxiety—cont'd

**Objective**

- Psychomotor agitation (fidgeting, jitteriness, restlessness)
- Tightened, wrinkled brow
- Strained (worried) facial expression
- Hypervigilance (scans environment)
- Startles easily
- Distractibility
- Sweaty palms
- Fragmented sleep patterns
- Tachycardia
- Tachypnea

### OUTCOME CRITERIA

- Patient effectively uses learned relaxation strategies.
- Patient demonstrates significant decrease in psychomotor agitation.
- Patient verbalizes reduction in tingling sensations in hands and feet.
- Patient is able to focus on the tasks at hand.
- Patient expresses positive, futuristic plans to family and staff.
- Patient's heart rate and rhythm remain within limits commensurate with physiological status.

### NURSING INTERVENTIONS *AND RATIONALE*

1. Continue to monitor the assessment parameters listed under "Defining Characteristics."
2. Instruct the patient in the following simple, effective relaxation strategies:
   - If not contraindicated cardiovascularly, tense and relax all muscles progressively from toes to head.
   - Perform slow, deep breathing exercises.
   - Focus on a single object or person in the environment.
   - Listen to soothing music or relaxation tapes with eyes closed.

   *Progressive toe-to-head relaxation releases the muscular tension that may be a stress-related effect resulting from the threat or change in the patient's health status and outcome of illness. Deep-breathing exercises provide slow, rhythmic, controlled breathing patterns that relax the patient and distract him or her from the effects of his or her illness and hospitalization. Focusing on a single object or person helps the patient dismiss the myriad of disorienting stimuli from his or her visual-perceptual field, which can have a dizzying, distorted effect. A clear sensorium allows him or her to feel more in control of his or her environment.* (Refer to the nursing management of Sensory-Perceptual Alterations, p. 489.) *Music or words expressed in soft, low tones tend to produce soothing, relaxing effects that counteract or inhibit escalating anxiety and provide respites from the patient's situational crisis. Closed eyes eliminate distracting, visual stimuli and promote a more restful environment.*
3. Actively listen to and accept the patient's concerns regarding the threats from his or her illness, outcome, and hospitalization. *Active listening and unconditional acceptance validate the patient as a worthwhile individual and assure him or her that his or her concerns, no matter how great, will be addressed. Knowledge that he or she has an avenue for ventilation will assuage anxiety.*
4. Help the patient distinguish between realistic concerns and exaggerated fears through clear, simple explanations. EXAMPLE STATEMENTS: "Your lab results show that you're doing OK right now." "The shortness of breath you're experiencing is not unusual." "The pain you described is expected and this medication will relieve it." *A patient who is informed about his or her progress and is reassured about expected symptoms and management of care will be better equipped to maintain a more realistic perspective of his or her illness and its outcome. Thus anxiety emanating from imagined or exaggerated fears will likely be assuaged or averted.*
5. Provide simple clarification of environmental events and stimuli that are not related to the patient's illness and care. EXAMPLE STATEMENTS: "That loud noise is coming from a machine that is helping another patient." "The visitor behind the curtain is crying because she's had an upsetting day." "That gurney is here to bring another patient to x-ray." *Clarification of events and stimuli that are unrelated to the patient helps to disengage him or her from the extant anxiety-provoking situations surrounding him or her, thus avoiding further anxiety and apprehension.*
6. Assist the patient in focusing on building on prior coping strategies to deal with the effects of his or her illness and care. EXAMPLE STATEMENTS: "What methods have helped you get through difficult times in the past?" "How can we help you use those methods now?" (See Ineffective Individual Coping care plan for interventions that assist patients to use coping strategies effectively.) *Use of previously successful coping strategies in conjunction with newly learned techniques arms the patient with an arsenal of weapons against anxiety, providing him or her with greater control over his or her situational crisis and decreased feelings of doom and despair.*
7. Give the patient permission to deny or suppress the effects of his or her illness and hospitalization with which he or she cannot cope or control. EXAMPLE STATEMENTS: "It's perfectly OK to ignore things you can't handle right now." "How can we help ease your mind during this time?" "What are some things or tasks that may help distract you?" *Adaptive denial can be helpful in reducing feelings of anxiety in patients with life-threatening illness. Bigus* reports that in studies of two groups of patients with myocardial infarction, the group that used adaptive denial demonstrated significantly fewer symptoms of state anxiety than those patients who failed to use it.* (Refer to the nursing management of Altered Sexuality Patterns on p. 453 for interventions with patients using adaptive denial vs. patients using maladaptive denial or no denial.)

*From Bigus KM: West J Nurs Res 3:150, 1981.

## Sexual Dysfunction

**Definition:** *The state in which an individual experiences a change in sexual function that is viewed as unsatisfying, unrewarding, or inadequate.*

### *Sexual Dysfunction Related to Activity Intolerance Secondary to Myocardial Infarction*

#### DEFINING CHARACTERISTICS

- Verbalized reluctance to resume pre-illness levels of sexual activity because of decrease in energy and increase in fatigue. EXAMPLE STATEMENT: "I won't be the same in bed after this setback. I just don't have the stamina."
- Chest pain, dyspnea, and increased heart rate during routine hospital activities, which patient assumes will occur during sexual activity. EXAMPLE STATEMENTS: "I get chest pain and out of breath just by moving around in my room and my heart speeds up when I exert myself. How is this going to affect my sex life?" "How will I know when I'm in danger of having another heart attack during sexual activity?"

#### OUTCOME CRITERIA

- Patient lists activities that are comparable in METs to energy expenditure and oxygen consumption during sexual activity, including orgasm. (see Table 4-1.)
- Patient states with accuracy the specific vocabulary that describes and contrasts the three types of chest pain (chest wall, anginal, and infarct), their individual symptoms, conditions that provoke them, and actions taken for relief.
- Patient demonstrates correct monitoring of pulse rate while performing activities comparable, according to METs, in energy expenditure to sexual intercourse.
- Patient states which medications may alter or decrease sexual desire or performance.
- Patient verbalizes understanding of activities and situations to avoid before and during sexual intercourse.
- Patient describes symptoms related to sexual activity and orgasm that are considered life-threatening and must be reported immediately to a physician.
- Patient participates in progressive cardiac rehabilitation program.
- Patient and partner express they have achieved a mutually gratifying pre-illness level of sexual function as measured by patient's increased energy and decreased fatigue, dyspnea, heart rate, and chest pain 6 weeks after myocardial infarction.

#### NURSING INTERVENTIONS *AND RATIONALE*

1. Continue to monitor the assessment parameters listed under "Defining Characteristics."
2. Review METs (Table 4-1) with the patient and partner and explain which activities are comparable to sexual activity in energy expenditure and oxygen consumption (3-4 METs) such as climbing two flights of stairs in 10 seconds, walking briskly (2½ miles in 1 hour), pushing light power mower, or pulling light golfbag.
3. Demonstrate monitoring of heart rate to be practiced by patient during activities that are equivalent to energy expenditure during intercourse and explain that coitus can be performed safely when heart rate is maintained within 110 to 120 beats/min without precipitating angina or severe shortness of breath.
4. Teach the patient the specific vocabulary that describes each type of chest pain, and ask him or her to associate each type of pain with its symptoms, provocation, and actions for relief such as the following:
   - *Chest wall pain.* SYMPTOMS: tightness in chest muscles, sore to touch, shortness of breath. *Caused by* "hunching" of back, which strains chest muscles and/or anxiety. ACTIONS: straighten back; relax chest muscles; take slow, deep breaths; and focus on idea that pain will go away. If not relieved within 5 minutes, notify physician.
   - *Anginal pain.* SYMPTOMS: jaw pain or substernal pain that may radiate to left arm and/or shoulder; may be felt as indigestion or toothache. Caused by increased stress (exercise, anger, extremes of hot or cold temperatures). ACTIONS: prevent by taking vasodilator before sex; should be relieved in minutes by use of vasodilator (nitroglycerin), cessation of sex, and rest. If pain persists or worsens, notify physician immediately.
   - *Infarct pain.* SYMPTOMS: severe, persistent, "crushing" chest pain may be accompanied by sweating, severe shortness of breath, and feeling of impending doom. *Caused by* inability of narrowed coronary arteries to meet oxygen needs of heart muscle. ACTIONS: notify physician and alert emergency facility immediately to obtain relief with narcotic-analgesics and oxygen.
5. Inform the couple that studies indicate the "patient-on-bottom" position during sex uses nearly as much energy as "patient-on-top" position but that isometric exercises (tightening of muscles, including heart) may increase heart rate more than safe parameters and should be avoided.
6. Construct a list of the patient's medications that may alter or decrease libido, performance, and/or sexual activity, and explain that the physician's adjusting the dose of some drugs may correct the problem.
7. Reassure the couple that safe sexual activity is possible, provided that situations that dangerously increase the workload of the heart are avoided before sexual activity. Such activities include ingesting a large meal, consuming alcohol either excessively or 3 hours before sexual activity, fatigue, and emotional outburst.

## Sexual Dysfunction—cont'd

8. Instruct the couple to avoid the following situations during sexual activity, and state the reasons why they should be avoided: anal intercourse, isometrics or "tightening" of muscles, extreme hot or cold temperatures, and sexual intercourse with a new partner.
9. Inform couple that if the following symptoms occur as a result of sexual activity, the physician should be notified immediately, *since it is a signal that the heart's workload is greater than its capacity to meet the body's energy demands:* shortness of breath that persists more than 5 minutes after orgasm, increased heart rate or palpitations that persist more than 5 minutes after orgasm, extreme fatigue the day after intercourse, insomnia the day after intercourse, and chest pain during or after intercourse that is unrelieved by measures listed in interventions for chest wall pain and anginal pain (may indicate infarct pain).
10. Teach patient that, while in the hospital, his or her exercise tolerance during sex will be ascertained by formal testing such as monitoring heart rate during treadmill tests, the use of calibrated bicycle ergometer, and before and after walking briskly down the hospital corridor.
11. Reassure patient and partner that compliance with treatment regimen and participation in rehabilitation program will reduce workload of the heart and promote mutually satisfying sexual activity, with increased energy and decreased fatigue, chest pain, and shortness of breath, within 4 to 6 weeks after myocardial infarction.

## *Sexual Dysfunction Related to Activity Intolerance Secondary to Chronic Lung Disease*

### DEFINING CHARACTERISTICS

- Patient and partner express the need to avoid or experience decreased frequency in sexual activities because of patient's dyspnea on exertion during all activities. (EXAMPLE STATEMENT: "It's too hard to breathe during any kind of exertion, so sex is probably out of the question.")
- Patient verbalizes anxiety or fear about life-threatening respiratory distress and increased heart rate during sexual activity. (EXAMPLE STATEMENT: "Sex is just not worth the risk to my life. I need to conserve my energy to survive.")
- Patient expresses feelings that increased mucus production, which is exacerbated by activities, including sex, may be repulsive to partner. (EXAMPLE STATEMENT: "My breath smells horrible with all this sputum, and it's worse during activities. How can anyone come close to me?")
- Patient avoids or rejects efforts by partner to kiss or embrace in the critical care unit.

### OUTCOME CRITERIA

- Patient demonstrates intimate behaviors with partner and masturbates, if feasible, while in critical care unit (affords patient the opportunity to monitor return of pulse and respiratory rate to normal after orgasm).
- Patient expresses willingness to engage in sexual intercourse after taking appropriate rest periods to conserve energy, decrease mucus production, and reduce dyspnea.
- Patient verbalizes desire to try alternative, energy-saving positions during sexual intercourse.
- Patient lists appropriate medications or treatments for use before sexual activity.
- Patient states knowledge of effects of drug therapy, alcohol consumption, and heavy meals on sexual activity.

### NURSING INTERVENTIONS *AND RATIONALE*

1. Continue to monitor the assessment parameters listed under "Defining Characteristics."
2. The nurse will inform the patient about the following:
   - Sexual intercourse will increase the pulse and respiratory rates, but they will normally return to baseline very quickly. (Demonstrate how to monitor pulse rate.)
   - Sexual intercourse with orgasm uses approximately the same amount of energy as climbing two flights of stairs in 10 seconds, walking briskly (2½ miles in 1 hour), pushing light mower, or pulling light golf bag. (See Table 4-1.)
   - The "patient-on-top" position, although shown in most studies to require nearly the same amount of energy expenditure as the "patient-on-bottom" position, should be avoided by the respiratory patient *because it may tend to produce more dyspnea. On the other hand, the "patient-on-bottom" position could lead to compression of the chest, which may also lead to shortness of breath.* Thus the following alternative positions should be tried:

   Side-to-side, rear, or front entry (by male) except for the hypoxemic individual *who may not be able to tolerate having head and upper chest in a flat position.* In this situation, *upright position augments ventilation and perfusion and improves oxygenation status.*

   Patient in chair with feet on floor and partner (female) astride.

*Continued.*

## Sexual Dysfunction—cont'd

Masturbation and oral-genital sex (if feasible). Remember that age, religion, cultural beliefs, and desire should be considered before suggesting these alternatives. Although oral-genital sex may be difficult because of the dyspnea, cough, and sputum production, it is up to the patient to determine how bothersome this is compared with the pleasure of sexual fulfillment. Some authorities believe that masturbation can begin in the critical care unit, depending on the couple's inclination and the condition of the patient. They believe that *patients who masturbate while in the critical care unit set the stage for a smoother transition toward resumption of "normal" or "near-normal" sexual function after discharge as their conditions allow.*

- *Holding, touching, and caressing are acceptable behaviors in the critical care unit. Also, whenever couples express anxiety about having sex when at home, they should be advised to relax, "cuddle up," and enjoy an intimate moment together at home.*
- *Inhaled bronchodilators can be used by patients with asthma before, during, and after sex to decrease anxiety and shortness of breath.*
- Taking medications 30 to 60 minutes before sexual activity *may decrease dyspnea.*
- Use of steroids and theophylline have no effect on sexual functioning. (In some instances, adjusting the dose with physician's advice may increase libido and potency.)
- If oxygen is used at home, increase the liter flow by 1 L/min during intercourse with the recommendation of the physician.
- Intercourse should be avoided after a heavy meal. *A full stomach can restrict ventilatory movement because of the raised diaphragm.*
- Excessive alcohol consumption decreases sexual function.
- Sexual intercourse is best initiated after a rest period such as in the morning hours, but if there is excessive sputum production at that time, it may be better to plan sexual activities for the afternoon after a nap.
- The use of a waterbed is recommended by some who believe that *there is decreased demand for energy during sexual intercourse because of the rhythm of the bed.*
- Attending a pulmonary rehabilitation program to learn about the techniques that aid breathing and conserve energy and about exerciese that can increase activity tolerance during sex is crucial after discharge.

## Altered Sexuality Patterns

**Definition:** *The state in which an individual experiences concern about his or her sexuality.*

### *Altered Sexuality Patterns Related to Fear of Death During Coitus Secondary to Myocardial Infarction*

#### DEFINING CHARACTERISTICS

- Patient and partner demonstrate behaviors indicating sexual intercourse is a threat to patient's cardiac integrity and life function (EXAMPLE STATEMENTS *[patient]:* "I guess I'll have to take life easy from now on." "My [sexual partner] and I will have to be satisfied with holding hands" [affect anxious, voice tremulous].)
- Partner demonstrates overprotective attitude toward patient, which invokes a shared sense of anxiety (sense of impending doom); partner verbalizes that patient "won't have to lift a finger from now on" (facial expression strained)
- Patient demonstrates grieving behaviors, indicating diminished sense of self-worth related to threat to sexual performance and perceived body image change, including the following:
  - Saddened affect (stares into space with bland facial expression)
  - Lack of interest in food, treatment, and exercise program
  - Apathy toward sexual information offered by nurses
  - Resistance to sexual partner's intimate attempts such as kissing and hugging
- Patient exhibits behaviors indicative of *maladaptive denial* (unconscious defense mechanism used to decrease anxiety and protect the ego against a painful, unacceptable reality—in this case fear of death and threat to sexual integrity) such as the following:
  - Lack of cooperation with staff (uses loud, "bullying" tones)
  - Nonparticipation in treatment and exercise program
  - Refusal to pace activities (states intentions to " . . . work, drink, smoke, and have sex as usual")
  - Strong rejection of information about sexuality

#### OUTCOME CRITERIA

- Patient demonstrates positive attitude with decreased anxiety (steady voice tone; calm body movement; eye contact when discussing illness, recovery, and sexual potential).
- Patient rejects overprotective behaviors of partner (feeds and grooms self). This defuses partner's anxiety and builds mutual confidence in future sex roles.
- Patient does the following:
  - Exhibits brightened affect (animated facial expression and expressive voice tone) and indicates interest in life and a positive self-esteem
  - Actively participates in treatment and exercise program and reflects acceptance of body image change and potential for sexual participation
  - Accepts sexual information offered by nurses about METs and repeats it accurately in a calm manner
  - Responds to intimate advances of sexual partner and indicates decreased fear of resuming sexual activity on discharge
- Patient does the following:
  - Refrains from using "bullying" behaviors (angry, demanding voice tone), and displays calm, cooperative attitude toward staff and sexual partner
  - Requests information about how safely to pace activities such as work, drink, cigarette smoking, and sex and repeats information accurately

#### NURSING INTERVENTIONS *AND RATIONALE*

1. Continue to monitor the assessment parameter listed under "Defining Characteristics."
2. Clarify any misconceptions about myocardial infarction, contrasting realistic concerns with irrational fears about future sexual function and performance (Refer to "Sexual Dysfunction related to activity intolerance secondary to myocardial infarction" for specific information about cardiac work load during sexual activity.)
3. Inform the patient and partner early in the rehabilitation program that activity and independence are crucial to the patient's emotional and physical recovery in which sexual function plays a role. The ability to feed oneself is one indication of such progress.
4. Do the following:
   - Use therapeutic communication skills to elicit feelings of fear and anxiety about the effect of sexual intercourse on the function of the heart muscle and the life of the patient.
   - Encourage and provide privacy for intimate behaviors between patient and partner and for masturbation, if feasible.
   - Provide clear, concise information about rationale for medical protocol and provide role-modeling of calm, controlled, adult behavior. *Knowledge provides power, which builds self-esteem and decreases anxiety. Use of adult behavior influences patient to respond in like manner.*
   - Praise the patient generously for participation in cardiac rehabilitation program, for pacing activities of daily living, for displays of intimacy, and for calm, controlled, adult behavior.
   - Discuss resumption of sexual activity in nonthreatening, matter-of-fact manner, beginning with discussion of the least personal activities such as gardening to the most personal areas. See box entitled "Sample Interview Guidelines." (EXAMPLE STATEMENT: "I'd like to discuss how you can safely incorporate activities, including sexual activity, back into your life.")

# Nursing Management of Sleep Alterations

## Sleep Pattern Disturbance

**Definition:** *Disruption of sleep time that causes a patient discomfort or interferes with the patient's desired life-style.*

### *Sleep Pattern Disturbance Related to Fragmented Sleep and/or Circadian Desynchronization*

#### DEFINING CHARACTERISTICS

- Decreased sleep during one block of sleep time
- Daytime sleepiness
- Sleep deprivation
  Less than one half normal total sleep time
  Decreased slow wave or REM sleep
- Anxiety
- Fatigue
- Restlessness
- Disorientation and hallucinations
- Combativeness
- Frequent wakenings
- Decreased arousal threshold
- Sleep is out of synchronization with biological rhythms, resulting in sleeping during the day and awakening at night

#### OUTCOME CRITERIA

- Patient's total sleep time approximates patient's norm.
- Patient is able to complete sleep cycles of 90 minutes without interruption.
- Patient has no delusions, hallucinations, illusions.
- Patient has reality-based thought content.
- Patient is oriented to four spheres.
- Majority of patient's sleep time will fall during low cycle of the circadian rhythm (normally at night).

#### NURSING INTERVENTIONS *AND RATIONALE*

1. Continue to monitor the assessment parameters listed under "Defining Characteristics."
2. Assess normal sleep pattern on admission and any history of sleep disturbance or chronic illness that may affect sleep or sedative/hypnotic use. Promote normal sleep activity while patient is in critical care unit. Assess sleep effectiveness by asking patient how his or her sleep in the hospital compares to sleep at home. (Refer to Sensory-Perceptual Alterations, p. 489, for the management of the acutely psychotic/suspicious patient.)
3. Minimize awakenings *to allow for at least 90-minute sleep cycles*. Continually assess the need to awaken the patient, particularly at night. Distinguish between essential and nonessential nursing tasks. Organize nursing care to allow for maximum amount of uninterrupted sleep while ensuring close monitoring of the patient's condition. Whenever possible, monitor physiological parameters without waking the patient. Coordinate awakenings with other departments such as respiratory therapy, laboratory, and x-ray *to minimize sleep interruptions*.
4. Minimize noise, particularly that of the staff and noisy equipment. Reduce the level of environmental stimuli. Refer to the nursing management of Sensory-Perceptual Alterations on p. 489 for interventions to minimize sensory overload.
5. Plan nap times to assist in equilibrating the normal total sleep time. Discourage or prevent catnaps (sleep lasting longer than 90 minutes at a time), because *these physically refresh the individual and thereby decrease the stimulus for longer sleep cycles in which REM sleep is obtained*. Early morning naps, however, may be beneficial in promoting REM sleep, because *a greater proportion of early morning sleep is allocated to REM activity*.
6. Promote comfort, relaxation, and a sense of well-being. Treat pain. Eliminate stressful situations before bedtime. Use of relaxation techniques, imagery, backrubs, or warm blankets may be helpful. Other interventions may include increased privacy or a private room. Individual patients may prefer quiet or may prefer the background noise of the television *to best promote sleep*.
7. Be aware of the effects of commonly used medications on sleep. *Many sedative and hypnotic medications decrease REM sleep*. Sedative and analgesic medications should not be withheld, but rather, drugs that minimally disrupt sleep should be used to complement comfort measures, with dosages reduced gradually as the medication is no longer necessary. Do not abruptly withdraw REM-suppressing medications, because *this can result in "REM rebound."*
8. Foods containing tryptophan, such as milk or turkey, may be appropriate because *these promote sleep*.
9. Be aware that the best treatment for sleep deprivation is prevention.
10. Facilitate staff awareness that sleep is essential and health promoting. Assess for the critical care unit sleep-reducing stimuli and work to minimize them.
11. Document amount of uninterrupted sleep per shift, especially sleep episodes lasting longer than 2 hours. This can be effectively documented as part of the 24-hour flow sheet and reported routinely, shift to shift. *Sleep pattern disturbance is diagnosed, treated, and resolved more efficiently when formally documented in this manner*.
12. Assist patient to maintain normal day-night cycles by decreasing lighting, noise, and sensory stimulation at night and critically evaluating the need to awaken the patient at night.
13. Activity during the daytime should be increased to stimulate wakefulness. Increased physical activity until 2 hours before bedtime is useful in *promoting naturally-induced sleep*. Limiting caffeine intake after early afternoon will promote sleep in the evening.
14. Do not schedule routine procedures at night.
15. Be aware that cardiac dysrhythmias can be precipitated by the decreased arousal threshold secondary to desynchronization.
16. If desynchronization occurs, plan for resynchronization by maintaining constancy in day-night pattern for at least 3 days (may require 5 to 12 days to reacclimatize). Plan for activities during the day *to stimulate wakefulness* and use comfort measures (comfortable body position, warm blankets, backrub, etc.) *to promote sleep* at night. Resynchronization is characteristically associated with chronic fatigue, malaise, and a decreased ability to perform life tasks.

# Nursing Management of Cardiovascular Alterations

## Decreased Cardiac Output

**Definition:** *The state in which the blood pumped by an individual's heart is so sufficiently reduced that it is inadequate to meet the needs of the body's tissues.*

### *Decreased Cardiac Output Related to Supraventricular Tachycardia*

#### DEFINING CHARACTERISTICS

- Sudden drop in blood pressure
- Atrial and/or ventricular rate >100
- Decreased mentation
- Decreased urine output
- Chest pain
- Dyspnea

#### OUTCOME CRITERIA

- Systolic blood pressure >100.
- Mean arterial pressure (MAP) is >80.
- Ventricular rate is <100.
- Sensorium is intact.
- Urine output is >30 ml/hr.

#### NURSING INTERVENTIONS *AND RATIONALE*

1. Continue to monitor the assessment parameters listed under "Defining Characteristics."
2. Carefully distinguish supraventricular tachycardia from ventricular tachycardia. Monitoring the patient in lead $MCL_1$ *may assist in distinguishing ventricular ectopy from aberrancy.*
3. Follow critical care emergency standing orders regarding the administration of supraventricular antidysrhythmic agents, such as verapamil, quinidine, procainamide, propranolol, edrophonium, digoxin, and phenylephrine.
4. Consider positioning patient supine *to increase preload.*
5. Identify precipitating factors when possible, such as emotional stress, caffeine, nicotine, and sympathomimetic drugs, and intervene to reduce or eliminate their effect.
6. Assess apical-radial pulse *to identify deficits indicating nonperfused beats.* Monitor amplitude of peripheral pulses *to ascertain perfusion to extremities.*
7. Monitor arterial blood pressure *to determine symptomatic decompensation.*
8. With physician collaboration, consider carotid sinus massage or Valsalva maneuver, *thereby increasing vagal tone.*
9. Anticipate possibility of synchronized cardioversion or overdrive pacing.
10. For atrial fibrillation that is either spontaneously, pharmacologically, or electrically converted, monitor for signs of cerebral, pulmonary, and/or peripheral thromboembolization as a result of liberation of mural thrombi.
11. If patient is hypoxemic, or if dysrhythmia is suspected to be a result of or exacerbated by ischemia, administer oxygen observing the following principles:
    - Without physician collaboration, liter flow should be no greater than 2 L/min via nasal prongs in patients whose pulmonary history is either unknown or reveals a pattern of chronic $CO_2$ retention. *Administration of oxygen at concentrations higher than 2 L/min via nasal prongs may induce $CO_2$ narcosis in patients who chronically retain $CO_2$.*
    - Oxygen should be administered with the goal of achieving a $PaO_2$ no greater than 95 mm Hg *to avoid toxic concentrations of oxygen.*
    - Observe caution when administering oxygen at an $FIO_2$ greater than 40% *in view of the higher risk for oxygen toxicity.*
12. Assess serum electrolyte levels, especially potassium and calcium, because *increased or decreased electrolyte levels may exacerbate the dysrhythmia or may impair treatment of the dysrhythmia.*

## Decreased Cardiac Output—cont'd

### *Decreased Cardiac Output Related to Relative Excess* of Preload and Afterload Secondary to Impaired Ventricular Contractility*

**DEFINING CHARACTERISTICS**

- Systolic blood pressure (SBP) <100
- Mean arterial pressure (MAP) <80
- Change in mentation
- Decreased urine output
- Cardiac index <2.5
- Pulmonary artery wedge pressure (PAWP) >15
- Pulmonary artery diastolic pressure (PADP) >15
- Bibasilar fluid crackles
- Faint peripheral pulses
- Ventricular gallop rhythm ($S_3$)
- Skin cool, pale, moist
- Activity intolerance

**OUTCOME CRITERIA**

- Cardiac index is 2.5-4.0.
- SBP is >90.
- MAP is >80.
- PAWP and PADP are <15.

**NURSING INTERVENTIONS *AND RATIONALE***

**The following interventions reduce preload**

1. Continue to monitor the assessment parameters listed under "Defining Characteristics."
2. Implement fluid restriction.
3. Double concentrate intravenous drug drips when possible *to decrease the amount of volume infused to the patient.*
4. Position patient with extremities dependent *to pool blood in the extremities, thus decreasing preload.*
5. With physician collaboration, administer diuretics.
6. Titrate venous vasodilators and inotropic drips, per protocol, to desired SBP, MAP, PAWP, and/or PADP. Withhold and/or change drip rate when SBP, MAP, PAWP, and/or PADP begin to drop.

**The following interventions reduce afterload**

1. Intervene to reduce anxiety and *thereby limit catecholamine release:* administer intravenous $MSO_4$ per protocol and titrate to MAP or SBP, relaxation techniques, imagery. (Refer to the nursing management of Anxiety on p. 448).
2. Titrate arterial vasodilators drips to attain desired SBP, PAWP, and/or PADP. Change drip rate when SBP, PAWP, and/or PADP stabilize or begin to drop.
3. Anticipate possibility of intraaortic balloon pumping.

**The following interventions reduce myocardial oxygen consumption**

1. Absolute bed rest *to decrease metabolic demand.*
2. Consider slackening activity restrictions if such restrictions precipitate anxiety. *Anxiety stimulates the sympathetic outpouring of catecholamines and thereby increases myocardial oxygen consumption.*
3. Ensure that patient and family understand routine of critical care unit and explain all care given to patient *to increase patient comfort level and to decrease catecholamine release associated with fear of being in an unknown environment.*

**Relative excess of preload and afterload refers not to an actual increase in these pressures, but rather to the inability of the ventricle to handle normal pressures because of impaired ventricular function. Therefore the normal pressures become "excessive" to the poorly functioning ventricle.*

### *Decreased Cardiac Output Related to Decreased Preload Secondary to Mechanical Ventilation With or Without PEEP*

**DEFINING CHARACTERISTICS**

- Sudden drop in SBP, PAWP, or PADP corresponding to the application of mechanical ventilation or PEEP, or changes in tidal volume delivery or level of PEEP.

**OUTCOME CRITERIA**

- SBP is >90, MAP is >80.
- PAWP and PAD are >6.

**NURSING INTERVENTIONS *AND RATIONALE***

1. Continue to monitor the assessment parameters listed under "Defining Characteristics."
2. Monitor vital organ perfusion (through assessment of urine output and mentation, for example) carefully, because *some degree of reduction in cardiac output will coexist with the successful application of mechanical ventilation and/or PEEP.*
3. Position patient supine *to increase preload and therefore cardiac output.*
4. With physician collaboration, consider increasing the administration of parenteral fluids to achieve ideal preload. (*The ideal preload may be that which existed before the application of mechanical ventilation and/or PEEP*).

## Decreased Cardiac Output—cont'd

### *Decreased Cardiac Output Related to Atrioventricular (AV) Heart Block*

**DEFINING CHARACTERISTICS**

- Systolic blood pressure <100
- Mean arterial pressure (MAP) <80
- Ventricular rate <60
- Decreased mentation or syncope
- Decreased urine output

**OUTCOME CRITERIA**

- Systolic blood pressure is >90.
- MAP is >80.
- Ventricular rate is >60.
- The patient is awake and responsive.
- Urine output is >30 ml/hr.

**NURSING INTERVENTIONS *AND RATIONALE***

**First-degree AV Block**

1. Continue to monitor the assessment parameters listed under "Defining Characteristics."
2. Monitor closely, measuring P-R intervals *to determine further prolongation, which would suggest progression of heart block.*
3. With physician collaboration, consider withholding supraventricular antidysrhythmic agents such as digitalis, quinidine, beta-blocking agents, and calcium channel blockers.

**Second-Degree AV Block—Mobitz I (Wenckebach pattern)**

1. Continue to monitor the assessment parameters listed under "Defining Characteristics."
2. Monitor for symptomatic decompensation resulting from slow ventricular rate (rare).
3. While symptomatic, position patient supine *to increase preload and therefore cardiac output.*
4. Monitor for progression to complete heart block.
5. With physician collaboration, consider withholding digitalis.
6. Eliminate sources of vagal stimulation. *Vagal stimulation increases the delay in conduction at the AV node.*

**Second-Degree AV Block—Mobitz II**

1. Continue to monitor the assessment parameters listed under "Defining Characteristics."
2. Monitor closely for symptomatic decompensation as a result of slow ventricular rate (common).
3. While symptomatic, position patient supine *to increase preload and therefore cardiac output.*
4. Monitor for progression of existing block, such as 2:1, 3:1, 4:1 conduction and for progression to complete heart block.
5. Follow critical care emergency standing orders regarding the administration of positive chronotropic agents, such as atropine or isoproterenol.
6. Anticipate possibility of pacemaker insertion.

**Third-Degree (Complete) AV Block**

1. Continue to monitor the assessment parameters listed under "Defining Characteristics."
2. Monitor closely for symptomatic decompensation resulting from slow ventricular rate (common).
3. While symptomatic, position patient supine *to increase preload and therefore cardiac output.*
4. Follow critical care emergency standing orders regarding the administration of isoproterenol.
5. Anticipate the necessity of pacemaker insertion or use of external pacemaker (for example, Pace-Aid).

### *Decreased Cardiac Output Related to Hemopericardium Secondary to Open Heart Surgery*

**DEFINING CHARACTERISTICS**

- Cardiac output <5
- Cardiac index <2.5
- Elevated PAWP, PADP, or CVP
- Narrowed pulse pressure
- Pulsus paradoxus
- Muffled heart sounds
- Distended neck veins
- Decreasing SBP or MAP
- Tachycardia
- Enlarged cardiac silhouette on chest film

**OUTCOME CRITERIA**

- Cardiac output is >5.
- Cardiac index is >2.5.
- PAWP, PADP, CVP are reduced to baseline.
- Crisp heart sounds are heard.
- SBP is >100, MAP is >80.
- Heart rate is reduced to baseline.
- Cardiac silhouette is reduced to baseline.

**NURSING INTERVENTIONS *AND RATIONALE***

1. Continue to monitor the assessment parameters outlined under "Defining Characteristics."
2. Monitor mediastinal tube drainage for sudden cessation and/or increase. *Either event is to be considered highly suggestive of impending cardiac tamponade.*
3. Milk mediastinal tubes per protocol *to ensure continual patency.*
4. Titrate vasodilator drips *to keep SBP below level at which graft(s) or anastomoses may leak or tear (usually SBP kept <150).*
5. Anticipate the necessity of either bedside pericardiocentesis or return to surgery.

## Decreased Cardiac Output—cont'd

### *Decreased Cardiac Output Related to Decreased Preload Secondary to Fluid Volume Deficit*

#### DEFINING CHARACTERISTICS

- CO <5
- CI <2.5
- PAWP, PADP, CVP less than normal or less than baseline
- Tachycardia
- Narrowed pulse pressure
- SBP <100
- Mean arterial pressure (MAP) <80
- Urine <30/hr
- Skin pale, cool, moist
- Apprehensiveness

#### OUTCOME CRITERIA

- CO is >5.
- CI is >2.5.
- PAWP, PADP, CVP are normal or back to baseline level.
- Pulse is normal or back to baseline.
- SBP is >90.
- MAP is >80.
- Urine is >30/hr.

#### NURSING INTERVENTIONS *AND RATIONALE*

**For Active Blood Loss**

1. Continue to monitor the assessment parameters listed under "Defining Characteristics." In addition, a serum lactate level >3 mosm is felt to represent cellular perfusion failure at its earliest stage.
2. Secure airway and administer oxygen.
3. Position patient supine with legs elevated *to increase preload and therefore cardiac output*. Avoid Trendelenburg's position because *this position causes abdominal viscera to exert pressure against the diaphragm, thereby limiting diaphragmatic descent and inhalation*. Consider low-Fowler's position with legs elevated for patients with head injury *to avoid increases in intracranial pressure*.
4. For fluid repletion use the 3:1 rule, replacing 3 parts of fluid for every unit of blood lost.
5. Administer solutions using the fluid challenge technique: Infuse precise amounts of fluid (usually 5 to 20 ml/min) over 10-minutes periods and monitor cardiac loading pressures serially to determine successful challenging. If the PAWP or PADP elevates more than 7 mm Hg above beginning level, the infusion should be stopped. If the PAWP or PADP rises only to 3 mm Hg above baseline, or falls, another fluid challenge should be given.
6. Assess for signs and symptoms of fluid overload once fluid replacement has begun. These may include elevations above normal of PAP or CVP levels, pulmonary crackles, or dyspnea.
7. Replete fluids first before considering use of vasopressors since *vasopressors increase myocardial oxygen consumption out of proportion to the reestablishment of coronary perfusion in the early phases of treatment.*
8. When blood is available or indicated, replace with fresh packed red cells and fresh-frozen plasma *to keep clotting factors intact.*
9. Move or reposition patient minimally *to decrease or limit tissue oxygen demands.*
10. Evaluate patient's anxiety level and intervene via patient education or sedation *to decrease tissue oxygen demands.*
11. Be alert to the possiblity of development of adult respiratory distress syndrome (ARDS) and/or disseminated intravascular coagulation (DIC) in the ensuing 72 hours.

**For Dehydration**

1. Continue to monitor the assessment parameters listed under "Defining Characteristics."
2. Position patient supine with legs elevated *to increase preload and therefore cardiac output.* Avoid Trendelenburg's position, because this position causes abdominal viscera to exert pressure against the diaphragm, therby limiting diaphragmatic descent and inhalation. Consider low-Fowler's position with legs elevated for patients with head injury *to avoid increases in intracranial pressure.*
3. Calculate the patient's 24-hour fluid requirements per BSA and replete with the appropriate electrolyte solution.
4. Administer solutions using the fluid challenge technique: Infuse precise amounts of fluid (usually 5 to 20 ml/min) over 10-minute periods and monitor cardiac loading pressure serially to determine successful challenging. If the PAWP, or PADP elevates more than 7 mm Hg above beginning level, the infusion should be stopped. If the PAWP or PADP rises only to 3 mm Hg above baseline, or falls, another fluid challenge should be given.
5. Assess for signs and symptoms of fluid overload once fluid replacement has begun. These may include elevations of PAP or CVP to above normal levels, pulmonary crackles, or dyspnea.
6. Replete fluids first before considering use of vasopressors since *vasopressors increase myocardial oxygen consumption out of proportion to the re-establishment of coronary perfusion in the early phase of treatment.*

## Decreased Cardiac Output—cont'd

### *Decreased Cardiac Output Related to Ventricular Tachycardia*

#### DEFINING CHARACTERISTICS

- Sudden drop in blood pressure
- Syncope
- Loss of consciousness
- Faint or absent peripheral pulses

#### OUTCOME CRITERIA

- Systolic blood pressure is >90.
- Mean arterial pressure (MAP) is >70.
- The patient is awake and responsive.
- Peripheral pulses are palpable.

#### NURSING INTERVENTIONS *AND RATIONALE*

1. Continue to monitor the assessment parameters listed under "Defining Characteristics."
2. Carefully distinguish ventricular tachycardia from supraventricular tachycardia. Monitoring the patient in lead $MCL_1$ *may assist in distinguishing ventricular ectopy from aberrancy.*
3. Monitor and treat the "warning dysrhythmias" (that is, >6 premature ventricular contractions [PVCs] per minute, multifocal PVCs, R on T phenomenon, couplets, bursts of ventricular tachycardia, bigeminy, trigeminy).
4. Assess serum electrolyte levels, especially potassium, because *increased or decreased electrolyte levels may exacerbate the dysrhythmia or may impair treatment of the dysrhythmia.*
5. Follow critical care emergency standing orders regarding the administration of ventricular antidysrhythmic agents, such as lidocaine, bretylium, and procainamide.
6. For asymptomatic ventricular tachycardia, treat with lidocaine. For symptomatic ventricular tachycardia, treat with synchronized cardioversion. For pulseless ventricular tachycardia, treat as ventricular fibrillation and defibrillate. (See ACLS algorithms in Appendix B.)
7. Position patient supine *to increase preload.*
8. Anticipate possibility that sporadic ventricular dysrhythmias may progress to ventricular tachycardia or ventricular fibrillation and be prepared to treat with implementation of synchronized cardioversion and defibrillation, respectively.
9. Anticipate possibility of cardiac standstill and activation of resuscitation protocol.
10. When safe rhythm is reestablished, carefully assess for femoral and carotid pulsations *to rule out electromechanical dissociation.*
11. Identify precipitating factors when possible, such as hypoxia, electrolyte abnormalities, drug toxicity (especially amrinone, digitalis, quinidine, disopyramide, procainamide, phenothiazines, tricyclic and tetracyclic antidepressants), or recent MI, and intervene to reduce or eliminate their effect.

### *Decreased Cardiac Output Related to Decreased Preload Secondary to Septicemia*

#### DEFINING CHARACTERISTICS

- Tachycardia >100
- Skin dry, warm, flushed (early stage); cold, clammy, cyanotic (late stage)
- CO, CI, elevated (early stage); CO, CI, decreased (late stage)
- PA pressures decreased (early stage), elevated (late stage)
- SBP, MAP, less than normal or baseline (early); profound hypotension (late stage)
- Urine output <30 ml/hr

#### OUTCOME CRITERIA

- Heart rate is normal or back to baseline.
- CO is >5, CI is >2.5, SBP is >90, MAP is >80.
- Urine output >30 ml/hr.

#### NURSING INTERVENTIONS *AND RATIONALE*

1. Continue to monitor the assessment parameters listed under "Defining Characteristics." In addition, a serum lactate level >3 mosm is felt to represent cellular perfusion failure at its earliest stage.
2. Secure airway and administer oxygen.
3. Position patient supine with legs elevated *to increase preload and therefore cardiac output in late-stage shock.*
4. Administer intravenous solutions as prescribed using the fluid challenge technique: Infuse precise amounts of fluid (usually 5 to 20 ml/min) over 10-minute periods and monitor cardiac loading pressures serially to determine successful challenging. If the PAWP or PADP elevates more than 7 mm Hg above beginning levels, the infusion should be stopped. If the PAWP or PADP rises only to 3 mm Hg above baseline, or falls, another fluid challenge should be given.
5. Assess for signs and symptoms of fluid overload once fluid replacement has begun. These may include elevations above normal of PAP or CVP levels, pulmonary crackles, or dyspnea.
6. With physician collaboration, administer intravenous antimicrobials and closely monitor their effectiveness and specific side effects. Carefully assess patient for hypersensitivity reaction to antimicrobials.
7. With physician collaboration, administer vasopressor agents and positive inotropic drugs *to maintain perfusion and cardiac output.*
8. With physician collaboration, administer steroids.

## Decreased Cardiac Output—cont'd

### *Decreased Cardiac Output Related to Vasodilation and Bradycardia Secondary to Sympathetic Blockade of Neurogenic (Spinal) Shock Following Spinal Cord Injury Above T-6 Level*

#### DEFINING CHARACTERISTICS

- Postural hypotension, such as turning from supine to prone
- SBP <90 mm Hg or below patient's norm
- Decreased PAP, PAD, and PCWP
- Decreased cardiac index
- Decreased SVR
- Bradycardia
- Cardiac dysrhythmias
- Decreased urinary output
- Hypothermia as a result of inability to retain body heat (See section on neurological alterations for the assessment and treatment of other neurological manifestations of spinal shock.)

#### OUTCOME CRITERIA

- SBP is >90 mm Hg or within patient's norm.
- Fainting/dizziness with position change is absent.
- <10 mm Hg DBP drop with position change.
- HR is 60-100 beats/min.
- <20 beats/min HR increase with position change.
- PAP is 4 to 6 mm Hg.
- PCWP is 4 to 12 mm Hg.
- PAD is 8 to 14 mm Hg.
- SVR is 950 to 1300 dynes/sec/cm.
- Cardiac index is 2.5 to 4.0.
- Urinary output is >30 ml/hr.
- Normothermia is present.

#### NURSING INTERVENTIONS *AND RATIONALE*

1. Continue to monitor the assessment parameters listed under "Defining Characteristics."
2. Implement measures *to prevent episodes of postural hypotension.*
   - Change patient's position slowly.
   - Apply antiembolic stockings *to promote venous return.*
   - Perform range of motion exercises every 2 hours *to prevent venous pooling.*
   - Collaborate with physical therapy regarding use of a tilt table *to progress patient from supine to upright position.*
3. Administer crystalloid intravenous fluids using fluid challenge technique: Infuse precise amounts of fluid (usually 5 to 20 ml/min) over 10-minute periods; monitor cardiac loading pressures serially to determine successful challenging.
4. Anticipate the administration of colloids.
5. Anticipate administration of vasopressors if fluid challenges ineffective.
6. Monitor cardiac rhythm. Be especially vigilant during vagal stimulating procedures such as suctioning because *serious bradycardia can result.*
7. Administer atropine per critical care emergency standing orders for symptomatic bradycardia.
8. Maintain normothermia by increasing temperature in patient's room and applying blankets. Avoid use of electronic warming devices *because of decreased peripheral blood flow and sensation.*

## Altered Tissue Perfusion

**Definition:** *The state in which the individual experiences a decrease in nutrition and oxygenation at the cellular level due to a deficit in arterial capillary blood supply.*

### *High Risk for Altered Peripheral Tissue Perfusion*

**RISK FACTORS**

- Vasopressor therapy

**DEFINING CHARACTERISTICS OF AN ACTUAL PROBLEM**

- Pale or cyanotic digits
- Ischemic pain
- Delayed capillary refill
- Weak peripheral pulses

**OUTCOME CRITERIA**

- Digits are free from pallor or cyanosis.
- Ischemic pain is absent.
- Capillary refill is immediate.
- Peripheral pulses are full and equal.

**NURSING INTERVENTIONS *AND RATIONALE***

1. Continue to monitor the assessment parameters listed under "Defining Characteristics."
2. Careful evaluation of the adequacy of peripheral perfusion is essential in patients receiving infusions of the following vasopressor drugs. In addition, *extravasation of these agents into tissues results in localized ischemic necrosis and therefore are infused through central lines when possible.* Dopamine infusions: At dosages >10 mcg/kg/min, alpha adrenergic receptors are stimulated, *producing moderate peripheral vasoconstriction;* at dosages >20 μg/kg/min, intense peripheral vasoconstriction results, *producing serious perfusion alterations.* Levarterenol bitartrate infusions: At all dosages alpha adrenergic receptors are stimulated, *producing the potential for perfusion alterations.*
3. Avoid high-dose vasopressor therapy. Titrate vasopressor drips to achieve and maintain SBP of 90 or MAP above 70. Further augmentation of SBP or MAP should be accomplished by means of other modalities.
4. Immediate physician notification is indicated at the earliest sign of peripheral perfusion alterations.

### *High Risk for Altered Peripheral Tissue Perfusion*

**RISK FACTORS**

- Orthopedic injury or manipulation of an extremity
- Orthopedic devices applied to an extremity

**DEFINING CHARACTERISTICS OF AN ACTUAL PROBLEM**

- Weak and/or unequal peripheral pulses
- Delayed capillary refill
- Ischemic pain distal to injury/manipulation/device
- Cool skin distal to injury/manipulation/device
- Paresthesias

**OUTCOME CRITERIA**

- Peripheral pulses are full and equal bilaterally.
- Capillary refill is equal bilaterally.
- There is no ischemic pain distal to injury/manipulation/device.
- There is equal skin temperature distal to injury/manipulation/device.
- Paresthesias are absent.

**NURSING INTERVENTIONS *AND RATIONALE***

1. Continue to monitor the assessment parameters listed under "Defining Characteristics."
2. Elevate extremity above heart level *to promote venous and lymphatic drainage, thereby reducing interstitial swelling.*
3. Apply ice over or beside area of injury or manipulation for the first 24 hours. Follow a schedule of ice on 20 minutes, off 20 minutes, repeat. *This optimizes the therapeutic effect of ice in prevention and/or reducing swelling.*
4. Maintain patency of wound drainage device *to prevent excessive interstitial swelling or blood accumulation.*
5. Assess dressings for fit and loosen if constrictive to superficial blood vessels.

## Activity Intolerance

**Definition:** *The state in which an individual has insufficient physiologic energy to endure or complete desired or required daily activities.*

### *Activity Intolerance Related to Postural Hypotension Secondary to Prolonged Immobility, Narcotics, Vasodilator Therapy*

#### DEFINING CHARACTERISTICS

- SBP drop >20, heart rate increase >20 on postural change
- Vertigo on postural change
- Syncope on postural change

#### OUTCOME CRITERIA

- SBP drop is <10, heart rate increase is <10 on postural change.
- Vertigo or syncope is absent on postural change.

#### NURSING INTERVENTIONS *AND RATIONALE*

1. Continue to monitor the assessment parameters listed under "Defining Characteristics."
2. *To increase muscular and vascular tone,* instruct and assist in the following bed exercises: straight leg raises, dorsiflexion/plantar flexion, and quadriceps setting and gluteal setting exercises.
3. Determine that the patient is hydrated to 24-hour fluid requirements per BSA *to increase preload and thus stroke volume and cardiac output.* Hydrate accordingly if not contraindicated by cardiac or renal disorders.
4. Assist with postural changes accomplished in increments:
   - Head of bed to 45 degrees and hold until patient is symptom free
   - Head of bed to 90 degrees and hold until patient is symptom free
   - Dangle until patient is symptom free
   - Stand until patient is symptom free and then ambulate patient
5. As soon as it is medically safe, assist patient to sit at bedside for meals.
6. When treating pain with narcotic analgesics, plan ambulation to occur well before peak action of the drug.

### *Activity Intolerance Related to Knowledge Deficit of Energy-Saving Techniques*

#### DEFINING CHARACTERISTICS

- Dyspnea on exertion
- Subjective fatigue on activity
- Heart rate elevations 30 beats above baseline on activity; heart rate 15 beats above baseline on activity for patients on beta blockers or calcium channel blockers

#### OUTCOME CRITERIA

- The patient has subjective tolerance of activity.
- Heart rate elevations are <20 beats above baseline on activity and are <10 beats above baseline on activity for patients on beta blockers or calcium channel blockers.

#### NURSING INTERVENTIONS *AND RATIONALE*

1. Continue to monitor the assessment parameters listed under "Defining Characteristics."
2. Teach and supervise energy-saving techniques based on the principle of performing work on exhalation, that is, standing up from a bed or chair, repositioning self in bed with or without help, reaching, washing face, brushing hair or teeth. *Inhalation is an active exercise requiring energy expenditure and oxygen consumption, whereas exhalation is passive. Performing work on exhalation increases the availability of energy for activity.*
3. To the extent possible, have the patient perform work while seated.
4. Teach and supervise muscle-toning exercises, *observing that a toned muscle uses less oxygen,* such as arm bends with elbows down, elbow bends with arms up, straight arm raises inward and outward, plantar flexion and dorsiflexion of the feet, straight leg raises.

## Activity Intolerance—cont'd

### *Activity Intolerance Related to Decreased Cardiac Output and/or Myocardial Tissue Perfusion Alterations*

#### DEFINING CHARACTERISTICS

- Heart rate elevations 30 beats above baseline on activity; heart rate elevations 15 beats above baseline upon activity for patients on beta blockers or calium channel blockers
- Heart rate elevations above baseline 5 minutes after activity
- Ischemic pain on activity
- Electrocardiographic changes on activity
- Subjective fatigue on activity

#### OUTCOME CRITERIA

- Heart rate elevations are <20 beats above baseline on activity and are <10 beats above baseline on activity for patients on beta blockers or calcium channel blockers.
- Heart rate returns to baseline 5 minutes after activity.
- Ischemic pain is absent on activity.
- The patient has subjective tolerance to activity.

#### NURSING INTERVENTIONS *AND RATIONALE*

1. Continue to monitor the assessment parameters listed under "Defining Characteristics."
2. Encourage active or passive range-of-motion exercises while the patient is in bed *to keep joints flexible and muscles stretched.* Teach patient to refrain from holding breath while performing exercises, *avoiding Valsalva maneuver.*
3. Encourage performance of muscle-toning exercises at least 3 times daily, *because a toned muscle uses less oxygen when performing work than an untoned muscle.*
4. Supervise progressive ambulation.
5. Teach patient pulse taking *to determine activity tolerance:* Take pulse for full minute before exercise, then for 10 seconds and multiply by 6 at exercise peak.

## High Risk for Infection

**Definition:** *The state in which the individual is at increased risk for being invaded by pathogenic organisms.*

### *High Risk for Infection*

#### RISK FACTOR

- Invasive monitoring devices

#### DEFINING CHARACTERISTICS OF AN ACTUAL PROBLEM

- Fever of undetermined origin
- Tachycardia
- Elevated white blood cells
- Reddened, inflamed catheter insertion sites
- Drainage from catheter insertion sites

#### OUTCOME CRITERIA

- Patient is afebrile.
- HR is within range of baseline.
- Catheter insertion sites are clear and dry.

#### NURSING INTERVENTIONS *AND RATIONALE*

NOTE: *The rationale for each of the following interventions is the avoidance of contamination and colonization of invasive lines and is based on national standards and supported with research.*

1. Continue to monitor the assessment parameters listed under "Defining Characteristics."
2. Practice handwashing consisting of 15 seconds using mechanical friction and soap and water before drawing blood or any line manipulation in which the closed system is interrupted.
3. Secure catheters to prevent piston movement (in and out).
4. Maintain an occlusive, sterile dressing. Gauze dressings over arterial lines are recommended.
5. Eliminate all nonessential stopcocks. When stopcocks are necessary, they should have as few ports as possible. Stopcocks should be replaced every 24 hours or when soiled, and they should be covered at all times.
6. A new anatomic site should be selected for each catheter inserted.
7. To the extent possible, limit blood drawing by obtaining all specimens at the same time.
8. Use uniform, prepackaged, sterile transducer/pressure monitoring and flush assembly.
9. Maintain a strict protocol for skin preparation. Clean the skin with iodofor after degreasing and defatting with acetone. Wear gloves, mask, and cap and use sterile drapes. A sterile gown should be worn when inserting central lines.
10. Use sterile normal saline as the flush solution.
11. Before obtaining a sample of blood, the stopcock port must be cleansed thoroughly with 70% alcohol with a sterile towel placed under the port being entered.
12. Transparent, occlusive dressing should be changed every 72 hours or when integrity is disrupted. Gauze dressings should be changed every 48 hours or sooner if soiled, saturated, or disrupted.
13. Catheters inserted in an emergency, without proper asepsis, should be removed and, if necessary, replaced under aseptic conditions.
14. At any sign of infection (localized pain, inflammation, sepsis, fever of undetermined origin), catheters should be removed and cultured.

# Nursing Management of Pulmonary Alterations

## Ineffective Airway Clearance

**Definition:** *The state in which an individual is unable to clear obstructions or secretions from the respiratory tract to maintain airway patency.*

### *Ineffective Airway Clearance Related to Excessive Secretions*

#### DEFINING CHARACTERISTICS

- Congested lung fields, audible mucus in airways
- Arterial partial pressure of oxygen ($PaO_2$) <predicted for age and a given fraction of inspired oxygen concentration ($FIO_2$)
- $PaCO_2$ >45 mm Hg

#### OUTCOME CRITERIA

- Cough produces thin mucus.
- Lungs are clear to auscultation.
- $PaO_2$ is equal to predicted for age.
- $PaCO_2$ of 35 to 45 mm Hg indicates adequate depth and rate of ventilation.

#### NURSING INTERVENTIONS *AND RATIONALE*

1. Continue to monitor the assessment parameters listed under "Defining Characteristics."
2. In the absence of cardiac or renal dysfunction, hydrate the 24-hour fluid requirements per body surface area (BSA) *to thin secretions. Adequate hydration is the most effective mucolytic.* Avoid caffeinated beverages, *because caffeine is a mild diuretic and can contribute to fluid loss.*
3. Monitor serum osmolality, *considering that an elevation may indicate need for further hydration.*
4. Provide humidification to airways through mask, room vaporizer, or other means *to assist in thinning secretions.* When artificial airway is present, ensure that humidification to airway is available and functioning properly. *Thick, tenacious secretions may mean insufficient fluid intake and/or insufficient external humidification.*
5. Instruct and supervise controlled cough technique. If controlled cough technique is not possible, consider huff coughing or quad coughing techniques.

*Controlled Cough Technique:*

a. Maximal inhalation—an effective cough is contingent on filling the lungs and airways distal to the mucus *so that the succeeding forced exhalation will propel the mucus up to the airways. Maximal inhalation also increases airway caliber; as a result, it is more likely that the air will pass distal to partially obstructing mucus or foreign matter.*
b. Hold breath 2 seconds—*this step permits the patient to prepare for exhalation and allows distribution of the inhaled air to the lung's periphery.*
c. Cough twice—*the first cough will loosen mucus, the second will propel the mucus. Further coughing may use excessive oxygen and energy at a time when the lung volume has already been expelled with the first two coughs, and the effort is thus wasted.*
d. Pause—just long enough to regain control.
e. Inhale by sniffing—sniffing is recommended, because *a deep inhalation through the mouth may drive loose mucus back down into the airways.*
f. Rest.

*Huff coughing:*

Huff coughing is a series of coughs produced with the glottis held open while saying the word, "huff." The sharp sound of a cough should not be produced with a huff cough, but the sound should be that of forced exhalation. Huff coughing may be helpful for COPD patients who have significant airway collapse on forced exhalation, because *huff coughing is associated with higher flow rates in these patients than in the normal closed-glottis approach to coughing. Furthermore, huff coughing may assist in moving secretions from the smaller airways into the main-stem bronchi or trachea where the controlled cough technique can be used for effective expectoration.*

## Ineffective Airway Clearance—cont'd

*Quad coughing:*

*Quad coughing is helpful in patients who have flaccid or weakened abdominal musculature. The most obvious example is the patient with paralysis or weakness caused by neuromuscular disorders.* Quad coughing calls for the nurse to push upward and inward on the abdomen, toward the diaphragm, while the patient exhales.

a. Position for optimal coughing by placing patient either in high-Fowler's position with knees drawn up and a brace for his or her feet or on side with knees drawn up. *High-Fowler's position promotes best diaphragmatic descent and maximal inhalation, which allow maximal cough. Drawn-up knees assist in abdominal muscle contraction, resulting in a stronger expulsive force and cough velocity.*
b. Assess sputum for color, consistency, and amount. *Yellow or green may mean chest infection; an increase in amount may mean a worsening condition.*
c. Assess for signs or symptoms of chest infection such as fever, tachycardia, yellow or green mucus (culture and sensitivity may be necessary), leukocytosis, increase in pulmonary crackles or wheezes on chest auscultation, and chest radiograph consistent with alveolar infiltrates.
d. If patient is hypoxemic, administer oxygen, observing the following principles:
   - Without physician's collaboration, liter flow should be no greater than 2 L/min in patients whose pulmonary history is unknown or reveals a pattern of chronic carbon dioxide retention, *because a high $FIO_2$ level in these patients may depress ventilatory drive.*
   - Oxygen should be administered with the goal of achieving a $PaO_2$ level no greater than 100 mm Hg. *A higher $PaO_2$ level is of little value and may necessitate using an $FIO_2$ higher than 40%, which can precipitate oxygen toxicity (see the section in Chapter 12, "Oxygen Toxicity").*
   - With physician's collaboration, consider the application of mechanical ventilation with positive end-expiratory pressure (PEEP) in patients whose hypoxemia is refractory to high concentrations of oxygen through mask or nasal prongs.

6. Reposition frequently (at least q2 hr) and dynamically *to mobilize secretions and to match ventilation with perfusion.*
7. With physician's collaboration, teach and supervise bronchial drainage with or without chest physiotherapy *to assist with the expulsion of retained secretions.*
8. Consider suctioning nasopharyngeal airway or artificial tracheal airway when secretions are audible.
9. Allow rest periods between coughing sessions, chest physiotherapy, or other demanding activities.
10. Consider breathing exercise sessions that incorporate sustained maximal inhalation of at least 10 per hour with or without the use of an incentive spirometer *to prevent atelectasis.*

## Ineffective Airway Clearance—cont'd

### *Ineffective Airway Clearance Related to Impaired Cough Secondary to Loss of Glottic Closure With Cuffed Endotracheal or Tracheostomy Tube*

#### DEFINING CHARACTERISTICS

- Lung fields congested on auscultation
- Weak, ineffectual cough

#### OUTCOME CRITERIA

- Cough is productive of thin mucus.
- Lung auscultation reveals mobilization of secretions with cough.

#### NURSING INTERVENTIONS *AND RATIONALE*

NOTE: *The ability to take a deep breath, close the glottis, and forcefully contract abdominal muscles is essential to an effective cough and subsequent airway clearance. An impairment in any of these abilities results in an ineffective airway clearance.*

1. Continue to monitor the assessment parameters listed under "Defining Characteristics."
2. Ensure that the inspired air source (at **any** $FIO_2$) is humidified, because *the artificial airway bypasses the body's normal humidification system.*
3. In the absence of cardiac or renal disease, hydrate to 24-hour fluid requirements per BSA *to thin secretions.*
4. In patients with reduced vital capacity resulting from weak abdominal and/or diaphragmatic musculature, teach and supervise abdominal muscle-tightening exercises and diaphragmatic breathing.
5. Position for optimal coughing by placing patient either in high-Fowler's position with knees drawn up or on side with knees drawn up. *High-Fowler's position promotes best diaphragmatic descent and maximal inhalation, which allow maximal cough. Drawn-up knees assist in abdominal muscle contraction, resulting in a stronger expulsive force and cough velocity.*
6. Practice coughing, simulating glottis effect:
   - Have patient take deep breath.
   - Place gloved finger over end of airway tube.
   - Have patient contract abdominal muscles.
   - Immediately remove finger.
7. Suction artificial airway as necessary per unit standards. Consider airway lavage, instilling 2 to 4 ml sterile sodium chloride solution during inhalation.
8. Suction oropharyngeally and obtain frequent cuff pressure measurements *to prevent aspiration of oropharyngeal secretions* (see the nursing management of High Risk for Aspiration on p. 476).

### *Ineffective Airway Clearance Related to Knowledge Deficit of Controlled Cough and Hydration Techniques*

#### DEFINING CHARACTERISTICS

- Frequent hospitalizations for exacerbations of underlying chronic lung disease
- Weak, ineffectual cough
- Congested lung fields on auscultation
- Thick, tenacious mucus

#### OUTCOME CRITERIA

- Lung auscultation reveals mobilization of secretions with cough.
- Patient demonstrates correct controlled cough technique.
- Cough is productive of thin mucus.

#### NURSING INTERVENTIONS *AND RATIONALE*

1. Continue to monitor the assessment parameters listed under "Defining Characteristics."
2. Have patient demonstrate usual technique of airway clearance *to ascertain method of coughing and to point out to the patient why his or her cough is ineffective.*
3. Teach controlled cough technique. Refer to the nursing management of Ineffective Airway Clearance related to excessive secretions on p. 466.
4. In the absence of cardiac or renal dysfunction, teach patient to increase fluid intake to at least his 24-hour fluid requirements per BSA *to keep secretions thin and easily expectorated.* Beverages should be decaffeinated and nonalcoholic.

## Ineffective Airway Clearance—cont'd

### *Ineffective Airway Clearance Related to Respiratory Muscle Dysfunction and Impaired Cough Secondary to Quadriplegia, Paraplegia, Guillain-Barré Syndrome, Myasthenia Gravis, and Others*

#### DEFINING CHARACTERISTICS

- Weak, ineffectual cough
- Lung fields congested to auscultation
- Observed weakness of respiratory muscle groups

#### OUTCOME CRITERIA

- Cough is productive.
- Secretions are thin and clear.

#### NURSING INTERVENTIONS *AND RATIONALE*

1. Continue to monitor the assessment parameters listed under "Defining Characteristics."
2. If hypoxemic, administer oxygen, observing principles detailed under "Ineffective Airway Clearance related to excessive secretions."
3. In the absence of cardiac or renal dysfunction, teach and provide hydration to 24-hour fluid requirements per BSA *to thin secretions and facilitate airway clearance.*
4. Assist with quad coughing, since *weakened or flaccid abdominal muscles will prevent effective cough.* Refer to the nursing management of Ineffective Airway Clearance related to excessive secretions on p. 466.
5. Position patient for most effective cough.
6. Consider chest physiotherapy (bronchial drainage and chest percussion) three to four times per day *to assist with the expulsion of retained secretions.*
7. Change position at least q2 hr *to prevent stasis of secretions and to match ventilation with perfusion.*

### *Ineffective Airway Clearance Related to Abdominal or Thoracic Pain*

#### DEFINING CHARACTERISTICS

- Congested lung fields, audible mucus in airways
- Weak, ineffectual cough

#### OUTCOME CRITERIA

- Lungs are clear to auscultation.
- Cough produces thin mucus.

#### NURSING INTERVENTIONS *AND RATIONALE*

1. Continue to monitor the assessment parameters listed under "Defining Characteristics."
2. Treat pain according to its etiology. Refer to the nursing management of Acute Pain on p. 485.
3. If hypoxemic, administer oxygen, observing principles detailed under "Ineffective Airway Clearance related to excessive secretions."
4. In the absence of cardiac or renal dysfunction, hydrate to 24-hour fluid requirements per BSA *to thin secretions and improve airway clearance.*
5. Emphasize diaphragmatic breathing in the patient with chest wall pain/incision and chest breathing in the patient with abdominal pain/incision. *This reduces tension on affected part and minimizes pain.*
6. Emphasize deep breathing exercises with sustained maximal inhalation. *They will stimulate an effective cough if, in fact, secretions are present in the airways. In addition, a more effective cough will be achieved because the high volumes of deep breathing will result in an increased velocity of expired air.*
7. Teach and provide incisional splinting, if appropriate, during breathing exercises in anticipation of cough stimulation and during coughing episodes.

## Ineffective Breathing Pattern

**Definition:** *The state in which an individual's inhalation and/or exhalation pattern does not enable adequate pulmonary inflation or emptying.*

### *Ineffective Breathing Pattern Related to Chronic Airflow Limitations*

#### DEFINING CHARACTERISTICS

- Use of accessory muscles of ventilation
- Reported and/or observed episodes of respiratory panic
- Chest breathing

#### OUTCOME CRITERIA

- Patient demonstrates pursed-lip and diaphragmatic breathing regularly and during episodes of respiratory panic.

#### NURSING INTERVENTIONS *AND RATIONALE*

1. Continue to monitor the assessment parameters listed under "Defining Characteristics."
2. Teach and supervise pursed-lip breathing. *Explain that this maneuver keeps airways open longer during exhalation and evacuates trapped air.* The procedure for pursed-lip breathing should be used along with diaphragmatic breathing during episodes of shortness of breath.
3. Teach and supervise diaphragmatic breathing. *Explain that this maneuver saves energy (the diaphragm uses oxygen more efficiently than the accessory muscles) and retrains the diaphragm to assume its normal percentage of the work of breathing.* Diaphragmatic breathing is useful in terminating episodes of acute shortness of breath but should *also* be incorporated into an hourly routine of muscle retraining.
4. During episodes of acute shortness of breath or respiratory panic, it is useful for the nurse to actually *breathe with* the patient, using pursed-lip and diaphragmatic breathing techniques. It is *not* useful during such an episode to instruct or encourage the use of these techniques. Statements such as, "Now slow down your breathing" or "Take nice big breaths for me," *do little to assist the patient in regaining control of his or her breathing pattern. In addition, concentration on techniques of breathing may serve the very beneficial function of distracting the patient from fear and panic.*

### *Ineffective Breathing Pattern Related to Modifiable Chest Wall Restrictions Secondary to Pneumothorax or Pleural Effusion*

#### DEFINING CHARACTERISTICS

- Shallow tachypnea
- Atelectatic crackles
- Diminished breath sounds
- Asymmetrical chest expansion

#### OUTCOME CRITERIA

- Respiratory rate at rest is $<20$.
- Atelectatic crackles are minimal or absent.
- Breath sounds are full and equal bilaterally.
- Chest expands symmetrically.

#### NURSING INTERVENTIONS *AND RATIONALE*

1. Continue to monitor the assessment parameters listed under "Defining Characteristics." In addition, check serial chest radiographs *to monitor resolution of underlying disorder.*
2. Treat pain, if present, according to cause. See the nursing management of Acute Pain, p. 485.
3. If the patient is hypoxemic, administer oxygen, observing the principles detailed under "Ineffective Breathing Pattern related to abdominal or thoracic pain."
4. Teach and supervise deep breathing with sustained maximal inspiration. *In the patient with a pneumothorax and a chest tube, this maneuver reexpands the lung and evacuates air (and fluid) from the pleural space into the chest drainage system. In the patient with a pleural effusion, this maneuver may reexpand atelectatic portions of the lung overlying the pleural effusion.*
5. Reposition the patient q2 hr, observing the "good lung down" principle *to limit pain, as well as to better match ventilation with perfusion* (refer to the nursing management of Impaired Gas Exchange related to ventilation-perfusion inequality, p. 474). Favor a head-of-bed up position *to facilitate diaphragmatic descent.*
6. Avoid coughing exercises unless there are audible secretions in the airways. *Coughing is painful and, if performed unnecessarily (as in the absence of secretions), may promote airway collapse or atelectasis.*
7. For assessment and maintenance of chest tubes and closed chest drainage systems, see Chapter 12.

## Ineffective Breathing Pattern—cont'd

### *Ineffective Breathing Pattern Related to Respiratory Muscle Deconditioning Secondary to Mechanical Ventilation*

#### DEFINING CHARACTERISTICS

- Hypercapnia
- Atelectatic crackles
- Use of accessory ventilatory muscles
- Anxious behaviors
- During spontaneous breaths, tidal volume less than predicted, diminished basilar breath sounds, decreased chest excursion, and tachypnea

#### OUTCOME CRITERIA

- Tidal volume is greater than or equal to that predicted.
- Breath sounds are clear from apices to bases.
- Normocapnia.

#### NURSING INTERVENTIONS *AND RATIONALE*

Continue to monitor the assessment parameters listed under "Defining Characteristics."

1. Assist the patient to distinguish spontaneous breaths from mechanically delivered breaths by helping him or her to identify the sensation of breathing *(this is lost when air bypasses the nasooropharynx)* through simple kinesthetic feedback: "The machine is giving you six breaths per minute; you are breathing on your own in between the machine breaths. Feel the difference between the machine's breaths and your own. You are working to make your own breaths as deep and full as the machine's."
2. Carefully snip excess length from the proximal end of the endotracheal tube *to decrease dead space and thereby decrease the work of breathing. Similarly, ensure that ventilator circuit tubings impose no excess dead space.*
3. Collaborate with physician about the application of pressure support to the mechanical ventilator or about the use of a ventilator which will not increase the work of breathing during the IMV or SIMV breaths. *There should be no excessive work of breathing on the part of the patient because of ventilator circuitry. Pressure support may decrease the work of breathing.*
4. Position patient in semi-Fowler's position *for best use of ventilatory muscles and to facilitate diaphragmatic descent.*
5. Confront patient's fear and support his or her confidence; provide progress reports frequently: "The volume of your breaths is steadily increasing and this has made your lungs clearer. Your hard work is paying off."
6. Avoid pharmacological sedation if possible. Consult with physician in selecting a sedative drug with minimal muscle relaxant effects.
7. With physician's collaboration, ensure that at least 50% of the diet's nonprotein caloric source is in the form of lipid (fat) vs. carbohydrates to prevent excess carbon dioxide accumulation. *Carbon dioxide is an end product of carbohydrate metabolism, and its excess accumulation in the bloodstream falsely suggests a reduction in the patient's alveolar ventilation. In addition, excess carbon dioxide increases the patient's ventilatory workload.*

## Ineffective Breathing Pattern—cont'd

### *Ineffective Breathing Pattern Related to Abdominal or Thoracic Pain*

#### DEFINING CHARACTERISTICS

- Atelectatic crackles
- Asymmetrical chest expansion caused by splinting
- Hypocapnia
- Diminished basiliar breath sounds, shallow breathing
- Presence of pain

#### OUTCOME CRITERIA

- Breath sounds are clear and equal bilaterally.
- Chest expands symmetrically.
- $Paco_2$ is 35 to 45 mm Hg.

#### NURSING INTERVENTIONS *AND RATIONALE*

1. Continue to monitor the assessment parameters listed under "Defining Characteristics."
2. Treat pain according to its cause. Refer to the nursing management of Acute Pain, p. 485.
3. If patient is hypoxemic, administer oxygen, observing the following principles:
   - Without physician's collaboration, liter flow should be no greater than 2 L/min in patients whose pulmonary history is unknown or reveals a pattern of chronic carbon dioxide retention because *a high $FIO_2$ in these patients may depress ventilatory drive.*
   - Oxygen should be administered with the goal of achieving a $PaO_2$ no greater than 95 mm Hg.
   - Observe caution when administering oxygen at $FIO_2$ greater than 40% *in view of the higher risk for oxygen toxicity.* With physician's collaboration, consider the application of mechanical ventilation with PEEP in patients whose hypoxemia is refractory to high concentrations of oxygen.

**The following interventions are appropriate for patients with thoracic pain**

1. Carefully distinguish between chest wall pain and the pain of myocardial ischemia. For example, ask the patient if this pain is his or her "usual" chest wall or incisional pain, palpate the chest wall to elicit the pain, and have the patient take a deep breath to elicit the pain. *These maneuvers will reasonable confirm the existence of chest wall or incisional pain vs. the pain of myocardial ischemia. If any doubt exists, a 12-lead electrocardiogram (ECG) should be obtained.*
2. Teach and supervise deep breathing or incentive spirometry with sustained maximal inhalation. The emphasis with these modalities should be on the diaphragmatic breathing technique *to increase abdominal expansion and decrease chest wall expansion, thereby decreasing pain.*
3. Reposition patient at least q2 hr, observing the "good lung down" principle (refer to the nursing management of Impaired Gas Exchange related to ventilation-perfusion inequality, p. 474). *This will result in decreased incidence of pain and better matching of ventilation with perfusion.*
4. Treat impaired coughing. See "Ineffective Airway Clearance related to abdominal and thoracic pain," p. 469.

**The following interventions are appropriate for patients with abdominal pain**

1. Teach and supervise deep breathing or incentive spirometry with sustained maximal inspiration. *The emphasis for these maneuvers should not be diaphragmatic breathing but chest breathing to decrease the incidence of abdominal pain.*
2. Reposition patient frequently and dynamically. Favor semi-Fowler's to high-Fowler's position *to maximize chest expansion.*

## Ineffective Breathing Pattern—cont'd

### *Ineffective Breathing Pattern Related to Unmodifiable Chest Wall Restrictions Secondary to Kyphoscoliosis or Obesity*

#### DEFINING CHARACTERISTICS

- Activity intolerance (that is, heart rate elevations 30 beats above baseline with activity [15 beats above baseline for patients on beta or calcium channel blockers]; heart rate elevations above baseline 5 minutes after activity; dyspnea)
- Shallow tachypnea

#### OUTCOME CRITERIA

- Patient has subjective and objective activity tolerance.

#### NURSING INTERVENTIONS *AND RATIONALE*

1. Continue to monitor the assessment parameters listed under "Defining Characteristics."
2. Prevent unnecessary exertion because *the patient's ventilatory reserve is limited.* Grade all activity to within the patient's tolerance as measured by heart rate elevations less than 30 beats above baseline with activity. Heart rate elevations less than 15 beats above baseline with activity indicates activity tolerance in patients receiving beta or calcium channel blockers.
3. If patient is hypoxemic, administer oxygen, observing the principles detailed under "Ineffective Breathing Pattern related to abdominal or thoracic pain." Ensure that oxygen is administered, especially during activity.
4. Teach and supervise energy-saving techniques (refer to the nursing management of Activity Intolerance related to knowledge deficit of energy-saving techniques on p. 463).
5. Teach and supervise diaphragmatic breathing. *Diaphragmatic breathing is especially effective in patients with unmodifiable chest wall restrictions because it allows an increase in the tidal volume through diaphragmatic descent, which is otherwise impossible through chest wall expansion.* Incorporate the sustained maximal inspiration maneuver when possible.
6. Reposition patient dynamically q2 hr, favoring semi-Fowler's to high-Fowler's position *to facilitate diaphragmatic descent.*
7. Ideally, position the patient sitting at the bedside with arms resting on a pillow on the overbed table. *This position eliminates splinting of the chest wall against any surface and thereby decreases chest wall restriction and work of breathing.*

## Impaired Gas Exchange

**Definition:** *The state in which an individual experiences a decreased passage of oxygen and/or carbon dioxide between the alveoli of the lungs and the vascular system.*

### *Impaired Gas Exchange Related to Ventilation-Perfusion Inequality Secondary to (Specify)*

#### DEFINING CHARACTERISTICS

**Definitive**

- $Pa_{O_2}$ <predicted for age
- $Pa_{CO_2}$ >45 mm Hg (hypercapnia)

**Presumptive**

- Confusion
- Somnolence
- Restlessness
- Irritability
- Inability to move secretions

#### OUTCOME CRITERIA

- $Pa_{O_2}$ is equal to predicted for age.
- $Pa_{CO_2}$ is 35 to 45 mm Hg or back to baseline for patient.
- Airways are clear of mucus.

#### NURSING INTERVENTIONS *AND RATIONALE*

1. Continue to monitor the assessment parameters listed under "Defining Characteristics." In addition, observe for physical signs and symptoms of tissue hypoxia (increased respiratory rate, visual disturbances, impairment of intellectual function, headache, lethargy, tachycardia, dysrhythmias) and hypercapnia (headache [usually occipital], asterixis, lethargy, confusion).
2. Administer oxygen, observing the following principles:
   - Without physician's collaboration, liter flow should be no greater than 2 L/min in patients whose pulmonary history is unknown or reveals a pattern of chronic carbon dioxide retention, because *a high $FI_{O_2}$ level in these patients may depress ventilatory drive.*
   - Oxygen should be administered with the goal of achieving a $Pa_{O_2}$ level no greater than 100 mm Hg. *A higher $Pa_{O_2}$ level is of little value and may necessitate an $FI_{O_2}$ level higher than 40% which can precipitate oxygen toxicity (see "Oxygen Toxicity" in Chapter 12).*
   - With physician's collaboration, consider the application of CPAP or mechanical ventilation with PEEP in patients whose hypoxemia is refractory to high concentrations of oxygen. *CPAP and PEEP accomplish alveolar hyperinflation, thereby increasing the surface area for gas exchange.*
3. In the absence of cardiac or renal dysfunction, hydrate to 24-hour fluid requirements per body surface area (BSA) *to thin secretions. Adequate hydration is the most effective mucolytic.* Avoid caffeinated beverages *because caffeine is a mild diuretic and can contribute to fluid loss.*
4. Monitor serum osmolality, *considering that an elevation may indicate need for further hydration.*
5. Provide humidification to airways through mask, room vaporizor, or other means *to assist in thinning secretions.* When artifical airway is present, ensure that humidification of airway is available and functioning properly. *Thick, tenacious secretions may indicate insufficient fluid intake and/or a need for external humidification.*
6. Consider suctioning if mucus is suspected within the trachea. If mucus is suspected within the main-stem or segmental bronchi, assist in its passage into the trachea through cough or chest physiotherapy. *Most studies have shown suctioning is effective only in evacuating mucus from the tracheal level; therefore every effort should be made to move mucus into the trachea before suctioning is attempted.* Always preoxygenate and postoxygenate the patient's airways as part of the suctioning technique *to prevent further decrease of the $Pa_{O_2}$ level as a result of suctioning.*
7. For a patient with unilateral lung disease, position him or her with the good lung down because *this will best match ventilation with perfusion and result in improved $Pa_{O_2}$.** (Exception: Place sick lung down in cases of lung abcess or unilateral interstitial pulmonary emphysema.)
8. For patient with bilateral lung disease, position with right lung down because *this lung is larger than the left lung and affords a greater area for ventilation and perfusion. Further, the cardiac output may be enhanced in the right lateral position.*
9. Evaluate arterial blood gas values obtained with the patient in various positions so that the position that results in the best oxygenation may be revealed.
10. Change the patient's position at least q2 hr, favoring those positions that allow the best oxygenation. Limit the time the patient spends in a position that compromises oxygenation. Avoid any position that seriously decreases the $Pa_{O_2}$.
11. When appropriate, instruct patient in controlled cough technique or huff or quad cough techniques, depending on the patient's cough ability.
12. Obtain order for incentive spirometry and instruct in its proper use *as a means to prevent atelectasis, which can further complicate or worsen impaired gas exchange.*
13. Evaluate need for chest physiotherapy.

*Blood flow (perfusion) in the lungs is gravity dependent. With the patient in the upright position, perfusion is greatest in the lung bases; in the left side-lying position, perfusion is greatest in the periphery of the left lung, and so forth. By positioning the patient with his or her "good lung down," one is redirecting the greatest amount of perfusion to that lung with the greatest amount of ventilation, thereby improving ventilation-perfusion ratios. Conversely, by positioning the patient with his or her "bad lung down," one is *wasting* perfusion on an underventilated lung.

## Impaired Gas Exchange—cont'd

### *Impaired Gas Exchange Related to Alveolar Hypoventilation Secondary to ______ (Specify)*

#### DEFINING CHARACTERISTICS

- $PaO_2$ <predicted for age
- Hypercapnia

#### OUTCOME CRITERIA

- $PaO_2$ is within limits of norm for age.
- $PaCO_2$ is 35 to 45 mm Hg.

#### NURSING INTERVENTIONS *AND RATIONALE*

1. Continue to monitor the assessment parameters listed under "Defining Characteristics." In addition, observe for physical signs and symptoms of tissue hypoxia (increased respiratory rate, visual disturbances, impairment of intellectual function, headache, lethargy, tachycardia, dysrhythmias) and hypercapnia (headache [usually occipital], asterixis, lethargy, confusion).
2. Administer oxygen, observing the principle detailed under "Impaired Gas Exchange related to ventilation-perfusion inequality."
3. Intervene deliberately to resolve the specific cause of the alveolar hypoventilation.

## High Risk for Aspiration

**Definition:** *The state in which an individual is at risk for entry of gastrointestinal secretions, oropharyngeal secretions, or solids or fluids into tracheobronchial passages.*

### *High Risk for Aspiration*

#### RISK FACTORS

- Reduced level of consciousness
- Depressed cough and gag reflexes
- Presence of tracheostomy or endotracheal tube
- Incomplete lower esophageal sphincter
- Gastrointestinal tubes
- Tube feedings
- Medication administration
- Situations hindering elevation of upper body
- Increased intragastric pressure
- Increased gastric residual
- Decreased gastrointestinal motility
- Delayed gastric emptying
- Impaired swallowing
- Facial/oral/neck surgery or trauma
- Wired jaws

#### DEFINING CHARACTERISTICS OF AN ACTUAL PROBLEM

**Early**
- Hypoxemia

**Later** (6 hours after aspiration)
- Dyspnea
- Wheezing, crackles
- Cough with pink, frothy fluid, resembling cardiogenic pulmonary edema
- Fever
- Tachycardia
- Hypotension
- Radiologic: patchy alveolar infiltrates in portions of lung dependent at time of aspiration
- Evidence of gastric contents in lùng secretions

#### OUTCOME CRITERIA

- Lungs are clear to auscultation.
- $Pao_2$ is proportional to that predicted for age and $Fio_2$.
- Lung secretions show no evidence of gastric contents.
- Patient is afebrile.

#### NURSING INTERVENTIONS *AND RATIONALE*

1. Continue to monitor the assessment parameters listed under "Defining Characteristics."
2. Auscultate bowel sounds and assess abdominal contour and girth. *Rule out hypoactive peristalsis and abdominal distention with gastric contents, thereby avoiding the heightened risk of esophageal reflux.*
3. Position patient with 30-degree head of bed elevation (lying on side, ideally) *to prevent gastric reflux through gravity*. Whenever head elevation is contraindicated, a right lateral decubitus position is recommended because *it facilitates passage of gastric contents across the pylorus.*
4. Suction and clear oropharyngeal secretions. For patients with cuffed tracheostomy or endotracheal tubes, suction oropharyngeally and obtain cuff pressure measurements *to limit aspiration of oropharyngeal secretions.*
5. Maintain patency and functioning of nasogastric suction apparatus.
6. Treat nausea promptly; consider obtaining physician's order for antiemetic *to prevent vomiting and resultant aspiration.*
7. With physician's collaboration, consider administration of oral antacids and $H_2$ receptor antagonists *to increase gastric pH and thereby limit chemical burn to lung tissue should aspiration occur.*

**The following interventions are also appropriate for patients receiving continuous or intermittent enteral tube feedings:**

1. Position patient with 45-degree head elevation at all times *to prevent gastric reflux across an epiglottis held open by the gastric tube.* If a head-down position becomes necessary at any time, interrupt the feeding 30 minutes to 1 hour before position change.
2. Check placement of feeding tube either by ausculation or radiographically at regular intervals (for example, before administering intermittent feedings, after position changes, and after suctioning, coughing episodes, or vomiting). *The feeding tube can migrate without demonstrating a change in its external position.*
3. Instill blue food coloring to feeding solutions *to assist identification of gastric contents in pulmonary secretions. Green, red, or yellow food dye is unacceptable because each resembles other body substances.*
4. If possible, aspirate enteral contents through feeding tube and measure residual amounts before intermittent feedings and at regular intervals during continuous feedings. Consider withholding intermittent feedings for residuals greater than 100 to 150 ml and interrupting continuous feedings for residual greater than 20% of the hourly rate.
5. With physician's collaboration, consider administering metoclopramide (Reglan) *to increase upper gastrointestinal motility and gastric sphincter tone and to decrease gastric volume.*

## High Risk for Aspiration—cont'd

**The following interventions are also appropriate for patients with impaired swallowing:**

1. Assess for classic indicators of impaired swallowing—drooling (especially persistence of drooling with head reclined), food retained in mouth, poor head and neck control, tongue pumping or excess mouth movement before swallowing, coughing during or after eating, breathy or "gurgly" voice, and slurred speech.
2. Initiate consult with in-house "swallowing team." This team may consist of a speech pathologist, occupational therapist, physical therapist, dietitian, and/or physical rehabilitation nursing and medical staff members. *Swallowing is not a reflex but a patterned response involving both voluntary and nonvoluntary components. It may, in some instances, be retrained after injury.*
3. Predict the patient's swallowing competence by assessing the symmetry and dynamics of tongue mobility. Have patient protrude his or her tongue and move it to the left and right. *The swallowing response consists of coordinated movements of the tongue, palate, pharynx, larynx, and esophagus. This response is initiated by the tongue; therefore competence in initiating the swallow may be partially predicted.*
4. Predict airway protection by asking the patient to cough and clear the throat. *A cough that is weak, "gurgly," or unobtainable indicates reduced airway closure, which is the reason for aspiration during the swallow.*
5. For the patient who is either being evaluated for swallowing difficulty or in whom swallowing is being reinitiated (for example, after tracheal extubation or prolonged NPO status), observe swallowing competence by placing 3 ml of water on the patient's tongue. The swallow should be initiated within 1 second of introducing water to the oral cavity. If response is delayed or no response occurs after three attempts, consider formal evaluation by "swallowing team" and initiate NPO status. *Water is hardest to swallow and easiet to aspirate; if swallowing is impaired sufficiently to result in pulmonary aspiration, the 3 ml of water is a safe medium with which to demostrate this impairment.*
6. When reasonable swallowing competence has been established, provide foods with the consistency of yogurt, ice cream, pudding, or custard. *Semisolids are more easily swallowed than either liquids or solids.*
7. Avoid introducing fluids into the patient's mouth with the use of a syringe. *This maneuver paritally bypasses the tongue, interfering with the swallowing response and therefore increasing the risk of aspiration.*

# Nursing Management of Neurological Alterations

## Altered Tissue Perfusion

**Definition:** *The state in which an individual experiences a decrease in nutrition and oxygenation at the cellular level due to a deficit in arterial capillary blood supply.*

### *Altered Cerebral Tissue Perfusion Related to Vasospasm Secondary to Subarachnoid Hemorrhage after Ruptured Intracranial Aneurysm or Arteriovenous Malformation*

NOTE: Vasospasm takes place in two phases. The acute phase occurs within minutes or hours of aneurysm rupture and serves as a protective mechanism by decreasing blood flow to the site and lessening the chance of rebleeding. Chronic vasospasm begins approximately 3 to 4 days after aneurysm rupture and persists for days to weeks. Early management of subarachnoid hemorrhage also includes aggressive treatment to prevent or combat vasospasm. Therefore this nursing management plan addresses the simultaneous management of subarachnoid hemorrhage and vasospasm.

#### DEFINING CHARACTERISTICS

**Subarachnoid hemorrhage**

- Aneurysm grading system according to Hunt and Hess
  - Grade I: minimal bleed
    - Asymptomatic or minimal headache
    - Slight nuchal rigidity
  - Grade II: mild bleed
    - Moderate-to-severe headache
    - Nuchal rigidity
    - Minimal neurological deficit (for example, possible cranial nerve palsies—oculomotor [cranial nerve III] most common; unilateral pupillary dilation, ptosis, and dysconjugate gaze)
  - Grade III: moderate bleed
    - Drowsiness
    - Confusion
    - Nuchal rigidity
    - Possible mild focal neurological deficits
  - Grade IV: moderate-to-severe bleed
    - Very decreased level of consciousness, stupor
    - Possible moderate-to-severe hemiparesis
    - Possible early posturing (decorticate or decerebrate)
  - Grade V: severe bleed
    - Profound coma
    - Posturing
    - Moribund appearance
- Pathological reflexes resulting from meningeal irritation:
  Kernig's sign: resistance to full extension of the leg at the knee when the hip is flexed
  Brudzinski's sign: flexion of the hip and knee during passive neck flexion
- Photophobia
- Nausea and vomiting

**Vasospasm related to subarachnoid hemorrhage**

- Worsening headache
- Confusion and decreasing level of consciousness
- Focal motor deficits such as unilateral weakness of extremities
- Speech deficits such as slurring, receptive or expressive aphasia
- Increasing BP

#### OUTCOME CRITERIA

- Patient is oriented to time, place, person, and situation.
- Pupils are equal and normoreactive.
- BP is within patient's norm.
- Motor function is bilaterally equal.

## Altered Tissue Perfusion—cont'd

- Headache, nausea, and vomiting are absent.
- Patient has no signs or symptoms of increased ICP and herniation as evidenced by ICP 0-15 mm Hg and by above criteria.
- Patient verbalizes importance of and displays compliance with reduced activity.

### NURSING INTERVENTIONS *AND RATIONALE*

1. Continue to monitor the assessment parameters listed under "Defining Characteristics." In addition, assess for indicators of increased ICP and brain herniation (see nursing management of Altered Cerebral Tissue Perfusion related to increased ICP). *ICP will increase during vasospasm only when caused by the edema resulting from brain infarction.*
2. Anticipate early surgical intervention for patients with grade I or II symptoms.
3. Maintain patent airway and adequate ventilation, and supply oxygen as ordered *to prevent hypoxemia and hypercarbia.*
4. Monitor ABG values and maintain $Pao_2$ >80 mm Hg and $Paco_2$ <45 mm Hg.
5. If hypertensive-hypervolemic therapy is prescribed, administer crystalloid and colloid IV fluids and monitor pulmonary capillary wedge pressure (PCWP), pulmonary artery diastolic pressure (PAD), systemic vascular resistance (SVR), and BP to achieve and maintain prescribed parameters. Systolic blood pressure is usually maintained at 150-160 mm Hg.
6. Monitor lung sounds and chest x-ray reports because *of the risk of pulmonary edema associated with fluid overload.*
7. Anticipate administration of calcium channel blockers such as nifedipine *to decrease peripheral vascular resistance and cause vasodilation.*
8. For patients in severe vasospasm, anticipate barbiturate administration *to decrease cerebral metabolic rate.*
9. Keep head of bed flat *to optimize cerebral perfusion.*
10. Rebleeding is a potential complication of aneurysm rupture; to PREVENT REBLEEDING, the following interventions constitute subarachnoid precautions:
    - Ensure bed rest in a quiet environment *to lessen external stimuli.*
    - Maintain darkened room *to lessen symptoms of photophobia.*
    - Restrict visitors and instruct them to keep conversation as nonstressful as possible.
    - Administer presribed sedatives as needed *to reduce anxiety and promote rest.*
    - Administer analgesics as prescribed *to relieve or lessen headache.*
    - Provide a soft, high-fiber diet and stool softeners *to prevent constipation, which can lead to straining and increased risk of rebleeding.*
    - Assist with activities of daily living (feeding, bathing, dressing, toileting).
    - Avoid any activity that could lead to increased ICP; ensure that the patient does not flex the hips beyond 90 degrees and avoids neck hyperflexion, hyperextension, or lateral hyperrotation *that could impede jugular venous return.*

## Altered Tissue Perfusion—cont'd

### *Altered Cerebral Tissue Perfusion Related to Increased Intracranial Pressure Secondary to Brain Trauma, Hemorrhage, Edema, Infection, Tumor, Stroke, Hydrocephalus*

#### DEFINING CHARACTERISTICS

- ICP >15 mm Hg, sustained for 15-30 minutes
- Headache
- Vomiting, with or without nausea
- Seizures
- Decrease in Glasgow Coma Scale of two or more points from baseline
- Alteration in level of consiousness, ranging from restlessness to coma
- Change in orientation: disoriented to time and/or place and/or person
- Difficulty or inability to follow simple commands
- Increasing systolic BP of more than 20 mm Hg with widening pulse pressure
- Bradycardia
- Irregular respiratory pattern (such as Cheyne-Stokes, central neurogenic hyperventilation, ataxic, apneustic)
- Change in response to painful stimuli (such as purposeful to inappropriate or absent response)
- Signs of impendig brain herniation, which, in addition to the above, may include the following:
  Hemiparesis or hemiplegia
  Hemisensory changes
  Unequal pupil size (1 mm or more difference)
  Failure of pupil to react to light
  Dysconjugate gaze and inability to move one eye beyond midline if third, fourth, or sixth cranial nerves involved
  Loss of oculocephalic or oculovestibular reflexes
  Possible decorticate or decerebrate posturing

#### OUTCOME CRITERIA

- ICP is ≤15 mm Hg.
- CPP is >60 mm Hg.
- Clinical signs of increased ICP as described above are absent.

#### NURSING INTERVENTIONS *AND RATIONALE*

1. Continue to monitor the assessment parameters listed under "Defining Characteristics."
2. Maintain adequate CPP.
   a. With physician's collaboration, maintain BP within patient's norm by administering volume expanders, vasopressors, or antihypertensives.
   b. Reduce ICP.
      - Elevate head of bed 30 to 45 degrees *to facilitate venous return.*
      - Maintain head and neck in neutral plane (avoid flexion, extension, or lateral rotation) *to enhance venous drainage from the head.*
      - Avoid extreme hip flexion.
      - With physician's collaboration, administer steroids, osmotic agents, and diuretics.
      - Drain CSF according to protocol if ventriculostomy in place.
      - Assist patient to turn and move self in bed (instruct patient to exhale while turning or pushing up in bed) *to avoid isometric contractions and Valsalva maneuver.*
3. Maintain patent airway, adequate ventilation, and supply oxygen *to prevent hypoxemia and hypercarbia.*
4. Monitor arterial blood gas (ABG) values and maintain $Pa{O_2}$ >80 mm Hg, $Pa{CO_2}$ at 25-35 mm Hg, and pH at 7.35-7.45.
5. Avoid suctioning beyond 10 seconds at a time; hyperoxygenate and hyperventilate before and after suctioning.
6. Plan patient care activities and nursing interventions around the patient's ICP response. Avoid unnecessary additional disturbances and allow patient up to 1 hour of rest between activities as frequently as possible. *Studies have shown the direct correlation between nursing care activities and increases in ICP.*
7. Maintain normothermia with external cooling or heating measures as necessary. Wrap hands, feet, and male genitalia in soft towels before cooling measures *to prevent shivering and frostbite.*
8. With physician's collaboration, control seizures with prophylactic and as necessary (PRN) anticonvulsants. *Seizures can greatly increase the cerebral metabolic rate.*
9. With physician's collaboration, administer sedatives, barbiturates, or paralyzing agents *to reduce cerebral metabolic rate.*
10. Counsel family members to maintain calm atmosphere and to avoid disturbing conversation (such as that about condition, pain, prognosis, family crisis, financial difficulties).
11. If signs of impending brain herniation are present, do the following:
    - Notify physician at once.
    - Be sure head of bed is elevated 45 degrees and patient's head is in neutral plane.
    - Slow mainline intravenous (IV) infusion to keep open rate.
    - If ventriculostomy catheter in place, drain CSF as ordered.
    - Prepare to administer osmotic agents and/or diuretics.
    - Prepare patient for emergency computed tomographic (CT) head scan and/or emergency surgery.

## Hypothermia

**Definition:** *The state in which an individual's body temperature is reduced below normal range.*

### *Hypothermia Related to Exposure to Cold Environment, Illness, Trauma (Including Spinal Cord Trauma), or Damage to the Hypothalamus*

#### DEFINING CHARACTERISTICS

- Core body temperature below 35° C (95° F)
- Skin cold to touch
- Slurred speech, incoordination
- At temperature below 33° C (91.4° F):
  Cardiac dysrhythmias (atrial fibrillation, bradycardia)
  Cyanosis
  Respiratory alkalosis
- At temperatures below 32° C (89.5° F):
  Shivering replaced by muscle rigidity
  Hypotension
  Dilated pupils
- At temperatures below 28°-29° C (82.4-84.2° F):
  Absent deep tendon reflexes
  Hypoventilation (3 to 4 breaths/min to apnea)
  Ventricular fibrillation possible
- At temperatures below 26°-27° C (78.8-80.6° F):
  Coma
  Flaccid muscles
  Fixed, dilated pupils
  Ventricular fibrillation to cardiac standstill
  Apnea

#### OUTCOME CRITERIA

- Core body temperature is greater than 35° C (95° F).
- Patient is alert and oriented.
- Cardiac dysrhythmias are absent.
- Acid-base balance is normal.
- Pupils are normoreactive.

#### NURSING INTERVENTIONS *AND RATIONALE*

NOTE: Rapid rewarming of a chronically hypothermic patient by active external measures can lead to peripheral vasodilation, resulting in further loss of body temperature; mobilization of blood containing high potassium; low pH, high $Pco_2$, and low $Po_2$ levels; profound hypotension; and fatal ventricular fibrillation. Keep in mind that children have been successfully resuscitated after immersion in cold water for 20 to 40 minutes.

1. Continue to monitor the assessment parameters listed under "Defining Characteristics." In addition, continuously monitor core body temperature with a low-reading thermometer.
2. Intubation and mechanical ventilation may be needed. Heated air or oxygen can be added *to help rewarm the body core.* Because carbon dioxide production is low, do not hyperventilate the hypothermic patient, because *this action may induce severe alkalosis and precipitate ventricular fibrillation.*
3. Apply cardiopulmonary resuscitation (CPR) and advanced cardiac life support until core body temperature is up to at least 29.5° C before determining that patient cannot be resuscitated.
4. Monitor ABG values to direct further therapy, and be sure that the pH, $Pao_2$, and $Paco_2$ are corrected for temperature.
5. For abrupt-onset hypothermia (for example, immersion in cold water, exposure to cold, wet climate, collapse in snow) rewarming can take place rapidly *because the pathophysiological changes associated with chronic hypothermia have not had time to evolve.*
   - Institute rapid, active rewarming by immersion in warm water (38°-43° C).
   - Apply thermal blanket at 36.6°-37.7° C. Some researchers suggest rewarming only the torso or trunk first, leaving the extremities exposed to room temperature. *This is to prevent early peripheral vasodilation with abrupt redistribution of intravascular volume. This also prevents colder blood trapped in the extremities from returning to the body core before the heart is rewarmed.*
   - Perform rapid core rewarming with heated (37°-43° C) IV infusion, hemodialysis, peritoneal dialysis, and colonic or gastric irrigation fluids.
6. Electrical defibrillation is usually successful in terminating ventricular fibrillation if the temperature is greater than 28° C.
7. Administer cardiac resuscitation drugs sparingly because *as the body warms, peripheral vasodilation occurs. Drugs that remain in the periphery are suddenly released, leading to a "bolus effect" that may cause fatal dysrhythmias.*
8. Monitor peripheral circulation because *gangrene of the fingers and toes is a common complication of accidental hypothermia.*
9. For chronic hypothermia, how aggressive the treatment is will depend on the setting, the underlying disease, and the body temperature. Concurrent treatment of the underlying disease processes is indicated.
   - Core temperatures greater than 33° C may be rewarmed either slowly or rapidly.
   - Coma in a patient with a temperature greater than 28° C is probably not caused by hypothermia. Look for other causes such as hypoglycemia, alcohol, narcotics, and head trauma and treat accordingly.
   - If patient is hyperglycemic, remember that insulin is ineffective at body temperatures below 30° C.
   - Restore intravascular volume cautiously *to avoid circulatory overloading of the hypothermic heart and to avoid precipitating pulmonary edema.* As circulation and a more normal temperature are restored, the patient may require large volumes of crystalloid and colloid fluids *to refill the dilated vascular bed.*

## Unilateral Neglect

**Definition:** *The state in which an individual is perceptually unaware of and inattentive to one side of the body.*

### *Unilateral Neglect Related to Perceptual Disruption Secondary to Stroke Involving the Right Cerebral Hemisphere*

#### DEFINING CHARACTERISTICS

**Major (must be present)**

- Neglect of involved body parts and/or extrapersonal space
- Denial of the existence of the affected limb or side of body

**Minor (may be present)**

- Denial of hemiplegia or other motor and sensory deficits
- Left homonymous hemianopsia
- Difficulty with spatial-perceptual tasks
- Left hemiplegia

#### OUTCOME CRITERIA

- Patient is safe and free from injury.
- Patient is able to identify safety hazards in the environment.
- Patient recognizes disability and describes physical deficits present (for example, paralysis, weakness, numbness).
- Patient demonstrates ability to scan the visual field to compensate for loss of function or sensation in affected limb(s).

#### NURSING INTERVENTIONS *AND RATIONALE*

1. Continue to monitor the assessment parameters listed under "Defining Characteristics."
2. Maintain patient safety: *Because of the patient's usually brief stay within the critical care unit, the emphasis is placed on patient safety. Therefore the environment is adapted to the patient's deficit.*
   - Position the patient's bed with the unaffected side facing the door.
   - Approach and speak to the patient from the unaffected side. If the patient must be approached from the affected side, announce your presence as soon as entering the room *to avoid startling the patient.*
   - Position the call light, bedside stand, and personal items on the patient's unaffected side.
   - If the patient will be assisted out of bed, simplify the environment *to eliminate hazards* by removing unnecessary furniture and equipment.
   - Provide frequent reorientation of the patient to the environment.
   - Observe the patient closely and anticipate his or her needs. In spite of repeated explanations, the patient may have difficulty retaining information about the deficits.
   - When patient is in bed, elevate his or her affected arm on a pillow *to prevent dependent edema and support the hand in a position of function.*
3. Assist the patient to recognize the perceptual defect.
   - Encourage the patient to wear any prescription corrective glasses or hearing aids *to facilitate communication.*
   - Instruct the patient to turn the head past midline to view the environment on the affected side.
   - Encourage the patient to look at the affected side and to stroke the limbs with the unaffected hand. Encourage handling of the affected limbs *to reinforce awareness of the affected side.*
   - Instruct the patient to always look for the affected extremity or extremities when performing simple tasks *to know where it is at all times.*
   - After pointing to them, have the patient name the affected parts.
   - Encourage the patient to use self-exercises (for example, lifting the affected arm with the good hand).
   - If the patient is unable to discriminate between the concepts of "right" and "left," use descriptive adjectives such as " the weak arm," "the affected leg," or "the good arm" to refer to the body. Use gestures not just words, to indicate right and left.

## Unilateral Neglect—cont'd

4. Collaborate with the patient, physician, and rehabilitation team to *design and implement a beginning rehabilitation program for use during critical care unit stay.*
   - Use adaptive equipment (braces, splints, slings) as appropriate.
   - Teach the patient the individual components of any activity separately, then proceed to integrate the component parts into a completed activity.
   - Instruct the patient to attend to the affected side, if able, and to assist with the bath or other tasks.
   - Use tactile stimulation *to reintroduce the arm or leg to the patient.* Rub the affected parts with different textured materials *to stimulate sensations (warm, cold, rough, soft).*
   - Encourage activities that required the patient to turn the head toward the affected side and retrain the patient to scan the affected side and environment visually.
   - If patient is allowed out of bed, cue him or her with reminders to scan visually when ambulating. Assist and remain in constant attendance because *the patient may have difficulty maintaining correct posture, balance, and locomotion.* There may be vertical-horizontal perceptual problems, with the patient leaning to the affected side to align with the perceived vertical. Provide sitting, standing, and balancing exercises before getting the patient out of bed.
   - Feeding: see "High Risk for Aspiration, risk factor: impaired swallowing," p. 476.
     a. Avoid giving patient any very hot food items that could cause injury.
     b. Place the patient in an upright sitting position if possible.
     c. Encourage the patient to feed himself or herself; if necessary, guide the patient's hand to the mouth.
     d. If the patient is able to feed himself or herself, place one dish at a time in front of the patient. When the patient is finished with the first, add another dish. Tell the patient what he or she is eating.
     e. Initially place food in the patient's visual field; then gradually move the food out of the field of vision and teach the patient to scan the entire visual field.
     f. When the patient has learned to visually scan the environment, offer a tray of food with various dishes.
     g. Instruct the patient to take small bites of food and to place the food in the unaffected side of the mouth.
     h. *To eliminate retained food in the affected side of the mouth,* teach the patient to sweep out these pockets of food with the tongue after every bite.
     i. After meals or oral medications, check the patient's oral cavity for pockets of retained material.
5. Initiate patient and family health teaching.
   - Assess to ensure that both the patient and the family understand the nature of the neurological deficits and the purpose of the rehabilitation plan.
   - Teach the proper application and use of any adaptive equipment.
   - Teach the importance of maintaining a safe environment and point out potential environmental hazards.
   - Instruct family members how to facilitate relearning techniques (for example, cueing, scanning visual fields).

## Dysreflexia

**Definition:** *The state in which an individual with a spinal cord injury at T-7 or above experiences a life-threatening uninhibited sympathetic response of the nervous system to a noxious stimulus.*

### *Dyreflexia Related to Excessive Autonomic Response to Certain Noxious Stimuli (i.e., Distended Bladder, Distended Bowel, Skin Irritation) Occurring in Patients With Cervical or High Thoracic (T-6 or above) Spinal Cord Injury*

#### DEFINING CHARACTERISTICS

**Major**

- Paroxysmal hypertension (sudden periodic elevated BP in which systolic pressure is greater than 140 mm Hg and diastolic pressure is greater than 90 mm Hg); for many spinal cord injury patients, a normal BP may be only 90/60
- Bradycardia (most common; pulse rate <60 beats per minute) or tachycardia (pulse rate >100 beats per minute)
- Diaphoresis (above the injury)
- Facial flushing
- Pallor (below the injury)
- Headache (a diffuse pain in different portions of the head and not confined to any nerve distribution area)

**Minor**

- Nasal congestion
- Engorgement of temporal and neck vessels
- Conjunctival congestion
- Chills without fever
- Pilomotor erection (goose bumps)
- Blurred vision
- Chest pain
- Metallic taste in mouth
- Horner's syndrome (constriction of the pupil, partial ptosis of the eyelid, enophthalmos, and sometimes loss of sweating over the affected side of the face)

#### OUTCOME CRITERIA

- Systolic BP is <140 mm Hg, and diastolic blood pressure is <90 mm Hg (or within patient's norm).
- Pulse rate is >60 or <100 beats per minute (or within patient's norm).
- Headache is absent.
- Nasal stuffiness, sweating, and flushing above level of injury are absent.
- Chills, goose bumps, and pallor below level of injury are absent.
- Patient verbalizes causes, prevention, symptoms, and treatment of condition.

#### NURSING INTERVENTIONS *AND RATIONALE*

1. Continue to monitor the assessment parameters listed under "Defining Characteristics."
2. Place on cardiac monitor and assess for bradycardia, tachycardia, or other dysrhythmias. *Disturbances of cardiac rate and rhythm can occur because of autonomic dysfunction associated with dysreflexia.*
3. Do not leave patient alone. One nurse monitors the blood pressure and patient status every 3 to 5 minutes while another provides treatment.
4. Place patient's head of bed to upright position *to decrease BP and promote cerebral venous return.*
5. Investigate for and remove offending cause of dysreflexia.
   a. Bladder
      - If catheter not in place, immediately catheterize patient.
      - Lubricate catheter with lidocaine jelly before insertion.
      - Drain 500 ml of urine and recheck BP.
      - If BP still elevated, drain another 500 ml of urine.
      - If BP declines after the bladder is empty, serial BP should be monitored closely because *the bladder can go into severe contractions, causing hypertension to recur.* With physician's collaboration, instill 30 ml tetracaine through the catheter *to decrease the flow of impulses from the bladder.*
      - If indwelling catheter in place, check for kinks or granular sediment that may indicate occlusion.
      - If plugged catheter is suspected, irrigate it gently with no more than 30 ml of sterile normal saline solution. If the bladder is in tetany, fluid will go in but will not drain out.
      - If unable to irrigate catheter, remove it, reinsert a new catheter, an proceed with its lubrication, drainage, and observation as stated above.
      - Atropine is sometimes administered *to relieve bladder tetany.*

   b. Bowel
      - Using glove lubricated with anesthetic ointment, check rectum for fecal impaction.
      - If impaction is felt, *to decrease flow of impulses from bowel,* insert anesthetic ointment into rectum 10 minutes before manual removal of impaction.
      - A low, hypertonic enema or a suppository may be given *to assist bowel evacuation.*

   c. Skin
      - Loosen clothing or bed linens as indicated.
      - Inspect skin for pimples, boils, pressure sores, and ingrown toenails and treat as indicated.
6. If symptoms of dysrelexia do not subside, have available the IV solutions and antihypertensive drugs of the physician's choosing (for example, hydralazine, phentolamine, diazoxide, sodium nitroprusside). Administer medications and monitor their effectiveness. Assess BP, pulse, and subjective and objective signs and symptoms.
7. Instruct patient about causes, symptoms, treatment, and prevention of dysreflexia.
8. Encourage patient to carry informational card to present to medical personnel in the event dysreflexia may be developing.

## Acute Pain

**Definition:** *The state in which an individual experiences and reports the presence of severe discomfort or an uncomfortable sensation.*

### *Acute Pain Related to Transmission and Perception of Cutaneous, Visceral, Muscular, or Ischemic Impulses Secondary to _______ (Specify)*

#### DEFINING CHARACTERISTICS

**Subjective**

- Patient verbalizes presence of pain
- Patient rates pain on scale of 1 to 10

**Objective**

- Increase in BP, pulse, and respirations
- Pupillary dilation
- Diaphoresis, pallor
- Skeletal muscle reactions (grimacing, clenching fists, writhing, pacing, guarding or splinting affected part)
- Apprehensive, fearful appearance

#### OUTCOME CRITERIA

NOTE: Outcome is highly variable, dependent on individual patient and pain circumstance factors.

- Patient verbalizes that pain is reduced to a tolerable level or is removed.
- Patient's pain rating on scale of 1 to 10 is lower.
- BP, heart rate, and respiratory rate return to baseline 5 minutes after administration of IV narcotic or 20 minutes after administration of intramuscular (IM) narcotic.

#### NURSING INTERVENTIONS *AND RATIONALE*

1. Continue to monitor the assessment parameters listed under "Defining Characteristics." In addition, monitor postural vital sign changes; determine hydration status and manage fluid volume deficit, if indicated, before administering narcotic analgesic.
2. Modify variables that heighten the patient's experience of pain.
   - Explain to the patient that frequent, detailed, and seemingly repetitive assessments will be conducted *to allow the nurse to better understand the patient's pain experience, not because the existence of pain is in question.*
   - Explain the factors responsible for pain production in the individual. Estimate the expected duration of the pain if possible.
   - Explain diagnostic and therapeutic procedures to the patient in relation to sensations the patient should expect to feel. *Preparatory sensory information enhances learning and retention of knowledge and decreases anxiety.*
   - Reduce the patient's fear of addiction by explaining the difference between drug tolerance and drug addiction. Drug tolerance is a physiological phenomenon in which a drug dose begins to lose effectiveness after repeated doses; drug dependence is a psychological phenomenon in which narcotics are used regularly for emotional, not medical reasons.
   - Instruct patient to ask for pain medication when pain is beginning and not to wait until it is intolerable.
   - Explain that the physician will be consulted if pain relief is inadequate with the present medication.
   - Instruct patient in the importance of adequate rest, especially when it reduces pain, *to maintain strength and coping abilities and to reduce stress.*
3. Perform pharmacological interventions.
   - For postsurgical or posttraumatic cutaneous, muscular, or visceral pain, perform the following:
     a. Medicate with narcotic maximally to break the pain cycle as long as level of consciousness and HR and BP are stable: Check patient's previous response to similar dosage and narcotic.

NOTE: First dose received postoperatively is usually reduced by one half *to evaluate patient's individual response to medication.*

   b. Continuous pain requires continuous analgesia.
      (1) Establish optimal analgesic dose that brings optimal pain relief.
      (2) Offer pain mediation at prescribed regular intervals rather than making patient ask for it.
   c. If administering medication on prn basis, give it when patient's pain is just beginning, rather than at its peak. Advise patient to intercept pain, not endure it, or it may take several hours and higher doses of narcotics to relieve pain, leading to a cycle of undermedication and pain alternating with overmedication and drug toxicity.
   d. Perform rehabilitation exercises (turn, deep breathe, leg exercises, ambulate) shortly before peak of drug effect because *this will be the optimal time for the patient to increase activity with the least risk of increasing pain.*
   e. In making the transition from IM or IV to by mouth (po) medications, try alternating them in the following pattern: IM, IM, po, IM, po, po, IM, po, po, po, IM, po . . . or IV, IV, IM, IV, IM, IM, IV, IM, IM, IM, IV, IM . . ..
   f. To assess effectiveness of pain medication, do the following:
      (1) Reevaluate pain 5 minutes after IV and 20 minutes after IM medication administration, observe patient's behavior, and ask patient to rate pain on scale of 1 to 10.
      (2) Collaborate with physician to add or delete other medications such as antiemetics, hypnotics, sedatives, or muscle relaxants that potentiate the action of analgesics.

Continued.

## Acute Pain—cont'd

(3) Observe for indicators of undertreatment: report of pain not relieved; observed restlessness, sleeplessness, irritability, and anorexia; decreased activity level.

(4) Indicators of overtreatment: hypotension or bradycardia; respiratory rate <10/min; excessive sedation.

g. If IV patient-controlled analgesia (PCA) is used, perform the following:

(NOTE: *Patient-controlled analgesia allows patients to administer small doses of their prescribed medication when they feel the need. Constant levels of the drug in the bloodstream mean lower doses can be used to obtain analgesia. Pain control is improved because the patient is in control and experiences less fear of unrelieved pain. Reduced net narcotic use is noted as is less sedation. Critical care patients appropriate for patient-controlled analgesia are those who are alert, such as burn patients, trauma patients without head injury, and some postoperative patients.)*

(1) Instruct the patient as follows: "When you have pain, instead of ringing for the nurse to receive pain medicine, push the button that activates the machine, and a small dose of pain medicine will be injected into your IV line. Give yourself only enough medicine to take care of your pain, but do not activate the machine for a dose if you start to feel sleepy. Try to balance the pain relief against sleepiness. If your pain medicine seems to stop working despite pushing the button several times, call the nurse to check your IV. If this is still a problem, the nurse will call your doctor."

(2) Monitor vital signs, especially BP and respiratory rate, every hour for the first 4 hours and assess postural heart rate and BP before initial ambulation.

(3) Monitor respirations every 2 hours while patient is on patient-controlled analgesia.

(4) If patient's respirations decrease to <10/min or if patient is overly sedated, anticipate IV administration of naloxone.

h. If epidural narcotic analgesia is used, do the following:

(NOTE: *The delivery of narcotics such as morphine by epidural route to specific receptors in the spinal cord selectively blocks pain impulses to the brain for up to 24 hours. Effective analgesia can be obtained without many of the negative side effects or serum narcotic concentrations. Critical care patients appropriate for epidural analgesia include postsurgical and trauma patients.)*

(1) Keep patient's head elevated 30 to 45 degrees after injection *to prevent respiratory depressant effects.*

(2) Observe closely for respiratory depression up to 24 hours after injection. Monitor respiratory rate every 15 minutes for 1 hour every 30 minutes for 7 hours, and every 1 hour for the remaining 16 hours.

(3) Assess for adequate cough reflex.

(4) Avoid use of other CNS depressants such as sedatives.

(5) Observe for reports of pruritis, nausea, or vomiting.

(6) Anticipate administration of naloxone for respiratory depression (and smaller doses of naloxone for pruritis).

(7) Assess for and treat urinary retention.

(8) Assess epidural catheter site for local infection. Keep catheter taped securely.

- For peripheral vascular ischemic pain (hypothetical vascular occlusion of leg), do the following:

a. Correctly identify and differentiate ischemic pain from other types of pain.

(NOTE: *Ischemic pain is usually a burning, aching pain made worse by exercise and lessened or relieved by rest. Eventually the pain occurs at rest. Coldness and pallor of extremity may be noted, especially if the limb is elevated above the heart level. Rubor and mottling of the skin may be evident from prolonged tissue anoxia and inability of damaged vessels to constrict. Eventually cyanosis and gangrenous tissue will be evident. Chronic ischemia leads to trophic changes in the limb such as flaking skin, brittle nails, hair loss, leg ulcers, and cellulitis.)*

## Acute Pain—cont'd

b. Administer pain medications and evaluate their effectiveness as previously described. Remember that the pain of ischemia is chronic and continuous and can make the patient irritable and depressed.

c. Treat the cause of the ischemic pain and institute measures to increase circulation to the affected part (see the nursing management of Altered Peripheral Tissue Perfusion, p. 462.)

4. Perform nonpharmalogic interventions.
   - Treat contributing factors and provide explanations (see intervention number 2 at beginning of this nursing management plan).
   - Apply comfort measures, using gate control theory.

   a. Use relaxation techniques such as back rubs, massage, warm baths. Use blankets and pillows *to support the painful part and reduce muscle tension*. Encourage slow, rhythmic breathing.

   b. Encourage progressive muscle relaxation techniques.
      (1) Instruct patient to inhale and tense (tighten) specific muscle groups, then relax the muscles as exhalation occurs.
      (2) Suggest an order for performing the tension-relaxation cycle (for example, start with facial muscles and move down body ending with toes).

   c. Encourage guided imagery
      (1) Ask patient to recall an experienced image that is very pleasurable and relaxing and involves at least two senses.
      (2) Have patient begin with rhythmic breathing and progressive relaxation, then travel mentally to the scene.
      (3) Have the patient slowly experience the scene—how it looks, sounds, smells, feels.
      (4) Ask patient to practice this imagery in private.
      (5) Instruct the patient to end the imagery be counting to three and saying, "Now I'm relaxed." If person does not end the imagery and falls asleep, the purpose of the technique is defeated.

   d. If TENS unit is prescribed by physician, do the following:

(NOTE: *TENS is a battery-operated unit that serves as a nerve stimulator. It produces mild, tingling sensations as it blocks incisional pain messages to the brain. It is sometimes used as part of the pain relief program for the postsurgical patient.)*

      (1) Take the TENS unit, patient pamphlet, and teaching electrodes to the patient before surgery to explain the process.
      (2) Apply electrodes to skin and instruct patient in proper use of unit. Let patient experience how the TENS unit should feel when activated. Refer to manufacturer's directions for proper application and operation of TENS unit.
      (3) Electrodes are usually placed by the physician on the skin alongside the operative incision at the close of the surgical procedure in the operating room. The unit is usually used for 3 to 5 days as an adjunct to medications.
      (4) When the patient is awake and alert, readjust the amplitude or output of the TENS unit to the patient's comfort as necessary. Keep the TENS unit on continuously unless ordered otherwise. Occasionally, percutaneous epidural nerve stimulation is used when more than one nerve root is involved in producing pain. Again, patients are able to control their pain by adjusting the rate and frequency of a millivoltage electrical current stimulator affixed externally.

   f. Assist with biofeedback, which represents a wide range of behavioral techniques that provide the patient with information about changes in body functions of which the person is usually unaware. For example, information used to reduce muscle contraction is obtained by an electromyogram recorded from body surface electrodes. Changes in blood flow are produced by monitoring skin temperature changes. The person using biofeedback tries to change the display of information in the desired direction by actions such as reducing muscle tension or reducing or altering blood flow to a particular area. The critical care nurse should be familiar with the theoretical concepts of biofeedback and should support the patient in maximizing pain control through whatever techniques are successful for that patient.

## Impaired Verbal Communication

**Definition:** *The state in which an individual experiences a decreased or absent ability to use or understand language in human interaction.*

### *Impaired Verbal Communication: Aphasia Related to Cerebral Speech Center Injury*

#### DEFINING CHARACTERISTICS

**Major (must be present)**

- Inappropriate or absent speech or responses to questions

**Minor (may be present)**

- Inability to speak spontaneously
- Inability to understand spoken words
- Inability to follow commands through gestures
- Difficulty or inability to understand written language
- Difficulty or inability to express ideas in writing
- Difficulty or inability to name objects

#### OUTCOME CRITERIA

- Patient is able to make basic needs known.

#### NURSING INTERVENTIONS *AND RATIONALE*

1. Continue to monitor the assessment parameters listed under "Defining Characteristics."
2. Obtain a speech pathology evaluation (if available) *to determine the extent of the patient's communication deficit (for example, if fluent, nonfluent, or global aphasia is involved).*
3. Have the speech therapist post a list of appropriate ways to communicate with the patient in the patient's room *so that all nursing personnel can be consistent in their efforts.*
4. Assess the patient's ability to comprehend, speak, read, and write.
   - Ask questions that can be answered with a yes or a no. If a patient answers yes to a question, ask the opposite (for example, "Are you hot?" "Yes." "Are you cold?" "Yes."). *This may help determine if in fact the patient understands what is being said.*
   - Ask simple, short questions and use gestures, pantomime, and facial expressions to give the patient additional clues.
   - Stand in the patient's line of vision, giving a good view of your face and hands.
   - Have the patient try to write with a pad and pencil. Offer pictures and alphabet letters at which to point.
   - Make flash cards with pictures or words depicting frequently used phrases (for example, glass of water, bedpan).
5. Maintain an uncluttered environment and decrease external distractions that could hinder communication.
6. Maintain a relaxed and calm manner and explain all diagnostic, therapeutic, and comfort measures before initiating them.
7. Do not shout or speak in a loud voice. *Hearing loss is not a factor in aphasia, and shouting will not help.*
8. Have only one person talk at a time. *It is more difficult for the patient to follow a multisided conversation.*
9. Use direct eye contact and speak directly to the patient in unhurried, short phrases.
10. Give one-step commands and directions, and provide cues through pictures or gestures.
11. Try to ask questions that can be answered with a yes or a no, and avoid topics that are controversial, emotional, abstract, or lengthy.
12. Listen to the patient in an unhurried manner and wait for his or her attempt to communicate.
    - Expect a time lag from when you ask the patient something until the patient responds.
    - Accept the patient's statement of essential words without expecting complete sentences.
    - Avoid finishing the sentence for the patient if possible.
    - Wait approximately 30 seconds before providing the word the patient may be attempting to find (except when the patient is very frustrated and needs something such as a bedpan quickly).
    - Rephrase the patient's message aloud *to validate it.*
    - Do not pretend to understand the patient's message if you do not.
13. Encourage the patient to speak slowly in short phrases and to say each word clearly.
14. Ask the patient to write the message, if able, or draw pictures if only verbal communciation is affected.
15. Observe the patient's nonverbal clues for validation (for example, answers "yes" but shakes head "no").
16. When handing an object to the patient, state what it is, since *hearing language spoken is necessary to stimulate language development.*
17. Explain what has happened to the patient and offer reassurance about the plan of care.
18. Verbally address the problem of frustration over inability to communicate and explain that patience is needed for both the nurse and the patient.
19. Maintain a calm, positive manner, and offer reassurance (for example, "I know this is very hard for you, but it will get better if we work on it together").
20. Talk to the patient as an adult. Be respectful and avoid talking down to the patient.
21. Do not discuss the patient's condition or hold conversations in the patient's presence without including him or her in the discussion. *This may be the reason some aphasic patients develop paranoid thoughts.*
22. Do not exhibit disapproval of emotional utterances or spontaneous use of profanity; instead, offer calm, quiet reassurance.
23. If the patient makes an error in speech, do not reprimand or scold but try to compliment the patient by saying, "That was a good try."
24. Delay conversation if the patient is tired. *The symptoms of aphasia worsen if the patient is fatigued, anxious, or upset.*
25. Be prepared for emotional outbursts and tears in patients who have difficulty in expressing themselves. The patient may become depressed, refuse treatment and food, ignore relatives, and push objects away. Comfort the patient with statements such as, "I know it's frustrating and you feel sad, but you are not alone. Other people who have had strokes have felt the way you do. We will be here to help you get through this."

## Sensory-Perceptual Alterations

**Definition:** *The state in which an individual experiences a change in the amount or patterning of incoming sitmuli accompanied by a dimished, exaggerated, distorted, or impaired response to such stimuli.*

### *Sensory-Perceptual Alterations Related to Sensory Overload, Sensory Deprivation, and Sleep Pattern Disturbance*

#### DEFINING CHARACTERISTICS

- Hallucinations
- Delusions
- Illusions
- Disorientation
- Short-term memory deficits
- Impaired abstraction

#### OUTCOME CRITERIA

- Patient has no evidence of hallucinations, delusions, or illusions.
- Results of reality testing are appropriate.
- Short-term memory is intact.
- Abstract reasoning is intact.

#### NURSING INTERVENTIONS *AND RATIONALE*

. Continue to monitor the assessment parameters listed under "Defining Characteristics." Determine and document the patient's dominant spoken language, his or her literacy, and the language(s) in which he or she is literate. Determine and document his or her premorbid degree of orientation, cognitive capabilities, and any sensory-perceptual deficits. *It is sometimes the case that people are not literate in their spoken language or, less frequently, that they are literate only in their second language. These situations can result in unfortunate errors in the appraisal of patients' ability to communicate in writing and in estimating the extent of their orientation. Similarly, assuming that patients were or were not fully oriented before critical care admission bases the nurse's assessment on possibly erroneous assumptions.*

**The following interventions are appropriate for patients with sensory overload:**

1. Initate each nurse-patient encounter by calling the patient by name and identifying yourself by name. *This fosters reality orientation and assists the patient in filtering irrelevant or impersonal conversation.*
2. Assess the patient's immediate physical environment from his or her viewpoint and explain equipment, its sounds, and its therapeutic purpose. Demonstrate audible and visual alarms and explain the possible alarm conditions. *This decreases alienation of the patient from the technological environment and reduces the inherent sense of fear and urgency accompanying alarm conditions.*
3. For each procedure performed, provide "preparatory sensory information," that is, explain procedures in relation to the sensations the patient will experience, including duration of sensations. *Preparatory sensory information enhances learning and lessens anticipatory anxiety.*
4. Limit noise levels. Certainly, audible alarms cannot and should not be silenced, and many critical, albeit noisy, activities must take place in the critical care area. It has been shown, however, that noise levels produced by clinical personnel exceed those levels designated as "acceptable" and are often greater than those generated by technological devices. Staff conversations should be kept soft enough that they are inaudible to the patient whenever possible. Critical care personnel should assume that everything said at or around a patient's bedside is intended for that patient's awareness and that it will be interpreted as pertaining to him or her. *As discussed below, conversations about the patient but not to him or her foster depersonalization and delusions of reference.*
5. Well-enforced noise limits should exist for nighttime.
6. Readjust alarm limits on physiological monitoring devices as the patient's condition changes (improves or deteriorates) *to lessen unnecessary alarm states.*
7. Consider use of head phones and audio cassette with patient's favorite and/or subliminal or classical music. *This can effectively filter out assaultive noise of the critical care environment and supplant it with familiar, soothing sounds and rhythms.*
8. Modify lighting. Day-night cycles should be simulated with environmental lighting. At no time should overhead fluorescent lights be abruptly turned on without either warning the patient, assisting him or her out of the supine position, and/or shielding his or her eyes with gauze or a face cloth. *Continuous bright lighting sustains anxiety and promotes circadian rhythm desynchronization.*
9. To the extent possible, shield patients from viewing urgent and emergent events in the critical care unit. *Resuscitation efforts, albeit difficult to conceal, engender fear in the patient and a sense of instability and vulnerability (for example, thoughts of "I'm next").* When such an event occurs, the nurse should endeavor to elicit the patient's cognitive and emotional reaction; thoughts, impressions, and feelings should be shared and misconceptions clarified. A useful approach for the nurse in this interchange is that of emphasizing the differences between the patient at hand and the one resuscitated (for example, "He was considerably older," "more unstable," "had serious lung disease").

*Continued.*

## Sensory-Perceptual Alterations—cont'd

10. Ensure patient's privacy, their modesty and, at the very least, their dignity. Physical exposure and nudity, although seeming to pale in importance alongside such priorities as physiologic assessment and stabilization, are primal indignities in all individuals. Patients should be kept minimally exposed. When, in the course of assessment and intervention, it becomes necessary to expose the patient, the nurse should first verbally apologize for this necessity. *To be naked is to feel vulnerable; to be vulnerable is to feel fearful. In this regard, fear is an emotional concomitant to critical care that is preventable through nursing intervention.*

**The following interventions are appropriate for patients with sensory deprivation:**

1. Provide reality orientation in four spheres (person, place, time, and situation) at more frequent intervals than when testing. Convey this information in the context of routine conversation. EXAMPLE STATEMENTS: "Mr. Clark, this is Tuesday morning and you're in University Hospital. Your heart surgery was yesterday morning and you're doing well. My name is Joe, and I'm your nurse today." *The patient is made to feel patronized by repetitions such as, "Do you know where you are?"* Given the effects of general anesthesia, narcotic analgesics, sedatives, and sleep, it if fully expected that some degree of disorientation will exist normally.
2. Ensure the patient's visual access to a calender. (Interestingly, the design of most state-of-the-art critical care units now reflects many of the principles of sensory stimulation. One such coronary care unit was designed with a large wall clock facing the patient. A patient who had spent more than a week in this unit later reflected that one of the most "distressing, frustrating" aspects of his stay in the coronary care unit was the monotonous, inescapable attention to the clock and its painfully slow documentation of the passing of time.)
3. Apprise the patient of daily news events and the weather.
4. Touch patients for the express purpose of communicating caring. Hold their hands, stroke their brows, rub the skin on an aspect of their arms. *Touch is the universal language of caring. In the setting of critical care, in which there is considerable physical body manipulation, it is useful and important to contrast assaultive touch with comforting touch.* Touch can be used as a technique for distraction from painful stimuli when used in conjunction with uncomfortable procedures. (IMPORTANT: See discussion of the use of touch in "Management of the Patient Experiencing Hallucinations" below).
5. Foster liberal visitation by family and significant others. Encourage significant others to touch the patient consistent with their individual comfort level and cultural norms.
6. Structure and identify opportunities for the patient to exercise decision-making skills, however small. *Although not so designated, patients with sensory alterations experience a type of "cognitive deprivation" as well. (Refer to the nursing management of Powerlessness on p. 445.)*
7. Assist patients to find meaning in their experiences. Explain the therapeutic purpose of all that they are asked to do for themselves and all that is done with them and for them. Avoid statements such as, "Will you turn to that side for me?" or "I need you to swallow this medication." *These statements implicitly convey that the maneuver has some value for the nurses versus the patients.* Similarly, use "thank you" judiciously. *This simple salutation, when used indiscriminately, suggests something was done to benefit the nurses and not the patients.* Patients need to find meaning and to identify their roles in the experience of critical illness and critical care. The sensations that constitute this experience and those that do not are made bearable and intelligible to patients when attached to the larger picture of their conditions, treatment, and progress.

**The following interventions are appropriate for patients with sleep pattern disturbances:**

For excellent management strategies of sleep pattern disturbance, refer to the nursing management of Sleep Alterations on p. 455.)

**The following interventions are appropriate for patients experiencing hallucinations:**

1. Approach the patient with a calm, matter-of-fact demeanor. *The goal of this interaction is for the nurse to demonstrate external control. This helps decrease the anxiety and fear that generally accompany hallucinations and allows the patient to feel safe. Anxiety is transferable.*
2. Address the patient by name. *This is a useful presentation of reality because self-identity is the last sphere of orientation to vanish.*
3. In responding to the patient's description of the hallucination, DO NOT deny, argue, or attempt to disprove the existance of the perceived event. *Statements such as, "There are no voices coming from that air vent" or, "Look, I'm brushing my hand across the wall, and there are no bugs" confuse the patient further, because the hallucination, although frightening, is his or her perceived reality.*
4. Express to the patient that your experiences are dissimilar, and acknowledge how frightening his or hers must be. EXAMPLE STATEMENT: "I don't hear (see, etc.) what you do, but I know how frightening such an experience must be to you. I'm Joe, your nurse, and I'm going to stay with you until the voices (etc.) go away." Remain with any patient who is experiencing a hallucination. *Feelings of fear and anxiety often acclerate when a patient is left alone. He or she needs someone to represent a nonthreatening reality. In addition, validating the patient's feelings demonstrates acceptance and sensitivity to the experience and promotes trust.*

*An exception is the patient who the nurse suspects is experiencing auditory hallucination, that is, hearing "voice commands." To ascertain that the voices are not telling the patient to harm himself, it is appropriate for the nurse to ask simply and concretely, "What are the voices saying?"

## Sensory-Perceptual Alterations—cont'd

5. DO NOT explore the content of the hallucination with the patient by asking about its nature or character. *The nurse is the patient's link with reality. Pursuit of a detailed description of a hallucination may signify to the patient that the nurse accepts his or her sensory distortion as factual. This may further confuse the patient and distance him or her more from reality.** The nurse can help bridge the gap between the patient's misperception and reality be addressing the feelings (such as fear, anxiety) and/or meanings (such as danger, death) engendered by the hallucination. Determination of how the misperception affects the patient emotionally, acknowledgment of those feelings, and a calm, controlled, matter-of-fact approach will *provide the trust and comfort he or she needs to tolerate this frightening experience*. In other words, deal with the intent more than the content of the hallucination. *The resultant decrease in anxiety will enable the patient to focus more accurately on his or her immediate environment.*
6. Talk concretely with the patient about things that are really happening. EXAMPLE STATEMENTS: "How does your chest incision feel this afternoon, Mr. Clark?" "Your sister Kate was here to see you, but you were sleeping. She went down to the cafeteria and will be back." "Your secretions are a little easier for you to cough up today." *Interpretation of reality-based stimuli by the nurse encourages the patient to focus on actual circumstances and discourages a preoccupation with sensory misperceptions.*
7. There may be circumstances in which it is appropriate for the nurse simply to distract the patient by changing the topic. This tactic is useful in situations of escalating anxiety and confusion or when all else fails. Topics should consist of basic themes that are universally understood and culturally congruent such as music, food, or weather. They may also be topics of special interest to the patient such as hobbies, crafts, or sports. Topics that evoke strong emotions such as politics, religion, or sexuality should be avoided with most patients. *This is especially true of the patient with reality distortions; sometimes hallucinations and delusions are expressions of repressed conflicts associated with religious, sexual, or aggressive issues. Pursuit of such subjects could increase confusion and anxiety.*
8. The use of touch: *Touch presents a nonthreatening external reality and can therefore be useful in the management of patients with sensory alterations. However, in the patient experiencing hallucinations (as well as delusions and illusions), touch can be readily misinterpreted as, for instance, aggression or pain, or it can actually provide the basis for a tactile illusion.* Therefore the use of touch as an intervention strategy should be avoided in any patient who evidences escalating anxiety or paranoid, suspicious, or mistrustful thoughts.
9. Types of hallucinations include the following: auditory—voices or running commentaries, with self-destructive messages; visual—persons or images that appear threatening; olfactory—smells that may be interpreted as poisonous gases; gustatory—tastes that seem peculiar or harmful; and tactile—touch that feels unusual or unnatural.
10. Specific management strategies for patients experiencing hallucinations.
    - Auditory hallucinations
      a. Patient behaviors: Head cocked as if listening to an unseen presence; lips moving.
      b. Therapeutic nurse responses: "Mr. Clark, you appear to be listenting to something." *If patient acknowledges voices:* "I don't hear any voices, but I know this is troubling you. The voices will go away. Nothing is going to harm you. I'm Joe, your nurse, and I'll be here with you."
      c. Nontherapeutic nurse responses: "Tell me about your conversations with these voices." "To whom do the voices belong—anyone you know?"
    - Visual hallucinations
      a. Patient behaviors: Staring into space as if focused on an unseen object; startled movements and anxious facial expression.
      b. Therapeutic nurse responses: "Mr. Clark, something seems to be troubling you. Tell me what it is." *If patient states he visualizes people, images, or the devil in his environment and implies a sense of danger,* respond, "There are only nurses and doctors here, Mr. Clark. I know this must be upsetting, but these images will go away. We're here with you in the hospital. Nothing will happen to you."
      c. Nontherapeutic nurse responses: "Describe the people you see. What are they wearing?" "What does the devil mean in your life? What about God?"

**The following interventions are appropriate for patients experiencing delusions:**

1. Explain all unseen noises, voices, and activity simply and clearly. *They readily feed a delusional system.* EXAMPLE STATEMENTS: "That is Dr. Smith. He's come to see you and other patients here in the hospital." "The voices and activity you hear are from the bedside of the patient behind this curtain. He's being helped by one of the nurses."
2. Avoid the "negative challenge" (for example, "Nobody here stole your belongings" or "Doctors and nurses do not harm people") of the patient's delusion. Similarly, avoid defending the referents of the patient's belief: "Nurses are good" and "Doctors mean well." *Remember, a delusion is a belief, albeit false, that cannot be changed with logic. To attempt this change is to challenge the patient's belief system and thereby escalate his or her anxiety, further blurring the boundaries between reality and the patient's internally based "logic."*

Continued.

## Sensory-Perceptual Alterations—cont'd

3. For the patient with persecutory delusions who refuses food, fluids, or medications because of a belief they have been poisoned or tainted, permit the refusal unless it is a life-threatening event. Try again in 20 minutes; allow the patient to choose an alternate selection of food or to read the label on the unit medication. Coercion, show of force, or engaging in complicated, logical justifications will only heighten the patient's suspiciousness and possibly reinforce the delusional belief. *When the patient feels more in control, he or she need not rely on the "paradoxical" quality of the delusion to equip him or her with a false sense of power. His or her power instead is derived from making reality-based decisions.*
4. Staff members should be particularly careful not to engage in unnecessary laughter or whispering among themselves within view of the delusional patient. *The delusional patient is hypervigilant, scanning the environment for evidence to corroborate or confirm his or her belief that staff members are colluding against him or her. Clearly, laughter and whispers easily suggest this belief, this delusion of reference. This rationale pertains to the patient experiencing hallucinations and/or illusions as well.*
5. Observe the principles detailed in the third intervention under the previous section describing interventions for the hallucinating patient.

**The following interventions are appropriate for patients experiencing illusions:**

1. As with the management of delusions, the nurse should simply and briefly interpret reality-based stimuli for the patient in a calm, matter-of-fact manner. *Seen and unseen noises, voices, activity, and people can provide the stimulus for a sensory misinterpretation, an illusion.*
2. The immediate environment of the patient should provide as low a level of stimulation as possible. Nursing interventions detailed previously under "Sensory Overload" are especially relevant here.
3. The theme of the nurse's verbal approach to the patient experiencing illusions is similar to that outlined for hallucinations and delusions: Address the feelings and meanings associated with the experience, not the content of the sensory misinterpretation.
   - Patient behaviors: Eyes darting, startled movements; frightened facial expression. "I know who you are. You're the devil come to take me to hell."
   - Therapeutic nurse responses: "I'm Joe, your nurse, I know this experience is troubling for you. You're in the hospital, and no one here will harm you."
   - Nontherapeutic nurse responses: "There are no such things as devils or angels." "Do you think the devil would be dressed in white?" *The first nontherapeutic nurse response carries a parental tone (for example, "You know better than that"), thus infantilizing the patient and adding to his or her feelings of powerlessness over the environment. The second nontherapeutic response reflects obvious logic, which is not in the patient's sensory domain; therefore it cannot be processed and only adds to his or her confused state.*
4. Observe the principles detailed under number 5, in interventions for patients experiencing hallucinations.

# Nursing Management of Renal Alterations

## Fluid Volume Deficit

**Definition:** *The state in which an individual experiences intravascular dehydration.*

### *Fluid Volume Deficit Related to Hyponatremia (Absolute Sodium Loss)*

#### DEFINING CHARACTERISTICS

- Central nervous system (CNS) symptoms: headache, lethargy, confusion, muscular weakness
- Postural hypotension
- Tachycardia
- Gastrointestinal (GI) symptoms: nausea, diarrhea, cramping
- Diaphoresis, cold and clammy skin
- Loss of skin turgor and elasticity
- Serum sodium <135 mEq/L
- Urinary specific gravity <1.010
- Elevated red blood cell and plasma protein levels

#### OUTCOME CRITERIA

- CNS symptoms (for example, headache, lethargy) are absent.
- Blood pressure and heart rate return to baseline.
- Skin turgor is normal.
- Serum sodium and urinary specific gravity levels are normal.

#### NURSING INTERVENTIONS *AND RATIONALE*

1. Continue to monitor the assessment parameters listed under "Defining Characteristics."
2. With physician's collaboration, replace fluid and sodium loss with normal saline solution or with hypertonic saline solution (3% or 5%).
3. Provide oral fluids such as juice or bouillon that are high in sodium.
4. Avoid the use of diuretics, especially thiazide and loop diuretics, because *they will further decrease sodium.*
5. If patient is ambulatory, protect from falls until CNS symptoms and/or postural hypotension clears.
6. If performing nasogastric suctioning, irrigate tube with normal saline solution, not water. In addition, carefully restrict ice chip intake; consider using iced saline solution chips. *Excessive intake of water dilutes serum sodium and can result in water intoxication.*

## Fluid Volume Deficit—cont'd

### *Fluid Volume Deficit Related to Active Blood Loss*

**DEFINING CHARACTERISTICS**

- Cardiac output <5 L/min
- Cardiac index <2.5 L/min
- Pulmonary capillary wedge pressure (PCWP), PAD, central venous pressure (CVP) less than normal or less than baseline
- Tachycardia
- Narrowed pulse pressure
- Systolic blood pressure <100 mm Hg
- Urinary output <30 ml/hour
- Pale, cool, moist skin
- Apprehensiveness

**OUTCOME CRITERIA**

- CO is >5 L/min and CI is <2.5 L/min.
- PCWP, PAD, and CVP are normal or back to baseline level.
- Pulse is normal or back to baseline.
- Systolic blood pressure is >90.
- Urinary output is >30 ml/hour.

**NURSING INTERVENTIONS *AND RATIONALE***

1. Continue to monitor the assessment parameters listed under "Defining Characteristics." In addition, a serum lactate level >2 mOsm/L is believed to represent cellular perfusion failure at its earliest stage.
2. Secure airway and administer high flow oxygen.
3. Place patient in supine position with legs elevated *to increase preload.* Consider using low-Fowler's position with legs elevated for patient with head injury.
4. For fluid repletion use the 3:1 rule, replacing three parts of fluid for every unit of blood lost.
5. Administer crystalloid solutions using the fluid challenge technique: infuse precise aliquots of fluid (usually 5 to 20 ml/min) over 10-minute periods; monitor cardiac loading pressures serially *to determine successful challenging.* If the PCWP or PAD elevates more than 7 mm Hg above beginning level, the infusion should be stopped. If the PCWP or PAD rises only to 3 mm Hg above baseline, or falls, another fluid challenge should be administered.
6. Replete fluids first before considering use of vasopressors, since *vasopressors increase myocardial oxygen consumption out of proportion to the reestablishment of coronary perfusion in the early phases of treatment.*
7. When blood is available or its need is indicated, replace it with fresh packed red cells and fresh frozen plasma *to keep clotting factors intact.*
8. Move or reposition patient minimally *to decrease or limit tissue oxygen demands.*
9. Evaluate patient's anxiety level and intervene through patient education or sedation *to decrease tissue oxygen demands.*
10. Be alert for the possiblity of adult respiratory distress syndrome (ARDS) development in the ensuing 72 hours.

### *Fluid Volume Deficit Related to Diarrhea, Wound Drainage*

**DEFINING CHARACTERISTICS**

- Dry mucous membranes and skin
- Weight loss in excess of 10%
- Acute thirst
- Hypotension
- Tachycardia
- Longitudinal wrinkling of the tongue
- Metabolic acidosis
- Serum electrolyte imbalances: hyperchloremia, hypokalemia
- Electrocardiogram (ECG) changes associated with hypokalemia

**OUTCOME CRITERIA**

- Mucous membranes are moist.
- Patient's weight returns to baseline.
- Patient's blood pressure returns to baseline.
- Patient's heart rate returns to baseline.
- Tongue is moist and nonwrinkled.
- Acid-base balance is normal.
- Serum electrolyte values are normal.

**NURSING INTERVENTIONS *AND RATIONALE***

1. Continue to monitor the assessment parameters listed under "Defining Characteristics."
2. With physician's collaboration, replace base and electrolyte losses.
3. With physician's collaboration, replace fluid loss with intravenous isotonic saline solution or dextrose and one-half normal saline solution.
4. Provide oral fluids such as juices that are high in electrolytes.
5. Provide oral potassium replacement according to serum potassium measurements as the metabolic acidosis is corrected.

## Fluid Volume Deficit—cont'd

### *Fluid Volume Deficit Related to Active Plasma Loss and Fluid Shift into Interstitium Secondary to Burns*

#### DEFINING CHARACTERISTICS

- PCWP, PAD, CVP less than normal or less than baseline
- Tachycardia
- Narrowed pulse pressure
- Systolic blood pressure <100 mm Hg
- Urinary output <30 ml/hour
- Increased hematocrit level

#### OUTCOME CRITERIA

- PCWP, PAD, and CVP levels are normal or back to baseline.
- Systolic blood pressure is >90 mm Hg.
- Urinary output is >30 ml/hour.
- The patient's hematocrit level is normal.

#### NURSING INTERVENTIONS *AND RATIONALE*

1. Continue to monitor the assessment parameters listed under "Defining Characteristics." In addition, inspect soft tissues *to determine the presence of edema*.
2. With physician's collaboration, administer intravenous (IV) fluid replacements (usually normal saline solution or lactated Ringer's solution) at a rate sufficient *to maintain urinary output >40 ml/hour*. Colloid solutions are avoided in the initial phases (but can be used later) *because of the possibility of increased edema formation as a result of the increased capillary permeability*.

## High Risk for Fluid Volume Excess

**Definition:** *The state in which an individual is at risk for experiencing intravascular fluid excess.*

### *High Risk for Fluid Volume Excess*

#### RISK FACTOR

- Renal failure

#### DEFINING CHARACTERISTICS OF AN ACTUAL PROBLEM

- Weight gain that occurs during a 24- to 48-hour period
- Dependent pitting edema
- Ascites in severe cases
- Fluid crackles on lung auscultation
- Exertional dyspnea
- Oliguria or anuria
- Hypertension
- Engorged neck veins
- Decrease in urinary osmolality as renal failure progresses

#### OUTCOME CRITERIA

Weight returns to baseline.

- Edema or ascites are absent or reduced to baseline.
- Lungs are clear to auscultation.
- Exertional dyspnea is absent.
- Blood pressure returns to baseline.
- Neck veins are flat.

#### NURSING INTERVENTIONS *AND RATIONALE*

1. Continue to monitor the assessment parameters listed under "Defining Characteristics."
2. Promote skin integrity of edematous areas by frequent repositioning and elevation of areas where possible. Avoid massaging pressure points or reddened areas of skin because *this results in further tissue trauma*.
3. Plan patient care to provide rest periods *to not heighten exertional dyspnea*.
4. Weigh patient daily at same time in same clothing, preferably with the same scale.
5. Instruct the patient about the correlation between fluid intake and weight gain, using commonly understood fluid measurements (for example, ingesting 4 cups [1000 ml] of fluid results in an approximate 2-pound weight gain in the anuric patient).

# Nursing Management of Gastrointestinal Alterations

## Altered Nutrition: More Than Body Requirements

**Definition:** *The state in which an individual experiences an intake of nutrients that exceeds metabolic needs.*

### *Altered Nutrition: More Than Body Protein-Calorie Requirements Related to Overfeeding of Exogenous Nutrients and/or Organ Dysfunction*

#### DEFINING CHARACTERISTICS

**Carbohydrate related**

- Blood glucose >150 mg%/dl
- Glycosuria >3+
- Increased urinary output with low specific gravity
- Progressive clinical symptoms: thirst, diuresis, weight loss, clouded sensorium, nausea, headache, poor skin turgor, hypotension, convulsions, coma
- Increased minute ventilation compared to baseline (increased $Pao_2$)
- Increased arterial partial pressure of carbon dioxide ($Pao_2$) compared to baseline before nutritional support was instituted
- Measured respiratory quotient >1
- >50% of nonprotein calories in nutritional support solution supplied as carbohydrate in ventilator-dependent patient

**Protein related**

- Blood urea nitrogen (BUN) greater than baseline
- BUN: creatinine ratio greater than 10:1
- Diuresis or oliguria
- Greater than normal levels of potassium, magnesium, or phosphate, indicative of renal dysfunction

**Lipid related**

- Lipemia
- Hyponatremia without other cause
- Serum triglyceride level >250 mg/dl
- Decreased platelets without other cause
- Use of fat emulsions at >2-4 mg/kg/hr
- Clinical complaints of nausea, vomiting, headache, altered taste, allergic response

#### OUTCOME CRITERIA

**Carbohydrate related**

- Blood glucose is <150 mg%/dl.
- Glycosuria is <2+.
- Fluid balance is evident.
- Clinical symptoms of progressive hyperglycemia are absent.
- $Paco_2$ of ventilator-dependent patients is in normal range.
- 30%-50% of nonprotein calories are administered as fat emulsion.
- Measured respiratory quotient is <1.

**Protein related**

- BUN is within normal limits.
- BUN: creatinine ratio is within normal limits.
- Urinary output is at least 30 ml/hr.
- Serum and urinary levels of potassium, phosphate, and magnesium are normal.

**Lipid related**

- There is no evidence of lipemia.
- Serum triglyceride levels are <250 mg/dl.
- Serum sodium level is >130 mg/dl.
- Platelets are within normal limits for patient.
- Infusion of fat emulsion is in range of 2-4 mg/kg/hr.
- Patient has no clinical complaints.

#### NURSING INTERVENTIONS *AND RATIONALE*

NOTE: The rationale for each of the following interventions is the prevention and/or identification of complications resulting from carbohydrate, protein, and/or lipid overfeeding.

**Carbohydrate related**

1. Assess serum glucose level on a daily basis; every 6-hour fingersticks for glucose may be needed.
2. Perform urinary testing for sugar every 6 hours.
3. Maintain infusion control of TPN or enteral infusion nutritional support infusion rates.
4. Maintain accurate intake and output, with tracking of fluid balance.
5. Observe and document clinical signs of progressive hyperglycemia.
6. Supplement with exogenous regular insulin as ordered.
7. Carefully observe and document ventilator-dependent patient's attempts at weaning.
8. Identify patients at risk early (for example, septic, diabetic, hypermetabolic, or elderly patients, renal or pancreatic insufficiencies, use of steroids.)
9. Obtain daily weights.
10. Gradually increase formula's or solution's hourly rates based on documented patient tolerance.

**Protein related**

1. Monitor serum values of BUN, creatinine, potassium, phosphate, magnesium.
2. Maintain accurate intake and output and measurement of fluid balance.
3. Obtain daily weights.
4. Perform daily assessment of sensorium

**Lipid related**

1. Monitor laboratory values (triglycerides, platelets).
2. Control infusion of fat emulsion at a rate no greater than 125 ml/hr for 10% solutions and 62 ml/hr for 20% solutions.
3. Observe patient for nausea, vomiting, altered taste, headache, allergic response.

## High Risk for Impaired Skin Integrity

**Definition:** *A state in which an individual's skin is at risk of being adversely affected.*

### *High Risk for Impaired Skin Integrity*

#### RISK FACTORS

**Mechanical factors**
- Immobility or reduced mobility
- Malnutrition (hypoalbuminemia)
- Incontinence
- Frequent or repetitive dressing changes
- Impaired cognition or sensorium
- Poor subcutaneous tissue support (for example, such as occurs with older patients or those receiving steroids)
- Irradiated skin
- Presence of immobilizing devices

**Fungal infections**
- Antibiotics
- Moisture (for example, such as occurs with incontinence, febrile states, damp dressings, pressure-relieving devices that prevent air circulation)
- Compromised host (such as occurs with diabetes, leukopenia)

**Chemical factors**
- Ileostomy, colostomy, or fistula
- Drain sites
- Incontinence
- Dressings that use harsh solutions
- Tube feedings
- Medications that can cause diarrhea

#### DEFINING CHARACTERISTICS OF AN ACTUAL PROBLEM

**Mechanical factors**
- Erythema over bony prominence
- Moist, denuded tissue under adhesives

**Fungal infection**
- Erythematous papular rash
- Moisture entrapped against skin

**Chemical factors**
- Erythematous rash surrounding orifice

#### OUTCOME CRITERIA

**Mechanical factors**
- No erythema is present over bony prominence.
- Skin under adhesives remains intact.

**Fungal infection**
- Papular rash does not develop.
- Moisture or drainage is not trapped against skin.

**Chemical factors**
- Skin around drain sites remains intact.
- No erosion develops around orifice.

#### NURSING INTERVENTIONS *AND RATIONALE*

1. Continue to monitor the assessment parameters listed under "Defining Characteristics."
2. Mechanical factors
   a. Prevent shear or friction.
      - Place genuine sheepskin under patient's hips when head elevated. *Sheepskin keeps patient's skin from sticking to sheets.*
      - Allow feet to rest against footboard when head elevated—*prevents sliding.*
      - Provide heel and elbow protectors—*prevent friction against sheets.*
      - Lift patient with lift sheet to reposition—*prevents sliding patient's body against sheets.*

   b. Prevent epidermal stripping.
      - Apply tape without tension—*avoids blistering.*
      - Use porous type—*allows moisture evaporation.*
      - Remove tape by peeling tape away from skin while stabilizing skin—*avoids traumatic removal of epidermis.*
      - Roll gauze or tubular stockinette to secure dressings—*avoids unnecessary use of adhesives on skin.*
      - Apply skin sealants or solid wafer skin barriers under adhesives. *Both provide a protective layer over skin for adherence of adhesive, thus serving as a second skin.*
      - Secure wound dressings with Montgomery straps—*provides another means of securing dressing without repeated tape applications so epidermal stripping can be avoided.*

   c. Prevent pressure.
      - Apply pressure-reducing support surface to bed (see below)—*redistributes weight.*

**Support surfaces that help prevent impaired skin integrity**

Pressure-reduction device
- Dense, convoluted foam with 3-inch base
- Air-filled devices
- Gel pads

Pressure-relief beds
- Low air loss (for example, Kin-Air; Flexi-Care)
- High air loss (for example, Clinitron)
  - Reposition patient every 2 hours or more often if bony prominence remains erythematous more than 15 minutes after pressure is relieved. *Frequent repositioning redistributes weight and allows capillary refill. Erythema unresolved within 15 minutes indicates tissue ischemia, which can progress to necrosis if pressure is unrelieved.*

*Continued.*

## High Risk for Impaired Skin Integrity—cont'd

- Use pressure-relief support surface if patient is unstable. *Pressure-relief device reduces pressure exerted against skin to less than capillary closing pressure so frequent repositioning to relieve pressure is not necessary.*

2. Fungal infections.
   a. Change dressings over drain site as frequently as needed—*keeps dressing from being saturated.*
   b. Apply skin sealant or solid wafer skin barrier under dressings and around drain site—*protects skin from moisture.*
   c. Dust skin folds with cornstarch or lay gauze (unfolded into skin folds—*absorbs moisture.*
3. Chemical factors.
   a. Maintain intact ostomy pouch over fistula and ostomy. *Change pouch routinely every 3 days or when leakage develops—prevents contact of effluent with skin.*
   b. Apply petrolatum-based ointment to perianal skin for treatment of incontinence—*prevents contct of effluent with skin.*
   c. Apply skin sealants or solid wafer skin barrier around drain sites or wounds—*prevents contact of effluent with skin.*
   d. Gently cleanse skin exposed to drainage with cotton balls and water—*prevents mechanical abrasion of jeopardized skin.*
   e. Use rectal pouch for diarrhea—*protects skin and contains effluent.*
   f. Rule out fecal impaction as source of diarrhea by performing digital examination. *Fecal impaction can function as an obstruction and can stimulate fluid shifts into bowel lumen to create diarrhea.*

# Nursing Management of Endocrine Alterations

## Fluid Volume Excess

**Definition:** *The state in which an individual experiences intravascular fluid excess.*

### *Fluid Volume Excess Related to Increased Secretion of ADH*

#### DEFINING CHARACTERISTICS

- Weight gain *without edema*
- Hyponatremia (dilutional)
- Decreased urinary output
- Urinary osmolality above normal, exceeding plasma osmolality
- Urinary specific gravity >1.030
- Evidence of water intoxication:
  - Fatigue
  - Headache
  - Abdominal cramps
  - Altered level of consciousness
  - Diarrhea
  - Seizures

#### OUTCOME CRITERIA

- Weight returns to baseline.
- Serum sodium is 135-145 mEq/L.
- Urinary output is >30 ml/hr.
- Urinary osmolality is 300-1400 mOsm/L.
- Urinary specific gravity is 1.005-1.030.
- Patient has no evidence of water intoxication.

#### NURSING INTERVENTIONS *AND RATIONALE*

1. Continue to monitor the assessment parameters listed under "Defining Characteristics." In addition, monitor patient closely for evidence of cardiac decompensation caused by excessive preload, that is, elevated pulmonary artery diastolic pressure (PADP) or pulmonary capillary wedge pressure (PCWP), tachycardia, lung congestion.
2. Anticipate administration of demeclocycline, lithium carbonate, furosemide, and/or narcotic agonists.
3. With physician's collaboration, administer intravenous hypertonic sodium chloride *to temporarily correct hyponatremia.*
4. Weigh patient daily at same time in same clothing, preferably with same scale.
5. Maintain fluid restriction.
6. Monitor hydration status.
7. Initiate seizure precautions, since *severe sodium deficit can result in seizures.*

## Fluid Volume Deficit

**Definition:** *The state in which an individual experiences an intravascular dehydration.*

### *Fluid Volume Deficit Related to Decreased Secretion of ADH*

#### DEFINING CHARACTERISTICS

- Polyuria (15 L per day)
- Serum sodium 145 mEq/L (particularly in patients who are not drinking to replace losses)
- Intense thirst
- Polydipsia (alert patients)
- Urinary specific gravity <1.005
- Urinary osmolality <300 mOsm/L
- Plasma osmolality >300 mOsm/L

#### OUTCOME CRITERIA

- Urinary volume, specific gravity, and osmolality are normal.
- Thirst is reduced.
- Plasma osmolality and serum sodium level are normal.

#### NURSING INTERVENTIONS *AND RATIONALE*

1. Continue to monitor the assessment parameters listed under "Defining Characteristics." In addition, monitor for signs of critical volume deficits, such as hypotension, fall in pulmonary artery pressures, tachycardia.
2. With physician's collaboration, administer intravenous electrolyte replacement solutions, because *critical electrolyte loss occurs along with water loss.* Replace losses milliliter for milliliter plus 50 ml/hr for insensible losses. Avoid replacement of losses with intravenous dextrose solutions because *of the risk of water intoxication.*
3. If he or she is alert, allow the patient to satisfy partially his or her replacement needs by drinking according to thirst. Caution should be observed regarding the patient's excessive ingestion of water (typically, the patient will crave iced water) because *of the risk of water intoxication.*
4. With physician's collaboration, administer vasopressin intravenously, intramuscularly, or per the nasal route.
5. For patients after hypophysectomy, teach the administration of vasopressin and its reportable side and toxic effects, the monitoring of intake and output measurement, and the documentation of daily weights.

# APPENDIXES

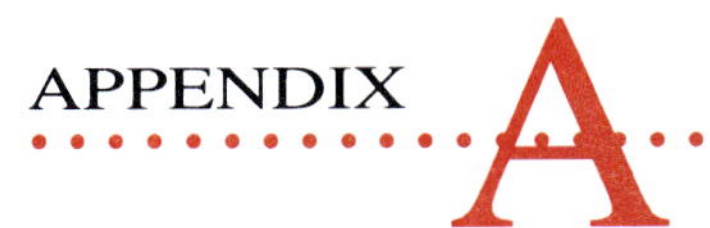

# North American Nursing Diagnosis Association's (NANDA) Taxonomy I Revised*

**PATTERN 1: EXCHANGING**

| | |
|---|---|
| 1.1.2.1 | Altered Nutrition: More Than Body Requirements |
| 1.1.2.2 | Altered Nutrition: Less Than Body Requirements |
| 1.1.2.3 | Altered Nutrition: Potential for More Than Body Requirements |
| 1.2.1.1 | High Risk for Infection |
| 1.2.2.1 | High Risk for Altered Body Temperature |
| 1.2.2.2 | Hypothermia |
| 1.2.2.3 | Hyperthermia |
| 1.2.2.4 | Ineffective Thermoregulation |
| 1.2.3.1 | Dysreflexia |
| 1.3.1.1 | Constipation |
| 1.3.1.1.1 | Perceived Constipation |
| 1.3.1.1.2 | Colonic Constipation |
| 1.3.1.2 | Diarrhea |
| 1.3.1.3 | Bowel Incontinence |
| 1.3.2 | Altered Urinary Elimination |
| 1.3.2.1.1 | Stress Incontinence |
| 1.3.2.1.2 | Reflex Incontinence |
| 1.3.2.1.3 | Urge Incontinence |
| 1.3.2.1.4 | Functional Incontinence |
| 1.3.2.1.5 | Total Incontinence |
| 1.3.2.2 | Urinary Retention |
| 1.4.1.1 | Altered (Specify Type) Tissue Perfusion (Renal, Cerebral, Cardiopulmonary, Gastrointestinal, Peripheral) |
| 1.4.1.2.1 | Fluid Volume Excess |
| 1.4.1.2.2.1 | Fluid Volume Deficit |
| 1.4.1.2.2.2 | High Risk for Fluid Volume Deficit |
| 1.4.2.1 | Decreased Cardiac Output |
| 1.5.1.1 | Impaired Gas Exchange |
| 1.5.1.2 | Ineffective Airway Clearance |
| 1.5.1.3 | Ineffective Breathing Pattern |
| 1.6.1 | High Risk for Injury |
| 1.6.1.1 | High Risk for Suffocation |
| 1.6.1.2 | High Risk for Poisoning |
| 1.6.1.3 | High Risk for Trauma |
| 1.6.1.4 | High Risk for Aspiration |
| 1.6.1.5 | High Risk for Disuse Syndrome |
| 1.6.2 | Altered Protection |
| 1.6.2.1 | Impaired Tissue Integrity |
| 1.6.2.1.1 | Altered Oral Mucous Membrane |
| 1.6.2.1.2.1 | Impaired Skin Integrity |
| 1.6.2.1.2.2 | High Risk for Impaired Skin Integrity |

**PATTERN 2: COMMUNICATING**

| | |
|---|---|
| 2.1.1.1 | Impaired Verbal Communication |

**PATTERN 3: RELATING**

| | |
|---|---|
| 3.1.1 | Impaired Social Interaction |
| 3.1.2 | Social Isolation |
| 3.2.1 | Altered Role Performance |
| 3.2.1.1.1 | Altered Parenting |
| 3.2.1.1.2 | High Risk for Altered Parenting |
| 3.2.1.2.1 | Sexual Dysfunction |
| 3.2.2 | Altered Family Processes |
| 3.2.3.1 | Parental Role Conflict |
| 3.3 | Altered Sexuality Patterns |

**PATTERN 4: VALUING**

| | |
|---|---|
| 4.1.1 | Spiritual Distress (Distress of the Human Spirit) |

**PATTERN 5: CHOOSING**

| | |
|---|---|
| 5.1.1.1 | Ineffective Individual Coping |
| 5.1.1.1.1 | Impaired Adjustment |
| 5.1.1.1.2 | Defensive Coping |
| 5.1.1.1.3 | Ineffective Denial |
| 5.1.2.1.1 | Ineffective Family Coping: Disabling |
| 5.1.2.1.2 | Ineffective Family Coping: Compromised |
| 5.1.2.2 | Family Coping: Potential for Growth |
| 5.2.1.1 | Noncompliance (Specify) |
| 5.3.1.1 | Decisional Conflict (Specify) |
| 5.4 | Health-Seeking Behaviors (Specify) |

*Reflects diagnoses and taxonomic structure approved up to and including the Eighth Conference on the Classification of Nursing Diagnoses, 1990.

## PATTERN 6: MOVING

6.1.1.1 Impaired Physical Mobility
6.1.1.2 Activity Intolerance
6.1.1.2.1 Fatigue
6.1.1.3 High Risk for Activity Intolerance
6.2.1 Sleep Pattern Disturbance
6.3.1.1 Diversional Activity Deficit
6.4.1.1 Impaired Home Maintenance Management
6.4.2 Altered Health Maintenance
6.5.1 Feeding Self-Care Deficit
6.5.1.1 Impaired Swallowing
6.5.1.2 Ineffective Breastfeeding
6.5.1.3 Effective Breastfeeding
6.5.2 Bathing/Hygiene Self-Care Deficit
6.5.3 Dressing/Grooming Self-Care Deficit
6.5.4 Toileting Self-Care Deficit
6.6 Altered Growth and Development

## PATTERN 7: PERCEIVING

7.1.1 Body Image Disturbance
7.1.2 Self-Esteem Disturbance
7.1.2.1 Chronic Low Self-Esteem
7.1.2.2 Situational Low Self-Esteem
7.1.3 Personal Identity Disturbance
7.2 Sensory/Perceptual Alterations (Specify) (Visual, Auditory, Kinesthetic, Gustatory, Tactile, Olfactory)
7.2.1.1 Unilateral Neglect
7.3.1 Hopelessness
7.3.2 Powerlessness

## PATTERN 8: KNOWING

8.1.1 Knowledge Deficit (Specify)
8.3 Altered Thought Processes

## PATTERN 9: FEELING

9.1.1 Pain
9.1.1.1 Chronic Pain
9.2.1.1 Dysfunctional Grieving
9.2.1.2 Anticipatory Grieving
9.2.2 High Risk for Violence: Self-Directed or Directed at Others
9.2.3 Post-Trauma Response
9.2.3.1 Rape-Trauma Syndrome
9.2.3.1.1 Rape-Trauma Syndrome: Compound Reaction
9.2.3.1.2 Rape-Trauma Syndrome: Silent Reaction
9.3.1 Anxiety
9.3.2 Fear

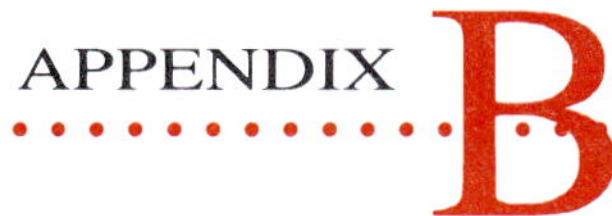

APPENDIX B



# ACLS Guidelines

Witnessed arrest | Unwitnessed arrest

Check pulse—if no pulse | Check pulse—if no pulse

Precordial thump

Check pulse—if no pulse

CPR until a defibrillator is available

Check monitor for rhythm—if VF or VT*

Defibrillate, 200 joules†

Defibrillate, 200-300 joules†

Defibrillate with up to 360 joules†

CPR if no pulse

Establish IV access

Epinephrine, 1:10,000, 0.5-1.0 mg IV push‡

Intubate if possible§

Defibrillate with up to 360 joules†

Lidocaine, 1 mg/kg IV push

Defibrillate with up to 360 joules†

Bretylium, 5 mg/kg IV push||

(Consider bicarbonate)¶

Defibrillate with up to 360 joules†

Bretylium, 10 mg/kg IV push||

Defibrillate with up to 360 joules†

Repeat lidocaine or bretylium

Defibrillate with up to 360 joules†

**Fig. B-1 Ventricular fibrillation (and pulseless ventricular tachycardia).** This sequence was developed to assist in teaching how to treat a broad range of patients with ventricular fibrillation (VF) or pulseless ventricular tachycardia (VT). Some patients may require care not specified herein. This algorithm should not be construed as prohibiting such flexibility. Flow of algorithm presumes that VF is continuing. CPR indicates cardiopulmonary resuscitation.

*Pulseless VT should be treated identically to VF.

†Check pulse and rhythm after each shock. If VF recurs after transiently converting (rather than persists without converting), use whatever energy level has previously been successful for defibrillation.

‡Epinephrine should be repeated every 5 minutes.

§Intubation is preferable. If it can be accomplished simultaenously with other techniques, then the earlier the better. However, defibrillation and epinephrine are more important initially if the patient can be ventilated without intubation.

||Some may prefer repeated doses of lidocaine, which may be given in 0.5-mg/kg boluses every 8 minutes to a total dose of 3 mg/kg.

¶Value of sodium bicarbonate is questionable during cardiac arrest, and it is not recommended for routine cardiac arrest sequence. Consideration of its use in a dose of 1 mEq/kg is appropriate at this point. Half of original dose may be repeated every 10 minutes if it is used. (Reproduced with permission from the American Heart Association: Textbook of advanced cardiac life support, 1987, The Association.)

Continue CPR

Establish IV access

Epinephrine, 1:10,000, 0.5-1.0 mg IV push*

Intubate when possible†

(Consider bicarbonate)‡

Consider hypovolemia,
cardiac tamponade,
tension pneumothorax,
hypoxemia,
acidosis,
pulmonary embolism

**Fig. B-2 Electromechanical dissociation.** This sequence was developed to assist in teaching how to treat a broad range of patients with electromechanical dissociation. Some patients may require care not specified herein. This algorithm should not be construed to prohibit such flexibility. Flow of algorithm presumes that electromechanical dissociation is continuing. CPR indicates cardiopulmonary resuscitation; IV, intravenous.
*Epinephrine should be repeated every 5 minutes.
†Intubation is preferable. If it can be accomplished simultaneously with other techniques, then the earlier the better. However, epinephrine is more important initially if the patient can be ventilated without intubation.
‡Value of sodium bicarbonate is questionable during cardiac arrest, and it is not recommended for routine cardiac arrest sequence. Consideration of its use in a dose of 1 mEq/kg is appropriate at this point. Half of original dose may be repeated every 10 minutes if it is used. (Reproduced with permission form the American Heart Association: Textbook of advanced cardiac life support, 1987, The Association.)

| **Unstable** | **Stable** |
|---|---|
| Synchronous cardioversion 75-100 joules | Vagal maneuvers |
| Synchronous cardioversion 200 joules | Verapamil, 5 mg IV |
| Synchronous cardioversion 360 joules | Verapamil, 10 mg IV (in 15-20 min) |
| Correct underlying abnormalities | |
| Pharmacological therapy + cardioversion | Cardioversion, digoxin, $\beta$-blockers, pacing as indicated |

If conversion occurs but PSVT recurs, repeated electrical cardioversion is *not* indicated. Sedation should be used as time permits.

**Fig. B-3 Paroxysmal supraventricular tachycardia (PSVT).** This sequence was developed to assist in teaching how to treat a broad range of patients with PSVT. Some patients may require care not specified herein. This algorithm should not be construed as prohibiting such flexibility. Flow of algorithm presumes PSVT is continuing. (Reproduced with permission from the American Heart Association: Textbook of advanced cardiac life support, 1987, The Association.)

**No Pulse**

Treat as VF

**Pulse Present**

| **Stable*** | **Unstable†** |
|---|---|
| $O_2$ | $O_2$ |
| IV access | IV access |
| Lidocaine, 1 mg/kg | (Consider sedation)§ |
| Lidocaine, 0.5 mg/kg every 8 min until VT resolves, or up to 3 mg/kg | Cardiovert 50 joules§, ‖ |
| | Cardiovert 100 joules§ |
| Procainamide, 20 mg/min until VT resolves, or up to 1,000 mg | Cardiovert 200 joules§ |
| | Cardiovert with up to 360 joules§ |
| Cardiovert as in unstable patients‡ | If recurrent, add lidocaine and cardiovert again starting at energy level previously successful; then procainamide or bretylium¶ |

**Fig. B-4 Sustained ventricular tachycardia (VT).** This sequence was developed to assist in teaching how to treat a broad range of patients with sustained VT. Some patients may require care not specified herein. This algorithm should not be construed as prohibiting such flexibility. Flow of algorithm presumes that VT is continuing. VF indicates ventricular fibrillation.

*If patient becomes unstable (see footnote † for definition) at any time, move to "Unstable" arm of algorithm.

†Unstable indicates symptoms (e.g., chest pain or dyspnea), hypotension (systolic blood pressure <90 mm Hg) congestive heart failure, ischemia, or infarction.

‡Sedation should be considered for all patients, including those defined in footnote † as unstable, except those who are hemodynamically unstable (e.g., hypotensive, in pulmonary edema, or unconscious).

§If hypotension, pulmonary edema, or unconsciousness is present, unsynchronized cardioversion should be done to avoid delay associated with synchronization.

‖In the absence of hypotension, pulmonary edema, or unconsciousness, a precordial thump may be employed before cardioversion.

¶Once VT has resolved, begin intravenous (IV) infusion of antiarrhythmic agent that has aided resolution of VT. If hypotension, pulmonary edema, or unconsciousness is present, use lidocaine if cardioversion alone is unsuccessful, followed by bretylium. In all other patients, recommended order of therapy is lidocaine, procainamide, and then bretylium. (Reproduced with permission from the American Heart Association: Textbook of advanced cardiac life support, 1987, The Association.)

If rhythm is unclear and possibly ventricular fibrillation, defibrillate as for VF. If asystole is present*

Continue CPR

Establish IV access

Epinephrine, 1:10,000, 0.5-1.0 mg IV push†

Intubate when possible‡

Atropine, 1.0 mg IV push (repeated in 5 min)

(Consider bicarbonate)§

Consider pacing

**Fig. B-5 Asystole (cardiac standstill).** This sequence was developed to assist in teaching how to treat a broad range of patients with asystole. Some patients may require care not specified herein. This algorithm should not be construed to prohibit such flexibility. Flow of algorithm presumes asystole is continuing. VF indicates ventricular fibrillation; IV, intravenous.

*Asystole should be confirmed in two leads.

†Epinephrine should be repeated every 5 minutes.

‡Intubation is preferable; if it can be accomplished simultaneously with other techniques, then the earlier the better. However, cardiopulmonary resuscitation (CPR) and use of epinephrine are more important initally if the patient can be ventilated without intubation. (Endotracheal epinephrine may be used.)

§Value of sodium bicarbonate is questionable during cardiac arrest, and it is not recommended for the routine cardiac arrest sequence. Consideration of its use in a dose of 1 mEq/kg is appropriate at this point. Half of original dose may be repeated every 10 minutes if it is used. (Reproduced with permission from the American Heart Association: Textbook of advanced cardiac life support, 1987, The Association.)

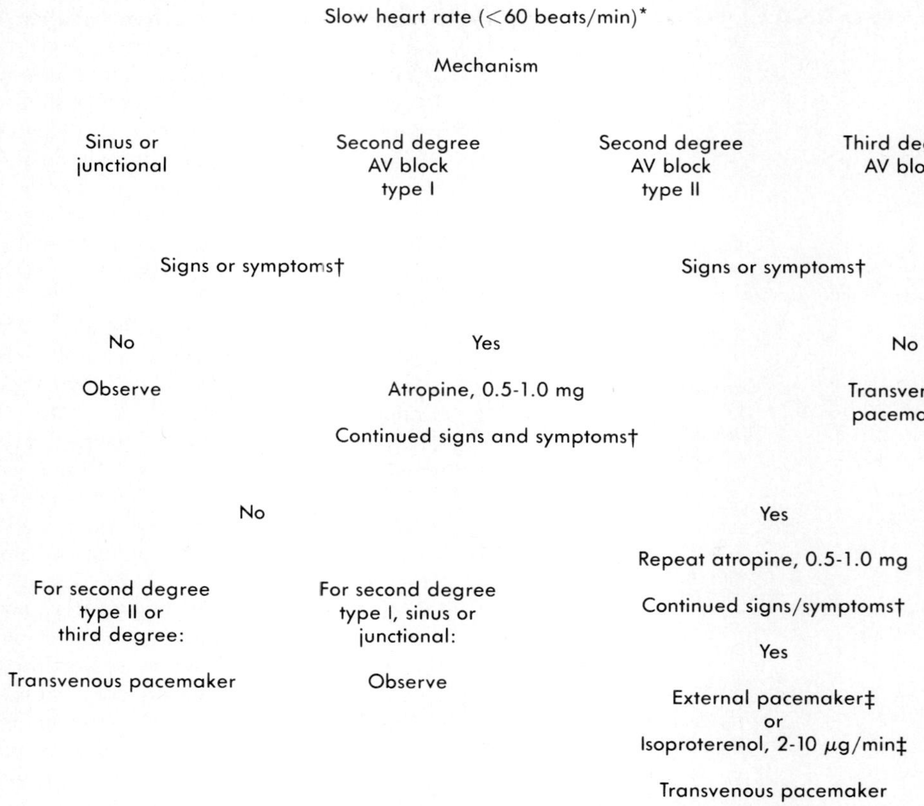

Slow heart rate (<60 beats/min)*

Mechanism

Sinus or junctional

Second degree AV block type I

Second degree AV block type II

Third degree AV block

Signs or symptoms†

Signs or symptoms†

No

Observe

Yes

Atropine, 0.5-1.0 mg

Continued signs and symptoms†

No

For second degree type II or third degree:

Transvenous pacemaker

For second degree type I, sinus or junctional:

Observe

Yes

Repeat atropine, 0.5-1.0 mg

Continued signs/symptoms†

Yes

External pacemaker‡
or
Isoproterenol, 2-10 μg/min‡

Transvenous pacemaker

No

Transvenous pacemaker

**Fig. B-6 Bradycardia.** This sequence was developed to assist in teaching how to treat a broad range of patients with bradycardia. Some patients may require care not specified herein. This algorithm should not be construed to prohibit such flexibility. AV indicates atrioventricular.
*A solitary chest thump or cough may stimulate cardiac electrical activity and result in improved cardiac output and may be used at this point.
†Hypotension (blood pressure <90 mm Hg), premature ventricular contractions, altered mental status or symptoms (e.g., chest pain or dyspnea), ischemia, or infarction.
‡Temporizing therapy. (Reproduced with permission from the American Heart Association: Textbook of advanced cardiac life support, 1987, The Association.)

Assess for need for
acute suppressive therapy

Rule out treatable cause
Consider serum potassium
Consider digitalis level
Consider bradycardia
Consider drugs

Lidocaine, 1 mg/kg

If not suppressed,
repeat lidocaine, 0.5 mg/kg every 2-5 min,
until no ectopy, or up to 3 mg/kg given

If not suppressed,
procainamide 20 mg/min
until no ectopy, or up to 1,000 mg given

If not suppressed,
and not contraindicated,
bretylium, 5-10 mg/kg over 8-10 min

If not suppressed,
consider overdrive pacing

Once ectopy resolved, maintain as follows:
After lidocaine, 1 mg/kg . . . lidocaine drip, 2 mg/min
After lidocaine, 1-2 mg/kg . . . lidocaine drip, 3 mg/min
After lidocaine, 2-3 mg/kg . . . lidocaine drip, 4 mg/min
After procainamide . . . procainamide drip, 1-4 mg/min (check blood level)
After bretylium . . . bretylium drip, 2 mg/min

**Fig. B-7 Ventricular ectopy: acute suppressive therapy.** This sequence was developed to assist in teaching how to treat a broad range of patients with ventricular ectopy. Some patients may require therapy not specified herein. This algorithm should not be construed as prohibiting such flexibility. (Reproduced from the American Heart Association: Textbook of advanced cardiac life support, 1987, The Association.)

# Index

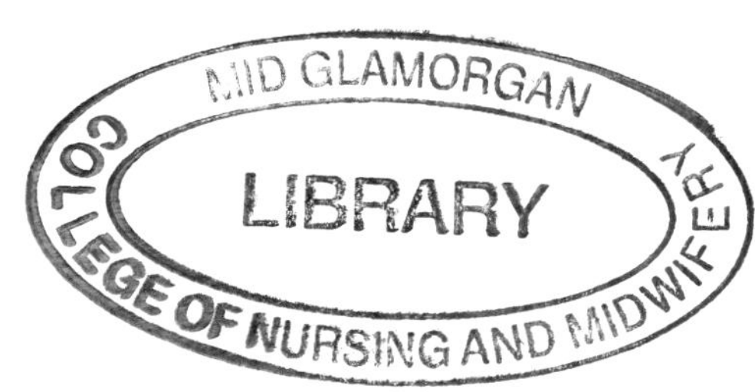

**E**

**J**



**K**

## U

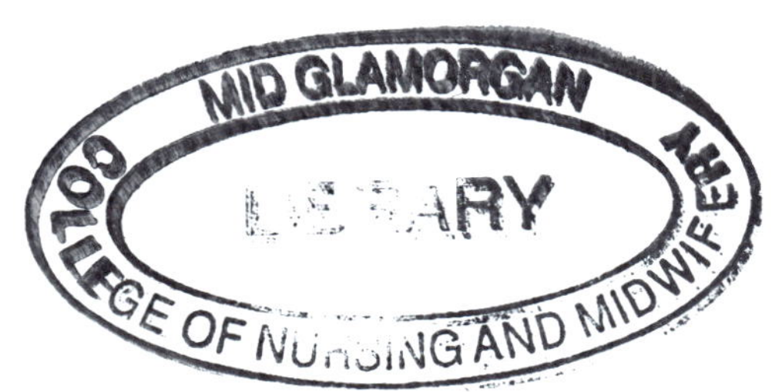
MID GLAMORGAN
LIBRARY
COLLEGE OF NURSING AND MIDWIFERY

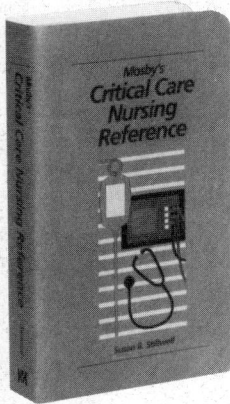

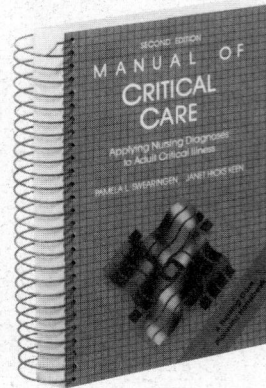